PEDIATRIC PARA[...]

	premie	new born	6 MO	YR	YR	YR	YR	YR	YR
WT (KG)	2.5-3.5 kg	3.5-4 kg	6-8 kg	10 kg	13-16 kg	20-25 kg	25-35 kg	40-50 kg	>50 kg
BAG VALVE MASK	Infant	Infant	Small Child	Small Child	Child	Child	Child/ S. Adult	Adult	Adult
NASAL AIRWAY	12 Fr	12 Fr	14-16 Fr	14-16 Fr	14-18 Fr	14-18 Fr	16-20 Fr	18-22 Fr	22-36 Fr
ORAL AIRWAY	Infant 50 mm	Small 60 mm	Small 60 mm	Small 60 mm	Small 70 mm	Small 70-80 mm	Med 80-90 mm	Med 90 mm	Med 90 mm
BLADE	MIL 0	MIL 0	MIL 1	MIL 1, MAC 2	MIL 1, MAC 2	MIL 2, MAC 3	MIL 2, MAC 3	MIL 2, MAC 3	MIL 2, MAC 3
ETT	2.5-3.0	3.0-3.5	3.5-4.0	4.0-4.5	4.5-5.0	5.0-5.5	5.5-6.0	6.0-6.5	7.0-8.0
LMA	1	1	1.5	2	2	2.5	2.5-3	3	4
GLIDESCOPE	1	1 or 2	2	2	3	3	3	3 or 4	3 or 4
IV CATH	22-24 ga	22-24 ga	20-24 ga	20-24 ga	18-22 ga	18-22 ga	18-22 ga	18-20 ga	16-20 ga
CVL	3 Fr	3-4 Fr	4 Fr	4-5 Fr	4-5 Fr	5 Fr	5 Fr	7 Fr	7 Fr
NGT/OGT	5 Fr	5-8 Fr	8 Fr	10 Fr	10-12 Fr	12-14 Fr	12-14 Fr	14-18 Fr	14-18 Fr
CHEST TUBE	10-12 F	10-12 Fr	12-18 Fr	16-20 Fr	16-24 Fr	20-28 Fr	20-32 Fr	28-38 Fr	28-42 Fr
FOLEY	6 Fr	8 Fr	8 Fr	8 Fr	8 Fr	8 Fr	8 Fr	10 Fr	12 Fr

ESTIMATED BLOOD PRESSURE BY AGE

MEASUREMENT	50th %	5th %
Systolic BP	90 + (age x 2)	60 (neonate); 70 (1mo-1 yr) 70 + (age x 2) (for 2-10 yrs) <90 (>10 yrs)
MAP	55 + (age x 1.5)	40 + (age x 1.5)

NORMAL VITAL SIGNS BY AGE

Age	HR (beats/min)	BP (mm Hg)	RR (breaths/min)
Premie	120-170	55-75/35-45 (gestational age approximates nml MAP)	40-70
0-3 mo	110-160	65-85/45-55	30-60
3-6 mo	100-150	70-90/50-65	30-45
6-12 mo	90-130	80-100/55-65	25-40
1-3 yrs	80-125	90-105/55-70	20-30
3-6 yrs	70-115	95-110/60-75	20-25
6-12 yrs	60-100	100-120/60-75	14-22
>12 yrs	60-100	100-120/70-80	12-18

ENDOTRACHEAL TUBE FORMULAS

Uncuffed ETT size: age (years)/4 +4; Cuffed ETT size: age (years)/4 +3
ETT depth (from lip to mid-trachea): ETT internal diameter (size) x 3

GLASGOW COMA SCALE

Activity	Score	Child/Adult	Score	Infant
Eye opening	4	Spontaneous	4	Spontaneous
	3	To speech	3	To speech/sound
	2	To pain	2	To pain
	1	None	1	None
Verbal	5	Oriented	5	Coos/babbles
	4	Confused	4	Irritable cry
	3	Inappropriate	3	Cries to pain
	2	Incomprehensible	2	Moans to pain
	1	None	1	None
Motor	6	Obeys commands	6	Normal spontaneous
	5	Localizes to pain	5	Withdraws to touch
	4	Withdraws to pain	4	Withdraws to pain
	3	Abnormal flexion	3	Abnormal flexion (decorticate)
	2	Abnormal extension	2	Abnormal extension (decerebrate)
	1	None	1	None

Adapted from Hunt B, Nelson K. The Johns Hopkins Children's Center Kids Kard, 2014.

IV INFUSIONS* $6 \times \dfrac{\text{Desired dose (mcg/kg/min)}}{\text{Desired rate (mL/hr)}} \times \text{Wt (kg)} = \dfrac{\text{mg drug}}{100 \text{ mL fluid}}$

Medication	Dose (mcg/kg/min)	Dilution in 100 mL D₅W	IV Infusion Rate
Alprostadil (prostaglandin E₁)	0.05–0.1	0.3 mg/kg	1 mL/hr = 0.05 mcg/kg/min
Amiodarone	5–15	6 mg/kg	1 mL/hr = 1 mcg/kg/min
DOPamine	2–20	6 mg/kg	1 mL/hr = 1 mcg/kg/min
DOBUTamine	2–20	6 mg/kg	1 mL/hr = 1 mcg/kg/min
EPINEPHrine	0.1–1	0.6 mg/kg	1 mL/hr = 0.1 mcg/kg/min
Lidocaine	20–50	6 mg/kg	1 mL/hr = 1 mcg/kg/min
Phenylephrine	0.05–2	0.3 mg/kg	1 mL/hr = 0.05 mcg/kg/min
Terbutaline	0.1–10	0.6 mg/kg	1 mL/hr = 0.1 mcg/kg/min
Vasopressin (pressor)	0.5–2 milliunits/kg/min	6 milliunits/kg	1 mL/hr = 1 milliunit/kg/min

* Standardized concentrations are recommended when available.

RESUSCITATION MEDICATIONS

Adenosine Supraventricular tachycardia	**0.1 mg/kg IV/IO RAPID BOLUS** (over 1-2 sec), Flush with 10 mL normal saline May repeat at 0.2 mg/kg IV/IO after 2 min Max first dose 6 mg, max subsequent dose 12 mg
Amiodarone Ventricular tachycardia Ventricular fibrillation	**5 mg/kg IV/IO** No Pulse: Push Undiluted Pulse: Dilute and give over 30 minutes Max first dose 300 mg, max subsequent dose 150 mg Monitor for hypotension
Atropine Bradycardia (increased vagal tone) Primary AV block	**0.02 mg/kg IV/IO, 0.04–0.06 mg/kg ETT** Max single dose 0.5 mg Repeat once if needed
Calcium chloride (10%) Hypocalcemia	**20 mg/kg IV/IO** Max dose 1 g
Dextrose	**<5 kg: 10% dextrose 10 mL/kg** **5-44 kg: 25% dextrose 4 mL/kg** **≥45 kg: 50% dextrose 2 mL/kg, max single dose 50 g = 100 mL**
Epinephrine Pulseless arrest Bradycardia (symptomatic) Anaphylaxis	**0.01 mg/kg (0.1 mL/kg) 1:10,000 IV/IO** every 3–5 min (max single dose 1 mg) **0.1 mg/kg (0.1 mL/kg) 1:1000 ETT** every 3–5 min (max single dose 2.5 mg) **Anaphylaxis: 0.01 mg/kg (0.01 mL/kg) of 1:1000 IM** (max 0.5 mg) in thigh every 15 min PRN Standardized/Autoinjector: <10 kg: 0.01 mg/kg (0.01 mL/kg) of 1:1000 IM 10-30 kg: 0.15 mg IM >30 kg: 0.3 mg IM
Insulin (Regular or Aspart) Hyperkalemia	**0.1 units/kg IV/IO with 1 g/kg of dextrose** Max single dose 10 units
Magnesium sulfate Torsades de pointes Hypomagnesemia	**50 mg/kg IV/IO** No Pulse: Push Pulse: Give over 15-20 minutes Max single dose 2 g Monitor for hypotension/bradycardia
Naloxone Opioid overdose Coma	**Respiratory Depression: 0.001-0.005 mg/kg/dose IV/IO/IM/SubQ** (max 0.08 mg first dose, may titrate to effect) **Full Reversal/Arrest Dose: 0.1 mg/kg IV/IO/IM/SubQ** (max dose 2 mg) ETT dose 2–3 times IV dose. May give every 2 min PRN
Sodium Bicarbonate (8.4%) Metabolic acidosis Hyperkalemia Tricyclic antidepressant overdose	**1 mEq/kg IV/IO** Dilute 1:1 with sterile water for <10 kg Hyperkalemia: Max single dose 50 mEq
Vasopressin	**0.5 units/kg/dose IV/IO** Max single dose 40 units

ETT Meds (NAVEL: naloxone, atropine, vasopressin, epinephrine, lidocaine)—dilute meds to 5 mL with NS, follow with positive-pressure ventilation.

Special thanks to LeAnn McNamara and Angela Helder, Clinical Pharmacy Specialists, for their expert guidance with IV infusion and resuscitation medications guidelines.

Adapted from Hunt B, Nelson K. The Johns Hopkins Children's Center Kids Kard, 2014, and the American Heart Association, PALS Pocket Card, 2010.

TWENTIETH
EDITION

THE
HARRIET LANE
HANDBOOK

A Manual for Pediatric House Officers

JOHNS HOPKINS
CHILDREN'S CENTER

THE HARRIET LANE HANDBOOK

A Manual for Pediatric House Officers

The Harriet Lane Service at
The Charlotte R. Bloomberg Children's Center of
The Johns Hopkins Hospital

EDITORS
Branden Engorn, MD
Jamie Flerlage, MD

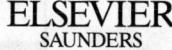

ELSEVIER
SAUNDERS

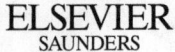

1600 John F. Kennedy Blvd.
Ste 1800
Philadelphia, PA 19103-2899

THE HARRIET LANE HANDBOOK, TWENTIETH EDITION   ISBN: 978-0-323-09644-7

Copyright © 2015 by Saunders, an imprint of Elsevier Inc.   International Edition: 978-0-323-11244-4

Previous editions copyrighted 2012, 2009, 2005, 2002, 2000, 1996, 1993, 1991, 1987, 1984, 1981, 1978, 1975, 1972, 1969 by Mosby, Inc., an affiliate of Elsevier Inc. All rights reserved.

Library of Congress Cataloging-in-Publication Data
Harriet Lane Service (Johns Hopkins Hospital), author.
The Harriet Lane handbook : a manual for pediatric house officers / the Harriet Lane Service, Children's Medical and Surgical Center of the Johns Hopkins Hospital ; editors, Jamie Flerlage, Branden Engorn. -- Twentieth edition.
     p. ; cm.
Preceded by the Harriet Lane handbook / editors, Megan M. Tschudy, Kristin M. Arcara. 19th ed. c2012.
Includes bibliographical references and index.
ISBN 978-0-323-09644-7 (pbk. : alk. paper)
I. Flerlage, Jamie, editor of compilation. II. Engorn, Branden, editor of compilation. III. Title.
[DNLM: 1. Pediatrics--Handbooks. WS 29]
RJ48
618.92--dc23   2014003506

Senior Content Strategist: Jim Merritt   *Publishing Services Manager:* Anne Altepeter
Content Development Manager: Lucia Gunzel   *Project Manager:* Cindy Thoms
Senior Content Development Specialist: Andrea Vosburgh   *Manager, Art and Design:* Steven Stave

Printed in the United States of America
Last digit is the print number: 9 8 7 6 5 4 3 2 1

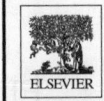

To all who use this book
May the work you do better the lives
of children everywhere.

To our patients
May we serve you well and learn
from you each day.

To our families
To Anne and Bob Laubisch and my
entire family, thank you for your endless
encouragement in my life that has allowed
me to follow my dreams.
To Jayne and Steven Engorn and my
entire family, thank you for teaching me
to work hard and never give up, and that
family gets us through both the good times
and the bad times.

To our spouses
To Tim Flerlage, my amazing husband
and best friend, thank you for your daily
support that allows me to do what I love,
and for that I am forever grateful.
To Kristin Moosmann Engorn, my
wonderful wife and best friend,
coming home to you is the perfect
ending to every day.

To our mentors
To Julia McMillan, may you know that
your mentorship has shaped our lives
and that you are the physician
we will always strive to be.
To George Dover, The Johns Hopkins
Children's Center will forever be indebted
to you for all the love, compassion,
dedication, and time that you have given
to enhance the lives of countless children
and families.

Preface

"Why this child? Why this disease? Why now?"

—**Barton Childs, MD**

The Harriet Lane Handbook was first developed in 1953 after Harrison Spencer (chief resident in 1950–1951) suggested that residents should write a pocket-sized "pearl book." As recounted by Henry Seidel, the first editor of *The Harriet Lane Handbook,* "Six of us began without funds and without [the] supervision of our elders, meeting sporadically around a table in the library of the Harriet Lane Home." The product of their efforts was a concise yet comprehensive handbook that became an indispensable tool for the residents of the Harriet Lane Home. Ultimately, Robert Cooke (department chief, 1956–1974) realized the potential of the handbook, and, with his backing, the fifth edition was published for widespread distribution by Year Book. Since that time, the handbook has been regularly updated and rigorously revised to reflect the most up-to-date information and clinical guidelines available. It has grown from a humble Hopkins resident "pearl book" to become a nationally and internationally respected clinical resource. Now translated into many languages, the handbook is still intended as an easy-to-use manual to help pediatricians provide current and comprehensive pediatric care.

Today, *The Harriet Lane Handbook* continues to be updated and revised *by* house officers *for* house officers. Recognizing the limit to what can be included in a pocket guide, additional information has been placed online and for use via mobile applications.

This symbol 🔗 throughout the chapters denotes online content in Expert Consult. The online-only content includes expanded text, tables, additional images, and other references.

In this edition, the following are just a few examples of the changes made to enhance the usefulness of the book, decrease the weight of white coat pockets everywhere, and reflect changes made in guidelines and management since the ninetheenth edition of the *The Harriet Lane Handbook:*

- Most notable, the **cover** has been changed from its traditional picture of the Johns Hopkins Dome to a photo of our new home, The Charlotte R. Bloomberg Children's Center. The change for this edition commemorates 100 years since the opening of the Harriet Lane Home, 20 editions of The Harriet Lane Handbook, and the beginning of the next century of pediatric care at Johns Hopkins Hospital.
- In the **Development, Behavior, and Mental Health** chapter, the content has been updated to reflect the changes in the new *Diagnostic and Statistical Manual of Mental Disorders,* Fifth Edition, most notably the diagnostic criteria for intellectual disability.
- In the **Procedures** chapter, links to the *New England Journal of Medicine* "Videos in Clinical Medicine" were added to the online content. Images for various procedures were updated.

- In the **Trauma, Burns, and Common Critical Care Emergencies** chapter, new additions include practice parameters for pediatric and neonatal septic shock as well as guidelines for the acute management of severe traumatic brain injury.
- The **Genetics** chapter has been divided for usability into two sections, metabolism and dysmorphology, and a table of collection information for common genetic tests was added.
- The photo atlas in the **Radiology** chapter has been expanded and improved.
- The majority of the **Formulary Adjunct** chapter content was moved to the relevant chapters.

The Harriet Lane Handbook, designed for pediatric house staff, was made possible by the extraordinary efforts of this year's senior resident class, the members of which balanced their busy schedules with authoring the chapters that follow. We are grateful to each of these residents along with their faculty advisors, who selflessly dedicated their time to improve the quality and content of this publication.The spirit of this handbook is our residents, who are the heart and soul of our department.

Chapter Title	Resident	Faculty Advisor
1. Emergency Management	Stephanie Chin-Sang, MD	Jennifer Anders, MD
2. Poisonings	Zachary Nayak, MD	Mitchell Goldstein, MD
	Jocelyn Ronda, MD	Suzanne Doyon, MD
3. Procedures	Bradley D. McCammack, MD	Jason Custer, MD
4. Trauma, Burns, and Common Critical Care Emergencies	Emily Krennerich, MD	Melissa J. Sacco, MD Dylan Stewart, MD
5. Adolescent Medicine	Natalie Spicyn, MD, MHS	Arik Marcell, MD, MPH
6. Analgesia and Procedural Sedation	Sean Barnes, MD, MBA	Myron Yaster, MD
7. Cardiology	Catherine B. Gretchen, MD Arpana S. Rayannavar, MD	Jane Crosson, MD William Ravekes, MD W. Reid Thompson, MD
8. Dermatology	Jing Fang, MD	Bernard Cohen, MD
9. Development, Behavior, and Mental Health	Melissa Kwan, MD	Mary Leppert, MB, BCh, BAO Emily Frosch, MD
10. Endocrinology	Teresa Mark, MD	David Cooke, MD
11. Fluids and Electrolytes	Emily Young Thomas, MD	Michael Barone, MD
12. Gastroenterology	Tina Navidi, MD	Darla Shores, MD
13. Genetics: Metabolism and Dysmorphology	Jessica Duis, MD	Ronald Cohn, MD Ada Hamosh, MD
14. Hematology	Radha Gajjar, MD Elizabeth Jalazo, MD	James Casella, MD Clifford Takemoto, MD Jeffrey Keffer, MD
15. Immunology and Allergy	Emily Braun, MD	Robert Wood, MD
16. Immunoprophylaxis	Jennifer Albon, MD	Ravit Boger, MD
17. Microbiology and Infectious Disease	Edith Dietz, MD Courtney Mangus, MD	Pranita Tamma, MD
18. Neonatology	Lauren Beard, MD	Sue Aucott, MD
19. Nephrology	Katie Shaw, MD	Jeffrey Fadrowski, MD

Chapter Title	Resident	Faculty Advisor
20. Neurology	Lisa Sun, MD	Thomas Crawford, MD Christopher Oakley, MD Eric Kossoff, MD
21. Nutrition and Growth	Michael Koldobskiy, MD Jenifer Thompson, MS, RD, CSP	Sybil Klaus, MD
22. Oncology	M. Eric Kohler, MD, PhD	Patrick Brown, MD
23. Palliative Care	Jessica Knight-Perry, MD	Nancy Hutton, MD
24. Pulmonology	Margaret Grala, MD	Laura Sterni, MD
25. Radiology	Jessica Knight-Perry, MD	Jane Benson, MD
26. Rheumatology	Steven C. Marek, MD	Sangeeta Sule, MD, PhD Edward Sills, MD
27. Blood Chemistries and Body Fluids	Branden Engorn, MD Jamie Flerlage, MD	Lori Sokoll, PhD
28. Biostatistics and Evidence-Based Medicine	Kari Bjornard, MD, MPH	Janet Serwint, MD, MPH
29. Drug Dosages	Carlton K.K. Lee, PharmD, MPH Branden Engorn, MD Jamie Flerlage, MD	
30. Formulary Adjunct	Sara Mixter, MD, MPH J. Deanna Wilson, MD	Carlton K.K. Lee, PharmD, MPH
31. Drugs in Renal Failure	Monica C. Mix, MD Branden Engorn, MD	Carlton K.K. Lee, PharmD, MPH Angela Helder, PharmD

The Formulary, which is undoubtedly the most used handbook section, is complete, concise, and up to date thanks to the efforts of Carlton K.K. Lee, PharmD, MPH. With each edition, he carefully updates, revises, and improves the section. His herculean efforts make the Formulary one of the most useful and cited pediatric drug reference texts available.

We truly are humbled to have the opportunity to build on the great work of the preceding editors: Drs. Henry Seidel, Harrison Spencer, William Friedman, Robert Haslam, Jerry Winkelstein, Herbert Swick, Dennis Headings, Kenneth Schuberth, Basil Zitelli, Jeffery Biller, Andrew Yeager, Cynthia Cole, Peter Rowe, Mary Greene, Kevin Johnson, Michael Barone, George Siberry, Robert Iannone, Veronica Gunn, Christian Nechyba, Jason Robertson, Nicole Shilkofski, Jason Custer, Rachel Rau, Megan Tschudy, and Kristin Arcara. Many of these previous editors continue to contribute to the learning and maturation of the Harriet Lane house staff. They all are true examples of outstanding clinicians, educators, and mentors.

An undertaking of this magnitude could not have been accomplished without the support and dedication of some extraordinary people. First, a thanks to Kathy Miller, who has been an unwavering constant in the face of change, an advocate for residents, and a huge help with *The Harriet Lane Handbook*. We offer our deepest gratitude to our chairman, George Dover, whose compassion for children, dedication to improvement, and endless hours of service continue to enhance the Johns Hopkins Children's Center and pediatric resident education. He has taught years of chief residents that "perfect is the evil of the good." Our special thanks go to our friends and mentors, Jeffrey Fadrowski and Barry Solomon, who have taught us that enthusiasm is a vector for change. Thank you to our program director, Janet Serwint, whose leadership continues to deeply enrich our lives. She is the example of excellence in patient care, scholarship, and education. Thank you for teaching us that "data is power." Finally, none of this would have been possible without Julia McMillan. She is a true academic pediatrician in every sense of the word. She is the consummate diagnostician who has shaped the careers of countless pediatricians. She will forever be the pediatrician we strive to emulate.

Residents

Ibukun Akinboyo
Martha Amoako
Julia Aziz
Nikita Barai
Benjamin Barnes
Carolyn Bramante
May Chen
Natalia Diaz-Rodriguez
Grace Milad Felix
Timothy Flerlage
Ashley Foster
Wendy Goldstein
Helen Hughes
Fatima Ismail
Allison Kaeding
Lauren Kahl
Jennifer Kamens
Jillian Kaskavage
Kathryn Lemberg
Iris Leviner
Sarah Mahoney
Marisa Matthys
Zwena McLeod
Melanie McNally
Steven Miller
Kathryn Neubauer
Benjamin Oldfield
Danna Qunibi
Jacqueline Salas
Laura Scott
Miranda Simon

Interns

Annika Barnett
Devika Bhushan
Danielle Bliss
Madeline Cayton
Sally Cohen-Cutler
Matthew Elrick
Caitlin Engelhard
Amy Franciscovich
Michelle Gontasz
Taryn Hill
Daniel Hindman
Jennifer Hoffmann
Geoffrey Kelly
Christopher Knoll
Jennifer Miller
Idoreyin Montague
Candice Nalley
Angela-Tu Nguyen
Olamide Olambiwonnu
Christina Peroutka
Kristal Prather
Kristina Pyclik
Anirudh Ramesh
Naomi Rios
Camille Robinson
Suzanne Rossi
Jessica Rubens
Philip Sacks
Shivang Shah
Amena Smith
Heather Wasik
Olivia Widger

Branden Engorn

Jamie Flerlage

Contents

PART I   Pediatric Acute Care

1   Emergency Management   3
    Stephanie Chin-Sang, MD

2   Poisonings   19
    Zachary Nayak, MD, and Jocelyn Ronda, MD

3   Procedures   27
    Bradley D. McCammack, MD

4   Trauma, Burns, and Common Critical Care Emergencies   61
    Emily Krennerich, MD

PART II   Diagnostic and Therapeutic Information

5   Adolescent Medicine   91
    Natalie Spicyn, MD, MHS

6   Analgesia and Procedural Sedation   111
    Sean Barnes, MD, MBA

7   Cardiology   127
    Catherine B. Gretchen, MD, and Arpana S. Rayannavar, MD

8   Dermatology   172
    Jing Fang, MD

9   Development, Behavior, and Mental Health   195
    Melissa Kwan, MD

10 Endocrinology   214
    Teresa Mark, MD

11 Fluids and Electrolytes   246
    Emily Young Thomas, MD

12 Gastroenterology   268
    Tina Navidi, MD

13 Genetics: Metabolism and Dysmorphology   284
    Jessica Duis, MD

14 Hematology   305
    Radha Gajjar, MD, and Elizabeth Jalazo, MD

15 Immunology and Allergy 334
    Emily Braun, MD

16 Immunoprophylaxis 350
    Jennifer Albon, MD

17 Microbiology and Infectious Disease 380
    Edith Dietz, MD, and Courtney Mangus, MD

18 Neonatology 415
    Lauren Beard, MD

19 Nephrology 438
    Katie Shaw, MD

20 Neurology 467
    Lisa Sun, MD

21 Nutrition and Growth 485
    Michael Koldobskiy, MD, PhD, and Jenifer Thompson, MS, RD, CSP

22 Oncology 523
    M. Eric Kohler, MD, PhD

23 Palliative Care 540
    Jessica Knight-Perry, MD

24 Pulmonology 549
    Margaret Grala, MD

25 Radiology 572
    Jessica Knight-Perry, MD

26 Rheumatology 602
    Steven C. Marek, MD

PART III Reference

27 Blood Chemistries and Body Fluids 621
    Branden Engorn, MD, and Jamie Flerlage, MD

28 Biostatistics and Evidence-Based Medicine 634
    Kari Bjornard, MD, MPH

PART IV   Formulary

29   Drug Dosages   645
*Carlton K.K. Lee, PharmD, MPH; Branden Engorn, MD;
and Jamie Flerlage, MD*

30   Formulary Adjunct   987
Sara Mixter, MD, MPH, and J. Deanna Wilson, MD

31   Drugs in Renal Failure   994
Monica C. Mix, MD, and Branden Engorn, MD

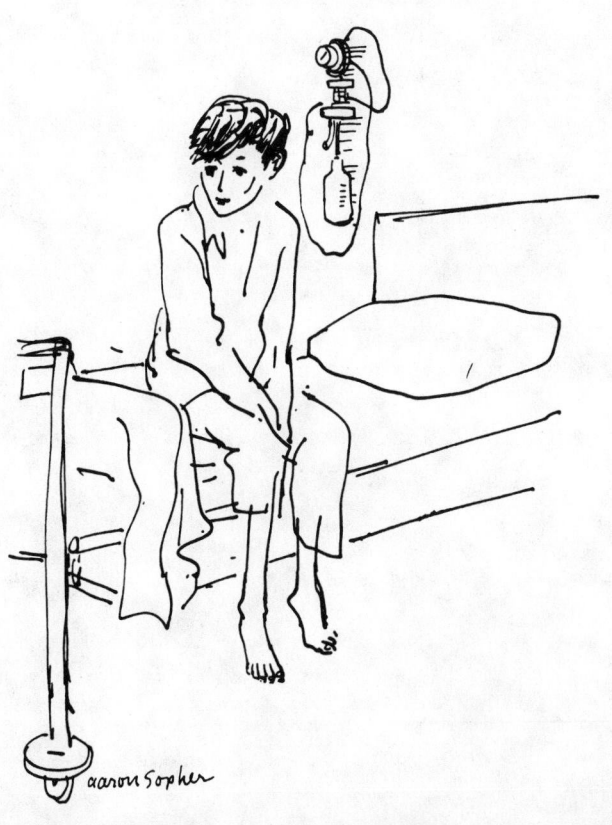

aaron Sopher

Chapter 1

Emergency Management

Stephanie Chin-Sang, MD

When approaching a patient in cardiopulmonary arrest, one must first and foremost focus on the A, B, C, D, and Es. The history, physical exam, and laboratory studies should closely follow a rapid primary assessment. **NOTE:** The 2010 American Heart Association Guidelines for Cardiopulmonary Resuscitation and Emergency Cardiovascular Care updates the 2005 guidelines by recommending that immediate chest compressions should be the first step in reviving **victims of sudden cardiac arrest,** so the new acronym C-A-B has come into use and is presented in this section. The original A-B-C pathway remains the accepted method for rapid assessment and management of any critically ill patient.[1]

See the 2010 AHA CPR guidelines.

I. INITIAL ASSESSMENT: C-A-B

A. Assess pulse: If infant/child is unresponsive and not breathing (gasps do not count as breathing), health care providers may take up to 10 seconds to feel for pulse (brachial in infant, carotid/femoral in child).[2]

1. **If pulseless,** immediately begin chest compressions (see Circulation, B.1).
2. **If pulse,** begin A-B-C pathway of evaluation.

II. AIRWAY[3-6]

A. Assessment

1. **Assess airway patency; think about obstruction:** Head tilt/chin lift (or jaw thrust if injury suspected) to open airway.
2. **Assess for spontaneous respiration:** If no spontaneous respirations, begin ventilating via rescue breaths, bag-mask, or endotracheal tube.
3. **Assess adequacy of respirations:**
a. Look for chest rise.
b. Recognize signs of distress (stridor, tachypnea, flaring, retractions, accessory muscle use, wheezes).

B. Management[3-12]

1. **Equipment**
a. Bag-mask ventilation with cricoid pressure may be used indefinitely if ventilating effectively (look at chest rise).
b. Use oral or nasopharyngeal airway in patients with obstruction:
   (1) Oral: Unconscious patients—measure from corner of mouth to mandibular angle.
   (2) Nasal: Conscious patients—measure tip of nose to tragus of ear.

   c. Laryngeal mask airway (LMA): Simple way to secure an airway (no laryngoscopy needed), especially in difficult airways; does not prevent aspiration.
2. **Intubation:** Indicated for (impending) respiratory failure, obstruction, airway protection, pharmacotherapy, or need for likely prolonged support
   a. Equipment (see page i): **SOAP** (**S**uction, **O**xygen, **A**irway Supplies, **P**harmacology)
     (1) Laryngoscope blade:
       (a) Miller (straight blade):
         (i) #00-1 for premature to 2 months
         (ii) #1 for 3 months to 3 years
         (iii) #2 for > 3 years
       (b) Macintosh (curved blade):
         (i) #2 for > 2 years
         (ii) #3 for > 8 years
     (2) Endotracheal tube (ETT):
       (a) Size determination: Internal diameter of ETT (mm) = (Age/4) + 4, or use length-based resuscitation tape to estimate.
       (b) Approximate depth of insertion in cm = ETT size × 3.
       (c) Uncuffed ETT for patients <8 years of age (note: cuffed tube can be used in children <8 y/o—see AHA guidelines for sizing recommendations).
       (d) Stylet should not extend beyond the distal end of the ETT.
       (e) Attach end-tidal CO_2 monitor as confirmation of placement and effectiveness of chest compressions if applicable.
     (3) Nasogastric tube (NGT): To decompress the stomach; measure from nose to angle of jaw to xiphoid for depth of insertion.
   b. Rapid sequence intubation (RSI) recommended for aspiration risk:
     (1) Preoxygenate with non-rebreather at 100% O_2 for minimum of 3 minutes:
       (a) Do not use positive-pressure ventilation (PPV) unless patient effort is inadequate.
       (b) Children have less oxygen/respiratory reserve than adults, owing to higher oxygen consumption and lower functional residual capacity.
     (2) See Fig. 1-1 and Table 1-1 for drugs used for RSI (adjunct, sedative, paralytic). Important considerations in choosing appropriate agents include clinical scenario, allergies, presence of neuromuscular disease, anatomic abnormalities, or hemodynamic status.
     (3) For patients who are difficult to mask ventilate or have difficult airways, may consider sedation without paralysis and the assistance of subspecialists (anesthesiology and otolaryngology).
   c. Procedure (attempts should not exceed 30 seconds):
     (1) Preoxygenate with 100% O_2.
     (2) Administer intubation medications (see Fig. 1-1 and Table 1-1).
     (3) Apply cricoid pressure to prevent aspiration (Sellick maneuver) during bag-valve-mask ventilation and intubation. (Note: Use of cricoid pressure is optional; no benefit has been demonstrated.)

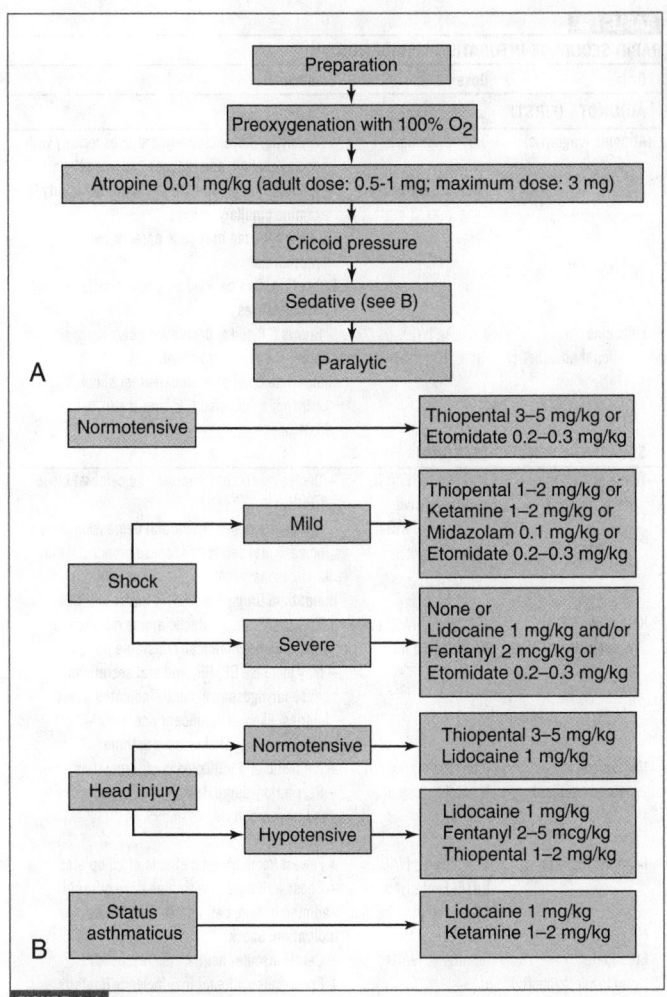

FIGURE 1-1

A, Treatment algorithm for intubation. **B,** Sedation options. *(Modified from Nichols DG, Yaster M, Lappe DG, et al [eds].* Golden Hour: The Handbook of Advanced Pediatric Life Support. *St Louis: Mosby; 1996:29.)*

TABLE 1-1

RAPID-SEQUENCE INTUBATION MEDICATIONS

Drug	Dose	Comments
ADJUNCTS (FIRST)		
Atropine (vagolytic)	0.01–0.02 mg/kg IV/IO Adult dose: 0.5-1.0 mg; max: 3 mg	+ Vagolytic; prevents bradycardia, especially with succinylcholine, and reduces oral secretions − Tachycardia, pupil dilation eliminates ability to examine pupillary reflexes Less than 0.1 mg may case paradoxical bradycardia **Indication:** Can be used as premedication in all circumstances
Lidocaine (optional anesthetic)	1 mg/kg IV/IO; max 100 mg/dose	+ Blunts ICP spike, decreased gag/cough; controls ventricular arrhythmias **Indication:** Good premedication for shock, arrhythmia, elevated ICP, and status asthmaticus
SEDATIVE-HYPNOTIC (SECOND)		
Thiopental (barbiturate)	3–5 mg/kg IV/IO if normotensive 1–2 mg/kg IV/IO if hypotensive	+ Decreases O_2 consumption and cerebral blood flow − Vasodilation and myocardial depression; may increase oral secretions, cause bronchospasm/laryngospasm (not to be used in asthma) **Indication:** Drug of choice for increased ICP
Ketamine (NMDA receptor antagonist)	1–2 mg/kg IV/IO or 4–10 mg/kg IM	+ Bronchodilation; catecholamine release may benefit hemodynamically unstable patients − May increase BP, HR, and oral secretions; may cause laryngospasm; contraindicated in eye injuries; likely insignificant rise in ICP **Indication:** Drug of choice for asthma
Midazolam (benzodiazepine)	0.05–0.1 mg/kg IV/IO Max total dose of 10 mg	+ Amnestic and anticonvulsant properties − Respiratory depression/apnea, hypotension, and myocardial depression **Indication:** Mild shock
Fentanyl (opiate)	1–5 mcg/kg IV/IO **NOTE:** Fentanyl is dosed in mcg/kg, not mg/kg.	+ Fewest hemodynamic effects of all opiates − Chest wall rigidity with high dose or rapid administration; cannot use with MAOIs **Indication:** Shock
Etomidate (imidazole/hypnotic)	0.3 mg/kg IV/IO	+ Cardiovascular neutral; decreases ICP − Exacerbates adrenal insufficiency (inhibits 11-beta hydroxylase) **Indication:** Patients with severe shock, especially cardiac patients
Propofol (sedative-hypnotic)	2 mg/kg IV/IO	+ Extremely quick onset and short duration; blood pressure lowering; good antiemetic − Hypotension and profound myocardial depression; contraindicated in patients with egg allergy **Indication:** Induction agent for general anesthesia

TABLE 1-1

RAPID-SEQUENCE INTUBATION MEDICATIONS (Continued)

Drug	Dose	Comments
PARALYTICS (NEUROMUSCULAR BLOCKERS) (THIRD)		
Succinylcholine (depolarizing)	1–2 mg/kg IV/IO 2–4 mg/kg IM	+ Quick onset (30–60 sec), short duration (3–6 min) make it an ideal paralytic − Irreversible; bradycardia in <5 years old or with rapid doses; increased risk of malignant hyperthermia; contraindicated in burns, massive trauma/muscle injury, neuromuscular disease, myopathies, eye injuries, renal insufficiency
Vecuronium (non-depolarizing)	0.1 mg/kg IV/IO	+ Onset 70–120 sec; cardiovascular neutral − Duration 30–90 min; must wait 30–45 min to reverse with glycopyrrolate and neostigmine **Indication:** When succinylcholine contraindicated or when longer-term paralysis desired
Rocuronium (non-depolarizing)	0.6–1.2 mg/kg IV/IO 1.8 mg/kg IM	+ Quicker onset (30–60 sec), shorter acting than vecuronium; cardiovascular neutral − Duration 30–60 min; may reverse in 30 min with gylcopyrrolate and neostigmine

+, Potential advantages; −, potential disadvantages or cautions; BP, blood pressure; HR, heart rate; ICP, intracranial pressure; MAOI, monoamine oxidase inhibitor.

(4) Use scissoring technique to open mouth.
(5) Hold laryngoscope blade in left hand. Insert blade into right side of mouth, sweeping tongue to the left out of line of vision.
(6) Advance blade to epiglottis. With straight blade, lift up, directly lifting the epiglottis to view cords. With curved blade, place tip in vallecula, elevate the epiglottis to visualize the vocal cords.
(7) If possible, have another person hand over the tube, maintaining direct visualization, and pass through cords until black marker reaches the level of the cords.
(8) Hold endotracheal tube firmly against the lip until tube is securely taped.
(9) Verify ETT placement: observe chest wall movement, auscultation in both axillae and epigastrium, end-tidal CO_2 detection (there will be a false-negative response if there is no effective pulmonary circulation), improvement in oxygen saturation, chest radiograph, repeat direct laryngoscopy to visualize ETT.
(10) If available, in-line continuous CO_2 detection should be used.

III. BREATHING[3,4,13,14]

A. Assessment

Once airway is secured, continually reevaluate ETT positioning (listen for breath sounds). Acute respiratory failure may signify **D**isplacement of the ETT, **O**bstruction, **P**neumothorax, or **E**quipment failure (DOPE).

B. Management

1. **Mouth-to-mouth or mouth-to-nose breathing:** provide two slow breaths (1 sec/breath) initially. For newborns, apply one breath for every three chest compressions. In infants and children, apply two breaths after 30 compressions (one rescuer) or two breaths after 15 compressions (two rescuers). Breaths should have adequate volume to cause chest rise.
2. **Bag-mask ventilation** is used at a rate of 20 breaths/min (30 breaths/min in infants) using the E-C technique:
a. Use non-dominant hand to create a C with thumb and index finger over top of mask. Ensure a good seal, but *do not* push down on mask. Hook remaining fingers around the mandible (*not* the soft tissues of the neck!), with the fifth finger on the angle creating an E, and lift the mandible up toward the mask.
b. Assess chest expansion and breath sounds.
c. Decompress stomach with orogastric or nasogastric tube with prolonged bag-mask ventilation.
3. **Endotracheal intubation:** See prior section.

IV. CIRCULATION[3-5,13]

A. Assessment

1. **Rate/rhythm:** Assess for bradycardia, tachycardia, abnormal rhythm, or asystole. Generally, bradycardia requiring chest compressions is <60 beats/min; tachycardia of >220 beats/min suggests tachyarrhythmia rather than sinus tachycardia.
2. **Perfusion:**
a. Assess pulses, capillary refill (<2 sec = normal, 2 to 5 sec = delayed, >5 sec suggests shock), mentation, and urine output (if Foley in place).
b. If one cannot identify a pulse within 10 seconds, initiate cardiopulmonary resuscitation (CPR).
3. **Blood pressure (BP):** Hypotension is a late manifestation of circulatory compromise. Can be calculated in children >1 year with

formula: Hypotension = Systolic BP< $[70 + (2 \times \text{Age in years})]$

B. Management (Table 1-2)[15]

1. **Chest compressions**
a. Press hard (⅓ to ½ anteroposterior [AP] diameter of chest) and fast (100-120 per minute) on backboard base with full recoil and minimal interruption.
b. Use end-tidal CO_2 to estimate effectiveness (<20 mmHg indicates inadequate compressions).
c. Use two-finger technique for infant if single rescuer available; otherwise, two thumbs with hands encircling chest is preferable.
2. **Use of automated external defibrillator (AED):** To determine whether rhythm is shockable, use an AED/defibrillator.

TABLE 1-2

MANAGEMENT OF CIRCULATION

	Location*	Rate (per min)	Compressions: Ventilation
Infants	1 fingerbreadth below intermammary line	>100	15:2 (2 rescuers) 30:2 (1 rescuer)
Pre-pubertal children	2 fingerbreadths below intermammary line	≥100	15:2 (2 rescuers) 30:2 (1 rescuer)
Adolescents/adults	Lower half of sternum	100	30:2 (1 or 2 rescuers)

*Depth of compressions should be one third to one half anteroposterior diameter of the chest.

3. **Resuscitation with poor perfusion and shock:**
a. Optimize oxygen delivery with supplemental O_2.
b. Support respirations to reduce work of patient.
c. Place intraosseous (IO) access immediately if in arrest and/or if intravenous (IV) access not obtained within 90 seconds.
d. Resuscitation fluids are lactated Ringer's or normal saline.
   (1) Give up to three 20-mL/kg boluses each within 5 minutes for a total of 60 mL/kg in the first 15 minutes after presentation, checking for hepatomegaly after each bolus.
   (2) 5- to 10-mL/kg bolus in patient with cardiac insufficiency.
   (3) Consider colloid such as albumin, plasma, packed red blood cells (PRBCs) if poor response to crystalloids.
e. Identify type of shock: Hypovolemia, cardiogenic (congenital heart disease, myocarditis, cardiomyopathy, arrhythmia), distributive (sepsis, anaphylaxis, neurogenic), obstructive (pulmonary embolus [PE], cardiac tamponade, tension pneumothorax).
f. Pharmacotherapy (See inside front cover and consider stress-dose corticosteroids and/or antibiotics if applicable.)

V. ALLERGIC EMERGENCIES (ANAPHYLAXIS)[16,17]

A. Definition

1. **A rapid-onset immunoglobulin (Ig) E–mediated systemic allergic reaction involving multiple organ systems, including two or more of the following:**
a. **Cutaneous/mucosal** (flushing, urticaria, pruritus, angioedema); seen in 90%
b. **Respiratory** (laryngeal edema, bronchospasm, dyspnea, wheezing, stridor, hypoxemia); seen in ≈70%
c. **Gastrointestinal (GI)** (vomiting, diarrhea, nausea, crampy abdominal pain); seen in ≈ -40% to 50%
d. **Circulatory** (tachycardia, hypotension, syncope); seen in ≈ -30% to 40%
2. **Initial reaction may be delayed for several hours AND symptoms may recur up to 72 hours after initial recovery.** Patients should therefore be observed for a minimum of 6 to 24 hours for late-phase symptoms.

B. Initial Management

1. **Remove/stop exposure to precipitating antigen.**

2. **Epinephrine** = mainstay of therapy. While performing ABCs, immediately give intramuscular (IM) epinephrine, 0.01 mg/kg (0.01 mL/kg) of 1:1000 subcutaneously (SQ) or IM (maximum dose 0.5 mg). Repeat every 5 minutes as needed. Site of choice is lateral aspect of the thigh, owing to its vascularity.
3. **Establish airway** and give O_2 and PPV as needed.
4. **Obtain IV access,** Trendelenburg position with head 30 degrees below feet, administer fluid boluses followed by pressors as needed.
5. **Histamine-1 receptor antagonist** such as diphenhydramine, 1 to 2 mg/kg via IM, IV, or oral (PO) route (maximum dose, 50 mg). Also consider a histamine-2 receptor antagonist (e.g., ranitidine).
6. **Corticosteroids** help prevent the late phase of the allergic response. Administer methylprednisolone in a 2-mg/kg IV bolus, followed by 2 mg/kg/day IV or IM, divided every 6 hours, or prednisone, 2 mg/kg PO once daily.
7. **Albuterol** 2.5 mg for <30 kg, 5 mg for >30 kg, for bronchospasm or wheezing. Repeat every 15 minutes as needed.
8. **Racemic epinephrine** 0.5 mL of 2.25% solution inhaled for signs of upper airway obstruction
9. Patient should be discharged with an **Epi-Pen** (>30 kg), **Epi-Pen Junior** (<30 kg), or comparable injectable epinephrine product with specific instructions on appropriate use, as well as an anaphylaxis action plan.

VI. RESPIRATORY EMERGENCIES[18]

The hallmark of upper airway obstruction is stridor, whereas lower airway obstruction is characterized by cough, wheeze, and a prolonged expiratory phase.

A. Asthma[19,20]

Lower airway obstruction resulting from triad of inflammation, bronchospasm, and increased secretions:
1. **Assessment:** Respiratory rate (RR), work of breathing, O_2 saturation, heart rate (HR), peak expiratory flow, alertness, color
2. **Initial management:**
a. Give O_2 to keep saturation >95%.
b. Administer inhaled β-agonists: Nebulized albuterol as often as needed.
c. Ipratropium bromide
d. Steroids: Methylprednisolone, 2 mg/kg IV/IM bolus, then 2 mg/kg/day divided every 6 hours; *or* prednisone/prednisolone, 2 mg/kg PO every 24 hours; requires minimum of 3 to 4 hours to take effect.
e. If air movement is still poor despite maximizing above therapy:
   (1) Epinephrine: 0.01 mg/kg (0.01 mL/kg) of 1:1000 subcutaneously (SQ) or IM (maximum dose 0.5 mg)
      (a) Bronchodilator, vasopressor, and inotropic effects
      (b) Short-acting (~15 min) and should be used as temporizing rather than definitive therapy

(2) Magnesium sulfate: 25 to 75 mg/kg/dose IV or IM (maximum 2 g) infused over 20 minutes.
   (a) Smooth muscle relaxant; relieves bronchospasm.
   (b) Many clinicians advise giving a saline bolus prior to administration, because hypotension may result.
   (c) Contraindicated if patient already has significant hypotension or renal insufficiency.
(3) Terbutaline: 0.01 mg/kg SQ (maximum dose 0.4 mg) every 15 minutes up to three doses.
   (a) Systemic β_2-agonist limited by cardiac intolerance.
   (b) Monitor continuous 12-lead electrocardiogram (ECG), cardiac enzymes, urinalysis (UA), and electrolytes.
3. **Further management:** If incomplete or poor response, consider obtaining an arterial blood gas value.
   NOTE: A normalizing Pco_2 is often a sign of impending respiratory failure.
a. Maximize and continue initial treatments.
b. Terbutaline 2 to 10 mcg/kg IV load, followed by continuous infusion of 0.1 to 4 mcg/kg/min titrated to effect in increments of 0.1 to 0.2 mcg/kg/min every 30 minutes depending on clinical response. Infusion should be started with lowest possible dose; doses as high as 10 mcg/kg/min have been used. Use appropriate cardiac monitoring in intensive care unit (ICU), as above.
c. A helium (≥70%) and oxygen mixture may be of some benefit in the critically ill patient but is more useful in upper airway edema. Avoid use in the hypoxic patient.
d. Methylxanthines (e.g., aminophylline) may be considered in the ICU setting but have significant side effects and have not been shown to affect intubation rates or length of hospital stay.
e. Noninvasive positive-pressure ventilation (e.g., BiPAP) may be used in patients with impending respiratory failure, both as a temporizing measure and to avoid intubation, but requires a cooperative patient with spontaneous respirations.
4. **Intubation** of those with acute asthma is dangerous and should be reserved for impending respiratory arrest.
a. Indications for endotracheal intubation include deteriorating mental status, severe hypoxemia, and respiratory or cardiac arrest.
b. Use lidocaine as adjunct and ketamine for sedative (see Fig. 1-1 and Table 1-1).
c. Consider using an inhaled anesthetic such as isoflurane.
5. **Hypotension:** Result of air trapping, hyperinflation, and therefore decreased pulmonary venous return. See Section IV.B.3 for management. Definitive treatment is reducing lower airway obstruction.

B. Upper Airway Obstruction[21-24]

Upper airway obstruction is most commonly caused by foreign-body aspiration or infection.

1. **Epiglottitis:** Most often affects children between 2 and 7 years, but may occur at any age. This is a true emergency involving cellulitis and edema of the epiglottis, aryepiglottic folds, and hypopharynx.
   a. Patient is usually febrile, anxious, and toxic appearing, with sore throat, drooling, respiratory distress, stridor, tachypnea, and *tripod positioning* (sitting forward supported by both arms, with neck extended and chin thrust out). Any agitation of the child may cause complete obstruction, so avoid invasive procedures/evaluation until airway is secured.
   b. Unobtrusively give O_2 (blow-by). Nothing by mouth, monitor with pulse oximetry, allow parent to hold patient.
   c. Summon epiglottitis team (most senior pediatrician, anesthesiologist, intensive care physician, and otolaryngologist in hospital).
   d. Management options:
      (1) If unstable (unresponsive, cyanotic, bradycardic) → emergently intubate.
      (2) If stable with high suspicion → take patient to operating room for laryngoscopy and intubation under general anesthesia.
      (3) If stable with moderate or low suspicion → obtain lateral neck radiographs to confirm.
   e. After airway is secure, obtain cultures of blood and epiglottic surface. Begin antibiotics to cover *Haemophilus influenzae* type B, *Streptococcus pneumoniae,* group A streptococci, *Staphylococcus aureus.*
   f. Epiglottitis may also be caused by thermal injury, caustic ingestion, or foreign body.
2. **Croup (laryngotracheobronchitis):** Most common in infants 6 to 36 months. Croup is a common syndrome involving inflammation of the subglottic area; presents with fever, barking cough, and stridor. Patients rarely appear toxic, as in epiglottitis.
   a. Mild (no stridor at rest): Treat with minimal disturbance, cool mist, hydration, antipyretics, and consider steroids.
   b. Moderate to severe:
      (1) The efficacy of mist therapy is not established.
      (2) Racemic epinephrine. After administering, observe for a minimum of 2 to 4 hours, owing to potential for rebound obstruction. Hospitalize if more than one nebulization required.
      (3) Dexamethasone, 0.3 to 0.6 mg/kg IV, IM, or PO once. Effect lasts 2 to 3 days. Alternatively, nebulized budesonide (2 mg) may be used, though little data exist to support its use, and some studies find it inferior to dexamethasone.
      (4) A helium-oxygen mixture may decrease resistance to turbulent gas flow through a narrowed airway.
   c. If a child fails to respond as expected to therapy, consider other etiologies (e.g., retropharyngeal abscess, bacterial tracheitis, subglottic stenosis, epiglottitis, foreign body). Obtain airway radiography, computed tomography (CT), and evaluation by otolaryngology or anesthesiology.

3. **Foreign-body aspiration:** Occurs most often in children 6 months to 3 years old. It frequently involves hot dogs, candy, peanuts, grapes, or balloons. Most events unwitnessed, so suspect this in children with sudden-onset choking, stridor, or wheezing.
a. If the patient is stable (i.e., forcefully coughing, well oxygenated), removal of the foreign body by bronchoscopy or laryngoscopy should be attempted in a controlled environment.
b. If the patient is unable to speak, moves air poorly, or is cyanotic:
   (1) Infant: Place infant over arm or rest on lap. Give five back blows between the scapulae. If unsuccessful, turn infant over and give five chest thrusts (*not* abdominal thrusts).
   (2) Child: Perform five abdominal thrusts (Heimlich maneuver) from behind a sitting or standing child.
   (3) After back, chest, and/or abdominal thrusts, open mouth using tongue-jaw lift and remove foreign body if visualized. Do not attempt blind finger sweeps. Magill forceps may be used to retrieve objects in the posterior pharynx. Ventilate if unconscious, and repeat sequence as needed.
   (4) If there is complete airway obstruction and the patient cannot be ventilated by bag-valve mask or ETT, consider percutaneous (needle) cricothyrotomy (Fig. 1-2).[4]

VII. NEUROLOGIC EMERGENCIES

A. Altered States of Consciousness[25]

1. **Assessment:** Range of mental status includes alert, confused, disoriented, delirious, lethargic, stuporous, and comatose.
a. History: Consider structural versus medical causes (Box 1-1). Obtain history of trauma, ingestion, infection, fasting, drug use, diabetes, seizure, or other neurologic disorder.
b. Examination: Assess HR, BP, respiratory pattern, Glasgow Coma Scale (Table 1-3), temperature, pupillary response, funduscopy (a late finding, absence of papilledema does not rule out increased intracranial pressure [ICP]), rash, abnormal posturing, and focal neurologic signs.
2. **Acute traumatic head injury:**[26]
a. Assess pupillary response:
   (1) Blown pupil: Elevate head of bed, hyperventilate, maintain blood pressure, administer hypertonic saline and/or mannitol.
3. **Management of coma:**
a. **A**irway (with cervical spine immobilization), **B**reathing, **C**irculation, **D**-stick, **O**xygen, **N**aloxone, **T**hiamine (ABC DON'T)
   (1) Naloxone, 0.1 mg/kg IV, IM, SQ, or ETT (maximum dose, 2 mg). Repeat as necessary, given short half-life (in case of opiate intoxication).
   (2) Thiamine, 100 mg IV (before starting glucose in adolescents, in case of alcoholism or eating disorder).
   (3) $D_{25}W$, 2 to 4 mL/kg IV bolus if hypoglycemia is present.

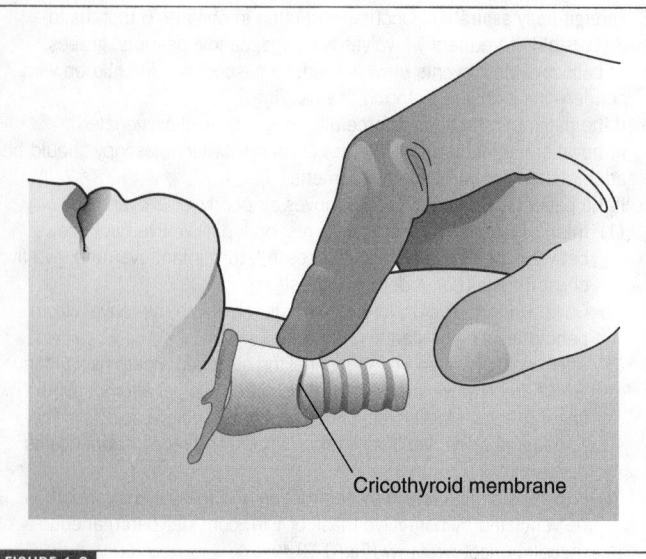

Cricothyroid membrane

FIGURE 1-2

Percutaneous (needle) cricothyrotomy. Extend neck, attach a 3-mL syringe to a 14- to 18-gauge intravenous catheter, and introduce catheter through cricothyroid membrane (inferior to thyroid cartilage, superior tocricoid cartilage). Aspirate air to confirm position. Remove syringe and needle, attach catheter to an adaptor from a 3.0-mm endotracheal tube, which can then be used for positive-pressure oxygenation. *(Modified from Dieckmann RA, Fiser DH, Selbst SM. Illustrated Textbook of Pediatric Emergency and Critical Care Procedures. St Louis: Mosby, 1997:118.)*

BOX 1-1

DIFFERENTIAL DIAGNOSIS OF ALTERED LEVEL OF CONSCIOUSNESS

I. Structural Causes

Vascular—e.g., cerebrovascular accident, cerebral vein thrombosis
Increased intracranial pressure—e.g., hydrocephalus, tumor, abscess, cyst, subdural empyema, pseudotumor cerebri
Trauma (intracranial hemorrhage, diffuse cerebral swelling, shaken baby syndrome)

II. Medical Causes

Anoxia
Hypothermia/hyperthermia
Metabolic—e.g., inborn errors of metabolism, diabetic ketoacidosis, hyperammonemia, uremia, hypoglycemia, electrolyte abnormality
Infection—e.g., sepsis, meningitis, encephalitis, subdural empyema
Seizure/postictal state
Toxins/ingestions
Psychiatric/psychogenic

Modified from Avner J. Altered states of consciousness. *Pediatr Rev.* 2006;27:331-337.

TABLE 1-3

COMA SCALES

Glasgow Coma Scale		Modified Coma Scale for Infants	
Activity	Best Response	Activity	Best Response
EYE OPENING			
Spontaneous	4	Spontaneous	4
To speech	3	To speech	3
To pain	2	To pain	2
None	1	None	1
VERBAL			
Oriented	5	Coo/babbles	5
Confused	4	Irritable	4
Inappropriate words	3	Cries to pain	3
Nonspecific sounds	2	Moans to pain	2
None	1	None	1
MOTOR			
Follows commands	6	Normal spontaneous movements	6
Localizes pain	5	Withdraws to touch	5
Withdraws to pain	4	Withdraws to pain	4
Abnormal flexion	3	Abnormal flexion	3
Abnormal extension	2	Abnormal extension	2
None	1	None	1

Data from Jennet B, Teasdale G. Aspects of coma after severe head injury. *Lancet*. 1977;1:878; and James HE. Neurologic evaluation and support in the child with an acute brain insult. *Pediatr Ann*. 1986;15:16.

b. Laboratory tests: Consider complete blood cell count (CBC), electrolytes, liver function tests, NH_3, lactate, toxicology screen (serum and urine; always include salicylate and acetaminophen levels), blood gas, serum osmolality, prothrombin time (PT)/partial thromboplastin time (PTT), and blood/urine culture. If patient is an infant or toddler, consider assessment of plasma amino acids, urine organic acids, and other appropriate metabolic workup.

c. If meningitis or encephalitis is suspected, consider lumbar puncture (LP) and start antibiotics and acyclovir.

d. Request emergency head CT after ABCs are stabilized; consider neurosurgical consultation and electroencephalogram (EEG) if indicated.

e. If ingestion is suspected, airway must be protected before GI decontamination (see Chapter 2).

f. Monitor Glasgow Coma Scale and reassess frequently (see Table 1-3).

B. Status Epilepticus[27,28]

See Chapter 20 for non-acute evaluation and management of seizures.

1. **Assessment:** Common causes of childhood seizures include electrolyte abnormalities, hypoglycemia, fever, subtherapeutic anticonvulsant levels, central nervous system (CNS) infections, trauma, toxic ingestion, and metabolic abnormalities. Consider specific patient history, such as

shunt malfunction in patient with ventriculoperitoneal shunt. Less common causes include vascular, neoplastic, and endocrine diseases.

2. **Acute management of seizures** (Table 1-4): If CNS infection is suspected, give antibiotics and/or acyclovir early.

3. **Diagnostic workup:** When stable, workup may include CT or magnetic resonance imaging, EEG, and LP.

TABLE 1-4

ACUTE MANAGEMENT OF SEIZURES

Time (min)	Intervention
0–5	Stabilize patient.
	Assess airway, breathing, circulation, and vital signs.
	Administer oxygen.
	Obtain IV or IO access.
	Consider hypoglycemia, thiamine deficiency, intoxication (dextrose, thiamine, naloxone may be given immediately if suspected).
	Obtain laboratory studies: consider glucose, electrolytes, calcium, magnesium, blood gas, CBC, BUN, creatinine, LFTs, toxicology screen, anticonvulsant levels, blood culture (if infection is suspected).
	Initial screening history and physical examination
5–15	Begin pharmacotherapy:
	Lorazepam (Ativan), 0.05–0.1 mg/kg IV/IM, max dose 2 mg
	Or
	Diazepam (Valium), 0.2–0.5 mg/kg IV (0.5 mg/kg rectally); max dose <5 y/o: 5 mg, >5 y/o: 10 mg
	May repeat lorazepam or diazepam 5–10 min after initial dose
15–25	If seizure persists, load with one of the following:
	1. Fosphenytoin* 15–20 mg PE/kg IV/IM at 3 mg PE/kg/min via peripheral IV line (maximum 150 mg PE/min). If given IM, may require mulitple dosing sites.
	2. Phenytoin† 15–20 mg/kg IV at rate not to exceed 1 mg/kg/min via central line
	3. Phenobarbital 15–20 mg/kg IV at rate not to exceed 1 mg/kg/min
25–40	If seizure persists:
	Levetiracetam 20–30 mg/kg IV at 5 mg/kg/min; or valproate 20 mg/kg IV at 5 mg/kg/min
	May give phenobarbital at this time if still seizing at 5 minutes and (fos) phenytoin previously used
	Additional phenytoin or fosphenytoin 5 mg/kg over 12 hr for goal serum level of 10 mg/L
	Additional phenobarbital 5 mg/kg/dose every 15–30 min (maximum total dose of 30 mg/kg; be prepared to support respirations)
40–60	If seizure persists,‡ consider pentobarbital, midazolam, or general anesthesia in intensive care unit. Avoid paralytics.

*Fosphenytoin dosed as phenytoin equivalent (PE).
†Phenytoin may be contraindicated for seizures secondary to alcohol withdrawal or most ingestions (see Chapter 2).
‡Pyridoxine 100 mg IV in infant with persistent initial seizure.
BUN, Blood urea nitrogen; CBC, complete blood cell count; CT, computed tomography; EEG, electroencephalogram; LFTs, liver function tests; IM, intramuscular; IO, intraosseus; IV, intravenous.
Modified from Abend, NS, Dlugos, DJ. Treatment of refractory status epilepticus: literature review and a proposed protocol. *Pediatr Neurol.* 2008;38:377.

REFERENCES

1. Field JM, Hazinski MF, Sayre MR, et al. 2010 American Heart Association guidelines for cardiopulmonary resuscitation and emergency cardiovascular care. *Circulation*. 2010:Nov 2;122(18 Suppl 3):S640-656.

2. Berg MD, Schexnayder SM, Chameides L, et al. Part 13: pediatric basic life support: 2010 American Heart Association guidelines for cardiopulmonary resuscitation and emergency cardiovascular care. *Circulation*. 2010;122(18 Suppl 3):S862-S875.

3. American Heart Association. Pediatric advanced life support. *Pediatrics*. 2006;117:e1005-e1028.

4. Nichols DG, Yaster M, Lappe DG, et al, eds. *Golden Hour: The Handbook of Advanced Pediatric Life Support*. St Louis: Mosby, 1996.

5. Ralston M, Hazinski MF, Zaritsky AL, et al, eds. *Pediatric Advanced Life Support Provider Manual*. Dallas: American Heart Association, Subcommittee on Pediatric Resuscitation, 2006.

6. Sagarin MJ, Barton ED, Chng YM, et al. Airway management by US and Canadian emergency medicine residents: a multicenter analysis of more than 6,000 endotracheal intubation attempts. *Ann Emerg Med*. 2005;46:328-336.

7. American Heart Association. Pharmacology. In: *Pediatric Advanced Life Support Provider Manual*. Dallas: American Heart Association, Subcommittee on Pediatric Resuscitation; 2006:228.

8. Sagarin MJ, Chiang V, Sakles JC, et al. Rapid sequence intubation for pediatric emergency airway management. *Pediatr Emerg Care*. 2002;18:417.

9. Zelicof-Paul A, Smith-Lockridge A, Schnadower D, et al. Controversies in rapid sequence intubation in children. *Curr Opin Pediatr*. 2005;17:355.

10. Sivilotti ML, Filbin MR, Murray HE, et al. Does the sedative agent facilitate emergency rapid sequence intubation? *Acad Emerg Med*. 2003;10:612.

11. Perry J, Lee J, Wells G. Rocuronium versus succinylcholine for rapid sequence induction intubation. *Cochrane Database Syst Rev*. 2003:CD002788.

12. Trethewy CE, Burrows JM, Clausen D, Doherty SR. Effectiveness of cricoid pressure in preventing gastric aspiration during rapid sequence intubation in the emergency department: study protocol for a randomised controlled trial *Trials*. Epub 2012 Feb 16;13;17.

13. Pediatric basic life support. *Circulation*. 2005;112:IV156.

14. Berg RA, Sanders AB, Kern KB, et al. Adverse hemodynamic effects of interrupting chest compressions for rescue breathing during cardiopulmonary resuscitation for ventricular fibrillation cardiac arrest. *Circulation*. 2001;104:2465.

15. Stevenson AG, McGowan J, Evans AL, et al. CPR for children: one hand or two? *Resuscitation*. 2005;64:205.

16. Sampson HA, Munoz-Furlong A. Second symposium on the definition and management of anaphylaxis: summary report—Second National Institute of Allergy and Infectious Disease/Food Allergy and Anaphylaxis Network symposium. *J Allergy Clin Immunol*. 2006;117:391-397.

17. Lee JM, Greenes DS. Biphasic anaphylactic reactions in pediatrics. *Pediatrics*. 2000;106:762.

18. Luten RC, Kissoon N. The difficult pediatric airway. In: Walls RM, ed. *Manual of Emergency Management*. 2nd ed. Philadelphia: Williams & Wilkins, 2004:236.

19. National Asthma Education and Prevention Program. *Expert Panel Report III: Guidelines for the Diagnosis and Management of Asthma*. Bethesda, MD: National Heart, Lung and Blood Institute; National Heart, Lung, and Blood Institute, 2007.

20. Carroll CL, Schramm CM. Noninvasive positive pressure ventilation for the treatment of status asthmaticus in children. *Ann Allergy Asthma Immunol.* 2006;96:454.

21. Cherry JD. Croup (laryngitis, laryngotracheitis, spasmodic croup, laryngotracheobronchitis, bacterial tracheitis, and laryngotracheobronchopneumonitis). In: Feigin RD, Cherry JD, Demmler H, et al, ed. *Textbook of Pediatric Infectious Diseases.* 6th ed. Philadelphia: Saunders, 2009:254.

22. Alberta Medical Association. Guideline for the diagnosis and management of croup. Alberta Clinical Practice Guidelines 2008. Published on the Alberta Medical Association Practice Guideline Website.

23. McMillan JA, Feigin RD, DeAngelis C, et al. Epiglottitis. In: *Oski's Pediatrics: Principles and Practice.* 4th ed. Philadelphia: Lippincott Williams & Wilkins, 2006.

24. Beharloo F, Veyckemans F, Francis C, et al. Tracheobronchial foreign bodies. Presentation and management in children and adults. *Chest.* 1999;115:1357.

25. Avner J. Altered states of consciousness. *Pediatr Rev.* 2006;27:331-337.

26. Kochanek PM, Carney N, Adelson PD, et al. American Academy of Pediatrics–Section on Neurological Surgery, American Association of Neurological Surgeons/Congress of Neurological Surgeons, Child Neurology Society, European Society of Pediatric and Neonatal Intensive Care, Neurocritical Care Society, Pediatric Neurocritical Care Research Group, Society of Critical Care Medicine, Paediatric Intensive Care Society UK, Society for Neuroscience in Anesthesiology and Critical Care, World Federation of Pediatric Intensive and Critical Care Societies. Guidelines for the acute medical management of severe traumatic brain injury in infants, children, and adolescents–second ed. *Pediatr Crit Care Med.* 2012;13 Suppl 1:S1-S82.

27. Abend NS, Dlugos DJ. Treatment of refractory status epilepticus: literature review and a proposed protocol. *Pediatr Neurol.* 2008;38:377.

28. Wheless JW. Treatment of status epilepticus in children. *Pediatr Ann.* 2004;33:377-383.

Chapter 2
Poisonings

Zachary Nayak, MD, and Jocelyn Ronda, MD

🔄 See additional content on Expert Consult

I. WEBSITES

American Association of Poison Control Centers: http://www.aapcc.org/dnn/Home.aspx

American Academy of Clinical Toxicology: http://www.clintox.org/index.cfm

Centers for Disease Control and Prevention, Section on Environmental Health: http://www.cdc.gov/Environmental/

II. INITIAL EVALUATION

A. History

1. **Exposure history**
a. Obtain history from witnesses and/or close contacts.
b. Route, timing, and number of exposures (acute, chronic, or repeated ingestion), prior treatments or decontamination efforts.[1,2]

2. **Substance identification**
a. Attempt to identify exact name of substance ingested and constituents, including product name, active ingredients, possible contaminants, expiration date, concentration, and dose.
b. Consult local poison control for pill identification: 1-800-222-1222.

3. **Quantity of substance ingested**
a. Attempt to estimate a missing volume of liquid or the number of missing pills from a container.

4. **Environmental information**
a. Accessible items in the house or garage; open containers; spilled tablets; household members taking medications, herbs, or other complementary medicines.[2]

B. Laboratory Findings

1. **Toxicology screens**: Includes amphetamines, barbiturates, cocaine, ethanol, and opiates (Table 2-1).
a. If a particular type of ingestion is suspected, verify that the agent is included in the toxicology test.[2]
b. When obtaining a urine toxicology test, consider measuring both aspirin and acetaminophen blood levels because these are common analgesic ingredients in many medications.[2]
c. Gas chromatography or gas mass spectroscopy can distinguish medications that may cause a false-positive toxicology screen.[3]

TABLE 2-1

URINE TOXICOLOGY SCREEN*

Agent	Time Detectable in Urine
Amphetamines	2–4 days; up to 15 days
Benzodiazepines	3 days (if short-term use); 4–6 weeks (if >1 year use)
Buprenorphine	3–4 days
Cannabinoids	2–7 days (occasional use); 21–30 days (chronic use)
Cocaine	12 hours (parent form); 12–72 hours (metabolites)
Codeine	2–6 days
Ethanol	2–4 hours; up to 24 hours
Heroin	2–4 days
Hydromorphone	2–4 days
Methadone	Up to 3 days
Methamphetamine	2–5 days (depends on urine pH)
Morphine	2–4 days (up to 14 days)
Phencyclidine (PCP)	2–8 days (occasional use); 30 days (regular use)

*Recognize drugs not detected by routine toxicology screens.

The length of detection of drugs of abuse in urine varies. The above periods of detection should only be considered rough estimates and depend upon the individual's metabolism, physical condition, fluid intake, frequency, and quantity of ingestion.[4]

C. Clinical Diagnostic Aids (Table EC 2-A)

III. TOXIDROMES (TABLE 2-2)

TABLE 2-2

TOXIDROMES

Drug Class	Signs and Symptoms	Causative Agents
Anticholinergic: "Mad as a hatter, red as a beet, blind as a bat, hot as a hare, dry as a bone."	Delirium, psychosis, paranoia, dilated pupils, thirst, hyperthermia, ↑HR, urinary retention	Antihistamines, phenothiazines, scopolamine, tricyclic antidepressants
Cholinergic: Muscarinic	Salivation, lacrimation, urination, defecation, ↑HR emesis, bronchospasm	Organophosphates
Cholinergic: Nicotinic	Muscle fasciculations, paralysis, ↑HR, ↑BP	Tobacco, black widow venom, insecticides
Opiates	Sedation, constricted pupils, hypoventilation, ↓BP	Opioids
Sympathomimetics	Agitation, dilated pupils, ↑HR, ↓BP, moist skin	Amphetamines, cocaine, albuterol, caffeine, PCP
Sedative/hypnotic	Depressed mental status, normal pupils, ↓BP	Benzodiazepines, barbiturates,
Serotonergic	Confusion, flushing, ↑HR, shivering, hyperreflexia, muscle rigidity, clonus	SSRIs (alone or in combination with other meds including MAOIs, tramadol, and TCAs)

IV. INGESTION AND ANTIDOTES (TABLE 2-3)

A. In general, the following are guidelines of supportive care for the management of ingestions.

1. **For hypotension,** patients often require aggressive fluid resuscitation or vasopressors.
2. **Treat hyperpyrexia with cooling measures.**
3. **For ingestions that cause seizure,** treat with benzodiazepines unless otherwise specified.
4. **Selective decontamination with activated charcoal.**
5. **Hemodialysis** may be indicated to remove a drug/toxin regardless of renal function or in cases of renal impairment.

B. Consult local poison control for further management at 1-800-222-1222. Consult Poisindex if available.

TABLE 2-3

COMMONLY INGESTED AGENTS[4]

Ingested Agent	Signs and Symptoms	Antidote[4]
Acetaminophen	See Section V	
Amphetamine	See sympathomimetics toxidrome in Table 2-3	Supportive care (see above)
Anticholinergics[1]	See anticholinergic toxidrome in Table 2-3	**Physostigmine:** See formulary for dosing
Anticholinesterase (insecticides, donepezil, mushrooms)	See cholinergic:muscarinic and cholinergic:nicotinic toxidrome in Table 2-3	**Atropine:** See formulary for dosing
Antihistamines[5]	See anticholinergic toxidrome in Table 2-3; paradoxical CNS stimulation, dizziness, seizures	Supportive care (see above)
Benzodiazepines[6,7]	Coma, dysarthria, ataxia, drowsiness, hallucinations, confusion, agitation, bradycardia, hypotension, respiratory depression	**Flumazenil:** See formulary for dosing
β-blockers[8-10]	Coma, seizures, altered mental status, hallucinations, bradycardia, congestive heart failure, hypotension, respiratory depression, bronchospasm, hypoglycemia	**Glucagon:** See formulary for dosing; see **insulin/dextrose** treatment in calcium channel blockers
Calcium channel blockers[9,10]	Seizures, coma, dysarthria, lethargy, confusion, cardiac arrhythmia, hypotension, pulmonary edema, hyperglycemia, flushing	**CaCl (10%):** See formulary for dosing **CaGluc (10%):** See formulary for dosing **Glucagon:** See formulary for dosing **Insulin/dextrose:** 1 U/kg bolus → infuse at 0.1–1 U/kg/hr; give with D25% 0.25 g/kg bolus → 0.5 g/kg/hr infusion

Continued

TABLE 2-3—cont'd

Ingested Agent	Signs and Symptoms	Antidote[4]
Clonidine[10]	Symptoms resemble an opioid tox-idrome. CNS depression, coma, lethargy, hypothermia, miosis, bradycardia, profound hypoten-sion, respiratory depression	See opioid antidote
Cocaine[11]	See sympathomimetics toxidrome in Table 2-3	Supportive care (see above)
Ecstasy[11]	Hallucinations, teeth grinding, hyperthermia, seizures	Supportive care (see above)
Ethanol[1,12]	See sedative/hypnotic toxidrome in Table 2-3	Supportive care (see above)
Ethylene glycol/metha-nol[1,12]	Similar to ethanol; additionally blurry or double vision, meta-bolic acidosis, abdominal pain	**Fomepizole:** See formulary for dosing. Alternatively, if not available, can use Ethanol (see formulary for dosing), but requires more monitoring than fomepizole.
Iron[13,14]	Vomiting, diarrhea, ↓BP, lethargy, renal failure	**Deferoxamine:** See formulary for dosing
Lead	See Section VI	
NSAIDs	Nausea, vomiting, epigastric pain, headache, GI hemor-rhage, renal failure	Supportive care (see above)
Opioids	See opioid toxidrome in Table 2-3	**Naloxone:** See formulary for dosing
Organophosphates	See cholinergic:muscarinic toxidrome in Table 2-3	If muscle fasciculations, respiratory depression, coma, use **Pralidoxime:** see formulary for dosing. **Atropine:** used for muscarinic effects (see anticholinesterase)
Salicylates[12]	GI upset, tinnitus, tachypnea, hyperpyrexia, dizziness, lethargy, dysarthria, seizure, coma, cerebral edema	Supportive care (see above)
Serotonin syndrome	Seizures, muscle rigidity, myoc-lonus, hyperpyrexia, flushing, rhabdomyolysis	**Cyproheptadine:** See formulary for dosing; for agitation: **Diazepam:** See formulary for dosing
Sulfonylureas[12]	Fatigue, dizziness, agitation, confusion, tachycardia, diaphoresis	**Dextrose:** 0.5–1 g/kg (2–4 mL/kg of D25W) After euglycemia achieved: **Octreotide:** 1–2 mcg/kg SQ Q6–12 hr if rebound hypoglycemia after dextrose
TCA[15,16]	Seizures, delirium, ventricular arrhythmias, hypotension	For wide QRS complex: **NaHCO₃:** 1–2 mEq/kg IV; goal serum pH 7.45–7.55, For torsades: **MgSulfate:** 50 mg/kg IV over 5–15 min (max dose 2 g)
Warfarin	Bleeding	**Phytonadione/Vitamin K₁:** See formulary for dosing

V. ACETAMINOPHEN OVERDOSE[4,17,18,19,20]

Metabolites are hepatotoxic. Reactive intermediates can cause liver necrosis.

A. Four Phases of Intoxication

1. **Phase 1 (first 24 hr):** nonspecific symptoms such as nausea, malaise, vomiting.
2. **Phase 2 (24 to 72 hr):** above symptoms resolve, RUQ pain and hepatomegaly develop. Increase in liver function tests, bilirubin levels, and prothrombin time.
3. **Phase 3 (72 to 96 hr):** return of nonspecific symptoms as well as evidence of liver failure (e.g., jaundice, hypoglycemia, coagulopathy).
4. **Phase 4 (4 days to 2 weeks):** recovery or death.

B. Treatment Criteria:

1. **Serum acetaminophen** concentration above the possible toxicity line on the Rumack-Matthew nomogram (Fig. 2-1).
2. **History of ingesting more than 200 mg/kg or 10 g** (whichever is less) and serum concentration not available or time of ingestion not known.

C. Antidotes: N-Acetylcysteine

1. **PO:** 140 mg/kg loading dose followed by 70 mg/kg Q4 hr for a total of 72 hours.
2. **IV:** 150 mg/kg N-acetylcysteine IV over 60 minutes followed by 12.5 mg/kg/hr x 4 hours followed by 6.25 mg/kg/hr x 16 hours for a total of 21 hours of infusion. Some patients may require more than 21 hours of N-acetylcysteine.
3. **Liver failure:** treat patients in liver failure with N-acetylcysteine IV, same dose as above. Continue 6.25 mg/kg/hr infusion until resolution of encephalopathy, decreasing aminotransferases and improvement in coagulopathy

VI. LEAD POISONINGS[21-23]

A. Etiologies: paint, dust, soil, drinking water, cosmetics, cookware, toys, and caregivers with occupations and/or hobbies utilizing lead-containing materials or substances.*

B. Definition: Centers for Disease Control and Prevention (CDC) defines an elevated blood lead level (BLL) as ≥5 mcg/dL.[21]

C. Overview of Symptoms by BLL:

1. **BLL >40 mcg/dL:** irritability, vomiting, abdominal pain, constipation, and anorexia.
2. **BLL >70 mcg/dL:** lethargy, seizure, and coma.

NOTE: Children may be asymptomatic with lead levels >100 mcg/dL.

C. Management (Tables 2-4, 2-5, and 2-6):

---

*Children aged 1 to 5 years are at greatest risk of lead poisoning.

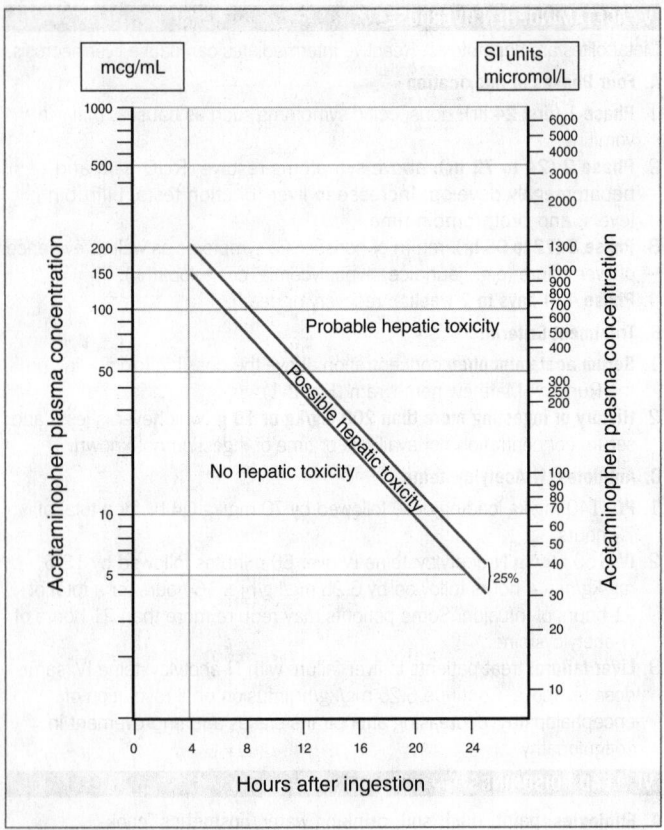

FIGURE 2-1

Semilogarithmic plot of plasma acetaminophen levels versus time. This nomogram is valid for use after acute ingestions of acetaminophen. The need for treatment cannot be extrapolated based on a level before 4 hours. *(Based on Pediatrics 55:871, 1975 and Micromedex.)*

CHELATION THERAPY

1. **Routine indication:** BLL ≥ 46 mcg/dL
2. **Overview of antidotes:**
A. **Succimer:** 10 mg/kg or 350 mg/m² PO Q8 hr x 5 days --> Q12 hr x 14 days
B. **Edetate (EDTA) calcium disodium:** 1000 mg/m²/24 hr IV infusion as an 8-24 hr infusion OR intermittent dosing divided Q12 hr x 5 days. May repeat course as needed after 2-4 days of no EDTA.

*Warning: Do not mistake edetate disodium for edetate calcium disodium. Edetate calcium disodium is used for the treatment of lead poisoning.

TABLE 2-4

MANAGEMENT OF LEAD POISONING[21]

Blood Lead Levels (BLL)	Recommended Guidelines
≥ 5 and <10 mcg/dL	1. Provide education about reducing environmental lead exposure and reducing dietary lead absorption.* 2. Perform environmental assessment in homes built before 1978. 3. Follow repeat blood lead testing guidelines (see Table 2-5).
≥ 10 and ≤45 mcg/dL	1. As above for BLL ≥ 5 and <10 2. Environmental investigation and lead hazard reduction 3. Complete history and exam 4. Iron level, complete blood cell count (CBC), abdominal radiography (if ingestion is suspected) with bowel decontamination if indicated 5. Neurodevelopmental monitoring
BLL ≥45 and ≤69 mcg/dL	1. As above for BLL ≤45 mcg/dL 2. Check free erythrocyte protoporphyrin. 3. Administer chelation therapy (See below).
BLL ≥70 mcg/dL	1. As above for BLL ≥45 mcg/dL 2. Hospitalize and commence chelation therapy.

*Iron, calcium, and vitamin C help minimize absorption of lead.

TABLE 2-5

REPEAT BLOOD LEAD TESTING GUIDELINES[21]

If Screening BLL is:	Time Frame of Confirmation of Screening BLL	Follow-Up Testing (After Confirmatory Testing)	Later Follow-Up Testing After BLL Declining
≥ 5–9 mcg/dL	1–3 months	3 months	6–9 months
10–19 mcg/dL	1 week–1 month*	1–3 months	3–6 months
20–24 mcg/dL	1 week–1 month*	1–3 months	1–3 months
25–44 mcg/dL	1 week–1 month*	2 weeks–1 month	1 month
45–59 mcg/dL	48 weeks	As soon as possible	
60–69 mcg/dL	24 hours		
>70 mcg/dL	Urgently		

*The higher the blood lead level (BLL) on the screening test, the more urgent the need for confirmatory testing.

C. **D-penicillamine:** 25-35 mg/kg/day PO in divided doses. Start at 25% of this dose and increase to full dose over 2-3 weeks. Do not give D-penicillamine to patients with a penicillin allergy.

3. **Non-routine indications:** patient with encephalopathy

A. **Give Dimercaprol (BAL):** 75 mg/m² IM Q4 hr x 5 days; immediately after second dose of BAL give EDTA 1500 mg/m²/day IV as a continuous infusion or 2-4 divided doses x 5 days

REFERENCES

1. Nelson L, Lewin N, Howland MA, et al. *Goldfrank's Toxicologic Emergencies.* 9th ed. New York: McGraw-Hill; 2010.
2. Dart RC, Rumack BH. Poisoning. In: Hay WW, Levin MJ, Sondheimer JM, et al, eds. *Current Pediatric Diagnosis and Treatment.* 19th ed. New York: McGraw-Hill; 2009:313-338.

3. Hoppe-Roberts JM. Poisoning mortality in United States: comparison of national mortality statistics and poison control center reports. *Ann Emerg Med.* 2000;35(5):440-448.

4. POISINDEX® System [Internet database]. Greenwood Village, Colo: Thomson Reuters (Healthcare) Inc. Updated periodically.

5. Scharman EJ, Erdman AR, Wax PM, et al. Diphenhydramine and dimenhydrinate poisoning: An evidence-based consensus guideline for out-of-hospital management. *Clin Toxicol (Phila).* 2006;44:205-223.

6. Isbister GK, O'Regan L, Sibbritt D, et al. Alprazolam is relatively more toxic than other benzodiazepines in overdose. *Br J Clin Pharmacol.* 2004;58(1):88-95.

7. Thomson JS. Use of flumazenil in benzodiazepine overdose. *Emerg Med J.* 2006;23:162.

8. Love JN, Howell JM, Klein-Schwartz W, et al. Lack of toxicity from pediatric beta-blocker exposure. *Hum Exp Toxicol.* 2006;25:341-346.

9. Shepard G. Treatment of poisoning caused by beta-adrenergic and calcium-channel blockers. *Am J Health-Syst Pharm.* 2006;63(19):1828-1835.

10. DeWitt CR, Waksman JC. Pharmacology, pathophysiology and management of calcium channel blocker and beta-blocker toxicity. *Toxicol Rev.* 2004;23:223-238.

11. Kaul P. Substance abuse. In: Hay WW, Levin MJ, Sondheimer JM, et al, eds. *Current Pediatric Diagnosis and Treatment.* 19th ed. New York: McGraw-Hill; 2009:137-151.

12. Henry K, Harris CR. Deadly ingestions. *Pediatr Clin North Am.* 2006;53:293-315.

13. Aldridge MD. Acute iron poisoning: What every pediatric intensive care unit nurse should know. *Dimens Crit Care Nurs.* 2007;26:43-48.

14. Manoguerra AS, Erdman AR, Booze LL, et al. Iron ingestion: an evidence-based consensus guideline for out-of-hospital management. *Clin Toxicol (Phila).* 2005;43:553-570.

15. Miller J. Managing antidepression overdoses. *Emerg Med Serv.* 2004;33:113-119.

16. Rosenbaum TG, Kou M. Are one or two dangerous? Tricyclic antidepressant exposure in toddlers. *J Emerg Med.* 2005;29:169-174.

17. Hanhan UA. The poisoned child in the pediatric intensive care unit. *Pediatr Clin North Am.* 2008;55:669-686.

18. White M, Liebelt EL. Update on antidotes for pediatric poisonings. *Pediatr Emerg Care.* 2006;22:740-749.

19. Calello D, Osterhoudt KC, Henretig FM. New and novel antidotes in pediatrics. *Pediatr Emerg Care.* 2006;22:523-530.

20. Kanter MZ. Comparison of oral and IV acetylcysteine in the treatment of acetaminophen poisoning. *Am J Health Syst Pharm.* 2006;63:1821-1827.

21. Advisory Committee on Childhood Lead Poisoning Prevention of the Centers for Disease Control and Prevention. Low level lead exposure harms children: A renewed call for primary prevention. http://www.cdc.gov/nceh/lead/ACCLPP/Final_Document_030712.pdf. Published January 2012.

22. American Academy of Pediatrics, Committee on Environmental Health. Lead exposure in children: prevention, detection, and management. *Pediatrics.* 2005;116:1036-1046.

23. Davoli CT, Serwint JR, Chisolm JJ. Asymptomatic children with venous lead levels >100 mcg/dL. *Pediatrics.* 1996;98:965-968.

Chapter 3
Procedures

Bradley D. McCammack, MD

I. GENERAL GUIDELINES

A. Consent

Before performing any procedure, it is crucial to obtain informed consent from the parent or guardian by explaining the procedure, the indications, any risks involved, and any alternatives. Obtaining consent for life-saving emergency procedures is unnecessary.

B. Risks

1. **All invasive procedures involve pain and risk for infection and bleeding.** Specific complications are listed by procedure.
2. **Sedation and analgesia should be planned in advance, and the risks of such explained to the parent and/or patient as appropriate.** In general, 1% lidocaine buffered with sodium bicarbonate is adequate for local analgesia. See Chapter 6 for Analgesia and Procedural Sedation guidelines. Also see the "AAP Guidelines for Monitoring and Management of Pediatric Patients During and After Sedation for Diagnostic and Therapeutic Procedures."[1]
3. **Universal precautions should be followed for all patient contact that exposes the health care provider to blood, amniotic fluid, pericardial fluid, pleural fluid, synovial fluid, cerebrospinal fluid (CSF), semen, or vaginal secretions.**
4. **Proper sterile technique is essential to achieving good wound closure, decreasing transmittable diseases, and preventing wound contamination.**
5. **Videos are available for some procedures via *New England Journal of Medicine's* "Videos in Clinical Medicine."** Links to videos will be listed in the respective sections when available.

II. BLOOD SAMPLING

A. Heelstick and Fingerstick[2]

1. **Indications:** Blood sampling in infants for laboratory studies unaffected by hemolysis
2. **Complications:** Infection, bleeding, osteomyelitis
3. **Procedure:**
a. Warm heel or finger.
b. Clean with alcohol.
   (1) Puncture heel using a lancet on the lateral part of the heel, avoiding the posterior area.
   (2) Puncture finger using a lancet on the palmar lateral surface of the finger near the tip.

c. Wipe away the first drop of blood, then collect the sample using a capillary tube or container.

d. Alternate between squeezing blood from the leg toward the heel (or from the hand toward the finger) and then releasing the pressure for several seconds.

B. External Jugular Puncture[3]

1. **Indications:** Blood sampling in patients with inadequate peripheral vascular access or during resuscitation

2. **Complications:** Infection, bleeding, pneumothorax

3. **Procedure** (Fig. 3-1):

a. Restrain infant securely. Place infant with head turned away from side of blood sampling. Position with towel roll under shoulders or with head over side of bed to extend neck and accentuate the posterior margin of the sternocleidomastoid muscle on the side of the venipuncture.

b. Prepare area in a sterile fashion.

c. The external jugular vein will distend if its most proximal segment is occluded or if the child cries. The vein runs from the angle of the mandible to the posterior border of the lower third of the sternocleidomastoid muscle.

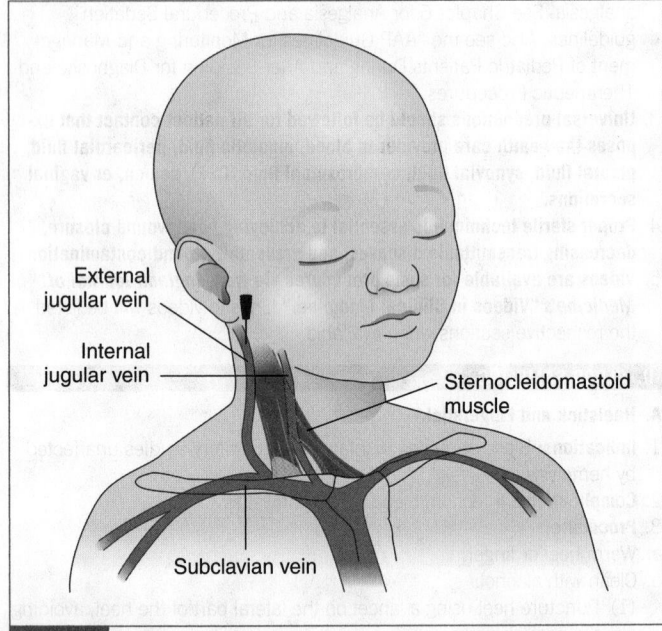

FIGURE 3-1

External jugular cannulation. *(From Dieckmann R, Fiser D, Selbst S. Pediatric Emergency and Critical Care Procedures. St. Louis: Mosby, 1997.)*

d. With continuous negative suction on the syringe, insert the needle at about a 30-degree angle to the skin. Continue as with any peripheral venipuncture.

e. Apply a sterile dressing, and put pressure on the puncture site for 5 minutes.

C. Femoral Artery and Femoral Vein Puncture[3,4]

1. **Indications:** Venous or arterial blood sampling in patients with inadequate vascular access or during resuscitation.

2. **Contraindications:** Femoral puncture is particularly hazardous in neonates and *not* recommended in this age group. There is also a risk in children for trauma to the femoral head and joint capsule. Avoid femoral punctures in children who have thrombocytopenia or coagulation disorders and in those who are scheduled for cardiac catheterization.

3. **Complications:** Infection, bleeding, hematoma of femoral triangle, thrombosis of vessel, osteomyelitis, septic arthritis of hip.

4. **Procedure** (Fig. 3-2):

a. Hold child securely in frog-leg position with the hips flexed and abducted. It may help to place a roll under the hips.

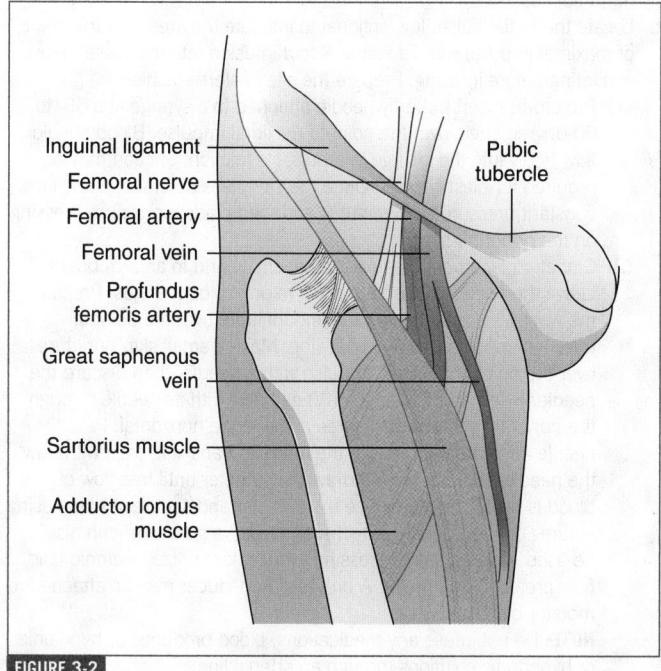

Inguinal ligament
Femoral nerve
Femoral artery
Femoral vein
Profundus femoris artery
Great saphenous vein
Sartorius muscle
Adductor longus muscle
Pubic tubercle

FIGURE 3-2

Femoral artery and vein anatomy. *(From Dieckmann R, Fiser D, Selbst S.* Pediatric Emergency and Critical Care Procedures. *St. Louis: Mosby, 1997.)*

b. Prepare area in sterile fashion.
c. Locate femoral pulse just distal to the inguinal crease (note that vein is medial to pulse). Insert needle 2 cm distal to the inguinal ligament and 0.5 to 0.75 cm into the groin. Aspirate while maneuvering the needle until blood is obtained.
NOTE: The right femoral vein is easier to cannulate than left owing to straighter path to inferior vena cava.
d. Apply direct pressure for minimum of 5 minutes.

D. Radial Artery Puncture and Catheterization[3,4]

1. **Indications:** Arterial blood sampling or frequent blood gases and continuous blood pressure monitoring in an intensive care setting.
2. **Complications:** Infection, bleeding, occlusion of artery by hematoma or thrombosis, ischemia if ulnar circulation is inadequate.
3. **Procedure:**
a. Before procedure, test adequacy of ulnar blood flow with the Allen test. Clench the hand while simultaneously compressing ulnar and radial arteries. The hand will blanch. Release pressure from the ulnar artery, and observe the flushing response. Procedure is safe to perform if entire hand flushes.
b. Locate the radial pulse. It is optional to infiltrate the area over the point of maximal impulse with lidocaine. Avoid infusion into the vessel by aspirating before infusing. Prepare the site in sterile fashion.
   (1) Puncture: Insert butterfly needle attached to a syringe at a 30- to 60-degree angle over the point of maximal impulse. Blood should flow freely into the syringe in a pulsatile fashion. Suction may be required for plastic tubes. Once the sample is obtained, apply firm, constant pressure for 5 minutes and then place a pressure dressing on the puncture site.
   (2) Catheter placement: Secure the patient's hand to an arm board. Leave the fingers exposed to observe any color changes. Prepare the wrist with sterile technique and infiltrate over the point of maximal impulse with 1% lidocaine. Make a small skin puncture over the point of maximal impulse with a needle, then discard the needle. Insert an intravenous (IV) catheter with its needle through the puncture site at a 30-degree angle to the horizontal. Pass the needle and catheter through the artery to transfix it, then withdraw the needle. Very slowly, withdraw the catheter until free flow of blood is noted, then advance the catheter and secure in place using sutures or tape. Seldinger technique using a guidewire can also be used. Apply a sterile dressing. Infuse heparinized isotonic fluid (per protocol) at 1 mL/hr. A pressure transducer may be attached to monitor blood pressure.
   NOTE: Do not infuse any medications, blood products, or hypotonic or hypertonic solutions through an arterial line.
   (3) Suggested size of arterial catheters based on weight:
      (a) Infant (<10 kg): 24G or 2.5Fr, 2.5 cm

    (b) Child (10 to 40 kg): 22G or 2.4Fr, 2.5 cm
    (c) Adolescent (>40 kg): 20G
4. **A video on radial artery catheterization is available on the New England Journal of Medicine's website.**
E. **Posterior Tibial and Dorsalis Pedis Artery Puncture**[4]
1. **Indications:** Arterial blood sampling when radial artery puncture is unsuccessful or inaccessible.
2. **Complications:** Infection, bleeding, ischemia if circulation is inadequate
3. **Procedure (see Section II.D for technique):**
a. Posterior tibial artery: Puncture the artery posterior to medial malleolus while holding foot in dorsiflexion.
b. Dorsalis pedis artery: Puncture the artery at dorsal midfoot between first and second toes while holding foot in plantar flexion.

III. VASCULAR ACCESS

A. **Peripheral Intravenous Placement**
1. **Indications:** To obtain access to peripheral venous circulation to deliver fluid, medications, or blood products.
2. **Complications:** Thrombosis, infection.
3. **Procedure:**
a. Choose IV placement site and prepare with alcohol.
b. Apply tourniquet and then insert IV catheter, bevel up, at angle almost parallel to the skin, advancing until a *flash* of blood is seen in the catheter hub. Advance the plastic catheter only, remove the needle, and secure the catheter.
c. After removing tourniquet, attach T connector filled with saline to the catheter, flush with normal saline (NS) to ensure patency of the IV line.
4. **A video on peripheral IV placement is available on the New England Journal of Medicine's website.**
B. **Central Venous Catheter Placement**[3,5-7]
1. **Indications:** To obtain emergency access to central venous circulation, monitor central venous pressure, deliver high-concentration parenteral nutrition or prolonged IV therapy, or infuse blood products or large volumes of fluid.
2. **Complications:** Infection, bleeding, arterial or venous perforation, pneumothorax, hemothorax, thrombosis, catheter fragment in circulation, air embolism.
3. **Ultrasound guidance:** Quickly becoming standard among health care facilities to aid placement of central venous catheters. It has been shown to reduce failure and complication rates when effectively implemented.
4. **Access sites:**
a. External jugular vein
b. Subclavian vein: Least common site in children owing to increased complications
c. Internal jugular vein: Contraindicated with elevated intracranial pressure
d. Femoral vein: Contraindicated with severe abdominal trauma

5. **Procedure:** Seldinger technique (Fig. 3-3)
a. Secure patient, prepare site, and drape according to the following guidelines for sterile technique[7]:
   (1) Wash hands.
   (2) Wear hat, mask, eye shield, sterile gloves, and sterile gown.

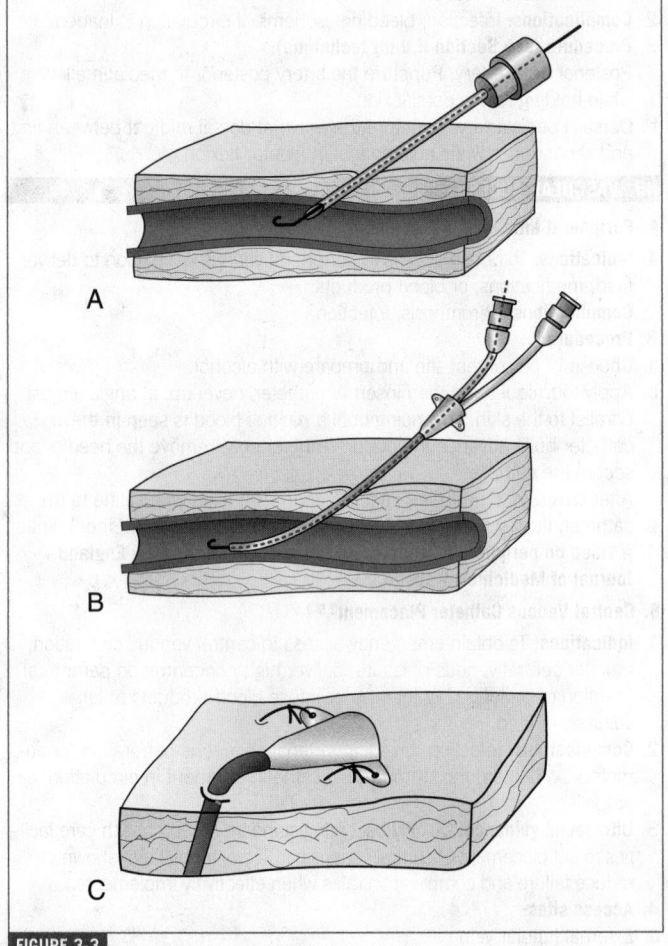

FIGURE 3-3

Seldinger technique. **A,** Guidewire is placed through introducer needle into lumen of vein. **B,** Catheter is advanced into vein lumen along guidewire. **C,** Hub of catheter is secured to skin with suture. *(Modified from Fuhrman B, Zimmerman J. Pediatric Critical Care. 4th ed. Philadelphia: Mosby, 2011.)*

    (3) Prep procedure site for 30 seconds (chlorhexidine), and allow to dry for an additional 30 seconds (in groin, scrub for 2 minutes, and allow to dry for 1 minute).

    (4) Use sterile technique to drape the site.

b. Insert needle, applying negative pressure to locate vessel.

c. When there is blood return, insert a guidewire through the needle into the vein. Watch cardiac monitor for ectopy.

d. Remove the needle, firmly holding the guidewire.

e. Slip a catheter that has been preflushed with sterile saline over the wire into the vein in a twisting motion. The entry site may be enlarged with a small skin incision or dilator. Pass the entire catheter over the wire until the hub is at the skin surface. Slowly remove the wire, secure the catheter by suture, and attach IV infusion.

f. Apply a sterile dressing over the site.

g. For neck vessels, obtain a chest radiograph to rule out pneumothorax.

h. A video on central venous catheterization is available on the New England Journal of Medicine's website.

6. **Approach:**

a. External jugular (see Fig. 3-1): Place patient in 15- to 20-degree Trendelenburg position. Turn the head 45 degrees to the contralateral side. Enter the vein at the point where it crosses the sternocleidomastoid muscle.

b. Internal jugular (Fig. 3-4): Place patient in 15- to 20-degree Trendelenburg position. Hyperextend the neck to tense the sternocleidomastoid muscle, and turn head away from the site of line placement. Palpate the sternal and clavicular heads of the muscle, and enter at the apex of the triangle formed. An alternative landmark for puncture is halfway between the sternal notch and tip of the mastoid process. Insert the needle at a 30-degree angle to the skin, and aim toward the ipsilateral nipple. When blood flow is obtained, continue with Seldinger technique. Right side is preferable because of straight course to right atrium, absence of thoracic duct, and lower pleural dome on right side. The internal jugular vein runs lateral to the carotid artery.

c. Subclavian vein (Fig. 3-5): Position child in Trendelenburg position with a towel roll under thoracic spine to hyperextend the back. Aim the needle under the distal third of the clavicle toward the sternal notch. When blood flow is obtained, continue with Seldinger technique.

    (1) A video on subclavian venous catheter placement is available on the New England Journal of Medicine's website.

d. Femoral vein (Fig. 3-6): Hold child securely with the hip flexed and abducted. Locate the femoral pulse just distal to the inguinal crease. In infants, vein is 5 to 6 mm *medial* to arterial pulse. In adolescents, vein is usually 10 to 15 mm *medial* to the pulse. Place the thumb of the nondominant hand on the femoral artery. Insert the needle medial to the thumb. The needle should enter the skin 2 to 3 cm distal to the inguinal ligament at a 30-degree angle to avoid entering the abdomen. When blood flow is obtained, continue with Seldinger technique.

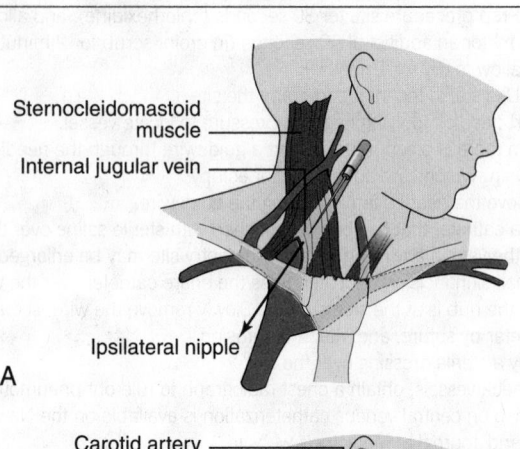

Sternocleidomastoid muscle

Internal jugular vein

Ipsilateral nipple

A

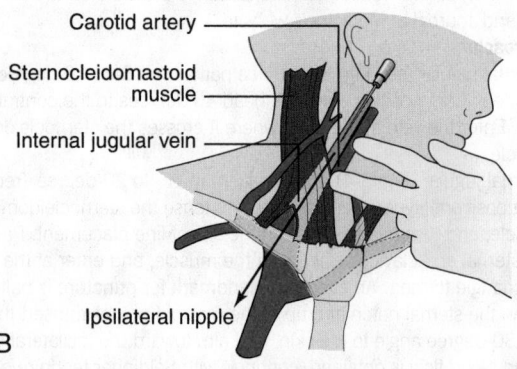

Carotid artery

Sternocleidomastoid muscle

Internal jugular vein

Ipsilateral nipple

B

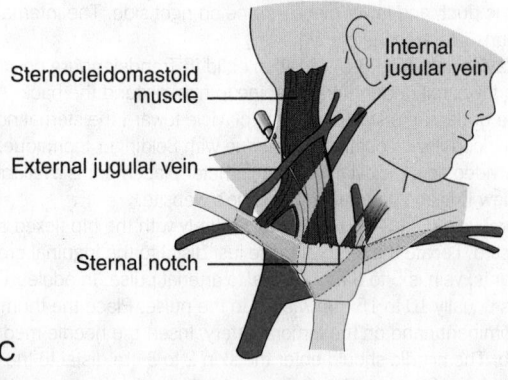

Sternocleidomastoid muscle

External jugular vein

Sternal notch

Internal jugular vein

C

FIGURE 3-4

Approaches to the internal jugular vein. Patient is supine in slight Trendelenburg position, with neck extended over a shoulder roll and head rotated away from side of approach. **A,** Middle approach. Introducer needle enters at apex of a triangle formed by the heads of the sternocleidomastoid muscle and clavicle and is directed toward the ipsilateral nipple at an angle of approximately 30 degrees with the skin. **B,** Anterior approach. Carotid pulse is palpated and may be slightly retracted medially. Introducer needle enters along anterior margin of sternocleidomastoid about halfway between sternal notch and mastoid process and is directed toward the ipsilateral nipple. **C,** Posterior approach. Introducer needle enters at the point where external jugular vein crosses posterior margin of sternocleidomastoid and is directed under its head toward sternal notch. *(Modified from Fuhrman B, Zimmerman J.* Pediatric Critical Care. *4th ed. Philadelphia: Mosby, 2011.)*

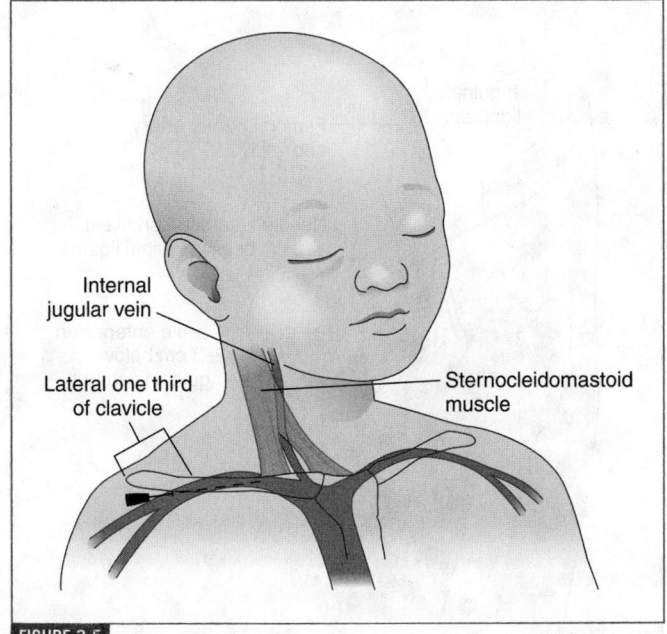

Internal jugular vein

Lateral one third of clavicle

Sternocleidomastoid muscle

FIGURE 3-5

Subclavian vein cannulation. *(From Dieckmann R, Fiser D, Selbst S.* Pediatric Emergency and Critical Care Procedures. *St. Louis: Mosby, 1997.)*

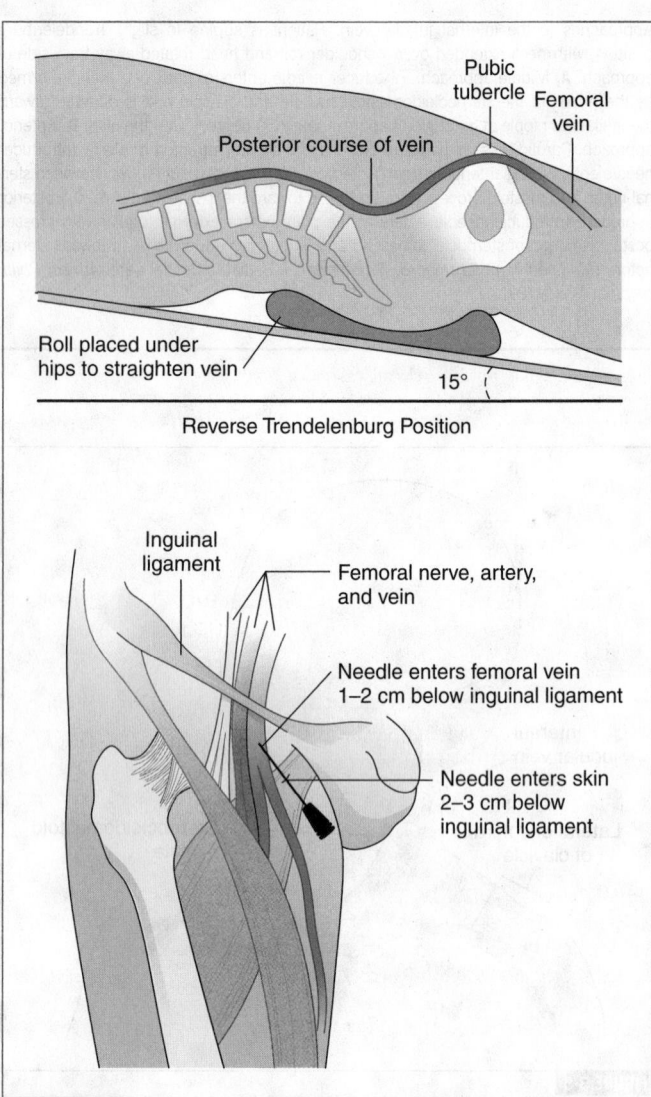

FIGURE 3-6

Femoral vein cannulation. *(From Dieckmann R, Fiser D, Selbst S.* Pediatric Emergency and Critical Care Procedures. *St. Louis: Mosby, 1997.)*

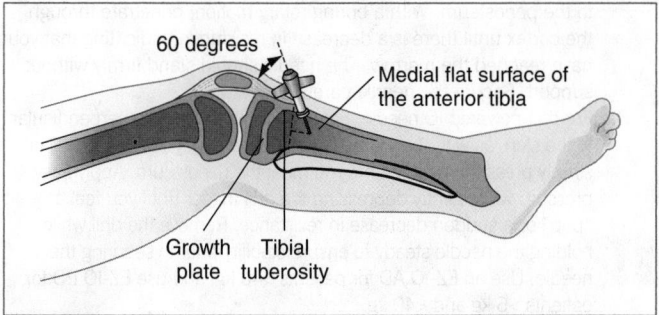

FIGURE 3-7

Intraosseous needle placement using standard anterior tibial approach. Insertion point is in the midline on medial flat surface of anterior tibia, 1 to 3 cm (2 fingerbreadths) below tibial tuberosity. *(From Dieckmann R, Fiser D, Selbst S. Pediatric Emergency and Critical Care Procedures. St. Louis: Mosby, 1997.)*

    (1) A video on femoral venous catheterization is available on the New England Journal of Medicine's website.

C. Intraosseous (IO) Infusion[3,4] (Fig. 3-7)

1. **Indications:** Obtain emergency access in children during life-threatening situations. This is very useful during cardiopulmonary arrest, shock, burns, and life-threatening status epilepticus. IO line can be used to infuse medications, blood products, or fluids. The IO needle should be removed once adequate vascular access has been established.

2. **Complications:**
a. Complications are rare, particularly with correct technique. Frequency of complications increases with prolonged infusions.
b. Extravasation of fluid from incomplete cortex penetration, infection, bleeding, osteomyelitis, compartment syndrome, fat embolism, fracture, epiphyseal injury.

3. **Sites of entry (in order of preference):**
a. Anteromedial surface of the proximal tibia, 2 cm below and 1 to 2 cm medial to the tibial tuberosity on the flat part of the bone (see Fig. 3-7)
b. Distal femur 3 cm above the lateral condyle in the midline
c. Medial surface of the distal tibia 1 to 2 cm above the medial malleolus (may be a more effective site in older children)
d. Anterosuperior iliac spine at an angle of 90 degrees to the long axis of the body

4. **Procedure:**
a. Prepare the selected site in sterile fashion if situation allows.
b. If the child is conscious, anesthetize the puncture site down to the periosteum with 1% lidocaine (optional in emergency situations).
c. Choose between manual IO or drill-powered IO insertion device:
    (1) For manual IO needle: Insert a 15- to 18-gauge IO needle perpendicular to skin at angle away from epiphyseal plate, and advance

to the periosteum. With a boring rotary motion, penetrate through the cortex until there is a decrease in resistance, indicating that you have reached the marrow. The needle should stand firmly without support. Secure the needle carefully.

(2) For drill-powered IO needle: Enter skin with the needle perpendicular to the skin, as with the manual needle, and gently power the drill or simply press the needle until you meet the periosteum. Apply easy pressure while gently depressing the drill trigger until you feel a "pop" or a sudden decrease in resistance. Remove the drill while holding the needle steady to ensure stability prior to securing the needle. Use an EZ-IO AD for patients >40 kg, and use EZ-IO PD for patients >6 kg and <40 kg.

d. Remove the stylet and attempt to aspirate marrow. (Note that it is not necessary to aspirate marrow.) Flush with 10 to 20 mL of crystalloid solution. Observe for fluid extravasation. Marrow can be sent for determination of glucose levels, chemistries, blood type and crossmatch, hemoglobin, blood gas analysis, and cultures.

e. Attach standard IV tubing. Any crystalloid, blood product, or drug that may be infused into a peripheral vein may also be infused into the IO space, but increased pressure (through pressure bag or push) is necessary for infusion. There is a high risk for obstruction if continuous high-pressure fluids are not flushed through the IO needle.

5. **A video on IO catheter placement is available on the New England Journal of Medicine's website.**

D. Umbilical Artery (UA) and Umbilical Vein (UV) Catheterization[3]

1. **Indications:** Vascular access (via UV), blood pressure (via UA), and blood gas (via UA) monitoring in critically ill neonates.

2. **Complications:** Infection, bleeding, hemorrhage, perforation of vessel; thrombosis with distal embolization; ischemia or infarction of lower extremities, bowel, or kidney; arrhythmia if catheter is in the heart; air embolus.

3. **Caution:** UA catheterization should never be performed if omphalitis or peritonitis is present. It is contraindicated in the presence of possible necrotizing enterocolitis or intestinal hypoperfusion.

4. **Line placement:**

a. Arterial line: Low line vs. high line.

(1) Low line: Tip of catheter should lie just above the aortic bifurcation between L3 and L5. This avoids renal and mesenteric arteries near L1, possibly decreasing the incidence of thrombosis or ischemia.

(2) High line: Tip of catheter should be above the diaphragm between T6 and T9. A high line may be recommended in infants weighing less than 750 g, in whom a low line could easily slip out.

b. UV catheters should be placed in the inferior vena cava above the level of the ductus venosus and the hepatic veins and below the level of the right atrium.

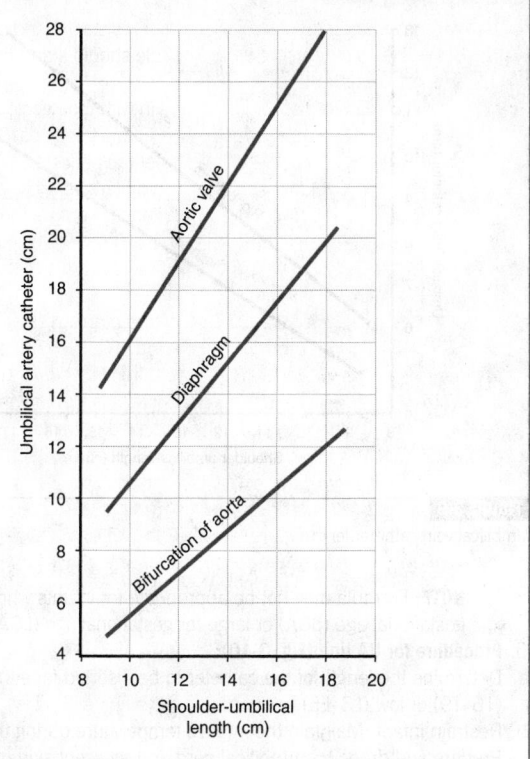

FIGURE 3-8

Umbilical artery catheter length.

c. Catheter length: Determine the length of catheter required using either a
   standardized graph or the regression formula. Add length for the height
   of the umbilical stump.
   (1) Standardized graph: Determine the shoulder-umbilical length
       by measuring the perpendicular line dropped from the tip of the
       shoulder to the level of the umbilicus. Use the graph in Fig. 3-8 to
       determine the arterial catheter length, and the graph in Fig. 3-9 to
       determine venous catheter length.
   (2) Birth weight (BW) regression formula:

   Low line : UA catheter length (cm) = BW (kg) + 7.

   High line : UA catheter length (cm) = [3 × BW (kg)] + 9

   UV catheter length (cm) = [0.5 × high line UA (cm)] + 1

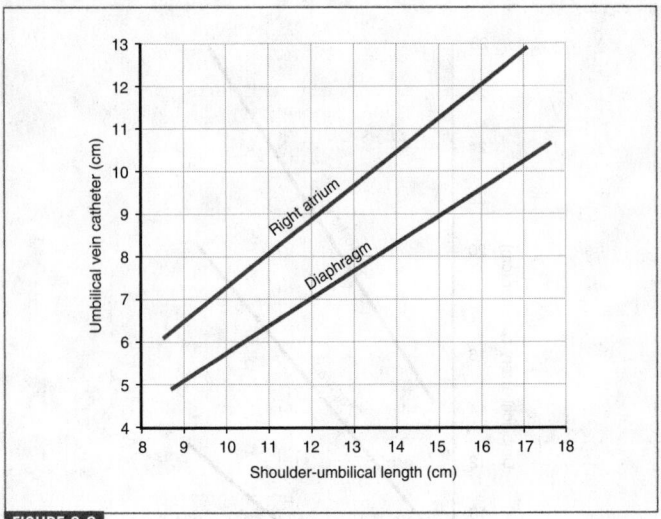

FIGURE 3-9

Umbilical vein catheter length.

> **NOTE:** Formula may not be appropriate for infants who are small for gestational age (SGA) or large for gestational age (LGA).

5. **Procedure for UA line (Fig. 3-10):**
a. Determine the length of the catheter to be inserted for either high (T6–T9) or low (L3–L5) position.
b. Restrain infant. Maintain the infant's temperature during the procedure. Prepare and drape the umbilical cord and adjacent skin using sterile technique.
c. Flush the catheter with sterile saline solution before insertion. Ensure there are no air bubbles in the catheter or attached syringe.
d. Place sterile umbilical tape around the base of the cord. Cut through the cord horizontally about 1.5 to 2 cm from the skin; tighten the umbilical tape to prevent bleeding.
e. Identify the one large, thin-walled umbilical vein and two smaller, thick-walled arteries. Use one tip of open, curved forceps to gently probe and dilate one artery. Use both points of closed forceps, and dilate artery by allowing forceps to open gently.
f. Grasp the catheter 1 cm from its tip with toothless forceps, and insert the catheter into the lumen of the artery. Aim the tip toward the feet, and gently advance the catheter to the desired distance. *Do not force.* If resistance is encountered, try loosening umbilical tape, applying steady and gentle pressure, or manipulating the angle of the umbilical cord to skin. Often the catheter cannot be advanced because of creation of a "false luminal tract." There should be good blood return when the catheter enters the iliac artery.

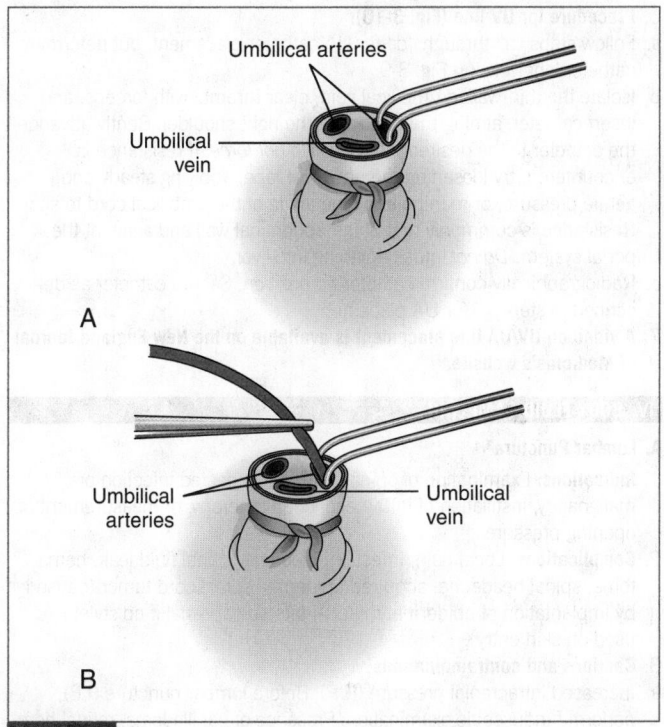

FIGURE 3-10

Placement of umbilical arterial catheter. **A,** Dilating lumen of umbilical artery. **B,** Insertion of umbilical artery catheter. **C,** Securing catheter to abdominal wall using bridge method of taping. *(From Dieckmann R, Fiser D, Selbst S. Pediatric Emergency and Critical Care Procedures. St. Louis: Mosby, 1997.)*

g. Radiographically confirm catheter tip position. Secure catheter with a suture through the cord, a marker tape, and a tape bridge. The catheter may be pulled back but *not* advanced once the sterile field is broken.

h. Observe for complications: Blanching or cyanosis of lower extremities, perforation, thrombosis, embolism, or infection. If any complications occur, the catheter should be removed.

i. Use isotonic fluids, which contain 0.5 units/mL of heparin. Never use hypo-osmolar fluids in the UA.

   NOTE: There are no definitive guidelines on feeding with a UA catheter in place. There is concern (up to 24 hours after removal) that the UA catheter or thrombus may interfere with intestinal perfusion. A risk-to-benefit assessment should be individualized.

6. **Procedure for UV line (Fig. 3-10):**
a. Follow steps "a" through "d" for UA catheter placement, but determine catheter length using Fig. 3-9.
b. Isolate the thin-walled umbilical vein, clear thrombi with forceps, and insert catheter, aiming the tip toward the right shoulder. Gently advance the catheter to the desired distance. *Do not force.* If resistance is encountered, try loosening the umbilical tape, applying steady and gentle pressure, or manipulating the angle of the umbilical cord to skin. Resistance is commonly met at the abdominal wall and again at the portal system. *Do not* infuse anything into liver.
c. Radiographically confirm catheter tip position. Secure catheter as described in step "g" for UA placement.
7. **A video on UV/UA line placement is available on the New England Journal of Medicine's website.**

IV. BODY FLUID SAMPLING

A. Lumbar Puncture[3,4]

1. **Indications:** Examination of spinal fluid for suspected infection or malignancy, instillation of intrathecal chemotherapy, or measurement of opening pressure.
2. **Complications:** Local pain, infection, bleeding, spinal fluid leak, hematoma, spinal headache, acquired epidermal spinal cord tumor (caused by implantation of epidermal material into spinal canal if no stylet is used on skin entry).
3. **Cautions and contraindications:**
a. Increased intracranial pressure (ICP): Before lumbar puncture (LP), perform funduscopic examination. Presence of papilledema, retinal hemorrhage, or clinical suspicion of increased ICP may be contraindications to the procedure. A sudden drop in intraspinal pressure by rapid release of CSF may cause fatal herniation. If LP is to be performed, proceed with extreme caution. Computed tomography (CT) may be indicated before LP if there is suspected intracranial bleeding, focal mass lesion, or increased ICP. A normal CT scan does not rule out increased ICP but usually excludes conditions that may put the patient at risk for herniation. Decision to obtain CT should not delay appropriate antibiotic therapy if indicated.
b. Bleeding diathesis: Platelet count >50,000/mm³ is desirable before LP, and correction of any clotting factor deficiencies can minimize risk for bleeding and subsequent cord or nerve root compression.
c. Overlying skin infection may result in inoculation of CSF with organisms.
d. LP should be deferred in an unstable patient, and appropriate therapy should be initiated, including antibiotics if indicated.
4. **Procedure:**
a. Apply local anesthetic cream if sufficient time is available.
b. Position child in either the sitting position (Fig. 3-11) or lateral recumbent position (Fig. 3-12), with hips, knees, and neck flexed. Keep shoulders and hips aligned (perpendicular to examining table in recumbent

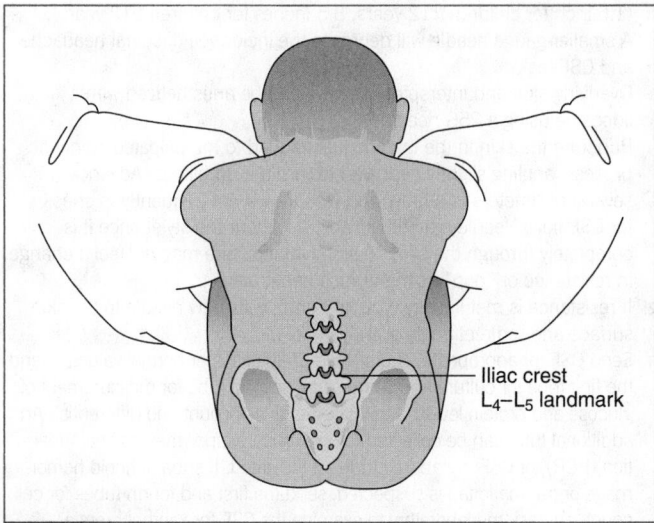

FIGURE 3-11

Lumbar puncture site in sitting position. (*From Dieckmann R, Fiser D, Selbst S.* Pediatric Emergency and Critical Care Procedures. *St. Louis: Mosby, 1997.*)

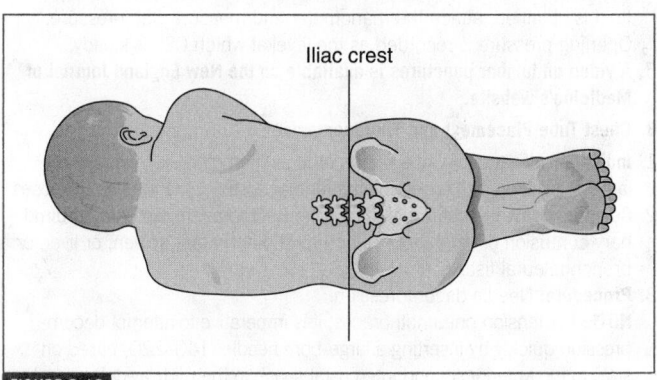

FIGURE 3-12

Lumbar puncture site in lateral (recumbent) position. (*From Dieckmann R, Fiser D, Selbst S.* Pediatric Emergency and Critical Care Procedures. *St. Louis: Mosby, 1997.*)

position) to avoid rotating the spine. *Do not* compromise a small infant's cardiorespiratory status with positioning.

c. Locate the desired intervertebral space (either L3-4 or L4-5) by drawing an imaginary line between the top of the iliac crests.

d. Prepare the skin in sterile fashion. Drape conservatively to make monitoring the infant possible. Use a 20G to 22G spinal needle with stylet

(1.5 inch for children <12 years, 3.5 inches for children ≥12 years). A smaller-gauge needle will decrease the incidence of spinal headache and CSF leak.

e. Overlying skin and interspinous tissue can be anesthetized with 1% lidocaine using a 25G needle.

f. Puncture the skin in the midline just caudad to the palpated spinous process, angling slightly cephalad toward the umbilicus. Advance several millimeters at a time, and withdraw stylet frequently to check for CSF flow. Needle may be advanced without the stylet once it is completely through the skin. In small infants, one may *not* feel a change in resistance or "pop" as the dura is penetrated.

g. If resistance is met initially (you hit bone), withdraw needle to the skin surface and redirect angle slightly.

h. Send CSF for appropriate studies (see Chapter 27 for normal values). Send the first tube for culture and Gram stain, second tube for measurement of glucose and protein levels, and last tube for cell count and differential. An additional tube can be collected for viral cultures, polymerase chain reaction (PCR), or CSF metabolic studies if indicated. If subarachnoid hemorrhage or traumatic tap is suspected, send the first and fourth tubes for cell count, and ask the laboratory to examine the CSF for xanthochromia.

i. Accurate measurement of CSF pressure can be made only with the patient lying quietly on his or her side in an unflexed position. It is not a reliable measurement in the sitting position. Once free flow of spinal fluid is obtained, attach the manometer and measure CSF pressure. Opening pressure is recorded as the level at which CSF is steady.

5. **A video on lumbar punctures is available on the New England Journal of Medicine's website.**

B. **Chest Tube Placement and Thoracentesis[3,6]**

1. **Indications:** Evacuation of a pneumothorax, hemothorax, chylothorax, large pleural effusion, or empyema for diagnostic or therapeutic purposes.

2. **Complications:** Infection, bleeding, pneumothorax, hemothorax, pulmonary contusion or laceration, puncture of diaphragm, spleen, or liver, or bronchopleural fistula.

3. **Procedure:** Needle decompression.
   NOTE: For tension pneumothoraces, it is imperative to attempt decompression quickly by inserting a large-bore needle (14G–22G, based on size) in the anterior second intercostal space in the midclavicular line. Insert needle over superior aspect of rib margin to avoid vascular structures.

a. When pleural space is entered, attach catheter to a three-way stopcock and syringe, and aspirate air.

b. Subsequent insertion of a chest tube is still necessary.

4. **Procedure (Fig. 3-13):** Chest tube insertion.
   (See inside front cover for chest tube sizes.)

a. Position child supine or with affected side up and arm restrained over the head.

b. Point of entry is the third to fifth intercostal space in the mid- to anterior axillary line, usually at the level of the nipple (avoid breast tissue).

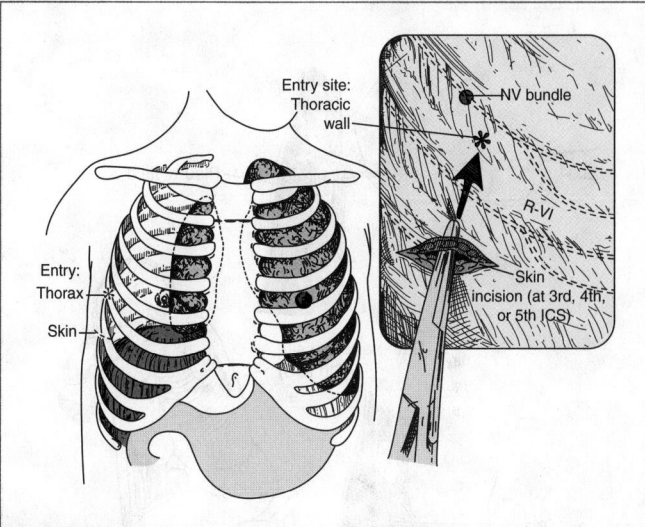

FIGURE 3-13

Technique for insertion of chest tube. ICS, Intercostal space; NV, neurovascular; R-VI, sixth rib. (*Modified from Fleisher G, Ludwig S. Pediatric Emergency Medicine. 3rd ed. Baltimore: Williams & Wilkins, 2000.*)

   c. Prepare and drape in sterile fashion.

   d. Patient may require sedation (see Chapter 6). Locally anesthetize skin, subcutaneous tissue, periosteum of rib, chest wall muscles, and pleura with 1% lidocaine.

   e. Make sterile 1- to 3-cm incision one intercostal space below desired insertion point, and bluntly dissect with a hemostat through tissue layers until the superior portion of the rib is reached, avoiding the neurovascular bundle on the inferior portion of the rib.

   f. Push hemostat over the top of the rib, through pleura, and into pleural space. Enter the pleural space cautiously and not deeper than 1 cm. Spread hemostat to open, place chest tube in clamp, and guide through entry site to desired distance.

   g. For a pneumothorax, insert tube anteriorly toward the apex. For a pleural effusion, direct tube inferiorly and posteriorly.

   h. Secure chest tube with purse-string sutures in which suture is first tied at the skin, then wrapped around the tube once and tied at the tube.

   i. Attach to a drainage system with 20 to 30 cm H_2O pressure.

   j. Apply a sterile occlusive dressing.

   k. Confirm position and function with chest radiograph.

5. **A video on chest tube insertion is available on the New England Journal of Medicine's website.**

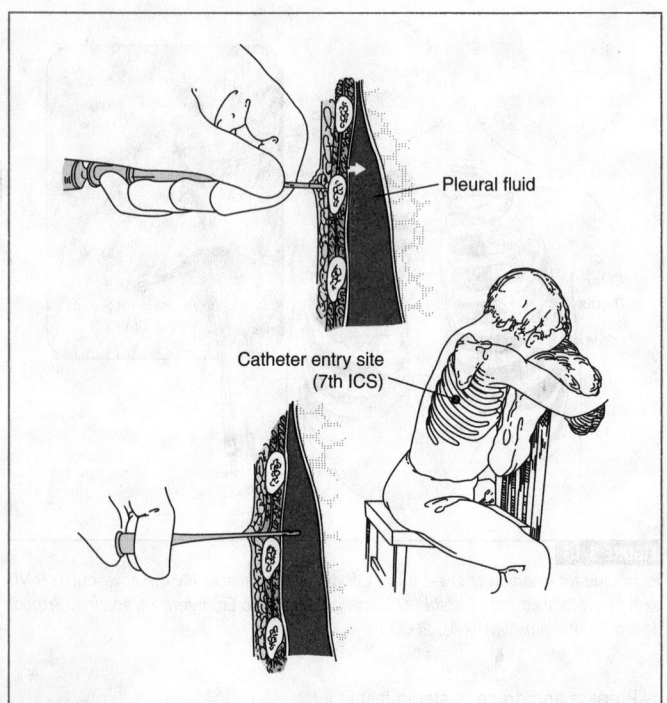

FIGURE 3-14

Thoracentesis. ICS, Intercostal space. (*Modified from Fleisher G, Ludwig S.* Pediatric Emergency Medicine. *3rd ed. Baltimore: Williams & Wilkins, 2000.)*

6. **Procedure:** Thoracentesis (Fig. 3-14)
a. Confirm fluid in pleural space by clinical examination and radiographs or ultrasonography.
b. If possible, place child in sitting position leaning over table; otherwise place supine.
c. Point of entry is usually in the seventh intercostal space and posterior axillary line.
d. Prepare and drape area in sterile fashion.
e. Anesthetize skin, subcutaneous tissue, rib periosteum, chest wall, and pleura with 1% lidocaine.
f. Advance an 18G–22G IV catheter or large-bore needle attached to a syringe onto the rib, and then "walk" over the superior aspect into the pleural space while providing steady negative pressure; often a popping sensation is generated. *Be careful to not advance too far into the pleural cavity.* If an IV or pigtail catheter (with guidewire) is used, the soft catheter may be advanced into the pleural space, aiming downward.

g. Attach syringe and stopcock device to remove fluid for diagnostic studies and symptomatic relief (see Chapter 27 for evaluation of pleural fluid).

h. After removing needle or catheter, place an occlusive dressing over the site and obtain a chest radiograph to rule out pneumothorax.

7. **A video on thoracentesis is available on the New England Journal of Medicine's website.**

C. Pericardiocentesis[3,6]

1. **Indications:** To obtain pericardial fluid in cardiac tamponade emergently or nonemergently for diagnostic or therapeutic purposes.

2. **Complications:** Bleeding, infection, puncture of cardiac chamber, cardiac dysrhythmia, hemopericardium or pneumopericardium, pneumothorax, hemothorax, cardiac arrest, death.

3. **Procedure (Figs. 3-15 and 3-16):**

a. Unless contraindicated, provide sedation and/or analgesia for the patient. Monitor electrocardiogram (ECG).

b. Place patient at a 30-degree angle (reverse Trendelenburg). Have patient secured.

c. Prepare and drape puncture site in sterile fashion. A drape across upper chest is unnecessary and may obscure important landmarks.

d. Anesthetize puncture site with 1% lidocaine.

e. Insert an 18G or 20G needle just to the left of the xiphoid process, 1 cm inferior to the bottom rib at about a 45-degree angle to the skin.

f. While gently aspirating, advance needle toward the patient's left shoulder until pericardial fluid is obtained.

g. Upon entering the pericardial space, clamp the needle with a hemostat at the skin edge to prevent further penetration. Attach a 30-mL syringe with a stopcock.

h. Gently and slowly remove the fluid. Rapid withdrawal of pericardial fluid can result in shock or myocardial insufficiency.

i. Send fluid for appropriate laboratory studies (see Chapter 27).

j. In nonemergent conditions, this is best performed under two-dimensional echocardiographic guidance.

4. **A video on pericardiocentesis is available on the New England Journal of Medicine's website.**

D. Paracentesis[4]

1. **Indications:** Percutaneous removal of intraperitoneal fluid for diagnostic or therapeutic purposes.

2. **Complications:** Bleeding, infection, puncture of viscera.

3. **Cautions:**

a. *Do not* remove a large amount of fluid too rapidly; hypovolemia and hypotension may result from rapid fluid shifts.

b. Avoid scars from previous surgery; localized bowel adhesions increase the chances of entering a viscus in these areas.

c. Urinary bladder should be empty to avoid perforation.

d. Never perform paracentesis through an area of cellulitis.

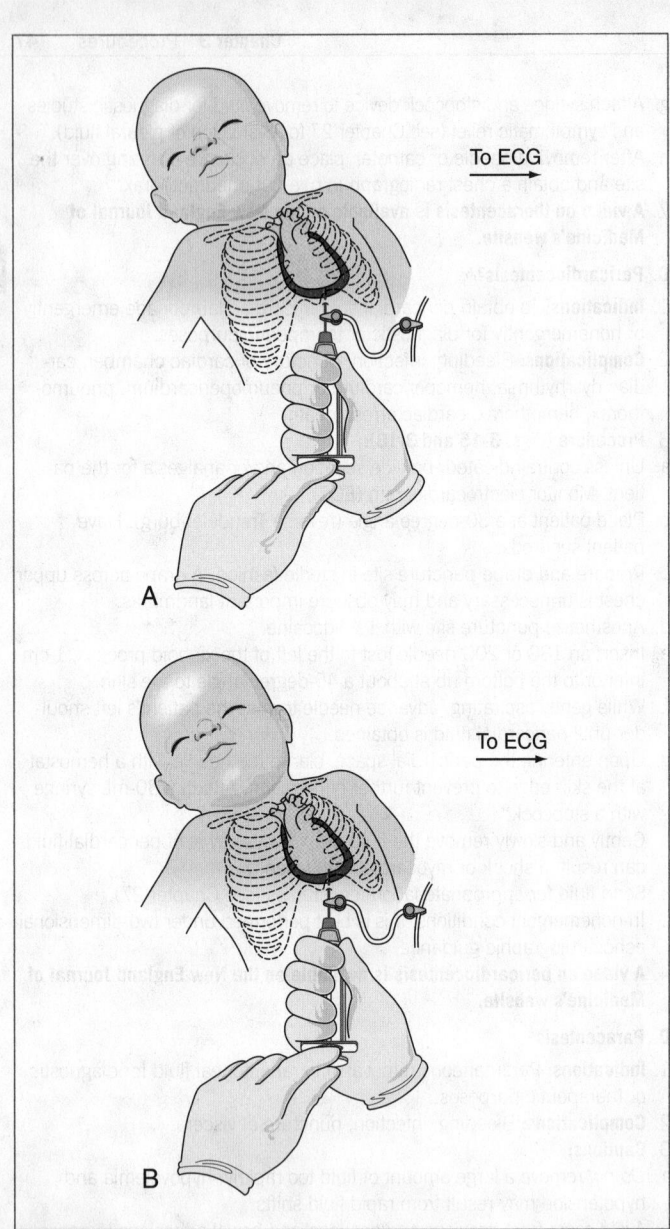

FIGURE 3-15

Subxiphoid approach for pericardiocentesis. **A,** Needle in pericardial sac with normal electrocardiogram (ECG). **B,** Needle in heart with current of injury pattern on ECG. (*From Dieckmann R, Fiser D, Selbst S. Pediatric Emergency and Critical Care Procedures. St. Louis: Mosby, 1997.*)

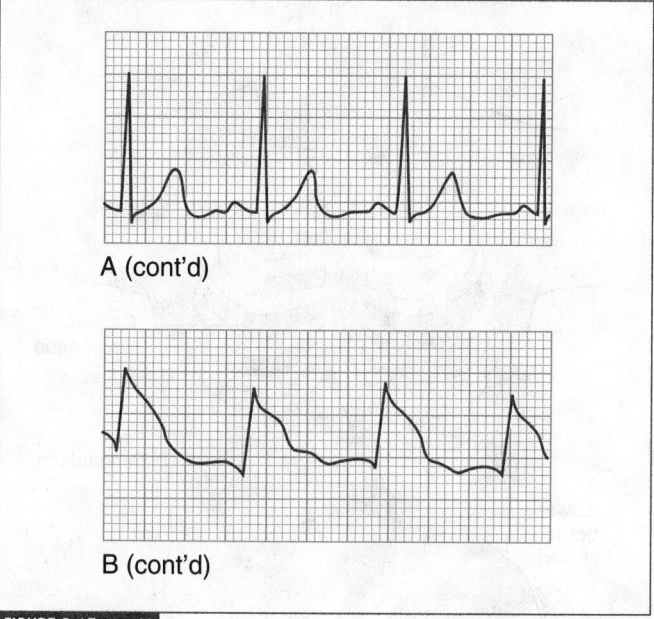

A (cont'd)

B (cont'd)

FIGURE 3-15, cont'd

4. **Procedure:**
a. Prepare and drape abdomen as for a surgical procedure. Anesthetize puncture site.
b. With patient in semisupine, sitting, or lateral decubitus position, insert a 16G to 22G IV catheter attached to a syringe in midline 2 cm below umbilicus. In neonates, insert just lateral to rectus muscle in the right or left lower quadrants, a few centimeters above inguinal ligament.
c. Aiming cephalad, insert needle at a 45-degree angle while one hand pulls the skin caudally until entering the peritoneal cavity. This creates a Z tract when the skin is released and the needle removed. Apply continuous negative pressure.
d. Once fluid appears in the syringe, remove introducer needle and leave catheter in place. Attach a stopcock and aspirate slowly until an adequate amount of fluid has been obtained for studies or symptomatic relief.
e. If, on entering the peritoneal cavity, air is aspirated, withdraw the needle immediately. Aspirated air indicates entrance into a hollow viscus. (In general, penetration of a hollow viscus during paracentesis does not lead to complications.) Repeat paracentesis with sterile equipment.
f. Send fluid for appropriate laboratory studies (see Chapter 27).
5. **A video on paracentesis is available on the New England Journal of Medicine's website.**

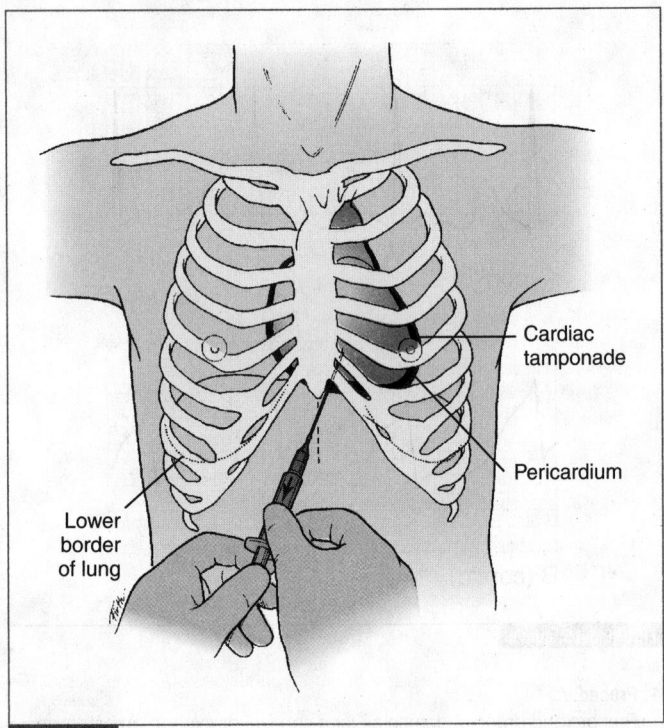

FIGURE 3-16

Insertion of needle for pericardiocentesis at junction of xiphoid and left costal margin, aiming toward left shoulder. *(Modified from Brundage SI, Scott BG, Karmy-Jones R, et al. Pericardiocentesis and pericardial window. In: Shoemaker WC, Velmahos BC, Demetriades D, eds. Procedures and Monitoring for the Critically Ill. Philadelphia: Saunders, 2002.)*

E. Urinary Bladder Catheterization[4]

1. **Indications:** To obtain urine for urinalysis and culture sterilely and to accurately monitor hydration status.
2. **Complications:** Hematuria, infection, trauma to urethra or bladder, intravesical knot of catheter (rarely occurs).
3. **Procedure:**
a. Infant/child should not have voided within 1 hour of procedure.
   NOTE: Catheterization is contraindicated in pelvic fractures, known trauma to the urethra, or blood at the meatus.
b. Prepare the urethral opening using sterile technique.
c. In males, apply gentle traction to the penis to straighten the urethra. In uncircumcised male infants, expose the meatus with gentle retraction of the foreskin. The foreskin has to be retracted only far enough to visualize the meatus.

d. Gently insert a lubricated catheter into the urethra. Slowly advance catheter until resistance is met at the external sphincter. Continued pressure will overcome this resistance, and the catheter will enter the bladder. In girls, the urethral orifice may be difficult to visualize, but it is usually immediately anterior to the vaginal orifice. Only a few centimeters of advancement is required to reach the bladder in girls. In boys, insert a few centimeters longer than the shaft of the penis.

e. Carefully remove the catheter once specimen is obtained, and cleanse skin of iodine.

f. If indwelling Foley catheter is inserted, inflate balloon with sterile water as indicated on bulb, then connect catheter to drainage tubing attached to urine drainage bag. Secure catheter tubing to inner thigh.

4. **A video on catheterization of the male urethra is available on the New England Journal of Medicine's website.**

5. **A video on catheterization of the female urethra is available on the New England Journal of Medicine's website.**

F. Suprapubic Bladder Aspiration[3]

1. **Indications:** To sterilely obtain urine for urinalysis and culture in children younger than 2 years (avoid in children with genitourinary tract anomalies, coagulopathy, or intestinal obstruction). Bypasses distal urethra, thereby minimizing risk for contamination.

2. **Complications:** Infection (cellulitis), hematuria (usually microscopic), intestinal perforation.

3. **Procedure (Fig. 3-17):**

a. Anterior rectal pressure in girls or gentle penile pressure in boys may be used to prevent urination during the procedure. Child should not have voided within 1 hour of procedure.

b. Restrain infant in the supine, frog-leg position. Prepare suprapubic area in sterile fashion.

c. The site for puncture is 1 to 2 cm above the symphysis pubis in the midline. Use a syringe with a 22G, 1-inch needle, and puncture at a 10- to 20-degree angle to the perpendicular, aiming slightly caudad.

d. Gently exert suction as the needle is advanced until urine enters syringe. The needle should not be advanced more than 1 inch. Aspirate urine with gentle suction.

e. Cleanse skin of iodine.

G. Soft Tissue Aspiration[8]

1. **Indications:** Cellulitis that is unresponsive to initial standard therapy, recurrent cellulitis or abscesses, immunocompromised patients in whom organism recovery is necessary and may affect antimicrobial therapy

2. **Complications:** Pain, infection, bleeding

3. **Procedure:**

a. Select site to aspirate at *point of maximal inflammation* (more likely to increase recovery of causative agent than leading edge of erythema or center).[8]

b. Cleanse area in sterile fashion.

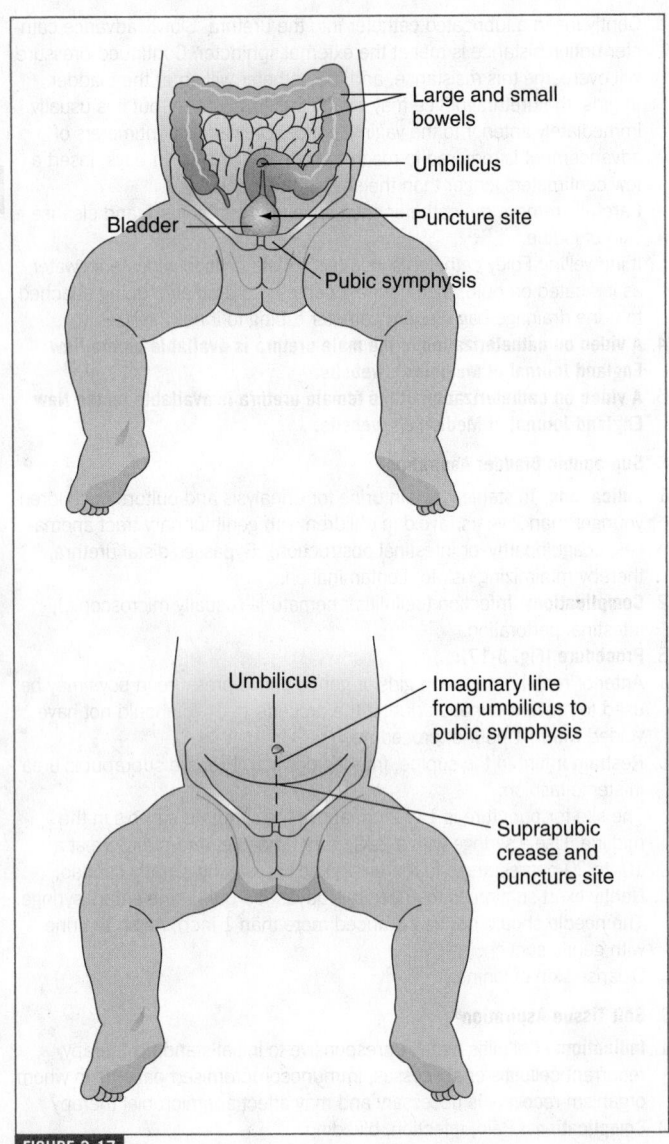

FIGURE 3-17

Landmarks for suprapubic bladder aspiration. *(From Dieckmann R, Fiser D, Selbst S. Pediatric Emergency and Critical Care Procedures. St. Louis: Mosby, 1997.)*

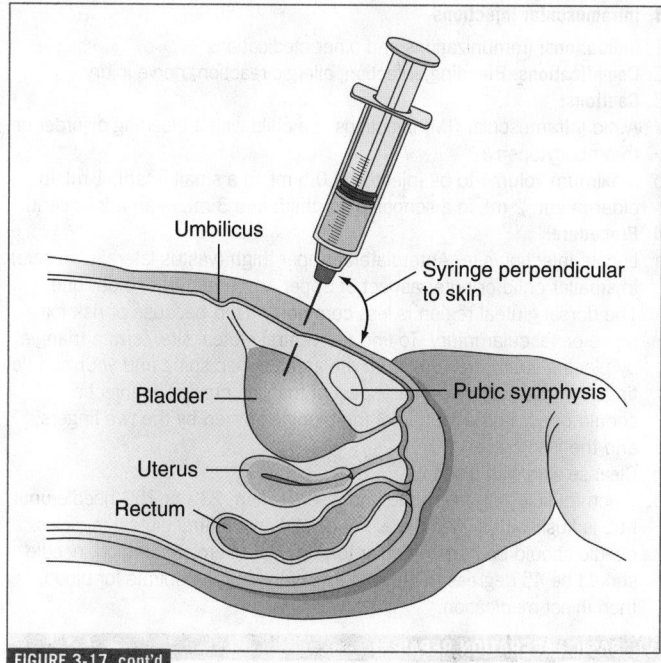

Umbilicus

Syringe perpendicular to skin

Bladder

Pubic symphysis

Uterus

Rectum

FIGURE 3-17, cont'd

c. Local anesthesia with 1% lidocaine is optional.
d. Fill tuberculin syringe with 0.1 to 0.2 mL of *nonbacteriostatic* sterile saline, and attach to needle.
e. Using 18G or 20G needle (22G for facial cellulitis), advance to appropriate depth and apply negative pressure while withdrawing needle.
f. Send fluid from aspiration for Gram stain and cultures. If no fluid is obtained, needle can be streaked on agar plate. Consider acid-fast bacillus (AFB) and fungal stains in immunocompromised patients.

V. IMMUNIZATION AND MEDICATION ADMINISTRATION[4]

A. Subcutaneous Injections

1. **Indications:** Immunizations and other medications
2. **Complications:** Bleeding, infection, allergic reaction, lipohypertrophy or lipoatrophy after repeated injections
3. **Procedure:**
a. Locate injection site: Upper outer arm or outer aspect of upper thigh.
b. Cleanse skin with alcohol.
c. Insert 0.5-inch, 25G or 27G needle into subcutaneous layer at a 45-degree angle to the skin. Aspirate for blood, then inject medication.

B. Intramuscular Injections

1. **Indications:** Immunizations and other medications
2. **Complications:** Bleeding, infection, allergic reaction, nerve injury
3. **Cautions:**
a. Avoid intramuscular (IM) injections in a child with a bleeding disorder or thrombocytopenia.
b. Maximum volume to be injected is 0.5 mL in a small infant, 1 mL in an older infant, 2 mL in a school-aged child, and 3 mL in an adolescent.
4. **Procedure:**
a. Locate injection site: Anterolateral upper thigh (vastus lateralis muscle) in smaller child or outer aspect of upper arm (deltoid) in older one. The dorsal gluteal region is less commonly used because of risk for nerve or vascular injury. To find the ventral gluteal site, form a triangle by placing your index finger on the anterior iliac spine and your middle finger on the most superior aspect of the iliac crest. The injection should occur in the middle of the triangle formed by the two fingers and the iliac crest.
b. Cleanse skin with alcohol.
c. Pinch muscle with free hand and insert 1-inch, 23G or 25G needle until hub is flush with skin surface. For deltoid and ventral gluteal muscles, needle should be perpendicular to skin. For anterolateral thigh, needle should be 45 degrees to the long axis of the thigh. Aspirate for blood, then inject medication.

VI. BASIC LACERATION REPAIR[3]

A. Suturing

1. **Techniques (Fig. 3-18):**
a. Simple interrupted
b. Horizontal mattress: Provides eversion of wound edges
c. Vertical mattress: For added strength in areas of thick skin or areas of skin movement; provides eversion of wound edges
d. Running intradermal: For cosmetic closures
2. **Procedure:**
   NOTE: Lacerations of the face, lips, hands, genitalia, mouth, or periorbital area may require consultation with a specialist. Ideally, lacerations at increased risk for infection (areas with poor blood supply, contaminated/crush injury) should be sutured within 6 hours of injury. Clean wounds in cosmetically important areas may be closed up to 24 hours after injury in the absence of significant contamination or devitalization. In general, bite wounds should not be sutured except in areas of high cosmetic importance (face). The longer sutures are left in place, the greater the scarring and potential for infection. Sutures in cosmetically sensitive areas should be removed as soon as possible. Sutures in high-tension areas (e.g., extensor surfaces) should stay in longer (Table 3-1).
a. Prepare child for procedure with appropriate sedation, analgesia, and restraint.

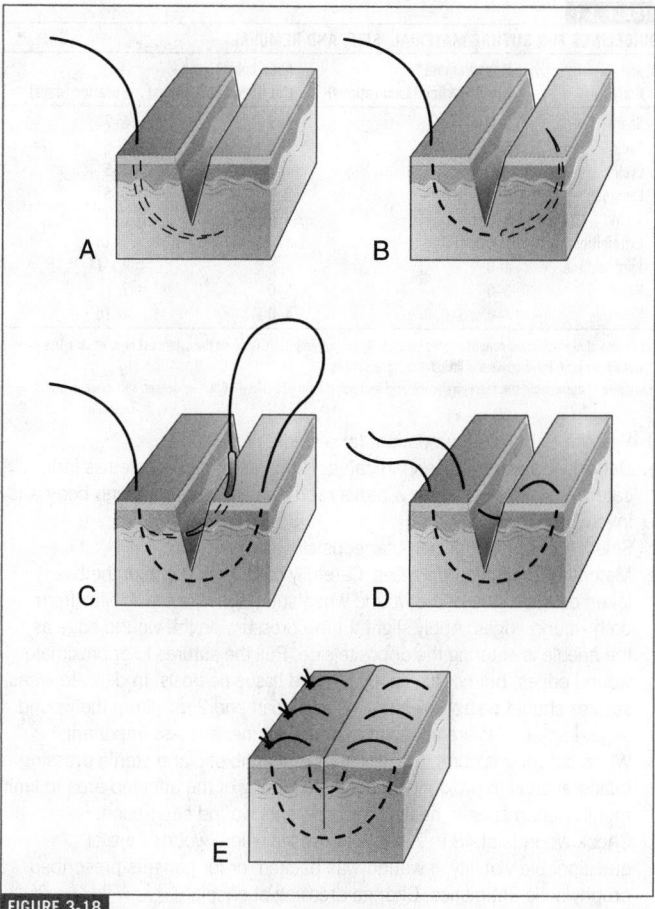

FIGURE 3-18

A–E, Vertical mattress suture. After initial placement of a simple interrupted stitch with a larger bite, make a backhand pass across the wound, taking small superficial bites. When knot is tied, edges of laceration should evert slightly. *(From Dieckmann R, Fiser D, Selbst S.* Pediatric Emergency and Critical Care Procedures. *St. Louis: Mosby, 1997.)*

b. Anesthetize the wound with topical anesthetic or with lidocaine bicarbonate by injecting the anesthetic into the subcutaneous tissues (see Formulary).

c. Forcefully irrigate the wound with copious amounts of sterile NS. Use at least 250 mL for smaller superficial wounds and more for larger wounds. This is the most important step in preventing infection. Avoid high-pressure irrigation of deep puncture wounds.

TABLE 3-1
GUIDELINES FOR SUTURE MATERIAL, SIZE, AND REMOVAL

Body Region	Monofilament* (for Superficial Lacerations)	Absorbable† (for Deep Lacerations)	Duration (days)
Scalp	5–0 or 4–0	4–0	5–7
Face	6–0	5–0	3–5
Eyelid	7–0 or 6–0	—	3–5
Eyebrow	6–0 or 5–0	5–0	3–5
Trunk	5–0 or 4–0	3–0	5–7
Extremities	5–0 or 4–0	4–0	7–10
Joint surface	4–0	—	10–14
Hand	5–0	5–0	7
Foot sole	4–0 or 3–0	4–0	7–10

*Examples of monofilament nonabsorbable sutures: Nylon, polypropylene. Good for the outermost layer of skin. Use 4–5 throws per knot. Polypropylene is good for scalp, eyebrows.
†Examples of absorbable sutures: Polyglycolic acid and polyglactin 910 (Vicryl). Good for deeper, subcuticular layers.

d. Prepare and drape the patient for a sterile procedure.
e. Debride the wound when indicated. Probe for foreign bodies as indicated. Consider obtaining a radiograph if a radiopaque foreign body was involved in the injury.
f. Select suture type for percutaneous closure (see Table 3-1).
g. Match layers of injured tissues. Carefully match the depth of the bite taken on each side of the wound when suturing. Take equal bites from both wound edges. Apply slight thumb pressure on the wound edge as the needle is entering the opposite side. Pull the sutures to approximate wound edges, but not too tightly to avoid tissue necrosis. In delicate areas, sutures should be approximately 2 mm apart and 2 mm from the wound edge. Larger bites are acceptable where cosmesis is less important.[3]
h. When suturing is complete, apply topical antibiotic and sterile dressing. If laceration is in proximity of a joint, splinting of the affected area to limit mobility often speeds healing and prevents wound separation.
i. Check wounds at 48 to 72 hours in cases where wounds are of questionable viability, if wound was packed, or for patients prescribed prophylactic antibiotics. Change dressing at check.
j. For hand lacerations, close skin only; *do not* use subcutaneous stitches. Elevate and immobilize the hand. Consider consulting a hand or plastics specialist.
k. Consider the child's need for tetanus prophylaxis (see Chapter 16, Table 16-3, for guidelines).
3. **A video on basic laceration repair is available on the New England Journal of Medicine's website.**
B. **Skin Staples**
1. **Indications:**
a. Best for scalp, trunk, extremities
b. More rapid application than sutures but can be more painful to remove
c. Lower rates of wound infection

2. **Contraindications:**
a. Not for areas that require meticulous cosmesis
b. Avoid in patients who require magnetic resonance imaging (MRI) or CT

3. **Procedure:**
a. Appose wound edges and staple.
b. Left in place for the same length of time as sutures (see Table 3-1).
c. To remove, use staple remover.

C. **Tissue Adhesives**

1. **Indications:**
a. For use with superficial lacerations with clean edges
b. Excellent cosmetic results, ease of application, and reduced patient anxiety
c. Lower rates of wound infection

2. **Contraindications:**
a. Not for use in areas under large amounts of tension (e.g., hands, joints).
b. Use caution with areas near the eye.

3. **Procedure:**
a. Use pressure to achieve hemostasis and clean the wound as explained previously.
b. Hold together wound edges.
c. Apply adhesive dropwise along the wound surface, avoiding applying adhesive to the inside of the wound. Hold in place for 20 to 30 seconds.
d. If the wound is malaligned, remove the adhesive with forceps and reapply.
e. Adhesive will slough off after 7 to 10 days.

VII. MUSCULOSKELETAL PROCEDURES

A. **Basic Splinting**[3]

1. **Indications:** to provide short-term stabilization of limb injuries
2. **Complications:** pressure sores, dermatitis, neurovascular impairment
3. **Procedure:**
a. Determine style of splint needed
b. Measure and cut fiberglass or plaster to appropriate length. If using plaster, upper-extremity splints require 8 to 10 layers, and lower-extremity splints require 12 to 14 layers.
c. Pad extremity with cotton Webril, taking care to overlap each turn by 50%. In prepackaged fiberglass splints, additional padding is not generally required. Bony prominences may require additional padding. Place cotton between digits if they are in a splint.
d. Immerse plaster slabs into room-temperature water until bubbling stops. Smooth out wet plaster slab, avoiding any wrinkles.
Warning: Plaster becomes hot after drying.
e. Position splint over extremity and wrap externally with gauze. When dry, an elastic wrap can be added.
f. Alternatively, wet one side of fiberglass until saturated. Roll or fold to remove excess water. Mold splint as indicated.

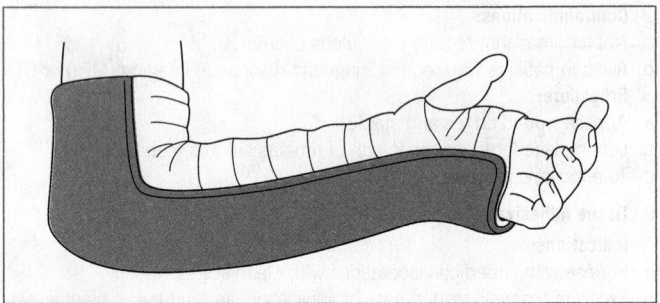

FIGURE 3-19

Long arm posterior splint.

NOTE: Using warm water will decrease drying time. This may result in inadequate time to mold splint. Turn edge of the splint back on itself to produce a smooth surface. Take care to cover the sharp edges of fiberglass. When dry, wrap with elastic bandage.

g. Use crutches or slings as indicated.

h. The need for orthopedic referral should be individually assessed.

B. Long Arm Posterior Splint (Fig. 3-19)

1. **Indications:** Immobilization of elbow and forearm injuries

C. Sugar Tong Forearm Splint (Fig. 3-20)

1. **Indications:** For distal radius and wrist fractures, to immobilize the elbow and minimize pronation and supination

D. Ulnar Gutter Splint

1. **Indications:** Nonrotated fourth or fifth (boxer) metacarpal metaphyseal fracture with less than 20 degrees of angulation, uncomplicated fourth and fifth phalangeal fracture.

2. **Assess for malrotation, displacement (especially Salter I–type fracture), angulation, and joint stability before splinting.**

3. **Procedure:** Elbow in neutral position, wrist in neutral position, metacarpophalangeal (MP) joint at 70 degrees, interphalangeal (IP) joint at 20 degrees. Apply splint in U shape from the tip of the fifth digit to 3 cm distal to the volar crease of the elbow. Splint should be wide enough to enclose the fourth and fifth digits.

E. Thumb Spica Splint

1. **Indications:** Nonrotated, nonangulated, nonarticular fractures of the thumb metacarpal or phalanx, ulnar collateral ligament injury (gamekeeper's or skier's thumb), scaphoid fracture or suspected scaphoid fracture (pain in anatomic snuff box).

2. **Procedure:** Wrist in slight dorsiflexion, thumb in some flexion and abduction, IP joint in slight flexion. Apply splint in U shape from tip of thumb to mid-forearm. Mold the splint along the long axis of the thumb so that

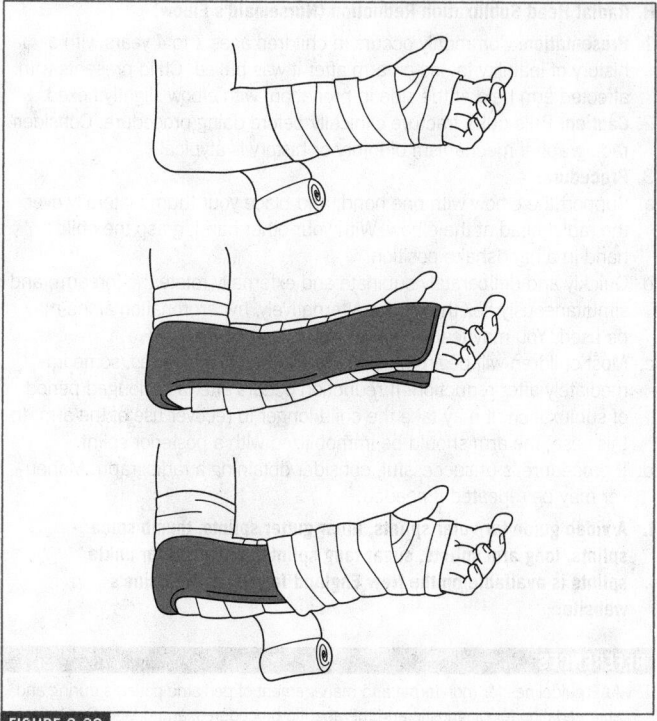

FIGURE 3-20

Sugar tong forearm splint.

thumb position is maintained. This will result in a spiral configuration along the forearm.

F. Volar Splint

1. **Indications:** Wrist immobilization.
2. **Procedure:** Wrist in slight dorsiflexion. Apply splint on palmar surface from the MP joint to 2 to 3 cm distal to the volar crease of the elbow. It is useful to curve the splint to allow the MP joint to rest at an 80- to 90-degree angle.

G. Posterior Ankle Splint

1. **Indications:** Immobilization of ankle sprains and fractures of the foot, ankle, and distal fibula.
2. **Procedure:** Measure leg for appropriate length of plaster. Splint should extend to base of toes and upper portion of the calf. A sugar tong (stirrup) splint can be added to increase stability for ankle fractures.

H. Radial Head Subluxation Reduction (Nursemaid's Elbow)

1. **Presentation:** Commonly occurs in children ages 1 to 4 years with a history of inability to use an arm after it was pulled. Child presents with affected arm held at the side in pronation, with elbow slightly flexed.

2. **Caution:** Rule out a fracture clinically before doing procedure. Consider radiograph if mechanism of injury or history is atypical.

3. **Procedure:**

a. Support the elbow with one hand, and place your thumb laterally over the radial head at the elbow. With your other hand, grasp the child's hand in a handshake position.

b. Quickly and deliberately supinate and externally rotate the forearm, and simultaneously flex the elbow. Alternatively, hyperpronation alone may be used. You may feel a click as reduction occurs.

c. Most children will begin to use the arm within 15 minutes, some immediately after reduction. If reduction occurs after a prolonged period of subluxation, it may take the child longer to recover use of the arm. In this case, the arm should be immobilized with a posterior splint.

d. If procedure is unsuccessful, consider obtaining a radiograph. Maneuver may be repeated if needed.

I. **A video guide for volar splints, ulnar gutter splints, thumb spica splints, long arm splints, sugar tong splints, and posterior ankle splints is available on the New England Journal of Medicine's website.**

REFERENCES

1. AAP guidelines for monitoring and management of pediatric patients during and after sedation for diagnostic and therapeutic procedures: an update. *Pediatrics.* 2006;118:2587-2602.

2. Barone MA. Pediatric procedures. In: *Oski's Pediatrics: Principles and Practice.* 4th ed. Philadelphia: Lippincott Williams & Wilkins; 2006:2671-2687.

3. Fleisher G, Ludwig S. *Textbook of Pediatric Emergency Medicine.* 6th ed. Baltimore: Williams & Wilkins, 2010.

4. Dieckmann R, Fiser D, Selbst S. *Illustrated Textbook of Pediatric Emergency and Critical Care Procedures.* St. Louis: Mosby, 1997.

5. Jain A, Haines L. *Ultrasound-Guided Critical Care Procedures. Critical Care Emergency Medicine.* New York: McGraw-Hill, 2012.

6. Nichols DG, Yaster M, Lappe DG, et al. *Golden Hour: The Handbook of Advanced Pediatric Life Support.* 2nd ed. St. Louis: Mosby, 1996.

7. Berenholtz SM, Pronovost PJ, Lipsett PA, et al. Eliminating catheter-related bloodstream infections in the intensive care unit. *Crit Care Med.* 2004;32:2014-2020.

8. Howe PM, Eduardo Fajardo J, Orcutt MA. Etiologic diagnosis of cellulitis: comparison of aspirates obtained from the leading edge and the point of maximal inflammation. *Pediatr Infect Dis J.* 1987;6:685–686.

Chapter 4

Trauma, Burns, and Common Critical Care Emergencies

Emily Krennerich, MD

🔵 See additional content on Expert Consult

I. TRAUMA: OVERVIEW[1]

A. Primary Survey

The primary survey includes assessment of the ABCs (airway, breathing, circulation) via the algorithm **CAB: C**irculation, **A**irway, and **B**reathing.[2] See Chapter 1 for a complete algorithm.

NOTE: The CAB sequence is currently in use by the American Heart Association as part of the Pediatric Advanced Life Support (PALS) algorithm. The Advanced Trauma Life Support (ATLS) algorithm developed by the American College of Surgeons continues to support the ABC sequence in the primary survey. Depending on the patient and the injury incurred, either sequence may be used during acute trauma stabilization.

B. Secondary Survey

Procedures used in a secondary survey are listed in Table 4-1 and include assessment of neurologic status using the quick screen **AVPU** (**A**lert, **V**ocal stimulation response, **P**ainful stimulation response, **U**nresponsive) or Glasgow Coma Scale (GCS). Remove all the patient's clothing, and perform a thorough head-to-toe examination. Remember to keep the child warm during the examination.

C. AMPLE History

Obtain an **AMPLE** history: **A**llergies, **M**edications, **P**ast illnesses, **L**ast meal, **E**vents preceding injury.

II. SPECIFIC TRAUMATIC INJURIES

A. Minor Closed Head Trauma[3]

1. **Head injury can be caused by penetrating trauma, blunt force, rotational acceleration, or acceleration-deceleration injury.** Closed head trauma (CHT) can lead to depressed or nondepressed skull fracture, epidural or subdural hematoma, cerebral contusion, brain edema, increased intracranial pressure (ICP), brain herniation, concussion (mild to moderate diffuse brain injury), and/or coma (diffuse axonal injury [DAI]). See Section III.B for treatment of elevated ICP associated with severe CHT.

2. **Evaluation:**

a. Physical examination (after CAB and cervical spine [C-spine] immobilization):

   (1) Assign GCS score (see Chapter 1).

TABLE 4-1

SECONDARY SURVEY

Organ System	Secondary Survey
Head	Scalp/skull injury
	Raccoon eyes: Periorbital ecchymoses; suggests orbital roof fracture
	Battle's sign: Ecchymoses behind pinna; suggests mastoid fracture
	Cerebrospinal fluid leak from ears/nose or hemotympanum suggests basilar skull fracture
	Pupil size, symmetry, and reactivity: Unilateral dilation of one pupil suggests compression of cranial nerve (CN) III and possible impending herniation; bilateral dilation of pupils is ominous and suggests bilateral CN III compression or severe anoxia and ischemia
	Corneal reflex
	Funduscopic examination for papilledema as evidence of increased intracranial pressure
	Hyphema
Neck	Cervical spine tenderness, deformity, injury
	Trachea midline
	Subcutaneous emphysema
	Hematoma
	Bruit
Chest	Clavicle deformity, tenderness
	Breath sounds, heart sounds
	Chest wall symmetry, paradoxical movement, rib deformity/fracture
	Petechiae over chest/head suggest traumatic asphyxia
Abdomen	Serial examinations to evaluate tenderness, distention, ecchymosis
	Shoulder pain suggests referred subdiaphragmatic process
	Orogastric aspirates with blood or bile suggest intraabdominal injury
	Splenic laceration suggested by left upper quadrant rib tenderness, flank pain, and/or flank ecchymoses "seatbelt sign"
Pelvis	Tenderness, symmetry, deformity, stability
Genitourinary	Laceration, ecchymoses, hematoma, bleeding
	Rectal tone, blood, displaced prostate
	Blood at urinary meatus suggests urethral injury; do not catheterize
Back	Log-roll patient to evaluate spine for step-off along spinal column
	Tenderness
	Open or penetrating wound
Extremities	Neurovascular status: Pulse, perfusion, pallor, paresthesias, paralysis, pain
	Deformity, crepitus, pain
	Motor/sensory examination
	Compartment syndrome: Pain out of proportion to expected; distal pallor/pulselessness
Neurologic	Quick screen: Alert, Vocal stimulation response, Painful stimulation response, Unresponsive (AVPU) or Glasgow Coma Scale
Skin	Capillary refill, perfusion
	Lacerations, abrasions, contusion

BOX 4-1

CATCH CLINICAL DECISION RULE FOR DETERMINING WHETHER HEAD CT IS NEEDED IN THE SETTING OF MINOR CLOSED HEAD TRAUMA[5]

If any one of the following findings in either category is present, obtain head CT.
High risk (likely need for neurologic intervention):
- GCS <15 at 2 hours after injury
- Suspected open or depressed skull fracture
- Worsening headache
- Irritability

Medium risk (brain injury likely will be evident on CT):
- Any sign of basal skull fracture (CSF leakage, hemotympanum, periorbital or mastoid ecchymosis)
- Large, boggy scalp hematoma
- Hazardous mechanism of injury (motor vehicle crash, fall from over 3 feet, fall down five or more stairs)

CSF, Cerebraospinal fluid; CT, computed tomography; GCS, Glasgow Coma Scale. Modified from CATCH: a clinical decision rule for the use of computed tomography in children with minor head injury. *CMAJ*. 2010;182:341-348.

(2) Obtain vital signs; pay special attention to Cushing triad (hypertension, bradycardia, irregular respiratory pattern) as an indication of increased intracranial pressure.

(3) Perform neurologic examination as part of secondary survey (see Table 4-1).

(4) If severe symptoms or vital sign changes are present, or if major CHT, follow procedures for emergency management of increased ICP and coma (see Section III.B).

(5) Rule out possible drug or alcohol ingestion/use as etiology of altered mental status.

b. Associated symptoms: Altered level or loss of consciousness (LOC), amnesia (before, during, or after the event), mental status change, behavior change, seizure activity, vomiting, headache, gait disturbance, visual change, or lethargy since event

c. Mechanism of injury:
(1) Linear forces: Less likely to cause LOC; more commonly lead to skull fractures, intracranial hematoma, or cerebral contusion.
(2) Rotational forces: Commonly cause LOC; occasionally associated with DAI.
(3) Suspect abuse if mechanism of injury is not consistent with sustained injuries.

3. **Management[4]:**
a. Evaluate C-spine (see Section II.B).
b. Consider if noncontrast computed tomography (CT) scan of head is indicated (Box 4-1).
(1) Most cases may be observed initially in the emergency department without neuroimaging.
(2) Vomiting or brief LOC is not an absolute indication for head CT.

c. Observe patient:
(1) Monitor for 4 to 6 hours to detect delayed signs/symptoms of intra-cranial injury. A symptom-free lucid period can precede variable degrees of acute-onset mental status change with epidural bleeds.
(2) Recommend continued observation at home, and counsel parents on indications to have the patient reevaluated by medical staff. Continued observation can occur in the hospital if patient is clinically unstable or if there are concerns about home environment (caregiver reliability, follow-up, etc.).
d. Consider hospitalizing patients with the following symptoms:
(1) Depressed or declining level of consciousness or prolonged unconsciousness (GCS 8–12)
(2) Focal neurologic deficit
(3) Increasing headache, persistent vomiting, or seizures
(4) Cerebrospinal fluid (CSF) otorrhea or rhinorrhea, hemotympanum, mastoid ecchymosis (Battle's sign), or periorbital ecchymosis (raccoon eyes)
(5) Linear skull fracture crossing the groove of the middle meningeal artery, a venous sinus of the dura, or the foramen magnum
(6) Depressed or compound skull fracture or fracture into the frontal sinus
(7) Bleeding disorder or patient on anticoagulation therapy
(8) Intoxication, illness, or injury obscuring neurologic state
(9) Suspected nonaccidental trauma
(10) Patient is unable to return to emergency department (ED) for reassessment
e. Concussions in sports-related injuries[6]:
(1) Definition: Trauma-induced alteration of consciousness that may or may not cause LOC
(2) Immediate signs: Change in playing ability, confusion, slowing, memory disturbance (including of events surrounding injury), incoordination, headache, dizziness, nausea, vomiting, and LOC
(3) Postconcussive symptoms: Headaches, fatigue, sleep disturbance, nausea/vomiting, vision changes, tinnitus, balance problems, emotional/behavioral changes, sensitivity to light or sound, and cognitive changes
(4) Management: Evaluate CAB, perform mental status assessment
(a) Grade of concussion less important than carefully tracking recovery course over time
(b) Return to play only if: No signs or symptoms during rest or exertion, normal neurologic examination, neuroimaging normal (if obtained)
(c) Consider neuropsychologic testing if history of multiple injuries, recovery not progressing as expected
(5) Refer to Centers for Disease Control and Prevention Guidelines: Concussion in Youth Sports: http://www.cdc.gov/concussion/Heads Up/youth.html

B. Neck Injuries[3]

See Chapter 25 (Radiology) for in-depth evaluation of cervical trauma and reading C-spine films.

1. **Immobilize C-spine before history and physical examination.** Infants generally have large occiputs, so use support under neck/shoulders to maintain neutral position and avoid neck flexion. If patient is seen after immobilization by an emergency respondent, attempt to clear clinically and consider radiographic studies based on findings.

2. **Radiographic studies:**
a. Posteroanterior (PA), lateral views (including C7), and odontoid view
b. Flexion and extension views of C-spine can be considered if:
   (1) Unstable C-spine injury not suspected.
   (2) PA and lateral views are normal, but bony tenderness is present.
   (3) Symptoms are present on palpation.
c. Magnetic resonance imaging (MRI) indicated to rule out direct spinal cord damage if neurologic symptoms persist and plain films are negative

3. **Clinically clear the C-spine:**
a. Patient must be awake, alert, and without a distracting injury or intoxication.
b. Palpate posterior neck for localized tenderness. If there is pain, maintain C-spine collar for immobilization until further evaluation can definitively rule out injury. If there is no pain, assess active and passive range of motion.

C. Blunt Thoracic and Abdominal Trauma[7]

1. **Anatomic considerations in children:** Pliable rib cage, solid organs proportionally larger than those of adults, underdeveloped abdominal musculature

2. **Common injuries:**
a. Thoracic: Pneumothorax, hemothorax, pulmonary contusion, fractures, damage to major blood vessels, heart, or diaphragm
b. Abdominal: Damage to spleen, liver, kidneys, pancreas, genitourinary (GU) system, or major blood vessels; hematomas within the gastrointestinal (GI) tract

3. **Evaluation:**
a. Careful history and physical examination
b. Laboratory studies:
   (1) Type and cross-match
   (2) Thoracic injury: Complete blood cell count (CBC), pulse oximetry; consider arterial blood gas (ABG)
   (3) Abdominal injury: CBC (follow serial hemoglobin values), electrolytes, liver function tests, amylase, lipase, urinalysis
c. Radiologic evaluation:
   (1) Chest radiograph, with or without chest CT with intravenous (IV) contrast, if patient is stable.
   (2) Abdominal CT with IV contrast if there is a concern based on history or physical examination (routine oral contrast *not* indicated; high false-negative rate for hollow viscus injury).

(3) Consider focused abdominal ultrasound when coexisting injuries (e.g., neurologic or significant orthopedic) prevent CT scan.

4. **Emergent treatment:**

a. If significant trauma is suspected or diagnosed, consult a pediatric surgeon.

b. Tension pneumothorax:
   (1) Signs: Marked respiratory distress, distended neck veins, contralateral tracheal deviation, diminished breath sounds, compromised systemic perfusion, trauma arrest
   (2) Treatment: Needle decompression, then chest tube placement directed toward lung apex (see Chapter 3)

c. Open pneumothorax (also known as "sucking chest wound"): Allows free flow of air between atmosphere and hemithorax. Cover defect with occlusive dressing (i.e., petroleum jelly gauze), give positive-pressure ventilation, and insert chest tube (see Chapter 3).

d. Hemothorax: Provide fluid resuscitation, followed by placement of a chest tube directed posteriorly and inferiorly.

e. Abdominal trauma: Penetrating trauma requires surgical evaluation and exploration. Nonoperative management may be possible in blunt trauma, even in the presence of intraabdominal bleeding. Bleeding from injured spleen, kidneys, or liver is often self-limited. The decision to pursue operative vs. nonoperative management should be made by a surgeon.

D. Orthopedic/Long Bone Trauma[8,9]

1. **Fractures:** Some fracture patterns are unique to children (Fig. 4-1). Growthplate injuries are classified by the Salter-Harris classification (Table 4-2). Because ligaments are stronger than bones or growth plates in children, dislocations and sprains are relatively uncommon, whereas growth-plate disruption and bone avulsion are more common. For basic splinting techniques, see Chapter 3.

2. **Compartment syndrome[1,9]:** Elevated muscle compartment pressure (due to space limitation by surrounding fascia) impairs blood flow, resulting in nerve and muscle damage.

a. Common causes include crush injury, fractures (most common: tibia), burns, infections (necrotizing fasciitis), or hemorrhage.

b. Marked by **6 Ps**: **P**ain (earliest symptom), **P**aresthesias, **P**allor, **P**oikilothermia, **P**aralysis, **P**ulselessness.
   (1) Unremitting pain, even after appropriate analgesia, is the most sensitive sign.
   (2) Pain with passive muscle stretch is a strong indicator.

c. Intercompartmental pressure measurement: Normal = 10 mmHg; symptoms occur with pressures 20 to 30 mmHg.

d. Management: Emergency fasciotomy within 6 hours of onset; absolutely indicated if pressure >30 mmHg.

e. Complications: Rhabdomyolysis. Follow urinalysis, creatine kinase (CK), electrolytes (risk for hyperkalemia). Consider saline resuscitation, urine alkalinization (with goal urine pH >6.5), or mannitol (0.25–0.5 g/kg).

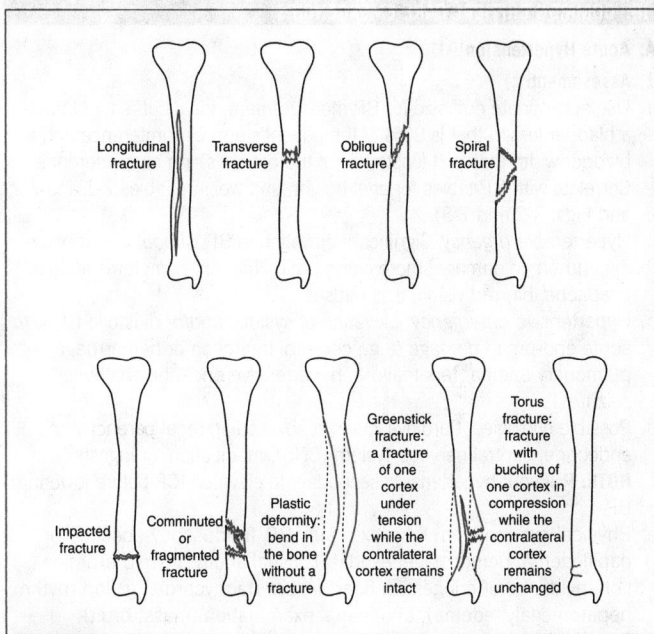

FIGURE 4-1

Fracture patterns unique to children. *(Modified from Ogden JA. Skeletal Injury in the Child. 3rd ed. Philadelphia: WB Saunders, 2000.)*

TABLE 4-2

SALTER-HARRIS CLASSIFICATION OF GROWTH PLATE INJURY

Class I	Class II	Class III	Class IV	Class V
Fracture along growth plate	Fracture along growth plate with metaphyseal extension	Fracture along growth plate with epiphyseal extension	Fracture across growth plate, including metaphysis and epiphysis	Crush injury to growth plate without obvious fracture
I	II	III	IV	V

III. COMMON CRITICAL CARE EMERGENCIES

A. Acute Hypertension[10,11]

1. **Assessment:**
   a. Use appropriate cuff size for BP measurement. Ideal cuff should have a bladder length that is 80% of the patient's arm circumference and a bladder width that is at least 40% of the patient's arm circumference. Correlate with BP tables for age, height, and weight (Tables 7-1 and 7-2 and Figs. 7-2 and 7-3).
   b. Hypertensive *urgency:* Significant elevation in BP *without* accompanying end-organ damage; more common in children. Symptoms include headache, blurred vision, and nausea.
   c. Hypertensive *emergency:* Elevation of systolic and/or diastolic BP *with* acute end-organ damage (e.g., cerebral infarction or hemorrhage, pulmonary edema, renal failure, hypertensive encephalopathy, or seizures).
   d. Possible etiologies: Cardiovascular, renovascular, renal parenchymal, endocrine, central nervous system (CNS), medication, or ingestion.
   NOTE: Rule out hypertension secondary to elevated ICP before lowering BP.
   e. Physical examination: Four-extremity BP, funduscopy (looking for papilledema, hemorrhage, exudate), visual acuity, thyroid examination, evidence of congestive heart failure (tachycardia, gallop rhythm, hepatomegaly, edema), abdominal examination (mass, bruit), thorough neurologic examination, evidence of virilization, cushingoid effect.
   f. Diagnostic evaluation:
      (1) Initial: Urinalysis, blood urea nitrogen, creatinine, electrolytes, chest radiograph, electrocardiogram (ECG).
      (2) Subsequent: Consider renin level, toxicology screen, thyroid and adrenal testing, urine catecholamines, abdominal ultrasound, renal Doppler ultrasound, head CT.

2. **Management:** After elevated ICP is ruled out, do not delay treatment pending further diagnostic workup.
   a. Hypertensive emergency:
      (1) Goal: Lower BP promptly but gradually to preserve cerebral auto-regulation (Table 4-3).
         (a) Mean arterial pressure (MAP) = 1/3 systolic + 2/3 diastolic BP
         (b) Lower by 1/3 of planned MAP reduction over first 6 hours, *then*
         (c) Lower by additional 1/3 over next 24 to 36 hours, *then*
         (d) Lower final 1/3 over next 48 hours
      (2) Consult nephrologist and/or cardiologist.
   b. Hypertensive urgency:
      (1) Goal: To lower MAP by 20% over 1 hour and return to baseline levels over 24 to 48 hours (Table 4-4).
      (2) Oral route may be adequate. Use of sublingual nifedipine is *not* recommended; a precipitous uncontrolled fall in BP may result.

TABLE 4-3

MEDICATIONS FOR HYPERTENSIVE EMERGENCY*

Drug	Onset (Route)	Duration	Interval to Repeat	Comments
Diazoxide (arteriole vasodilator)	1–5 min (IV)	Variable (2–12 hr)	15–30 min	May cause edema, hyperglycemia
Hydralazine (arteriole vasodilator)	5–20 min (IV)	2–6 hr	4–6 hr	May cause reflex tachycardia, prolonged hypotension, nausea
INFUSIONS				
Nitroprusside (arteriole and venous vasodilator)	<30 sec (IV)	Very short	30–60 min	Requires ICU setting; follow thiocyanate level
Labetalol (α-, β-blocker)	1–5 min (IV)	Variable (≈6 hr)	10 min	May require ICU setting
Nicardipine (calcium channel blocker)	1 min (IV)	3 hr	15 min	May cause edema, headache, nausea, vomiting

*See Formulary for dosing.
ICU, Intensive care unit; IV, intravenous.

TABLE 4-4

MEDICATIONS FOR HYPERTENSIVE URGENCY*

Drug	Onset (Route)	Duration	Interval to Repeat	Comments
Enalapril	15 min (IV)	12–24 hr	8–24 hr	May cause hyperkalemia, hypoglycemia
Minoxidil	30 min (PO)	2–5 days	4–8 hr	Contraindicated in pheochromocytoma

*See Formulary for dosing.
IV, Intravenous; PO, per os (oral).

B. Increased Intracranial Pressure[12,13,14]

See Chapter 20 for evaluation and management of hydrocephalus.

1. **Assessment:**
a. Obtain history regarding trauma, prior shunt or other neurologic surgical or medical condition, vomiting, fever, headache, neck pain, unsteadiness, seizure, vision change, gaze preference, and change in mental status. In infants, look for irritability, vomiting, poor feeding, lethargy, and bulging fontanelle.
b. Physical examination:
   (1) Evaluate vital signs for Cushing triad (hypertension, bradycardia, irregular respiratory pattern) as a sign of increasing intracranial pressure.
   (2) Thorough neurologic examination: Attention to photophobia, pupillary response, papilledema, cranial nerve dysfunction (especially

paralysis of upward gaze or abduction), neck stiffness, neurologic deficit, abnormal posturing, altered mental status, or evidence of trauma.

c. Laboratory studies: CBC, electrolytes, glucose, toxicology screen, blood culture. Lumbar puncture (LP) is contraindicated due to herniation risk if cause is obstructive.

2. **Management:** Elevate head of bed 30 degrees. Patient should be midline with neck straight to maximize venous drainage from the head. Keep life-saving stabilizing devices in place, but be certain cervical collars and medical devices do not obstruct jugular venous drainage. Obtain emergent neurosurgical consult and head CT. Do not lower BP if elevated ICP is suspected. Immobilize C-spine if trauma is suspected.

a. Stable patient (responsive, stable vital signs, no focal findings): Apply cardiorespiratory monitor.

b. Unstable patient:
   (1) Give normal saline or hyperosmolar solutions for maintenance fluids.
   (2) For temporary reduction of ICP give 3% NaCl bolus (range, 2 to 5 mL/kg). Maintain serum osmolarity goal of <360 mOsm/L.
      (a) Alternatively, can use mannitol 0.25 g/kg with max single dose of 12.5 g. Can increase dose to 1 g/kg, although high dose mannitol can produce significant hypotension due to osmotic diuresis, so consider giving fluid bolus at same time. If using mannitol, remember to place a Foley catheter.
   (3) Reserve hyperventilation for acute management; keep partial pressure of carbon dioxide ($Paco_2$) at 30 to 35 mmHg. Provide controlled neuroprotective intubation as outlined in Table 1-1, and consider advanced neuromonitoring for evaluation of cerebral ischemia.
   (4) In traumatic brain injury (TBI), consider controlled moderate hypothermia (32° to 33°C).

c. Do not delay antibiotics if meningitis suspected.

d. In space-occupying lesions (tumors, abscesses), consider dexamethasone to reduce cerebral edema (in consultation with a neurosurgeon). Otherwise, corticosteroids are not recommended for children with TBI.

e. Consider epinephrine or phenylephrine infusion to maintain systemic pressure above ICP.

$$\text{Cerebral perfusion pressure (CPP)} = \text{MAP} - \text{ICP}$$

Goal minimum CPP is 40 mmHg in children with TBI.

f. Prevent hyperthermia: Goal is body temperature <37.5°C.

g. Consider consult for prophylactic seizure control to reduce incidence of early posttraumatic seizures in children with TBI.

h. Avoid hypotension, hypoxia, hypercarbia, and hypovolemia.

C. Shock[15,16]

1. **Definition:** Physiologic state characterized by inadequate oxygen and nutrient delivery to meet tissue demands. See Table 4-5 for categorization.

a. Compensated shock: Body maintains perfusion to vital organs. This clinical state may be hard to detect because BP changes are a late finding in young children. Tachycardia may be present and is often the most sensitive vital sign change.

b. Decompensated shock: Poor perfusion, tachycardia, hypotension.

2. **Causes (see Table EC 4-A):**

a. Hypovolemic shock.

b. Distributive shock (including septic, anaphylactic, and neurogenic shock).

c. Cardiogenic shock.

d. Obstructive shock (including cardiac tamponade, tension pneumothorax, massive pulmonary embolism).

3. **Management (Fig. 4-2):** Always treat underlying cause.

D. Respiratory Failure[15]

1. **Definition:** Failure of the lungs to exchange oxygen and/or carbon dioxide

2. **Causes:**

a. Neurologic: Muscle weakness, altered sensorium, CNS impairment

b. Obstruction: Foreign body, inflammation

c. Parenchymal disease: Pneumonia, pulmonary edema, acute respiratory distress syndrome (ARDS), asthma

d. Mechanical: Abnormal chest wall, trauma

3. **Management:**

a. Noninvasive positive-pressure ventilation

b. Intubation and mechanical ventilation (see Chapter 1 for discussion of intubation)

4. **Types of ventilatory support:**

a. Volume limited:
   (1) Delivers a preset tidal volume to a patient, regardless of pressure required
   (2) Risk for barotrauma reduced by pressure alarms and pressure pop-off valves that limit peak inspiratory pressure (PIP)

b. Pressure limited:
   (1) Gas flow is delivered to the patient until a preset pressure is reached and then held for the set inspiratory time (reduces the risk for barotrauma).
   (2) Useful for neonatal and infant ventilatory support (<10 kg), where the volume of gas being delivered is small in relation to the volume of compressible air in the ventilator circuit, which makes reliable delivery of a set tidal volume difficult.

c. High-frequency ventilation
   See additional content on Expert Consult.[17]

5. **Ventilator parameters:**

a. PIP: Peak pressure attained during the respiratory cycle

b. Positive end-expiratory pressure (PEEP): Airway pressure maintained between inspiratory and expiratory phases; prevents alveolar collapse during expiration, decreases work of reinflation, and improves gas exchange

TABLE 4-5

CATEGORIZATION OF HEMORRHAGE AND SHOCK IN PEDIATRIC TRAUMA PATIENTS[22,23]

System	Class I: Compensated Shock, Very Mild Hemorrhage (<15% Blood Volume Loss)	Class II: Compensated Shock, Mild Hemorrhage (15%–30% Blood Volume Loss)	Class III: Decompensated Shock, Moderate Hemorrhage (30%–40% Blood Volume Loss)	Class IV: Cardiopulmonary Failure, Severe Hemorrhage (>40% Blood Volume Loss)
Cardiovascular	Normal heart rate	Mild tachycardia	Moderate tachycardia	Severe tachycardia
	Normal peripheral pulses	Normal or weak peripheral pulses	Weak or absent peripheral pulses	Absent peripheral pulses
	Strong central pulses	Strong central pulses	Weak central pulses	Weak or absent central pulses
	Normotension to slight hypertension	Normotension to slight hypotension	Frank hypotension	Profound hypotension
	No acidosis	Mild acidosis	Moderate acidosis	Severe acidosis
Respiratory	Normal respiratory rate	Mild tachypnea	Moderate tachypnea	Severe tachypnea, bradypnea, or apnea
Neurologic	Slight anxiety	Mild anxiety, confusion, combative	Severe anxiety, confusion, lethargy	Severe confusion, obtundation, lethargy, comatose
Integumentary	Warm extremities, pink	Cool extremities, mottling	Cool extremities, mottling, or pallor	Cold extremities, pallor, or cyanosis
	Normal capillary refill (<2 sec)	Poor capillary refill (>2 sec)	Delayed capillary refill (>3 sec)	Prolonged capillary refill (>5 sec)
Excretory	Normal urine output	Mild oliguria, increased specific gravity	Marked oliguria, increased blood urea nitrogen	Severe oliguria or anuria

Modified from Fleisher GR, Ludwig S, ed. *Textbook of Pediatric Emergency Medicine*. 5th ed. Philadelphia: Lippincott Williams & Wilkins; 2006.

Initial management:

- Early recognition based on vital sign and physical examination changes is key
- Establish access via large-bore IV or IO
- Start high-flow oxygen via facemask or nasal cannula, even in the absence of respiratory distress

First 5–15 minutes:

- Rapidly push 20 mL/kg isotonic saline or colloid
  - Each 20 mL/kg should be given in 5 minutes or less
  - Many patients require total of 60 mL/kg, some may require up to 200 mL/kg within the first hour of shock
  - Continue until perfusion improves or signs of fluid overload such as pulmonary crackles or hepatomegaly develop
- Correct hypoglycemia and hypocalcemia
- Start broad-spectrum IV antibiotics

At 15 minutes without reversal of shock:

- Start inotrope via second IV/IO access site
  - Cold shock—dopamine 2 to 20 mcg/kg/min or epinephrine 0.05 to 1 mcg/kg/min
  - Warm shock—norepinephrine 0.05 to 2 mcg/kg/min
- Consider securing airway with early intubation and mechanical ventilation

At 60 minutes without reversal of shock:

- Give hydrocortisone 2 mg/kg (max 100 mg) in patients at risk for adrenal insufficiency or patients who are unresponsive to pressors
- Consider transfer to pediatric intensive care unit

Note:

It is very important to prepare for each step in advance to be able to complete the recommended interventions within the first hour of recognized shock.

FIGURE 4-2

Emergency management of pediatric shock—first hour. *(From Brierley J, Carcillo JA, Choong K, et al. Clinical practice parameters for hemodynamic support of pediatric and neonatal septic shock: 2007 update from The American College of Critical Care Medicine. Crit Care Med. 2009;37:666-688.)*

c. Rate (intermittent mandatory ventilation) or frequency (Hz): Number of mechanical breaths delivered per minute, or rate of oscillations in HFOV

d. Inspired oxygen concentration (Fio_2): Fraction of oxygen present in inspired gas

e. Inspiratory time (Ti): Length of time spent in the inspiratory phase of the respiratory cycle

f. Tidal volume (V_T): Volume of gas delivered during inspiration

g. Power (ΔP): Amplitude of the pressure waveform in HFOV

h. Mean airway pressure ($\overline{PAW}$): Average pressure over entire respiratory cycle

6. **Modes of operation:**

a. Intermittent mandatory ventilation (IMV): A preset number of breaths are delivered each minute. Patient can take breaths on his or her own, but the ventilator may cycle on during a patient breath.

b. Synchronized IMV (SIMV): Similar to IMV, but the ventilator synchronizes delivered breaths with inspiratory effort and allows the patient to finish expiration before cycling on. More comfortable for patient than IMV.

c. Assist control ventilation (AC): Every inspiratory effort by the patient triggers a ventilator-delivered breath at the set V_T. Ventilator-initiated breaths are delivered when the spontaneous rate falls below the backup rate.

d. Pressure support ventilation (PSV): Inspiratory effort opens a valve, allowing airflow at a preset positive pressure. Patient determines rate and inspiratory time. May be used in combination with other modes of operation. Determine effectiveness of ventilation by monitoring tidal volumes.

e. Noninvasive positive-pressure ventilation (NIPPV): Respiratory support provided through face mask.

    (1) Continuous positive airway pressure (CPAP): Delivers airflow (with set Fio_2) to maintain a set airway pressure

    (2) Bilevel positive airway pressure (BiPAP): Delivers airflow to maintain set pressures for inspiration and expiration

7. **Initial ventilator settings:**

a. Volume limited:

    (1) Rate: Approximately normal range for age (see Table 24-1).

    (2) V_T: Approximately 8 to 10 mL/kg.

    (3) Ti: Generally use inspiration-to-expiration (I/E) ratio of 1:2. More prolonged expiratory phases are required for obstructive diseases to avoid air trapping.

    (4) Fio_2: Selected to maintain targeted oxygen saturation and partial pressure of arterial oxygen (Pao_2).

b. Pressure limited:

    (1) Rate: Approximately normal range for age (see Table 24-1).

    (2) PEEP: Start with 3 to 5 cm H_2O and increase as clinically indicated. Monitor for decreases in cardiac output with increasing PEEP.

    (3) PIP: Set at pressure required to produce adequate chest wall movement (approximate this using hand-ventilating and manometry).

    (4) Fio_2: Selected to maintain targeted oxygen saturation and Pao_2.

c. HFOV

See additional content on Expert Consult.

8. **Further ventilator management:**

a. Follow patient closely with pulse oximetry, end-tidal carbon dioxide measurements, and clinical assessment. Confirm findings with ABGs, and adjust ventilator parameters as indicated (Table 4-6).

b. In cases of ARDS or other condition of poor compliance or air leaks, permissive hypercapnia and V_T of 5 mL/kg should be used to avoid barotrauma.

c. Parameters for initiating high-frequency ventilation:

   (1) Oxygenation index (OI) >40 (see Section III.G for calculation of OI)

   (2) Inability to provide adequate oxygenation or ventilation with conventional ventilator

d. Parameters predictive of successful extubation:

   (1) $Paco_2$ appropriate for patient

   (2) PIP generally 14 to 16 cm H_2O

   (3) PEEP 2 to 3 cm H_2O (infants) or 5 cm H_2O (children)

   (4) IMV 2 to 4 breaths/min (infants); children may be weaned to CPAP or pressure support

   (5) Fio_2 <40% (maintaining Pao_2 >70)

   (6) Adequate air leak around endotracheal tube in cases of airway edema or stenosis

   (7) Maximum negative inspiratory pressure (NIF) >20 to 25 cm H_2O

   (8) Minimal secretions

E. Status Epilepticus (See Chapter 1)

F. Status Asthmaticus (See Chapter 1)

G. Critical Care Reference Data

1. **Minute ventilation (V_E):**

$$V_E = \text{Respiratory rate} \times \text{Tidal volume } (V_T)$$

a. $V_E \times Paco_2 = \text{constant}$ (for volume-limited ventilation)

b. Normal $V_T = 8$ to 10 mL/kg

TABLE 4-6

EFFECTS OF VENTILATOR SETTING CHANGES

Ventilator Setting Changes	Typical Effects on Blood Gases	
	$Paco_2$	Pao_2
↑ PIP	↓	↑
↑ PEEP	↑	↑
↑ Rate (IMV)	↓	Minimal ↑
↑ I:E ratio	No change	↑
↑ Fio_2	No change	↑
↑ Flow	Minimal ↓	Minimal ↑
↑ Power (in HFOV)	↓	No change
↑ PAW (in HFOV)	Minimal ↓	↑

Fio_2, Fraction of inspired oxygen; HFOV, high-frequency oscillatory ventilation; I:E, inspiratory/expiratory ratio; IMV, intermittent mechanical ventilation; Pao_2, partial pressure of arterial oxygen; $Paco_2$, partial pressure of carbon dioxide; PAW, mean airway pressure; PEEP, positive end-expiratory pressure; PIP, peak inspiratory pressure.

2. **Alveolar gas equation:**

$$P_{AO_2} = P_{IO_2} - (Pa_{CO_2}/R)$$

$$P_{IO_2} = F_{IO_2} \times (P_B - 47\,mmHg)$$

a. P_{IO_2} = partial pressure of inspired O_2 minus 150 mmHg at sea level on room air.
b. R = respiratory exchange quotient (CO_2 produced/O_2 consumed) = 0.8.
c. Pa_{CO_2} = partial pressure of alveolar CO_2 minus partial pressure of arterial CO_2 (Pa_{CO_2}).
d. P_B = atmospheric pressure = 760 mmHg at sea level. Adjust for high-altitude environment.
e. Water vapor pressure = 47 mmHg.
f. P_{AO_2} = partial pressure of O_2 in the alveoli.
3. **Alveolar-arterial oxygen gradient (A-a gradient):**

$$A - a\ gradient = P_{AO_2} - Pa_{O_2}$$

a. Obtain ABG, measuring Pa_{O_2} and Pa_{CO_2} with patient on 100% F_{IO_2} for at least 15 minutes.
b. Calculate the P_{AO_2} and then the A-a gradient.
c. The larger the gradient, the more serious the respiratory compromise. A normal gradient is 20 to 65 mmHg on 100% O_2 or 5 to 20 mmHg on room air.
4. **Oxygenation Index (OI):**

$$OI = \frac{Mean\ airway\ pressure\,(cm\ H_2O)\ \times FiO_2 \times 100}{Pa_{O_2}}$$

OI >35 for 5 to 6 hours is one criterion for ECMO (extracorporeal membrane oxygen) support.
See more critical care reference data on Expert Consult.

IV. ANIMAL BITES[3,18]

A. Wound Considerations

1. **High infection risk:** Puncture wounds, crush injury, bites over hand, foot, genitalia, or joint surface, bites from a cat or human, wounds in asplenic or immunocompromised patients, wounds with care delayed >12 hours
2. **Special considerations:**
a. Deep bites: Possibility of foreign body or fracture—consider radiographs (especially hand or scalp)
b. Periorbital bites: Possibility of corneal abrasion, lacrimal duct involvement, or other ocular damage—consider ophthalmologic evaluation
c. Hand: Site most prone to infection—follow for development of osteomyelitis
d. Nose: Evaluate for cartilage injury

3. **Animal species (Table 4-7)**

B. Management

1. **Wound hygiene:**

a. Irrigate with copious amounts (at least 100 mL/cm of laceration) of sterile saline using high-pressure syringe irrigation. Do not irrigate puncture wounds. Do not soak the wound. Do not use alcohol or peroxide to clean.

b. Debride devitalized tissue and evaluate for foreign bodies.

c. Consider surgical debridement/exploration for extensive wounds, wounds involving metacarpophalangeal joint, and cranial bites by a large animal.

d. Culture only if evidence of infection is present.

2. **Closure:**

a. Avoid closing wounds of high infection risk (see Section IV.A). Exception: Cat bites on the face or scalp may be closed.

b. Wounds that involve tendons, joints, deep fascia, or major vasculature should be evaluated by a plastic or hand surgeon and, if indicated, closed in the operating room.

c. Suturing: When indicated, closure should be done with minimal simple interrupted nylon sutures that are as superficial as possible. Loosely approximate wound edges. Use prophylactic antibiotics.

(1) Head and neck: Can usually be safely sutured (with exceptions noted) after copious irrigation and wound debridement if within 6 to 8 hours of injury and no signs of infection. Facial wounds often require primary closure for cosmetic reasons; good vascular supply lowers infection risk.

TABLE 4-7

ANIMAL BITES

Animal	Common Organism(s)	Special Considerations
Dog	*Staphylococcus aureus* *Pasteurella multocida* *Streptococcus* spp. *Capnocytophaga canimorsus* Anaerobes	Crush injury
Cat	*Pasteurella multocida* *Staphylococcus aureus* *Moraxella catarrhalis* *Bartonella henselae*	Deep puncture wound Often associated with fulminant infection, abscess, and/or osteomyelitis Slow to respond to treatment
Human	*Streptococcus viridans* *Staphylococcus aureus* Anaerobes *Eikenella corrodens* Hepatitis B and C HIV (rare, associated with blood in biter's saliva)	Consider child abuse, especially if intercanine distance >3 cm High infection and complication rate
Rodent	*Streptobacillus moniliformis* *Spirillum minus*	Low incidence of secondary infection Rat-bite fever—occurs rarely

(2) Hands: In large wounds, subcutaneous dead space should be closed with minimal absorbable sutures, with delayed cutaneous closure in 3 to 5 days if there is no evidence of infection.

3. **Antibiotics:** Prophylactic antibiotics are indicated in cases of high infection risk, as listed in Section IV.A. See Chapter 17 for appropriate antibiotic therapies and treatment course.

4. **Rabies and tetanus prophylaxis:** Always give postexposure prophylaxis when animal is a skunk, raccoon, bat, fox, woodchuck, or other carnivore. For other cases, see Chapter 16.

5. **Imaging:** Obtain if bite is extensive, on the hand or closed fist, and after a "mauling" injury. Imaging can reveal fracture, air in joint space, or a foreign body in the wound.

6. **Disposition:**

a. Outpatient care: Obtain careful follow-up of all bite wounds within 24 to 48 hours, especially those requiring surgical closure. Extremity wounds, especially of the hands, should be immobilized in position of function and kept elevated. Wounds should be kept clean and dry.

b. Inpatient care: Consider hospitalization for observation and parenteral antibiotics for significant human bites, immunocompromised or asplenic hosts, deep or severe infections, bites associated with systemic complaints, bites with significant functional or cosmetic morbidity, and/or unreliable follow-up or care by parent/guardian.

7. **Infected wound:** Subtle pain and tenderness may be the first sign of infection. Wounds that subsequently become infected may require drainage and debridement, possibly under anesthesia. Adjust antibiotic therapy according to Gram stain and culture results.

V. BURNS[1,3,19]

A. Evaluation of Pediatric Burns (Tables 4-8 and 4-9)

NOTE: Depending on the extent and type of burn, severity may progress over the first few days after injury; complete daily assessment necessary until burn has declared itself.

B. Burn Mapping

Calculate total body surface area (TBSA) burned (Fig. 4-3): Based only on percentage of superficial and deep partial-thickness burns plus full-thickness burns.

C. Emergent Management of Pediatric Burns

1. **Acute stabilization:**

a. Circulation:

(1) Start Parkland formula (Fig. 4-4) IV fluid resuscitation with normal saline for burns >15% BSA, or with any evidence of smoke inhalation.

b. Airway with C-spine stabilization

(1) Assess airway for signs of inhalation injury or respiratory distress: Soot in nares, carbonaceous sputum, stridor.

TABLE 4-8

THERMAL INJURY

Type of Burn	Description/Comment
Flame	Most common type of burn worldwide; when clothing burns, the heat exposure is prolonged, and the severity increased.
Scald/contact	Mortality for full-thickness scald burns is similar to that in flame burns when total body surface area involved is equivalent; see Fig. 4-3.
Chemical	Tissue is damaged by protein coagulation or liquefaction rather than hyperthermic activity.
Electrical	Injury is often extensive, involving skeletal muscle and other tissues in addition to the skin damage. Extent of damage may not be initially apparent. The tissues with the least resistance are most heat sensitive; bone offers the most resistance, nerve tissue the least. Cardiac arrest due to passage of current through the heart can occur.
Inhalation	Present in 30% of victims of major flame burns and increases mortality. Consider when there is evidence of fire in enclosed space. Signs include singed nares, facial burns, charred lips, carbonaceous secretions, posterior pharynx edema, hoarseness, cough, or wheezing.
Cold injury/frostbite	Freezing results in direct tissue injury. Toes, fingers, ears, and nose are commonly involved. Initial treatment includes rewarming in tepid (105°–110°F) water for 20–40 minutes. Excision of tissue should not be done until complete demarcation of nonviable tissue has occurred.

TABLE 4-9

BURN CLASSIFICATION

Superficial	Injury to epidermis only
	Characterized by erythema, pain, includes sunburn or minor scalds
	Patients with only superficial burns do not usually require intravenous fluid replacement
	Not included in estimate of surface area burned
	Generally heals on its own without scarring in 3–5 days
Superficial partial thickness	Damages but does not destroy epidermis and dermis
	Characterized by intense pain, blisters, pink to cherry-red skin, moist and weepy
	Nails, hair, sebaceous glands, and nerves intact
	Can progress to deep partial- or full-thickness burn
	Spontaneous reepithelialization in 2–3 weeks
Deep partial thickness	Injury to epidermis and dermis
	Characterized by intense pain, dry and white in color
	Can result in disruption of nails, hair, sebaceous glands
	May cause scarring; skin grafting usually required
Full thickness	Injury involves all layers of skin, characterized by charred black color, ± areas dry or white
	Pain may be intense or absent, depending on nerve ending involvement
	Causes scarring; skin grafting required

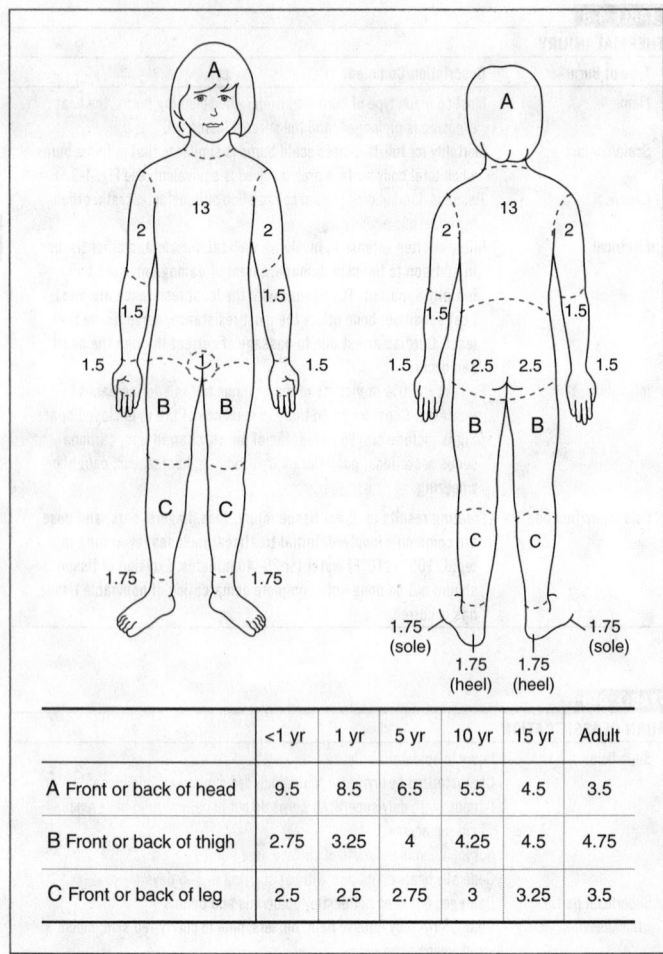

	<1 yr	1 yr	5 yr	10 yr	15 yr	Adult
A Front or back of head	9.5	8.5	6.5	5.5	4.5	3.5
B Front or back of thigh	2.75	3.25	4	4.25	4.5	4.75
C Front or back of leg	2.5	2.5	2.75	3	3.25	3.5

FIGURE 4-3

Burn assessment chart. All numbers are percentages. *(From Barkin RM, Rosen P. Emergency Pediatrics: A Guide to Ambulatory Care. 6th ed. St Louis: Mosby, 2003.)*

    (2) Establish definitive airway early: Consider intubation for >30% TBSA burned.

    NOTE: Avoid use of succinylcholine more than 24 hours from time of injury.

c. Breathing:

    (1) Inhalation injury: Assume carbon monoxide poisoning with severe and/or closed-space burns.

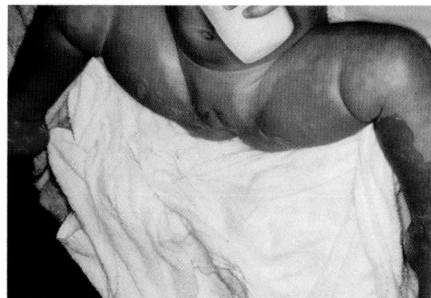

FIGURE 4-5

Infant whose lower extremities and buttocks have been burned when immersed in hot water. *(From Zitelli B, Davis H. Atlas of Pediatric Physical Diagnosis. 5th ed. St Louis: Mosby, 2008.)*

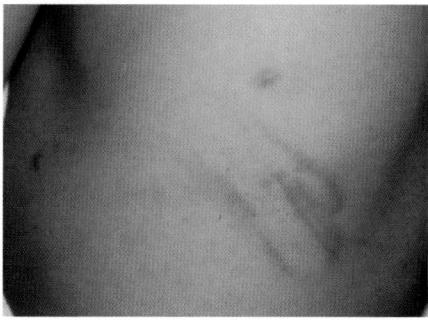

FIGURE 4-6

Child who has been beaten with a looped cord. *(From Zitelli B, Davis H. Atlas of Pediatric Physical Diagnosis. 5th ed. St Louis: Mosby, 2008.)*

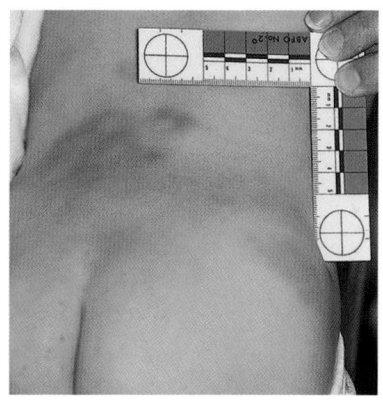

FIGURE 4-7

Child with suspicious bruising on lower back. *(From Zitelli B, Davis H. Atlas of Pediatric Physical Diagnosis. 5th ed. St Louis: Mosby, 2008.)*

Toddler slapped in the face, with linear hand marks visible. *(From Zitelli B, Davis H. Atlas of Pediatric Physical Diagnosis. 5th ed. St Louis: Mosby; 2008.)*

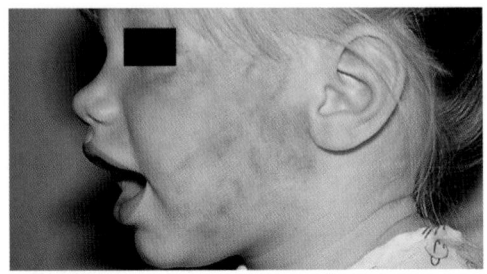

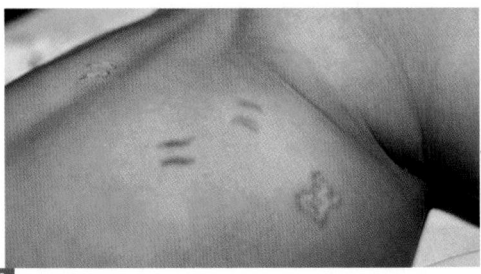

Skin burned with hot cigarette lighter. *(From Zitelli B, Davis H. Atlas of Pediatric Physical Diagnosis. 5th ed. St Louis: Mosby, 2008.)*

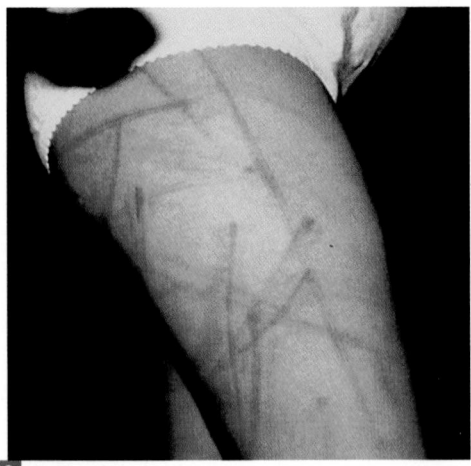

Child beaten with a switch. *(From Zitelli B, Davis H. Atlas of Pediatric Physical Diagnosis. 5th ed. St Louis: Mosby, 2008.)*

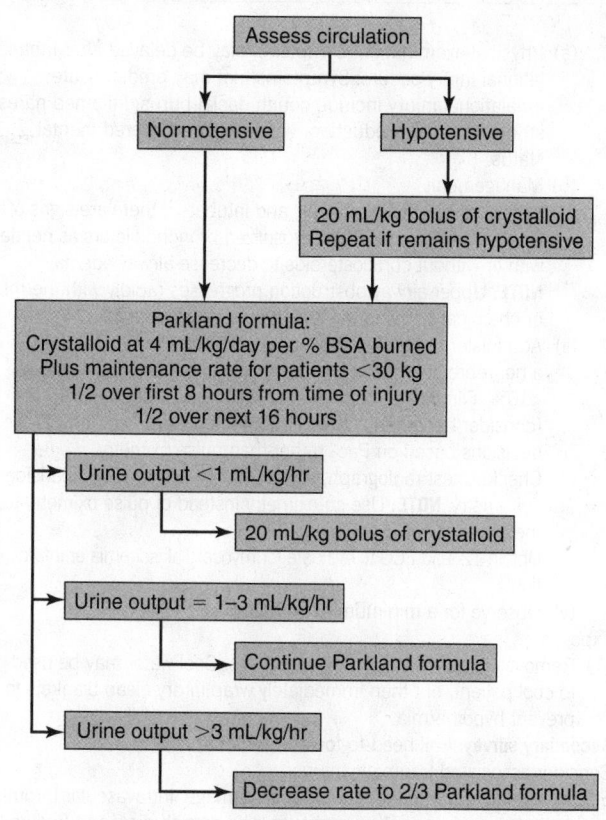

Assess circulation

Normotensive | Hypotensive

Hypotensive → 20 mL/kg bolus of crystalloid
Repeat if remains hypotensive

Parkland formula:
Crystalloid at 4 mL/kg/day per % BSA burned
Plus maintenance rate for patients <30 kg
1/2 over first 8 hours from time of injury
1/2 over next 16 hours

Urine output <1 mL/kg/hr → 20 mL/kg bolus of crystalloid

Urine output = 1–3 mL/kg/hr → Continue Parkland formula

Urine output >3 mL/kg/hr → Decrease rate to 2/3 Parkland formula

1) Consider central venous access for burns >25% BSA.

2) Use the Parkland formula as a guideline to estimate fluid need. Requirements decrease by 25% to 50% after first 24 hours. Monitor weight, serum electrolytes, urine output, nasogastric losses to determine concentrations and rates.

3) Consider adding colloid after 18 to 24 hours (albumin, 1 g/kg/day) to maintain serum albumin >2 g/dL.

4) Withhold potassium generally for the first 48 hours because of a large release of potassium from damaged tissues. To manage electrolytes most effectively, monitor urine electrolytes twice weekly and replace urine losses accordingly.

FIGURE 4-4

Fluid management of life-threatening burns. (Modified from Nichols DG, Yaster M, Lappe DG, et al. Golden Hour: The Handbook of Pediatric Advanced Life Support. St Louis: Mosby, 1996:460.)

(a) Physical examination: Symptoms may be delayed after inhalational injury occurs. Symptoms that may predict acute inhalational injury include cough, facial burns, inflamed nares, stridor, sputum production, wheezing, and altered mental status.

(b) Management:

(i) Assess stability of the airway, and intubate if there are signs of airway compromise. Give aerosolized bronchodilators as needed with or without corticosteroids to decrease airway edema. **NOTE:** Upper airway obstruction progresses rapidly with thermal or chemical burns to the face, nares, or oropharynx.

(ii) Administer humidified 100% supplemental oxygen through a nonrebreather mask until carboxyhemoglobin (COHb) level <10%. Elimination half-life of COHb is dependent on Pao_2 (consider hyperbaric O_2 if pH <7.4 and COHb elevated). Make decisions based on Pao_2 rather than pulse oximetry.

(iii) Check: Chest radiograph, ABGs with co-oximetry, and bedside spirometry. **NOTE:** Use co-oximetry instead of pulse oximetry to measure oxyhemoglobin.

(iv) Obtain 12-lead ECG to evaluate for myocardial ischemia or infarction.

(v) Observe for a minimum of 24 hours.

d. Exposure:

(1) Remove clothes to stop burning process. Cool water may be used to cool patient, but then immediately wrap in dry clean blankets to prevent hypothermia.

2. **Secondary survey:** Full head-to-toe assessment.

a. Consider associated traumatic injuries.

b. Electrical injury can produce deep tissue damage, intravascular thrombosis, cardiac and respiratory arrest, cardiac arrhythmias, and fractures secondary to muscle contraction. Look for exit site in electrical injury.

3. **Assess for signs of compartment syndrome,** especially after fluid resuscitation has begun.

4. **GI burns:** Place gastric tube for decompression; begin prophylaxis for Curling stress ulcers with histamine-2 receptor blockers, proton-pump inhibitor, and/or antacids.

5. **Eye:** Ophthalmologic evaluation as necessary. Use topical ophthalmic antibiotics if abrasions are present.

6. **GU:** Consider Foley catheter to monitor urine output during fluid resuscitation phase.

7. **Pain management:** IV narcotic therapy often necessary for pain control.

8. **Special considerations:**

a. Tetanus immunoprophylaxis for patients with < three prior tetanus toxoid doses (including DTaP, DT, Td, or Tdap; patients with unknown tetanus prophylaxis history; or patients with ≥ three prior tetanus toxoid doses, but last dose >5 years prior [see Chapter 16]).

b. Chemical burns: Wash away or neutralize chemicals: brush dry chemical away and flush with copious warmed water.

D. Further Management of Pediatric Burns

1. **Inpatient management:**

a. Indications:

   (1) Any partial-thickness burn >10% TBSA

   (2) Any full-thickness burn

   (3) Circumferential burns

   (4) Electrical, chemical, or inhalation injury

   (5) Burns of critical areas, such as face, hands, feet, perineum, or joints

   (6) Patient with underlying chronic illness, suspicion of abuse, or unsafe home environment

b. Outpatient management:

   (1) Indications: If burn is <10% total TBSA and does not meet previous criteria for inpatient management

   (2) Management:

       (a) Clean with warm saline or mild soap and water. Debride open wounds and necrotic tissue.

       (b) Apply topical antibacterial agent such as bacitracin; cover with nonadherent dressing. See Box EC 4-A on Expert Consult.

       (c) Clean daily as mentioned previously, then change dressing. Premedicate with pain medication 30 minutes before each dressing change.

       (d) Oral antibiotics not indicated.

       (e) Follow-up within 1 week is recommended.

c. Burn prevention: Install smoke detectors outside every bedroom and on each floor, install carbon monoxide detectors, and keep water heater temperature set <49°C (<120°F).

VI. CHILD ABUSE

A. Introduction

A multidisciplinary approach is warranted in cases of suspected abuse and neglect. The multidisciplinary team should include medical providers, law enforcement, social service workers, and prosecutors. Although particular populations are especially vulnerable (children with special healthcare needs and infants), children from all walks of life can be abused, so an approach to evaluating injuries should be applied uniformly.

B. Management[3,20,21]

The medical professional should suspect, diagnose, treat, report, and document all cases of child abuse, neglect, or maltreatment. It is the role of the physician to report any suspected case of abuse, regardless of whether there is proof of abuse.

1. **Suspect:** Increase suspicion if there is inappropriate parental response, inadequate history of injury, a mechanism inconsistent with physical findings, evidence of neglect or failure to thrive, evidence of disturbed

emotions or expressions in a child, prior history of suspicious events, or parental substance abuse.

NOTE: A delay in seeking medical attention may increase suspicion of abuse, but this alone does not necessarily indicate abuse.

2. **Diagnose:** Concerning injuries. Attempt to correlate all physical findings with history; photodocument if possible (Figs. 4-5 to 4-10, color insert).

a. Bruises: Shape of bruises is important. Be suspicious of bruises in protected areas (chest, abdomen, back, buttocks).

   (1) Inflicted: Located in unusual places, patterned, multiple bruises or bruises in different stages of healing, bruises that do not fit the history and developmental stage.

   (2) Accidental: Usually located at bony surfaces such as shins, cheek, or forehead; bruises are in the same stage of healing; history fits the bruise.

b. Bites: Shape, size, and location are important. Intercanine distance of >3 cm is suggestive of human bites, which generally crush more than lacerate.

c. Burns: Signs concerning for child maltreatment include multiple burn sites, well-demarcated edges, stocking/glove distributions, absence of splash marks, symmetrically burned buttocks and/or lower legs, mirror image burns of extremities, symmetrical involvement of palms or soles, spared inguinal or other flexural creases, central sparing over buttocks or perineum, parent denial that the lesion is a burn, parent attributing the cause of the burn to a sibling, and delay in seeking medical attention.

d. Bleeding:

   (1) Evaluation for retinal hemorrhages should be performed by an ophthalmologist. Retinoschisis or retinal hemorrhages that are too numerous to count, multilayered, or continue to the periphery of the retina are virtually pathognomonic for abusive head trauma.

   (2) Duodenal hematomas are suspicious for nonaccidental blunt trauma; may lead to upper GI obstruction.

e. Fractures: Certain fracture types are suspicious for nonaccidental trauma (Table 4-10).

f. Abusive head trauma (AHT): Findings may include retinal hemorrhages, subdural hematomas, long bone or rib fractures, and CNS dysfunction (e.g., seizure, apnea, lethargy secondary to intracranial injury).

g. Sexual abuse:

   (1) If abuse is suspected to have occurred within 72 hours for a child younger than age 12 or within 120 hours for a child older than 12, defer interview and GU examination at presenting facility and urgently involve a multidisciplinary team with expertise in evaluation of sexual abuse if available. Avoid collection of laboratory specimens without input from this team. Nonacute examinations falling outside of the above time windows should be deferred to a child advocacy center.

   (2) Genital examination should be performed by trained forensic specialist, owing to anatomic variability (especially of hymen).

TABLE 4-10	
SKELETAL INJURY IN NONACCIDENTAL TRAUMA	
Skeletal injury	Correlate mechanism of injury with physical finding; rule out any underlying bony pathology.
Long bones	Classic fracture is the epiphyseal/metaphyseal fracture, seen as a "bucket handle" or "corner" fracture at the end of long bones. This fracture is often secondary to jerking/shaking of a child's limb but can also be caused by natural shearing forces.
	Spiral fractures may be suspicious of abuse but can be seen with rotational forces (e.g., "toddler's fracture" of tibia).
Ribs	Posterior nondisplaced rib fractures are usually due to severe squeezing of the rib cage. May not be visible on plain film until callus formation.
Skull	Fractures >3 mm wide, complex fractures, bilateral fractures, and nonparietal fractures suggest forces greater than those sustained from minor household trauma.

(3) Normal genital examination does not rule out abuse; 95% of examinations are normal in cases of abuse.

3. **Useful studies:**
a. Skeletal survey is suggested to evaluate suspicious bony trauma in any child; these studies are mandatory for children <2 years of age (see Chapter 25 for components).
b. Bone scan may be indicated to identify early or difficult-to-detect fractures.
c. Noncontrast head CT is useful for visualizing intracranial hemorrhage but unreliable for detection of skull fractures.
d. MRI may identify lesions not detected by CT (e.g., posterior fossa injury and diffuse axonal injury).
e. Dilated indirect ophthalmoscopy by an ophthalmologist is important for accurate detection of retinal hemorrhages in suspected AHT.
4. **Treat:** Medical stabilization is primary goal. Prevention of further injuries is the long-term goal.
5. **Report:** All healthcare providers are required by law to report suspected child maltreatment to the local police and/or child welfare agency. Suspicion supported by objective evidence is criterion for reporting and should first be discussed with not only the entire medical team but also the family. The professional who makes such reports is immune from any civil or criminal liability.
6. **Document:** Write legibly, carefully documenting the following: reported and suspected history and mechanisms of injury, any history given by the victim in his or her own words (use quotation marks), information provided by other providers or services, and physical examination findings, including drawings of injuries and details of dimensions, color, shape, and texture. Always consider early use of police crime laboratory photography to document injuries.

REFERENCES

1. Marx J, Hockberger R, Walls R. *Rosen's Emergency Medicine: Concepts and Clinical Practice.* 7th ed. St Louis: Mosby, 2009.
2. Field JM, Hazinski MF, Sayre MR, et al. American Heart Association guidelines for cardiopulmonary resuscitation and emergency cardiovascular care science. *Circulation.* 2010;122(suppl 3):18.
3. Fleisher GR, Ludwig S, eds. *Textbook of Pediatric Emergency Medicine.* 5th ed. Philadelphia: Lippincott Williams & Wilkins, 2006.
4. Mehta S. Neuroimaging for paediatric minor closed head injuries. *Paediatr Child Health.* 2007;12:482-484.
5. Osmond MH, Klassen TP, Wells GA, et al. Pediatric Emergency Research Canada (PERC) Head Injury Study Group. CATCH: a clinical decision rule for the use of computed tomography in children with minor head injury. *CMAJ.* 2010;182:341-348.
6. Kirkwood MW, Yeates KO, Wilson PE. Pediatric sport-related concussion: a review of the clinical management of an oft-neglected population. *Pediatrics.* 2006;117:1359-1371.
7. Sanchez J, Paidas C. Childhood trauma: now and in the new millennium. *Surg Clin North Am.* 1999;79:1503-1535.
8. Green NE. *Skeletal Trauma in Children.* 3rd ed. Philadelphia: WB Saunders, 2003.
9. Canale ST. *Campbell's Operative Orthopedics.* 10th ed. St Louis: Mosby, 2003.
10. Pickering TG, Hall JE, Appel LJ, et al. Recommendations for blood pressure measurement in humans and experimental animals: part 1: blood pressure measurement in humans: a statement for professionals from the Subcommittee of Professional and Public Education of the American Heart Association Council on High Blood Pressure Research. *Circulation.* 2005;111:697-716.
11. Offiah A, van Rijn RR, Perez-Rossello JM, et al. Skeletal imaging of child abuse (non-accidental injury). *Pediatr Radiol.* 2009;39:461-470.
12. Nichols DG, Yaster M, Lappe DG, et al. *Golden Hour: The Handbook of Advanced Pediatric Life Support.* 2nd ed. St Louis: Mosby, 1996.
13. Walker PA, Harting MT, Baumgartner JE, et al. Modern approaches to pediatric brain injury therapy. *J Trauma.* 2009;67(suppl 2):S120-S712.
14. Kochanek PM, Carney N, Adelson PD, et al. American Academy of Pediatrics–Section on Neurological Surgery, American Association of Neurological Surgeons/Congress of Neurological Surgeons, Child Neurology Society, European Society of Pediatric and Neonatal Intensive Care, Neurocritical Care Society, Pediatric Neurocritical Care Research Group, Society of Critical Care Medicine, Paediatric Intensive Care Society UK, Society for Neuroscience in Anesthesiology and Critical Care, World Federation of Pediatric Intensive and Critical Care Societies. Guidelines for the acute medical management of severe traumatic brain injury in infants, children, and adolescents—second edition. *Pediatr Crit Care Med.* 2012;13(suppl 1):S1-S82.
15. Rogers M. *Textbook of Pediatric Intensive Care.* 4th ed. Baltimore: Williams & Wilkins, 2008.
16. Biban P, Gaffuri M, Spaggiari S, et al. Early recognition and management of septic shock in children. *Pediatr Rep.* 2012;4:e13.
17. Mesiano G, Davis GM. Ventilatory strategies in the neonatal and paediatric intensive care units. *Paediatr Respir Rev.* 2008;9:281-288.
18. Thomas N, Brook I. Animal bite-associated infections: microbiology and treatment. *Exp Rev Anti Infect Ther.* 2011;9:215-226.

19. Barkin RM, Rosen P. *Emergency Pediatrics: A Guide to Ambulatory Care*. 6th ed. St Louis: Mosby, 2003.
20. Kellogg N. The evaluation of sexual abuse in children. *Pediatrics*. 2005;116:506-512.
21. Sato Y. Imaging of nonaccidental head injury. *Pediatr Radiol*. 2009;39(suppl 2):S230-S235.
22. Waltzman ML, Mooney DP. Major trauma. In: Fleisher GR, Ludwig S, Henretig FM, eds. *Textbook of Pediatric Emergency Medicine*. Philadelphia: Lippincott Williams & Wilkins, 2006:1354.
23. Hazinski MF, Barkin RM. Shock. In: Barkin RM, ed. *Pediatric Emergency Medicine: Concepts and Clinical Practice*. St Louis: Mosby-Yearbook, 1997:118.

59. Holcomb JB, Rose T. Compensated pediatric... in Trauma care. J Trauma. 2003; 55:...

60. Bickell WH. Fluid resuscitation in the... blunt or penetrating... Surgery. 2002; 51:553-812.

61. Stein Y. Handling of plasma... fresh frozen plasma in trauma. J Trauma. 2002; 52:...

62. Wilson RF, Morris DC... in trauma vic... Philadelphia, PA: Lippincott-...

63. Hess JR... and Patient Emergency Medicine Clinics. Philadelphia, PA: ... 2001;33...

64. Rosenfeld ME. Burn shock to cardiac... trauma. Emergency medicine... Burn and management. Philadelphia, PA: 1997;178.

PART II

DIAGNOSTIC AND THERAPEUTIC INFORMATION

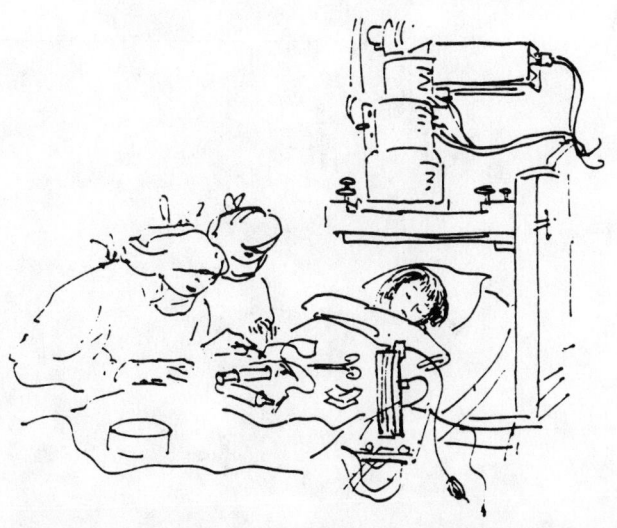

Chapter 5

Adolescent Medicine

Natalie Spicyn, MD, MHS

See additional content on Expert Consult

I. WEBSITES

A. Websites for Clinicians

American Academy of Pediatrics (AAP) section on adolescent health: http://www.aap.org/sections/adolescenthealth

Adolescent development: http://www.aacap.org

Sexual and reproductive health, including minor consent laws: http://www.guttmacher.org/sections/adolescents.php

B. Websites for Patients

Sexual health: http://www.ashastd.org

Drug abuse: http://teens.drugabuse.gov

II. INTRODUCTION TO ADOLESCENT HEALTH

A. Pubertal Development[1-5]

1. **Pubic hair** (for males and females); (Table 5-1)
2. **Female breast development** (Fig. 5-1)
3. **Male genital development** (Table 5-2). Also see Table 10-16 for testicular volumes
4. **Gynecomastia in males**
   a. Generally occurs in middle–late stages of puberty.
   b. Etiology: Breast growth stimulated by estradiol.
   c. Prevalence: Occurs in 50% of boys (50% unilateral, 50% bilateral).
   d. Clinical course: Regression usually occurs over 2-year period.
   e. Physical examination: With patient supine, palpate breast looking for glandular or fibroglandular breast tissue beneath nipple and areola, comparing to the lateral breast tissue to distinguish true gynecomastia from adiposity, pseudogynecomastia, or a pathologic etiology. A testicular examination should also be performed.
   f. Treatment: Often no treatment is necessary. Severe or nonregressing cases may warrant surgical referral.
5. **Precocious puberty:** Onset of secondary sexual characteristics before age 8 in girls and age 9 in boys.
6. **Delayed puberty:** Lack of secondary sexual development by age 14 (see Figure 10-5 for more information on the approach to a child with delayed puberty).

B. Psychosocial Development (Table EC 5-A available on Expert Consult).

TABLE 5-1

PUBIC HAIR TANNER STAGING

Tanner Stage	Appearance
1	No hair
2	Sparse, downy hair at base of symphysis pubis
3	Sparse, coarse hair across symphysis pubis
4	Adult hair quality, fills in pubic triangle, no spread to thighs
5	Adult quality and distribution including spread to medial thighs

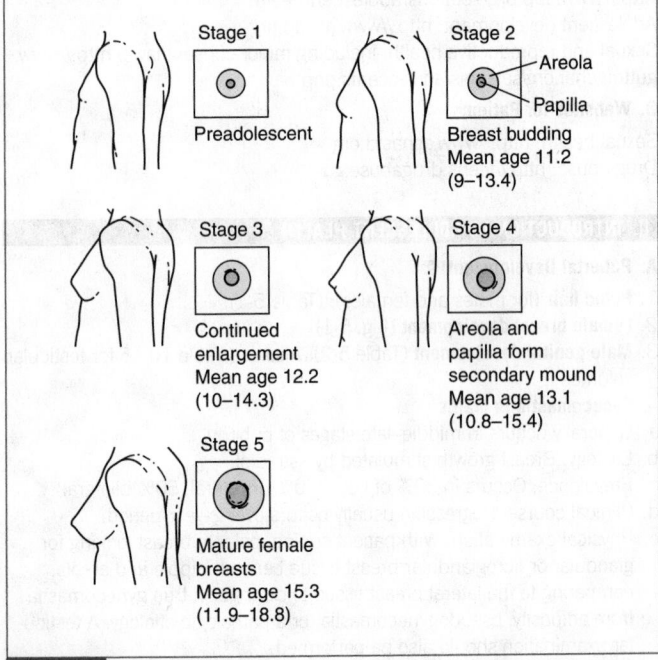

FIGURE 5-1

Tanner stages of breast development in females. *(Modified from Johnson TR, Moore WM. Children Are Different: Developmental Physiology. 2nd ed. Columbus, Ohio, Ross Laboratories, 1978. Mean age and range [2 standard deviations around mean] from Joffe A. Introduction to adolescent medicine. In McMillan JA, DeAngelis CD, Feigin RD, et al, eds. Oski's Pediatrics: Principles and Practice. 4th ed. Philadelphia: Lippincott Williams & Wilkins, 2006:549-550.)*

TABLE 5-2

GENITAL DEVELOPMENT (MALE)

Stage	Comment (±2 Standard Deviations Around Mean Age)
1	Prepubertal
2	Enlargement of scrotum and testes; skin of scrotum reddens and changes in texture; little or no enlargement of penis; mean age 11.4 yr (9.5–13.8 yr)
3	Enlargement of penis, first mainly in length; further growth of testes and scrotum; mean age 12.9 yr (10.8–14.9 yr)
4	Increased size of penis with growth in breadth and development of glans; further enlargement of testes and scrotum and increased darkening of scrotal skin; mean age 13.8 yr (11.7–15.8 yr)
5	Genitalia adult in size and shape; mean age 14.9 yr (13–17.3 yr)

Data from Joffe A. Introduction to adolescent medicine. In McMillan JA, DeAngelis CD, Feigin RD, et al, eds. *Oski's Pediatrics: Principles and Practice.* 4th ed. Philadelphia: Lippincott Williams & Wilkins, 2006:546-557.

C. Psychosocial and Medicosocial History[6,7,27]

HEADSSS[3,4,6]: Brief instrument that screens for psychosocial factors that impact adolescent mental and physical health (Box 5-1)

BOX 5-1

HEADSSS ASSESSMENT

(H)OME: Household composition, family dynamics and relationships, living and sleeping arrangements, recent changes, any periods of homelessness, running away from home

(E)DUCATION/(E)MPLOYMENT/(E)ATING: School performance, attendance, suspensions; attitude toward school; favorite, most difficult, best subjects; special educational needs; goals for the future; afterschool job or other work history (see Section III.C, Review of Systems, for eating/nutrition questions)

(A)CTIVITIES: Friendships with same or opposite sex, ages of friends, best friend, dating, recreational activities, physical activity, sports participation, hobbies and interests

(D)RUGS: Personal use of tobacco, alcohol, illicit drugs, anabolic steroids; peer substance use; family substance use and attitudes; if personal use, determine frequency, quantity, binge, injury with use; consider use of **CRAFFT** questionnaires (Box 5-2)

(S)EXUALITY: See Box EC 5-A for the "Five Ps" of the sexual history; additional helpful information includes age at first sex, number of lifetime and current partners, ages of partners, recent change in partners; knowledge of emergency contraception and sexually transmitted infection/human immunodeficiency virus (STI/HIV) prevention; prior testing for STI/HIV, prior pregnancies, abortions; ever fathered a child; history of nonconsensual intimate physical contact or sex

(S)UICIDE/DEPRESSION: Feelings about self, both positive and negative; history of depression or other mental health problems; sleep problems (difficulty getting to sleep, early waking); changes in appetite or weight; anhedonia; irritability; anxiety; current or prior suicidal thoughts or attempts; other self-harming or injurious behavior

(S)AFETY: Feeling unsafe at home, at school, or in the community; bullying; guns in the home; weapon carrying, what kinds of weapons; fighting; arrests; gang membership

---

BOX 5-2

CRAFFT QUESTIONNAIRE[27]

C—Have you ever ridden in a **C**AR driven by someone (or yourself) who was "high" or had been using alcohol or drugs?

R—Do you ever use alcohol or drugs to **R**ELAX, feel better about yourself, or fit in?

A—Do you ever use alcohol/drugs while you are **A**LONE?

F—Do your family or **F**RIENDS ever tell you that you should cut down on your drinking or drug use?

F—Do you ever **F**ORGET things you did while using alcohol or drugs?

T—Have you gotten into **T**ROUBLE while you were using alcohol or drugs?

NOTE: Answering yes to two or more questions is a positive screen.

III. ADOLESCENT HEALTH MAINTENANCE

Bright Futures Guidelines for Health Supervision of Adolescents[8]
(Box EC 5-B on Expert Consult)

A. Confidentiality

Adolescents are concerned about the confidentiality of their interactions with healthcare providers. Laws governing minors' ability to consent to health care vary by state and type of service. More information can be found at the Guttmacher Institute's website (http://www.guttmacher.org/statecenter/spibs/spib_OMCL.pdf).

B. Chief Complaint

Hidden agenda: Adolescents may state a chief complaint that is not always the real concern for the visit. Upon initiating a visit, reviewing the reason for the visit ("What brings you in today?" "Is there anything else?") can reveal the actual reason.

C. Review of Systems (Areas of Emphasis with an Adolescent)

1. **Nutrition:** Dietary habits, including skipped meals, special diets, purging methods, recent weight gain or loss
2. **Skin:** Acne, moles, rashes, warts
3. **Genitourinary:** Dysuria, urgency, frequency, discharge, bleeding
4. **Menstrual:** Menarche, frequency, duration, pain, menometrorrhagia

D. Family History[3,4]

Including psychiatric disorders, suicide, alcoholism or substance abuse, and chronic medical conditions or familial risk factors (hypertension, diabetes, cholesterol, blood clot, heart attack, stroke, cancer, asthma, tuberculosis, HIV).

E. Physical Examination (Most Pertinent Aspects)[3,4,8-10]

Whenever possible, examine patient in a gown to ensure a complete and thorough examination.

1. **Height, weight (calculate body mass index [BMI]), and blood pressure with percentiles.**
2. **Dentition and gums** (smokeless tobacco use, enamel erosion from induced vomiting).

3. **Skin:** Acne (type and distribution of lesions), atypical nevi, acanthosis nigricans, scars, piercings, tattoos
4. **Thyroid**
5. **Spine:** Routine screening for idiopathic scoliosis is not recommended owing to unfavorable balance of risks and benefits, but clinicians should be prepared to evaluate scoliosis if incidentally discovered or the patient or parent expresses concern.

   More information about assessment and treatment of scoliosis is available on Expert Consult.
6. **Breasts:** Sexual maturity rating for females (see Fig. 5-1), masses (females); gynecomastia (males)
7. **Genitalia:** For both male and female genital examinations, talk patients through examination, commenting on normal findings. Touch a nongenital part of body first, examine painful areas last. Avoid lengthy discussions while patients are undressed and in a compromising position. Consider use of a chaperone.
a. Male:
   (1) Visual inspection for sexual maturity rating for hair (Table 5-2, see Table 10-16) and signs of STI (e.g., warts, lice, ulcers, discharge)
   (2) Genital examination for sexual maturity rating for testicles (see Table 10-16) and identification of masses, hydrocele, varicocele, hernias
b. Female:
   (1) External examination: Visual inspection of perineum (warts, ulcers, rashes, pubic lice, trauma, discharge) and sexual maturity rating for hair (Tanner stage, see Table 5-1).
   (2) Internal examination (pelvic examination): Indications include vaginal discharge (assess cervix for mucopurulent discharge, friability, large ectropion, foreign body); lower abdominal or pelvic pain; urinary symptoms in a sexually active female; menstrual disorders (amenorrhea, abnormal vaginal bleeding, or dysmenorrhea refractory to medical therapy); consideration of intrauterine device or diaphragm (not necessary before prescription of other methods of contraception); and suspected or reported sexual abuse or rape (refer to a specialized center if not trained and equipped to appropriately document evidence of trauma and collect forensic specimens).
c. Anal inspection for patients engaging in anal sex.

F. Screening Laboratory Tests and Procedures[8,11-16]

1. **A dearth of research and evidence for screening examinations for adolescence** has led to variability in guidelines for topics such as screening for dyslipidemia, iron-deficiency anemia, diabetes, and tuberculosis. Updated guidelines issued by various organizations

may be accessed at the listed sites; recommendations that follow are largely based on CDC guidelines:

a. Bright Futures[8]: http://brightfutures.aap.org

b. CDC: http://www.cdc.gov/HealthyYouth/index.htm

c. U.S. Preventive Services Task Force (USPSTF): http://www.uspreventive servicestaskforce.org/tfchildcat.htm

2. **Adolescents may legally consent to medical care for STIs without parental notification** in all 50 states and Washington, D.C., but providers should be aware of barriers to confidentiality related to medical billing and explanation of benefits by insurance companies.

CDC STI screening guidelines for sexually active adolescents are as follows[17]:

a. HIV: Routine screening recommended starting at age 13, with subsequent tests at least annually for all persons at high risk.[13] Rescreening for both HIV and syphilis 3–4 months after a documented STI. Remember that screening (antibody) testing will not pick up acute infection, so if concerned about the clinical syndrome of acute HIV infection, ribonucleic acid (RNA) testing should be ordered.

b. Syphilis: Routine screening recommended annually for persons at risk.

c. Chlamydia and gonorrhea:
   (1) *Chlamydia trachomatis* (CT): Routine screening in sexually active persons < age 25. For males, screening especially recommended in high prevalence communities and/or settings (e.g., STI clinics, adolescent clinics, correctional facilities).
   (2) *Neisseria gonorrhoeae* (GC) testing recommended for all sexually active female adolescents. Among young men who have sex with men (YMSM), at least annual testing is also recommended, with attention to site of collection (urine for insertive partner, rectal swab for receptive partner, pharyngeal swab for receptive partner in oral intercourse).
   (3) Female: Self- or provider-collected vaginal nucleic acid amplification test (NAAT) is preferred method to screen for CT/GC; self-collected specimens may have higher patient acceptability. Vaginal swabs are as sensitive and specific as cervical samples; urine samples are less so.
   (4) Male: Urine NAAT is preferred method to screen for CT/GC. Sexually active adolescent males are considered. YMSM specifically for GC.
   (5) Patients who test positive for chlamydia should be rescreened 3–4 months after treatment; rates of reinfection are high.[14]
   (6) Patients with gonorrhea: Consider test of cure 3–4 weeks later if patients did not receive CDC-recommended or alternative antibiotic regimens.

d. Other STIs:
   (1) Routine screening of asymptomatic adolescents not recommended for other STIs (e.g., trichomoniasis, herpes simplex virus [HSV], hepatitis A and B viruses [HAV, HBV], human papillomavirus [HPV]).
   (2) Refer to CDC guidelines for specific additional recommendations for STI screening among YMSM who might require more thorough evaluation.

3. **Cervical cancer cytologic analysis** (Papanicolaou [Pap] smear)[11,12]:
a. *Immunocompetent:* Regardless of age of sexual debut, cervical cancer screening with Pap smear should not begin until a woman is 21 years old. Subsequent tests should be done every 3 years. Cytologic evaluation only should be used; HPV testing is indicated until age 30.
b. *HIV+ or immunosuppressed (e.g., organ transplant recipient, systemic lupus erythematosus patient, poorly controlled diabetic):* Every 6 months in first year after HIV diagnosis or after sexual debut if immunosuppressed; thereafter, annually.
c. In immunocompetent adolescents, risk of adverse pregnancy outcomes outweighs benefits of screening and treatment, given the low rate of cervical cancer and high rate of resolution of HPV infections. However, immunocompetent adolescents who have had abnormal cytologic study results may be treated according to Table EC 5-B (available on Expert Consult). Immunosuppressed adolescents with abnormal cytologic results should be referred for further management.

G. Immunizations

Refer to Chapter 16 for dosing, route, formulation, and schedules.

IV. PREPARTICIPATION PHYSICAL EVALUATION (PPE)[18,19]

PPE is an opportunity to screen for risks related to participation in sports but is also an opportunity to deliver adolescent clinical preventive services, because this may be a young person's only visit during adolescence.

A. Medical History

Includes information about chronic conditions/medications (including performance-enhancing agents), hospitalizations/surgeries, use of protective equipment during sports participation, allergies (especially those associated with anaphylaxis, respiratory compromise, or exercise-induced), and immunizations (HBV; measles, mumps, rubella [MMR]; tetanus; varicella).
NOTE: See Chapter 7, Table 7-14, and Table EC 7-D for further information about PPE screening and exercise restrictions with cardiac disease.

B. Review of Systems and Physical Examination

   (Physical examination items in italics.)

1. **Height and weight**
2. **Vision:** Visual problems, corrective lenses, visual acuity, pupil equality
3. **Cardiac:** History of congenital heart disease; syncope, dizziness, or chest pain during exercise; history of high blood pressure or heart murmurs; family history of heart disease; history of disqualification or limited participation in sports because of a cardiac problem; *blood pressure, heart rate and rhythm, pulses (including radial/femoral lag), auscultation of heart sounds, murmurs—both standing and supine*
4. **Respiratory:** Asthma, coughing, wheezing, or dyspnea during exercise
5. **Abdomen:** *Organomegaly* and single kidney are contraindications for contact sports

6. **Genitourinary:** Age at menarche, last menstrual period, regularity of menstrual periods, number of periods in the last year, longest interval between periods, dysmenorrhea; *palpation of abdomen, palpation of testicles, examination of inguinal canals*

7. **Orthopedic:** Previous injuries that have limited sports participation or required medical intervention; screening orthopedic examination (Fig. EC 5-C available on Expert Consult). Consider checking vitamin D levels if history of a fracture with minor trauma.

8. **Neurology:** History of significant head injury/concussion, numbness or tingling of extremities, severe headaches, seizure disorder (although not an absolute contraindication to contact sports if well controlled, seizure within past 6 months should raise concern prior to clearance, particularly for those engaged in water sports)

9. **Skin:** Rashes; *evidence of contagious infections (e.g., varicella or impetigo)*

10. **Psychosocial:** Weight control and body image, stressors at home or in school, use or abuse of drugs and alcohol; *attention to signs of eating disorders, including oral ulcerations, eroded tooth enamel, edema, lanugo hair, calluses or ulcerations on knuckles*

V. SEXUAL HEALTH[9,20-25]

A. Sexual Orientation

Adolescents may explore a variety of sexual activities (penile-vaginal, anal, or oral intercourse) but not equate behaviors with sexual identity or orientation (e.g., heterosexual, homosexual, bisexual). Conversely, adolescents may self-identify with a particular sexual orientation but not be sexually active.

B. Gender Identity

Refers to an individual's self-awareness as male or female:

1. **Transgender:** An individual whose gender identity (internal sense) or gender expression (behavior, etc.) differs from the biological sex assigned at birth

2. **Transvestite:** An individual who derives pleasure from dressing in clothing of the opposite sex

3. **Gender identity is unrelated to sexual orientation;** transgender or transvestite individuals may feel themselves to be heterosexual, homosexual, or bisexual

C. Contraception

1. Special considerations in adolescents

a. Barriers may include confidentiality concerns, fear of the pelvic examination, and fear of side effects (e.g., weight gain, bleeding, etc.).

b. Adherence and continuation rates in adolescents are superior with long-acting reversible contraception (LARC) methods such as the intrauterine device and etonogestrel implant.

c. Counseling should include discussion of need for barrier method to prevent STIs, as well as tips for increasing adherence.

2. **Methods of contraception** (Fig. 5-2)

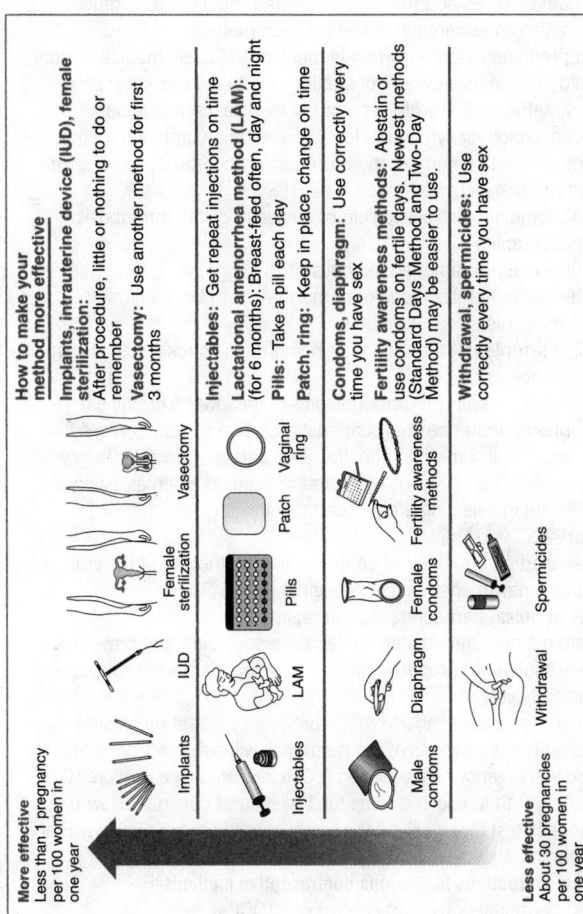

More effective
Less than 1 pregnancy per 100 women in one year

Less effective
About 30 pregnancies per 100 women in one year

Implants | IUD | Female sterilization | Vasectomy

Injectables | LAM | Pills | Patch | Vaginal ring

Male condoms | Diaphragm | Fertility awareness methods

Female condoms

Withdrawal | Spermicides

How to make your method more effective

Implants, intrauterine device (IUD), female sterilization:
After procedure, little or nothing to do or remember
Vasectomy: Use another method for first 3 months

Injectables: Get repeat injections on time
Lactational amenorrhea method (LAM): (for 6 months): Breast-feed often, day and night
Pills: Take a pill each day
Patch, ring: Keep in place, change on time

Condoms, diaphragm: Use correctly every time you have sex
Fertility awareness methods: Abstain or use condoms on fertile days. Newest methods (Standard Days Method and Two-Day Method) may be easier to use.

Withdrawal, spermicides: Use correctly every time you have sex

FIGURE 5-2

Comparing effectiveness of family planning methods. (*From World Health Organization Department of Reproductive Health and Research [WHO/RHR] and Johns Hopkins Bloomberg School of Public Health/Center for Communication Programs [CCP], Knowledge for Health Project. Family Planning: A Global Handbook for Providers (2011 Update). Baltimore, Geneva: CCP and WHO, 2011.)*

3. **Contraception selection and initiation:**

a. Selecting a contraceptive method[22]

Please refer to the CDC's Medical Eligibility Criteria (http://www.cdc.gov/mmwr/pdf/rr/rr59e0528.pdf) for any relative or absolute contraindications for each hormonal contraceptive method based on an individual's medical comorbidities and the CDC's Selected Practice Recommendations for minimum requirements to start each method.

   (1) To appropriately start a hormonal method, the basic medical history should include assessment of clotting risk, blood pressure, pregnancy status, and any other pertinent medical comorbidities.

   (2) Related to clotting symptoms for a person on a combined method, a mnemonic to remember the more serious complications of combined hormonal contraception is ACHES[23]:

      (a) **A**bdominal pain (pelvic vein or mesenteric vein thrombosis, pancreatitis)

      (b) **C**hest pain (pulmonary embolism)

      (c) **H**eadaches (thrombotic or hemorrhagic stroke, retinal vein thrombosis)

      (d) **E**ye symptoms (thrombotic or hemorrhagic stroke, retinal vein thrombosis)

      (e) **S**evere leg pain (thrombophlebitis of the lower extremities)

   (3) To support adherence and continuation, use a patient-centered approach, review method effectiveness, and provide anticipatory guidance regarding side effects of each method when assisting an adolescent in selecting a new contraceptive method.

b. Quick start[25]

Defined as starting a method of contraception on the day of the visit (not waiting until a new menstrual cycle begins) (Fig. 5-3)

Principles of quick-start contraception regimens:

   (1) Initiate method immediately to decrease confusion and prevent patient's failure to properly initiate contraception during subsequent menstrual cycle.

   (2) Rule out pregnancy; advise that a pregnancy test at quick-start initiation is not conclusive, but hormones will not affect pregnancy.

   (3) Provide emergency contraception (EC) if indicated (see Section V.C.5).

   (4) Counsel youth to use condoms for 1 week and obtain a follow-up pregnancy test in 4 weeks if the method was initiated after day 6 of the menstrual cycle.

4. **Patient use instructions for various contraceptive methods**[22-24]

a. Combined hormonal oral contraceptive pills (OCPs):

   (1) Take one pill at the same time each day (within a 4-hour window).

   (2) The first pill should be taken either on the day of the visit (quick start) or between the first and seventh day after the start of the menstrual period (most commonly Sunday).

   (3) Some pill packs have 28 pills, others have 21 pills. When the 28-day pack is empty, immediately start taking pills from a new

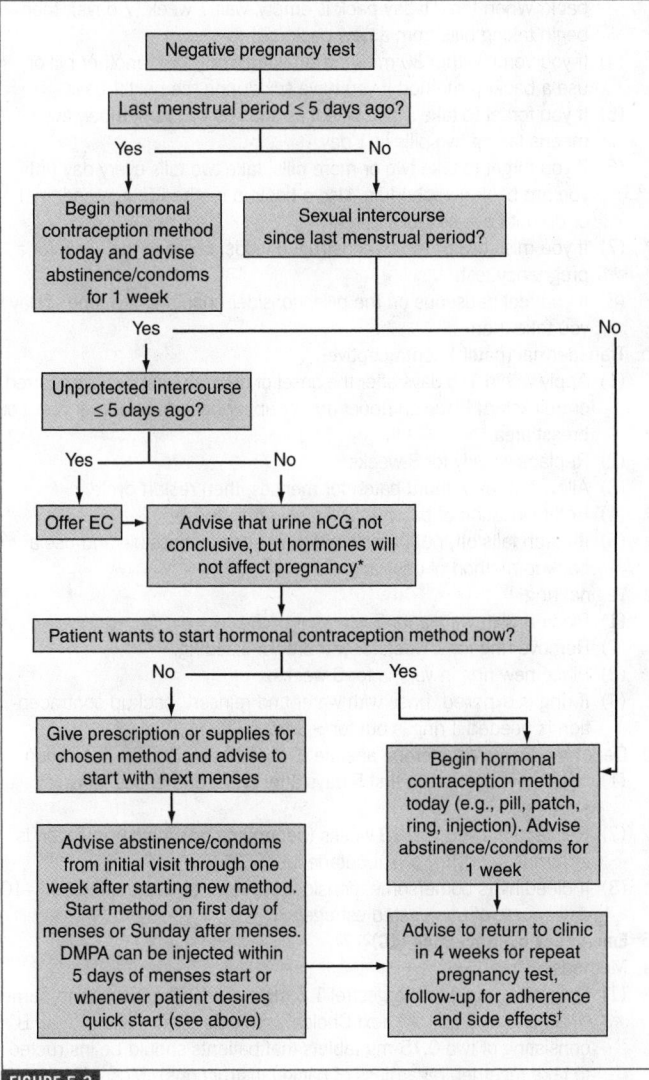

FIGURE 5-3

Algorithm for quick-start initiation of contraception. EC, Emergency contraception; hCG, human chorionic gonadotropin. *Pregnancy tests may take 2–3 weeks after sex to be accurate. †Consider pregnancy test at second depot medroxyprogesterone acetate (DMPA [Depo-Provera]) injection if quick-start regimen was used and patient failed 4-week follow-up visit. *(Modified from Zieman M, Hatcher RA, Cwiak C, et al. A Pocket Guide to Managing Contraception. Tiger, Georgia: Bridging the Gap Foundation, 2010:142.)*

pack. When the 21-day pack is empty, wait 1 week (7 days), then begin taking pills from a new pack.

(4) If you vomit within 30 minutes of taking a pill, take another pill or use a backup method if you have sex during the next 7 days.

(5) If you forget to take a pill, take it as soon as you remember, even if it means taking two pills in 1 day.

(6) If you forget to take two or more pills, take two pills every day until you are back on schedule. Use a backup method (e.g., condoms) or do not have sex for 7 days.

(7) If you miss two or more menstrual periods, come to the clinic for a pregnancy test.

(8) If you feel nauseous on the pills, consider changing the time of day you take them.

b. Transdermal (patch) contraceptive:

(1) Apply within 1–5 days after the onset of menses (first day is preferred) or quickstart. Place on upper arm or upper back but not over chest or breast area.

(2) Replace weekly for 3 weeks.

(3) Allow 1 week without patch for menses, then restart cycle.

(4) Rotate location of patch to avoid skin irritation.

(5) If patch falls off, put on new patch as soon as possible and use a backup method of contraception.

c. Vaginal ring:

(1) Place ring in vagina for 3 weeks.

(2) Remove ring for 1 week for withdrawal bleeding.

(3) Place new ring in vagina for 3 weeks.

(4) If ring is expelled, rinse with water and reinsert; backup contraception is needed if ring is out for > 3 hours.

d. Depot medroxyprogesterone acetate (DMPA [Depo-Provera]) injection:

(1) Initial injection within first 5 days after onset of menses (or quick start; see Fig. 5-3)

(2) Reinjection every 11–13 weeks (depending on whether injection is intramuscular [IM] or subcutaneous [SQ])

(3) If bleeding is bothersome, consider asking your doctor about a 7–10 day course of conjugated estrogen.

5. **Emergency contraception (EC)**[21,22]

a. Methods:

(1) Progestin only: Levonorgestrel 1.5 mg orally (PO) once (brand name "Plan B One Step" or "Next Choice" with older formulation; "Plan B" consisting of two 0.75-mg tablets that patients should be instructed to take together, regardless of packet instructions). Most efficacious within 72 hours of coitus but effective through 120 hours; ulipristal has superior efficacy in the 72–120 hour window.

(2) Selective progesterone receptor modulator: Ulipristal 30 mg PO once.

(3) Combined hormonal: Known as the "Yuzpe method," involves counseling patients to take two doses of OCPs, with each dose containing

at least 100 mcg of ethinyl estradiol and at least 500 mcg of levo-norgestrel (either 8 total tablets: 4 at a time, 12 hours apart, or for more precise instructions for a particular combination pill; refer to www.ec.princeton.edu). Consider prescribing an antiemetic, such as metoclopramide or meclizine, for use 1 hour before first dose.

    (4) Copper intrauterine device (IUD) may be inserted within 5 days of coitus.

b. Mechanism of action: Mixed hormonal or progestin-only methods work by interfering with or delaying ovulation and do not interfere with established pregnancy. Ulipristal, likewise, works by delaying ovulation, but it may result in first-trimester fetal loss.

c. Guidelines and instructions for use:

    (1) Counseling about EC should be a routine part of anticipatory guidance for all female and male adolescents. Levonorgestrel methods are available over the counter—no prescription necessary—but must be requested directly from the pharmacist by persons aged 17 or older in all 50 states. Advance prescriptions should be considered for all teens aged 16 and younger, regardless of current sexual activity. Ulipristal requires a prescription regardless of patient age.

    (2) EC should be taken as soon as possible; there is a linear relationship between efficacy and the time from intercourse to treatment.

    (3) If using progestin or mixed hormonal EC, taking the EC dose should not be delayed for pregnancy test, given diminishing efficacy over time to dosing. However, possibility of pregnancy *must* be excluded before ulipristal dosing.

    (4) Discuss proper use of regular, reliable birth control for the future, especially for patients frequently using EC.

    (5) May be combined with other ongoing methods of birth control.

        (a) OCPs may be started 24 hours after progestin-only or combined hormonal EC dosing has been completed. DMPA may be given the same day.

        (b) Expert opinion varies regarding initiation of hormonal contraception after ulipristal use (from 7–14 days); a barrier method should be used for the remainder of the cycle.

    (6) No absolute limit of EC frequency during a cycle.

    (7) Perform pregnancy test if no menses within 3 weeks of progestin-only or combined hormonal methods, or if menses more than 1 week late with ulipristal.

    (8) Advise patients to schedule a primary care medical visit after EC usage (pregnancy test and appropriate STI testing or treatment).

d. Contraindications:

    (1) For progestin-only regimens: Pregnancy, given lack of efficacy with potential for side effects; no evidence of teratogenicity.

    (2) For ulipristal: Pregnancy, given potential for first-trimester fetal loss; no evidence of teratogenicity.

(3) For estrogen-containing regimens: Same as those for OCPs, but use over time has shown that such stringent restrictions for single use are unnecessary. History of previous thrombosis is not a contraindication for single use, but progestin-only methods are preferred.

D. Follow-up Recommendations[8]

Two or three follow-up visits per year to monitor patient compliance, blood pressure, and side effects

E. Vaginal Infections, Genital Ulcers, and Warts[16]

See Chapter 17 for discussion of infection with chlamydia, gonorrhea, pelvic inflammatory disease, syphilis, and HIV. See Formulary for treatment dosage information. After diagnosis of STI, encourage patient to refrain from intercourse until full therapy is complete, partner is treated, and all visible lesions are resolved.

1. **Diagnostic features of vaginal infections** (Table 5-3) can assist in differentiating normal vaginal discharge from bacterial vaginosis, trichomoniasis, and yeast vaginitis.
2. **Diagnostic features of various genital lesions,** as well as management of warts and ulcers, are presented in Table 5-4.

VI. MENTAL HEALTH

A. Anxiety, Depression, and Bipolar Disorder

Please refer to Disorders of Mental Health, Chapter 9, Section IX.

B. Suicidality[30]

1. **Suicide is a leading cause of mortality among adolescents.** Risk factors include male sex, American Indian/Alaska Native racial background, bisexual or homosexual orientation, isolation or living alone, history of acute stressor or recent loss, family history of suicide, personal or family history of suicide attempt, personal or parental mental health problems, physical or sexual abuse, substance use, and firearms in the home (even if properly stored and secured).
2. **Screening questions for suicidal ideation are best asked after initial questioning regarding stressors, mood, and depressive symptoms.** Remember that irritability, vague or multiple somatic complaints, and behavioral problems may indicate depression in an adolescent.
3. **In addition to risk factors above,** assessment of suicidal risk should also include whether the adolescent has a plan, the potential lethality of the plan, access to means to carry out the plan, and whether the plan has ever been rehearsed.
4. **Any adolescent with risk factors and a suicide plan should be considered an imminent risk and not be allowed to leave the office.** Providers should contact local crisis support resources and undertake immediate consultation with a mental health professional; potential courses of action must

TABLE 5-3

DIAGNOSTIC FEATURES AND MANAGEMENT OF VAGINAL INFECTIONS

	No Infection	Yeast Vaginitis	Trichomoniasis	Bacterial Vaginosis
Etiology	—	*Candida albicans* and other yeasts	*Trichomonas vaginalis*	*Gardnerella vaginalis*, anaerobic bacteria, mycoplasma
Typical symptoms	None	Vulvar itching, irritation, ↑ discharge	Malodorous frothy discharge, vulvar itching	Malodorous, slightly ↑ discharge
Discharge				
Amount	Variable; usually scant	Scant to moderate	Profuse	Moderate
Color*	Clear or white	White	Yellow-green	Usually white or gray
Consistency	Nonhomogenous, floccular	Clumped; adherent plaques	Homogenous	Homogenous, low viscosity; smoothly coats vaginal walls
Vulvar/vaginal inflammation	No	Yes	Yes	No
pH of vaginal fluid†	Usually < 4.5	Usually < 4.5	Usually > 5.0	Usually > 4.5
Amine ("fishy") odor with 10% potassium hydroxide (KOH)	None	None	May be present	Present
Microscopy‡	Normal epithelial cells; *Lactobacillus* predominates	Leukocytes, epithelial cells, yeast, mycelia, or pseudomycelia in 40%–80% of cases	Leukocytes; motile trichomonads seen in 50%–70% of symptomatic patients, less often if asymptomatic	Clue cells, few leukocytes; *Lactobacillus* outnumbered by profuse mixed flora (nearly always including *G. vaginalis* plus anaerobes)
Usual treatment (see Formulary)	None	Oral fluconazole; intravaginal azoles	Metronidazole or tinidazole	Oral/intravaginal metronidazole or clindamycin
Management of sex partners	None	None	Treatment recommended	None

*Color of discharge is determined by examining vaginal discharge against the white background of a swab.

†pH determination is not useful if blood is present.

‡To detect fungal elements, vaginal fluid is digested with 10% KOH before microscopic examination; to examine for other features, fluid is mixed (1:1) with physiologic saline.

NOTE: Refer to Formulary for dosing information.

From Workowski KA, Berman S. Sexually transmitted diseases treatment guidelines, 2010. *MMWR Recomm Rep.* 2010;59(RR-12):1–110.

5

TABLE 5-4

DIAGNOSTIC FEATURES AND MANAGEMENT OF GENITAL ULCERS AND WARTS

Infection	Clinical Presentation	Presumptive Diagnosis	Definitive Diagnosis	Treatment/Management of Sex Partners
Genital herpes	Grouped vesicles, painful shallow ulcers	Tzanck preparation with multinucleated giant cells	HSV PCR	No known cure. Prompt initiation of therapy shortens duration of first episode. For severe recurrent disease, initiate therapy at start of prodrome or within 1 day. Transmission can occur during asymptomatic periods. See Formulary for dosing of acyclovir, famciclovir, or valacyclovir.
Chancroid	Etiology: *Haemophilus ducreyi* Painful genital ulcer, tender, suppurative inguinal adenopathy	No evidence of *Treponema pallidum* (syphilis) on darkfield microscopy or serologic testing; negative HSV	Use of special media (not widely available in United States); sensitivity < 80%	Single dose: Azithromycin 1 g orally OR Cegriaxone 250 mg IM Partners should be examined and treated, regardless of whether symptoms are present, or if they have had sex within 10 days preceding onset of patient's symptoms. Syphilis is a common copathogen with chancroid.
Primary syphilis	Indurated, well-defined, usually single painless ulcer or chancre; nontender inguinal adenopathy	Nontreponemal serologic test: VDRL, RPR, or STS	Treponemal serologic test: FTA-ABS or MHA-TP, darkfield microscopy or direct fluorescent antibody tests of lesion exudates or tissue	Parenteral penicillin G (see Chapter 17 for preparation(s), dosage, and length of treatment.) Treat presumptively for persons exposed within 3 months preceding the diagnosis of primary syphilis in a sex partner or who were exposed >90 days preceding the diagnosis and in whom serologic tests may not be immediately available or follow-up is uncertain.

Continued

TABLE 5-4
DIAGNOSTIC FEATURES AND MANAGEMENT OF GENITAL ULCERS AND WARTS—(Continued)

Infection	Clinical Presentation	Presumptive Diagnosis	Definitive Diagnosis	Treatment/Management of Sex Partners
HPV infection (genital warts)	Single or multiple soft, fleshy, papillary or sessile, painless growths around anus, vulvovaginal area, penis, urethra, or perineum; no inguinal adenopathy	Typical clinical presentation	Papanicolaou smear revealing typical cytologic changes	Treatment does not eradicate infection. Goal: Removal of exophytic warts. Exclude cervical dysplasia before treatment. Patient-administered therapies include podofilox and imiquimod cream. Clinician-applied therapies include podophyllin 10%–25% in compound tincture of benzoin, bichloroacetic or trichloroacetic acid, surgical removal, and cryotherapy with liquid nitrogen or cryoprobe. Podofilox, imiquimod, and podophyllin are contraindicated in pregnancy. Period of communicability unknown.

NOTE: Chancroid, lymphogranuloma venereum (LGV), and granuloma inguinale should be considered in the differential diagnosis of genital ulcers if the clinical presentation is atypical and tests for herpes and syphilis are negative.

FTA-ABS, Fluorescent treponemal antibody absorbed; HPV, human papillomavirus; HSV, herpes simplex virus; IM, intramuscular; MHA-TP, microhemagglutination assay for antibody to *Treponema pallidum*; RPR, rapid plasma reagin; STS, serologic test for syphilis; VDRL, Venereal Disease Research Laboratory.

Modified from Workowski KA, Berman S. Sexually transmitted diseases treatment guidelines, 2010. *MMWR Recomm Rep.* 2010;59(RR-12):1-110.

be individualized but include same-day mental health appointment, transfer to a psychiatric emergency room, and psychiatric hospitalization.

5. **Any adolescent with risk factors but no suicide plan or preparation should be considered moderate risk.** He or she should be provided with an immediate plan for behavioral health treatment, information about emergency resources, and ideas for coping strategies.

C. School Problems

Please refer to Chapter 9 for more information on learning disabilities (Medical Evaluation of Developmental Disorders) and attention deficit hyperactivity disorder (ADHD) (see Table 9-7).

D. Substance Use[29]

1. **Spectrum of substance use behavior:** Ranges from experimentation to limited use to dependence
2. **Drugs of abuse and acute toxidromes:** See Chapter 2
3. **Screening, brief intervention, and referral to treatment (SBIRT)**
   a. **S**ubstance use screening: Any alcohol, marijuana, other drugs in the past 12 months? If yes, administer full CRAFFT questionnaire (see Box 5-2). If no, administer only "Car" question (Ever ridden in a car with a driver who had used alcohol or drugs?)
   b. **B**rief **I**ntervention: stratify risk based on responses to screening questions.
      (1) Low risk (abstinent): Reinforce decisions with praise and anticipatory guidance regarding riding in a car with a driver under the influence.
      (2) Yes to "Car" question: Counsel, encourage safety plan, consider Contract for Life (http://www.sadd.org/contract.htm).
      (3) Moderate risk (CRAFFT negative): Advise to stop using the substance, educate regarding health risks of continued use, praise personal attributes.
      (4) High risk (CRAFFT ≥ 2): Conduct in-depth assessment using motivational enhancement techniques, conduct brief negotiated interview, or refer as appropriate.
   c. **R**eferral to **T**reatment: Further evaluation by a specialist in mental health/addiction can guide referral to an appropriate level of care.
4. **Levels of care**
   a. Substance use treatment may be delivered in a variety of settings, ranging from outpatient therapy to partial hospital to inpatient or residential treatment.
   b. Considerations for detoxification: Medical management of symptoms of withdrawal, particularly pertinent to teens dependent on alcohol, opioids, or benzodiazepines. **NOTE:** Detoxification is not equivalent to substance abuse treatment; once acute withdrawal symptoms have been managed, engage patient in a treatment program.

VII. TRANSITIONING ADOLESCENTS INTO ADULT CARE

All adolescents, particularly those with special healthcare needs or chronic conditions, benefit from careful attention to the process of transitioning to adult care. Resources for how to approach and organize the transition process are available at http://www.medicalhomeinfo.org/how/care_delivery/transitions.aspx.

REFERENCES

1. Kulin H, Muller J. The biological aspects of puberty. *Pediatr Rev.* 1996;17:75-86.
2. Muir A. Precocious puberty. *Pediatr Rev.* 2006;27:373-381.
3. Joffe A. Introduction to adolescent medicine. In: McMillan JA, DeAngelis CD, Feigan RD, et al, eds. *Oski's Pediatrics: Principles and Practice.* 4th ed. Philadelphia: Lippincott Williams & Wilkins, 2006:546-557.
4. Rosen DS, Neinstein LS. Preventive healthcare for adolescents. In: Neinstein LS, ed. *Adolescent Healthcare: A Practical Guide.* 4th ed. Philadelphia: Lippincott Williams & Wilkins, 2002:82-117.
5. Rosen D. Physiologic growth and development during adolescence. *Pediatr Rev.* 2004;25:194-200.
6. Fishman M, Bruner A, Adger H. Substance abuse among children and adolescents. *Pediatr Rev.* 1997;18:397-398.
7. Gutgesell M, Payne N. Issues of adolescent psychological development in the 21st century. *Pediatr Rev.* 2004;25:79-85.
8. Knight JE, Sherritt L, Shrier LA, et al. Validity of the CRAFFT substance abuse screening test among adolescent clinic patients. *Arch Pediatr Adolesc Med.* 2002;156:607-614.
9. American Academy of Pediatrics. *Bright Futures Guidelines for Health Supervision of Infants, Children, and Adolescents.* 3rd ed. Elk Grove, Village, IL: AAP, 2008.
10. Marcell AV, Wibbelsman C, Siegel WM, et al. Male adolescent sexual and reproductive health care. *Pediatrics.* 2011;128:e1658.
11. Braverman P, Breech L. Gynecologic examination for adolescents in the pediatric office setting. *Pediatrics.* 2010;126:583-590.
12. Weinstein S, Dolan L, Cheng J. Adolescent idiopathic scoliosis. *Lancet.* 2008;371:1527-1534.
13. Stewart D, Skaggs D. Consultation with the specialist: adolescent idiopathic scoliosis. *Pediatr Rev.* 2006;27:299-306.
14. American College of Obstetricians and Gynecologists. Cervical cancer in adolescents: screening, evaluation, and management. Committee Opinion No. 463. *Obstet Gynecol.* 2010;116:469-472.
15. ACS-ASCCP-ASCP Cervical Cancer Guideline Committee. Screening guidelines for the prevention and early detection of cervical cancer. *Ca Cancer J Clin.* 2012;62:147-172.
16. Branson BM, Handsfield H, et al. Revised recommendations for HIV testing of adults, adolescents, and pregnant women in health care settings. *MMWR Recomm Rep.* 2006;55:1-12.
17. Gaydos CA. Nucleic acid amplification tests for gonorrhea and chlamydia: practice and applications. *Infect Dis Clin North Am.* 2005;19:367-386.
18. Association of Public Health Laboratories. Laboratory diagnostic testing for *Chlamydia trachomatis* and *Neiserria gonorrhoeae*: Expert Consultation Meeting Summary Report. January 13-15, 2009:1-6; Atlanta, GA.
19. Workowski KA, Berman S. Sexually transmitted diseases treatment guidelines, 2010. *MMWR Recomm Rep.* 2010;59(RR-12):1-110.
20. Centers for Disease Control and Prevention. Sexually Transmitted Diseases Treatment Guidelines, 2010. Special Populations. Available at http://www.cdc.gov/std/treatment/2010/specialpops.htm#adolescents.

5

21. U.S. Preventive Services Task Force. *Screening for Idiopathic Scoliosis in Adolescents*. Available at http://www.uspreventiveservicestaskforce.org/uspstf/ uspsaisc.htm 2004; 1-3.

22. Andrews JS. Making the most of the sports physical. *Contemp Pediatr*. 1997;14:188.

23. Frankowski BL. Committee on Adolescence. Sexual orientation and adolescents. *Pediatrics*. 2004;113:1827-1832.

24. Committee on Adolescence. Emergency contraception. *Pediatrics*. 2012;130:1174.

25. Centers for Disease Control and Prevention. Division of Reproductive Health, National Center for Chronic Disease Prevention and Health Promotion. U.S. medical eligibility criteria for contraceptive use, 2010. *MMWR Morb Mortal Wkly Rep*. 2010;59:1-84.

26. Calderoni ME, Coupey SM. Combined hormonal contraception. *Adolesc Med*. 2005;16:517-537.

27. Burkett AM. Progestin-only contraceptives and their use in adolescents: clinical options and medical indications. *Adolesc Med Clin*. 2005;16:553-567.

28. Zurawin RK, Ayensu-Coker L. Innovations in contraception: a review. *Clin Obstet Gynecol*. 2007;50:425-439.

29. Shain BM. Suicide and suicide attempts in adolescents. *Pediatrics*. 2007;120:669-676.

30. Committee on Substance Abuse. Substance use screening, brief intervention, and referral to treatment for pediatricians. *Pediatrics*. 2011;128:e1330.

Chapter 6

Analgesia and Procedural Sedation

Sean Barnes, MD, MBA

⊗ See additional content on Expert Consult

I. WEB RESOURCES

International Association for the Study of Pain: http://childpain.org/
American Pain Society: http://www.ampainsoc.org/
American Society of Anesthesiologists: http://www.asahq.org/

II. PAIN ASSESSMENT

A. Infant[1]

1. **Physiologic responses seen primarily in acute pain; subsides with continuing/chronic pain.** Characterized by oxygen desaturation, crying, diaphoresis, flushing or pallor, and increases in blood pressure, heart rate, and respiratory rate.

2. **Behavioral response (Table 6-1):**
   a. Observe characteristics and duration of cry, facial expressions, visual tracking, body movements, and response to stimuli.
   b. Neonatal Infant Pain Scale (NIPS): Behavioral assessment tool for the preterm neonate and full-term neonate up to 6 weeks after birth.
   c. FLACC scale (Table 6-2): Measures and evaluates pain interventions by quantifying pain behaviors like **F**acial expression, **L**eg movement, **A**ctivity, **C**ry, and **C**onsolability, with scores ranging from 0–10.[2] Revised FLACC scale reliable for children with cognitive impairment.[3]

B. Preschooler

In addition to physiologic and behavioral responses, the **FACES** pain rating scale can be used to assess pain intensity in children as young as 3 years of age (Fig. 6-1).

C. School-Age and Adolescent

Evaluate physiologic and behavioral responses; ask about description, location, and character of pain. Starting at age 7, children can use the standard pain rating scale (0 is no pain and 10 is the worst pain ever experienced).

III. ANALGESICS[1,4]

A. Nonopioid Analgesics

Weak analgesics with antipyretic activity are commonly used to manage mild to moderate pain of nonvisceral origin. Administer alone or in

TABLE 6-1

DEVELOPMENTAL RESPONSES TO PAIN

Stage	Age	Response
Infant	<6 mo	No expression of anticipatory fear. Level of anxiety reflects that of the parent.
	6–18 mo	Anticipatory fear of painful experiences begins to develop.
Preschooler	18–24 mo	Verbalization. Children express pain with words such as "hurt" and "boo-boo."
	3 yr	Localization and identification of external causes. Children more reliably assess their pain but continue to depend on visual cues for localization and are unable to understand a reason for pain.
School-age child	5–7 yr	Cooperation. Children have improved understanding of pain and ability to localize it and cooperate.

Data from Yaster, M, et al. Cognitive Development Aspects of Pain in School-Age Children. Pain In Infants, Children, and Adolescents. 1993; 65-74.

TABLE 6-2

FLACC PAIN ASSESSMENT TOOL

FACE

0—No particular expression or smile
1—Occasional grimace or frown, withdrawn, disinterested
2—Frequent to constant frown, quivering chin, clenched jaw

LEGS

0—Normal position or relaxed
1—Uneasy, restless, tense
2—Kicking or legs drawn up

ACTIVITY

0—Lying quietly, normal position, moves easily
1—Squirming, shifting back and forth, tense
2—Arched, rigid, or jerking

CRY

0—No cry (awake or asleep)
1—Moans or whimpers, occasional complaint
2—Crying steadily, screams or sobs, frequent complaints

CONSOLABILITY

0—Content, relaxed
1—Reassured by occasional touching, hugging, or being talked to; distractible
2—Difficult to console or comfort

Modified from Manworren R, Hynan L. Clinical validation of FLACC: preverbal patient pain scale. *Pediatr Nurs.* 2003;29:140-146.

combination with opiates. Drugs, routes of administration, and specific comments are as follows:

1. **Acetaminophen (by mouth [PO]/per rectum [PR]/intravenous [IV]):** Weak analgesic with no anti-inflammatory activity; no platelet inhibition or gastrointestinal (GI) irritation. Hepatotoxicity with high doses.
2. **Aspirin (PO/PR):** Associated with platelet inhibition and GI irritation. Avoid in pediatrics, owing to risk of Reye syndrome.

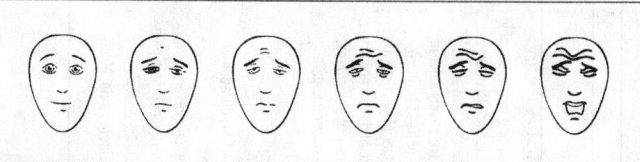

FIGURE 6-1

Faces pain scale. *(From Hicks CL, von Baeyer CL, Spafford PA, et al. The Faces Pain Scale-Revised: toward a common metric in pediatric pain measurement. Pain. 2001;93:173-183. With instructions and translations as found on the website: http://www.usask.ca/childpain/fpsr/. This Faces Pain Scale-Revised has been reproduced with permission of the International Association for the Study of Pain [IASP]. The figure may not be reproduced for any other purpose without permission.)*

3. **Choline magnesium trisalicylate (PO):** No platelet inhibition. Also associated with Reye syndrome.
4. **Nonsteroidal anti-inflammatory drugs (NSAIDs):** Ibuprofen (PO), ketorolac (IV/intramuscular [IM]/PO), naproxen (PO)
   a. Especially useful for sickle cell, bony, rheumatic, and inflammatory pain
   b. Associated with GI symptoms (epigastric pain, gastritis, GI bleeding): Recommend histamine-2-receptor blocker concurrently with prolonged use
   c. Other adverse effects: Interference with platelet aggregation, bronchoconstriction, hypersensitivity reactions, and azotemia. May interfere with bone healing. Should be avoided in patients with severe renal disease, dehydration, or heart failure.
   NOTE: Ketorolac is a potent analgesic (1 mg/kg IV is equivalent to 0.1 mg/kg morphine). Only parenteral NSAID available.
   See the quick reference to analgesics drugs in Table EC 6-A on Expert Consult.
B. **Opioids (Table 6-3)**
1. **Produce analgesia by binding mu receptors in the brain and spinal cord**
2. **Most flexible and widely used analgesics for moderate and severe pain**
3. **Side effects:** Pruritus, nausea, vomiting, constipation, urine retention, and (rarely) respiratory depression and hypotension
4. **Morphine:** Gold standard of this drug class
C. **Local Anesthetics[4-7]**

   Administered topically or subcutaneously into peripheral nerves (e.g., digital nerve, penile nerve block) or centrally (epidural/spinal). They act by temporarily blocking nerve conduction at the sodium channel.
1. **For all local anesthetics, 1% solution = 10 mg/mL**
2. **Topical local anesthetics** (Table 6-4)[8]
3. **Injectable local anesthetics** (Table 6-5):
   a. Infiltration of the skin at the site: Used for painful procedures such as wound closure, IV line placement, or lumbar puncture

TABLE 6-3

COMMONLY USED OPIATES

Drug	Route; Equi-analgesic Doses (mg/kg/dose)	Onset (min)	Duration (hr)	Side Effects	Comments
Codeine	PO; 1.2	30–60	3–4	• Can cause severe nausea and vomiting • Histamine release	**No longer recommended in pediatrics;** 3%–5% of population overmetabolize, potentially leading to catastrophic overdose. Converted in liver to morphine (10%). Newborns and 10% of U.S. population cannot make this conversion.
Fentanyl	IV; 0.001 Transdermal; 0.001 Transmucosal; 0.01	1–2 12 15	0.5–1 2–3	• Pruritus • Bradycardia • Chest wall rigidity with doses >5 mcg/kg (but can occur at all doses); treat with naloxone or neuromuscular blockade	Rarely causes cardiovascular instability (relatively safer in hypovolemia, congenital heart disease, or head trauma). Respiratory depressant effect much longer (4 hr) than analgesic effect. Levels of unbound drug are higher in newborns. Most commonly used opioid for short, painful procedures, but transdermal route is more effective in chronic pain situations.
Hydromorphone	IV/SQ; 0.015 PO; 0.02–0.1	5–10 30–60	3–4	• Less sedation, nausea, pruritus than morphine.	
Methadone	IV; 0.1 PO; 0.1	5–10 30–60	4–24 4–24		Initial dose may produce analgesia for 3–4 hr; duration of action is increased with repeated dosing.
Morphine	IV; 0.1 IM/SQ; 0.1–0.2 PO; 0.3–0.5	5–10 10–30 30–60	3–4 4–5 4–5	• Seizures in neonates • Can cause significant histamine release	The gold standard against which all other opioids are compared. Available in sustained-release form for chronic pain.
Oxycodone	PO; 0.1	30–60	3–4		Available in sustained-release form for chronic pain. Much less nauseating than codeine.

IM, Intramuscular; IV, intravenous; PO, by mouth; SQ, subcutaneous.
Modified from Yaster M, Cote C, Krane E, et al. *Pediatric Pain Management and Sedation Handbook.* St Louis: Mosby, 1997:29-50.

TABLE 6-4

COMMONLY USED TOPICAL LOCAL ANESTHETICS[8]

	Components	Indications	Peak Effect	Duration*	Cautions†
EMLA	Lidocaine 2.5% Prilocaine 2.5%	Intact skin only Venipuncture, circumcision, LP, abscess drainage, BMA	60 min	90 min	Methemoglobinemia: not for use in patients predisposed to methemoglobinemia (e.g., G6PD deficiency, some medications) Infants <3 mo of age: use sparingly (up to 1 g is safe)
LMX	Lidocaine 4%	Same as EMLA	30 min	60 min	Same as EMLA
LET	Lidocaine 4% Epinephrine 0.1% Tetracaine 0.5% Can be mixed with cellulose to create a gel	Safe for nonintact skin Lacerations Not for use in contaminated wounds	30 min	45 min	Vasoconstriction: contraindicated in areas supplied by endarteries (e.g., pinna, nose, penis, digits) Avoid contact with mucus membranes
Viscous lidocaine	Lidocaine 2% May be mixed with Maalox and Benadryl elixir in a 1:1:1 ratio for palatability	Safe for nonintact skin Mucous membranes (e.g., urethral catheter placement, mucositis)	10 min	30 min	Overuse can lead to life-threatening toxicity Not to be used for teething

*Approximate.
†Maximum lidocaine dose is 5 mg/kg.
BMA, Bone marrow aspiration; EMLA, eutectic mixture of local anesthetics; G6PD, glucose-6-phosphate dehydrogenase; LP, lumbar puncture.

TABLE 6-5

COMMONLY USED INJECTABLE LOCAL ANESTHETICS[1,5]

Agent	Concentration (%) (1% solution = 10 mg/mL)	Max dose (mg/kg)	Onset (min)	Duration (hr)
Lidocaine	0.5–2	5	3	0.5–2
Lidocaine with epinephrine	0.5–2	7	3	1–3
Bupivicaine	0.25–0.75	2.5	15	2–4
Bupivicaine with epinephrine	0.25–0.75	3	15	4–8
Ropivacaine	0.2–0.5	3.5	15	2–4

NOTE: Max volume = (max mg/kg × weight in kg)/(% solution × 10).
Data from St Germain Brent A. The management of pain in the emergency department. *Pediatr Clin North Am.* 2000;47:651-679; and Yaster M, Cote C, Krane E, et al. *Pediatric Pain Management and Sedation Handbook.* St Louis: Mosby, 1997:51-72.

b. To reduce stinging from injection, use a small needle (27- to 30-gauge). Alkalinize anesthetic: Add 1 mL (1 mEq) sodium bicarbonate to 9 mL lidocaine (or 29 mL bupivacaine), use lowest concentration of anesthetic available, warm solution (between 37° and 42° C), inject anesthetic slowly, and rub skin at injection site first.

c. To enhance efficacy and duration, add epinephrine to decrease vascular uptake. **Never use local anesthetics with epinephrine in areas supplied by end arteries (e.g., pinna, digits, nasal tip, penis).**

d. Toxicity: Central nervous system (CNS) and cardiac toxicity are of greatest concern. CNS symptoms are seen before cardiovascular collapse. Progression of symptoms: Perioral numbness, dizziness, auditory disturbances, muscular twitching, unconsciousness, seizures, coma, respiratory arrest, cardiovascular collapse. It is important to calculate the volume limit of the local anesthetic and always draw up less than the maximum volume (see Formulary for maximum doses). Lipid emulsion therapy and possibly cardiopulmonary bypass may be required for systemic toxicity. If concerned for systemic toxicity, please contact an anesthesiologist.
NOTE: Bupivicaine is associated with more severe cardiac toxicity than lidocaine.

D. Nonpharmacologic Measures of Pain Relief[9,10]

1. **Sucrose for neonates (Sweet Ease):**

a. Indications: Procedures like heel sticks, immunizations, venipuncture, IV line insertion, arterial puncture, insertion of a Foley catheter, and lumbar puncture in neonates and infants. Strongest evidence exists for infants 0–1 month of age,[9] but more recent evidence suggests efficacy up to 12 months.[10]

b. Procedure: administer up to 2 mL of 24% sucrose into the infant's mouth by syringe or from a nipple/pacifier ~ 2 minutes before procedure.
NOTE: Effective doses in very low-birth-weight infants may be as low as 0.05–0.1 mL 24% sucrose, and in term neonates may be as high as 2 mL 24% sucrose.

c. May be given for more than one procedure within a relatively short period of time but should not be administered more than twice in 1 hour.
NOTE: Studies have suggested potential adverse neurocognitive effects with many repeated doses.[10]

d. Effectiveness has been most often studied with adjunctive pacifier/nipple and parental holding, which may contribute to stress/pain alleviation.

e. Avoid use if patient is under nothing by mouth (NPO) restrictions.

2. **Parental presence**
3. **Distraction with toys**
4. **Child life specialists strongly encouraged**

IV. PATIENT-CONTROLLED ANALGESIA

A. Definition

Patient-controlled analgesia (PCA) is a device that enables a patient to receive continuous (basal) opioids and/or self-administer small supplemental

TABLE 6-6					
ORDERS FOR PATIENT-CONTROLLED ANALGESIA					
Drug	Basal Rate (mcg/kg/hr)	Bolus Dose (mcg/kg)	Lockout Period (min)	Boluses (hr)	Max Dose (mcg/kg/hr)
Morphine	10–30	10–30	6–10	4–6	100–150
Hydromorphone	3–5	3–5	6–10	4–6	15–20
Fentanyl	0.5–1	0.5–10	6–10	2–3	2–4

Data from Yaster M, Cote C, Krane E, et al. *Pediatric Pain Management and Sedation Handbook.* St Louis: Mosby, 1997:100.

doses (bolus) of analgesics on an as-needed basis. In children younger than 6 years (or physically/mentally handicapped), a family member, caregiver, or nurse may administer doses (i.e., surrogate PCA, PCA by proxy, or parent/nurse-controlled analgesia).

B. Indications

Moderate to severe pain of acute or chronic nature. Commonly used in sickle cell disease, postsurgery, posttrauma, burns, and cancer. Also for preemptive pain management (e.g., to facilitate dressing changes).

C. Routes of Administration

IV, SQ, or epidural

D. Agents (Table 6-6)

E. Complications

1. **Pruritus, nausea, constipation, urine retention, excessive drowsiness, respiratory depression.**
2. **Consider a low-dose naloxone (Narcan) infusion (1 mcg/kg/hr) to reduce pruritus and nausea.**

V. OPIOID TAPERING[4]

A. Indication

Tapering schedule is required if the patient has received frequent opioid analgesics for >5–10 days, owing to development of dependence and potential for withdrawal.

B. Withdrawal

1. **See Box 18-1 for symptoms of opiate withdrawal.**
2. **Onset of signs and symptoms:** 6–12 hours after last dose of morphine, 36–48 hours after last dose of methadone.
3. **Duration:** 7–14 days; peak intensity reached within 2–4 days.

C. Guidelines

1. **Conversion:** Convert all drugs to a single equi-analgesic member of that group (Table 6-7).
2. **PCA wean:** Change drug dosing from continuous/intermittent IV infusion to PO bolus therapy around the clock. If on PCA, administer first PO dose, then stop basal infusion 30–60 minutes later. Keep bolus doses,

TABLE 6-7
RELATIVE POTENCIES AND EQUIVALENCE OF OPIOIDS

Drug	Morphine Equivalence Ratio	IV Dose (mg/kg)	Equivalent PO Dose (mg/kg)
Meperidine	0.1	1	1.5–2
Methadone	0.25–1*	0.1	0.1
Morphine	1	0.1	0.3–0.5
Hydromorphone	5–7	0.015	0.02–0.1
Fentanyl	80–100	0.001	NA

*Morphine-to-methadone conversion in tolerant/dependent patient is variable. We recommend starting at the lowest conversion ratio, 0.25.

NOTE: Removing a transdermal fentanyl patch does not stop opioid uptake from the skin; fentanyl will continue to be absorbed for 12–24 hr after patch removal (fentanyl 25-mcg patch administers 25 mcg/hr of fentanyl).

IV, Intravenous; NA, not applicable; PO, by mouth.

From Yaster M, Cote C, Krane E, et al. *Pediatric Pain Management and Sedation Handbook*. St Louis: Mosby, 1997:40.

but reduce by 25%–50%. Discontinue PCA if no boluses are required in next 6 hours, increase PO dose, or add adjuvant analgesic (e.g., NSAID).

3. **Slow dose decrease:** During an intermittent IV/PO wean, decrease total daily dose by 10%–20% of original dose every 1–2 days (e.g., to taper a morphine dose of 40 mg/day, decrease the daily dose by 4–8 mg every 1–2 days).

4. **Oral regimen:** If not done previously, convert IV dosing to equivalent PO administration 1–2 days before discharge, and continue titration as outlined previously.

5. **Adjunctive therapy:** α_2-Agonists (e.g., clonidine, dexmedetomidine)

a. Clonidine in combination with opioid has been shown to decrease length of time needed for opioid weaning in neonatal abstinence syndrome, with few short-term side effects. Long-term safety has yet to be thoroughly investigated.[11]

b. Limited data exist evaluating use of oral clonidine in iatrogenic opioid abstinence syndrome in critically ill patients, but both transdermal clonidine and dexmedetomidine have shown promise.[12]

c. Several studies have examined use of clonidine in treating opioid dependence, but insufficient data exist to support its routine use outside of possibly the neonatal setting.[13]

D. **Examples (Box 6-1)**

VI. PROCEDURAL SEDATION[1,4-7,14]

A. **Definitions**

1. **Mild sedation (anxiolysis):** Intent is anxiolysis with maintenance of consciousness. Practically, obtained when a single drug is given once at a low dose (not chloral hydrate). Mild sedation can easily progress to deep sedation and general anesthesia.

BOX 6-1

EXAMPLES OF OPIOID TAPERING

EXAMPLE 1

Patient on morphine patient-controlled analgesia (PCA) to be converted to oral (PO) morphine with home weaning.

For example: morphine PCA basal rate = 2 mg/hr, average bolus rate = 0.5 mg/hr

Step 1: Calculate daily dose: basal + bolus = (2 mg/hr × 24 hr) + (0.5 mg/hr × 24 hr) = 60 mg intravenous (IV) morphine

Step 2: Convert according to drug potency: morphine IV/morphine oral = approx 3:1 potency; 3 × 60 mg = 180 mg PO morphine

Step 3: Prescribe 90 mg BID or 60 mg TID; wean 10%–20% of original dose (30 mg) every 1–2 days

EXAMPLE 2

Patient on morphine PCA to be converted to transdermal fentanyl. Morphine PCA basal rate = 2 mg/hr. No boluses.

Step 1: Convert according to drug potency: fentanyl/morphine = approx 100:1 potency; 2 mg/hr morphine = 2000 mcg/hr morphine = 20 mcg/hr fentanyl

Step 2: Prescribe 25-mcg fentanyl patch (delivers 25 mcg/hr fentanyl)

Step 3: Stop IV morphine 8 hr after patch is applied; prescribe second patch at 72 hr

Step 4: Prescribe as-needed (PRN) IV morphine with caution

Data from Yaster M, Cote C, Krane E, et al. *Pediatric Pain Management and Sedation Handbook.* St Louis: Mosby, 1997:29-50.

2. **Moderate sedation:** Formerly known as *conscious sedation*. A controlled state of depressed consciousness during which airway reflexes and airway patency are maintained. Patient responds appropriately to age-appropriate commands ("Open your eyes.") and light touch. Practically, obtained any time a combination of sedative-hypnotic and analgesic is used. Moderate sedation can easily progress to deep sedation and general anesthesia.

3. **Deep sedation:** A controlled state of depressed consciousness during which airway reflexes and airway patency may not be maintained, and the child is unable to respond to physical or verbal stimuli. Practically, required for most painful procedures in children. The following IV drugs always produce deep sedation: propofol, etomidate, thiopental, methohexital. Deep sedation can progress to general anesthesia.

4. **Dissociative sedation:** Unique state of sedation achieved with ketamine. Deep level of depressed consciousness, but airway reflexes and patency are generally maintained.

See the Quick Reference to Sedative-Hypnotic Drugs in Table EC 6-A.

B. Preparation

1. Patient should be **NPO** for solids and clear liquids (Table 6-8 shows current American Society of Anesthesiologists recommendations). See Fig. EC 6-A on Expert Consult for more information on fasting recommendations.

2. **Written informed consent**

TABLE 6-8

FASTING RECOMMENDATIONS FOR ANESTHESIA

Food Type	Minimum Fasting Period (hr)
Clear liquids	2
Breast milk	4
Nonhuman milk, formula	6
Solids	8

Data from Practice guidelines for preoperative fasting and the use of pharmacologic agents to reduce the risk of pulmonary aspiration: application to healthy patients undergoing elective procedures. A report by the American Society of Anesthesiologists Task Force on Preoperative Fasting and Use of Pharmacologic Agents to Reduce the Risk of Pulmonary Aspiration [Online]. http://www.asahq.org/publicationsAndServices/NPO.pdf.

3. **Focused patient history:**
   a. Allergies and medications
   b. Airway (asthma, acute respiratory disease, reactive airway disease), airway obstruction (mediastinal mass, history of noisy breathing, obstructive sleep apnea), craniofacial abnormalities (e.g., Pfeiffer, Crouzon, Apert, Pierre Robin syndromes), recent upper respiratory infection (suggests increased risk of laryngospasm)
   c. Aspiration risk (neuromuscular disease, esophageal disease, altered mental status, obesity, pregnancy)
   d. Prematurity, comorbidities, and adverse reactions to sedatives and anesthesia
4. **Physical examination:** With specific attention to head, ears, eyes, nose, and throat (HEENT); lungs; cardiac examination; and neuromuscular function. Assess ability to open mouth and extend neck. If risk for moderate sedation is too high, consider an anesthesia consultation and general anesthesia.
5. **Determine American Society of Anesthesiologists Physical Status Classification:** See Table EC 6-B on Expert Consult. Class I and II patients are generally good candidates for mild, moderate, or deep sedation outside of the operating room.[15]
6. **Have an emergency plan ready:** Make sure qualified backup personnel and equipment are close by.
7. **Personnel:** Two providers are required. One provider should perform the procedure, and a separate provider should monitor the patient during sedation and recovery.
8. **Ensure IV access.**
9. **Have airway/intubation equipment available** (see Chapter 1).
10. **Medications** to have available: Those for rapid sequence intubation (see Chapter 1) or emergencies (e.g., epinephrine, atropine)
11. **Antagonist** *(reversal)* **agents** should be readily available (e.g., naloxone, flumazenil).

C. Monitoring
1. **Vital signs:** Obtain baseline vital signs (including pulse oximetry). Continuously monitor heart rate and oxygen saturation; intermittently monitor

blood pressure and respiratory rate. Record vital signs at least every 5 minutes until patient returns to presedation level of consciousness.
NOTE: Complications most often occur 5–10 minutes after administration of IV medication and immediately after a procedure is completed (when stimuli associated with the procedure are removed).[7]

2. **Airway:** Frequently assess airway patency and adequacy of ventilation through capnography, auscultation, or direct visualization.

D. Pharmacologic Agents

1. **Goal of sedation:** To tailor drug combination to provide levels of analgesia, sedation-hypnosis, and anxiolysis deep enough to facilitate procedure but shallow enough to avoid loss of airway reflexes.

2. **CNS, cardiovascular, and respiratory depression** are potentiated by combining sedative drugs and/or opioids and by rapid drug infusion. Titrate to effect.

3. **Common sedative/hypnotic agents** (Box 6-2):
   Also see Tables 6-3 and 6-9 for more information on opiates and barbiturates/benzodiazepines.

BOX 6-2

PROPERTIES OF COMMON SEDATIVE-HYPNOTIC AGENTS

SEDATING ANTIHISTAMINES (DIPHENHYDRAMINE, HYDROXYZINE)

- Mild sedative-hypnotics with antiemetic and antipruritic properties; used for sedation and treatment of opiate side effects
- No anxiolytic or analgesic effects

BARBITURATES

- Contraindicated in patients with porphyria; suitable only for nonpainful procedures.
- No anxiolytic or analgesic effects

BENZODIAZEPINES

- Reversible with flumazenil.
- + Anxiolytic effects; no analgesic effects

OPIOIDS

- Reversible with naloxone
- + Analgesic effects; no anxiolytic effects

KETAMINE[1,5,9]

- Phencyclidine derivative that causes potent dissociative anesthesia, analgesia, and amnesia
- Nystagmus indicates likely therapeutic effect
- Vocalizations/movement may occur even with adequate sedation
- Results in "dissociative sedation" by any route
- Onset: IV, 0.5–2 min; IM, 5–10 min; PO/PR, 20–45 min
- Duration: IV, 20–60 min; IM, 30–90 min; PO/PR, 60–120+ min
- *CNS effects:* Increased ICP, emergence delirium with auditory, visual, and tactile hallucinations
- *Cardiovascular effects:* Inhibits catecholamine reuptake, causing increased HR, BP, SVR, PVR, direct myocardial depression

Continued

BOX 6-2

PROPERTIES OF COMMON SEDATIVE-HYPNOTIC AGENTS (Continued)

KETAMINE (Continued)

- ***Respiratory effects:*** Bronchodilation (useful in asthmatics), increased secretions (can result in laryngospasm), maintenance of ventilatory response to hypoxia, relative maintenance of airway reflexes
- ***Other effects:*** Increased muscle tone, myoclonic jerks, increased IOP, nausea, emesis
- **Contraindications:** Increased ICP, increased IOP, hypertension, preexisting psychotic disorders

PROPOFOL

- For purpose of deep sedation or general anesthesia, give 0.5–1 mg/kg IV bolus, followed by 50–100 mcg/kg/min infusion
- Rapid onset and brief recovery (5–15 min), antiemetic, and euphoric
- Caution: Respiratory depression, apnea, hypotension
- + Anxiolytic. No analgesic effects

DEXMEDETOMIDINE*

- Give 0.5–2 mcg/kg IV load over 10 min, followed by 0.2–1 mcg/kg/hr infusion.
- Extremely rapid onset and brief recovery (5–15 min) antiemetic and euphoric.
- Does not cause respiratory depression or apnea.
- + Anxiolytic and analgesic effects.
- Dexmedetomidine can also be given intranasally (1–2 mcg/kg). It will take 30–60 min to attain natural sleep, and patients will briefly awaken with stimulation. Can cause hypotension and bradycardia. Increased cost compared with other medications.

DEXMEDETOMIDINE AND KETAMINE*

- Most effective regimen appears to be use of bolus dose of both agents, dexmedetomidine (1 mcg/kg) and ketamine (1–2 mg/kg), to initiate sedation.
- This can then be followed by a dexmedetomidine infusion (1–2 mcg/kg/hr) with supplemental bolus doses of ketamine (0.5–1 mg/kg) as needed.

*These examples reflect commonly used current protocols at the Johns Hopkins Children's Center; variations are found at other institutions. See Formulary for dosing recommendations.
BP, Blood pressure; CNS, central nervous system; HR, heart rate; ICP, intracranial pressure; IM, intramuscular; IOP, intraocular pressure; IV, intravenous; PO, oral; PR, rectal; PVR, pulmonary vascular resistance; SVR, systemic vascular resistance.
Data from Yaster M, Cote C, Krane E, et al. *Pediatric Pain Management and Sedation Handbook.* St Louis: Mosby, 1997:376-382; St Germain Brent A. The management of pain in the emergency department. *Pediatr Clin North Am.* 2000;47:651-679; and Cote CJ, Lerman J, Todres ID, et al. *A Practice of Anesthesia for Infants and Children.* Philadelphia: WB Saunders, 2001.

4. **Reversal agents:**
a. Naloxone: Opioid antagonist. See Box 6-3 for Narcan administration protocol.
b. Flumazenil: Benzodiazepine antagonist. See Formulary for dosing details.

E. **Discharge Criteria**[15]

1. **Airway is patent and cardiovascular function is stable.**
2. **Easy arousability; intact protective reflexes (swallow and cough, gag reflex).**

TABLE 6-9

COMMONLY USED BENZODIAZEPINES* AND BARBITURATES:1,5,14

Drug Class	Duration of Action	Drug	Route	Onset (min)	Duration (hr)	Comments
Benzodiazepines	Short	Midazolam (Versed)	IV	1–3	1–2	• Has rapid and predictable onset of action, short recovery time
			IM/IN	5–10		• Causes amnesia
			PO/PR	10–30		• Results in mild depression of hypoxic ventilatory drive
	Intermediate	Diazepam (Valium)	IV (painful)	1–3	0.25–1	• Poor choice for procedural sedation
			PR	7–15	2–3	• Excellent for muscle relaxation or prolonged sedation
			PO	30–60	2–3	• Painful on IV injection
	Long	Lorazepam (Ativan)	IV	1–5	3–4	• Faster onset than midazolam
			IM	10–20	3–6	• Poor choice for procedural sedation
			PO	30–60	3–6	• Ideal for prolonged anxiolysis, seizure treatment
Barbiturates	Short	Methohexital	PR†	5–10	1–1.5	• PR form used as sedative for nonpainful procedures
	Intermediate	Pentobarbital	IV	1–10	1–4	• Predictable sedation and immobility for nonpainful procedures
			IM	5–15	2–4	• Minimal respiratory depression when used alone
			PO/PR	15–60	2–4	• Associated with slow wake up and agitation

*Use IV solution for PO, PR, and IN administration. Rectal diazepam gel (Diastat) is also available.
†IV administration produces general anesthesia; only PR should be used for sedation.
IM, Intramuscular; IN, intranasal; IV, intravenous; PO, by mouth; PR, per rectum.
Data from Yaster M, Cote C, Krane E, et al. *Pediatric Pain Management and Sedation Handbook.* St Louis: Mosby, 1997:345-374; St Germain Brent A. The management of pain in the emergency department. *Pediatr Clin North Am.* 2000;47:651-679; and Cote CJ, Lerman J, Todres ID, et al. *A Practice of Anesthesia for Infants and Children.* Philadelphia: WB Saunders, 2001.

6

BOX 6-3

NALOXONE (NARCAN) ADMINISTRATION

INDICATIONS: PATIENTS REQUIRING NALOXONE (NARCAN) USUALLY MEET ALL OF THE FOLLOWING
CRITERIA*

- Unresponsive to physical stimulation
- Shallow respirations or respiratory rate <8 breaths/min†
- Pinpoint pupils

PROCEDURE

1. **Stop opioid administration** (as well as other sedative drugs), start the **ABCs**
   (**A**irway, **B**reathing, **C**irculation), and call for **HELP.**
2. **Dilute naloxone:** Mix 0.4 mg (1 ampule) of naloxone with 9 mL of normal saline
   (final concentration 0.04 mg/mL = 40 mcg/mL)
3. (If child < 40 kg, dilute 0.1 mg (one-fourth ampule) in 9 mL of normal saline to
   make 0.01 mg/mL solution = 10 mcg/mL)
4. **Administer and observe response:** Administer dilute naloxone *slowly* (1–2 mcg/kg/
   dose IV over 2 min). Observe patient response.
5. **Titrate to effect:** Within 1–2 min, patient should open eyes and respond. If not,
   continue until a total dose of 10 mcg/kg is given. If no response is obtained,
   evaluate for other cause of sedation/respiratory depression.
6. **Discontinue naloxone administration:** Discontinue naloxone as soon as patient
   responds (e.g., takes deep breaths when directed).
7. **Caution:** Another dose of naloxone may be required within 30 min of first dose
   (duration of action of naloxone is shorter than that of most opioids).
8. **Monitor patient:** Assign a staff member to monitor sedation/respiratory status and
   remind patient to take deep breaths as necessary.
9. **Alternative analgesia:** Provide nonopioids for pain relief. Resume opioid administration at half the original dose when the patient is easily aroused and respiratory
   rate is >9 breaths/min.

*Patients with significant opiate exposure (sickle cell, cancer) should be carefully evaluated for the
need for naloxone. Reversal of analgesia could produce hypertension, tachycardia, ventricular arrhythmias, and pulmonary edema. If necessary, give at the lowest dose possible and titrate carefully.
†Respiratory rates that require naloxone vary according to infant's/child's usual rate.
Modified from McCaffery M, Pasero C. *Pain: Clinical Manual.* St Louis: Mosby, 1999:269-270.

---

3. **Ability to talk and sit up unaided** (if age appropriate).
4. **Alternatively, for very young or intellectually disabled children,** goal is to
   return as close as possible to presedation level of responsiveness.
5. **Adequate hydration.**
6. **Recovery after sedation protocols** varies but typically ranges from
   60–120 minutes.

F. **Examples of Sedation Protocols (Tables 6-10 and 6-11)**

TABLE 6-10

EXAMPLES OF SEDATION PROTOCOLS*

Protocol/Doses	Comments
Ketamine (1 mg/kg/dose IV × 1–3 doses)	Lowest rates of adverse events when ketamine used alone‡
Ketamine + midazolam + atropine ("ketazolam")	Atropine = antisialogogue
IV route:	Midazolam = counter emergence delirium
Ketamine 1 mg/kg/dose × 1–3 doses	
Midazolam 0.05 mg/kg × 1 dose	
Atropine 0.02 mg/kg × 1 dose	
IM route: combine (use smallest volume possible)	
Ketamine 1.5–2 mg/kg	
Midazolam 0.15–0.2 mg/kg	
Atropine 0.02 mg/kg	
Midazolam + fentanyl	High likelihood of respiratory depression
Midazolam 0.1 mg/kg IV × 3 doses PRN	
Fentanyl 1 mcg/kg IV × 3 doses PRN	Infuse fentanyl no more frequently than Q3 min

*These examples reflect commonly used current protocols at the Johns Hopkins Children's Center; variations are found at other institutions.

‡Green, SM, Roback MG, Krauss B, et al. Predictors of emesis and recovery agitation with emergency department ketamine sedation: an individual-patient data meta-analysis of 8,282 children. *Ann Emerg Med.* 2009;54:171-180.

Modified from Yaster M, Cote C, Krane E, et al. *Pediatric Pain Management and Sedation Handbook.* St Louis: Mosby, 1997.

TABLE 6-11

SUGGESTED ANALGESIA AND SEDATION PROTOCOLS

Pain Threshold	Procedure	Suggested Choices
Nonpainful	CT/MRI/EEG/ECHO	Midazolam*
Mild	Phlebotomy/IV	EMLA
	LP	EMLA (± midazolam)
	Pelvic exam	Midazolam
	Minor laceration, well vascularized	LET
	Minor laceration, not well vascularized	Lidocaine
Moderate	BM aspiration	EMLA (± midazolam)
	Arthrocentesis	Lidocaine (local) for cooperative child or ketamine† for uncooperative child
	Fracture reduction	Ketamine
	Major laceration	Ketamine or fentanyl + midazolam
	Burn debridement	Ketamine or fentanyl + midazolam
	Long procedures (>30 min)	Consider general anesthesia
Severe	Fracture reduction	Ketamine
	Long procedures (>30 min)	Consider general anesthesia

*Caution for antiepileptics for EEG.

†Ketamine should not be chosen with head injury or open globe eye injury.

BM, Bone marrow; CT, computed tomography; ECHO, echocardiogram; EEG, electroencephalogram; EMLA, eutectic mixture of local anesthetics; LP, lumbar puncture; LET, lidocaine, epinephrine, tetracaine; MRI, magnetic resonance imaging.

Modified from Yaster M, Cote C, Krane E, et al. *Pediatric Pain Management and Sedation Handbook.* St Louis: Mosby, 1997:551-552.

6

REFERENCES

1. Yaster M, Cote C, Krane E, et al. *Pediatric Pain Management and Sedation Handbook.* St Louis: Mosby, 1997.
2. Manworren R, Hynan L. Clinical validation of FLACC: preverbal patient pain scale. *Pediatr Nurs.* 2003;29:140-146.
3. Malviya S, Voepel-Lewis T. The revised FLACC observational pain tool: improved reliability and validity for pain assessment in children with cognitive impairment. *Paediatr Anaesth.* 2006;16:258-265.
4. Yaster M, Maxwell LG. Pediatric regional anesthesia. *Anesthesiology.* 1989;70:324-338.
5. St Germain Brent A. The management of pain in the emergency department. *Pediatr Clin North Am.* 2000;47:651-679.
6. Krauss B, Green S. Procedural sedation and analgesia in children. *Lancet.* 2006;367:766-780.
7. Krauss B, Green SM. Sedation and analgesia for procedures in children. *N Engl J Med.* 2000;342:938.
8. Zempsky W, Cravero J. Relief of pain and anxiety in pediatric patients in emergency medical systems. *Pediatrics.* 2004;114:1348-1356.
9. Stevens B, Yamada J, Ohlsson A. Sucrose for analgesia in newborn infants undergoing painful procedures (review). *Cochrane Database Syst Rev.* 2010;1:CD00106.
10. Harrison D, Stevens B, Bueno M, et al. Efficacy of sweet solutions for analgesia in infants between 1 and 12 months of age: a systematic review. *Arch Dis Child.* 2010;95:406-413.
11. Agthe AG, Kim GR, Mathias KB, et al. Clonidine as an adjunct therapy to opioids for neonatal abstinence syndrome: a randomized, controlled trial. *Pediatrics.* 2009;123:e849-e856.
12. Honey BL, Benefield RJ, Miller JL, et al. α2-Receptor agonists for treatment and prevention of iatrogenic opioid abstinence syndrome in critically ill patients. *Ann Pharmacother.* 2009;43:1506-1511.
13. Gowing L, Farrell M, Ali R, et al. Alpha-2 adrenergic agonists for the management of opioid withdrawal (review). *Cochrane Database Syst Rev.* 2009;3:CD002024.
14. Cote CJ, Lerman J, Todres ID. *APractice of Anesthesia for Infants and Children.* 4th ed Philadelphia: WB Saunders, 2008.
15. American Academy of Pediatrics Committee on Drugs. Guidelines for monitoring and management of pediatric patients during and after sedation for diagnostic and therapeutic procedures: an update. *Pediatrics.* 2006;118:2587-2602.
16. Agrawal D, Manzi SF, Gupta R, Krauss B. Preprocedural fasting state and adverse events in children undergoing procedural sedation and analgesia in a pediatric emergency department. *Ann Emerg Med.* 2003;42:636-646.

Chapter 7

Cardiology

Catherine B. Gretchen, MD, and
Arpana S. Rayannavar, MD

See additional content on Expert Consult

I. WEBSITES

http://www.pted.org
http://www.murmurlab.org

II. THE CARDIAC CYCLE (FIG. 7-1)

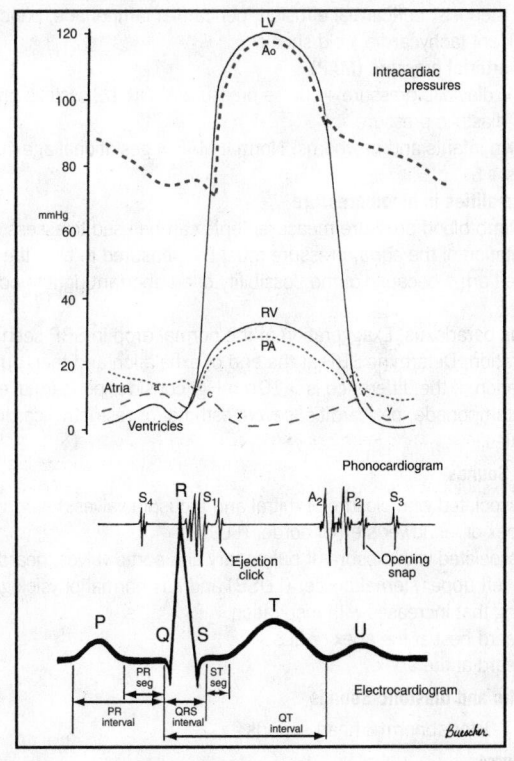

FIGURE 7-1

The cardiac cycle.

III. PHYSICAL EXAMINATION

A. Heart Rate

Refer to Table 7-4 for normal heart rate (HR) by age.

B. Blood Pressure

1. **Blood pressure:**
a. Blood pressure norms (systolic blood pressure [SBP], diastolic blood pressure [DBP]) by age[1,2]: Tables 7-1 and 7-2; Figs. 7-2, 7-3, and 7-4 For blood pressure norms for preterm infants, see Expert Consult: Table EC 7-A.
2. **Pulse pressure** = systolic pressure − diastolic pressure.
a. Wide pulse pressure (>40 mmHg): Differential diagnosis includes aortic insufficiency, arteriovenous fistula, patent ductus arteriosus, thyrotoxicosis, warm shock.
b. Narrow pulse pressure (<25 mmHg): Differential diagnosis includes aortic stenosis, pericardial effusion, pericardial tamponade, pericarditis, significant tachycardia, cold shock.
3. **Mean arterial pressure (MAP)**
a. MAP = diastolic pressure + (pulse pressure/3) OR 1/3 systolic pressure + 2/3 diastolic pressure.
b. Preterm infants and newborns: Normal MAP = gestational age in weeks + 5.
4. **Abnormalities in blood pressure**
a. Four-limb blood pressure measurements can be used to assess for coarctation of the aorta; pressure must be measured in both the right and left arms because of the possibility of an aberrant right subclavian artery.
b. Pulsus paradoxus: Exaggeration of the normal drop in SBP seen with inspiration. Determine SBP at the end of exhalation and then during inhalation; if the difference is > 10 mmHg, consider pericardial effusion, tamponade, pericarditis, severe asthma, or restrictive cardiomyopathies.

C. Heart Sounds

1. S_1: Associated with closure of mitral and tricuspid valves; heard best at the apex or left lower sternal border (LLSB).
2. S_2: Associated with closure of pulmonary and aortic valves; heard best at the left upper sternal border (LUSB) and has normal physiologic splitting that increases with inspiration.
3. S_3: Heard best at the apex or LLSB.
4. S_4: Heard at the apex.

D. Systolic and Diastolic Sounds

See Box 7-1 for abnormal heart sounds.[3]

E. Murmurs[4]

More information at http://www.murmurlab.org. Clinical characteristics summarized in Table 7-3.[3]

TABLE 7-1

BLOOD PRESSURE LEVELS FOR THE 50TH, 90TH, 95TH, AND 99TH PERCENTILES OF BLOOD PRESSURE FOR GIRLS AGE 1–17 YEARS BY PERCENTILES OF HEIGHT[2]

Age, yr	BP Percentile†	SBP, mmHg							DBP, mmHg						
		Percentile of Height*							Percentile of Height*						
		5th	10th	25th	50th	75th	90th	95th	5th	10th	25th	50th	75th	90th	95th
1	50th	83	84	85	86	88	89	90	38	39	39	40	41	41	42
	90th	97	97	98	100	101	102	103	52	53	53	54	55	55	56
	95th	100	101	102	104	105	106	107	56	57	57	58	59	59	60
	99th	108	108	109	111	112	113	114	64	64	65	65	66	67	67
2	50th	85	85	87	88	89	91	91	43	44	44	45	46	46	47
	90th	98	99	100	101	103	104	105	57	58	58	59	60	61	61
	95th	102	103	104	105	107	108	109	61	62	62	63	64	65	65
	99th	109	110	111	112	114	115	116	69	69	70	70	71	72	72
3	50th	86	87	88	89	91	92	93	47	48	48	49	50	50	51
	90th	100	100	102	103	104	106	106	61	62	62	63	64	64	65
	95th	104	104	105	107	108	109	110	65	66	66	67	68	68	69
	99th	111	111	113	114	115	116	117	73	73	74	74	75	76	76
4	50th	88	88	90	91	92	94	94	50	50	51	52	52	53	54
	90th	101	102	103	104	106	107	108	64	64	65	66	67	67	68
	95th	105	106	107	108	110	111	112	68	68	69	70	71	71	72
	99th	112	113	114	115	117	118	119	76	76	76	77	78	79	79
5	50th	89	90	91	93	94	95	96	52	53	53	54	55	55	56
	90th	103	103	105	106	107	109	109	66	67	67	68	69	69	70
	95th	107	107	108	110	111	112	113	70	71	71	72	73	73	74
	99th	114	114	116	117	118	120	120	78	78	79	79	80	81	81

Continued

TABLE 7-1

BLOOD PRESSURE LEVELS FOR THE 50TH, 90TH, 95TH, AND 99TH PERCENTILES OF BLOOD PRESSURE FOR GIRLS AGE 1–17 YEARS BY PERCENTILES OF HEIGHT (Continued)

Age, yr	BP Percentile	SBP, mmHg							DBP, mmHg						
		Percentile of Height*							Percentile of Height*						
		5th	10th	25th	50th	75th	90th	95th	5th	10th	25th	50th	75th	90th	95th
6	50th	91	92	93	94	96	97	98	54	54	55	56	56	57	58
	90th	104	105	106	108	109	110	111	68	68	69	70	71	72	72
	95th	108	109	110	111	113	114	115	72	72	73	74	74	75	76
	99th	115	116	117	119	120	121	122	80	80	80	81	82	83	83
7	50th	93	93	95	96	97	99	99	55	56	56	57	58	58	59
	90th	106	107	108	109	111	112	113	69	70	70	71	72	72	73
	95th	110	111	112	113	115	116	116	73	74	74	75	76	76	77
	99th	117	118	119	120	122	123	124	81	81	82	82	83	84	84
8	50th	95	95	96	98	99	100	101	57	57	57	58	59	60	60
	90th	108	109	110	111	113	114	114	71	71	71	72	73	74	74
	95th	112	112	114	115	116	118	118	75	75	75	76	77	78	78
	99th	119	120	121	122	123	125	125	82	82	83	83	84	86	86
9	50th	96	97	98	100	101	102	103	58	58	58	59	60	61	61
	90th	110	110	112	113	114	116	116	72	72	72	73	74	75	75
	95th	114	114	115	118	118	119	120	76	76	76	77	78	79	79
	99th	121	121	123	124	125	127	127	83	83	84	84	85	87	87
10	50th	98	99	100	102	103	104	105	59	59	59	60	61	62	62
	90th	112	112	114	115	116	118	118	73	73	73	74	75	76	76
	95th	116	116	117	119	120	121	122	77	77	77	78	79	80	80

TABLE 7-1

BLOOD PRESSURE LEVELS FOR THE 50TH, 90TH, 95TH, AND 99TH PERCENTILES OF BLOOD PRESSURE FOR GIRLS AGE 1–17 YEARS BY PERCENTILES OF HEIGHT (Continued)

Age, yr	BP Percentile†	SBP, mmHg							DBP, mmHg						
		5th	10th	25th	50th	75th	90th	95th	5th	10th	25th	50th	75th	90th	95th
11	99th	123	123	125	126	127	129	129	84	84	85	86	86	87	88
	50th	100	101	102	103	105	106	107	60	60	60	61	62	63	63
	90th	114	114	116	117	118	119	120	74	74	74	75	76	77	77
	95th	118	118	119	121	122	123	124	78	78	78	79	80	81	81
	99th	125	125	126	128	129	130	131	85	85	86	87	87	88	89
12	50th	102	103	104	105	107	108	109	61	61	61	62	63	64	64
	90th	116	116	117	119	120	121	122	75	75	75	76	77	78	78
	95th	119	120	121	123	124	125	126	79	79	79	80	81	82	82
	99th	127	127	128	130	131	132	133	86	86	87	88	88	89	90
13	50th	104	105	106	107	109	110	110	62	62	62	63	64	65	65
	90th	117	118	119	121	122	123	124	76	76	76	77	78	79	79
	95th	121	122	123	124	126	127	128	80	80	80	81	82	83	83
	99th	128	129	130	132	133	134	135	87	87	88	89	89	90	91
14	50th	106	106	107	109	110	111	112	63	63	63	64	65	66	66
	90th	119	120	121	122	124	125	125	77	77	77	78	79	80	80
	95th	123	123	125	126	127	129	129	81	81	81	82	83	84	84
	99th	130	131	132	133	135	136	136	88	88	89	90	90	91	92
15	50th	107	108	109	110	111	113	113	64	64	64	65	66	67	67
	90th	120	121	122	123	125	126	127	78	78	78	79	80	81	81
	95th	124	125	126	127	129	130	131	82	82	82	83	84	85	85

Continued

TABLE 7-1

BLOOD PRESSURE LEVELS FOR THE 50TH, 90TH, 95TH, AND 99TH PERCENTILES OF BLOOD PRESSURE FOR GIRLS AGE 1–17 YEARS BY PERCENTILES OF HEIGHT (Continued)

Age, yr	BP Percentile†	SBP, mmHg							DBP, mmHg						
		Percentile of Height*							Percentile of Height*						
		5th	10th	25th	50th	75th	90th	95th	5th	10th	25th	50th	75th	90th	95th
	99th	131	132	133	134	136	137	138	89	89	90	91	91	92	93
16	50th	108	108	110	111	112	114	114	64	64	65	66	66	67	68
	90th	121	122	123	124	126	127	128	78	78	79	80	81	81	82
	95th	125	126	127	128	130	131	132	82	82	83	84	85	85	86
	99th	132	133	134	135	137	138	139	90	90	90	91	92	93	93
17	50th	108	109	110	111	113	114	115	64	65	65	66	67	67	68
	90th	122	122	123	125	126	127	128	78	79	79	80	81	81	82
	95th	125	126	127	129	130	131	132	82	83	83	84	85	85	86
	99th	133	133	134	136	137	138	139	90	90	91	91	92	93	93

*Height percentile determined by standard growth curves.

†Blood pressure percentile determined by a single measurement.

Adapted from National High Blood Pressure Education Program Working Group on High Blood Pressure in Children and Adolescents. The fourth report on the diagnosis, evaluation, and treatment of high blood pressure in children and adolescents. *Pediatrics.* 2004;114(2 Suppl):555-576.

TABLE 7-2

BLOOD PRESSURE LEVELS FOR THE 50TH, 90TH, 95TH, AND 99TH PERCENTILES OF BLOOD PRESSURE FOR BOYS AGE 1–17 YEARS BY PERCENTILES OF HEIGHT[2]

| | | SBP, mmHg | | | | | | | DBP, mmHg | | | | | | |
| | | Percentile of Height* | | | | | | | Percentile of Height* | | | | | | |
Age, yr	BP Percentile[†]	5th	10th	25th	50th	75th	90th	95th	5th	10th	25th	50th	75th	90th	95th
1	50th	80	81	83	85	87	88	89	34	35	36	37	38	39	39
	90th	94	95	97	99	100	102	103	49	50	51	52	53	53	54
	95th	98	99	101	103	104	106	106	54	54	55	56	57	58	58
	99th	105	106	108	110	112	113	114	61	62	63	64	65	66	66
2	50th	84	85	87	88	90	92	92	39	40	41	42	43	44	44
	90th	97	99	100	102	104	105	106	54	55	56	57	58	58	59
	95th	101	102	104	106	108	109	110	59	59	60	61	62	63	63
	99th	109	110	111	113	115	117	117	66	67	68	69	70	71	71
3	50th	86	87	89	91	93	94	95	44	44	45	46	47	48	48
	90th	100	101	103	105	107	108	109	59	59	60	61	62	63	63
	95th	104	105	107	109	110	112	113	63	63	64	65	66	67	67
	99th	111	112	114	116	118	119	120	71	71	72	73	74	75	75
4	50th	88	89	91	93	95	96	97	47	48	49	50	51	51	52
	90th	102	103	105	107	109	110	111	62	63	64	65	66	66	67
	95th	106	107	109	111	112	114	115	66	67	68	69	70	71	71
	99th	113	114	116	118	120	121	122	74	75	76	77	78	79	79
5	50th	90	91	93	95	96	98	98	50	51	52	53	54	55	55
	90th	104	105	106	108	110	111	112	65	66	67	68	69	69	70
	95th	108	109	110	112	114	115	116	69	70	71	72	73	74	74
	99th	115	116	118	120	121	123	123	77	78	79	80	81	82	82
6	50th	91	92	94	96	98	99	100	53	53	54	55	56	57	57
	90th	105	166	108	110	111	113	113	68	68	69	70	71	72	72
	95th	109	110	112	114	115	117	117	72	72	73	74	75	76	76
	99th	116	117	119	121	123	124	125	80	80	81	82	83	84	84

Continued

TABLE 7-2

BLOOD PRESSURE LEVELS FOR THE 50TH, 90TH, 95TH, AND 99TH PERCENTILES OF BLOOD PRESSURE FOR BOYS AGE 1–17 YEARS BY PERCENTILES OF HEIGHT (Continued)

Age, yr	BP Percentile†	SBP, mmHg							DBP, mmHg						
		Percentile of Height*							Percentile of Height*						
		5th	10th	25th	50th	75th	90th	95th	5th	10th	25th	50th	75th	90th	95th
7	50th	92	94	95	97	99	100	101	55	55	56	57	58	59	59
	90th	106	107	109	111	113	114	115	70	70	71	72	73	74	74
	95th	110	111	113	115	117	118	119	74	74	75	76	77	78	78
	99th	117	118	120	122	124	125	126	82	82	83	84	85	86	86
8	50th	94	95	97	99	100	102	102	56	57	58	59	60	60	61
	90th	107	109	110	112	114	115	116	71	72	72	73	74	75	76
	95th	111	112	114	116	118	119	120	75	76	77	78	79	79	80
	99th	119	120	122	123	125	127	127	83	84	85	86	87	87	88
9	50th	95	96	98	100	102	103	104	57	58	59	60	61	61	62
	90th	109	110	112	114	115	117	118	72	73	74	75	76	76	77
	95th	113	114	116	118	119	121	121	76	77	78	79	80	81	81
	99th	120	121	123	125	127	128	129	84	85	86	87	88	88	89
10	50th	97	98	100	102	103	105	106	58	59	60	61	61	62	63
	90th	111	112	114	115	117	119	119	73	73	74	75	76	77	78
	95th	115	116	117	119	121	122	123	77	78	79	80	81	81	82
	99th	122	123	125	127	128	130	130	85	86	86	88	88	89	90
11	50th	99	100	102	104	105	107	107	59	59	60	61	62	63	63
	90th	113	114	115	117	119	120	121	74	74	75	76	77	78	78
	95th	117	118	119	121	123	124	125	78	78	79	80	81	82	82
	99th	124	125	127	129	130	132	132	86	86	87	88	89	90	90
12	50th	101	102	104	106	108	109	110	59	60	61	62	63	63	64
	90th	115	116	118	120	121	123	123	74	75	75	76	77	78	79
	95th	119	120	122	123	125	127	127	78	79	80	81	82	82	83
	99th	126	127	129	131	133	134	135	86	87	88	89	90	90	91

TABLE 7-2

BLOOD PRESSURE LEVELS FOR THE 50TH, 90TH, 95TH, AND 99TH PERCENTILES OF BLOOD PRESSURE FOR BOYS AGE 1–17 YEARS BY PERCENTILES OF HEIGHT (Continued)

Age, yr	BP Percentile[†]	SBP, mmHg							DBP, mmHg						
		Percentile of Height*							Percentile of Height*						
		5th	10th	25th	50th	75th	90th	95th	5th	10th	25th	50th	75th	90th	95th
13	50th	104	105	106	108	110	111	112	60	60	61	62	63	64	64
	90th	117	118	120	122	124	125	126	75	75	76	77	78	79	79
	95th	121	122	124	126	128	129	130	79	79	80	81	82	83	83
	99th	128	130	131	133	135	136	137	87	87	88	89	90	91	91
14	50th	106	107	109	111	113	114	115	60	61	62	63	64	65	65
	90th	120	121	123	125	126	128	128	75	76	77	78	79	79	80
	95th	124	125	127	128	130	132	132	80	80	81	82	83	84	84
	99th	131	132	134	136	138	139	140	87	88	89	90	91	92	92
15	50th	109	110	112	113	115	117	117	61	62	63	64	65	66	66
	90th	122	124	125	127	129	130	131	76	77	78	79	80	80	81
	95th	126	127	129	131	133	134	135	81	81	82	83	84	85	85
	99th	134	135	136	138	140	142	142	88	89	90	91	92	93	93
16	50th	111	112	114	116	118	119	120	63	63	64	65	66	67	67
	90th	125	126	128	130	131	133	134	78	78	79	80	81	82	82
	95th	129	130	132	134	135	137	137	82	83	83	84	85	87	87
	99th	136	137	139	141	143	144	145	90	90	91	92	93	94	94
17	50th	114	115	116	118	120	121	122	65	66	66	67	68	69	70
	90th	127	128	130	132	134	135	136	80	80	81	82	83	84	84
	95th	131	232	134	136	138	139	140	84	85	86	87	87	88	89
	99th	139	140	141	143	145	146	147	92	93	93	94	95	96	97

*Height percentile determined by standard growth curves.

[†]Blood pressure percentile determined by a single measurement.

Adapted from National High Blood Pressure Education Program Working Group on High Blood Pressure in Children and Adolescents: The fourth report on the diagnosis, evaluation, and treatment of high blood pressure in children and adolescents. *Pediatrics* 2004;114(2 Suppl):555–576.

7

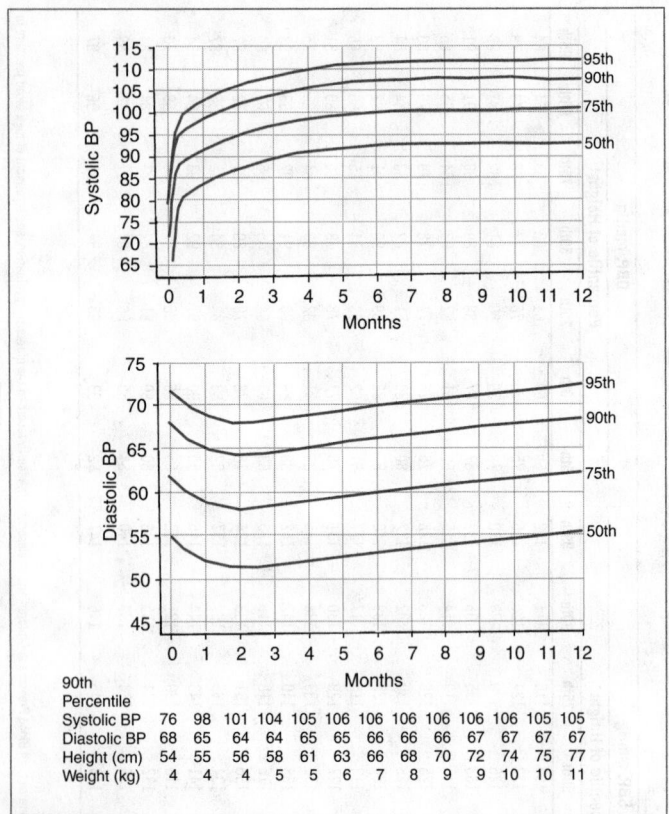

FIGURE 7-2

Age-specific percentiles of blood pressure (BP) measurements in boys from birth to 12 months of age; Korotkoff phase IV (K4) used for diastolic BP. *(From Task Force on Blood Pressure Control in Children. Report of the Second Task Force on Blood Pressure Control in Children. Pediatrics. 1987;79:1-25.)*

1. **Grading of heart murmurs:** Intensified by states of higher cardiac output (e.g., anemia, anxiety, fever, exercise)[3]
   a. Grade I: Barely audible
   b. Grade II: Soft but easily audible
   c. Grade III: Moderately loud but not accompanied by a thrill
   d. Grade IV: Louder, associated with a thrill
   e. Grade V: Audible with a stethoscope barely on the chest
   f. Grade VI: Audible with a stethoscope off the chest

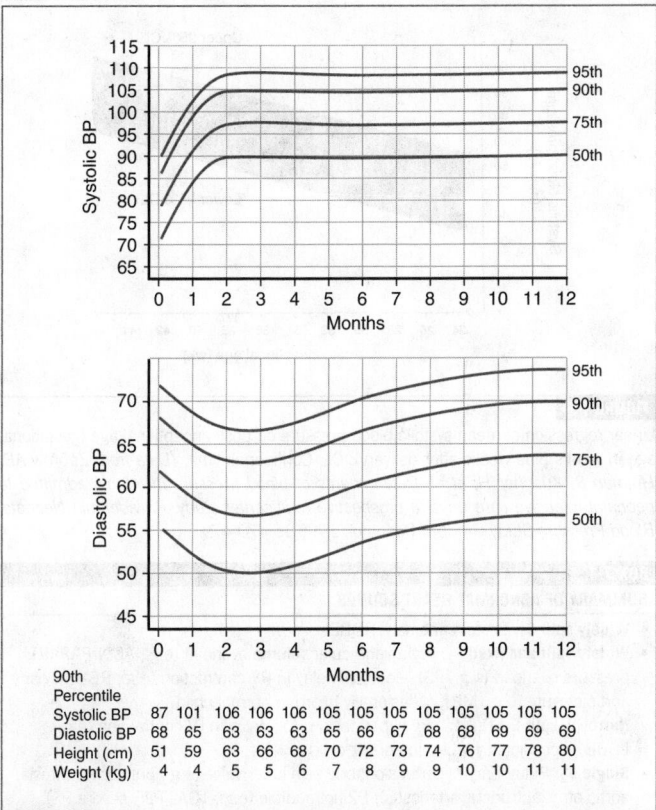

FIGURE 7-3

Age-specific percentile of blood pressure (BP) measurements in girls from birth to 12 months of age; Korotkoff phase IV (K4) used for diastolic BP. *(From Task Force on Blood Pressure Control in Children. Report of the Second Task Force on Blood Pressure Control in Children. Pediatrics. 1987;79:1-25.)*

2. **Benign heart murmurs:**
a. Caused by a disturbance of the laminar flow of blood; frequently produced as the diameter of the blood's pathway decreases and velocity increases.
b. Present in > 80% of children sometime during childhood, most commonly beginning at age 3 to 4 years.
c. Accentuated in high-output states, especially with fever and anemia.
d. Normal electrocardiogram (ECG) and radiographic findings.
   NOTE: ECG and chest radiograph are not routinely useful or cost-effective screening tools for distinguishing benign from pathologic murmurs.

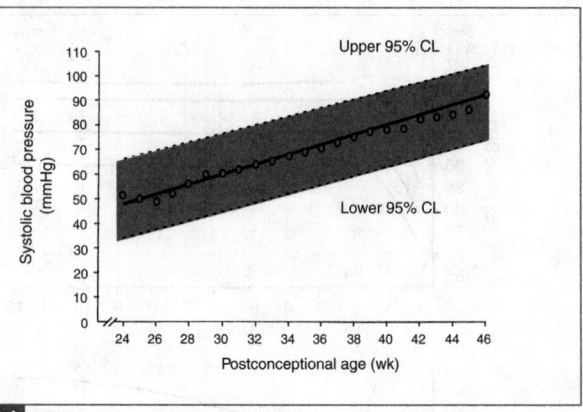

FIGURE 7-4

Linear regression of mean systolic blood pressure on postconceptional age (gestational age in weeks plus weeks after delivery). CL, Confidence limit. *(Data from Zubrow AB, Hulman S, Kushner H, et al. Determinants of blood pressure in infants admitted to neonatal intensive care units: a prospective multicenter study. Philadelphia Neonatal Blood Pressure Study Group. J Perinatol. 1995;15:470-479.)*

BOX 7-1

SUMMARY OF ABNORMAL HEART SOUNDS

- **Widely split S_1:** Ebstein anomaly, RBBB
- **Widely split and fixed S_2:** Right ventricular volume overload (e.g., ASD, PAPVR), pressure overload (e.g., PS), electrical delay in RV contraction (e.g., RBBB), early aortic closure (e.g., MR), occasionally heard in normal child
- **Narrowly split S_2:** Pulmonary hypertension, AS, delay in LV contraction (e.g., LBBB), occasionally heard in normal child
- **Single S_2:** Pulmonary hypertension, one semilunar valve (e.g., pulmonary atresia, aortic atresia, truncus arteriosus), P2 not audible (e.g., TGA, TOF, severe PS), severe AS, occasionally heard in normal child
- **Paradoxically split S_2:** Severe AS, LBBB, Wolff-Parkinson-White syndrome (type B)
- **Abnormal intensity of P2:** Increased P2 (e.g., pulmonary hypertension), decreased P2 (e.g., severe PS, TOF, TS)
- **S_3:** Occasionally heard in healthy children or adults or may indicate dilated ventricles (e.g., large VSD, CHF)
- **S_4:** Always pathologic; decreased ventricular compliance
- **Ejection click:** Heard with stenosis of the semilunar valves, dilated great arteries in the setting of pulmonary or systemic hypertension, idiopathic dilation of the PA, TOF, persistent truncus arteriosus
- **Midsystolic click:** Heard at the apex in mitral valve prolapse
- **Diastolic opening snap:** Rare in children; associated with TS/MS

AS, Aortic stenosis; ASD, atrial septal defect; CHF, congestive heart failure; LBBB, left bundle-branch block; MR, mitral regurgitation; MS, mitral stenosis; PA, pulmonary artery; PAPVR, partial anomalous pulmonary venous return; PS, pulmonary stenosis; RBBB, right bundle-branch block; RV, right ventricular; TGA, transposition of the great arteries; TOF, tetralogy of Fallot; TS, tricuspid stenosis; VSD, ventricular septal defect.
Modified from Park MK. *Pediatric Cardiology for Practitioners.* 5th ed. St Louis: Mosby; 2008:25.

3. **Likely pathologic murmur** when one or more of the following are present: Symptoms; cyanosis; systolic murmur that is loud (grade ≥3/6), harsh, pansystolic, or long in duration; diastolic murmur; abnormal heart sounds; presence of a click; abnormally strong or weak pulses.
4. **Systolic and diastolic heart murmurs** (Box 7-2)

TABLE 7-3

COMMON INNOCENT HEART MURMURS

Type (Timing)	Description of Murmur	Age Group
Classic vibratory murmur (Still's murmur; systolic)	Maximal at LMSB or between LLSB and apex Grade 2–3/6 in intensity Low-frequency vibratory, twanging string, groaning, squeaking, or musical	3–6 yr; occasionally in infancy
Pulmonary ejection murmur (systolic)	Maximal at LUSB Early to midsystolic Grade 1–3/6 in intensity Blowing in quality	8–14 yr
Pulmonary flow murmur of newborn (systolic)	Maximal at LUSB Transmits well to left and right chest, axilla, and back Grade 1–2/6 in intensity	Premature and full-term newborns Usually disappears by 3–6 mo
Venous hum (continuous)	Maximal at right (or left) supraclavicular and infraclavicular areas Grade 1–3/6 in intensity Inaudible in supine position Intensity changes with rotation of head and disappears with compression of jugular vein.	3–6 yr
Carotid bruit (systolic)	Right supraclavicular area over carotids Grade 2–3/6 in intensity Occasional thrill over carotid	Any age

LLSB, Left lower sternal border; LMSB, left middle sternal border; LUSB, left upper sternal border.
From Park MK. *Pediatric Cardiology for Practitioners.* 5th ed. St Louis: Mosby; 2008:36.

BOX 7-2

SYSTOLIC AND DIASTOLIC HEART MURMURS

I. RUSB

Aortic valve stenosis (supravalvar, subvalvar)
Aortic regurgitation

II. LUSB

Pulmonary valve stenosis
Atrial septal defect
Pulmonary ejection murmur, innocent
Pulmonary flow murmur of newborn
Pulmonary artery stenosis
Aortic stenosis
Coarctation of the aorta
Patent ductus arteriosus

Continued

BOX 7-2

SYSTOLIC AND DIASTOLIC HEART MURMURS (Continued)

Partial anomalous pulmonary venous return (PAPVR)
Total anomalous pulmonary venous return (TAPVR)
Pulmonary regurgitation

III. LLSB

Ventricular septal defect, including atrioventricular septal defect
Vibratory innocent murmur (Still's murmur)
HOCM (IHSS)
Tricuspid regurgitation
Tetralogy of Fallot
Tricuspid stenosis

IV. Apex

Mitral regurgitation
Vibratory innocent murmur (Still's murmur)
Mitral valve prolapse
Aortic stenosis
HOCM (IHSS)
Mitral stenosis

The location at which various murmurs may be heard. *Diastolic murmurs are in italics.* HOCM, Hypertrophic obstructive cardiomyopathy; IHSS, idiopathic hypertrophic subaortic stenosis; LLSB, left lower sternal border; LUSB, left upper sternal border; RUSB, right upper sternal border.

From Park MK. *Pediatric Cardiology for Practitioners.* 5th ed. St Louis: Mosby; 2008:30.

IV. ELECTROCARDIOGRAPHY

A. Basic Electrocardiography Principles

1. **Lead placement** (Fig. 7-5)
2. **ECG complexes** (see Fig. 7-1)
   a. P wave: Represents atrial depolarization
   b. QRS complex: Represents ventricular depolarization
   c. T wave: Represents ventricular repolarization
   d. U wave: May follow T wave, representing late phases of ventricular repolarization
3. **Systematic approach for evaluating ECGs** (Table 7-4 shows normal ECG parameters)[3,5]:
   a. Rate
      (1) Standardization: Paper speed is 25mm/sec. One small square = 1mm = 0.04 sec. One large square = 5mm = 0.2 sec. Amplitude standard: 10mm = 1 mV
      (2) Calculation: HR (beats per minute) = 60 divided by the average R-R interval in seconds, or 1500 divided by the R-R interval in millimeters
   b. Rhythm
      (1) Sinus rhythm: Every QRS complex is preceded by a P wave, normal PR interval (although PR interval may be prolonged, as in first-degree atrioventricular [AV] block), and normal P-wave axis (upright P in lead I and aVF).

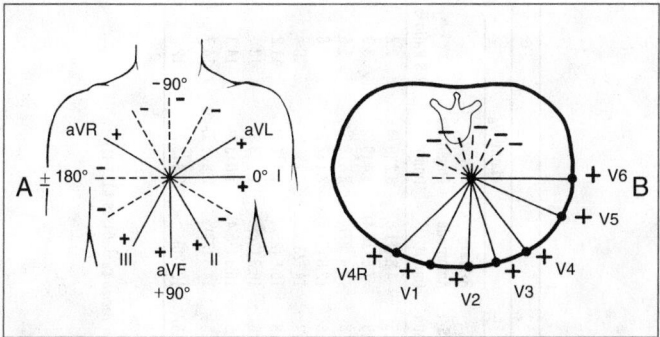

FIGURE 7-5

A, Hexaxial reference system. **B,** Horizontal reference system. *(Modified from Park MK, Guntheroth WG.* How to Read Pediatric ECGs. *4th ed. Philadelphia: Mosby; 2006:3.)*

    (2) There is normal respiratory variation of the R-R interval without morphologic changes of the P wave or QRS complex.
c. Axis: Look at the direction of the QRS in leads I and aVF. Determine quadrant and compare with age-matched normal values (Fig. 7-6; see Table 7-4).
d. Intervals (PR, QRS, QTc): See Table 7-4 for normal PR and QRS intervals. The QTc is calculated using the Bazett formula:

$$QTc = QT\ (sec)\ measured/ \sqrt{R\text{-}R}$$
(average 3 measurements taken from same lead)

    R-R interval should extend from the R wave in the QRS complex where you are measuring QT to the preceding R wave. Normal values for QTc are:
    (1) 0.44 sec is 97th percentile for infants 3–4 days old[6]
    (2) ≤0.45 sec in all males >1 week of age and prepubescent females
    (3) ≤0.46 sec for postpubescent females
e. P-wave size and shape: Normal P wave should be <0.10 sec in children, <0.08 sec in infants, with amplitude <0.3 mV (3 mm in height, with normal standardization)
f. R-wave progression: Generally a normal increase in R-wave size and decrease in S-wave size from leads V_1 to V_6 (with dominant S waves in right precordial leads and dominant R waves in left precordial leads), representing dominance of left ventricular forces. However, newborns and infants have a normal dominance of the right ventricle.
g. Q waves: Normal Q waves usually <0.04 sec in duration and <25% of total QRS amplitude. Q waves are <5 mm deep in left precordial leads and aVF and ≤8 mm deep in lead III for children <3 years of age.

TABLE 7.4

NORMAL PEDIATRIC ELECTROCARDIOGRAM (ECG) PARAMETERS

Age	Heart Rate (bpm)	QRS Axis*	PR Interval (sec)†	QRS Duration (sec)*	Lead V₁ R-Wave Amplitude (mm)†	Lead V₁ S-Wave Amplitude (mm)†	Lead V₁ R/S Ratio	Lead V₆ R-Wave Amplitude (mm)†	Lead V₆ S-Wave Amplitude (mm)†	Lead V₆ R/S Ratio
0–7 days	95–160 (125)	+30 to 180 (110)	0.08–0.12 (0.10)	0.05 (0.07)	13.3 (25.5)	7.7 (18.8)	2.5	4.8 (11.8)	3.2 (9.6)	2.2
1–3 wk	105–180 (145)	+30 to 180 (110)	0.08–0.12 (0.10)	0.05 (0.07)	10.6 (20.8)	4.2 (10.8)	2.9	7.6 (16.4)	3.4 (9.8)	3.3
1–6 mo	110–180 (145)	+10 to +125 (+70)	0.08–0.13 (0.11)	0.05 (0.07)	9.7 (19)	5.4 (15)	2.3	12.4 (22)	2.8 (8.3)	5.6
6–12 mo	110–170 (135)	+10 to +125 (+60)	0.10–0.14 (0.12)	0.05 (0.07)	9.4 (20.3)	6.4 (18.1)	1.6	12.6 (22.7)	2.1 (7.2)	7.6
1–3 yr	90–150 (120)	+10 to +125 (+60)	0.10–0.14 (0.12)	0.06 (0.07)	8.5 (18)	9 (21)	1.2	14 (23.3)	1.7 (6)	10
4–5 yr	65–135 (110)	0 to +110 (+60)	0.11–0.15 (0.13)	0.07 (0.08)	7.6 (16)	11 (22.5)	0.8	15.6 (25)	1.4 (4.7)	11.2
6–8 yr	60–130 (100)	−15 to +110 (+60)	0.12–0.16 (0.14)	0.07 (0.08)	6 (13)	12 (24.5)	0.6	16.3 (26)	1.1 (3.9)	13
9–11 yr	60–110 (85)	−15 to +110 (+60)	0.12–0.17 (0.14)	0.07 (0.09)	5.4 (12.1)	11.9 (25.4)	0.5	16.3 (25.4)	1.0 (3.9)	14.3
12–16 yr	60–110 (85)	−15 to +110 (+60)	0.12–0.17 (0.15)	0.07 (0.10)	4.1 (9.9)	10.8 (21.2)	0.5	14.3 (23)	0.8 (3.7)	14.7
>16 yr	60–100 (80)	−15 to +110 (+60)	0.12–0.20 (0.15)	0.08 (0.10)	3 (9)	10 (20)	0.3	10 (20)	0.8 (3.7)	12

*Normal range and (mean).
†Mean and (98th percentile).
Adapted from Park MK. *Pediatric Cardiology for Practitioners.* 5th ed. St Louis: Mosby; 2008; and Davignon A et al. Normal ECG standards for infants and children. *Pediatr Cardiol.* 1979;1:123-131.

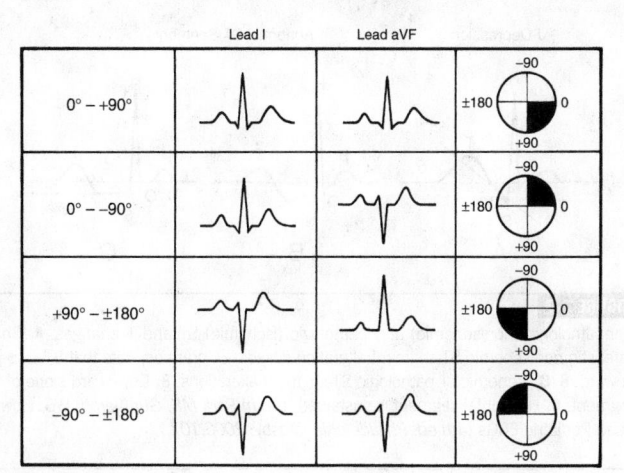

	Lead I	Lead aVF	
0° – +90°			
0° – –90°			
+90° – ±180°			
–90° – ±180°			

FIGURE 7-6

Locating quadrants of mean QRS axis from leads I and aVF. *(From Park MK, Guntheroth WG. How to Read Pediatric ECGs. 4th ed. Philadelphia: Mosby; 2006:17.)*

TABLE 7-5

NORMAL T-WAVE AXIS

Age	V_1, V_2	AVF	I, V_5, V_6
Birth–1 day	±	+	±
1–4 days	±	+	+
4 days to adolescent	–	+	+
Adolescent to adult	+	+	+

+, T wave positive; –, T wave negative; ±, T wave normally either positive or negative.

h. ST-segment (Fig. 7-7): ST-segment elevation or depression >1 mm in limb leads and >2 mm in precordial leads is consistent with myocardial ischemia or injury. **Note:** J-depression is an upsloping of the ST segment and a normal variant.

i. T wave:
   (1) Inverted T waves in V_1 and V_2 can be normal in children up to adolescence (Table 7-5).
   (2) Tall, peaked T waves may be seen in hyperkalemia.
   (3) Flat or low T waves may be seen in hypokalemia, hypothyroidism, normal newborns, and myocardial/pericardial ischemia and inflammation.

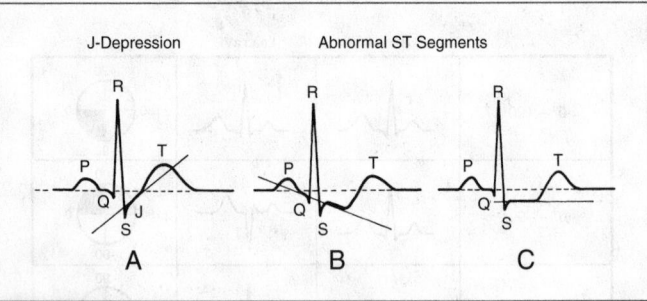

FIGURE 7-7

Nonpathologic (nonischemic) and pathologic (ischemic) ST and T changes. **A,** Characteristic nonischemic ST-segment alteration called *J-depression*; note that ST slope is upward. **B–C,** Ischemic or pathologic ST-segment alterations. **B,** Downward slope of ST segment. **C,** Horizontal segment is sustained. *(From Park MK, Guntheroth WG. How to Read Pediatric ECGs. 4th ed. Philadelphia: Mosby; 2006:107.)*

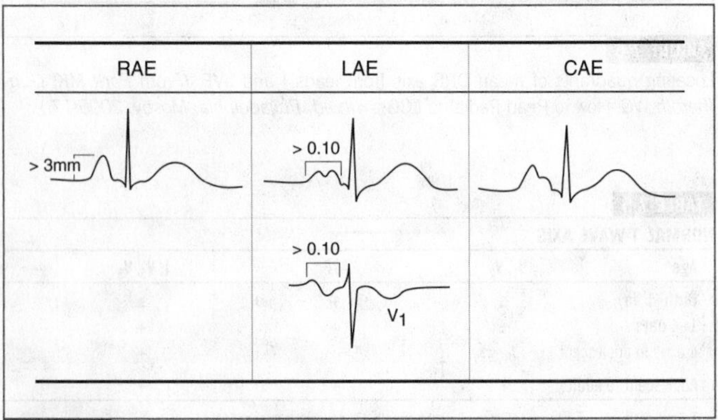

FIGURE 7-8

Criteria for atrial enlargement. CAE, Combined atrial enlargement; LAE, left atrial enlargement; RAE, right atrial enlargement. *(From Park MK. Pediatric Cardiology for Practitioners. 5th ed. St Louis: Mosby; 2008:53.)*

　　j. Hypertrophy/enlargement
　　　　(1) Atrial enlargement (Fig. 7-8)
　　　　(2) Ventricular hypertrophy: Diagnosed by QRS axis, voltage, and R/S ratio (Box 7-3; see also Table 7-4)
B. ECG Abnormalities
　1. **Nonventricular arrhythmias** (Table 7-6; Figs. 7-9 and 7-10)[7]
　2. **Ventricular arrhythmias** (Table 7-7; Fig. 7-11)
　3. **Nonventricular conduction disturbances** (Fig. 7-12 and Table 7-8)[8]
　4. **Ventricular conduction disturbances** (Table 7-9)

BOX 7-3

VENTRICULAR HYPERTROPHY CRITERIA

RIGHT VENTRICULAR HYPERTROPHY (RVH) CRITERIA

Must Have at Least One of the Following:
Upright T wave in lead V_1 after 3 days of age to adolescence
Presence of Q wave in V_1 (QR or QRS pattern)
Increased right and anterior QRS voltage (with normal QRS duration):
  R in lead V_1, >98th percentile for age
  S in lead V_6, >98th percentile for age
Right ventricular strain (associated with inverted T wave in V_1 with tall R wave)

LEFT VENTRICULAR HYPERTROPHY (LVH) CRITERIA

Left ventricular strain (associated with inverted T wave in leads V_6, I, and/or aVF)
Supplemental Criteria:
Left axis deviation (LAD) for patient's age
Volume overload (associated with Q wave >5 mm and tall T waves in V_5 or V_6)
Increased QRS voltage in left leads (with normal QRS duration):
R in lead V_6 (and I, aVL, V_5), >98th percentile for age
S in lead V_1, >98th percentile for age

TABLE 7-6

NONVENTRICULAR ARRHYTHMIAS

Name/Description	Cause	Treatment
SINUS		
TACHYCARDIA		
Normal sinus rhythm with HR >95th percentile for age (usually infants: <220 beats/min and children: <180 beats/min)	Hypovolemia, shock, anemia, sepsis, fever, anxiety, CHF, PE, myocardial disease, drugs (e.g., β-agonists, albuterol, caffeine, atropine)	Address underlying cause
BRADYCARDIA		
Normal sinus rhythm with HR <5th percentile for age	Normal (especially in athletic individuals), increased ICP, hypoxia, hyperkalemia, hypercalcemia, vagal stimulation, hypothyroidism, hypothermia, drugs (e.g., opioids, digoxin, β-blockers), long QT	Address underlying cause; if symptomatic, refer to inside back cover for bradycardia algorithm
SUPRAVENTRICULAR*		
PREMATURE ATRIAL CONTRACTION (PAC)		
Narrow QRS complex; ectopic focus in atria with abnormal P-wave morphology	Digitalis toxicity, medications (e.g., caffeine, theophylline, sympathomimetics), normal variant	Treat digitalis toxicity; otherwise no treatment needed
ATRIAL FLUTTER		
Atrial rate 250–350 beats/min; characteristic sawtooth or flutter pattern with variable ventricular response rate and normal QRS complex	Dilated atria, previous intra-atrial surgery, valvular or ischemic heart disease, idiopathic in newborns	Synchronized cardioversion or overdrive pacing; treat underlying cause

TABLE 7-6		
NONVENTRICULAR ARRHYTHMIAS (Continued)		
Name/Description	**Cause**	**Treatment**
ATRIAL FIBRILLATION		
Irregular; atrial rate 350–600 beats/min, yielding characteristic fibrillatory pattern (no discrete P waves) and irregular ventricular response rate of about 110–150 beats/min with normal QRS complex	Wolff-Parkinson-White syndrome and those listed previously for atrial flutter (except not idiopathic), alcohol exposure, familial	Synchronized cardioversion; then may need anticoagulation pretreatment
SVT		
Sudden run of three or more consecutive premature supraventricular beats at >220 beats/min(infant) or >180 beats/min (child), with narrow QRS complex and absent/abnormal P wave; either sustained (>30 sec) or nonsustained	Most commonly idiopathic but may be seen in congenital heart disease (e.g., Ebstein anomaly, transposition)	Vagal maneuvers, adenosine; if unstable, need immediate synchronized cardioversion (0.5 J/kg up to 1 J/kg). Consult cardiologist. See "Tachycardia with Poor Perfusion" or "Tachycardia with Adequate Perfusion" algorithms in back of handbook.
I. AV Reentrant: Presence of accessory bypass pathway, in conjunction with AV node, establishes cyclic pattern of reentry independent of SA node; most common cause of nonsinus tachycardia in children (see Wolff-Parkinson-White syndrome, Table 7-9 and Fig. 7-10)		
II. Junctional: Automatic focus; simultaneous depolarization of atria and ventricles yields invisible P wave or retrograde P wave	Cardiac surgery, idiopathic	Adjust for clinical situation; consult cardiology
III. Ectopic atrial tachycardia: Rapid firing of ectopic focus in atrium	Idiopathic	AV nodal blockade, ablation
NODAL ESCAPE/JUNCTIONAL RHYTHM		
Abnormal rhythm driven by AV node impulse, giving normal QRS complex and invisible P wave (buried in preceding QRS or T wave) or retrograde P wave (negative in lead II, positive in aVR); seen in sinus bradycardia	Common after surgery of atria	Often requires no treatment. If rate is slow enough, may require pacemaker.

*Abnormal rhythm resulting from ectopic focus in atria or AV node, or from accessory conduction pathways. Characterized by different P-wave shape and abnormal P-wave axis. QRS morphology usually normal. See Figures 7-9, 7-10.[6]

AV, Atrioventricular; CHF, congestive heart failure; HR, heart rate; ICP, intracranial pressure; PE, pulmonary embolism; SA, sinoatrial; SVT, supraventricular tachycardia.

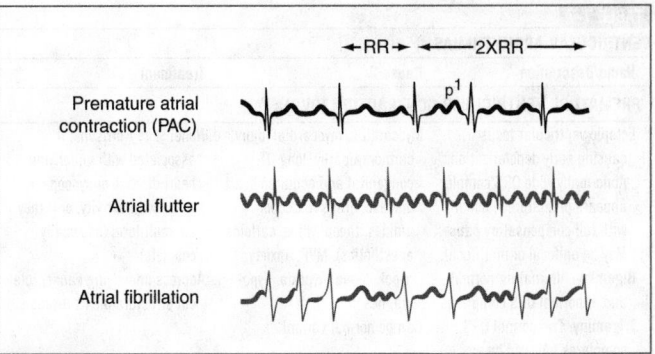

FIGURE 7-9

Supraventricular arrhythmias. p¹, Premature atrial contraction. *(From Park MK, Guntheroth WG.* How to Read Pediatric ECGs. *4th ed. Philadelphia: Mosby; 2006:129.)*

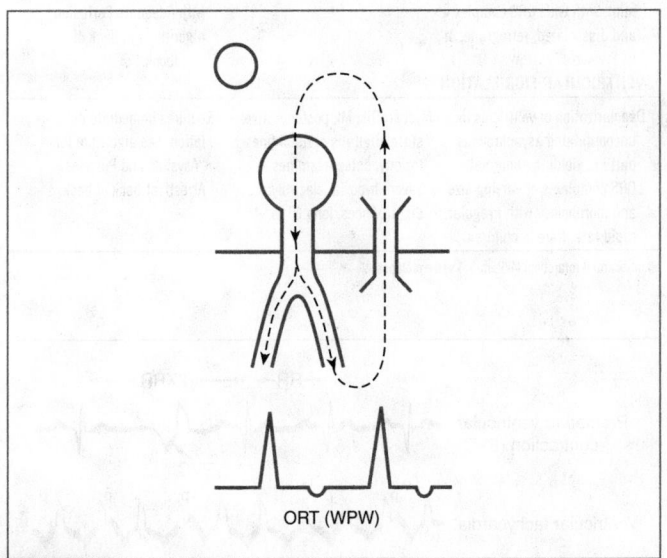

FIGURE 7-10

Supraventricular tachycardia pathway: Mechanism for orthodromic reentry tract (ORT), (i.e., Wolff-Parkinson-White [WPW]). Diagram shows sinoatrial (SA) node *(upper left circle)*, with atrioventricular (AV) node *(above horizontal line)* and bundle branches crossing to ventricle *(below horizontal line)*. *(Adapted from Walsh EP. Cardiac arrhythmias. In: Fyler DC,ed.* Nadas' Pediatric Cardiology. *Philadelphia: Hanley & Belfus; 1992:384.)*

TABLE 7-7

VENTRICULAR ARRHYTHMIAS

Name/Description	Cause	Treatment
PREMATURE VENTRICULAR CONTRACTION (PVC)		
Ectopic ventricular focus causing early depolarization. Abnormally wide QRS complex appears prematurely, usually with full compensatory pause. May be unifocal or multifocal. **Bigeminy:** Alternating normal and abnormal QRS complexes. **Trigeminy:** Two normal QRS complexes followed by an abnormal one. **Couplet:** Two consecutive PVCs.	Myocarditis, myocardial injury, cardiomyopathy, long QT, congenital and acquired heart disease, drugs (catechol-amines, theophylline, caffeine, anesthetics), MVP, anxiety, hypokalemia, hypoxia, hypo-magnesemia. Can be normal variant.	None. More worrisome if associated with underlying heart disease or syncope, if worse with activity, or if they are multiform (especially couplets). Address underlying cause, rule out structural heart disease.
VENTRICULAR TACHYCARDIA		
Series of three or more PVCs at rapid rate (120–250 beats/min), with wide QRS complex and dissociated, retrograde, or no P wave	See causes of PVCs (70% have underlying cause).	See "Tachycardia with Poor Perfusion" and "Tachycardia with Adequate Perfusion" algorithms in back of handbook.
VENTRICULAR FIBRILLATION		
Depolarization of ventricles in uncoordinated asynchronous pattern, yielding abnormal QRS complexes of varying size and morphology with irregular, rapid rate. Rare in children.	Myocarditis, MI, postoperative state, digitalis or quinidine toxicity, catecholamines, severe hypoxia, electrolyte disturbances, long QT	Requires immediate defibril-lation. See algorithm for "Asystole and Pulseless Arrest" at back of book.

MI, Myocardial infarction; MVP, mitral valve prolapse.

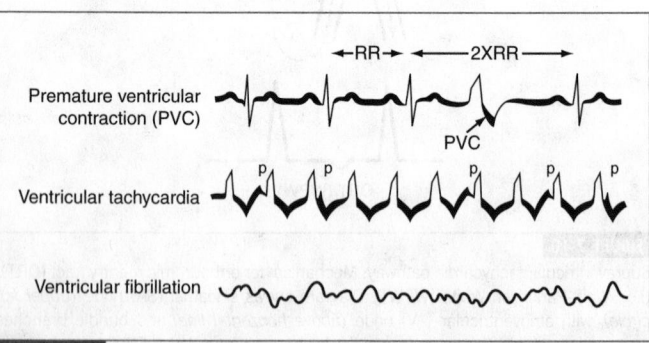

FIGURE 7-11

Ventricular arrhythmias. p, p wave, RR, R-R interval. (*From Park MK, Guntheroth WG. How to Read Pediatric ECGs. 4th ed. Philadelphia: Mosby; 2006:138.*)

FIGURE 7-12

Conduction blocks. p, p wave; R, QRS complex. *(From Park MK, Guntheroth WG. How to Read Pediatric ECGs. 4th ed. Philadelphia: Mosby; 2006:141.)*

TABLE 7-8

NONVENTRICULAR CONDUCTION DISTURBANCES

Name/Description*	Cause	Treatment
FIRST-DEGREE HEART BLOCK		
Abnormal but asymptomatic delay in conduction through AV node, yielding prolongation of PR interval	Acute rheumatic fever, tickborne (i.e., Lyme) disease, connective tissue disease, congenital heart disease, cardiomyopathy, digitalis toxicity, postoperative state, normal children	No specific treatment except address the underlying cause
SECOND-DEGREE HEART BLOCK: MOBITZ TYPE I (WENCKEBACH)		
Progressive lengthening of PR interval until a QRS complex is not conducted. Common finding in asymptomatic teenagers.	Myocarditis, cardiomyopathy, congenital heart disease, postoperative state, MI, toxicity (digitalis, β-blocker), normal children, Lyme disease, lupus	Address underlying cause, or none needed
SECOND-DEGREE HEART BLOCK: MOBITZ TYPE II		
Loss of conduction to ventricle without lengthening of the PR interval. May progress to complete heart block.	Same as for Mobitz type I	Address underlying cause; may need pacemaker
THIRD-DEGREE (COMPLETE) HEART BLOCK		
Complete dissociation of atrial and ventricular conduction, with atrial rate faster than ventricular rate. P wave and PP interval regular; RR interval regular and much slower.	Congenital due to maternal lupus or other connective tissue disease	If bradycardic and symptomatic, consider pacing; see bradycardia algorithm at back of book.

*High-degree AV block: Conduction of atrial impulse at regular intervals, yielding 2:1 block (two atrial impulses for each ventricular response), 3:1 block, etc.

AV, Atrioventricular; MI, myocardial infarction.

TABLE 7-9

VENTRICULAR CONDUCTION DISTURBANCES

Name/Description	Criteria	Causes/Treatment
RIGHT BUNDLE-BRANCH BLOCK (RBBB)		
Delayed right bundle conduction prolongs RV depolarization time, leading to wide QRS.	1. Prolonged or wide QRS with terminal slurred R′ (m-shaped RSR′ or RR′) in V_1, V_2, aVR 2. Wide and slurred S wave in leads I and V_6	ASD, surgery with right ventriculotomy, occasionally seen in normal children
LEFT BUNDLE-BRANCH BLOCK (LBBB)		
Delayed left bundle conduction prolongs septal and LV depolarization time, leading to wide QRS with loss of usual septal signal; there is still a predominance of left ventricle forces. Rare in children.	1. Wide negative QS complex in lead V_1 with loss of septal R wave 2. Wide R or RR′ complex in lead V_6 with loss of septal Q wave	Hypertension, ischemic or valvular heart disease, cardiomyopathy
WOLFF-PARKINSON-WHITE (WPW)		
Atrial impulse transmitted via anomalous conduction pathway to ventricles, bypassing AV node and normal ventricular conduction system. Leads to early and prolonged depolarization of ventricles. Bypass pathway is a predisposing condition for SVT.	1. Shortened PR interval 2. Delta wave 3. Wide QRS	Acute management of SVT if necessary as previously described; consider ablation of accessory pathway if recurrent SVT. All patients need cardiology referral.

ASD, Atrial septal defect; LV, left ventricle; RV, right ventricle; SVT, supraventricular tachycardia.

C. ECG Findings Secondary to Electrolyte Disturbances, Medications, and Systemic Illnesses (Table 7-10)[7,20]

D. Long QT

1. **Diagnosis:**
a. In general, QTc is similar in males and females from birth until late adolescence (0.37–0.44 sec).
b. In adults, prolonged QTc is > 0.45 sec for males and > 0.45–0.46 sec for females.
c. In approximately 10% of cases, patients may have a normal QTc on ECG. Patients may also have a family history of long QT with unexplained syncope, seizure, or cardiac arrest without prolongation of QTc on ECG.
d. Treadmill exercise test may prolong the QTc and will sometimes incite arryhthmias.
2. **Complications:** Associated with ventricular arrhythmias (torsades de pointes), syncope, and sudden death
3. **Management:**
a. Congenital long QT: β-blockers and/or defibrillators; rarely require cardiac sympathetic denervation or cardiac pacemakers

TABLE 7-10

SYSTEMIC EFFECTS ON ELECTROCARDIOGRAM

	Short QT	Long QT-U	Prolonged QRS	ST-T Changes	Sinus Tachycardia	Sinus Bradycardia	AV Block	Ventricular Tachycardia	Miscellaneous
CHEMISTRY									
Hyperkalemia			X	X			X	X	Low-voltage Ps; peaked Ts
Hypokalemia		X		X					
Hypercalcemia	X					X	X	X	
Hypocalcemia		X			X		X		
Hypermagnesemia							X		
Hypomagnesemia		X							
DRUGS									
Digitalis	X			X		T	X	T	
Phenothiazines		T						T	
Phenytoin	X						X		
Propranolol	X					X	T		
Tricyclics		T	T	T	T		T	T	
Verapamil						X	X		

Continued

TABLE 7-10

SYSTEMIC EFFECTS ON ELECTROCARDIOGRAM (Continued)

	Short QT	Long QT-U	Prolonged QRS	ST-T Changes	Sinus Tachycardia	Sinus Bradycardia	AV Block	Ventricular Tachycardia	Miscellaneous
MISCELLANEOUS									
CNS injury		X		X	X	X	X		
Friedreich ataxia				X	X				Atrial flutter
Duchenne muscular dystrophy					X	X			Atrial flutter
Myotonic dystrophy			X	X	X		X		
Collagen vascular disease				X			X	X	
Hypothyroidism						X			Low voltage
Hyperthyroidism			X	X	X		X		
Lyme disease			X				X		
Holt-Oram, maternal lupus							X		

CNS, Central nervous system; T, present only with drug toxicity; X, present.

Adapted from Garson A Jr. *The Electrocardiogram in Infants and Children: A Systematic Approach.* Philadelphia: Lea & Febiger; 1983:172; and Walsh EP. Cardiac arrhythmias. In: Fyler DC, Nadas A,eds. *Pediatric Cardiology.* Philadelphia: Hanley & Belfus; 1992:141-143.

b. Acquired long QT: Treatment of arrhythmias, discontinue precipitating drug, correction of metabolic abnormalities

E. Hyperkalemia: ECG changes dependent on serum K+level; may have normal ECG with level between 2.5 and 6

1. **Serum K+ <2.5:** Depressed ST segment, diphasic T wave
2. **Serum K+ >6:** Tall T wave
3. **Serum K+ >7.5:** Long PR interval, wide QRS, tall T wave
4. **Serum K+ >9:** Absent P wave, sinusoidal

F. Myocardial Infarction (MI) in Children

1. **Etiology:** Anomalous origin or aberrant course of a coronary artery, Kawasaki disease, congenital heart disease (presurgical and postsurgical), and dilated cardiomyopathy. Less often associated with hypertension, lupus, myocarditis, cocaine ingestion, and use of adrenergic drugs (e.g., β-agonists used for asthma). Rare in children.
2. **Frequent ECG findings in children with acute MI[9,10]** (Fig. 7-13):
a. New-onset wide Q waves (>0.035 sec) seen within first few hours (persist over several years)
b. ST-segment elevation (>2 mm) seen within first few hours
c. Diphasic T waves seen within first few days (becoming sharply inverted, then normalizing over time)
d. Prolonged QTc interval (>0.44 sec) with abnormal Q waves

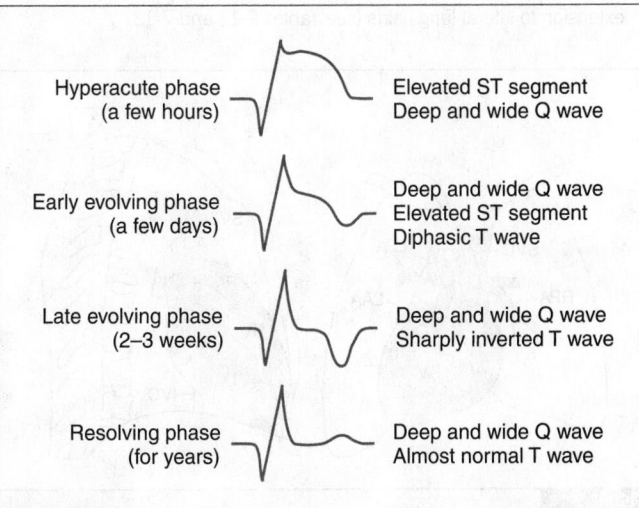

Hyperacute phase (a few hours) — Elevated ST segment / Deep and wide Q wave

Early evolving phase (a few days) — Deep and wide Q wave / Elevated ST segment / Diphasic T wave

Late evolving phase (2–3 weeks) — Deep and wide Q wave / Sharply inverted T wave

Resolving phase (for years) — Deep and wide Q wave / Almost normal T wave

FIGURE 7-13

Sequential changes during myocardial infarction. (*From Park MK, Guntheroth WG. How to Read Pediatric ECGs. 4th ed. Philadelphia: Mosby; 2006:115.*)

e. Deep, wide Q waves in leads I, aVL, or V$_6$, without Q waves in II, III, aVF, suggest anomalous origin of the left coronary artery.

3. **Other criteria:**

a. Elevated creatine kinase (CK)/MB fraction: Not specific for acute MI in children

b. Cardiac troponin I: More sensitive indicator of early myocardial damage in children.[10] Becomes elevated within hours of cardiac injury, persists for 4–7 days, is specific for cardiac injury.

V. IMAGING

A. Chest Radiograph

Please see Chapter 25 for more information on the chest radiograph.

1. **Evaluate the heart:**

a. Size: Cardiac shadow should be <50% of thoracic width (maximal width between inner margins of ribs, as measured on a posteroanterior radiograph during inspiration)

b. Shape: Can aid in diagnosis of chamber/vessel enlargement and some congenital heart disease (Fig. 7-14)

c. Situs (levocardia, mesocardia, dextrocardia)

2. **Evaluate the lung fields:**

a. Decreased pulmonary blood flow: Seen in pulmonary or tricuspid stenosis/atresia, TOF, pulmonary hypertension (peripheral pruning)

b. Increased pulmonary blood flow: Seen as increased pulmonary vascular markings (PVMs) with redistribution from bases to apices of lungs and extension to lateral lung fields (see Tables 7-12 and 7-13)

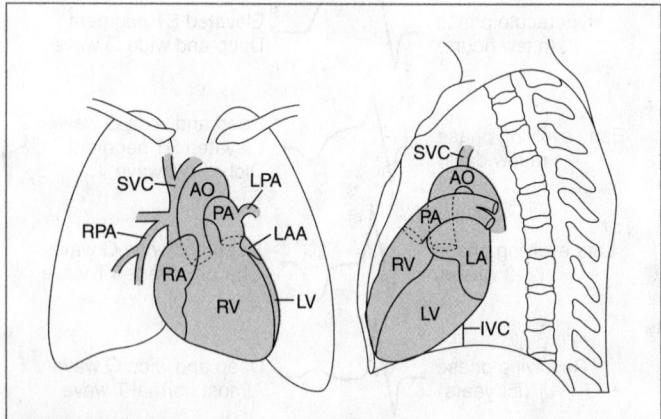

FIGURE 7-14

Radiologic contours of the heart. AO, Aorta; IVC, inferior vena cava; LA, left atrium; LAA, left atrial appendage; LPA, left pulmonary artery; LV, left ventricle; PA, pulmonary artery; RA, right atrium; RPA, right pulmonary artery; RV, right ventricle; SVC, superior vena cava.

c. Venous congestion, or congestive heart failure (CHF): Increased PVMs centrally, interstitial and alveolar pulmonary edema (air bronchograms), septal lines, and pleural effusions (see Tables 7-12 and 7-13)

3. **Evaluate the trachea:** Usually bends slightly to the right above the carina in normal patients with a left-sided aortic arch. A perfectly straight or left-bending trachea suggests a right aortic arch, which may be associated with other defects (TOF, truncus arteriosus, vascular rings, chromosome 22 microdeletion).

4. **Skeletal anomalies:**
a. Rib notching (e.g., from collateral vessels in patients >5 years of age with coarctation of the aorta)
b. Sternal abnormalities (e.g., Holt-Oram syndrome, pectus excavatum in Marfan, Ehlers-Danlos, and Noonan syndromes)
c. Vertebral anomalies (e.g., VATER/VACTERL syndrome: **V**ertebral anomalies, **A**nal atresia, **T**racheoesophageal fistula, **R**adial and **R**enal, **C**ardiac, and **L**imb anomalies)

B. Echocardiography

1. **Approach:**
a. Transthoracic echocardiography (TTE): Does not require general anesthesia, is simpler to perform than transesophageal echocardiography (TEE), but does have limitations in some patients (e.g., uncooperative, obese, or those with suspected endocarditis)
b. TEE: Uses an ultrasound transducer on the end of a modified endoscope to view the heart from the esophagus and stomach, allowing for better imaging of intracardiac structures. TEE allows for better imaging in obese and intraoperative patients and is also useful for visualizing very small lesions, such as some vegetations.

2. **Shortening fraction:** Very reliable index of left ventricular function. Normal values range from 30%–45%, depending on age.[11]
For more information on echocardiography see Expert Consult, Chapter 7.

C. Cardiac Catheterization

See Fig. EC 7-A for diagram of normal pressure values.

VI. CONGENITAL HEART DISEASE

A. Pulse Oximetry Screening for Critical Congenital Heart Disease

1. **Recommended after 24 hours of life or as late as possible if earlier discharge from the nursery.** There is a lower false-positive rate after 24 hours of life.

2. **Screening recommended on the right hand and on one foot,** either in parallel or direct sequence.

3. **Screening result would be considered positive if:**
a. Any oxygen saturation measure is < 90%.
b. Oxygen saturation is <95% in both extremities on 3 measures, each separated by 1 hour.

c. There is a >3% absolute difference in oxygen saturation between the right hand and foot on 3 measures, each separated by 1 hour.

B. Common Syndromes Associated with Cardiac Lesions (Table 7-11)

C. Acyanotic Lesions (Table 7-12)

D. Cyanotic Lesions (Table 7-13)

An oxygen challenge test is used to evaluate the etiology of cyanosis in neonates. Obtain baseline arterial blood gas (ABG) with saturation at $Fio_2 = 0.21$, then place infant in an oxygen hood at $Fio_2 = 1$ for a minimum of 10 min, and repeat ABG. In cardiac disease, there will not be a significant change in Pao_2 following the oxygen challenge test.

Note: Pulse oximetry will not be useful for following the change in oxygenation once the saturations reach 100% (approximately $Pao_2 > 90$ mmHg).[11-14]

1. See Table EC 7-B for **interpretation of oxygen challenge test.**
2. Table 7-14 shows acute **management of hypercyanotic spells in TOF.**

TABLE 7-11

MAJOR SYNDROMES ASSOCIATED WITH CARDIAC DEFECTS

Syndrome	Dominant Cardiac Defect
CHARGE	TOF, truncus arteriosus, aortic arch abnormalities
DiGeorge	Aortic arch anomalies, TOF, truncus arteriosus, VSD, PDA
Trisomy 21	Atrioventricular septal defect, VSD
Marfan	Aortic root dilation, mitral valve prolapse
Loeys-Dietz	Aortic root dilation with higher risk of rupture at smaller dimensions
Noonan	Supravalvular pulmonic stenosis, LVH
Turner	COA, bicuspid aortic valve, aortic root dilation as a teenager
Williams	Supravalvular aortic stenosis, pulmonary artery stenosis
FAS	Occasional: VSD, PDA, ASD, TOF
IDM	TGA, VSD, COA, cardiomyopathy
VATER/VACTERL	VSD
VCFS	Truncus arteriosus, TOF, pulmonary atresia with VSD, TGA, interrupted aortic arch

ASD, Atrial septal defect; CHARGE, a syndrome of associated defects including **C**oloboma of the eye, **H**eart anomaly, choanal **A**tresia, **R**etardation, and **G**enital and **E**ar anomalies; COA, coarctation of aorta; FAS, fetal alcohol syndrome; IDM, infant of diabetic mother; LVH, left ventricular hypertrophy; PDA, patent ductus arteriosis; TGA, transposition of the great arteries; TOF, tetralogy of Fallot; VATER/VACTERL, association of **V**ertebral anomalies, **A**nal atresia, **C**ardiac anomalies, **T**racheo**e**sophageal fistula, **R**enal/radial anomalies, **L**imb defects; VCFS, velocardiofacial syndrome; VSD, ventricular septal defect.

Adapted from Park MK. *Pediatric Cardiology for Practitioners.* 5th ed. St Louis: Mosby; 2008:10-12.

TABLE 7-12

ACYANOTIC CONGENITAL HEART DISEASE

Lesion Type	% of CHD/Examination Findings	CDG Findings	Chest Radiograph Findings
Ventricular septal defect (VSD)	2–5/6 holosystolic murmur, loudest at the LLSB, ± systolic thrill ± apical diastolic rumble with large shunt With large VSD and pulmonary hypertension, S_2 may be narrow	*Small VSD:* Normal *Medium VSD:* LVH ± LAE *Large VSD:* BVH ± LAE, pure RVH	May show cardiomegaly and increased PVMs, depending on amount of left-to-right shunting
Atrial septal defect (ASD)	Wide, fixed split S_2 with grade 2–3/6 SEM at the LUSB May have mid-diastolic rumble at LLSB	*Small ASD:* Normal *Large ASD:* RAD and mild RVH or RBBB with RSR′ in V_1	May show cardiomegaly with increased PVMs if hemodynamically significant ASD
Patent ductus arteriosus (PDA)	40%–60% in VLBW infants 1–4/6 continuous "machinery" murmur loudest at LUSB Wide pulse pressure	*Small–moderate PDA:* Normal or LVH *Large PDA:* BVH	May have cardiomegaly and increased PVMs, depending on size of shunt (see Chapter 18 Section IX.A for treatment)
Atrioventricular septal defects	Most occur in Down syndrome Hyperactive precordium with systolic thrill at LLSB and loud S_2 ± grade 3–4/6 holosystolic regurgitant murmur along LLSB ± systolic murmur of MR at apex ± mid-diastolic rumble at LLSB or at apex ± gallop rhythm	Superior QRS axis RVH and LVH may be present	Cardiomegaly with increased PVMs
Pulmonary stenosis (PS)	Ejection click at LUSB with valvular PS—click intensity varies with respiration, decreasing with inspiration and increasing with expiration S_2 may split widely with P_2 diminished in intensity SEM (2–5/6) ± thrill at LUSB with radiation to back and sides	*Mild PS:* Normal *Moderate PS:* RAD and RVH *Severe PS:* RAE and RVH with strain	Normal heart size with normal to decreased PVMs
Aortic stenosis (AS)	Systolic thrill at RUSB, suprasternal notch, or over carotids Ejection click that does not vary with respiration if valvular AS Harsh SEM (2–4/6) at second RICS or third LICS, with radiation to neck and apex ± early diastolic decrescendo murmur due to AR Narrow pulse pressure if severe stenosis	*Mild AS:* Normal *Moderate–severe AS:* LVH ± strain	Usually normal

TABLE 7-12

ACYANOTIC CONGENITAL HEART DISEASE (Continued)

Lesion Type	% of CHD/Examination Findings	CDG Findings	Chest Radiograph Findings
Coarctation of aorta may present as: 1. Infant in CHF 2. Child with HTN 3. Child with murmur	Male/female ratio of 2:1 2–3/6 SEM at LUSB, radiating to left interscapular area Bicuspid valve is often associated, so may have systolic ejection click at apex and RUSB BP in lower extremities will be lower than in upper extremities. Pulse oximetry discrepancy of >5% between upper and lower extremities is also suggestive of coarctation.	*In infancy:* RVH or RBBB *In older children:* LVH	Marked cardiomegaly and pulmonary venous congestion. Rib notching from collateral circulation usually not seen in children younger than 5 years because collaterals not yet established.

AR, Aortic regurgitation; ASD, atrial septal defect; BP, blood pressure; BVH, biventricular hypertrophy; CHD, congenital heart disease; CHF, congestive heart failure; HTN, hypertension; LAE, left atrial enlargement; LICS, left intercostal space; LLSB, left lower sternal border; LUSB, left upper sternal border; LVH, left ventricular hypertrophy; MR, mitral regurgitation; PVM, pulmonary vascular markings; RAD, right axis deviation; RAE, right atrial enlargement; RBBB, right bundle-branch block; RICS, right intercostal space; RUSB, right upper sternal border; RVH, right ventricular hypertrophy; SEM, systolic ejection murmur; VLBW, very low birth weight (i.e. <1500 g); VSD, ventricular septal defect.

TABLE 7-13

CYANOTIC CONGENITAL HEART DISEASE

Lesion	Examination Findings	ECG Findings	Chest Radiograph Findings
Tetralogy of Fallot: 1. Large VSD 2. RVOT obstruction 3. RVH 4. Overriding aorta Degree of RVOT obstruction will determine whether there is clinical cyanosis. If PS is mild, there will be a left-to-right shunt, and child will be acyanotic. Increased obstruction leads to increased right-to-left shunting across VSD, and child will be cyanotic.	Loud SEM at LMSB and LUSB and a loud, single $S_2 \pm$ thrill at LMSB and LLSB. *Tet spells:* Occur in young infants. As RVOT obstruction increases or systemic resistance decreases, right-to-left shunting across VSD occurs. May present with tachypnea, increasing cyanosis, and decreasing murmur. See Table 7-14 for treatment.	RAD and RVH	Boot-shaped heart with normal heart size ± decreased PVMs

TABLE 7-13

CYANOTIC CONGENITAL HEART DISEASE (Continued)

Lesion	Examination Findings	ECG Findings	Chest Radiograph Findings
Transposition of great arteries	Nonspecific. Extreme cyanosis. Loud, single S$_2$. No murmur unless there is associated VSD or PS.	RAD and RVH (due to RV acting as systemic ventricle). Upright T wave in V$_1$ after age 3 days may be only abnormality.	Classic finding: "egg on a string" with cardiomegaly; possible increased PVMs
Tricuspid atresia: Absent tricuspid valve and hypoplastic RV and PA. Must have ASD, PDA, or VSD to survive.	Single S$_2$ + grade 2–3/6 systolic regurgitation murmur at LLSB if VSD is present. Occasional PDA murmur.	Superior QRS axis; RAE or CAE and LVH	Normal or slightly enlarged heart size; may have boot-shaped heart
Total anomalous pulmonary venous return Instead of draining into LA, pulmonary veins drain into the following locations. Must have ASD or PFO for survival: 1. *Supracardiac (most common):* SVC 2. *Cardiac:* Coronary sinus or RA 3. *Subdiaphragmatic:* IVC, portal vein, ductus venosus, or hepatic vein 4. *Mixed type*	Hyperactive RV impulse, quadruple rhythm, S$_2$ fixed and widely split, 2–3/6 SEM at LUSB, and mid-diastolic rumble at LLSB	RAD, RVH (RSR' in V$_1$). May see RAE	Cardiomegaly and increased PVMs; classic finding is "snowman in a snowstorm," but this is rarely seen until after age 4 months.

OTHER

Cyanotic CHDs that occur at a frequency of <1% each include pulmonary atresia, Ebstein anomaly, truncus arteriosus, single ventricle, and double outlet right ventricle			

ASD, Atrial septal defect; CAE, common atrial enlargement; ECG, electrocardiogram; IVC, inferior vena cava; LA, left atrium; LLSB, left lower sternal border; LMSB, left mid-sternal border; LUSB, left upper sternal border; LVH, left ventricular hypertrophy; PA, pulmonary artery; PDA, patent ductus arteriosus; PFO, patent foramen ovale; PVM, pulmonary vascular markings; PS, pulmonary stenosis; RA, right atrium; RAD, right-axis deviation; RAE, right atrial enlargement; RV, right ventricle; RVH, right ventricular hypertrophy; RVOT, right ventricular outflow tract; SEM, systolic ejection murmur; SVC, superior vena cava; VSD, ventricular septal defect.

TABLE 7-14

TREATMENT OPTIONS FOR TET SPELLS

Treatment	Rationale
INITIAL OPTIONS	
Calm child	Decreases PVR
Encourage knee-chest position	Decreases venous return and increases SVR
Oxygen	Reduces hypoxemia, decreases PVR
Intravenous fluids	Provides volume resuscitation
Morphine (morphine sulfate 0.1–0.2 mg/kg SQ or IM)	Decreases venous return, decreases PVR, relaxes infundibulum. Do *not* try to establish IV access initially; use SQ route.
IF THERE IS NO RESPONSE TO INITIAL MEASURES	
Phenylephrine (0.02 mg/kg IV)	Increases SVR
Propranolol (0.01–0.25 mg/kg slow IV push)	Has negative inotropic effect on infundibular myocardium; may block drop in SVR
Ketamine 1–3 mg/kg	Increases SVR and sedates
OTHER	
Correct anemia	Increases delivery of oxygen to tissues
Correct pathologic tachyarrhythmias	May abort hypoxic spell
Infuse glucose	Avoids hypoglycemia from increased utilization and depletion of glycogen stores

IM, Intramuscular; IV, intravenous; PVR, peripheral venous resistance; SQ, subcutaneous; SVR, systemic vascular resistance.
From Park MK. *Pediatric Cardiology for Practitioners.* 5th ed. St Louis: Mosby; 2008:239.

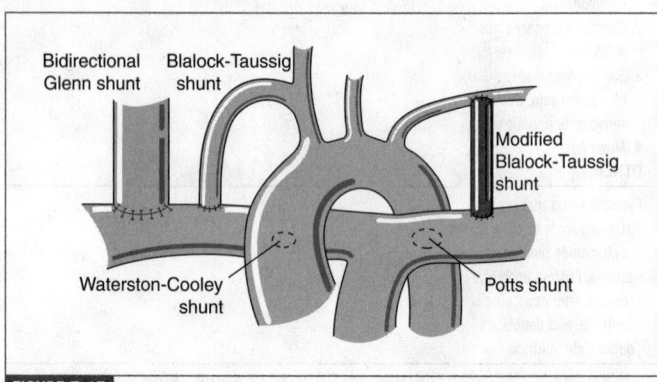

FIGURE 7-15

Schematic diagram of cardiac shunts.

E. Surgeries and Other Interventions (Fig. 7-15)

1. **Atrial septostomy:** Creates an intra-atrial opening to allow for mixing or shunting between atria of systemic and pulmonary venous blood. Used for transposition of the great arteries (TGA), tricuspid, mitral, tricuspid and pulmonary atresia, and sometimes total anomalous pulmonary venous return. Most commonly performed percutaneously with a balloon-tipped catheter (Rashkind procedure).

2. **Palliative systemic-to–pulmonary artery shunts,** such as the Blalock-Taussig shunt (subclavian artery to pulmonary artery [PA]): Use systemic arterial flow to increase pulmonary blood flow in cardiac lesions with impaired pulmonary perfusion (e.g., TOF, hypoplastic right heart, tricuspid atresia, pulmonary atresia)

3. **Palliative superior vena cava–to–pulmonary artery shunts,** such as the Glenn shunt, also known as the *hemi-Fontan* (superior vena cava [SVC] to the right pulmonary artery [RPA]): Directs a portion of the systemic venous return directly into the pulmonary blood flow as an intermediate step to a Fontan procedure. This procedure is usually performed outside the neonatal period, when there is lower pulmonary vascular resistance.

4. **Fontan procedure:** Performed after the Glenn shunt; involves anastomosis of the right atria and/or inferior vena cava (IVC) to pulmonary arteries via conduits; separates systemic and pulmonary circulations in patients with functionally single ventricles (tricuspid atresia, hypoplastic left heart syndrome)

5. **Norwood procedure:** Used for hypoplastic left heart syndrome

a. Stage 1 (neonatal period): To provide systemic blood flow, anastomosis of the proximal main pulmonary artery (MPA) is made to the aorta, with aortic arch reconstruction and patch closure of the distal MPA. To provide pulmonary blood flow, a modified right Blalock-Taussig shunt (subclavian artery to RPA) or Sano modification (RV to PA conduit) is performed. An atrial septal defect is created if needed to decompress the left atrium and allow for adequate left-to-right flow. Expected O_2 saturations: 75%–85%.

b. Stage 2 (3–6 months of age): Bidirectional Glenn shunt or hemi-Fontan to reduce volume overload of single right ventricle. Expected O_2 saturations: 80%–85%.

c. Modified Fontan (age 18 mo–4 yr): Needed to completely separate systemic and pulmonary circulations. Restores normal O_2 saturation, with expected O_2 saturation >92%.

6. **Arterial switch procedure**: Used for repair of TGA. Connects aorta to left ventricle and pulmonary artery to right ventricle. Procedure also involves reconnecting coronary arteries to aorta.

7. **Ross procedure:** Pulmonary root autograft for aortic stenosis; autologous pulmonary valve replaces aortic valve, and aortic or pulmonary allograft replaces pulmonary valve.

VII. ACQUIRED HEART DISEASE

A. Endocarditis

1. **Common causative organisms:** About 70% of causes of endocarditis are streptococcal species (*Streptococcus viridans,* enterococci); 20% are staphylococcal species (*Staphylococcus aureus, Staphylococcus epidermidis*); 10% are other organisms (*Haemophilus influenzae,* gram-negative bacteria, fungi).

2. **Clinical findings:** New heart murmur, recurrent fever, splenomegaly, petechiae, fatigue, Osler nodes (tender nodules at fingertips), Janeway lesions (painless hemorrhagic areas on palms or soles), splinter hemorrhages, and Roth spots (retinal hemorrhages)

B. Bacterial Endocarditis Prophylaxis

See Table 7-15 for antibiotic choices and Box 7-4 for cardiac conditions requiring prophylaxis.[15]

1. **All dental procedures** that involve treatment of gingival tissue or periapical region of the teeth or oral mucosal perforation

2. **Invasive procedures** that involve incision or biopsy of respiratory mucosa, such as tonsillectomy and adenoidectomy

3. **Not recommended** for genitourinary or gastrointestinal tract procedures; solely for bacterial endocarditis prevention

C. Myocardial Disease

1. **Dilated cardiomyopathy:** End result of myocardial damage, leading to atrial and ventricular dilation with decreased systolic contractile function of the ventricles

a. Etiology: Infectious, toxic (alcohol, anthracyclines), metabolic (hypothyroidism, muscular dystrophy), immunologic, collagen vascular disease, nutritional deficiency (kwashiorkor, beriberi)

b. Symptoms: Fatigue, weakness, shortness of breath

c. Examination: Look for signs of CHF (e.g., tachycardia, tachypnea, rales, cold extremities, jugular venous distention, hepatomegaly, peripheral edema, S_3 gallop, displacement of point of maximal impulse to the left and inferiorly)

d. Chest radiograph: Generalized cardiomegaly, pulmonary congestion

e. ECG: Sinus tachycardia, left ventricular hypertrophy (LVH), possible atrial enlargement, arrhythmias, conduction disturbances, ST-segment and T-wave changes

TABLE 7-15

PROPHYLACTIC REGIMENS FOR DENTAL AND RESPIRATORY TRACT PROCEDURES

Drug	Dosing* (not to exceed adult dose)
Amoxicillin[†]	Adult: 2 g; Child: 50 mg/kg PO
Ampicillin	Adult: 2 g; Child: 50 mg/kg IM/IV
Cefazolin or ceftriaxone[‡]	Adult: 1 g; Child: 50 mg/kg IM/IV
Cephalexin[‡]	Adult: 2 g; Child: 50 mg/kg PO
Clindamycin	Adult: 600 mg; Child: 20 mg/kg PO/IM/IV
Azithromycin/clarithromycin	Adult: 500 mg; Child: 15 mg/kg PO

*Oral (PO) medications should be given 1 hour before procedure; intramuscular/intravenous (IM/IV) medications should be given within 30 min prior to procedure.

†Standard general prophylaxis.

‡Cephalosporins should not be used in persons with intermediate-type hypersensitivity reaction to penicillins or ampicillin.

Adapted from Wilson W, Taubert KA, Gewitz M, et al. Prevention of infective endocarditis: Guidelines from the American Heart Association: A guideline from the American Heart Association Rheumatic Fever, Endocarditis, and Kawasaki Disease Committee, Council on Cardiovascular Disease in the Young, and the Council on Clinical Cardiology, Council on Cardiovascular Surgery and Anesthesia, and the Quality of Care and Outcomes Research Interdisciplinary Working Group. *Circulation.* 2007;116:1736-1754.

BOX 7-4

CARDIAC CONDITIONS FOR WHICH ANTIBIOTIC PROPHYLAXIS IS RECOMMENDED FOR DENTAL, RESPIRATORY TRACT, INFECTED SKIN, SKIN STRUCTURES, OR MUSCULOSKELETAL TISSUE PROCEDURES

- Prosthetic cardiac valve
- Previous bacterial endocarditis
- Congenital heart disease (CHD)—Limited to the following conditions*
  - Unrepaired cyanotic defect, including palliative shunts and conduits
  - Completely repaired CHD with prosthetic material/device (placed by surgery or catheterization), during first 6 months after procedure†
  - Repaired CHD with residual defects at or adjacent to the site of prosthetic patch or device (which inhibit endothelialization)
  - Cardiac transplantation patients who develop cardiac valvulopathy

*Conditions associated with the highest risk of adverse outcome from endocarditis.
†Endothelialization process of prosthetic material occurs within 6 months after the procedure.
Adapted from Wilson W, Taubert KA, Gewitz M, et al. Prevention of infective endocarditis: Guidelines from the American Heart Association: A guideline from the American Heart Association Rheumatic Fever, Endocarditis, and Kawasaki Disease Committee, Council on Cardiovascular Disease in the Young, and the Council on Clinical Cardiology, Council on Cardiovascular Surgery and Anesthesia, and the Quality of Care and Outcomes Research Interdisciplinary Working Group. *Circulation.* 2007;116:1736-1754.

---

f. Echocardiography: Enlarged ventricles (increased end-diastolic and end-systolic dimensions) with little or no wall thickening; decreased shortening fraction

g. Treatment: Management of CHF (digoxin, diuretics, vasodilation, angiotensin-converting enzyme [ACE] inhibitors, rest). Consider anticoagulants to decrease risk for thrombus formation.

2. **Hypertrophic cardiomyopathy:** Abnormality of myocardial cells leading to significant ventricular hypertrophy, particularly of left ventricle, with small to normal ventricular dimensions. Increased contractile function but impaired filling secondary to stiff ventricles. The most common type is asymmetrical septal hypertrophy, also called *idiopathic hypertrophic subaortic stenosis* (IHSS), with varying degrees of obstruction. A 4%–6% incidence of sudden death in children and adolescents with hypertrophic obstructive cardiomyopathy (HOCM).

a. Etiology: Genetic (autosomal dominant, 60% of cases) or sporadic (40% of cases)

b. Symptoms: Easy fatigability, anginal pain, shortness of breath, occasional palpitations

c. Examination: Usually in adolescents or young adults; signs include left ventricular heave, sharp upstroke of arterial pulse, murmur of mitral regurgitation, midsystolic ejection murmur along left midsternal border (LMSB) that increases in intensity in the standing position (in patients with midcavity left ventricular obstruction)

d. Chest radiograph: Globular-shaped heart with left ventricular enlargement

e. ECG: LVH, prominent Q waves (septal hypertrophy), ST-segment and T-wave changes, arrhythmias

f. Echocardiography: Extent and location of hypertrophy, obstruction, increased contractility

g. Treatment: Moderate restriction of physical activity, administration of negative inotropes (β-blocker, calcium channel blocker) to help improve filling and subacute bacterial endocarditis prophylaxis. If at increased risk for sudden death, may consider implantable defibrillator. If symptomatic with subaortic obstruction, may benefit from myectomy.

3. **Restrictive cardiomyopathy:** Myocardial or endocardial disease (usually infiltrative or fibrotic) resulting in stiff ventricular walls, with restriction of diastolic filling but normal contractile function. Results in atrial enlargement. Associated with a high mortality rate. Very rare in children.

a. Etiology: Scleroderma, amyloidosis, sarcoidosis, mucopolysaccharidosis

b. Treatment: Supportive, poor prognosis. Diuretics, anticoagulants, calcium channel blockers, pacemaker for heart block, cardiac transplantation if severe.

4. **Myocarditis:** Inflammation of myocardial tissue

a. Etiology: Viral (coxsackievirus, echovirus, adenovirus, poliomyelitis, mumps, measles, rubella, cytomegalovirus, HIV, arbovirus, influenza); bacterial, rickettsial, fungal, or parasitic infection; immune-mediated disease (Kawasaki disease, acute rheumatic fever); collagen vascular disease; toxin-induced

b. Symptoms: Nonspecific and inconsistent, depending on severity of disease. Variably anorexia, lethargy, emesis, lightheadedness, cold extremities, shortness of breath.

c. Examination: Look for signs of CHF (tachycardia, tachypnea, jugular venous distention, rales, gallop, hepatomegaly); occasionally a soft systolic murmur or arrhythmia may be noted.

d. Chest radiograph: Variable cardiomegaly and pulmonary edema

e. ECG: Low QRS voltages throughout (<5 mm), ST-segment and T-wave changes (e.g., decreased T-wave amplitude), prolongation of QT interval, arrhythmias (especially premature contractions, first- or second-degree AV block)

f. Laboratory tests: CK, troponin

g. Echocardiography: Enlargement of heart chambers, impaired left ventricular function

h. Treatment: Bed rest, diuretics, inotropes (dopamine, dobutamine, milrinone), digoxin, gamma globulin (2 g/kg over 24 hours), ACE inhibitors, possibly steroids. May require heart transplantation if no improvement (≈20%–25% of cases)

D. Pericardial Disease

1. **Pericarditis:** Inflammation of visceral and parietal layers of pericardium

a. Etiology: Viral (especially echovirus, coxsackievirus B), tuberculosis, bacterial, uremic, neoplastic, collagen vascular, post-MI or postpericardiotomy, radiation induced, drug induced (e.g., procainamide, hydralazine), or idiopathic

b. Symptoms: Chest pain (retrosternal or precordial, radiating to back or shoulder, pleuritic in nature, alleviated by leaning forward, aggravated by supine position), dyspnea

c. Examination: Pericardial friction rub, distant heart sounds, fever, tachypnea

d. ECG: Diffuse ST-segment elevation in almost all leads (representing inflammation of adjacent myocardium); PR-segment depression

e. Treatment: Often self-limited. Treat underlying condition and provide symptomatic treatment with rest, analgesia, and antiinflammatory drugs

2. **Pericardial effusion:** Accumulation of excess fluid in pericardial sac

a. Etiology: Associated with acute pericarditis (exudative fluid) or serous effusion resulting from increased capillary hydrostatic pressure (e.g., CHF), decreased plasma oncotic pressure (e.g., hypoproteinemia), and increased capillary permeability (transudative fluid)

b. Symptoms: Can present with no symptoms, dull ache in left chest, abdominal pain, or symptoms of cardiac tamponade (see later)

c. Examination: Muffled distant heart sounds, dullness to percussion of posterior left chest (secondary to atelectasis from large pericardial sac), hemodynamic signs of cardiac compression

d. Chest radiograph: Globular symmetrical cardiomegaly

e. ECG: Decreased voltage of QRS complexes, electrical alternans (variation of QRS axis with each beat secondary to swinging of heart within pericardial fluid)

f. Echocardiography shows extent and location of hypertrophy, obstruction, increased contractility

g. Treatment: Address underlying condition. Observe if asymptomatic; use pericardiocentesis if there is sudden increase in volume or hemodynamic compromise. Nonsteroidal antiinflammatory drugs (NSAIDs) or steroids may be of benefit, depending on etiology.

3. **Cardiac tamponade:** Accumulation of pericardial fluid under high pressure, causing compression of cardiac chambers, limiting filling, and decreasing stroke volume and cardiac output

a. Etiology: Same as pericardial effusion; most commonly associated with viral infection, neoplasm, uremia, and acute hemorrhage

b. Symptoms: Dyspnea, fatigue, cold extremities

c. Examination: Jugular venous distention, hepatomegaly, peripheral edema, tachypnea, rales (from increased systemic and pulmonary venous pressure), hypotension, tachycardia, pulsus paradoxus (decrease in systolic blood pressure by >10 mmHg with each inspiration), decreased capillary refill (from decreased stroke volume and cardiac output), quiet precordium, and muffled heart sounds

d. ECG: Sinus tachycardia, decreased voltage, electrical alternans

e. Echocardiography: Right ventricle collapse in early diastole, right atrial/left atrial collapse in end-diastole and early systole

f. Treatment: Pericardiocentesis with temporary catheter left in place if necessary (see Chapter 3, Figs. 3-15 and 3-16); pericardial window or stripping if it is a recurrent condition

E. Kawasaki Disease

Acute febrile vasculitis of unknown etiology, common in children < 8 years of age, and the leading cause of acquired heart disease in children in developed countries

1. **Etiology:** Unknown; thought to be immune regulated in response to infectious agents or environmental toxins
2. **Diagnosis:**
a. Typical Kawasaki disease: Based on clinical criteria. These include high fever lasting 5 days or more, plus at least 4 of the following 5 criteria:
    (1) Bilateral painless bulbar conjunctival injection without exudate
    (2) Erythematous mouth and pharynx, strawberry tongue, or red cracked lips
    (3) Polymorphous exanthem (may be morbilliform, maculopapular, or scarlatiniform)
    (4) Swelling of hands and feet, with erythema of palms and soles
    (5) Cervical lymphadenopathy (>1.5 cm in diameter), usually single and unilateral
b. Atypical/incomplete Kawasaki disease: A suspicion of Kawasaki but with fewer of the criteria required for diagnosis. Even without all criteria, there is a risk for coronary artery abnormalities.
    (1) More often seen in infants. Echocardiography should be considered in any infant < 6 months with fever > 7 days duration, laboratory evidence of systemic inflammation, and no other explanation for the febrile illness.
    (2) See Fig. 7-16 for evaluation of incomplete Kawasaki disease.
    (3) Supplemental laboratory criteria: Albumin ≤ 3.0 g/dL, anemia for age, elevation of alanine aminotransferase, platelets after 7 days ≥ 450,000 / mm^3, white blood cell count ≥ 15,000 / mm^3, and urine white blood cells/hpf ≥ 10.
3. **Other clinical findings:** Often associated with extreme irritability, abdominal pain, diarrhea, vomiting. Also seen are arthritis and arthralgias, hepatic enlargement, jaundice, acute acalculous distention of the gallbladder, carditis, aseptic meningitis (50% of those undergoing LP).
4. **Laboratory findings:** Leukocytosis with left shift, neutrophils with vacuoles or toxic granules, elevated C-reactive protein (CRP) or erythrocyte sedimentation rate (ESR) (seen acutely), thrombocytosis (after first week, peaking at 3 weeks), normocytic and normochromic anemia, sterile pyuria (33%), increased transaminases (40%), hyperbilirubinemia (10%)
5. **Subacute phase (11–25 days after onset of illness):** Resolution of fever, rash, and lymphadenopathy. Often, desquamation of the fingertips or toes and thrombocytosis occur.
    Cardiovascular complications: If untreated, 20%–25% develop coronary artery aneurysms and dilation in subacute phase (peak prevalence occurs about 2–4 weeks after onset of disease; rarely appears after 6 weeks) and are at risk for coronary thrombosis acutely and coronary stenosis chronically. Carditis; aortic, mitral, and tricuspid regurgitation; pericardial effusion; CHF; MI; left ventricular dysfunction; and ECG changes may also occur.

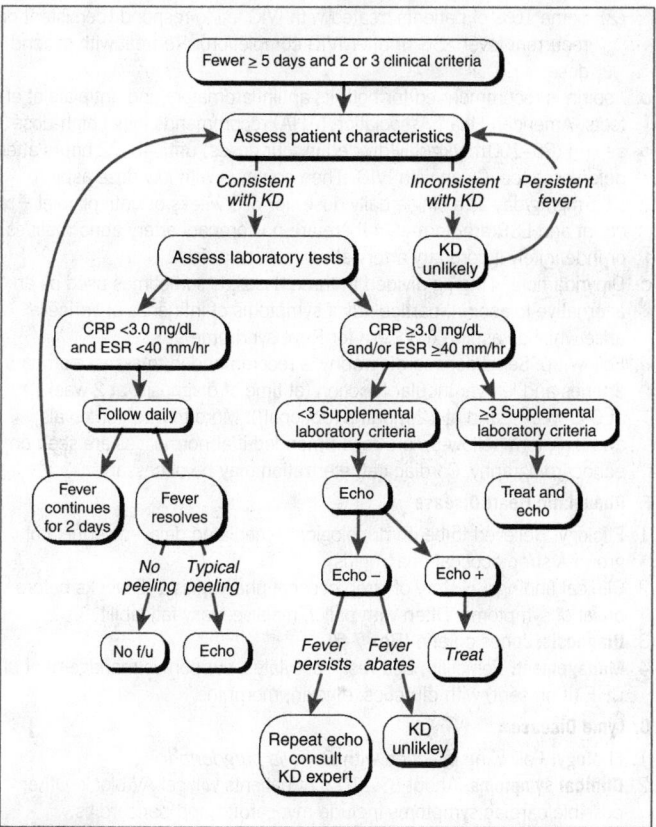

FIGURE 7-16

Evaluation of incomplete Kawasaki disease *(KD)*. CRP, C-reactive protein; echo, echo-cardiogram; ESR, erythrocyte sedimentation rate; f/u, follow-up. *(From Newburger JW, Takahashi M, Gerber MA, et al. Diagnosis, treatment, and long term management of Kawasaki disease. Circulation. 2004;110:2747-2771.)*

6. **Convalescent phase:** ESR, CRP, and platelet count return to normal. Those with coronary artery abnormalities are at increased risk for MI, arrhythmias, and sudden death.
7. **Management** (also see Table EC 7-C)[16]
   a. Intravenous immunoglobulin (IVIG)
      (1) Shown to reduce incidence of coronary artery dilation to <3% and decrease duration of fever if given in the first 10 days of illness. Current recommended regimen is a single dose of IVIG, 2 g/kg over 10–12 hours.

(2) Some 10% of patients treated with IVIG fail to respond (persistent or recurrent fever ≥36 hr after IVIG completion). Re-treat with second dose.

b. Aspirin is recommended for both its antiinflammatory and antiplatelet effects. American Heart Association (AHA) recommends initial high-dose aspirin (80–100 mg/kg/day divided in four doses) until 48–72 hours after defervescence. Given with IVIG. Then continue with low-dose aspirin (3–5 mg/kg/day as a single daily dose) for 6–8 weeks or until platelet count and ESR are normal (if there are no coronary artery abnormalities) or indefinitely if coronary artery abnormalities persist.

c. Dipyridamole, 4 mg/kg divided in three doses, is sometimes used as an alternative to aspirin, particularly if symptoms of influenza or varicella arise while on aspirin (concern for Reye syndrome).

d. Follow-up: Serial echocardiography is recommended to assess coronary arteries and left ventricular function (at time of diagnosis, at 2 weeks, at 6–8 weeks, and at 12 months [optional]). More frequent intervals and long-term follow-up are recommended if abnormalities are seen on echocardiography. Cardiac catheterization may be necessary.

F. Rheumatic Heart Disease

1. Etiology: Believed to be immunologically mediated delayed sequela of group A streptococcal pharyngitis

2. Clinical findings: History of streptococcal pharyngitis 1–5 weeks before onset of symptoms. Often with pallor, malaise, easy fatigability.

3. **Diagnosis:** Jones criteria (Box 7-5)

4. **Management:** Penicillin, bed rest, salicylates, supportive management of CHF (if present) with diuretics, digoxin, morphine

G. Lyme Disease

1. **Etiology:** Following infection with *Borrelia burgdorferi*

2. **Clinical symptoms:** About 8%–10% of patients will get AV block. Other possible cardiac symptoms include myocarditis and pericarditis.

VIII. EXERCISE RECOMMENDATIONS FOR CONGENITAL HEART DISEASE

See Table EC 7-D for exercise recommendations for congenital heart disease.[17]

IX. LIPID MONITORING RECOMMENDATIONS

A. Screening of Children and Adolescents[18]

1. **Universal screening** of non-fasting non-HDL cholesterol in children 9–11 years old (prior to onset of puberty) and again in individuals 17–21 years

2. **Targeted screening** should occur in children 2–8 years old and adolescents 12–16 years old, with two fasting lipid profiles (between 2 weeks and 3 months apart, results averaged) for the following risk factors:

a. Moderate or high-risk medical condition (history of prematurity, VLBW, congenital heart disease (repaired or nonrepaired), recurrent urinary

BOX 7-5

GUIDELINES FOR DIAGNOSIS OF INITIAL ATTACK OF RHEUMATIC FEVER (JONES CRITERIA)

Major Manifestations	Minor Manifestations
Carditis	Clinical findings:
Polyarthritis	Arthralgia
Chorea	Fever
Erythema marginatum	Laboratory findings:
Subcutaneous nodule	Elevated acute phase reactants (erythrocyte sedimentation rate, C-reactive protein)
	Prolonged PR interval

Plus

Supporting evidence of antecedent group A streptococcal infection

Positive throat culture or rapid streptococcal antigen test

Elevated or rising streptococcal antibody titer

NOTE: If supported by evidence of preceding group A streptococcal infection, the presence of two major manifestations or of one major and two minor manifestations indicates a high probability of acute rheumatic fever.

tract infections, known renal or urologic malformations, family history of congenital renal disease, solid organ transplant, malignancy or bone marrow transplant, treatment with drugs known to raise blood pressure, other systemic illness associated with hypertension (neurofibromatosis, tuberous sclerosis), evidence of elevated intracranial pressure

b. Have other cardiovascular risk factors (diabetes, hypertension, body mass index [BMI] ≥ 95th percentile, smoke cigarettes)

c. Have a family history of early cardiovascular disease (CVD) or severe hypercholesterolemia

  (1) Parent or grandparent who is < 55 years old (males) or < 65 years old (females) and had suffered a myocardial infarction or sudden death, undergone a coronary artery procedure, or who otherwise had evidence of coronary atherosclerosis, peripheral vascular disease, or cerebrovascular disease

  (2) Parent with total cholesterol ≥ 240 mg/dL or known dyslipidemia

B. Goals for Lipid Levels in Childhood

1. Total cholesterol

a. Acceptable (<170 mg/dL): Repeat measurement in 3–5 years

b. Borderline (170–199 mg/dL): Repeat cholesterol and average with previous measurement. If <170, repeat in 3–5 years. If ≥170, obtain lipoprotein analysis.

c. High (≥200 mg/dL): Obtain lipoprotein analysis

2. Low-density lipoprotein (LDL) cholesterol

a. Acceptable (<110 mg/dL)

b. Borderline (110–129 mg/dL)

c. High (≥130 mg/dL)

C. Management of Hyperlipidemia[18]

1. **Normal and borderline elevated LDL levels:** Education, risk factor intervention including diet, smoking cessation, and an exercise program. For borderline levels, reevaluate in 1 year.
2. **High LDL levels:** Examine for secondary causes (liver, thyroid, renal disorders) and familial disorders. Initiate low-fat, low-cholesterol diet; reevaluate in 6 months. **Note:** For LDL cholesterol > 250 or triglyceridemia >500, refer directly to a lipid specialist.
3. **Drug therapy:** Should be considered in children >10 years of age after failure of 6- to 12-month trial of diet therapy as follows:
a. LDL >190 mg/dL without other cardiovascular disease risk factors
b. LDL >160 mg/dL with risk factors (diabetes, obesity, hypertension, positive family history of premature CVD)
c. LDL >130 mg/dL in children with diabetes mellitus
d. Bile acid sequestrants and statins are the usual first-line drugs for treatment in children.
4. **Persistently high triglycerides (>150 mg/dL) and reduced HDL (<35 mg/dL):** Evaluate for secondary causes (diabetes, alcohol abuse, renal or thyroid disease). Treatment is diet and exercise.

X. CARDIOVASCULAR SCREENING

A. Sports[19]

There is no established mandated preparticipation sports screening. There is a recommended history and physical examination screening from the American Heart Association (AHA). Routine ECGs are not required unless there is suspicion of underlying cardiac disease (Box EC 7-A).

B. Attention Deficit/Hyperactivity Disorder (ADHD)

1. **Obtain a good patient and family history as well as physical examination.**
2. **There is not an increased risk of sudden cardiac death** in children without cardiac disease taking ADHD medications. There is no consensus on universal ECG screening. ECGs should be obtained in those who screen with positive answers on history, polypharmacy, tachycardia while on medications, and history of significant cardiac disease. If a patient has significant heart disease or concern for cardiac disease, have patient evaluated by a pediatric cardiologist.

REFERENCES

1. Zubrow AB, Hulman S, Kushner H, et al. Determinants of blood pressure in infants admitted to neonatal intensive care units: a prospective multicenter study. Philadelphia Neonatal Blood Pressure Study Group. *J Perinatol.* 1995;15:470.
2. National High Blood Pressure Education Program Working Group on High Blood Pressure in Children and Adolescents. The fourth report on the diagnosis, evaluation, and treatment of high blood pressure in children and adolescents. *Pediatrics.* 2004;114(2 Suppl):555-576.
3. Park MK. *Pediatric Cardiology for Practitioners.* 5th ed. St Louis: Mosby; 2008.

4. Sapin SO. Recognizing normal heart murmurs: a logic-based mnemonic. *Pediatrics.* 1997;99:616-619.

5. Davignon A, Rautaharju P, Boisselle E, et al. Normal ECG standards for infants and children. *Pediatr Cardiol.* 1979;1:123-131.

6. Schwartz PJ, Stramba-Badiale M, Segantini A, et al. Prolongation of the QT interval and the sudden infant death syndrome. *N Engl J Med.* 1998;338:1709-1714.

7. Garson A Jr. *TheElectrocardiogram in Infants and Children: A Systematic Approach.* Philadelphia: Lea & Febiger; 1983.

8. Park MK, Guntheroth WG. *How to Read Pediatric ECGs.* 4th ed. Philadelphia: Mosby; 2006.

9. Towbin JA, Bricker JT, Garson A Jr. Electrocardiographic criteria for diagnosis of acute myocardial infarction in childhood. *Am J Cardiol.* 1992;69:1545-1548.

10. Hirsch R, Landt Y, Porter S, et al. Cardiac troponin I in pediatrics: normal values and potential use in assessment of cardiac injury. *J Pediatr.* 1997;130:872-877.

11. Colan SD, Parness IA, Spevak PJ, et al. Developmental modulation of myocardial mechanics: age- and growth-related alterations in afterload and contractility. *J Am Coll Cardiol.* 1992;19:619-629.

12. Lees MH. Cyanosis of the newborn infant: recognition and clinical evaluation. *J Pediatr.* 1970;77:484-498.

13. Kitterman JA. Cyanosis in the newborn infant. *Pediatr Rev.* 1982;4:13-24.

14. Jones RW, Baumer JH, Joseph MC, et al. Arterial oxygen tension and response to oxygen breathing in differential diagnosis of heart disease in infancy. *Arch Dis Child.* 1976;51:667-673.

15. Wilson W, Taubert KA, Gewitz M, et al. Prevention of infective endocarditis: guidelines from the American Heart Association: a guideline from the American Heart Association Rheumatic Fever, Endocarditis, and Kawasaki Disease Committee, Council on Cardiovascular Disease in the Young, and the Council on Clinical Cardiology, Council on Cardiovascular Surgery and Anesthesia, and the Quality of Care and Outcomes Research Interdisciplinary Working Group. *Circulation.* 2007;116:1736-1754.

16. Newburger JW, Takahashi M, Gerber MA, et al. Diagnosis, treatment, and long term management of Kawasaki disease. *Circulation.* 2004;110:2747-2771.

17. Maron BJ, Zipes DP. Introduction: eligibility recommendations for competitive athletes with cardiovascular abnormalities. *J Am Coll Cardiol.* 2005;45: 1313-1375.

18. Expert Panel on Integrated Guidelines for Cardiovascular Health and Risk Reduction in Children and Adolescents: Summary Report. *Pediatrics.* 2011;128:S213-S256.

19. Maron BJ, Thompson PD, Ackerman MJ, et al. Recommendations and considerations related to preparticipation screening for cardiovascular abnormalities in competitive athletes: 2007 update: a scientific statement from the American Heart Association Council on Nutrition, Physical Activity, and Metabolism: endorsed by the American College of Cardiology Foundation. *Circulation.* 2007;115:1643-1655.

20. Walsh EP. Cardiac arrhythmias. In: Fyler DC, Nadas A, eds. *Pediatric Cardiology.* Philadelphia: Hanley & Belfus; 1992:384.

Chapter 8

Dermatology

Jing Fang, MD

I. WEBSITE

Dermatology Image Atlas: http://www.dermatlas.org
NOTE: Please refer to the color plates in this chapter for photographic examples of dermatologic findings.

II. EVALUATION AND CLINICAL DESCRIPTIONS OF SKIN FINDINGS

A. Primary Skin Lesions (Fig. 8-1)

1. **Macule:** Small flat lesion with altered color (<1 cm)
2. **Patch:** Large macule (>1 cm), also used to describe large macule with scale
3. **Papule:** Elevated, well-circumscribed lesion (<1 cm)
4. **Plaque:** Large papule (>1 cm)
5. **Nodule:** Mass located in dermis or subcutaneous fat (may be solid or soft)
6. **Tumor:** Large nodule
7. **Vesicle:** Blister with transparent fluid
8. **Bulla:** Large vesicle
9. **Wheal:** Erythematous, well-circumscribed, raised, edematous lesion that appears and disappears quickly

B. Secondary Skin Lesions (see Fig. 8-1)

1. **Scale:** Small, thin plate of horny epithelium
2. **Pustule:** Well-circumscribed elevated lesion filled with pus
3. **Crust:** Exudative mass consisting of blood, scale, and pus from skin erosions or ruptured vesicles/papules
4. **Ulcer:** Erosion of dermis and cutis, with clearly defined edges
5. **Scar:** Formation of new connective tissue after damage to epidermis and cutis, eaving permanent change in skin
6. **Excoriation:** Surface marks, often linear secondary to scratching
7. **Fissure:** Linear skin crack with inflammation and pain

III. SKIN LUMPS: DIAGNOSIS AND TREATMENT (FIGS. 8-2 TO 8-13)

A. Hemangiomas (Fig. 8-2, color)

1. **Pathogenesis:** Benign vascular tumor of infancy, with a phase of rapid proliferation (densely packed endothelial cells form small capillaries, and subsequent vessels develop from existing vasculature), followed by phase of spontaneous involution.
2. **Clinical presentation:**
a. Not fully formed at birth. Some newborns may demonstrate pale macules with threadlike telangiectasias that later develop into hemangiomas.

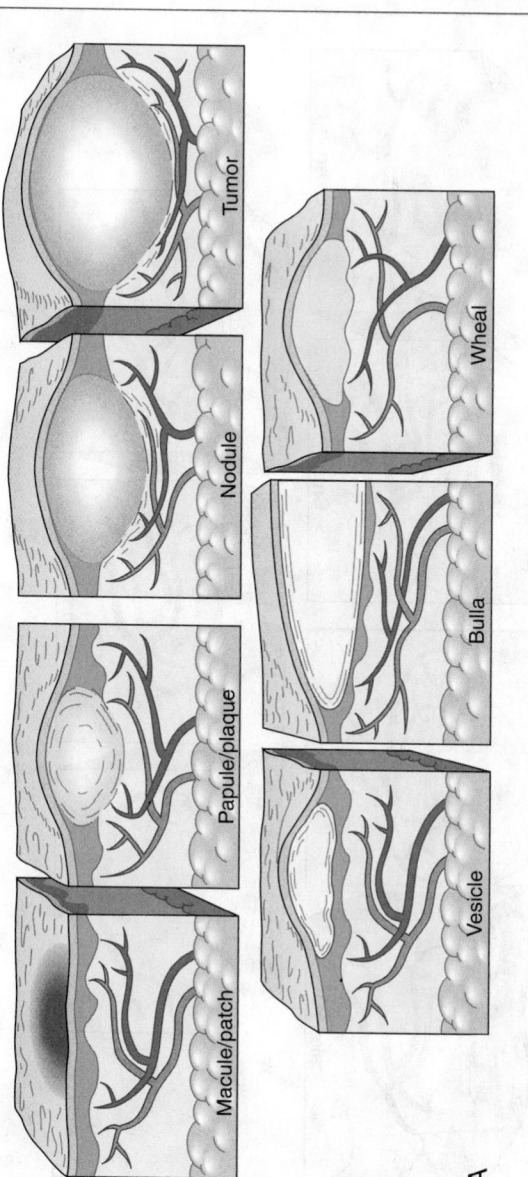

Continued

FIGURE 8-1

Pattern diagnosis. **A,** Primary skin lesions.

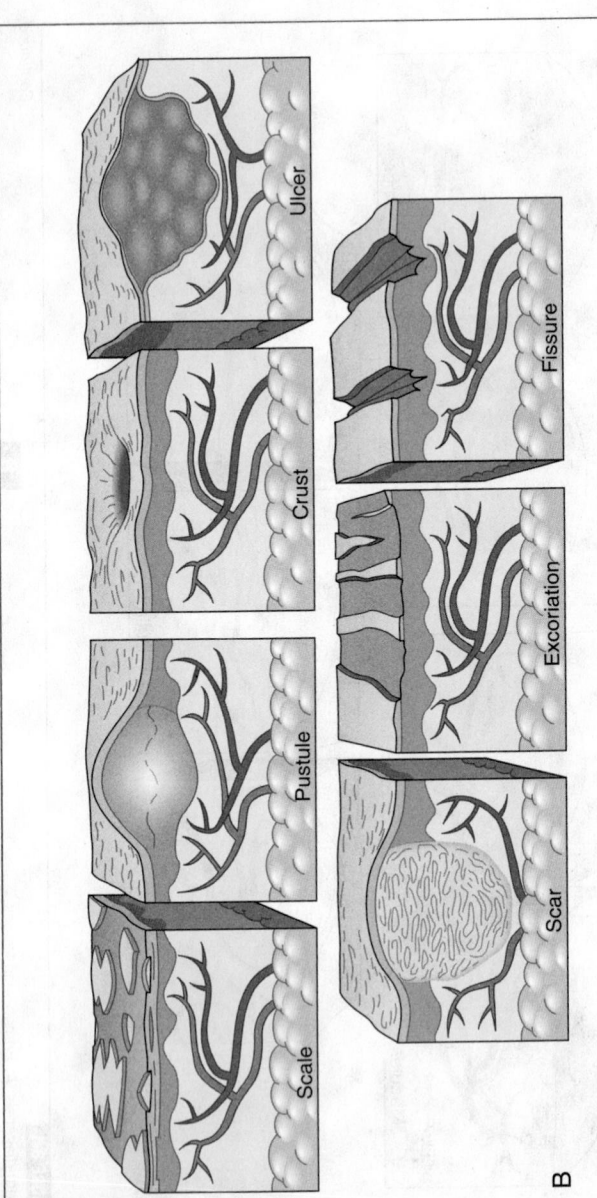

FIGURE 8-1: cont'd

B, Secondary skin lesions. *(From Cohen BA. Pediatric Dermatology. 2nd ed. St Louis: Mosby, 1999:5.)*

b. Superficial usually noted first, but most with both superficial and deep components.
   (1) Superficial: Bright red papule, nodule, plaque
   (2) Deep: Firm, rubbery nodule/tumor, often with overlying blue-purple discoloration
c. Size: Range from a few millimeters to many centimeters.
d. After involution, can have residual skin changes, including scarring and atrophy.

3. **Incidence:** Most common tumor of infancy. Low birth weight highest risk factor; increased risk in Caucasian infants (5%–10%, less common in other ethnic groups), premature infants, and females.

4. **Natural history:** Most occur within 2 days to 2 months of life. Undergo rapid growth phase in first few months, with 80% peaking by 3 months. Many begin to regress by 6 months, with rate of 10% complete involution per year (i.e., 50% or more completely involuted by 5 years).

5. **Diagnosis:** Usually diagnosed clinically. Atypical clinical findings, growth pattern, and equivocal imaging should prompt tissue biopsy to exclude other neoplasms or unusual vascular malformations.

6. **Complications:**
a. Ulceration: Most common complication. Can be extremely painful and will scar. Can also bleed and become superinfected.
b. Bleeding: Usually minimal, can be stopped with direct pressure.
c. Visual obstruction: From periorbital hemangiomas, especially involving upper medial eyelid. Require evaluation by an ophthalmologist.
d. Airway obstruction: Seen with airway hemangiomas. Infants with lesions in a beard distribution (i.e., chin, lower lip, mandible, anterior neck) are at greater risk. May have hoarseness, stridor, cough, and cyanosis.
e. Otitis externa: From ear hemangiomas that obstruct the auditory canal.
f. Deformation/destruction of important cosmetic structures: From especially large lesions (i.e., ear, nasal septum, vermillion border).
g. Rare complications:
   (1) Kasabach-Merritt phenomenon: Associated with hemangiopericytomas, tufted angiomas, or kaposiform hemangioendotheliomas, not true infantile hemangiomas. Rare complication due to platelet trapping within rapidly growing vascular tumor. Characterized by severe thrombocytopenia, coagulopathy, and variable degree of hemolytic anemia. Differentiated from benign hemangiomas by their deep red-blue appearance, marked firmness, and histologic appearance.
   (2) PHACES syndrome: **P**osterior cranial fossa malformations (as well as multiple other cerebral arteriovenous anomalies), large segmental facial **H**emangiomas, **A**rterial lesions, **C**ardiac abnormalitites (aortic coarctation, other anomalies of the aortic and mesenteric vessels), **E**ye abnormalities, **S**ternal cleft anomalies/supraumbilical raphes.[1]
   (3) Visceral hemangiomas: Usually hepatic hemangiomas; most are asymptomatic and can be observed without imaging. Rarely, can cause massive hepatosplenomegaly and heart failure. Associated

with segmental hemangiomas and multiple cutaneous hemangiomas, although may be isolated lesions.

(4) Sacral syndrome: Tethered cord, spinal, anorectal, and urogenital anomalies, associated with lumbosacral hemangiomas. Require evaluation with magnetic resonance imaging (MRI).

7. **Management:**

a. Most require no intervention. Decision to treat should be based on location, size, pattern, age of patient, and risk of complications. Photo documentation is used to follow the growth and regression process.

b. Treatment of clinically significant infantile hemangiomas[2]:

(1) Propranolol:

(a) Considered an off-label use. There is no U.S. Food and Drug Administration (FDA)-approved medical treatment for infantile hemagiomas, but propranolol is now accepted by pediatric dermatologists as the standard of care. Should be initiated under careful supervision of a pediatric dermatologist or other practitioner experienced in management.

(b) Patients should be clinically screened for cardiac disease. Electrocardiogram (ECG) and/or echocardiogram are not required but obtained only when indicated (e.g., heart murmur, suspected cardiac/other vascular anomalies).

(c) Inpatient treatment: Infants < 2 months or those deemed at risk for complications from oral propranolol should be admitted for 48 hours for initiation of therapy.

(i) Goal dosing: 2 mg/kg/day. Recommend starting with 1 mg/kg/day divided TID for 24 hours, then increasing to 2 mg/kg/day divided TID for 24 hours.
Side effects: Bradycardia, hypotension, hypoglycemia.
Blood pressure and heart rate should be monitored 1 hour after each dose. Blood glucose should be checked as indicated for unexpected changes in behavior (e.g., jitteriness, somnolence).

(ii) Child can be discharged if six doses of medication are tolerated without complications. Pediatrician should be notified at time of discharge.

(d) Outpatient treatment: Healthy infants >2 months can start therapy in a supervised clinic setting. Initial clinic visit should be 2 hours long.

(i) Goal dosing: 2 mg/kg/day. Give initial dose in clinic. Recommend starting with 1 mg/kg/day divided TID for 5 days, then increase to 1.5 mg/kg/day divided TID for another 5 days, and finally after day 10, increase to 2 mg/kg/day divided TID. Vital signs should be monitored before starting first dose, then Q30 min until discharge from clinic.
Parents should be trained during visit to check heart rate and assess for signs of hypoglycemia.

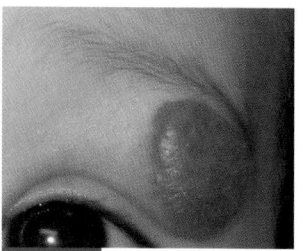

FIGURE 8-2

Infantile hemangioma.

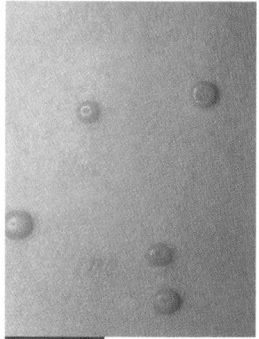

FIGURE 8-3

Molluscum contagiosum. *(From Cohen BA. Pediatric Dermatology. 3rd ed. St Louis: Mosby, 2005:126.)*

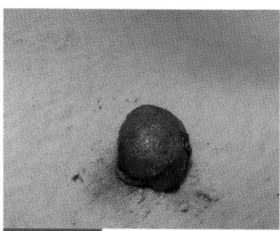

FIGURE 8-4

Pyogenic granuloma. *(From Cohen BA. Dermatology Image Atlas. Available at http://www.dermatlas.org/, 2001.)*

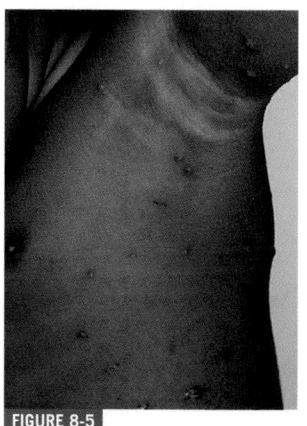

FIGURE 8-5

Scabies.

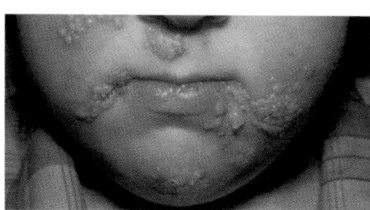

FIGURE 8-7

Herpetic gingivostomatitis. *(From Cohen BA. Pediatric Dermatology. 3rd ed. St Louis: Mosby, 2005: 103.)*

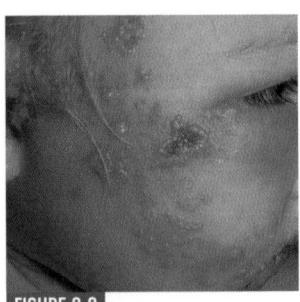

FIGURE 8-8

Herpes zoster. *(From Cohen BA. Pediatric Dermatology. 3rd ed. St Louis: Mosby, 2005:106.)*

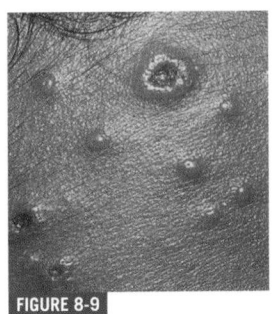

FIGURE 8-9

Varicella. *(From Cohen BA. Pediatric Dermatology. 3rd ed. St Louis: Mosby, 2005:104.)*

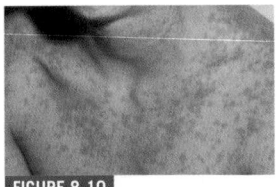

FIGURE 8-10

Measles. *(From Cohen BA. Pediatric Dermatology. 3rd ed. St Louis: Mosby, 2005:166.)*

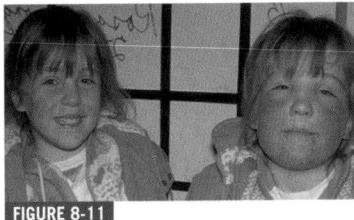

FIGURE 8-11

Fifth disease. *(From Cohen BA. Pediatric Dermatology. 3rd ed. St Louis: Mosby, 2005:167.)*

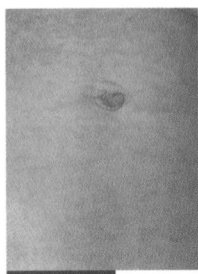

FIGURE 8-12

Roseola. *(From Cohen BA. Pediatric Dermatology. 3rd ed. St Louis: Mosby, 2005: 168.)*

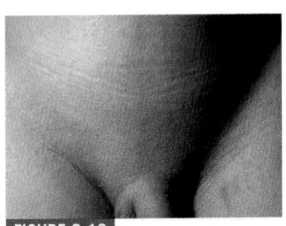

FIGURE 8-13

Scarlet fever. *(From Cohen BA. Dermatology Image Atlas. Available at http://www.dermatlas.org, 2001.)*

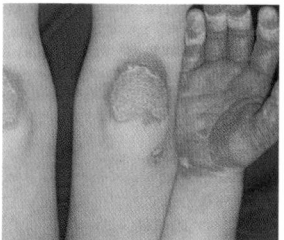

FIGURE 8-15

Psoriasis. *(From Cohen BA.* Pediatric Dermatology. *3rd ed. St Louis: Mosby, 2005:67.)*

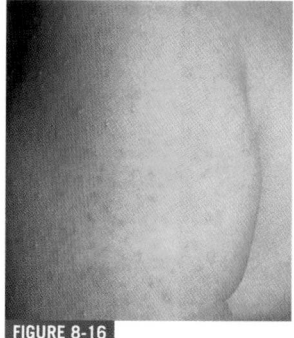

FIGURE 8-16

Keratosis pilaris. *(From Cohen BA.* Pediatric Dermatology. *3rd ed. St Louis: Mosby, 2005:81.)*

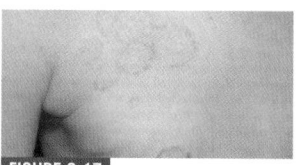

FIGURE 8-17

Tinea corporis. *(From Cohen BA.* Pediatric Dermatology. *3rd ed. St Louis: Mosby, 2005:94.)*

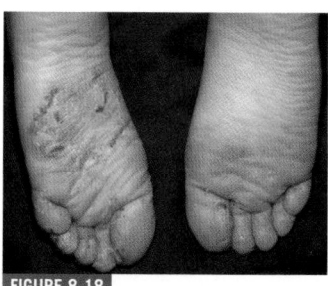

FIGURE 8-18

Tinea pedis. *(From Cohen BA.* Dermatology Image Atlas. *Available at http://www.dermatlas.org, 2001.)*

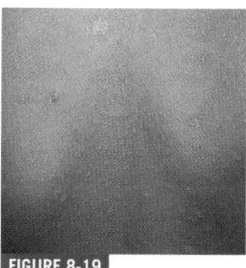

FIGURE 8-19

Pityriasis rosea. *(From Cohen BA.* Pediatric Dermatology. *3rd ed. St Louis: Mosby, 2005:87.)*

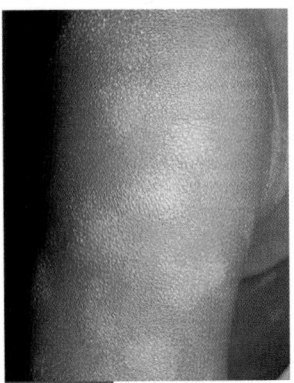

FIGURE 8-20

Pityriasis alba. *(From Cohen BA.* Pediatric Dermatology. *3rd ed. St Louis: Mosby, 2005:82.)*

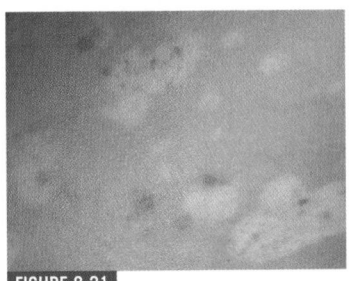

FIGURE 8-21

Postinflammatory hyperpigmentation. *(From Cohen BA.* Atlas of Pediatric Dermatology. *St Louis: Mosby, 1993.)*

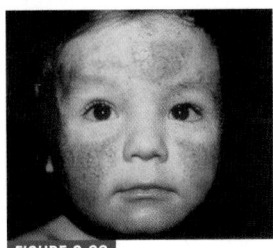

FIGURE 8-22

Infantile eczema. *(From Cohen BA.* Pediatric Dermatology. *3rd ed. St Louis: Mosby, 2005:79.)*

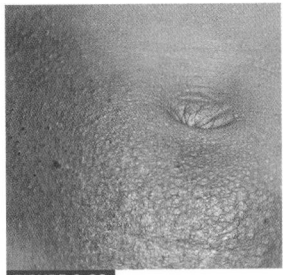

FIGURE 8-23

Childhood eczema. *(From Cohen BA.* Dermatology Image Atlas. *Available at www.med.jhu.edu/peds/dermatlas, 2001.)*

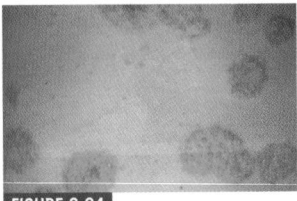

FIGURE 8-24

Nummular eczema. *(From Cohen BA.* Pediatric Dermatology. *3rd ed. St Louis: Mosby, 2005:80.)*

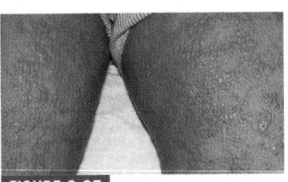

FIGURE 8-25

Follicular eczema. *(From Cohen BA.* Pediatric Dermatology. *3rd ed. St Louis: Mosby, 2005:80.)*

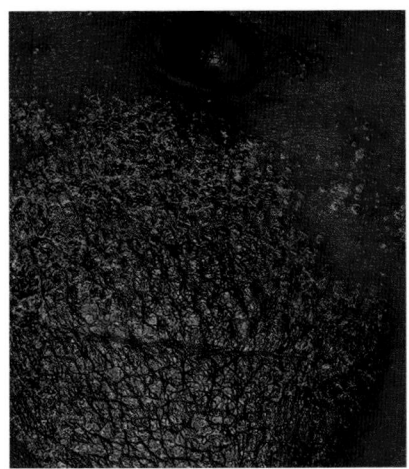

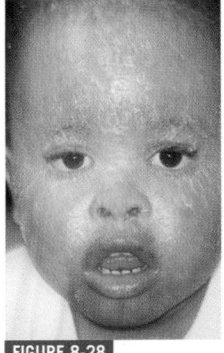

FIGURE 8-26
Childhood eczema with lesion in suprapubic area. *(From Cohen BA.* Pediatric Dermatology. *3rd ed. St Louis: Mosby, 2005, Fig. 3.20c.)*

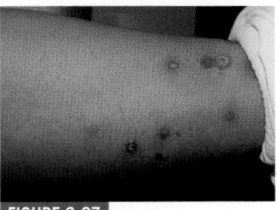

FIGURE 8-27
Papular urticaria. *(From Cohen BA.* Dermatology Image Atlas. *Available at http://www.dermatlas.org, 2001.)*

FIGURE 8-28
Congenital ichthyosis erythroderma. *(From Cohen BA.* Pediatric Dermatology. *3rd ed. St Louis: Mosby, 2005:79.)*

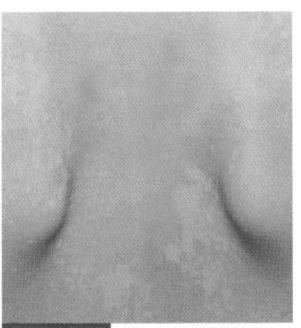

FIGURE 8-29
Tinea versicolor. *(From Cohen BA.* Atlas of Pediatric Dermatology. *St Louis: Mosby, 1993.)*

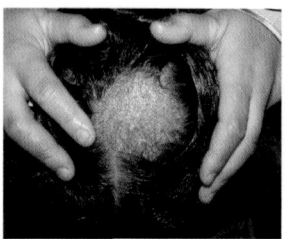

FIGURE 8-30

Tinea capitis. *(From Cohen BA.* Atlas of Pediatric Dermatology. *St Louis: Mosby, 1993.)*

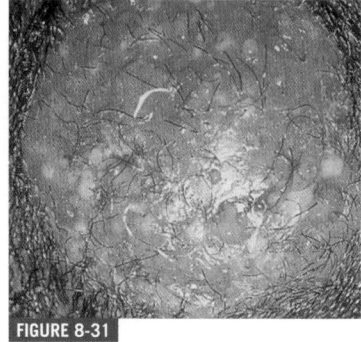

FIGURE 8-31

Kerion. *(From Cohen BA.* Pediatric Dermatology. *3rd ed. St Louis: Mosby, 2005:207.)*

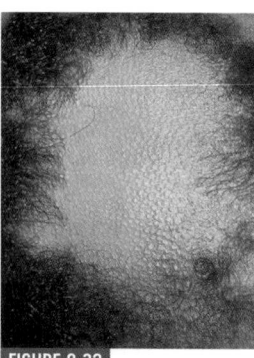

FIGURE 8-32

Alopecia areata. *(From Cohen BA.* Pediatric Dermatology. *3rd ed. St Louis: Mosby, 2005:208.)*

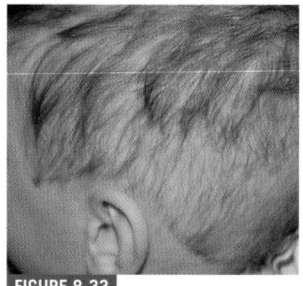

FIGURE 8-33

Telogen effluvium. *(From Cohen BA.* Dermatology Image Atlas. *Available at www.med.jhu.edu/peds/dermatlas, 2001.)*

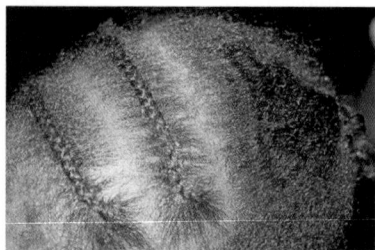

FIGURE 8-34

Traction alopecia. *(From Cohen BA.* Pediatric Dermatology. *3rd ed. St Louis: Mosby, 2005: 209.)*

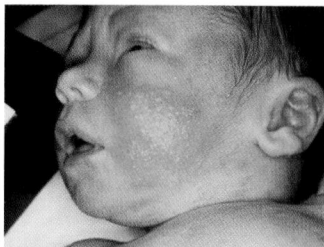

FIGURE 8-36

Erythema toxicum neonatorum. *(From Cohen BA. Pediatric Dermatology. 2nd ed. St Louis: Mosby, 1999:18.)*

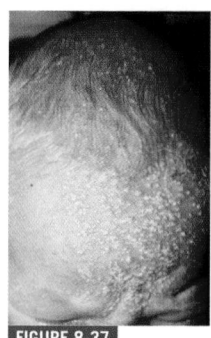

FIGURE 8-37

Transient neonatal pustular melanosis. *(From Cohen BA. Pediatric Dermatology. 3rd ed. St Louis: Mosby, 2005:20.)*

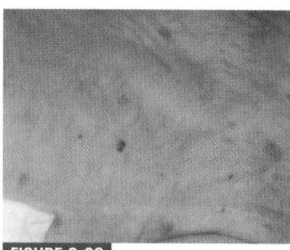

FIGURE 8-38

Hyperpigmentation from resolving transient neonatal pustular melanosis. *(From Cohen BA. Pediatric Dermatology. 3rd ed. St Louis: Mosby, 2005:20.)*

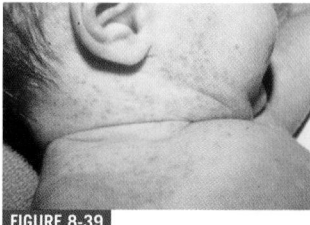

FIGURE 8-39

Miliaria rubra. *(From Cohen BA. Pediatric Dermatology. 3rd ed. St Louis: Mosby, 2005:22.)*

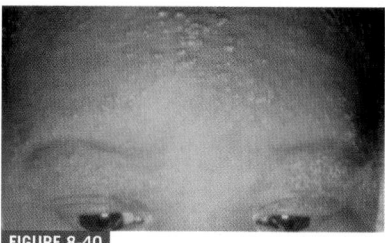

FIGURE 8-40

Milia. *(From Cohen BA. Pediatric Dermatology. 3rd ed. St Louis: Mosby, 2005:22.)*

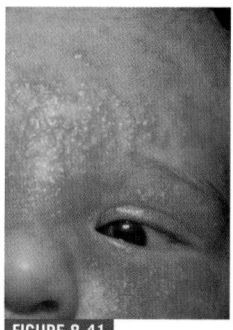

FIGURE 8-41

Neonatal acne. *(From Cohen BA. Pediatric Dermatology. 3rd ed. St Louis: Mosby, 2005:23.)*

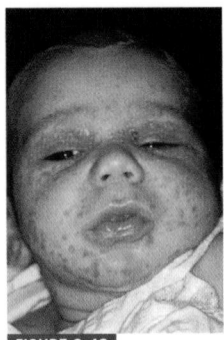

FIGURE 8-42
Seborrheic dermatitis. (*From Cohen BA*. Pediatric Dermatology. *3rd ed. St Louis: Mosby, 2005:33.*)

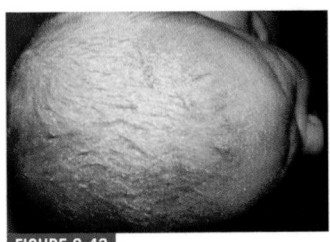

FIGURE 8-43
Seborrheic dermatitis. (*From Cohen BA. Pediatric Dermatology. 3rd ed. St Louis: Mosby, 2005:33.*)

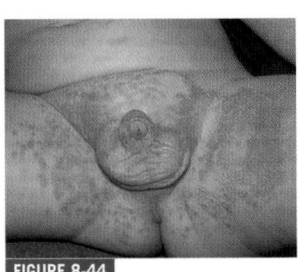

FIGURE 8-44
Diaper candidiasis. (*From Cohen BA. Pediatric Dermatology. 3rd ed. St Louis: Mosby, 2005:34.*)

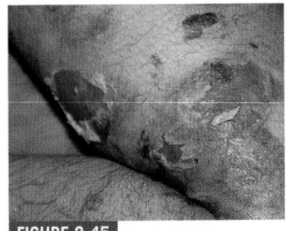

FIGURE 8-45
Pemphigus vulgaris. (*From Cohen BA. Dermatology Image Atlas. Available at www. dermatlas.org, 2001.*)

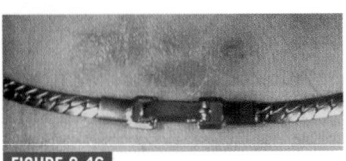

FIGURE 8-46
Allergic contact dermatitis. (*From Cohen BA. Pediatric Dermatology. 3rd ed. St Louis: Mosby, 2005:75.*)

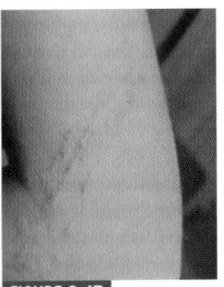

FIGURE 8-47
Poison ivy. (*From Cohen BA. Dermatology Image Atlas. Available at http://www.med. jhu.edu/peds/dermatlas, 2001.*)

(e) Average length of treatment is 6–9 months. Most patients can be tapered from propranolol at their first birthday; tapering can be monitored over 10–14 days. Younger infants tend to have a longer treatment course owing to higher rates of rebounds. Significant rebound should be treated by restarting medication.

(2) Steroids: No randomized trials to compare propranolol and systemic oral corticosteroids, but retrospective data suggest propranolol is more effective and has fewer adverse effects.

(3) Topical timolol: Efficacy noted in superficial hemangiomas and treatment duration > 3 months.

B. Warts

1. **Pathogenesis:** Caused by more than 100 types of human papillomavirus (HPV). Spread by skin-to-skin contact.

2. **Clinical presentation:**

a. Common warts: Skin-colored, rough, minimally scaly papules and nodules found most commonly on the hands, although can occur anywhere on the body. Can be solitary or multiple, range from a few millimeters to several centimeters, and may form large plaques or a confluent linear pattern secondary to autoinoculation. May be persistent in immunocompromised patients.

b. Flat warts: Occur over the hands, arms, and face; usually <2 mm wide. Often present in clusters.

c. Plantar warts: Occur on soles of feet. Can be painful; appear as inward-growing, hyperkeratotic plaques and papules. Trauma on weight-bearing surfaces results in small black dots (petechiae from thrombosed vessels on the surface of the wart).

d. Anogenital warts: See Chapter 5.

3. **Management**[3]:

a. Spontaneous resolution occurs in >75% of warts in otherwise healthy individuals within 3 years. No treatment clearly better than placebo, except for topical salicylic acid.

b. Keratolytics (i.e., topical salicylates): Work by removing excess scale within and around warts and by triggering an inflammatory reaction. Particularly effective in combination with adhesive tape occlusion; response may take 4–6 months.

c. Destructive techniques: Not more effective than placebo. Can be painful and cause scarring, so not recommended in children.

C. Molluscum Contagiosum (Fig. 8-3, color)

1. **Pathogenesis:** Caused by large DNA poxvirus. Spread by skin-to-skin contact.

2. **Clinical presentation:** Dome-shaped, often umbilicated, translucent to white papules that range from 1 mm to 1 cm. May be pruritic and can be surrounded with erythema, resembling eczema. Can occur anywhere except palms and soles, most commonly on the trunk and intertriginous

areas. Can occur in the genital area and lower abdomen when obtained as a sexually transmitted infection.

3. **Management:** Most spontaneously resolve within a few months and do not require intervention. Treatment may cause scarring and not more effective than placebo. Recurrences common. Monitor for secondary bacterial infection.

D. Pyogenic Granuloma (Lobular Capillary Hemangioma) (Fig. 8-4, color)

1. **Clinical presentation:** Benign vascular tumor, appears as small bright red papule that grows over several weeks to months into sessile or pedunculated papule with a "collarette" or scale. Usually no bigger than 1 cm. Can bleed profusely with minor trauma and can ulcerate. Rarely spontaneously regresses. Seen in all ages; average age of diagnosis 6 months to 10 years. Located on head and neck, sometimes in oral mucosa.

2. **Management:** Treatment usually required, given frequent bleeding and ulceration.

a. Shave excision or curettage with cautery of base: Recommended for pedunculated lesions.

b. Surgical excision: May be necessary for large or unusual lesions, but recurrence rates are high.

c. Laser therapy: Can be used for small pyogenic granulomas but may require 2 to 3 treatments.

E. Scabies (Fig. 8-5, color)

1. **Pathogenesis:** Caused by the mite *Sarcoptes scabiei*. Spread by skin-to-skin contact and through fomites; can live for 2 days away from a human host. Female mites burrow under the skin at a rate of 2 mm/day and lay eggs as they tunnel (up to 25 eggs).

2. **Clinical presentation:** Intial lesion is a small, erythematous papule that is easy to overlook. Can have burrows (elongated, edematous papulovesiscles, often with a pustule at the advancing border), which are pathognomonic. Most commonly located in interdigital webs, wrist folds, elbows, axilla, buttocks, and belt line. Burrows are most dramatic in patients who are unable to scratch (e.g., infants). Disseminated eczematous eruption results in generalized severe pruritus, especially at night. Can become nodular, particularly in intertriginous areas, or be susceptible to superinfection due to frequent excoriations.

3. **Treatment**[4]:

a. Permethrin cream: 5% cream applied to affected areas of skin, including under fingernails, face, and scalp. Rinse off after 8–14 hours. Can repeat in 7–10 days.

b. Ivermectin (off-label use): 200 mcg/kg oral dose; can repeat in 2 weeks. Efficacy comparable to permethrin cream.

F. Reactive Erythema (Figs. 8-6 to 8-13)

1. **Clinical presentation:** Group of disorders characterized by erythematous patches, plaques, and nodules that vary in size, shape, and distribution.

2. **Etiology:** Represent cutaneous reaction patterns triggered by endogenous and environmental factors.

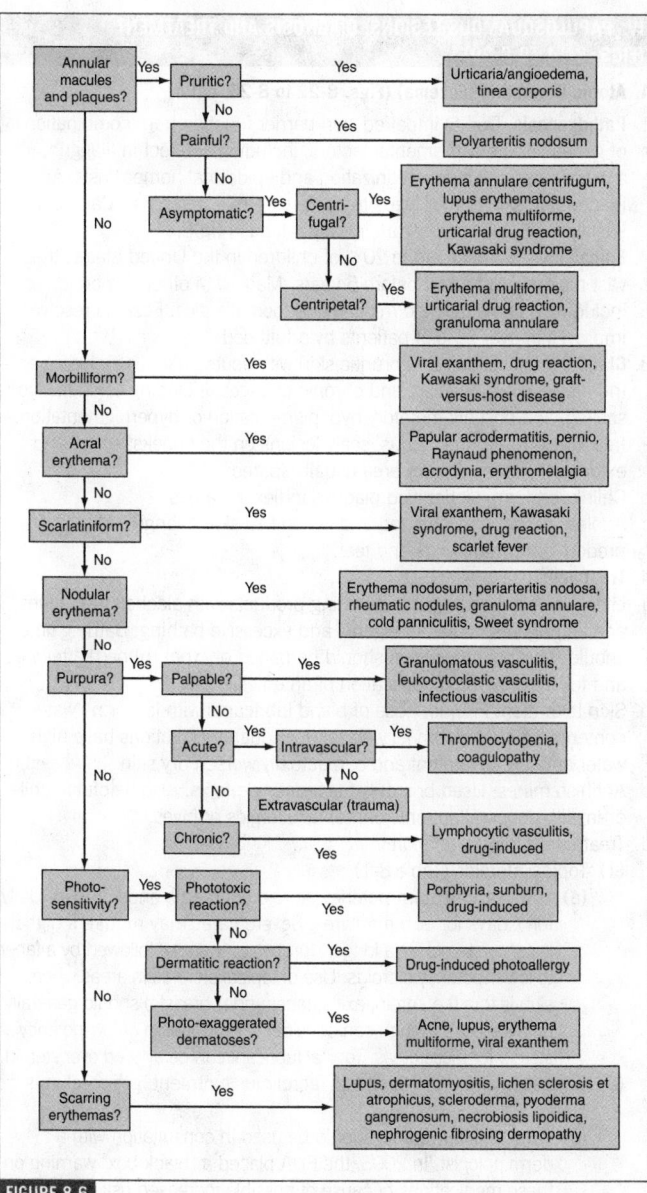

FIGURE 8-6

Reactive erythema. *(Modified from Cohen BA.* Atlas of Pediatric Dermatology. *3rd ed. St Louis: Mosby, 2005:196.)*

IV. PAPULOSQUAMOUS LESIONS: DIAGNOSIS AND TREATMENT (FIGS. 8-14 TO 8-29)

A. Atopic Dermatitis (Eczema) (Figs. 8-22 to 8-26, color)

1. **Pathogenesis:** Due to impaired skin barrier function from combination of genetic and environmental factors, including a defect in filaggrin, a protein essential for keratinization and epidermal homeostasis. An inadequate skin barrier leads to transepidermal water loss. Can be associated with elevated serum immunoglobulin (Ig)E.

2. **Epidemiology:** Affects up to 20% of children in the United States, the vast majority with onset before 5 years. Many with other comorbidities including asthma, allergic rhinitis, and food allergies. Eczema resolves or improves in over 75% of patients by adulthood.

3. **Clinical presentation:** Dry, pruritic skin with acute changes including erythema, vesicles, crusting, and chronic changes, including lichenification, scaling, and postinflammatory hypopigmentation or hyperpigmentation.

a. Infantile form: Erythematous, scaly lesions on the cheeks, scalp, and extensor surfaces. Diaper area usually spared.

b. Childhood form: Lichenified plaques in flexural areas.

c. Adolescence: More localized and lichenified skin changes. May be predominantly on hands and feet.

4. **Treatment**[5]:

a. Lifestyle: Avoiding triggers, including products with alcohol, fragrances, and astringents, sweat, allergens, and excessive bathing. Bathing time should be <5 minutes, skin should be patted dry (not rubbed) afterward and followed by rapid application of an emollient.

b. Skin hydration: Frequent use of bland lubricants with low or no water content (e.g., petroleum jelly, Vaseline, Aquaphor). Lotions have high water and low oil content and can actually worsen dry skin.

c. Antihistamines: Used primarily for sedating effects. Also helpful in children with concomitant environmental allergies or hives.

d. Treatment for inflammation:

   (1) Topical steroids (Table 8-1):

      (a) Low- and medium-potency steroid ointments once or twice daily for 7 days for eczema flares. Severe flares may require a higher-potency steroid for a longer duration of therapy, followed by a taper to lower-potency steroids. Use of topical steroids in areas where skin is thin (i.e., groin, axilla, face, under breasts) should generally be avoided, although can consider short duration of low-potency steroid for these areas. Topical lubricant can be applied over steroid.

   (2) Topical calcineurin inhibitors: Tacrolimus ointment, pimecrolimus cream

      (a) Second-line therapy; should be used in consultation with a dermatologist. In 2006, the FDA placed a "black box" warning on these medications because of possible increased risk of cancer, although no data confirm this as yet, and long-term safety studies are pending.[6]

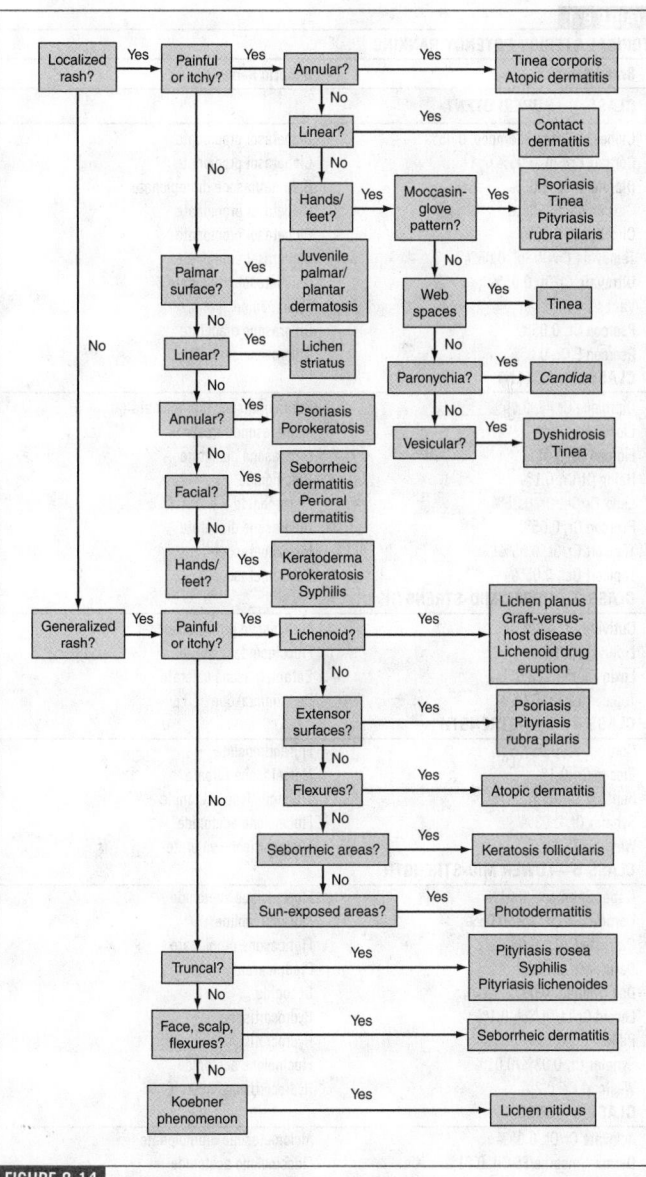

FIGURE 8-14

Papulosquamous disorders algorithm. *(Modified from Cohen BA. Atlas of Pediatric Dermatology. 3rd ed. St Louis: Mosby, 2005:97.)*

TABLE 8-1	
TOPICAL STERIOD POTENCY RANKING	
Brand Name	**Generic Name**
CLASS 1—SUPERPOTENT	
Clobex Lt/Spray/Shampoo, 0.05%	Clobetasol propionate
Cormax Cr/Sol, 0.05%	Clobetasol propionate
Diprolene Ot, 0.05%	Betamethasone dipropionate
Olux E Foam, 0.05%	Clobetasol propionate
Olux Foam, 0.05%	Clobetasol propionate
Temovate Cr/Ot/Sol, 0.05%	Clobetasol propionate
Ultravate Cr/Ot, 0.05%	Halobetasol propionate
Vanos Cr, 0.1%	Fluocinonide
Psorcon Ot, 0.05%	Diflorasone diacetate
Psorcon E Ot, 0.05%	Diflorasone diacetate
CLASS 2—POTENT	
Diprolene Cr AF, 0.05%	Betamethasone dipropionate
Elocon Ot, 0.1%	Mometasone furoate
Florone Ot, 0.05%	Diflorasone diacetate
Halog Ot/Cr, 0.1%	Halcinonide
Lidex Cr/Gel/Ot, 0.05%	Fluocinonide
Psorcon Cr, 0.05%	Diflorasone diacetate
Topicort Cr/Ot, 0.25%	Desoximetasone
Topicort Gel, 0.05%	Desoximetasone
CLASS 3—UPPER MID-STRENGTH	
Cutivate Ot, 0.005%	Fluticasone propionate
Lidex-E Cr, 0.05%	Fluocinonide
Luxiq Foam, 0.12%	Betamethasone valerate
Topicort LP Cr, 0.05%	Desoximetasone
CLASS 4—MID-STRENGTH	
Cordran Ot, 0.05%	Flurandrenolide
Elocon Cr, 0.1%	Mometasone furoate
Kenalog Cr/Spray, 0.1%	Triamcinolone acetonide
Synalar Ot, 0.03%	Flucinolone acetonide
Westcort Ot, 0.2%	Hydrocortisone valerate
CLASS 5—LOWER MID-STRENGTH	
Capex Shampoo, 0.01%	Fluocinolone acetonide
Cordran Cr/Lt/Tape, 0.05%	Flurandrenolide
Cutivate Cr/Lt, 0.05%	Fluticasone propionate
Derm Atop Cr, 0.1%	Prednicarbate
Des Owen Lt, 0.05%	Desonide
Locoid Cr/Lt/Ot/Sol, 0.1%	Hydrocortisone
Pandel Cr, 0.1%	Hydrocrotisone
Synalar Cr, 0.03%/0.01%	Flucinolone acetonide
Westcort Cr, 0.2%	Hydrocortisone valerate
CLASS 6—MILD	
Aclovate Cr/Ot, 0.05%	Alclometasone dipropionate
Derma-Smoothe/FS Oil, 0.01%	Fluocinolone acetonide
Desonate Gel, 0.05%	Desonide
Synalar Cr/Sol, 0.01%	Fluocinolone acetonide
Verdeso Foam, 0.05%	Desonide

TABLE 8-1	
TOPICAL STERIOD POTENCY RANKING (Continued)	
Brand Name	**Generic Name**
CLASS 7—LEAST POTENT	
Cetacort Lt, 0.5%/1%	Hydrocortisone
Cortaid Cr/Spray/Ot	Hydrocortisone
Hytone Cr/Lt, 1%/2.5%	Hydrocortisone
Micort-HC Cr, 2%/2.5%	Hydrocortisone
Nutracort Lt, 1%/2.5%	Hydrocortisone
Synacort Cr, 1%/2.5%	Hydrocortisone

National Psoriasis Foundation: Available at http://www.psoriasis.org/netcommunity/sublearn03_mild_potency. Accessed August 16, 2010.

5. **Complications**[7]:
a. Bacterial superinfection: Usually *Staphyloccus aureus*, sometimes group A *Streptococcus*. Depending on extent of infection, can be treated with topical mupirocin to systemic antibiotics. Can also take diluted bleach baths once to twice a week (mix 1/4 to 1/2 cup of bleach in full tub of lukewarm water and soak for 10 minutes, then rinse off with fresh water).
b. Eczema herpeticum superinfection with herpes simplex virus 1 (HSV-1) or -2, can cause severe systemic infection. Presents as vesiculopustular lesions with central punched-out erosions that do not respond to oral antibiotics. Must be treated systemically with acyclovir/valacyclovir. Should be evaluated by ophthalmologist if there is concern for eye involvement.

B. **Papular Urticaria (Fig. 8-27, color)**
1. **Pathogenesis:** Caused by insect bite-induced hypersensitivity (IBIH), usually from fleas, mosquitos, or bedbugs. Due to delayed type IV hypersensitivity reactions.
2. **Clinical presentation/epidemiology:** Summarized by the SCRATCH principles[8]:
Symmetric eruption: Exposed areas and scalp commonly affected. Spares diaper region, palms, and soles.
Cluster: Appear as "meal clusters" or "breakfast, lunch, dinner," which are linear or triangular groupings of lesions. Associated with bedbugs and fleas.
Rover not required: A remote animal exposure or lack of pet at home does not rule out IBIH.
Age: Tends to peak by 2 years of age. Not seen in newborn period. Most tend to develop tolerance by age 10.
Target lesions: Characteristic of IBIH, especially in more darkly pigmented patients. Also, **T**ime: emphasize chronic nature of eruption and need for patience and watchful waiting.
Confused pediatrician/parent: Diagnosis often met with disbelief by parent and/or referring pediatrician.
Household: Because of the nature of hypersensitivity, usually only affects one family member in the household.

3. **Management (the 3 Ps):**
   Prevention: Wear protective clothing, use insect repellent when outside, launder bedding and mattress pads for bedbugs, and maximize flea control for pets.
   Pruritus control: Topical steroids or antihistamines may be of some benefit.
   Patience: IBIH can be frustrating because of its persistent, recurrent nature. Ensure patients that their symptoms will resolve and they will eventually develop tolerance.

C. **Ichthyosis (Fig. 8-28, color)**

1. **Pathogenesis:** Diverse group of hereditary skin disorders of keratinization defects. Includes congenital ichthyosiform erythroderma, lamellar ichthyosis, epidermolytic ichthyosis, ichthyosis vulgaris, harlequin ichthyosis, and X-linked ichthyosis.

2. **Management:** Symptoms can be asymptomatic/mild to life-threatening. Basic management is aggressive skin hydration with emollients. Refer to dermatologist if therapy does not work, diagnosis is unclear, or there are other complications. Genetic markers available for many variants.

D. **Tinea Versicolor (Fig. 8-29, color)**

1. **Pathogenesis:** Caused by *Malassezia* (previously *Pityrosporum*), a lipid-dependent yeast. Exacerbated by hot/humid weather, hyperhidrosis, topical skin oil use. Not associated with poor hygiene. Not contagious.

2. **Clinical presentation:** Macules or patches that are hypopigmented, hyperpigmented, or erythematous. Hypopigmented areas tend to be more prominent in the summer because affected areas do not tan. Lesions often have a fine scale and can be mildly pruritic but are usually asymptomatic.

3. **Diagnosis:** Potassium hydroxide (KOH) microscopy reveals hyphae and yeast cells that appear like "spaghetti and meatballs."

4. **Treatment:** Topical antifungals (miconazole, oxiconazole, ketoconazole) or selenium sulfide are effective. Given the risk of hepatotoxicity, oral azole antifungals are reserved for resistant or widespread disease (oral terbinafine not effective). Pigmentation changes may take months to resolve despite successful treatment.

E. **Tinea Corporis[9]**

1. **Pathogenesis:** Caused by *Trichophyton* (anthropophilic) and *Microsporum* (zoophilic) species. Other species rarely involved. Can be spread through direct contact and fomites, especially in sports where there is close contact (e.g., wrestling).

2. **Clinical presentation:** Pruritic, erythematous, annular patch or plaque with central clearing and a scaly raised border. Typically affects glabrous skin (smooth and bare).

3. **Diagnosis:** Usually diagnosed clinically, but a KOH preparation or fungal culture can be used to help guide diagnosis.

4. **Treatment:** Topical antifungals (terbinafine, azole antifungals) until the lesion resolves, plus 1–2 additional weeks. Widespread eruption may require oral antibiotics.

V. HAIR LOSS: DIAGNOSIS AND TREATMENT (FIGS. 8-30 TO 8-34)

A. Tinea Capitis (Fig. 8-30, color)

1. **Pathogenesis:** Mostly caused by *Trichophyton tonsurans* (but *Trichophyton violeum and Trichophyton sudanese* clinically similar); sometimes *Microsporum canis*. Can be spread through contact and fomites.
2. **Epidemiology:** Usually occurs in young children, 1–10 years of age. African-American children more commonly affected, perhaps owing to the structure of their hair, but any age and any ethnicity can be affected.
3. **Clinical presentation:**
a. Black dot tinea capitis: Most common. Slowly growing, erythematous, scaling patches. These areas develop alopecia, and black dots are visible on scalp where hair has broken off.
b. Gray patch ("seborrheic dermatitis") tinea capitis: Erythematous, scaling, well-demarcated patch that grows centrifugally. Hair breaks off a few millimeters above scalp and takes on a gray/frosted appearance.
c. Kerion (Fig. 8-31, color): Complication of tinea capitis or tinea corporis. Type IV delayed hypersensitivity reaction to fungal infection. Appear as raised, boggy/spongy lesions, often tender and covered with exudate. Can be associated with posterior cervical lymphadenopathy.
4. **Diagnosis:** Can be made clinically, since oral antifungal therapy is indicated, but tinea capitis should be confirmed by examining KOH preparation under direct microscopic examination or culture of broken-off and surrounding hair.
5. **Treatment**[9]: First-line therapy includes oral griseofulvin for 10–12 weeks (which should be taken with fatty foods for improved absorption) and terbinafine, which is administered for 6 weeks. Topical antifungals will not be curative. All family members, particularly other children, should be examined carefully for subtle infection and treated. Selenium sulfide 2.5% shampoo may shorten the period of shedding of fungal organisms and reduce infection of unaffected family members.
Kerion: Same treatment as above. Patients with intractable pruritus or intense edema should be treated with oral steroids for 2–3 weeks to reduce risk of further scarring or permanent hair loss. Bacterial cultures should be sent in children with fever and signs of cellulitis, and treatment should be initiated with systemic antistaphylococcal antibiotics.

B. Alopecia Areata (Fig. 8-32, color)

1. **Clinical presentation:** Chronic inflammatory (probably autoimmune) disease that starts with small bald patches and normal-appearing underlying skin. New lesions may demonstrate subtle erythema and be pruritic. Bald patches may enlarge to involve large areas of the scalp or other hair-bearing areas. Many experience good hair regrowth within 1–2 years, although most will relapse. A minority progress to total loss of all scalp (alopecia totalis) and/or body hair (alopecia universalis).
2. **Diagnosis:** Usually clinical diagnosis. Biopsy is necessary in rare cases.

3. **Treatment**[10]: First-line therapy is topical and occasionally intralesional steroids. Minoxidil, anthralin, contact sensitization, and ultraviolet light therapy are second line. No evidence-based data that any therapy is better than placebo, so treatments with significant risk of toxicity should be avoided, particularly in children. Older children, adolescents, and young adults with long-standing localized areas of hair loss have the best prognosis.

C. **Telogen Effluvium (Fig. 8-33, color)**

1. **Pathogenesis:** Most common cause of diffuse hair loss, usually after stressful state (major illnesses or surgery, pregnancy, severe weight loss). Mature hair follicles switch prematurely to the telogen (resting) state, with shedding within 3 months.

2. **Clinical presentation:** Diffuse hair thinning 3 months after stressful event. May not be clinically obvious to an outsider until more than 20% of hair is lost.

3. **Treatment:** Self-limited, regrowth usually occurs over the next few months.

D. **Traction Alopecia (Fig. 8-34, color)**

1. **Pathogenesis:** Result of hairstyles that apply tension for long periods of time.

2. **Clinical presentation:** Noninflammatory linear areas of hair loss at margins of hairline, part line, or scattered regions, depending on hairstyling procedures used.

3. **Treatment:** Avoidance of styling products or styles that result in traction. If traction remains for long periods, condition may progress to permanent scarring hair loss.

E. **Trichotillomania**

1. **Pathogenesis:** Alopecia due to compulsive urge to pull out one's own hair, resulting in irregular areas of incomplete hair loss. Alopecia notable mainly on the scalp; can involve eyebrows and eyelashes. Onset is usually after age 10 and should be distinguished from hair pulling in younger children that resolves without treatment in most cases.

2. **Clinical presentation:** Characterized by hair of differing lengths; area of hair loss can be unusual in shape.

3. **Treatment:** Many cases require behavioral modification. Adolescents may benefit from psychiatric evaluation; condition can be associated with anxiety, depression, and obsessive-compulsive disorder.

VI. ACNE VULGARIS

A. **Pathogenesis:**

1. **Blockade of follicular opening from hyperkeratinization**

2. **Increased sebum production**

3. **Proliferation of *Propionibacterium acnes***

4. **Inflammation**

5. **Risk factors:** Androgens, family history, and stress. No strong evidence that dietary habits affect acne.

B. Clinical presentation:

1. **Noninflammatory lesions**

a. Closed comedo (whitehead): Accumulation of sebum and keratinous material, resulting in white/skin-colored papules without surrounding erythema.

b. Open comedo (blackhead): Dilated follicles packed with keratinocytes, oils, and melanin.

2. **Inflammatory lesions:** Papules, pustules, nodules, cysts. Typically appear later in the course of acne and vary from 1- to 2-mm micropapules to nodules >5 mm. Nodulocystic presentations are more likely to lead to permanent scarring and/or hyperpigmentation.

C. Classification: Used to estimate severity, but not always practical in a clinical setting

1. **Mild:** <20 comedones, <15 inflammatory lesions, or total <30

2. **Moderate:** 20–100 comedones, 15–50 inflammatory lesions, or total 30–125

3. **Severe:** >100 comedones, >50 inflammatory lesions, >5 cysts, or total >125

4. **Clinician should also consider** the number of skin areas involved and extent in each area (e.g., face, back, chest, and occasionally arms, legs, scalp)

D. Treatment[11,12] (Table 8-2 and Table 8-3)

1. **Skin care:** Gentle nonabrasive cleaning. Avoid picking or popping lesions. Vigorous scrubbing and abrasive cleaners can worsen acne.

2. **Topical retinoids:** First-line therapy for mild to moderate acne. Normalize follicular keratinization and decrease inflammation. A small amount should be applied as a thin layer to all affected areas. Can cause irritation and dryness of skin. Retinoids should probably be used at a different time of day than benzoyl peroxide to minimize risk of irritation, especially when therapy is initiated.

3. **Topical antimicrobials:**

a. Erythromycin, clindamycin, dapsone. Avoid topical antibiotics as monotherapy, and probably should not be used when an oral antibiotic is already being used.

b. Benzoyl peroxide (BPO): Oxidizing agent with antibacterial and mild anticomedolytic properties. Decreases antibiotic resistance when used with oral antibiotics. Can bleach hair, clothing, towels. Washes may be most convenient formulation, because they can be rinsed off in the shower.

c. Azelaic acid.

4. **Oral antibiotics:** First line for moderate to severe inflammatory acne. Avoid oral antibiotics as monotherapy, owing to increased antibiotic resistance. Doxycycline and minocycline are first line (although it is difficult to obtain 100-mg formulations of doxycycline). Use with BPO and/or topical retinoids. Try to limit length of therapy, and reassess clinically at 6–12 weeks.

5. **Oral contraceptives:** Good alternative for females who have sudden onset of moderate to severe acne and have not responded to conventional first-line therapy. Should not be used as monotherapy. Reduces sebum production and androgen levels.

TABLE 8-2

TOPICAL AND SYSTEMIC ANTIBIOTICS USED TO TREAT ACNE

Antibiotic	Characteristics
TOPICAL	
Erythromycin	*Propionibacterium acnes* very sensitive; least lipophilic
Clindamycin	*P. acnes* very sensitive; more lipophilic than erythromycin but less than benzoyl peroxide (BPO)
BPO +erythromycin	*P. acnes* very sensitive; most lipophilic topical agent; less irritating than BPO alone
BPO +clindamycin	Similar to characteristics for BPO + erythromycin
Azelaic acid	*P. acnes* sensitive; minimal lipophilia; can reduce abnormal desquamation
Metronidazole	*P. acnes* not sensitive; has antiinflammatory properties
BPO +glycolic acid	Glycolic acid may enhance penetration and reduce abnormal desquamation
SYSTEMIC	
Doxycycline	Lipophilic; *P. acnes* very sensitive; can cause photosensitivity, gastrointestinal (GI) upset, esophagitis, pseudotumor cerebri; must be taken with food
Minocycline	Lipophilic; *P. acnes* very sensitive; more expensive; less photosensitivity and GI upset, can cause drug hypersensitivity syndrome, lupus-like syndrome, rare staining of skin and teeth
Tetracycline	*P. acnes* sensitive; inexpensive; can cause photosensitivity, GI upset, pseudotumor cerebri, tooth discoloration, and inhibited skeletal growth. Limit use in pregnant women and children <8 years. Must be taken on empty stomach.
Erythromycin	*P. acnes* resistance emerging; inexpensive; can cause GI upset; safe for young children and pregnant women
Trimethoprim-sulfamethoxazole	Lipophilic; *P. acnes* very sensitive; severe erythema multiforme and toxic epidermal necrolysis limit use; potential alternative for patients allergic to other antibiotics
Clindamycin	Somewhat lipophilic; *P. acnes* very sensitive; pseudomembranous colitis limits use

From Leyden JJ. Therapy for acne vulgaris. *N Engl J Med.* 1997;16:1156-1162.

6. **Oral isotretinoin (Accutane):** Reserved for patients with severe nodular, cystic, or scarring acne who do not respond to traditional therapy. Should be managed by a dermatologist. Significantly decreases sebum production, inflammation, *P. acnes*, and can diminish scarring. Most patients have complete resolution of their acne after 16–20 weeks of use.

a. Side effects:

   (1) Teratogenicity: Patients and physicians are mandated by the FDA to comply with iPledge, a computerized risk management program designed to eliminate fetal exposure to isotretinoin. Female patients of child-bearing potential must use two forms of birth control and routinely get pregnancy tests.

   (2) Hepatoxicity, hyperlipidemia, and bone marrow suppression. A complete blood cell count (CBC), fasting lipid profile, and liver function tests should be obtained before initiation of therapy and repeated at 4 and 8 weeks.

   (3) Other: Myalgias, visual changes, pseudotumor cerebri.

TABLE 8-3

ACNE TREATMENT ALGORITHM

	Acne Severity						
	Mild		**Moderate**		**Severe**		
	Comedonal	Papular/Pustular	Papular/Pustular	Nodular	Nodular	Nodular/Conglobate	Severe
First-line treatment	Topical retinoid	Topical retinoid + Topical antibiotic	Oral antibiotic + Topical retinoid +/− BPO	Oral antibiotic + Topical retinoid +/− BPO	Oral isotretinoin		Oral isotretinoin
Alternative treatments	Alternative topical retinoid OR Azelaicacid	Alternativet opical antimicro-bialagent + Alternative topical retinoid OR Azelaic acid	Alternative oral antibiotic + Alternative topical retinoid +/− BPO	Oral isotretinoin OR Alternative oral antibiotic + Alternative topical retinoid +/− BPO	High-dose oral antibiotic + Topical retinoid +BPO		High-dose oral antibiotic + Topical retinoid +BPO
Alternative treatments for females			Oralanti-androgen + Topical retinoid +/− Topical antimicrobial	Oral antiandrogen + Topical retinoid +/− Oral antibiotic +/− Topical antimicrobial	High-dose oral antiandrogen + Topical retinoid +/− Topical antimicrobial		High-dose oral antiandrogen + Topical retinoid +/− Topical antimicrobial
Maintenance treatment	Topical retinoid		Topical retinoid +/− BPO				

BPO, Benzoyl peroxide.

Modified from Golinick H, Cunliffe W, Berson D, et al. Management of acne: areport from a Global Alliance to Improve Outcomes in Acne. *J Am Acad Dermatol.* 2003;49(suppl 1):S1-S37.

8

VII. COMMON NEONATAL DERMATOLOGIC CONDITIONS (FIGS. 8-35 TO 8-44)

A. Erythema Toxicum Neonatorum (ETN) (Fig. 8-36, color)

Most common rash of full-term infants; incidence declines with lower birth weight and prematurity. Appears as small erythematous macules and papules that evolve into pustules on erythematous bases. Rash occurs most often by 24–48 hours of life but can be present at birth or emerge as late as 2–3 weeks. Self-limited, resolves within 5–7 days; recurrences possible. Pustular fluid reveals eosinophils.

B. Transient Neonatal Pustular Melanosis (Figs. 8-37 and 8-38, color)

More commonly affects full-term infants with darker pigmentation. At birth, appears as small pustules on nonerythematous bases that rupture and leave erythematous/hyperpigmented macules with a collarette of scale. Self-limited; macules fade over weeks to months. Pustular fluid reveals neutrophils.

C. Miliaria (Heat Rash, Prickly Heat) (Fig. 8-39, color)

Common newborn rash associated with warmer climates, incubator use, or occlusion with clothes/dressings. Appears as small erythematous papules or pustules usually on face, scalp, or intertriginous areas. Due to obstruction of eccrine sweat ducts in the stratum corneum. Rash resolves when infant is placed in cooler environment or tight clothing/dressings are removed.

D. Milia (Fig. 8-40, color)

Common newborn rash. Appears as 1- to 3-mm white/yellow papules, frequently found on nose and face; due to retention of keratin and sebaceous materials in pilosebaceous follicles. Self-limited, resolves within first few weeks of life.

E. Neonatal Acne (Fig. 8-41, color)

Seen in 20% of infants. Appears as inflammatory papules or pustules without comedones, usually on face and scalp. Secondary to effect of maternal and endogenous androgens on infant's sebaceous glands. Peaks around 1 month, resolves within a few months, usually without intervention. Does not increase risk of acne as an adolescent.

F. Seborrheic Dermatitis (Cradle Cap) (Figs. 8-42 and 8-43, color)

Common rash characterized by erythematous plaques with greasy yellow scales. Located in areas rich with sebaceous glands, such as scalp, cheeks, ears, eyebrows, intertriginous areas, diaper area. Unknown etiology. Can be seen in newborns, more commonly in infants 1–4 months old. Self-limited and resolves within a few weeks to months. Can remove scales on scalp with soft brush/fine comb. In more severe cases, antifungal shampoos or low-potency topical steroid can shorten the course.

G. Mongolian Spots

Most common pigmented lesion of newborns, usually seen in babies with darker skin tone. Appear as blue/gray macules without definite

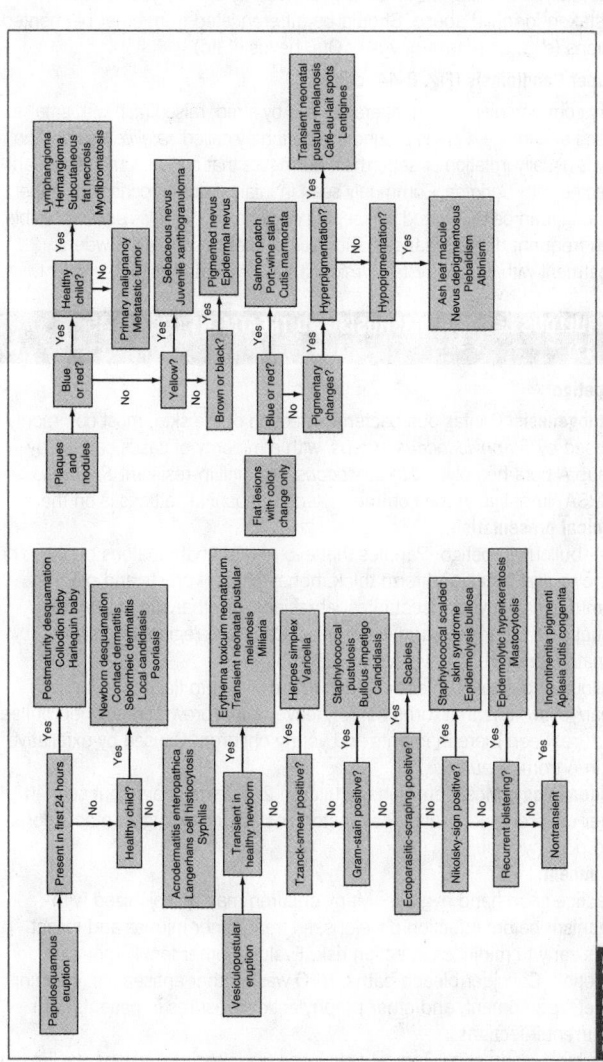

FIGURE 8-35

Evaluation of neonatal rashes. *(Modified from Cohen BA. Atlas of Pediatric Dermatology. 3rd ed. St Louis: Mosby, 2005:62.)*

borders, frequently seen on sacral regions or shoulders. Due to delayed disappearance of dermal melanocytes. Spots typically fade within first few years of life, with majority resolved by age 10 years. Can be mistaken for child abuse. Should be differentiated from other pigmented lesions (e.g., blue nevi, nevus of Ota, nevus of Ito).

H. Diaper Candidiasis (Fig. 8-44, color)

Very common diaper rash, characterized by a red, raised rash with small raised and infected areas around the periphery called *satellite lesions*. Etiology is usually irritation or seborrheic dermatitis that can become secondarily infected with *Candida*. Commonly seen in infancy during periods of diaper wearing. Can be minimized by keeping diaper area clean, as dry as possible, with frequent diaper changes and topical agents such as powders. Treatment with topical nystatin, miconazole, or clotrimazole is sufficient.

VIII. BULLOUS LESIONS: DIAGNOSIS AND TREATMENT (FIGS. 8-45 TO 8-47)

A. Impetigo

1. **Pathogenesis:** Contagious bacterial infection of the skin, most commonly caused by *Staphylococcus aureus*, with a minority of cases caused by group A beta-hemolytic *Streptococcus*. Methicillin-resistant *S. aureus* (MRSA) impetigo in the community and in hospital settings is on the rise.

2. **Clinical presentation:**

a. Non-bullous impetigo: Papules that evolve into erythematous pustules or vesicles that break and form thick, honey-colored crusts and plaques. Commonly overlying insect bites, abrasions, or other site of trauma. Usually found on face and extremities. Can have regional lymphadenopathy, but rare to have systemic symptoms.

b. Bullous impetigo: Painless vesicles that evolve into flaccid bullae with clear/yellow fluid that turns darker; leave yellow/brown crust when bullae rupture. Seen more in infants and young children. Caused by exfoliative toxin A from *S. aureus*.

3. **Epidemiology:** Most common in children 2–5 years of age, but seen in older children and adults. Risk factors include crowding, contact sports, and poor hygiene.

4. **Treatment:**

a. Practice good hand hygiene. Many children may be colonized with organism before infection develops, so treat minor injuries and insect bites early to minimize infection risk. Evaluate other family members for infection. Consider bleach baths, BPO wash, other antiseptics, cleaning athletic equipment, and other prophylactic measures in patients with recurrent infections.

b. Non-bullous impetigo: Topical antibiotics (mupirocin) if lesions are limited

c. Bullous impetigo or widespread non-bullous impetigo: Oral antibiotics with gram-positive coverage; consider MRSA coverage (dicloxacillin, cephalexin, clindamycin).

B. Autoimmune Bullous Diseases

1. **Very rare in children** but should be considered if bullous lesions do not respond to standard therapy. Suspicion for any of the following should warrant referral to a dermatologist for diagnosis and management.

2. **Pemphigus vulgaris (Fig. 8-45, color):**
   a. Pathogenesis: IgG autoantibodies to adhesion molecules desmoglein-1 and desmoglein-3, which interrupts integrity of epidermis and/or mucosa and results in extensive blister formation.
   b. Clinical presentation: Flaccid bullae that start in the mouth and spread to face, scalp, trunk, extremities, and other mucosal membranes. Positive Nikolsky sign. Ruptured blisters are painful and prone to secondary infection. Can lead to impaired oral intake if there is significant oral mucosal involvement.
   c. Treatment: Immunosuppressants (systemic glucocorticoids, rituximab, intravenous immunoglobulin [IVIG])

3. **Pemphigus foliaceus:**
   a. Pathogenesis: IgG autoantibodies to desmoglein-1. Antibodies bind to the same antigen as in bullous impetigo and staphylococcal scalded skin syndrome, so lesions are superficial and rupture easily. Can be triggered by certain drugs, including thiol compounds and penicillins.
   b. Clinical presentation: Scaling, crusting erosions on erythematous base that appear on face, scalp, trunk, and back. No mucosal involvement. Lesions are more superficial than in pemphigus vulgaris.
   c. Treatment: Immunosuppressants

4. **Bullous pemphigoid:**
   a. Pathogenesis: Autoantibodies to the epithelial basement membrane that results in an inflammatory cascade and causes separation of epidermis from dermis and epithelium from subepithelium.
   b. Clinical presentation: Prodrome of inflammatory lesions that progresses into large (1–3 cm), tense, extremely pruritic bullae on trunk, flexural regions, and intertriginous areas. A minority have oral mucosal lesions. Negative Nikolsky sign.
   c. Treatment: Immunosuppressants.

5. **Dermatitis herpetiformis:**
   a. Pathogenesis: Strong genetic predisposition and link to gluten intolerance/celiac disease. IgA deposits found in dermal papillae.
   b. Clinical presentation: Symmetric, intensely pruritic papulovesicles clustered on extensor surfaces.
   c. Treatment: Dapsone, strict gluten-free diet.

C. Burns (see Chapter 4)

D. Contact Dermatitis

1. **Irritant dermatitis:** Exposure to physical, chemical, or mechanical irritants to the skin. Top two causes in children are dry skin dermatitis and diaper dermatitis.

2. **Allergic dermatitis (Fig. 8-46, color):**
a. Pathogenesis: T-cell–mediated immune reaction in response to an environmental trigger that comes into contact with the skin. After initial exposure causes sensitization, an allergic response occurs with subsequent exposures.
b. Allergens: Common antigens are *Toxicodendron* spp. (poison ivy, poison oak, poison sumac). Also nickel, cobalt, gold, dyes, formaldehyde.
c. Clinical presentation: Pruritic erythematous dermatitis that can progress to a chronic stage involving scaling, lichenification, and pigmentary changes. Initial reaction occurs after a sensitization period of 7–10 days in susceptible individuals. Antigen reexposure causes a more rapid reactivation reaction.
   (1) Poison ivy (Fig. 8-47, color): Exposure to urushiol, the allergenic substance in poison ivy, causes streaks of erythematous papules, pustules, and vesicles. Highly pruritic, can become edematous, especially if rash is on face or genitals. In extreme cases, anaphylaxis can occur.
3. **Diagnosis:** Careful history taking. Patch testing may also be helpful.
4. **Treatment:**
a. Remove causative agent. For poison ivy contact, remove clothing and wash skin with mild soap and water as soon as possible.
b. Mild dermatitis: Topical steroids.
c. Widespread or severe dermatitis: Systemic steroids for 2–3 weeks. There is no role for short courses of steroids (e.g., Medrol dose pack), because eruption will flare when drug is stopped.

REFERENCES

1. Hartemink DA, Chiu YE, Drolet BA, Kerschner JE. PHACES syndrome: a review. *Int J Pediatr Otorhinolaryngol.* 2009;73:181-187.
2. Drolet BA, Frommelt PC, Chamlin SL, et al. Initiation and use of propranolol for infantile hemangioma: report of a consensus conference. *Pediatrics.* 2013;131:128-140.
3. Kwok CS, Gibbs S, Bennett C. Topical treatment for cutaneous warts. *Cochrane Database Syst Rev.* 2012:9 CD001781.
4. Hicks MI, Elston DM. Scabies. *Dermatol Ther.* 2009;22:279-292.
5. McAleer MA, Flohr C, Irvine AD. Management of difficult and severe eczema in childhood. *BMJ.* 2012;23:345.e4770.
6. Patel TS, Greer SC, Skinner RB Jr. Cancer concerns with topical immunomodulators in atopic dermatitis: overview of data and recommendations to clinicians. *Am J Clin Dermatol.* 2007;8:189-194.
7. Boquniewicz M, Leung DY. Recent insights into atopic dermatitis and implications for management of infectious complications. *J Allergy Clin Immunol.* 2010;125:4-13.
8. Hernandez RG, Cohen BA. Insect bite-induced hypersensitivity and the SCRATCH principles: a new approach to papular urticaria. *Pediatrics.* 2006;118:e189-e196.
9. Andrews MD, Burns M. Common tinea infections in children. *Am Fam Physician.* 2008;77:1415-1420.
10. Alkhalifah A, Alsantali A, Wang E, et al. Alopecia areata update: part II. Treatment. *J Am Acad Dermatol.* 2010;62:191-202.
11. Zaenglein AL, Thiboutot DM. Expert committee recommendations for acne management. *Pediatrics.* 2006;118:1188-1199.
12. Archer CB, Cohen SN, Baron SE. Guidance on the diagnosis and clinical management of acne. *Clin Exp Dermatol.* 2012;37(suppl 1):1-6.

Chapter 9

Development, Behavior, and Mental Health

Melissa Kwan, MD

🔵 See additional content on Expert Consult

I. WEBSITES

ADHD: www.chadd.org
ADHD Medication Guide: www.ADHDMedicationGuide.com
American Academy of Pediatrics—Developmental and Behavioral Pediatrics: www.dbpeds.org
Disability Programs and Services: www.disability.gov
Learning Disabilities Association of America: www.ldanatl.org
Intellectual Disability: www.thearclink.org
Bright Futures: www.brightfutures.org
National Early Childhood Technical Assistance Center: www.nectac.org
Reach Out and Read: www.reachoutandread.org
Child and Adolescent Psychiatry Practice Parameters: www.aacap.org
Mental health patient and provider handouts: www.nimh.nih.gov

II. INTRODUCTION

A. Development

1. **Development can be divided into five major streams:** Visual-motor, language, motor, social, and adaptive.
2. **Abnormal development** in one stream increases the risk for abnormality in another and should prompt a careful assessment of all streams.
3. **Developmental diagnosis** is a functional description and classification and does not specify an etiology or medical diagnosis.
4. **Developmental assessment** is based on the premise that milestone acquisition occurs at a specific rate in an orderly and sequential manner.
a. A good milestone is one that can easily be assessed by parents or a provider, and also one that occurs in a narrow time window.
b. When development is not progressing normally, the pattern of abnormal development may include delay, deviancy, and/or dissociation.

III. DEFINITIONS[1]

A. Developmental Quotient (DQ)

1. **A calculation that reflects the rate of development** in any given stream and represents the percentage of normal development present at the time of testing.
DQ = (Developmental Age/Chronologic Age) × 100
2. **Two separate developmental assessments** over time are more predictive than a single assessment.

195

B. Delay

1. **Performance significantly below average (DQ < 70) in a given area of skill.** May occur in a single stream or several streams.

C. Deviancy

1. **Atypical development within a single stream,** such as developmental milestones occurring out of sequence. Deviancy does not necessarily imply abnormality but should alert one to the possibility that problems may exist. Example: An infant who rolls at an early age may have abnormally increased tone.

2. **Deviancy may also denote emergence of a presentation that is not typically part of the developmental sequence.**
   Example: A toddler showing no interest in peers.

D. Dissociation

1. **A substantial difference in the rate of development between two or more streams.**
   Example: Motor delay relative to cognition seen in some children with cerebral palsy.

E. Gross Motor Skills

1. **Descriptions of posture and locomotion**—in general, how a child moves from one location to another.

F. Fine-Motor and Visual-Motor Problem-Solving Skills

1. **Upper extremity and hand manipulative abilities and hand-eye coordination.** These skills depend to some degree on an intact motor substrate and require a given level of nonverbal cognitive ability.

G. Language

1. **The ability to understand and communicate with another person.**

2. **In the absence of a communication disorder or significant hearing impairment,** language development represents the best predictor of intellectual performance.

H. Social Skills

1. **Communicative in origin and represent the cumulative impact of language comprehension and problem-solving skills.** Social behaviors might be considered the functional expression resulting from the interaction of these two streams of development.

I. Adaptive Skills

1. **Skills concerned with self-help or activities of daily living.**

IV. GUIDELINES FOR NORMAL DEVELOPMENT AND BEHAVIOR

A. Developmental Milestones (Table 9-1)

B. Reach Out and Read Milestones of Early Literacy (Table 9-2)

C. Age-Appropriate Behavioral Issues in Infancy and Early Childhood (Table 9-3)

TABLE 9-1

DEVELOPMENTAL MILESTONES

Age	Gross Motor	Visual-Motor/Problem-Solving	Language	Social/Adaptive
1 mo	Raises head from prone position	Visually fixes, follows to midline, has tight grasp	Alerts to sound	Regards face
2 mo	Holds head in midline, lifts chest off table	No longer clenches fists tightly, follows object past midline	Smiles socially (after being stroked or talked to)	Recognizes parent
3 mo	Supports on forearms in prone position, holds head up steadily	Holds hands open at rest, follows in circular fashion, responds to visual threat	Coos (produces long vowel sounds in musical fashion)	Reaches for familiar people or objects, anticipates feeding
4 mo	Rolls over, supports on wrists, shifts weight	Reaches with arms in unison, brings hands to midline	Laughs, orients to voice	Enjoys looking around
6 mo	Sits unsupported, puts feet in mouth in supine position	Unilateral reach, uses raking grasp, transfers objects	Babbles, ah-goo, razz, lateral orientation to bell	Recognizes that someone is a stranger
9 mo	Pivots when sitting, crawls well, pulls to stand, cruises	Uses immature pincer grasp, probes with forefinger, holds bottle, throws objects	Says "mama, dada" indiscriminately, gestures, waves bye-bye, understands "no"	Starts exploring environment, plays gesture games (e.g., pat-a-cake)
12 mo	Walks alone	Uses mature pincer grasp, can make a crayon mark, releases voluntarily	Uses two words other than "mama, dada" or proper nouns, jargoning (runs several unintelligible words together with tone or inflection), one-step command with gesture	Imitates actions, comes when called, cooperates with dressing
15 mo	Creeps up stairs, walks backward independently	Scribbles in imitation, builds tower of 2 blocks in imitation	Uses 4–6 words, follows one-step command without gesture	15–18 mo: uses spoon and cup
18 mo	Runs, throws objects from standing without falling	Scribbles spontaneously, builds tower of 3 blocks, turns two or three pages at a time	Mature jargoning (includes intelligible words), 7–10 word vocabulary, knows 5 body parts	Copies parent in tasks (sweeping, dusting), plays in company of other children
24 mo	Walks up and down steps without help	Imitates stroke with pencil, builds tower of 7 blocks, turns pages one at a time, removes shoes, pants, etc.	Uses pronouns (I, you, me) inappropriately, follows two-step commands, 50-word vocabulary, uses 2-word sentences	Parallel play

Continued

TABLE 9-1
DEVELOPMENTAL MILESTONES (Continued)

Age	Gross Motor	Visual-Motor/Problem-Solving	Language	Social/Adaptive
3 yr	Can alternate feet going up steps, pedals tricycle	Copies a circle, undresses completely, dresses partially, dries hands if reminded, unbuttons	Uses minimum of 250 words, 3-word sentences, uses plurals, knows all pronouns, repeats two digits	Group play, shares toys, takes turns, plays well with others, knows full name, age, gender
4 yr	Hops, skips, alternates feet going down steps	Copies a square, buttons clothing, dresses self completely, catches ball	Knows colors, says song or poem from memory, asks questions	Tells "tall tales," plays cooperatively with a group of children
5 yr	Skips alternating feet, jumps over low obstacles	Copies triangle, ties shoes, spreads with knife	Prints first name, asks what a word means	Plays competitive games, abides by rules, likes to help in household tasks

From Capute AJ, Biehl RF. Functional developmental evaluation: prerequisite to habilitation. *Pediatr Clin North Am.* 1973;20:3; Capute AJ, Accardo PJ. Linguistic and auditory milestones during the first two years of life: a language inventory for the practitioner. *Clin Pediatr.* 1978;17:847; and Capute AJ, Shapiro BK, Wachtel RC, et al. The Clinical Linguistic and Auditory Milestone Scale (CLAMS): identification of cognitive defects in motor delayed children. *Am J Dis Child.* 1986;140:694. Rounded norms from Capute AJ, Palmer FB, Shapiro BK, et al. Clinical Linguistic and Auditory Milestone Scale: prediction of cognition in infancy. *Dev Med Child Neurol.* 1986;28:762.

TABLE 9-2
REACH OUT AND READ MILESTONES OF EARLY LITERACY

Age	Motor	Cognitive
6–12 mo	Reaches for books, turns pages with help	Looks at pictures, pats pictures
12–18 mo	Carries book, holds book with help, turns several board pages at a time	Points to pictures with a single finger, points to specific items on page, gives book to adult
18–24 mo	Turns one board page at a time	Repeats and retells parts of known stories
24–36 mo	Begins to turn paper pages	Looks at favorite books on own, repeats and retells whole phrases and stories, associates pictures with text of story
3 yr	Turns paper pages easily	Growing attention span, recites favorite stories, begins to identify single letters
4 yr and older	Writes name	Uses past tense and plurals, answers "what will happen next"

From Reach Out and Read National Center: www.reachoutandread.org.

TABLE 9-3

AGE-APPROPRIATE BEHAVIORAL ISSUES IN INFANCY AND EARLY CHILDHOOD

Age	Behavioral Issue	Symptoms	Guidance
1–3 mo	Colic	Paroxysms of fussiness/crying, 3+ hr per day, 3+ days per wk, may pull knees up to chest, pass flatus	Crying usually peaks at 6 wk and resolves by 3–4 mo. Prevent overstimulation; swaddle infant; use white noise, swing, or car rides to soothe. Avoid medication and formula changes. Encourage breaks for the primary caregiver.
3–4 mo	Trained night feeding	Night awakening	Comfort quietly, avoid reinforcing behavior (i.e., avoid night feeds). Do not play at night. Introducing cereal or solid food does not reduce awakening. Develop a consistent bedtime routine. Place baby in bed while drowsy and not fully asleep.
9 mo	Stranger anxiety/separation anxiety	Distress when separated from parent or approached by a stranger	Use a transitional object (e.g., special toy, blanket); use routine or ritual to separate from parent; may continue until 24 mo but can reduce in intensity.
	Developmental night waking	Separation anxiety at night	Keep lights off. Avoid picking child up or feeding. May reassure verbally at regular intervals or place a transitional object in crib.
12 mo	Aggression	Biting, hitting, kicking in frustration	Say "no" with negative facial cues. Begin time out (1 minute per year of age). No eye contact or interaction, place in a nonstimulating location. May restrain child gently until cooperation is achieved.
	Need for limit setting	Exploration of environment, danger of injury	Avoid punishing exploration or poor judgment. Emphasize child-proofing and distraction.
18 mo	Temper tantrums	Occur with frustration, attention-seeking rage, negativity/refusal	Try to determine cause, react appropriately (i.e., help child who is frustrated, ignore attention-seeking behavior). Make sure child is in a safe location.
24 mo	Toilet training	Child needs to demonstrate readiness: shows interest, neurologic maturity (i.e., recognizes urge to urinate or defecate), ability to walk to bathroom and undress self, desire to please/imitate parents, increasing periods of daytime dryness.	Age range for toilet training is usually 2–4 yr. Give guidance early; may introduce potty seat but avoid pressure or punishment for accidents. Wait until the child is ready. Expect some periods of regression, especially with stressors.

Continued

TABLE 9-3

AGE-APPROPRIATE BEHAVIORAL ISSUES IN INFANCY AND EARLY CHILDHOOD (Continued)

Age	Behavioral Issue	Symptoms	Guidance
24–36 mo	New sibling	Regression, aggressive behavior	Allow for special time with parent, 10–20 min daily of one-on-one time exclusively devoted to the older sibling(s). Child chooses activity with parent. No interruptions. May not be taken away as punishment.
36 mo	Nightmares	Awakens crying, may or may not complain of bad dream	Reassure child, explain that he or she had a bad dream. Leave bedroom door open, use a nightlight, demonstrate there are no monsters under the bed. Discuss dream the following day. Avoid scary movies or television shows.
	Night terrors	Agitation, screaming 1–2 hr after going to bed. Child may have eyes open but not respond to parent. May occur at same time each night.	May be familial, not volitional. *Prevention:* For several nights, awaken child 15 min before terrors typically occur. Avoid overtiredness. *Acute:* Be calm; speak in soft, soothing, repetitive tones; help child return to sleep. Protect child against injury.

From Dixon SD, Stein MT. *Encounters with Children: Pediatric Behavior and Development*. St Louis: Mosby, 2000.

V. DEVELOPMENTAL SCREENING AND EVALUATION

A. Developmental Screening Guidelines

1. **Developmental surveillance should be included in every well-child visit, and any concerns should be addressed immediately.** Many parents do not differentiate between development and behavior, and many delays manifest through behavior.

a. Do you have any concerns about your child's development? Behavior? Learning?

b. What changes have you seen in your child's development since our last visit?

c. How old would you say your child acts?

2. **Developmental surveillance should occur at every well-child visit.** Standardized developmental screening should be administered at 9-month, 18-month, and 30-month well-child visits. If a 30-month visit is not possible, this screening can be done at the 24-month visit.

3. **Specific screening for autism should occur at the 18-month and 24-month visits.**[2]

B. Commonly Used Developmental Screening and Assessment Tools

1. **Appropriate screening tests vary with age and suspected diagnosis.** Significant delays on screening merit referral for formal assessment. Several developmental screening and assessment tools are available (Table 9-4).

TABLE 9-4

DEVELOPMENTAL AND MENTAL HEALTH SCREENING TESTS BY DIAGNOSIS

Diagnosis	Screening Tests	Age	Administration Time	Completed By	Weblink
Cognitive/motor development	Ages and Stages Questionnaire (ASQ)	4–60 mo	10–15 min	Parent	http://www.agesandstages.com
	Parents Evaluation of Developmental Status (PEDS)	0–8 yr	2–10 min	Parent	http://www.pedstest.com
	Denver II Developmental Screening Test	0–6 yr	10–12 min	Clinician	
	Capute Scales (CAT/CLAMS)	3–36 mo	15–20 min	Clinician	
Autism spectrum disorders	Modified Checklist for Autism in Toddlers (M-CHAT)	16–48 mo	5–10 min	Parent	http://www.firstsigns.org/downloads/m-chat.PDF
	Childhood Autism Rating Scale (CARS)	>2 yr	20–30 min	Clinician	
Attention deficit/hyperactivity disorder (ADHD)	Vanderbilt Scales Connors Scales	6–12 yr	10–15 min	Parent and teachers	http://www.brightfutures.org/mentalhealth/pdf/professionals/bridges/adhd.pdf
Mental health	Pediatric Symptom Checklist (PSC)	4–18 yr	5–10 min	Parent or child/adolescent	http://psc.partners.org/psc_english.pdf
Depression	Center for Epidemiological Studies Depression Scale for Children (CES-DC)		5–10 min	Child/adolescent	http://www.brightfutures.org/mentalhealth/pdf/professionals/bridges/ces_dc.pdf

CAT, Clinical Adaptive Test; CLAMS, Clinical Linguistic and Auditory Milestone Scale.
Partially modified from American Academy of Pediatrics. Identifying infants and young children with developmental disorders in the medical home: an algorithm for developmental surveillance and screening. *Pediatrics.* 2006;118:405–420.

9

2. **Capute Scales:** Assessment tools that give quantitative DQs for visual-motor/ problem-solving, and language abilities. The CLAMS (Clinical Linguistic and Auditory Milestone Scale) was developed for assessing language milestones from birth to age 36 months. The CAT (Clinical Adaptive Test) consists of problem-solving items for ages birth–36 months, adapted from standardized infant psychological tests.

3. **Denver II Developmental Assessment:** Tool for screening the apparently normal child from 0–6 years of age. Screens in four areas: personal-social, fine motor, gross motor, and language. For children born before 38 weeks' gestation, age should be corrected for prematurity up to age 2 years. A child fails a Denver screen if he or she has two or more delays noted. Indications for referral are a failed test or a classification of untestable on two consecutive screenings.

4. **Ages and Stages Questionnaire (ASQ):** Parent-based questionnaire for children aged 4–60 months. Benefits of parent-based questionnaires include increased time efficiency (parents can fill these out while waiting) and providing an opportunity to document milestones that are difficult to assess in the office or that children are less likely to perform in an unfamiliar setting.

5. **Parents' Evaluation of Developmental Status (PEDS):** Parent-based questionnaire for children up to 8 years of age.

6. **Goodenough-Harris Draw-a-Person Test:** Give the child a pencil and a sheet of blank paper. Instruct the child to "draw a person; draw the best person you can." Use scoring guidelines to assess drawing and compare with norms for age. See Box EC 9-A on Expert Consult.

7. **Gesell figures (Fig. 9-1):** Examiner *should not* demonstrate drawing figures for the child.

8. **Gesell block skills (Fig. 9-2):** Examiner *should* demonstrate block structures for the child. Fig. 9-2 includes developmental age at which each structure can usually be accomplished.

VI. MEDICAL EVALUATION OF DEVELOPMENTAL DISORDERS

A. History

1. **Prenatal and birth:** Toxins, trauma, prematurity, infection
2. **Past medical problems:** Trauma, infection, medication
3. **Developmental history:** Timing of milestone achievement, delayed skills, and loss of skills in all streams
4. **Behavioral history:** Social skills, eye contact, affection, hyperactivity, impulsivity, inattention, distractibility, self-regulation, perseveration, worries/ avoidance, stereotypies, peculiar habits
5. **Educational history:** Need for special services, retention, established educational plans
6. **Family history:** Developmental disabilities, late talkers or walkers, trouble with education, attention deficit/hyperactivity disorder (ADHD), seizures, tics

B. Physical Examination

1. **General:** Height, weight, head circumference, cardiac murmurs, midline defects

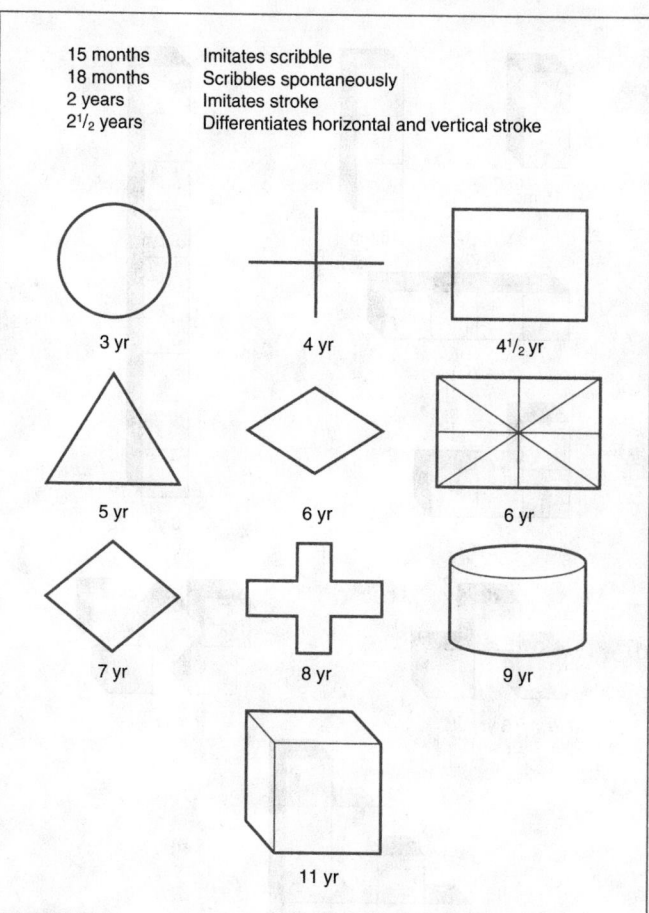

15 months	Imitates scribble
18 months	Scribbles spontaneously
2 years	Imitates stroke
2½ years	Differentiates horizontal and vertical stroke

FIGURE 9-1

Gesell figures. *(From Illingsworth RS. The Development of the Infant and Young Child, Normal and Abnormal. 5th ed. Baltimore: Williams & Wilkins, 1972:229-232; and Cattel P. The Measurement of Intelligence of Infants and Young Children. New York: Psychological Corporation, 1960:97-261.)*

2. **Review for dysmorphic features.**
3. **Age-directed neurologic examination:** Examination tailored to patient's age, including primitive reflexes for infants. See Tables EC 9-A and 9-B on Expert Consult.

C. **Laboratory Investigations, Imaging Studies, Other Tests**
1. **Audiologic testing:** Indicated for all children with global developmental delay or any delay in communication or language.

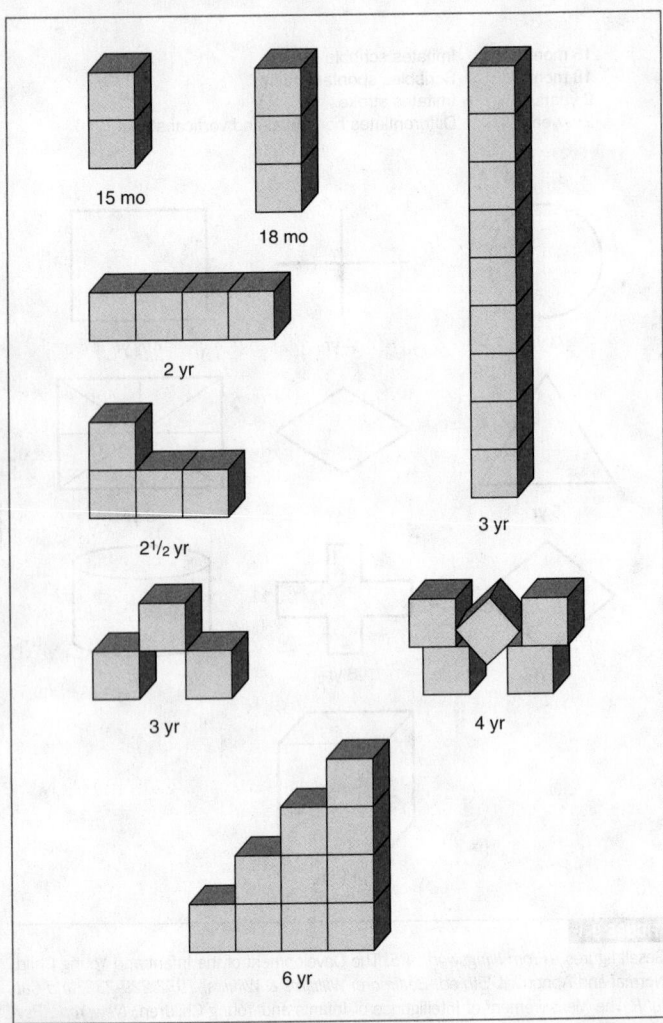

15 mo

18 mo

2 yr

2½ yr

3 yr

3 yr

4 yr

6 yr

FIGURE 9-2

Block skills. *(From Capute AJ, Accardo PJ*. The Pediatrician and the Developmentally Disabled Child: A Clinical Textbook on Mental Retardation. *Baltimore: University Park Press, 1979:122.)*

2. **Neuroimaging:** Consider if child has an abnormal neurologic examination or there is concern about head circumference growth velocity.

3. **Electroencephalogram:** If there is a history of seizure or concern about epilepsy syndrome

4. **Genetic studies may be considered based on individual history, family history, or physical examination:**

a. Microarray is the genetic test with the highest diagnostic yield and is considered the first-line cytogenetic test, although its cost should be carefully considered relative to its benefit to the family.

b. Karyotyping should be reserved for patients having signs of specific chromosomal syndromes (e.g., trisomy 13, 18, or 21).

c. Males with a history suggestive of X-linked inheritance may be considered for testing of one or more X-linked dominant (XLD) genes or screening of the entire X chromosome.

d. Females with severe impairment may be screened for MeCP2 mutations, regardless of whether the specific clinical features of Rett syndrome are present.

5. **Metabolic studies may be considered based on individual history, family history, or physical examination:**

a. Have a higher suspicion in children whose parents are consanguineous or have had children with similar problems or unexplained death or fetal demise.

b. These children may have multiple organ system dysfunction, failure to thrive, dietary selectivity, unusual odors, hearing loss, or episodic symptoms (seizures or encephalopathy).[3]

VII. DISORDERS OF DEVELOPMENT

A. **Intellectual Disability**

1. **Previously known as *mental retardation*, intellectual disability (ID) is characterized by three criteria:** deficits in intellectual functioning, deficits in adaptive functioning, and onset of these deficits during the developmental period. The adaptive deficit has to be in one or more domains of activites of daily living. (Note: Adaptive functioning determines level of support an individual needs, thereby defining the level of ID per DSM-5; Table 9-5.)

B. **Communication Disorders**

1. **Can be subdivided into language disorders, pragmatic communication disorders, and speech production disorders.**

2. **Differential diagnosis includes the previous disorders as well as intellectual disability, hearing loss, and autism or autism spectrum disorder.**

C. **Learning Disabilities (LDs)**

1. **A heterogeneous group of disorders that manifest as significant difficulties in one or more of seven areas (as defined by the federal government):** basic reading skills, reading comprehension, oral expression, listening comprehension, written expression, mathematic calculation, and mathematic reasoning.

TABLE 9-5

SEVERITY LEVELS FOR INTELLECTUAL DISABILITY (INTELLECTUAL DEVELOPMENTAL DISORDER)

Severity Level	Conceptual Domain	Social Domain
Mild	For preschool children, there may be no obvious conceptual differences. For school-age children and adults, there are difficulties in learning academic skills involving reading, writing, arithmetic, time, or money, with support needed in one or more areas to meet age-related expectations. In adults, abstract thinking, executive function (i.e., planning, strategizing, priority setting, and cognitive flexibility), and short-term memory, as well as functional use of academic skills (e.g., reading, money management) are impaired. There is a somewhat concrete approach to problems and solutions compared with age-mates.	Compared with typically developing age-mates, the individual is immature in social interactions (e.g., difficulty in accurately perceiving peers' social cues). Communication, conversation, and language are more concrete or immature than expected for age. There may be difficulties regulating emotion and behavior in age-appropriate fashion; these difficulties are noticed by peers in social situations. There is limited understanding of risk in social situations; social judgment is immature for age, and the person is at risk of being manipulated by others (gullibility).
Moderate	All through development, the individual's conceptual skills lag markedly behind those of peers. For preschoolers, language and preacademic skills may develop slowly. For school-age children, progress in reading, writing, mathematics, and understanding of time and money occurs slowly across the school years and is markedly limited compared with that of peers. For adults, academic skill development is typically at an elementary level, and support is required for all use of academic skills in work and personal life. Ongoing assistance on a daily basis is needed to complete conceptual tasks of day-to-day life, and others may take over these responsibilities fully for the individual.	The individual shows marked differences from peers in social and communicative behavior across development. Spoken language is typically a primary tool for social communication but is much less complex than that of peers. Capacity for relationships is evident in ties to family and friends, and the individual may have successful friendships across life and sometimes romantic relations in adulthood. However, individuals may not perceive or interpret social cues accurately. Social judgment and decision-making abilities are limited, and caretakers must assist the person with life decisions. Friendships with typically developing peers are often affected by communication or social limitations. Significant social and communicative support is needed in work settings for success.
Severe	Attainment of conceptual skills is limited. The individual generally has little understanding of written language or of concepts involving numbers, quantity, time, and money. Caretakers provide extensive supports for problem solving throughout life.	Spoken language is quite limited in terms of vocabulary and grammar. Speech may be single words or phrases and may be supplemented through augmentative means. Speech and communication are focused on the here and now within everyday events. Language is used for social communication more than for explication. Individuals understand simple speech and gestural communication. Relationships with family members and familiar others are a source of pleasure and help.

TABLE 9-5

SEVERITY LEVELS FOR INTELLECTUAL DISABILITY (INTELLECTUAL DEVELOPMENTAL DISORDER) (Continued)

Severity Level	Conceptual Domain	Social Domain
Profound	Conceptual skills generally involve the physical world rather than symbolic processes. The individual may use objects in goal-directed fashion for self-care, work, and recreation. Certain visuospatial skills (e.g., matching and sorting based on physical characteristics) may be acquired. However, co-occurring motor and sensory impairments may prevent functional use of objects.	The individual has very limited understanding of symbolic communication in speech or gesture. He or she may understand some simple instructions or gestures. The individual expresses his or her own desires and emotions largely through nonverbal, nonsymbolic communication. The individual enjoys relationships with well-known family members, caretakers, and familiar others, and initiates and responds to social interactions through gestural and emotional cues. Co-occurring sensory and physical impairments may prevent many social activities.

Reprinted with permission from the American Psychiatric Association. *Diagnostic and Statistical Manual of Mental Disorders.* 5th ed. Arlington, VA: APA, 2013.

2. **Specific LDs are diagnosed when** the individual's achievement on standardized tests in a given area is substantially below that expected for age, schooling, and level of intelligence.[4]

D. Cerebral Palsy (CP)

1. **A disorder of movement and posture** resulting from a permanent nonprogressive lesion of the immature brain.

2. **Manifestations may change with brain growth and development.**

3. **The diagnosis of CP is made at a mean age of 13 months.**

4. **CP is classified in terms of physiologic and topographic characteristics as well as severity** (Table 9-6).[5] Classification is important because different classifications often have very different etiologies and associated deficits.

E. Autism Spectrum Disorders (ASDs)

See the *Diagnostic and Statistical Manual of Mental Disorders,* 5th edition (DSM-5) for full diagnostic criteria.[6] For more detailed guidelines on evaluating for ASDs, see the American Academy of Pediatrics (AAP) practice guidelines.[7] Essential features are impaired social interaction and communication and a restricted group of activities and interests, with stereotyped behaviors, rituals, or mannerisms. Onset of abnormal functioning occurs in the early developmental period. A large proportion of autistic children function in the range of intellectual disability. Siblings of children with autism appear to be at greater risk, and males are disproportionately affected. Assessment scales like the Modified Checklist for

TABLE 9-6	

CLINICAL CLASSIFICATION OF CEREBRAL PALSY[5]

Type	Pattern of Involvement
I. SPASTIC (INCREASED TONE, CLASPED KNIFE, CLONUS, FURTHER CLASSIFIED BY DISTRIBUTION)	
Hemiplegia	Ipsilateral arm and leg; arm worse than leg
Diplegia	Legs primarily affected
Quadriplegia	All four extremities impaired; legs worse than arms
Double hemiplegia	All four extremities; arms notably worse than legs
Monoplegia	One extremity, usually upper; probably reflects a mild hemiplegia
Triplegia	One upper extremity and both lower; probably represents a hemiplegia plus a diplegia or incomplete quadriplegia
II. EXTRAPYRAMIDAL (LEAD PIPE OR CANDLE WAX RIGIDITY, VARIABLE TONE, ± CLONUS)	
Choreoathetosis, rigidity, dystonia	Complex movement/tone disorders reflecting basal ganglia pathology
Ataxia, tremor	Movement and tone disorders reflecting cerebellar origin
Hypotonia	Usually related to diffuse, often severe cerebral and/or cerebellar cortical damage

From Capute AJ, Accardo PJ, eds. *Cerebral Palsy: Developmental Disabilities in Infancy and Childhood.* 2nd ed. vol 2. Baltimore: Paul H. Brookes, 1996:83-86.

Autism in Toddlers (M-CHAT) and Childhood Autism Rating Scale (CARS) are available for screening (see Table 9-4).

VIII. DISORDERS OF MENTAL HEALTH

A. Overview

1. **Screening for mental health issues should occur at all routine well-child visits from early childhood through adolescence,** including history of mood symptoms and any behavioral issues.
2. **The Pediatric Symptom Checklist (PSC) is a general mental health checklist for ages 4–18 years that is filled out by a parent** and can be found in Table 9-4. It screens for a broad array of mental health disorders, including conduct disorders, attention disorders, depression, anxiety, and adjustment disorders. See the DSM-5 for a more complete list of psychiatric diagnoses and full diagnostic criteria.[6]

B. Attention Deficit/Hyperactivity Disorder (ADHD)

1. **Epidemiology:**
a. Affected 9.5% (5.4 million) of children in the United States in 2007.[8]
b. Majority of children continue to meet diagnostic criteria through adolescence, and ADHD does not remit after onset of puberty. Symptoms may last through adulthood, with significant impairment noted.
2. **Assessment:**
a. Diagnostic criteria: Inattention, impulsivity/hyperactivity that are more frequent and severe than typically observed in children of the same developmental age. Symptoms must persist for at least 6 months, occur

TABLE 9-7	
COMMONLY USED DRUGS	
Antidepressants/Anxiolytics*	**Antipsychotics***
Fluoxetine (Prozac)	Aripiprazole (Abilify)
Sertraline (Zoloft)	Haloperidol (Haldol)
Escitalopram (Lexapro)	Risperidone (Risperdal)
Mirtazapine (Remeron)	Quetiapine (Seroquel)

*For more drug information, indications, and dosing please refer to the Formulary (Chapter 29).

    before the age of 12 years, and be evident in two or more settings. See DSM-5 for updated diagnostic criteria.[6,9]

b. Screen all children aged 4–18 who have academic and/or behavioral issues, and for comorbid conditions (oppositional defiant disorder [ODD], conduct disorder, depression, anxiety).[10]

c. Diagnosis is made using history, observation, and behavioral checklists such as the Vanderbilt Assessment Scale (see Table 9-4).

d. If the medical history is unremarkable, no further laboratory or neurologic testing (e.g., computed tomography [CT], positron emission tomography [PET], electroencephalogram [EEG]) are required.

e. Psychological and neuropsychological testing are not required for diagnosis but recommended if other academic or developmental concerns are present.[9]

3. **Treatment:** Studies show pharmacologic treatment works best with behavioral treatment as an adjunct.

a. Before starting a stimulant medication, history should be taken to exclude cardiac symptoms, Wolff-Parkinson-White syndrome, sudden death in the family, hypertrophic cardiomyopathy, and long QT syndrome.[10]

    (1) See ADHD Medication Guide for recommended pharmacologic treatments. Also see Table 9-7.

C. Anxiety Disorders

1. **Epidemiology:**

a. One of the most common mental health issues that presents in the general pediatric setting. An estimated 15%–20% of children and adolescents are affected, with onset most often before age 25.[11]

b. Children may develop new anxiety disorders over time and are at higher risk for anxiety and depressive disorders than adults. They are also at risk for social, family, and academic impairments.

2. **Assessment:**

a. Presentation:

    (1) May present with fear or worry and not recognize their fear as unreasonable.

    (2) Commonly have somatic complaints of headache and stomachache

        (a) Crying, irritability, and angry outbursts are an expression of fear and effort to avoid anxiety-provoking stimulus.

    (3) Screening: Pediatric Anxiety Rating Scale (PARS), SCARED, and Spence Children's Anxiety Scale

3. **Categories:** See DSM-5 for specific criteria for each disorder.[12]

a. Generalized anxiety disorder

b. Separation anxiety disorder

c. Social anxiety disorder

d. Posttraumatic stress disorder

e. Obsessive-compulsive disorder

f. Selective mutism

g. Specific phobia

h. Panic disorder

i. Agorophobia

j. Substance/medication-induced anxiety disorder

4. **Treatment:**

a. Best results obtained with a combination of pharmacotherapy (Table 9-7) and psychotherapy with cognitive-behavioral therapy (CBT).[12]

D. Depressive Disorders

1. **Epidemiology:**

a. Major depressive disorder: 2% of children, 4%–8% of adolescents

b. Sub-clinical symptoms: 5%–10% of children

c. Most common comorbid conditions:

    (1) Anxiety disorders

    (2) Disruptive disorders

    (3) ADHD

    (4) Substance use (adolescents)

2. **Assessment:**

a. Major depression:

    (1) Five or more symptoms for at least 2 weeks, and one of the five must be either depressed/irritable mood or anhedonia.

    (2) Symptoms cause significant impairment in functioning.

    (3) Not due to substance use or a medical condition.

    (4) No history of manic episodes.[13]

3. **Treatment:**

a. May be initiated in primary care setting or may require a referral depending on severity.

b. Literature shows that antidepressant medications (Table 9-7) and CBT combined are the most effective treatment, followed by medication alone, then CBT alone.

c. Selective serotonin reuptake inhibitors (SSRIs) have a black box warning concerning a possible increase in suicidal thoughts or behaviors in children and adolescents after initiation of medication. Patients should be followed closely for the first 2–4 weeks, then every other week thereafter. SSRIs can be initiated in the primary care setting.[14]

d. Refer to the Physicians Med Guide prepared by the American Psychological Association (APA) and American Academy of Child and Adolescent Psychiatry (AACAP) for guidelines regarding medication use for depression in adolescent patients.[14]

E. Substance Abuse Disorder

1. **Epidemiology:**

a. Lifetime diagnosis of alcohol abuse: 0.4%–9%

b. Lifetime diagnosis of alcohol dependence: 0.6%–4.3%

c. Lifetime diagnosis of drug abuse or dependence: 3.3%–9.8%

d. Common comorbid conditions: Disruptive behavior disorders, mood disorders, anxiety disorders

2. **Assessment** (Box 9-1):

a. Establish standards of confidentiality.

b. CRAFFT Questionnaire (Box 9-2).

c. Evaluate for age of onset of use; progression of use for specific substances; circumstances, frequency, and variability of use; and types of agents used.

d. Determine treatment goals and readiness for change.

e. Toxicology workup should be part of any routine evaluation where substance abuse is concerned.

3. **Treatment:**

a. Families should be involved with treatment.

b. Medications can be used to manage withdrawal symptoms and/or cravings.

BOX 9-1

SIGNS AND SYMPTOMS OF SUBSTANCE ABUSE[15]

- Acute change in mood, behavior, and cognition
- Mood: Depression to euphoria
- Behavior: Disinhibition, lethargy, hyperactivity, agitation, somnolence, and hypervigilance
- Cognition: Impaired concentration, changes in attention span, perceptual and overt disturbances in thinking (e.g., delusions)
- Impairment in psychosocial and academic functioning (family conflict/dysfunction, interpersonal conflict, academic failure)
- Deviant or risk-taking behavior

BOX 9-2

CRAFFT QUESTIONNAIRE

C—Have you ever ridden in a **C**AR driven by someone (or yourself) who was "high" or had been using alcohol or drugs?

R—Do you ever use alcohol or drugs to **R**ELAX, feel better about yourself, or fit in?

A—Do you ever use alcohol/drugs while you are **A**LONE?

F—Do your family or **F**RIENDS ever tell you that you should cut down on your drinking or drug use?

F—Do you ever **F**ORGET things you did while using alcohol or drugs?

T—Have you gotten into **T**ROUBLE while you were using alcohol or drugs?

NOTE: Answering yes to two or more questions is a positive screen.

c. Treatment of comorbid conditions should occur at the same time.[15]
d. Find a treatment center at: www.SAMSHA.org.

IX. REFERRAL AND INTERVENTION

A. State Support

1. **The Individuals with Disabilities Education Act (IDEA)** requires states to provide early intervention services to children.
2. **Early intervention services eligibility criteria vary from state to state.** The National Early Childhood Technical Assistance Center (www.nectac.org) provides information about criteria in each state.

B. Recommendations

1. **Facilitate communication between family and school.**
2. **Advocate for appropriate services, and regularly monitor their effectiveness.**
3. **Medical workup when indicated.**
4. **Provide pharmacologic intervention as needed.**
5. **Refer to an appropriate specialist when indicated.**

REFERENCES

1. Capute AJ, Shapiro BK, Palmer FB. Spectrum of developmental disabilities: continuum of motor dysfunction. *Orthop Clin North Am.* 1981;12:15-21.
2. American Academy of Pediatrics. Identifying infants and young children with developmental disorders in the medical home: an algorithm for developmental surveillance and screening. *Pediatrics.* 2006;118:405-420.
3. Michelson DJ, Shevell MI, Sherr EH, Moeschler JB, Gropman AL, Ashwal S. Evidence report: genetic and metabolic testing on children with global developmental delay: report of the Quality Standards Subcommittee of the American Academy of Neurology and the Practice Committee of the Child Neurology Society. *Neurology.* 2011;77:1629-1635.
4. Shapiro BK, Gallico RP. Learning disabilities. *Pediatr Clin North Am.* 1993;40:491-505.
5. Capute AJ, Accardo PJ, eds. 2nd ed. *Cerebral Palsy: Developmental Disabilities in Infancy and Childhood.* vol 2. Baltimore: Paul H. Brookes, 1996.
6. American Psychiatric Association. *Diagnostic and Statistical Manual of Mental Disorders: Text Revision.* 5th ed. Arlington, VA: APA; 2013.
7. Johnson CP, Myers SM. American Academy of Pediatrics. Identification and evaluation of children with autism spectrum disorders. *Pediatrics.* 2007;120: 1183-1215.
8. Centers for Disease Control and Prevention (CDC). Increasing prevalence of parent-reported attention-deficit/hyperactivity disorder among children—United States, 2003 and 2007. *MMWR Morb Mortal Wkly Rep.* 2010;59:1439-1443.
9. Practice parameter for the assessment and treatment of children and adolescents with attention-deficit/hyperactivity disorder. *J Am Acad Child Adolesc Psychiatry.* 2007;46:894-921.
10. Subcommittee on Attention-Deficit/Hyperactivity Disorder, Steering Committee on Quality Improvement and Management, Wolraich M, Brown L, Brown RT, et al. ADHD: clinical practice guideline for the diagnosis, evaluation, and treatment of attention-deficit/hyperactivity disorder in children and adolescents. *Pediatrics.* 2011;128:1007-1022.

11. Beesdo K, Knappe S, Pine DS. Anxiety and anxiety disorders in children and adolescents: developmental issues and implications for DSM-5. *Psychiatr Clin North Am.* 2009;32:483-524.
12. Connolly SD, Bernstein GA; Work Group on Quality Issues. Practice parameter for the assessment and treatment of children and adolescents with anxiety disorders. *J Am Acad Child Adolesc Psychiatry.* 2007;46:267-283.
13. Birmaher B, Brent D; AACAP Work Group on Quality Issues. Practice parameter for the assessment and treatment of children and adolescents with depressive disorders. *J Am Acad Child Adolesc Psychiatry.* 2007;46:1503-1526.
14. Physicians Med Guide. The Use of Medication in Treating Childhood and Adolescent Depression: Information for Physicians. Available at http://www.parentsmedguide.org/physiciansmedguide.htm. Prepared by the American Psychiatric Association and the American Academy of Child and Adolescent Psychiatry. October 7, 2009.
15. Bukstein OG, Bernet W, Arnold V, Work Group on Quality Issues, et al. Practice parameter for the assessment and treatment of children and adolescents with substance use disorders. *J Am Acad Child Adolesc Psychiatry.* 2005;44:609-621.

Chapter 10

Endocrinology

Teresa Mark, MD

See additional content on Expert Consult

I. WEBSITES

Children with Diabetes (www.childrenwithdiabetes.com)
American Diabetes Association (www.diabetes.org)
International Society for Pediatric and Adolescent Diabetes (www.ispad.org)
Pediatric Endocrine Society (www.lwpes.org)

II. DIABETES

A. Evaluation and Diagnosis[1-3]

1. Diagnostic criteria (must meet 1 of 4):
a. Symptoms for diabetes (polyuria, polydipsia, or weight loss) and random blood glucose ≥ 200 mg/dL
b. Fasting blood glucose (FPG = no caloric intake for at least 8 hours) ≥ 126 mg/dL*
c. Oral glucose tolerance test (OGTT) with a 2-hour postload blood glucose ≥ 200 mg/dL*
d. Hemoglobin A_{1c}(HbA$_{1c}$) ≥ 6.5%

2. Defining increased risk: FPG 100–125, 2-hour post OGTT 140–199, HbA$_{1c}$ 5.7%–6.4%†

3. Interpreting HbA$_{1c}$: Estimates average blood glucose for the past 3 months; 6% approximately equals an average of 130 mg/dL, each additional 1% ≈ 30 mg/dL more

4. Oral glucose tolerance test:
a. Pretest preparation:
   (1) Calorically adequate diet required for 3 days before the test, with 50% of total calories taken as carbohydrate.
   (2) Delay test 2 weeks after illness.
   (3) Discontinue all hyperglycemic and hypoglycemic agents (e.g., salicylates, diuretics, oral contraceptives, phenytoin).
b. Procedure: Give 1.75 g/kg (maximum 75 g) oral (PO) glucose after a 12-hour fast, allowing up to 5 minutes for ingestion. Mix glucose with water and lemon juice as a 20% dilution. Quiet activity is permissible during the OGTT. Draw blood samples at 0 and 120 minutes after ingestion.

---

*In the absence of symptoms of hyperglycemia, these values should be repeated on another day.
†These values are for adults; equivalent values not yet determined in children.

c. Interpretation: 2-hour blood glucose < 140 mg/dL = normal; 140–199 mg/dL = impaired glucose tolerance; ≥200 mg/dL = diabetes mellitus (DM).

B. Diabetes Classification[1,2]

1. **Type I or type II (most common types, polygenic):**
a. Patient characteristics (Table 10-1)
b. Laboratory characteristics:
    (1) Islet cell autoantibodies: (GAD-65, insulin, islet cell antibodies) suggestive of type 1. However, ≈15% of children with type 1 diabetes will not have autoantibodies to a specific islet cell antigen and ≈5% will not have any detectable islet cell autoantibodies.
    NOTE: Some children with type 2 diabetes will have measurable islet cell autoantibodies.
    (2) Ketoacidosis: Usually associated with type 1 but does not exclude type 2 (see Sections C and D). Recurrent ketosis, especially diabetic ketoacidosis (DKA), in a type 2 patient should prompt reevaluation of classification.
    (3) C-peptide: In a type 1 patient, a measurable level >2 years after diagnosis should prompt reevaluation of classification.
    (4) Insulin and C-peptide: Often unhelpful in initial classification. At presentation, levels usually low in type 1, but there is significant overlap with type 2.

2. **Other forms of diabetes[4,5]:**
a. Monogenic diabetes: 1%–2% of DM cases. Due to single-gene mutations, typically relating to insulin production or release. Identifying the gene can have clinical significance.
b. Maturity-onset diabetes of youth (MODY):
    (1) Suspect if autosomal dominant inhertance pattern of early-onset (<25 years) diabetes, insulin independence, absent diabetes mellitus type 2 (DM2) phenotype (nonobese), preservation of C-peptide.
    (2) Six well-described subtypes: MODY1 and MODY3, which are due to mutations in transcription factors for insulin production, are responsive to sulfonylureas.

TABLE 10-1
CHARACTERISTICS SUGGESTIVE OF TYPE 1 VS. TYPE 2 DIABETES AT PRESENTATION

Characteristic	Type 1	Type 2
Onset	Usually prepuberty	Usually postpuberty
Polydipsia and polyuria	Present for days to weeks	Absent or present for weeks to months
Ethnicity	Caucasian	African American, Hispanic, Asian, Native American
Weight	Weight loss	Obese
Other physical findings		Acanthosis nigricans
Family history	Autoimmune diseases	Type 2 diabetes
Ketoacidosis	More common	Less common

c. Neonatal diabetes (NDM):
   (1) Defined as DM onset < 6 months of age
   (2) Rare: 1:160000–260000 lives births, typically a de novo mutation
   (3) May be transient (50% recur) or permanent
   (4) Subset respond to sulfonylureas
d. Other causes of DM: Diseases of exocrine pancrease due to pancreatitis, trauma, infection, invasive disease (cystic fibrosis [CF], hemochromatosis). Can also be drug or chemically induced.

C. Diabetic Ketoacidosis[6,7]

1. **Definition:** Hyperglycemia, ketonemia, ketonuria, and metabolic acidosis (pH < 7.30, bicarbonate < 15 mEq/L)
2. **Assessment:**
a. History: In *suspected* diabetic, determine whether there is a history of polydipsia, polyuria, polyphagia, weight loss, vomiting, or abdominal pain, as well as history of infection or inciting event. In a *known* diabetic, also determine the usual insulin regimen, timing and amount of last dose.
b. Examination: Assess for dehydration, Kussmaul respirations, fruity breath, change in mental status, and current weight.
c. Laboratory tests: See Fig. 10-1. Also consider HbA_{1c} to assess for chronic hyperglycemia (normal values are 4.5%–5.9%). In a new-onset diabetic, consider islet cell antibodies, insulin antibodies, thyroid antibodies, thyroid function tests, and celiac screen (endomesial antibody or tissue transglutaminase and total immunoglobulin [Ig]A).
3. **Management:** See Fig. 10-1. Because fluid and electrolyte requirements of patients in DKA vary greatly, the following guidelines are a starting point; therapy must be individualized based on patient dynamics.
a. Acidosis: pH is an indicator of insulin deficiency; if acidosis is not resolving, patient may need more insulin. **NOTE:** Initial insulin administration may cause transient worsening of acidosis as potassium is driven into cells in exchange for hydrogen ions.
b. Hyperglycemia: Blood glucose is an indicator of hydration status.
4. **Cerebral edema:** Most severe complication of DKA. Overly aggressive hydration and rapid correction of hyperglycemia may play a role in its development.
5. **Insulin requirements:** Once DKA is resolved, patient will need to be started on a regimen of subcutaneous (SQ) insulin. See Table 10-2 for calculations (also see Table 10-3). Insulin doses are subsequently adjusted based on actual blood sugars. Initially check blood sugars before meals (QAC), at bedtime (QHS), and at 2 AM.

D. Type II Diabetes Mellitus[8-10]

1. **Prevalence:** Increasing among children, especially among African Americans, Hispanics, and Native Americans. Increase is related to increased prevalence of childhood obesity.
2. **Etiology:** Abnormality in glucose levels caused by insulin resistance and insulin secretory defect.

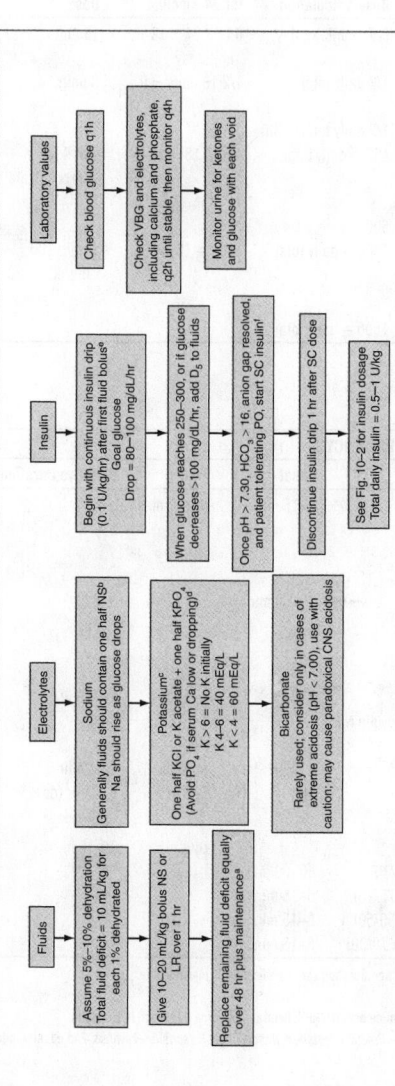

Fluids	Electrolytes	Insulin	Laboratory values

Fluids
- Assume 5%–10% dehydration
  Total fluid deficit = 10 mL/kg for each 1% dehydrated[a]
- Give 10–20 mL/kg bolus NS or LR over 1 hr[a]
- Replace remaining fluid deficit equally over 48 hr plus maintenance[a]

Electrolytes

Sodium
- Generally fluids should contain one half NS[b]
  Na should rise as glucose drops

Potassium[c]
- One half KCl or K acetate + one half KPO₄ (Avoid PO₄ if serum Ca low or dropping)[d]
  K > 6 = No K initially
  K 4–6 = 40 mEq/L
  K < 4 = 60 mEq/L

Bicarbonate
- Rarely used; consider only in cases of extreme acidosis (pH < 7.00), use with caution; may cause paratoxical CNS acidosis

Insulin
- Begin with continuous insulin drip (0.1 U/kg/hr) after first fluid bolus[e]
  Goal glucose
  Drop = 80–100 mg/dL/hr
- When glucose reaches 250–300, or if glucose decreases >100 mg/dL/hr, add D₅ to fluids
- Once pH > 7.30, HCO₃⁻ > 16, anion gap resolved, and patient tolerating PO, start SC insulin[f]
- Discontinue insulin drip 1 hr after SC dose
- See Fig. 10–2 for insulin dosage
  Total daily insulin = 0.5–1 U/kg

Laboratory values
- Check blood glucose q1h
- Check VBG and electrolytes, including calcium and phosphate, q2h until stable, then monitor q4h
- Monitor urine for ketones and glucose with each void

[a]Additional fluids may be needed if there is a large negative fluid balance in the first hours of treatment due to the osmotic diuresis when serum glucose is high.
[b]Some DKA protocols recommend using NS rather than half NS during part of the replacement period in an effort to further decrease risk of cerebral edema.
[c]Patients with DKA are total body K⁺ depleted and are at risk for severe hypokalemia during DKA therapy. However, serum K⁺ levels may be normal or elevated as a result of the shift of K⁺ to the extracellular compartment in the setting of acidosis.
[d]Phosphate is depleted in DKA and will drop further with insulin therapy. Consider replacing half of K as KPO₄ for first 8 hr, then all as KCl. Excessive phosphate may induce hypocalcemic tetany.
[e]Lower dose insulin infusions can be considered in very young patients.
[f]Some protocols recommend also waiting for urine ketones to decrease or clear before starting SC insulin.

FIGURE 10-1

Management of diabetic ketoacidosis. (*Modified from Cooke DW, Plotnick L. Management of diabetic ketoacidosis in children and adolescents.* Pediatr Rev. 2008;29:431-436.)

10

TABLE 10-2

SUBCUTANEOUS INSULIN DOSING

	Insulin	Dose Calculation	Sample Calculation for 24-kg child	Dose
Total daily dose		0.5–1 unit/kg/day	0.75 x 24 = 18 units/day	18 units
Basal	Glargine OR Detemir	1/2 daily total 1/2 daily total ÷ BID	1/2 18 units = 9	9 units
Carbohydrate coverage ratio	Lispro, aspart OR Regular	450 ÷ daily total 500 ÷ daily total	450 ÷ 18 = 25	1 unit: 25 g carbohydrate
Correction factor	Lispro, aspart OR Regular	1800 ÷ daily total 1500 ÷ daily total	1800 ÷ 18 = 100	1 unit: 100 mg/dL > 120

TABLE 10-3

CURRENTLY AVAILABLE INSULIN PRODUCTS

Insulin*	Onset	Peak	Effective Duration
Rapid acting Lispro (Humalog) Aspart (Novo Log) Glulisine (Apidra)	5–15 min	30–90 min	5 hr
Short Acting Regular U100 Regular U500 (concentrated)	30–60 min	2–3 hr	5–8 hr
Intermediate acting Isophane insulin (NPH, Humulin N/Novolin N)	2–4 hr	4–10 hr	10–16 hr
Long acting Glargine (Lantus) Detemir (Levemir)	2–4 hr† Slow	No peak 6–8 hr	20–24 hr 6–24 hr (dose related)
Premixed 70% NPH/30% regular (Humulin 70/30) 75% NPL/25% lispro (Humalog Mix 75/25) 50% NPL/50% lispro (Humalog Mix 50/50) 70% NPA/30% aspart (Novo Log Mix 70/30)	30–60 min 5–15 min 5–15 min 5–15 min	Dual	10-16 hr

*Assuming 0.1–0.2 U/kg per injection. Onset and duration vary significantly by injection site.
†Time to steady state.
NPA, Insulin aspart protamine (neutral protamine aspart); NPH, neutral protamine Hagedom; NPL, insulin.
Modified from American Diabetes Association. *Practical Insulin: A Handbook for Prescribing Providers,* 2nd ed. Alexandria, Va: American Diabetes Association, 2007.

3. **Presentation:** Although not typical, can present in ketoacidosis (chronic high glucose impairs β-cell function and increases peripheral insulin resistance).

4. **Screening:**

a. Consider screening by measuring fasting blood glucose levels in children who are overweight (body mass index > 85th percentile for age and gender) *and* have two of the following risk factors:

   (1) Family history of type 2 DM in a first- or second-degree relative

   (2) Race/ethnicity: African American, Native American, Hispanic, or Asian or Pacific Islander

   (3) Signs associated with insulin resistance (acanthosis nigricans, hypertension, dyslipidemia, polycystic ovarian disease)

b. Begin at age 10 years or onset of puberty (whichever occurs first), and repeat every 2 years.

c. Based on adult data, HbA_{1c} may be used as a screening tool: HbA_{1c} = 5.7%–6.4% indicates increased risk of future diabetes; 6.0%–6.5% is abnormal and indicates need for further testing (OGTT, fasting plasma glucose); >6.5% is diagnostic of diabetes.

5. **Treatment:** See Fig. 10-2.

E. **Monitoring**

1. **Glucose control:** Daily blood glucoses; HbA_{1c} level every 3 months

2. **Other involved organ systems:** Annual eye examinations and regular screening for hypertension, proteinuria, and hyperlipidemia (monitor Q2 yr with goals of low-density lipoprotein [LDL] < 100 mg/dL, high-density [HDL] > 35 mg/dL, triglycerides [TGs] < 150 mg/dL)

III. THYROID FUNCTION[11-13]

A. **Thyroid Tests[12,14,15]**

1. **Interpretation of thyroid function tests (Table 10-4):** See reference values for age (Table 10-5). Remember that preterm infants have different ranges (Table 10-6).

2. **Thyroid scan:** Used to study thyroid structure and function. Localizes ectopic thyroid tissue and hyperfunctioning and nonfunctioning thyroid nodules.

3. **Technetium uptake:** Measures uptake of technetium by thyroid gland. Levels are increased in Grave's disease and decreased in Hashitoxicosis and hypothyroidism (except dyshormonogenesis, when levels may be increased).

B. **Hypothyroidism (Table 10-7)**

1. **Can be congenital or acquired.** See Table 10-7 for characteristics and types of hypothyroidism.

2. **Hypothyroidism and obesity[16]:** Moderate elevations in thyroid-stimulating hormone (TSH [4–10 mIU/L]), with normal or slightly elevated triiodothyronine (T_3) and thyroxine (T_4) are seen in 10%–23% of obese children and adolescents. In these individuals, there does not appear to be a

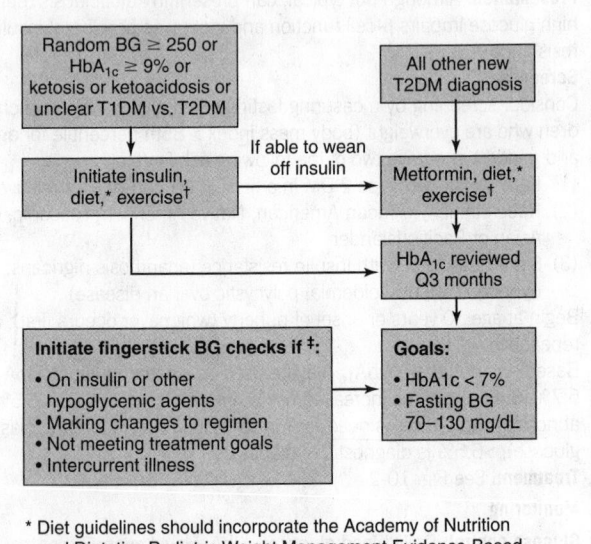

FIGURE 10-2

Treament decision tree for managment of type 2 diabetes (T2DM) in children and adolescents. (*Modified from Copeland KC, Silverstein J, Moore KR, et al. Clinical practice guideline: management of newly diagnosed type 2 diabetes mellitus (T2DM) in children and adolescents. Pediatrics. 2013;131:364-382.*)

TABLE 10-4

THYROID FUNCTION TESTS: INTERPRETATION

Disorder	TSH	T₄	Free T₄
Primary hyperthyroidism	L	H	High N to H
Primary hypothyroidism	H	L	L
Hypothalamic/pituitary hypothyroidism	L, N, H*	L	L
TBG deficiency	N	L	N
Euthyroid sick syndrome	L, N, H*	L	L to low N
TSH adenoma or pituitary resistance	N to H	H	H
Compensated hypothyroidism†	H	N	N

*Can be normal, low, or slightly high.
†Treatment may not be necessary.

H, High; L, low; N, normal; T₄, thyroxine; TBG, thyroxine-binding globulin; TSH, thyroid-stimulating hormone.

TABLE 10-5

AGE-BASED NORMAL VALUES FOR ROUTINE THYROID FUNCTION TESTS[14]

Age	Free T_4 (ng/dL)	TSH (mIU/L)	T_4 (mcg/dL)	T_3 (ng/dL)	Reverse T_3 (ng/dL)	TBG (mcg/mL)
Day of birth	0.94–4.39	2.43–24.3	5.85–18.68	19.53–266.26	19.53–358.70	19.17–44.7
1 wk	0.96–4.08	0.58–5.58*	5.90–18.58	20.83–265.61	19.53–338.52	19.16–44.68
1 mo	1.00–3.44	0.58–5.57*	6.06–18.27	25.39–264.31	19.53–283.84	19.12–44.59
3 mo	1.04–2.86	0.58–5.57*	6.39–17.66	36.46–259.75	19.53–197.90	19.02–44.35
6 mo	1.07–2.44	0.58–5.56*	6.75–17.04	51.43–252.59	19.53–137.36	18.87–44
1 yr	1.10–2.19	0.57–5.54	7.10–16.16	74.87–240.87	18.23–85.93	18.56–43.28
2 yr	1.11–2.05	0.57–5.51	7.16–14.98	103.51–228.50	16.93–55.99	17.94–41.82
5 yr	1.08–1.93	0.56–5.41	6.39–12.94	131.50–212.23	13.02–35.81	16–37.3
8 yr	1.04–1.87	0.55–5.31	5.72–11.71	130.85–202.46	11.72–30.60	14.2–33.09
12 yr	0.99–1.81	0.53–5.16	5.08–10.58	119.78–192.70	11.07–27.99	12.54–29.24
15 yr	1.03–1.77	0.52–5.05	4.84–10.13	110.02–184.88	10.42–27.34	11.96–27.89
18 yr	0.93–1.73	0.51–4.93		101.56–179.03	10.42–26.04	

*Some labs report the reference range upper limit for TSH for children up to 12 months of age as 8.35 mU/L.

T_3, Triiodothyronine; T_4, thyroxine; TBG, thyroxine-binding globulin; TSH, thyroid-stimulating hormone.

NOTE: If age-specific reference ranges are provided by the laboratory running the assay, please refer to those ranges. The above ranges are modified from Lem AJ, de Rijke YB, van Toor H, et al. Serum thyroid hormone levels in healthy children from birth to adulthood and in short children born small for gestational age. *J Clin Endocrinol Metab.* 2012;97:3170-3178.

10

TABLE 10-6

MEAN TSH AND T_4 OF PRETERM AND TERM INFANTS 0–28 DAYS[15]

Age ± SD	Cord (Day 0)	Day 7	Day 14	Day 28
T_4 (mcg/dL)				
23–27*	5.44 ± 2.02	4.04 ± 1.79	4.74 ± 2.56	6.14 ± 2.33
28–30	6.29 ± 2.02	6.29 ± 2.10	6.60 ± 2.25	7.46 ± 2.33
31–34	7.61 ± 2.25	9.40 ± 3.42	9.09 ± 3.57	8.94 ± 2.95
>37	9.17 ± 1.94	12.67 ± 2.87	10.72 ± 1.40	9.71 ± 2.18
FT_4 (ng/dL)				
23–27	1.28 ± 0.41	1.47 ± 0.56	1.45 ± 0.51	1.50 ± 0.43
28–30	1.45 ± 0.43	1.82 ± 0.66	1.65 ± 0.44	1.71 ± 0.43
31–34	1.49 ± 0.33	2.14 ± 0.57	1.96 ± 0.43	1.88 ± 0.46
>37	1.41 ± 0.39	2.70 ± 0.57	2.03 ± 0.28	1.65 ± 0.34
TSH (mIU/L)				
23–27	6.80 ± 2.90	3.50 ± 2.60	3.90 ± 2.70	3.80 ± 4.70
28–30	7.00 ± 3.70	3.60 ± 2.50	4.90 ± 11.2	3.60 ± 2.50
31–34	7.90 ± 5.20	3.60 ± 4.80	3.80 ± 9.30	3.50 ± 3.40
>37	6.70 ± 4.80	2.60 ± 1.80	2.50 ± 2.00	1.80 ± 0.90

*Weeks gestational age.

FT_4, Free thyroxine; T_4, thyroxine; TSH, thyroid-stimulating hormone.

Data modified from Williams FL, Simpson J, Delahunty C, et al. Collaboration from The Scottish Preterm Thyroid Group: Developmental trends in cord and postpartum serum thyroid hormones in preterm infants. *J Clin Endocrinol Metab.* 2004;89:5314-5320.

TABLE 10-7

HYPOTHYROIDISM

Disease and Clinical Symptoms	Onset	Etiology	Management	Follow-up
PRIMARY/CONGENITAL				
Large fontanelles, lethargy, constipation, hoarse cry, hypotonia, hypothermia, jaundice	Symptoms usually develop within first 2 weeks of life; almost always present by 6 weeks. Some infants may be relatively asymptomatic if the cause is other than absence of the thyroid gland. Treated patients are still at risk for developmental delay.	Primary hypothyroidism: Most common cause is defect of fetal thyroid development. Other causes include TSH receptor mutation or thyroid dyshormonogenesis. *OR* Central hypothyroidism: Deficiency of thyrotropin-releasing hormone (TRH) or thyrotropin (TSH).	Goal is to achieve T_4 in the upper half of normal range. In primary hypothyroidism, TSH should be kept <5. A minority of infants maintain persistently high TSH despite correction of T_4. Replacement with L-thyroxine as soon as diagnosis is confirmed.	Monitor T_4 and TSH at the end of weeks 1 and 2 of therapy and 3–4 weeks after any dose change. If levels are adequate, follow every 1–3 months during the first 12 months.
ACQUIRED				
Growth deceleration; other signs may include coarse, brittle hair, dry, scaly skin, delayed tooth eruption, cold intolerance	Can occur as early as the first 2 years of life.	Hashimoto thyroiditis (diagnosis supported by presence of antithyroglobulin or antimicrosomal antibodies). Head/neck radiation. Central hypothyroidism (pituitary/hypothalamic insult).	Replacement with L-thyroxine.	As for primary/congenital. After 2 years, monitor levels every 6–12 months as dose changes become less frequent.

NOTE: Thyroid hormone levels in premature infants are lower than those seen in full-term infants. Further, the TSH surge seen at approximately 24 hours of age in full-term babies does not appear in preterm infants. In this population, lower levels are associated with increased illness, but the effect of replacement therapy remains controversial.

L-thyroxine, Levothyroxine; TSH, thyroid-stimulating hormone.

benefit to treating with thyroxine. Values tend to normalize with weight loss, suggesting they are the result, rather than the cause, of obesity in these individuals. Could consider testing for thyroid antibodies to further clarify whether there is true thyroid dysfunction.

3. **Newborn screening for hypothyroidism**[13,17]**:** Mandated in all 50 states. Measures a combination of TSH and T_4, based on the particular state's algorithm; 1:25 abnormal tests are confirmed. Congenital hypothyroidism has prevalence of 1:3000–4000 U.S. infants. If abnormal results are found, clinicians should follow recommendations of American College of Medical Genetics—ACT sheets and Algorithm for confirmation testing. See Chapter 13 for further resources on newborn screening.

   NOTE: Because of the risk of inducing adrenal crisis if adrenocorticotropic hormone (ACTH) deficiency is present, *do not* begin treatment of central hypothyroidism until normal ACTH/cortisol functionis documented.

C. Hyperthyroidism

1. **General:**
   a. Symptoms: Hyperactivity, irritability, altered mood, insomnia, heat intolerance, increased sweating, pruritus, tachycardia, palpitations, fatigue, weakness, weight loss despite increased appetite (or weight gain), increased stool frequency, oligomenorrhea or amenorrhea, fine tremor, hyperreflexia, hair loss.
   b. Epidemiology: Prevalence increases with age, beginning in adolescence; 4:1 female-to-male predominance.
   c. Etiology: Most common cause in childhood is Graves disease (see later). Other causes: Subacute thyroiditis, factitious hyperthyroidism (intake of exogenous hormone), TSH-secreting pituitary tumor (rare). Pituitary resistance to thyroid hormone (compensatory rise in T_4, but TSH remains within normal range).
   d. Laboratory findings: ↑ T_4, ↑ T_3, usually ↓ TSH. Further tests include TSH receptor–stimulating antibody, thyroid-stimulating immunoglobulin (TSI), antithyroglobulin and antimicrosomal antibodies, free T_4, and free T_3.

2. **Graves disease:**
   a. Physical examination: Diffuse goiter, a feeling of grittiness and discomfort in the eye, retrobulbar pressure or pain, eyelid lag or retraction, periorbital edema, chemosis, scleral injection, exophthalmos, extraocular muscle dysfunction, localized dermopathy, and lymphoid hyperplasia.
   b. Epidemiology: Peak incidence, age 11–15 years; 5:1 female-to-male ratio. Family history of autoimmune thyroid disease.
   c. Etiology: Autoimmune (positive TSI; may also have low titers of thyroglobulin ± microsomal antibodies).
   d. Laboratory findings: ↑ T_4, ↑ T_3, ↓ TSH (↑ iodine 123 [^{123}I] uptake distinguishes from Hashimoto thyroiditis).
   e. Treatment and monitoring: Methimazole (inhibits formation of thyroid hormone). Propylthiouracil (PTU) should not be used as first-line treatment in children, owing to higher risk of liver dysfunction than with

methimazole. PTU can be considered for those with mild reactions to
methimazole. Radioactive iodine (^{131}I) or surgical thyroidectomy are
options for initial treatment or refractory cases. Follow symptoms and T_4
and TSH levels.

3. **Hashimoto thyroiditis:**
a. Presentation: ± Initial hyperthyroidism, followed by eventual thyroid
burnout and hypothyroidism.
b. Etiology: Autoimmune (significantly elevated thyroglobulin and/or microsomal antibody).
c. Laboratory findings: Mild to moderate ↑ T_4 (^{123}I uptake distinguishes from
Graves).
d. Treatment: Hyperthyroid phase is usually self-limited; patient may eventually need thyroid replacement. Propranolol if symptomatic.

4. **Thyroid storm:**
a. Presentation: Acute onset of hyperthermia, tachycardia, and restlessness. May progress to delirium, coma, and death.
b. Treatment: Propranolol is used to relieve signs and symptoms of thyrotoxicosis. Potassium iodide may also be used for acute hyperthyroid
management. Long-term management as for Graves disease.

5. **Neonatal thyrotoxicosis:**
a. Presentation: Microcephaly, frontal bossing, intrauterine growth
retardation (IUGR), tachycardia, systolic hypertension leading to widened
pulse pressure, irritability, failure to thrive, exophthalmos, goiter, flushing,
vomiting, diarrhea, jaundice, thrombocytopenia, and cardiac failure or
arrhythmias. Onset from immediately after birth to weeks.
b. Etiology: Occurs exclusively in infants born to mothers with Graves disease. Caused by transplacental passage of maternal TSI. Occasionally,
mothers are unaware they have Graves. Even if a mother has received
definitive treatment (thyroidectomy or radiation therapy), passage of TSI
remains possible.
c. Treatment and monitoring: Propranolol for symptom control. Methimazole to lower thyroxine levels. Digoxin may be indicated for heart failure.
Disease usually resolves by age 6 months.

IV. PARATHYROID GLAND FUNCTION AND VITAMIN D

A. Parathyroid Gland
1. **Parathyroid hormone (PTH) function:** Increases serum calcium by
increasing bone resorption, increasing calcium and magnesium reuptake in the kidney, increasing phosphorus excretion in the kidney, and
increasing 25-hydroxyvitamin D conversion to 1,25-dihydroxyvitamin D
in order to increase calcium absorption in the intestine.

2. **Hypoparathyroidism:**
a. Presentation: Asymptomatic or mild muscle cramps to hypocalcemic
tetany, prolonged QTc, and convulsions.
b. Etiology: Results from a decrease in PTH due to decreased function
or absence of the parathyroid gland. This can be due to transient

hypoparathyroidism in infants, autoimmune disease, DiGeorge syndrome, iatrogenic removal of the parathyroid gland during other surgical procedures. Pseudohypoparathyroidism results from PTH resistance and is distinguished by normal or elevated PTH.

c. Laboratory findings: ↓ PTH; ↓ serum Ca^{2+}, ↑ serum phosphorus, normal/↓ alkaline phosphatase, ↓ 1,25-OH–vitamin D_3

d. Treatment and monitoring: Calcium supplementation for documented hypocalcemia, vitamin D supplementation with calcitriol. Carefully monitor serum calcium and phosphorus during therapy. Monitor urine calcium levels to avoid hypercalciuria.

3. **Hyperparathyroidism:**

a. Presentation: Hypercalcemia leading to vomiting, constipation, abdominal pain, weakness, paresthesias, malaise, and bone pain. Uncommon in childhood.

b. Etiology: Primary hyperparathyroidism is uncommon in children and is usually due to overproduction secondary to adenoma or hyperplasia. Adenomas can be associated with multiple endocrine neoplasia (MEN) syndromes (see Expert Consult, Box EC 10-A). Secondary hyperparathyroidism is more common; develops in response to hypocalcemic states like renal failure or rickets.

c. Laboratory findings, primary: ↑ PTH, ↑ serum Ca^{2+}; ↓ serum phosphorus; normal/↑ alkaline phosphatase. In secondary hyperparathyroidism, Ca^{2+} normal/↓.

d. Treatment for hypercalcemia associated with primary hyperparathyroidism: Hydration is mainstay of treatment; enhances calciuria. Furosemide may be used with caution with adequate hydration. Hydrocortisone (1 mg/kg Q6 hr), reduces intestinal absorption of calcium. Calcitonin transiently opposes bone resorption. In severe hypercalcemia, bisphosphates may be considered. Surgical removal of parathyroid glands (may result in hypoparathyroidism).

B. **Vitamin D Deficiency (Table 10-8)[18-20]**

1. **Current recommendations suggest 600 IU/day in children >12 months of age to meet daily requirements.**

TABLE 10-8

VITAMIN D DEFICIENCY

Disease, Clinical Symptoms, and Onset	Etiology	Evaluation	Management
Rickets (infancy/childhood): Failure of adequate bone mineralization, leading to soft bones/skeletal deformities	Decreased dietary intake Inadequate exposure to sunlight Increased melanin Impaired renal function	↓ 25-OH vitamin D	Supplementation for: • Breast-fed infants • Those with celiac disease, cystic fibrosis, Crohn's disease, pancreatic deficiency
Osteomalacia (adults): Bone pain and muscle weakness	Fat malabsorption (celiac disease, cystic fibrosis, Crohn's disease)		Repletion per Formulary

VITAMIN D, 25-HYDROXYVITAMIN D[18-20]

25-Hydroxyvitamin D	Value (ng/mL)
Deficiency	<10–15*
Insufficiency	15–20
Optimal level	>20–30†

*Values <10–15 have been associated with bone changes found in rickets.

†Controversy exists regarding optimal 25-hydroxyvitamin D level. Some experts recommend a level >30 ng/mL as optimal. Johns Hopkins Laboratory uses 30 ng/mL as cutoff for normal.

NOTE: 1,25-Dihydroxyvitamin D is the physiologically active form, but 25-hydroxyvitamin D is the value to monitor for vitamin D deficiency because this approximates body stores of vitamin D. Cutoffs are not yet well defined.

2. **The definition and consequences of vitamin D deficiency and insufficiency is an evolving field.** See Table 10-9 for suggested ranges of 25-hydroxyvitamin D.

V. ADRENAL FUNCTION[21-23]

A. Adrenal Insufficiency

1. **Etiology:**

a. Common causes: Congenital adrenal hyperplasia (CAH) and chronic glucocorticoid treatment (suppression of ACTH secretion)

b. Other causes: Addison disease and hypothalamic or pituitary disease secondary to tumors, surgery, radiation therapy, or congenital defects

2. **Evaluation:**

a. AM cortisol level (see Table 10-10 for interpretation)

b. ACTH stimulation test:

   (1) Purpose: Measures ability of the adrenal gland to produce cortisol in response to ACTH. Most useful in diagnosis of adrenal insufficiency.

   (2) Interpretation: Normally, a rise in serum cortisol follows ACTH administration. With ACTH deficiency or prolonged adrenal suppression, there is no rise in cortisol after a single ACTH dose. Blunted cortisol response can be indicative of CAH. Lack of response after 3 consecutive days of ACTH stimulation is pathognomonic of Addison disease.

   (3) Standard-dose ACTH stimulation test (250 mcg intravenously; cortisol measured at 30 minutes. Used to evaluate for primary adrenal insufficiency, although may be used to evaluate for central adrenal insufficiency:

      (a) For evaluation of primary adrenal insufficiency:
          <18 mcg/dL: Highly suggestive of adrenal insufficiency
          >18 mcg/dL: Normal (rules out adrenal insufficiency)

      (b) For evaluation of central adrenal insufficiency:
          <16 mcg/dL: Highly suggestive of adrenal insufficiency
          16–30 mcg/dL: Adrenal insufficiency less likely but not excluded
          >30 mcg/dL: Normal (rules out adrenal insufficiency)

(4) Low-dose ACTH stimulation test (1 mcg/1.73 m²); cortisol measured at 30 minutes. Used to evaluate for central adrenal insufficiency, where it may have higher sensitivity than standard-dose test:

Level <16 mcg/dL: Suggestive of adrenal insufficiency

Level 16–22 mcg/dL: Adrenal insufficiency less likely but not excluded

Level >22 mcg/dL: Adrenal insufficiency unlikely

NOTE: No test for adrenal insufficiency has perfect sensitivity or specificity, so results must be interpreted in the individual clinical context.

c. Mineralocorticoid deficiency confirmed with ↑ renin and ↓ aldosterone

3. **Congenital adrenal hyperplasia**[22,23]:

a. Group of autosomal recessive disorders characterized by a defect in one of the enzymes required in the synthesis of cortisol from cholesterol (Fig. 10-3). Cortisol deficiency results in oversecretion of ACTH and hyperplasia of the adrenal cortex.

TABLE 10-10

CORTISOL, 8AM

Interpretation	Cortisol (mcg/dL)
Suggestive of adrenal insufficiency	<5 mcg/dL
Indeterminate	5–14 mcg/dL
Adrenal insufficiency unlikely	>14 mcg/dL

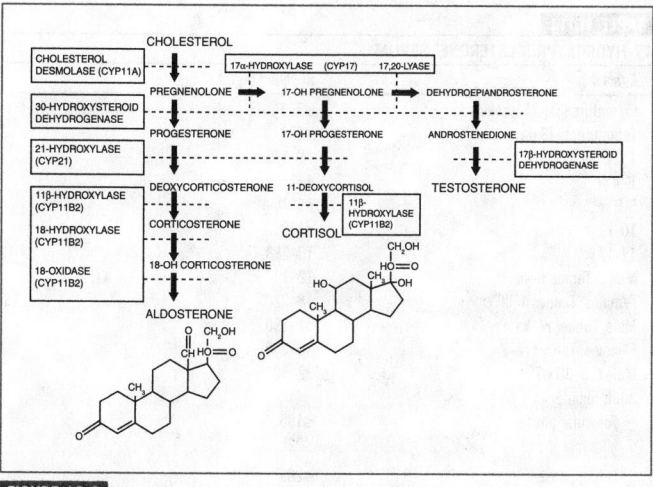

FIGURE 10-3

Biosynthetic pathway for steroid hormones. *(From Marshall I, Nimkarn S, New MI. Endocrine hypertension in childhood. Available at www.endotext.org/pediatrics/pediatrics9/index.html. Accessed December 21, 2007.)*

b. Most common cause of ambiguous genitalia in females.

c. 21-Hydroxylase deficiency accounts for 90% of cases.

d. The enzymatic defect results in impaired synthesis of adrenal steroids beyond the enzymatic block and overproduction of the precursors before the block. Two major classifications:

  (1) Classic (complete enzyme deficiency):

    (a) Occurs with or without salt loss.

    (b) Symptoms occur in the absence of stress.

    (c) Adrenal crisis in untreated patients occurs at 1–2 weeks of life, with signs and symptoms of adrenal insufficiency rarely occurring before 3–4 days of life. (Non–salt-losing forms have a less severe risk for adrenal crisis, owing to preservation of mineralocorticoid synthesis.)

    (d) Diagnosis: Elevated 17-hydroxyprogesterone (17-OHP) levels (often on newborn screen) (Table 10-11).

    (e) Elevated testosterone in girls and androstenedione in girls and boys.

    (f) For apparent male infants presenting with classic CAH, a karyotype should be evaluated to rule out the possibility of a severely masculinized female infant.

  (2) Nonclassic or simple virilizing form (partial enzyme deficiency):

    (a) Adrenal insufficiency tends to occur only under stress; manifests as androgen excess after infancy (precocious pubarche, irregular menses, hirsutism, acne, advanced bone age).

TABLE 10-11

17-HYDROXYPROGESTERONE, SERUM

Age	Baseline (ng/dL)
Premature (31–35 weeks)	≤360
Term infants (3 days)	≤420
1–12 mo	11–170
1–4 yr	4–115
5-9 yr	≤90
10-13 yr	≤169
14-17 yr	16–283
Males, Tanner II–III	12–130
Females, Tanner II–III	18–220
Male, Tanner IV–V	51–190
Females, Tanner IV–V	36–200
Male (18–30 yr)	32–307
Adult female	
Follicular phase	≤185
Midcycle phase	≤225
Luteal phase	≤285

Reference ranges from Quest Diagnostics LC/MS assay (liquid chromatography/tandem mass spectroscopy). For preterm infants or infants born small for gestational age, see Olgemöller B, Roscher AA, Liebl B, et al. Screening for congenital adrenal hyperplasia: adjustment of 17-hydroxyprogesterone cut-off values to both age and birth weight markedly improves the predictive value. *J Clin Endocrinol Metab.* 2003;88:5790-5794.

(b) Morning 17-OHP levels may be elevated, but diagnosis may require an ACTH stimulation test. A significant rise in the 17-OHP level 60 minutes after ACTH injection is diagnostic. Cortisol response will be decreased.

(3) Newborn screen:

(a) Measures 17-OHP on filter paper; can be artificially elevated due to prematurity, sickness, stress; 2% specific, resulting in 98% false-positive rate

(b) Results: If 17-OHP 40–100 ng/mL, repeat. If higher, check electrolytes and serum 17-OHP. If K ↑ and Na ↓, initiate treatment with hydrocortisone.

4. **Primary adrenal insufficiency** (Addison disease):[24]

a. Syndrome of weakness, fatigue, and hyperpigmentation due to insufficient mineralocorticoid and glucocorticoid production, with compensatory ACTH overproduction. Because of its nonspecific presentation, can be missed in older children.

b. Autoimmune destruction of adrenal glands is the most common cause outside of infancy. In children, it may be part of autoimmune polyendocrine syndrome type 1 (APS-1), which also includes hypoparathyroidism and chronic mucocutaneous candidiasis. Individuals with autoimmune Addison disease should also be screened for other endocrinopathies.

5. **Management of adrenal insufficiency (for relative potency of steroids see Table 10-12)**

TABLE 10-12

POTENCY OF VARIOUS THERAPEUTIC STEROIDS (SET RELATIVE TO POTENCY OF CORTISOL)

Steroid	Glucocorticoid Effect* (in mg of cortisol per mg of steroid)	Mineralocorticoid Effect† (in mg of cortisol per mg of steroid)
Cortisol (hydrocortisone)	1	1
Cortisone acetate (oral)	0.8	0.8
Cortisone acetate (intramuscular)	0.8	0.8
Prednisone	4	0.25
Prednisolone	4	0.25
Methyl prednisolone	5	0.4
Betamethasone	25	0
Triamcinolone	5	0
Dexamethasone	30	0
9α–fluorocortisone (fludrocortisone)	15	200
Deoxycorticosterone (DOC) acetate	0	20
Aldosterone	0.3	200–1,000

*To determine cortisol equivalent of a given steroid dose, multiply dose of steroid by corresponding number in column for glucocorticoid or mineralocorticoid effect. To determine dose of a given steroid based on desired cortisol dose, divide desired hydrocortisone dose by corresponding number in the column.

†Total physiologic replacement for salt retention is usually 0.1 mg Florinef, regardless of patient size.

Modified from Sperling MA. *Pediatric Endocrinology*, 3rd ed. Philadelphia: Saunders, 2008:476.

a. Glucocorticoid maintenance:
   (1) Adrenal insufficiency—replacement of physiologic glucocorticoid production: 6–18 mg/m^2/day ÷ TID hydrocortisone PO or 1.5–3.5 mg/m^2/day prednisone ÷ BID (or equivalent glucocorticoid dose of another steroid). Typically, lower doses are required for central adrenal insufficiency, intermediate doses for primary adrenal insufficiency, and higher doses for CAH. Consultation with an endocrinologist is recommended.
   (2) Doses are often titrated to preserve normal skeletal growth and rate of skeletal maturation, and in CAH to suppress production of excess androgen.
b. Mineralocorticoid maintenance:
   (1) These patients should have ready access to salt.
   (2) For salt-losing forms of adrenal insufficiency (e.g., CAH, Addison disease): 0.1 mg/m^2/day (typical range: 0.05–0.15 mg) oral (PO) fludrocortisone acetate once daily is recommended. (**NOTE:** Intravenous [IV] hydrocortisone at 50 mg/m^2/day will supply a maintenance amount of mineralocorticoid activity. Synthetic steroids such as prednisone and dexamethasone do not supply appropriate mineralocorticoid effects.)
   (3) Infants also require 1–2 g (17–34 mEq) of sodium supplementation per day.
   (4) Always monitor blood pressure and electrolytes when supplementing mineralocorticoids.
c. Stress-dose glucocorticoids:
   (1) Glucocorticoid dosage should increase in patients with fever or other illness to mimic normal physiologic cortisol response to stress.
   (2) Minor ambulatory illness stress dose: 30–50 mg/m^2/day of hydrocortisone PO ÷ TID or 6–10 mg/m^2/day prednisone PO ÷ BID.
   (3) Major stress (surgery/severe illness/adrenal crisis): Hydrocortisone 50 mg/m^2 IV bolus, then 25–100 mg/m^2/day IV (as a continuous infusion) or intramuscular (IM) injection of 25 mg/m^2/dose Q6 hr

6. **Acute adrenal crisis:**
a. Often precipitated by acute illness, trauma, surgery, or exposure to excess heat.
b. Presentation: Emesis, diarrhea, dehydration, hypotension, metabolic acidosis, shock.
c. Laboratory values: Often hypoglycemia, hyponatremia, and hyperkalemia. In addition, serum cortisol and aldosterone are decreased, and ACTH and renin are elevated. In infants with CAH, 17-OHP is increased. **NOTE:** Performing these studies before steroid administration is useful to confirm the diagnosis, but treatment should not be delayed.
d. Management includes rapid volume expansion to support blood pressure, sufficient dextrose to maintain blood glucose, close monitoring of electrolytes, and corticosteroid administration.
   (1) Give 50 mg/m^2 of hydrocortisone by IV bolus (rapid estimate: infants = 25 mg; children = 50–100 mg), followed by 50 mg/m^2/24 hr by continuous drip (preferable) or divided Q3–4 hr.

(2) Hydrocortisone and cortisone are the only glucocorticoids that provide the necessary mineralocorticoid effects.

7. **Cushing syndrome:**[25]

a. Signs and symptoms (including rapid weight gain with central obesity, buffalo hump, moon face, striae, thinning of skin and other membranes, hypertension) associated with elevated cortisol levels and overexposure to glucocorticoids (either endogenous or exogenous). Relatively rare in children, with most cases resulting from iatrogenic causes.

b. Cushing evaluation:

(1) 24-hour urine collection for excess cortisol (normal value range by mass spectrometry: ≤27–30 ng/mL).

(2) Salivary cortisol level: Measured at 11 PM (*spit in a tube*); levels are akin to free serum cortisol. Normal range is <0.2 mcg/dL.

(3) Dexamethasone suppression test:

(a) Dexamethasone suppresses secretion of ACTH by the normal pituitary, decreasing endogenous production of cortisol. Useful in determining the etiology of glucocorticoid or androgen overproduction.

(b) Overnight dexamethasone suppression test: Measure serum cortisol at 8 AM; preceded by 1 mg of dexamethasone PO given at 11 PM the night before. Level <1.8 mcg/dL (50 nmol/L) is within normal range of suppression.

NOTE: Random cortisol is not useful in evaluation for Cushing syndrome.

B. Adrenal Medulla—Pheochromocytoma[26-28]

1. **Pheochromocytoma only accounts for ≈1% of pediatric hypertension.** Often associated with syndromes: MEN IIa and IIb, Von Hippel-Lindau, neurofibromatosis (NF)1, familial paraganglioma syndrome.

2. **Evaluation for pheochromocytoma should involve imaging and laboratory workup.** See Expert Consult, Chapter 10, for additional information about plasma concentrations of free, fractionated metanephrines.

3. **Measurement of free, fractionated metanephrines in plasma:**

a. Use: Detection of pheochromocytoma

b. Upper limits of normal: Somewhat assay dependent

(1) One study suggests upper normal limits to be metanephrines, 0.3 nmol/L; normetanephrines, 0.6 nmol/L.[27]

(2) A pediatric study suggests metanephrines for boys, 0.52; girls, 0.37 nmol/L; normetanephrines for boys, 0.53; girls, 0.42 nmol/L.[28]

VI. POSTERIOR PITUITARY GLAND—VASOPRESSIN[29]

A. Syndrome of Inappropriate Antidiuretic Hormone Secretion (SIADH)

1. **Presentation:** Hyponatremia (Na^+ < 135 mEq/L) with inappropriately concentrated urine in the setting of euvolemia or mild hypervolemia

2. **Etiology:** Central nervous system (CNS) trauma, CNS infection, CNS or other types of surgery, particularly tonsillectomy and adenoidectomy, pneumonia

3. **Laboratory findings:** ↓ serum Na^+ and Cl^- with normal HCO_3^-, hypouricemia, inappropriately concentrated urine

4. **Treatment:** Correct hyponatremia slowly with fluid restriction (≈10% rise in Na^+ per 24 hours). *In the setting of coma or seizures,* use hypertonic saline to rapidly correct Na^+ to ≈ 120–125 mEq/L. Definitive therapy: identify and treat the underlying cause

B. Diabetes Insipidus (DI)[23]

1. **General:** Inability to concentrate urine

a. Presentation: Infants may present with failure to thrive, vomiting, constipation, unexplained fevers. In more severe cases, severe dehydration, hypovolemic shock, and seizure may occur.

b. Etiology: May be central or nephrogenic (see below).

c. Diagnosis: Water deprivation test. Vasopressin test differentiates between central and nephrogenic DI.

   (1) Water deprivation test:

      (a) Purpose: Determines ability to concentrate urine; useful in diagnosis of DI. Risk of dehydration and hypernatremia, so careful supervision is required.

      (b) Method:

         (i) Begin test after a 24-hour period of adequate hydration and stable weight.

         (ii) Obtain a baseline weight after bladder emptying.

         (iii) Restrict fluids. Measure body weight and urine specific gravity and volume hourly.

         (iv) Check serum Na and urine and serum osmolality Q2 hr. (Hematocrit and blood urea nitrogen [BUN] levels may also be obtained but are not critical.) Monitor carefully to ensure fluids are not ingested during the test.

         (v) Terminate test if weight loss approaches 5%.

      (c) Interpretation:

         (i) Normal individuals and those with psychogenic DI: Urine will be concentrated to 500–1400 mOsm/L; plasma osmolality will be 288–291 mOsm/L. Urine specific gravity rises to at least 1.010, urine-to-plasma osmolality ratio is >2, urine volume decreases significantly, and there should be no appreciable weight loss. Urine osmolarity > 1000 mOsm/L (or > 600 mOsm/L for >1 hour) generally excludes a diagnosis of DI.

         (ii) Central or nephrogenic DI: Specific gravity remains < 1.005. Urine osmolality remains <150 mOsm/L, with no significant reduction of urine volume. Weight loss of up to 5% usually occurs. At the end of the test, serum osmolality > 290 mOsm/L, Na > 150 mEq/L, and a rise of BUN and hematocrit provide evidence the patient has DI.

   (2) Vasopressin test:

      (a) Purpose: Used to differentiate between central (ADH-deficient) and nephrogenic DI

(b) Method: Vasopressin given subcutaneously (1 U/m^2), preferably at the end of water deprivation test. Urine output, urine specific gravity, and water intake are monitored.

(c) Interpretation:

(i) Central DI: Patients concentrate their urine (>1.010), demonstrate a reduction of urine volume and decreased fluid intake in response to exogenous vasopressin

(ii) Nephrogenic DI: No significant change in fluid intake, urine volume, or specific gravity

(iii) Psychogenic DI: Continued fluid intake, decreased urine output, and increased specific gravity

2. **Central DI:**

a. Etiology: Caused by vasopressin deficiency, associated with CNS injury, including trauma and tumors. After trauma to axons of vasopressin-containing neurons, a temporary or permanent DI may result. Owing to the initial edema occurring in the area of the hypothalamus and pituitary, a short-lived period (2–5 days) of DI is observed. This is succeeded by a stage of SIADH as dying neurons release vasopressin. The final stage results in permanent DI if a significant number of neurons are injured.

b. Laboratory findings: Low urine specific gravity (<1.005), low urine osmolarity (50–200), low vasopressin (<0.5 pg/mL)

c. Treatment: IV, PO, SQ, or nasal desmopressin acetate (DDAVP); titrate dosage to urine output. Goal is ≥1-hour period of diuresis per day that stimulates thirst. Monitor electrolytes. Infants are often not treated with DDAVP because of difficulty monitoring input and output. Rather, they can be treated with increased free water and salt restriction.

3. **Nephrogenic DI:**

a. Etiology: Caused by renal tubular resistance to vasopressin; genetic or acquired

b. Laboratory findings: Low urine specific gravity (<1.005), low urine osmolarity (50–200 mOsm/L)

c. Treatment: Increase free water and a low-salt diet

VII. GROWTH AND SEXUAL DEVELOPMENT[29-38]

A. Growth

1. **Target height range:** Calculated as midparental stature ± 2 SD (1 SD = 2 inches)

a. Midparental stature for boys: (Paternal height + maternal height + 5 inches)/2

b. Midparental stature for girls: (Paternal height + maternal height − 5 inches)/2

2. **Short stature (Fig. 10-4):**

a. Definition: Height less than 3rd percentile, decreasing growth velocity, height percentile below target height range.

b. Differential diagnosis: Constitutional growth delay (CGD) and familial short stature (FSS) must be distinguished from pathologic causes of short stature.

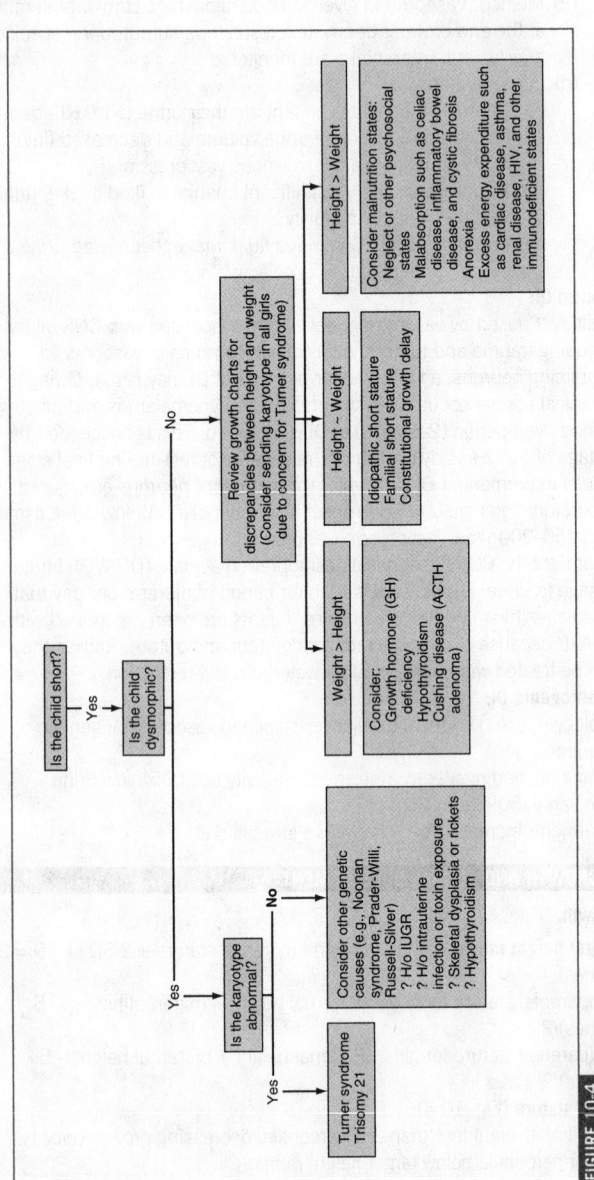

FIGURE 10-4
Differential diagnosis of short stature.

(1) FSS: Characterized by slow growth rate during the first 2–3 years of life, followed by a low-normal growth velocity. Bone age x-rays may be within normal limits for age.

(2) CGD: Typically characterized by similar growth charts as those with FSS, but a delay in onset of puberty and skeletal maturation allows for a period of catch-up growth. Family history of delayed puberty is often present. Bone age x-rays may be delayed for age.

(3) Pathologic short stature (see Fig. 10-4).

c. Initial evaluation: Detailed history/physical examination, evaluation of growth curves and pubertal stage. Initial screening tests include complete blood cell count (CBC), liver function tests, electrolytes, erythrocyte sedimentation rate, and urinalysis (including pH and specific gravity). Also consider thyroid function tests, serum insulin-like growth factor (IGF)-1 (Table 10-13) and IGF-binding protein-3 (IGFBP-3), tissue transglutaminase for celiac disease, bone age (radiograph of left wrist and hand), and karyotype (in girls). Consider a skeletal survey in a patient with disproportionate features.

3. **Tall stature:** Most common cause is familial tall stature or precocious puberty. Bone age may be helpful.

4. **Obesity:** A growing problem in pediatric population. Although the majority do not have endocrine etiology, two disease categories may be addressed when approaching the obese patient:

a. Hypothyroidism: May be evaluated with serum thyroid function tests

TABLE 10-13

INSULIN-LIKE GROWTH FACTOR 1 (IGF-1)

Age (years)	Male (ng/mL)	Females (ng/mL)
<1	≤142	≤185
1–1.9	≤134	≤175
2–2.9	≤135	≤178
3–3.9	30–155	38–214
4–4.9	28–181	34–238
5–5.9	31–214	37–272
6–6.9	38–253	45–316
7–7.9	48–298	58–367
8–8.9	62–347	76–424
9–9.9	80–398	99–483
10–10.9	100–449	125–541
11–11.9	123–497	152–593
12–12.9	146–541	178–636
13–13.9	168–576	200–664
14–14.9	187–599	214–673
15–15.9	201–609	218–659
16–16.9	209–602	208–619
17–17.9	207–576	185–551

NOTE: A clearly normal IGF-1 level argues against growth hormone (GH) deficiency, except in young children, where there is considerable overlap between normals and those with GH deficiency.

Reference ranges from Quest Diagnostics LC/MS (liquid chromatography/tandem mass spectrometry) assay.

b. Cushing syndrome: Unlikely without linear growth failure in addition to obesity (see Section V for laboratory testing details)

5. **Polycystic ovarian syndrome (PCOS):**

a. Syndrome of hyperandrogenism and menstrual dysfunction

b. Diagnostic criteria:

(1) Hyperandrogenism: Clinical characteristics are hirsutism, acne, and female pattern alopecia. Biochemical characteristic is elevated free testosterone, calculated from total serum testosterone and sex hormone binding protein (SHBG).

(2) Menstrual dysfunction: Amenorrhea or oligomenorrhea.

(3) Polycystic ovaries: Ultrasound (US) characteristics are increased ovarian volume (reliable in adolescents via transabdominal US) or follicular phase with ≥12 follicles measuring 2–9 mm (reliable via transvaginal US only).

c. Management:

(1) Weight reduction and other lifestyle changes increase SHBG (thus decreasing free testosterone) can restore ovulation, and increase insulin sensitivity.

(2) Treatment of hirsutism/acne: Hormonal contraceptives.

(3) Insulin-sensitizing agents (e.g., metformin) may help mitigate metabolic consequences.

(4) Prevention of endometrial hyperplasia (increased risk of endometrial cancer) by intermittent induction of menstruation or prevention of endometrial proliferation by hormonal contraception.

B. Sexual Development

1. **Delayed puberty:** For girls, no pubertal development by age 14 years, or >5 years between thelarche and adrenarche. Primary amenorrhea: no menarche by age 16 years in the presence of secondary sexual characteristics, or no menarche and no secondary sexual characteristics by age 14 years. For boys, no testicular enlargement by age 14 years, or >5 year for genital development.

a. Delayed puberty may be divided according to luteinizing hormone (LH) (Table 10-14) and follicle-stimulating hormone (FSH) levels (Table 10-15):

(1) **Hypergonadotropic hypogonadism** (high LH and FSH): Primary gonadal failure, possibly due to Turner or Klinefelter syndromes, androgen insensitivity, tumor, chemotherapy.

(2) **Hypogonadotropic hypogonadism** (low or normal LH/FSH): May be due to constitutional delay or central gonadotropin deficiency. Of the latter cause, etiologies include Kallman syndrome (most common cause of isolated gonadotropin deficiency), CNS tumors, hypopituitarism.

b. Evaluation of delayed puberty may also be divided into the following categories (Fig. 10-5):

(1) Constitutional delay

(2) Hypopituitarism

(3) Chromosomal abnormality

TABLE 10-14

LUTEINIZING HORMONE

Age	Males (mIU/mL)	Females (mIU/mL)
0–2 yr	Not established	Not established
3–7 yr	≤0.26	≤0.26
8–9 yr	≤0.46	≤0.69
10–11 yr	≤3.13	≤4.38
12–14 yr	0.23–4.41	0.04–10.80
15–17 yr	0.29–4.77	0.97–14.70
Tanner Stages	**Males (mIU/mL)**	**Females (mIU/mL)**
I	≤0.52	≤0.15
II	≤1.76	≤2.91
III	≤4.06	≤7.01
IV–V	0.06–4.77	0.10–14.70

Reference values are from Quest Diagnostics immunoassay. For more information visit www.questdiagnostics.com.

TABLE 10-15

FOLLICLE-STIMULATING HORMONE

Age	Male (mIU/mL)	Female (mIU/mL)
0–4 yr	Not established	Not established
5–9 yr	0.21–4.33	0.72–5.33
10–13 yr	0.53–4.92	0.87–9.16
14–17 yr	0.85–8.74	0.64–10.98

Reference values are from Quest Diagnostics immunoassay. For more information visit www.questdiagnostics.com.

10

c. Initial evaluation: LH and FSH, bone age, and thyroid studies. A gonad-otropin-releasing hormone (GnRH) stimulation test can be obtained to rule out hypogonadotropic hypogonadism.

d. GnRH stimulation test:[39]
   (1) Measures pituitary luteinizing hormone (LH) and FSH reserve: Helpful in the differential diagnosis of precocious or delayed sexual development.
   (2) Method: Give 20 mcg/kg GnRH analog (Leuprolide) SQ, and measure LH and FSH levels at 0 and 60 minutes.
   (3) Interpretation: Prepubertal children should show no or minimal increase in LH and FSH in response to GnRH. A rise of LH to > 3.3–5.0 IU/L is evidence of central puberty.

2. **Precocious puberty:** Traditionally defined as any sign of secondary sexual maturation before age 8 years in girls and age 9 years in boys. More recent data suggest early puberty may not warrant extensive evaluation or intervention if it occurs after age 6 years in African-American girls or after age 7 years in Caucasian girls.

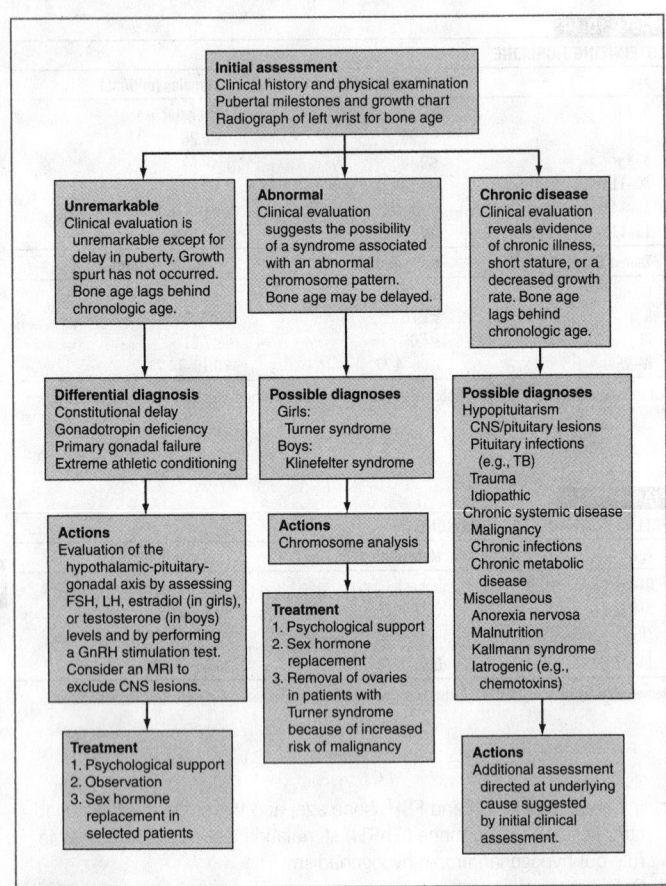

FIGURE 10-5

An approach to the child presenting with delayed puberty. CNS, Central nervous system; FSH, follicle-stimulating hormone; GnRH, gonadotropin-releasing hormone; LH, luteinizing hormone; MRI, magnetic resonance imaging; TB, tuberculosis.[37] *(From Blondell R, Foster MB, Dave KC. Disorders of puberty. Am Family Phys. 1999;60: 209-218.)*

a. Central, true, isosexual, *or* complete precocious puberty (CPP): Involves premature activation of hypothalamic-pituitary-gonadal axis, leading to increased GnRH and therefore increased LH/FSH; five times more likely to occur in females and often represents an idiopathic variant of normal puberty. In the majority of males with CPP, a CNS insult or structural anomaly is the cause.

TABLE 10-16	
ESTRADIOL	
Age	Level (pg/mL)
Prepubertal children	<25
Men	6–44
Women	
Luteal phase	26–165
Follicular phase	None detected–266
Midcycle	118–355
Adult women on OCP	None detected–102

NOTE: Normal infants have elevated estradiol at birth, which decreases to prepubertal values during the first week of life. Estradiol levels increase again between age 1 and 2 months and return to prepubertal values by age 6–12 months.

OCP, Oral contraceptive pill.

Values from JHH Laboratories.

  b. Peripheral *or* pseudoprecocious puberty: GnRH-independent puberty; involves adrenal, gonadal, ectopic, or exogenous sources of hormone production. Most common causes are CAH, adrenal tumors, McCune-Albright syndrome, gonadal tumors, human chorionic gonadotropin (hCG)-producing tumors, and exogenous sex hormones. Hypothyroidism can also cause GnRH-independent precocity. Penile length is disproportionately greater than testicular size in pseudo-precocious puberty, whereas testicular volume is disproportionately greater than penile size in normal puberty and CPP.

  c. Initial evaluation: Begin with history (assessing for premature thelarche/adrenarche) physical examination, and growth curves.

    (1) Bone age (generally >2 years in advance of chronologic age in long-standing precocious puberty due to action of sex hormones)

    (2) Assess degree of estrogenization or virilization: Check plasma estradiol or plasma testosterone/dehydroepiandrosterone (DHEAS), respectively. Check basal and/or GnRH-stimulated LH levels (see Table 10-14), estradiol measurement in girls (Table 10-16), testosterone levels in boys (Tables 10-17 and 10-18), 17-OHP levels (Table 10-11), DHEA levels (Tables 10-19 and 10-20), and urinary 17-ketosteroids.

    (3) Imaging: Magnetic resonance imaging (MRI) of the brain may help identify a CNS lesion. In girls, pelvic ultrasonography may identify ovarian cysts, whereas in boys it may detect nonpalpable Leydig-cell tumors and should be considered in cases of asymmetric testicular volume or peripheral precocious puberty. For normal testicular size and volume see Table 10-21.

3. **Ambiguous genitalia:**

a. Clinical findings in a neonate suspicious for ambiguous genitalia: Anogenital ratio > 0.5 (distance between anus and posterior fourchette divided by distance between anus and base of clitoris), phallus length < 1.9 cm (mean newborn length: 2.5 SD), clitoromegaly (length > 1 cm), nonpalpable gonads in an apparent male, and hypospadias associated with separation of scrotal sacs or undescended testis.

TABLE 10-17

TESTOSTERONE, TOTAL SERUM

Age	Male (ng/dL)	Female (ng/dL)
Cord blood	17–61	16–44
1–10 days	≤187	≤24
1–3 mo	72–344	≤17
3–5 mo	≤201	≤12
5–7 mo	≤59	≤13
7–12 mo	≤16	≤11
1–5.9 yr	≤5	≤8
6–7.9 yr	≤25	≤20
8–10.9 yr	≤42	≤35
11–11.9 yr	≤260	≤40
12–13.9 yr	≤420	≤40
14–17.9 yr	≤1000	≤40
≥18 (adult)	250–1100	2–45
Tanner Stage		
Stage I	≤5	≤8
Stage II	≤167	≤24
Stage III	21–719	≤28
Stage IV	25–912	≤31
Stage V	110–975	≤33

NOTE: Normal testosterone/dihydrotestosterone (T/DHT) ratio is <18 in adults and older children, <10 in neonates.
T/DHT ratio >20 suggests 5-alpha-reductase deficiency or androgen insensitivity syndrome.

Reference ranges from Quest Diagnostics LC/MS (liquid chromatography/tandem mass spectrometry) assay.

TABLE 10-18

TESTOSTERONE, FREE

Age	Male (pg/mL)	Female (pg/mL)
5.9–9 yr	≤5.3	0.2–5.0
10–13.9 yr	0.7–52	0.1–7.4
14–17.9 yr	18–111	0.5–3.9
18–69 yr	35–155	0.1–6.4

Reference ranges from Quest Diagnostics LC/MS (liquid chromatography/tandem mass spectrometry) assay.

TABLE 10-19

DEHYDROEPIANDROSTERONE (DHEA), UNCONJUGATED

Age	ng/dL
1–5 yr	≤377
6–9 yr	19–592
10–13 yr	42–1067
14–17 yr	137–1489
Adult male	61–1636
Adult female	102–1185

Reference ranges from Quest Diagnostics LC/MS (liquid chromatography/tandem mass spectrometry) assay.

TABLE 10-20

DEHYDROEPIANDROSTERONE SULFATE (DHEA-S)

Age	Male (mcg/dL)	Female (mcg/dL)
<1 mo	≤316	15–261
1–6 mo	≤58	≤74
7–11 mo	≤26	≤26
1–3 yr	≤15	≤22
4–6 yr	≤27	≤34
7–9 yr	≤91	≤92
10–13 yr	≤138	≤148
14–17 yr	38–340	37–307
Tanner Stages (ages 7–17)		
I	≤49	≤46
II	≤81	15–133
III	22–126	42–126
IV	33–177	42–241
V	110–370	45–320

Reference values from Quest Diagnostics assay. For more information see www.questdiagnostics.com.

TABLE 10-21

TESTICULAR SIZE

Tanner Stage (Genital)	Length (cm) (Mean ± SD)	Volume (mL)
I	2.0 ± 0.5	2
II	2.7 ± 0.7	5
III	3.4 ± 0.8	10
IV	4.1 ± 1.0	20
V	5.0 ± 0.5	29

NOTE: Testicular volume of >4 mL or a long axis >2.5 cm is evidence that pubertal testicular growth has begun.
SD, Standard deviation.

b. Etiology: Most common cause is CAH (see Section IV.A.3). Other causes: testicular regression syndrome, androgen insensitivity, testosterone biosynthesis disorders, and chromosomal abnormalities.

c. Diagnosis: Based on karyotype, measurement of gonadotropins (LH, FSH), adrenal steroids (cortisol, 17-OHP, and ACTH stimulation test), testosterone precursors (DHEA, androstenedione), testosterone, dihydrotestosterone (DHT), and hCG stimulation test (see hCG stimulation test on Expert Consult). **NOTE:** Best test for 5-alpha-reductase deficiency is the testosterone-to-DHT ratio.

d. **Cryptorchidism:**

(1) Prevalence: 3% of term male infants. About 50% of cryptorchid testicles descend by age 3 months and 80% by 12 months. Neoplasm occurs in 48.9% of individuals with untreated cryptorchidism, and 25% of those tumors occur in the contralateral testis.

(2) Evaluation: Rule out virilized female with a karyotype. hCG stimulation test can be used to differentiate cryptorchidism from anorchia. Human chorionic gonadotropin (hCG) stimulation test:

   (a) Measures capacity for testosterone biosynthesis; useful in differentiation of cryptorchidism (undescended testes) from anorchia (absent testes).

   (b) Method: Give 1000 units of intravenous (IV) or intramuscular (IM) hCG for 3 days, and measure serum testosterone and dihydrotestosterone on day 0 and day 4.

   (c) Interpretation: Testosterone level >100 ng/dL in response to hCG stimulation is evidence for adequate testosterone biosynthesis. In cryptorchidism, testosterone rises to adult levels after hCG administration; in anorchia, there is no rise.

(3) Treatment: Removal of trapped testicle at 1 year of life.

VIII. NEONATAL HYPOGLYCEMIA EVALUATION[40]

A. Neonatal Hypoglycemia and Glucagon Stimulation Test[40]

1. **Definition of hypoglycemia:** Serum glucose level insufficient to meet metabolic requirements; can vary with perinatal stress, birth weight, and maternal factors. For practical purposes, value is defined as <45 mg/dL. **NOTE:** Bedside glucometer is inaccurate at levels <40 mg/dL; stat serum glucose must be sent.

2. **Symptoms:** Abnormal cry, seizures, apnea, hypotonia, bradycardia, hypothermia.

3. **Treatment:** Do not delay while awaiting serum glucose results:

a. Plasma glucose 25–45 mg/dL (1.4–2.5 mM), asymptomatic: breast feed or nipple/gavage with formula

b. Plasma glucose level <25 mg/dL (<1.4 mM) ± symptoms, asymptomatic infants who do not tolerate enteral feeding, or symptomatic infants:

   (1) Give IV bolus of glucose 0.25 g/kg (2.5 mL/kg of 10% glucose, or 1 mL/kg of 25% glucose) over 1–2 minutes.

   (2) Continue IV glucose at a rate of 6–8 mg/kg/min (3.6–4.8 mL/kg/hr of 10% glucose).

   (3) Monitor blood glucose Q30–60 min, and increase glucose delivery by 1–2 mg/kg/min if blood glucose is consistently <50 mg/dL.

4. **If serum glucose is consistently <45 mg/dL:** Further endocrine workup warranted. At the time of hypoglycemia (serum glucose <45 mg/dL), obtain serum levels of glucose, insulin, growth hormone, free fatty acids, and β-hydroxybutyrate.

5. **Glucagon stimulation test:** At the time of hypoglycemia, obtain above laboratory tests, administer glucagon, and obtain serum glucose levels Q10 min × 4. Repeat growth hormone and cortisol levels 30 minutes after documented hypoglycemia.

a. A rise in glucose secondary to glucagon ≥30 mg/dL along with elevated insulin levels, low serum levels of free fatty acids and β-hydroxybutyrate, and a glucose requirement >8 mg/kg/min suggests a diagnosis of hyperinsulinemia.

b. Hypoglycemia with midline defects and micropenis in a male suggest hypopituitarism, supported by low serum levels of growth hormone and cortisol at the time of hypoglycemia.

IX. ADDITIONAL NORMAL VALUES

Please note that normal values may differ among laboratories because of variation in technique and type of assay used.

See Expert Consult, Chapter 10, for normal values of:

Table EC 10-A, Dihydrotestosterone (DHT)

Table EC 10-B, Catecholamines, urine

Table EC 10-C, Catecholamines, plasma

Table EC 10-D, Insulin-like growth factor binding protein

Table EC 10-E, Mean stretched penile length

Table EC 10-F, Androstenedione, serum

REFERENCES

1. American Diabetes Association. Diagnosis and classification of diabetes mellitus. *Diabetes Care.* 2012;35:S64.
2. Craig ME, Hattersley A, Donaghue KC. ISPAD Clinical Practice Consensus Guidelines 2009 Compendium: definition, epidemiology and classification of diabetes in children and adolescents. *Pediatr Diabetes.* 2009;10(suppl 12):3-12.
3. International Expert Committee report on the role of the A1c assay in the diagnosis of diabetes. *Diabetes Care.* 2009;32:1327-1334.
4. Hattersley A, Bruining J, Shield J, et al. ISPAD Clinical Practice Consensus Guidelines 2009. The diagnosis and management of monogenic diabetes in children. *Pediatr Diabetes.* 2009;10:33-42.
5. Steck AK, Winter WE. Review on monogenic diabetes. *Curr Opin Endocrinol Diabetes Obes.* 2011;18:252-258.
6. Cooke DW, Plotnick L. Management of diabetic ketoacidosis in children and adolescents. *Pediatr Rev.* 2008;29:431-436.
7. Dunger DB, Sperling MA, Acerini CL, European Society for Paediatric Endocrinology, Lawson Wilkins Pediatric Endocrine Society, et al. European Society for Paediatric Endocrinology/Lawson Wilkins Pediatric Endocrine Society consensus statement on diabetic ketoacidosis in children and adolescents. *Pediatrics.* 2004;113:e133-e140.
8. Alberti G, Zimmet P, Shaw J, et al. Type 2 diabetes in the young: the evolving epidemic: the International Diabetes Federation consensus workshop. *Diabetes Care.* 2004;27:1798-1811.
9. Rosenbloom AL, Silverstein JH, Amemiya S. ISPAD Consensus Practice Consensus Guidelines 2009 Compendium: type 2 diabetes in children and adolescents. *Pediatr Diabetes.* 2009;10(suppl 12):17-32.
10. Copeland KC, Silverstein J, Moore KR, et al. Management of newly diagnosed type 2 diabetes mellitus (T2DM) in children and adolescents. *Pediatrics.* 2013;131:364-382.
11. Fisher DA. The thyroid. In: Rudolph CD, Rudolph AM, Lister GE, et al, eds. *Rudolph's Pediatrics.* New York: McGraw-Hill, 2011.
12. Fisher DA. Thyroid function and dysfunction in premature infants. *Pediatr Endocrinol Rev.* 2007;4:317-328.
13. Büyükgebiz A. Newborn screening for congenital hypothyroidism. *J Pediatr Endocrinol Metab.* 2006;19:1291-1298.

14. Lem AJ, de Rijke YB, van Toor H, et al. Serum thyroid hormone levels in healthy children from birth to adulthood and in short children born small for gestational age. *J Clin Endocrinol Metab*. 2012;97:3170-3178.

15. Williams FL, Simpson J, Delahunty C, Collaboration from the Scottish Preterm Thyroid Group, et al. Developmental trends in cord and postpartum serum thyroid hormones in preterm infants. *J Clin Endocrinol Metab*. 2004;89:5314-5320.

16. Reinehr T. Thyroid function in the nutritionally obese child and adolescent. *Curr Opin Pediatr*. 2011;23:415-420.

17. Screening for Congenital Hypothyroidism: US Preventive Services Task Force Reaffirmation Recommendation. *Ann Family Med*. 2008;6:166.

18. Ross AC, Manson JE, Abrams SA, et al. The 2011 report on dietary reference intakes for calcium and vitamin D from the Institute of Medicine: what clinicians need to know. *J Clin Endocrinol Metab*. 2010;96:53-58.

19. Greer FR. Defining vitamin D deficiency in children: beyond 25-OH vitamin D serum concentrations. *Pediatrics*. 2009;124:1471-1473.

20. Misra M, Pacaud D, Petryk A, Drug and Therapeutics Committee of the Lawson Wilkins Pediatric Endocrine Society, et al. Vitamin D deficiency in children and its management: review of current knowledge and recommendations. *Pediatrics*. 2008;122:398-417.

21. Stewart PM. The adrenal cortex. In: Melmed S, Polonsky KS, Reed Larsen P, et al, ed. *Williams Textbook of Endocrinology*. Philadelphia: Saunders, 2011.

22. American Academy of Pediatrics, Section on Endocrinology and Committee on Genetics. Technical report: congenital adrenal hyperplasia. *Pediatrics*. 2000;106:1511-1518.

23. Autal Z, Zhou P. Congenital adrenal hyperplasia: diagnosis, evaluation and management. *Pediatr Rev*. 2009;30:e49-e57.

24. Autal Z, Zhou P. Addison disease. *Pediatr Rev*. 2009:30:491-493.

25. Stratakis CA. Cushing syndrome in pediatrics. *Endocrinol Metab Clin North Am*. 2012;41:793-803.

26. Edmonds S, Fein DM, Gurtman A. Pheochromocytoma. *Pediatr Rev*. 2011;32:308-310.

27. Lenders JWM, Pacak K, Walther MM, et al. Biomedical diagnosis of pheochromocytoma: which test is best? *JAMA*. 2002;287:1427-1434.

28. Weise M, Merke DP, Pacak K, et al. Utility of plasma free metanephrines for detecting childhood pheochromocytoma. *J Clin Endocrinol Metab*. 2002;87:1955-1960.

29. Robinson AG, Verbalis JG. Posterior pituitary. In: Melmed S, Polonsky KS, Reed Larsen P, et al, eds. *Williams Textbook of Endocrinology*. Philadelphia: Saunders, 2011.

30. Plotnick L, Miller R. Growth, growth hormone, and pituitary disorders. In: McMillan J, ed. *Oski's Pediatrics: Principles and Practice*. Philadelphia: Lippincott Williams & Wilkins, 2006:2084-2092.

31. Mac Gillivray MH. The basics for the diagnosis and management of short stature: a pediatric endocrinologist's approach. *Pediatr Ann*. 2000;29:570-575.

32. Norman RJ, Dewailly D, Legro RS, et al. Polycystic ovary syndrome. *Lancet*. 2007;370:685-697.

33. Styne DM. New aspects in the diagnosis and treatment of pubertal disorders. *Pediatr Endocrinol*. 1997;44:505-529.

34. Kaplowitz PB. Delayed puberty. *Pediatr Rev*. 2010;31:189-195.

35. Carel JC, Leger J. Clinical practice. Precocious puberty. *N Engl J Med*. 2008;358:2366-2377.

36. American Academy of Pediatrics, Committee on Genetics, Sections on Endocrinology and Urology. Evaluation of newborn with developmental anomalies of the external genitalia. *Pediatrics.* 2000;106:138-142.
37. Blondell R, Foster MB, Dave KC. Disorders of puberty. *Am Family Phys.* 1999;60:209-218.
38. Master-Hunter T, Heiman DL. Amenorrhea: evaluation and treatment. *Am Family Phys.* 2006;73:1374-1382.
39. Carel JC, Eugster EA, Rogol A, et al. Consensus statement on the use of gonadotropin-releasing hormone analogs in children. *Pediatrics.* 2009;123:e752-e762.
40. Cooke DW. Metabolism and endocrinology. In: Seidel HM, Rosenstein BJ, Pathak A, eds. *Primary Care of the Newborn.* 4th ed. Philadelphia: Mosby, 2006.

Chapter 11

Fluids and Electrolytes

Emily Young Thomas, MD

See additional content on Expert Consult

I. OVERALL GUIDANCE IN FLUID AND ELECTROLYTE MANAGEMENT

A. Goals

Fluid therapy is an essential component of the care of hospitalized children. The basic principles should be followed whether providing oral or parenteral fluids. Appropriate fluid management involves the calculation and administration of water volume and electrolyte concentration of:

1. **Maintenance requirements**
2. **Initial deficit repletion**
3. **Ongoing losses**

B. The purpose of this chapter is to help one understand:

1. **Proper water and electrolyte needs to maintain homeostasis** - see Section II.A. Although calculations demonstrate that ¼ normal saline (0.225% NaCl) supplies maintenance solute needs, the majority of acutely ill pediatric patients have solute needs beyond maintenance requirements (see Section II.B.2).
2. **Potential complications of using ¼ normal saline (NS) in an acutely ill patient.** An increased number of case studies have reported complications from using ¼ NS for acutely ill patients, most notably hospital-acquired hyponatremia.[1-4]
3. **How the clinical context of an individual patient, rather than dogma, should dictate the proper fluid therapy for a child.**
   a. For example, a child who is being hospitalized before surgery and is otherwise well only requires maintenance fluids; ¼ NS may be an appropriate choice.
   b. Postoperatively, however, this same child will likely have developed deficits or conditions that increase the release of antidiuretic hormone (ADH), so one should strongly reconsider using ¼ NS in this patient. For more conditions that increase ADH release, please see Box EC 11-A.[1]

II. MAINTENANCE REQUIREMENTS

Maintenance requirements are the amount of water and electrolytes lost during normal basal metabolism. Metabolism creates two byproducts, heat and solute, that must be eliminated to maintain homeostasis. The amount of heat dissipated through insensible water losses and the amount of solute excreted in urine are directly related to caloric expenditure.

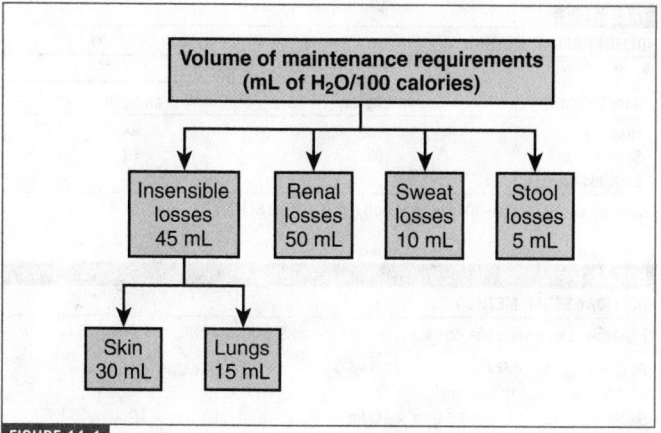

For each 100 calories metabolized in 24 hours, about 55–60 mL of fluid is required to provide for insensible losses as well as basal stool and sweat losses, and 50 mL of fluid is required for the kidneys to excrete an ultrafiltrate of plasma at 300 mOsm/L without having to concentrate the urine. *(Modified from Roberts KB. Fluids and electrolytes: parenteral fluid therapy. Pediatr Rev. 2001;22:380-387.)*

Metabolic demands do not increase in direct proportion to body mass (weight) across the continuum. The metabolic rate per kg body weight declines with age; an infant generates significantly more solute and heat per kg than a child or adolescent. To correctly calculate maintenance needs, it is necessary to determine calories burned (Fig. 11-1).[5]

A. Maintenance Volume: Caloric Calculations

There are three basic methods to calculate maintenance fluid volume needs:

1. **Basal calorie method:** Useful for all ages, types of body habitus, and clinical states
   a. Determine the child's estimated energy requirements based on age and activity level (see Table 21-2).
   b. Adjust caloric expenditure needs by various factors as described in Chapter 21.
   c. For each 100 calories metabolized in 24 hours, the average patient will need 100–120 mL H_2O, 2–4 mEq Na^+, and 2–3 mEq K^+.
2. **Holliday-Segar method** (Table 11-1 and Box 11-1)[6]: Estimates caloric expenditure in fixed-weight categories and makes the same assumption for water and electrolyte needs based on 100 kcal burned as above (refer to A.1.c of this section)
   NOTE: The Holliday-Segar method is not suitable for neonates <14 days old; generally it overestimates fluid needs in neonates compared with the caloric expenditure method. (See Chapter 18 for further neonatal fluid management.)

TABLE 11-1

HOLLIDAY-SEGAR METHOD

Body Weight	Water	
	mL/kg/day	mL/kg/hr
First 10 kg	100	≈4
Second 10 kg	50	≈2
Each additional kg	20	≈1

To calculate needed electrolytes: Na^+ 3 mEq/100 mL H_2O; Cl^- 2 mEq/100 mL H_2O; K^+ 2 mEq/100 mL H_2O.

BOX 11-1

HOLLIDAY-SEGAR METHOD

Example: Determine the correct fluid rate for an 8-year-old child weighing 25 kg:

First 10 kg:	4 mL/kg/hr × 10 kg = 40 mL/hr	100 mL/kg/day × 10 kg = 1000 mL/day
Second 10 kg:	2 mL/kg/hr × 10 kg = 20 mL/hr	50 mL/kg/day × 10 kg = 500 mL/day
Each additional 1 kg:	1 ml/kg/hr × 5 kg = 5 mL/hr	20 mL/kg/day × 5 kg = 100 mL/day
	Answer: 65 mL/hr	Answer: 1600 mL/day

TABLE 11-2

STANDARD VALUES FOR USE IN BODY SURFACE AREA (BSA) METHOD

H_2O	1500 mL/m²/24 hr
Na^+	30–50 mEq/m²/24 hr
K^+	20–40 mEq/m²/24 hr

m² = meters squared.

3. **Body surface area (BSA) method:** Based on the assumption that caloric expenditure is related to body surface area (BSA) (Table 11-2).[7,8] It should not be used for children <10 kg. See BSA calculation in Formulary Adjunct Figure 30-1.

B. Maintenance Solute

1. **For the purposes of fluid calculation,** fluid lost via insensible losses through the skin and respiratory tract can be considered electrolyte free. Urine represents the primary source of electrolyte loss, with variability based on the kidney's ability to dilute and concentrate. Average electrolyte requirements per 100 mL H_2O are seen in the legend of Table 11-1, with the addition of 5%–10% dextrose (depending on need) to prevent ketosis.
   Solute needs can thus be met by administering D_5¼ NS with 20 mEq/L KCl.

2. **Cautions regarding 1/4 NS fluid administration:** Many hospitalized patients have water and electrolyte deficits and may retain free water owing to various disease processes. Prior or ongoing losses of water or electrolytes require further volume and electrolyte deficit calculations

and appropriate adjustment of replacement fluids in their management (see Table 11-6).

III. DEFICIT REPLETION[8]

The following equations are numbered and can be used to calculate fluid management per Fig. 11-2, based on the amount of fluid/electrolytes lost before a patient's hospital presentation.

A. Water Deficit Volume

1. **Calculated assessment:** Most precise method of assessing fluid deficit is weight loss. If this is not known, clinical observation may be used:

Water deficit (L) = pre-illness weight (kg) − illness weight (kg)

(Equation A.1)

% Dehydration = (pre-illness weight − illness weight)/pre-illness weight × 100%

2. **Clinical assessment** (Table 11-3)[9,10]**:** Each 1% dehydration corresponds to 10 mL/kg fluid deficit

B. Solute Deficit Based on Solute Fluid Deficit (Isonatremic Dehydration)

Fluid losses from intracellular and extracellular compartments are used to determine electrolyte deficit and replacement.

NOTE: These calculations hold true for isonatremic dehydration. To calculate solute deficit in hypernatremic dehydration, see Section E.

1. **Extracellular fluid compartment:** ≈20% of the body's weight (40% in the newborn), divided 3:1 between interstitial and intravascular compartments, respectively.[11]

2. **In dehydration,** there are variable losses from the extracellular and intracellular compartments. The percentage deficit from these compartments is based on the total duration of illness.

a. Illness <3 days: 80% (0.8) extracellular fluid (ECF) deficit, 20% (0.2) intracellular fluid (ICF) deficit

b. Illness ≥3 days: 60% (0.6) ECF deficit, 40% (0.4) ICF deficit

3. **Composition of intracellular and extracellular fluid:** Shown in Table 11-4.

4. **Na^+ deficit:** Amount of Na^+ lost from the Na^+-containing ECF compartment during the dehydration period. Intracellular Na^+ is negligible as a proportion of total and can be disregarded (see Table 11-4).

Na^+ deficit (mEq) = fluid deficit (L) × proportion from ECF × Na^+ concentration (mEq/L) in ECF (Equation F.1)

A 25-kg (pre-illness weight) child who has been ill >3 days is 9% dehydrated, with serum [Na^+] 137 mEq/L:

$$\text{Fluid deficit} = (90\,\text{mL/kg})\,(25\,\text{kg}) = 2250\,\text{mL}$$

$$Na^+\ \text{deficit} = (2.25\,\text{L})\,(0.6)\,(137\,\text{mEq/L}) = 184\,\text{mEq}$$

Isonatremic Dehydration

	EQ	First 8 hours	Next 16 hours
Fluid deficit volume	A.1	Replace 1/2 of calculated deficits divided evenly over 8 hours.	Replace remaining 1/2 of calculated deficits divided evenly over 16 hours.
Na$^+$ deficit	F.1		
K$^+$ deficit	F.2		
Maintenance		To be given in addition to above calculated deficits at hourly rate.	

Hyponatremic Dehydration

	EQ	First 8 hours	Next 16 hours
Fluid deficit volume	A.1	Replace 1/2 of calculated deficits divided evenly over 8 hours.	Replace remaining 1/2 of calculated deficits divided evenly over 16 hours.
Na$^+$ deficit	F.1		
Excess Na$^+$ deficit	F.3		
K$^+$ deficit	F.2		
Maintenance		To be given in addition to above calculated deficits at hourly rate.	

Hypernatremic Dehydration

	EQ	First 8 hours	Next 16 hours	Next 24 hours
Free water deficit	F.4	Replace 1/2 of deficit over first 24 hours.		Replace remaining 1/2 of calculated deficit over next 24 hours.
Solute fluid deficit	F.5	Replace 1/2 of calculated deficits divided evenly over 8 hours.	Replace remaining 1/2 of calculated deficits divided evenly over 16 hours.	
Solute Na$^+$ deficit	F.6			
Solute K deficit	F.7			
Maintenance		To be given in addition to above calculated deficits at hourly rate.		

FIGURE 11-2

Fluid and solute replacement in isonatremic, hyponatremic, and hypernatremic dehydration.

TABLE 11-3

CLINICAL OBSERVATIONS IN DEHYDRATION*

	Older Child		
	3% (30 mL/kg)	6% (60 mL/kg)	9% (90 mL/kg)
	Infant		
	5% (50 mL/kg)	10% (100 mL/kg)	15% (150 mL/kg)
EXAMINATION			
Dehydration	Mild	Moderate	Severe
Skin turgor	Normal	Tenting	None
Skin (touch)	Normal	Dry	Clammy
Buccal mucosa/lips	Dry	Dry	Parched/cracked
Eyes	Normal	Deep set	Sunken
Tears	Present	Reduced	None
Fontanelle	Flat	Soft	Sunken
Mental status	Alert		Lethargic/obtunded
Pulse rate	Normal	Slightly increased	Increased
Pulse quality	Normal	Weak	Feeble/impalpable
Capillary refill	Normal	≈2-3 seconds	>3 seconds
Urine output	Normal/mild oliguira	Mild oliguria	Severe oliguria

*Serum sodium concentration affects the clinical manifestations of dehydration, such as skin turgor and mucous membranes. For example, hyponatremia exaggerates instability, and hypernatremia maintains intravascular volume at the expense of intracellular volume.

TABLE 11-4

INTRACELLULAR AND EXTRACELLULAR FLUID COMPOSITION

	Intracellular (mEq/L)	Extracellular (mEq/L)
Na^+	20	133–145
K^+	150	3–5
Cl^-	—	98–110
HCO_3^-	10	20–25
PO_4^{3-}	110–115	5
Protein	75	10
% Body weight	80	15 (interstitial), 5 (intravascular)

5. **K^+ deficit:** Amount of K^+ lost from the K^+-containing ICF compartment during the dehydration period. Extracellular K^+ is negligible as a proportion of total and can be disregarded (see Table 11-4).

$$K^+ \text{deficit (mEq)} = \text{fluid deficit (L)} \times \text{proportion from ICF} \times K^+ \text{concentration (mEq/L) in ICF} \quad \text{(Equation F.2)}$$

A 25-kg (pre-illness weight) child who has been ill >3 days and is 9% dehydrated:

$$K^+ \text{ deficit} = (2.25 \text{ L})(0.4)(150 \text{mEq/L}) = 135 \text{ mEq}$$

C. Excess Electrolyte Deficits

The amount of additional Na^+ or K^+ deficit calculated based on serum laboratory findings. Typically calculated in hyponatremic dehydration.

$$mEq\ required = [\text{concentration desired}\ (mEq/L) - \text{concentration present}\ (mEq/L) \\ \times fD \times weight\ (kg,\ pre\text{-}illness)$$

(Equation F.3)

fD = distribution factor as fraction of body weight (L/kg): HCO_3^- (0.4 − 0.5); Cl^- (0.2 − 0.3); Na^+ (0.6 − 0.7)

A 25-kg (pre-illness weight) child who has been ill >3 days and is 9% dehydrated, with serum [Na+] 117 mEq/L:

$$\text{Excess } Na^+ \text{ deficit} = (135\ mEq/L - 117\ mEq/L)\ (0.6)\ (25\ kg) = 270\ mEq$$

D. Free Water Deficit (FWD)

The amount of additional free water loss in a patient with **hypernatremic dehydration**. Based on estimates that it requires 4 mL/kg to decrease serum Na^+ by 1 mEq/L. **NOTE:** If serum Na^+ is >170, estimate decreases to 3 mL/kg.

$$FWD\ (mL) = 4\ mL/kg \times \text{pre-illness weight}\ (kg) \times [\text{concentration present}\ (mEq/L) \\ - \text{concentration desired}\ (mEq/L)]$$

(Equation F.4)

A 25-kg (pre-illness weight) child who has been ill >3 days and is 9% dehydrated, with serum [Na$^+$] 160 mEq/L:

$$FWD = (4\ mL/kg)\ (25\ kg)\ (160\ mEq/L - 145\ mEq/L) = 1500\ mL$$

E. Solute Fluid Deficit (SFD)

The amount of additional fluid volume loss beyond free water loss in a patient with **hypernatremic dehydration**. The SFD is subsequently used to calculate Na^+ and K^+ deficits in these patients.

$$SFD = \text{total fluid deficit} - FWD$$

(Equation F.5)

A 25-kg (pre-illness weight) child who has been ill >3 days and is 9% dehydrated, with serum [Na$^+$] 160 mEq/L:

$$\text{Total fluid deficit} = (90\ mL/kg)\ (25\ kg) = 2250\ mL$$

$$SFD = 2250\ mL - 1500\ mL = 750\ mL$$

$$\text{Solute } Na^+ \text{ deficit}\ (mEq/L) = SFD\ (L) \times \text{proportion from ECF} \\ \times Na^+ \text{concentration}\ (mEq/L)\ \text{in ECF}$$

(Equation F.6)

$$\text{Solute } Na^+ \text{ deficit} = (0.75\ L)\ (0.6)\ (145\ mEq/L) = 65\ mEq$$

Solute K^+ deficit (mEq/L) = SFD (L) × proportion from ICF × K^+ concentration (mEq/L) in ICF

(Equation F.7)

Solute K^+ deficit = (0.75 L) (0.4) (150 mEq/L) = 45 mEq

F. Deficit Replacement Strategy

1. **Phase I:** Rapid fluid resuscitation with isotonic fluid (NS or lactated Ringers [LR])
   a. Should be reserved for patients with need for rapid volume expansion (see Chapter 1). Generally, administration of isotonic fluid expands intravascular volume without causing significant fluid shifts, but overadministration of isotonic fluids can be dangerous in patients with hyperosmolarity (e.g., diabetic ketoacidosis [DKA] with hyperglycemia).
   b. Recognize that a bolus of 20 mL/kg represents only a 2% body weight replacement. A child calculated to be above 2% dehydrated will not be sufficiently repleted after an initial single bolus.
   c. Consider subtracting fluid and electrolytes given during resuscitation from the total deficits when calculating replacement of fluid and electrolytes.

2. **Phase II:** Deficit repletion, maintenance, and ongoing losses
   After initial stabilization, the remaining deficit is replaced over the next 24–48 hours. Replace half of the remaining deficit over the first 8 hours and the second half over the following 16 hours (with the exception of free water deficit, which is replaced over 48 hours), in addition to the previously calculated maintenance fluid rate. See Fig. 11-2 for calculation of fluid and solute replacement in isonatremic, hyponatremic, and hypernatremic dehydration.
   a. **Hyponatremic dehydration:** Excess Na^+ loss (Na^+ < 130 mEq/L). Rapid correction of serum Na^+ could result in central pontine myelinolysis and should be reserved for symptomatic patients. In asymptomatic patients, the rate of rise should not exceed 0.5–1 mEq/L per hour, or 10–12 mEq/L in 24 hours.
   b. **Isonatremic dehydration:** Proportional losses of Na and free water (Na^+ 130–149 mEq/L).
   c. **Hypernatremic dehydration:** Excess free water loss (Na^+ > 150 mEq/L). Avoid dropping the serum Na^+ by >15 mEq/L per 24 hours to minimize the risk of cerebral edema.
   d. See Tables EC 11-A, 11-B, and 11-C for sample calculations of fluid and solute replacement in isonatremic, hyponatremic, and hypernatremic dehydration.

G. Calculation of Appropriate Fluids

After completing the previous calculations for the patient, divide the desired amount of each solute by the total volume of fluid required to calculate the concentration of fluid and additives. Choose the appropriate corresponding fluid from Table 11-5, and add any other necessary solute components.

TABLE 11-5

COMPOSITION OF FREQUENTLY USED PARENTERAL AND ORAL REHYDRATION FLUIDS

	D% CHO (g/100 mL)	Protein* (g/100 mL)	Cal/L	Na+ (mEq/L)	K+ (mEq/L)	Cl− (mEq/L)	HCO3−† (mEq/L)	Ca2+ (mEq/L)	mOsm/L
PARENTERAL FLUID									
D5W	5	—	170	—	—	—	—	—	252
D10W	10	—	340	—	—	—	—	—	505
NS (0.9% NaCl)	—	—	—	154	—	154	—	—	308
½ NS (0.45% NaCl)	—	—	—	77	—	77	—	—	154
D5 ¼ NS (0.225% NaCl)	5	—	170	34	—	34	—	—	329
3% NaCl	—	—	—	513	—	513	—	—	1027
8.4% sodium bicarbonate (1 mEq/mL)	—	—	—	1000	—	—	1000	—	2000
Ringer's solution	0–10	—	0–340	147	4	155.5	—	≈4	—
Lactated Ringer's	0–10	—	0–340	130	4	109	28	3	273
Amino acid 8.5% (Travasol)	—	8.5	340	3	—	34	52	—	880
Plasmanate	—	5	200	110	2	50	29	—	300
Albumin 25% (salt poor)	—	25	1000	100–160	—	<120	—	—	—
Intralipid‡	2.25	2.25	1100	2.5	0.5	4.0	—	—	258–284
ORAL FLUID									
Pedialyte	2.5	—	—	45	20	35	30	—	250
WHO Solution	2	—	—	90	20	80	30	—	310
Rehydralyte	2.5	—	—	75	20	65	30	—	310

TABLE 11-5

COMPOSITION OF FREQUENTLY USED PARENTERAL AND ORAL REHYDRATION FLUIDS (Continued)

	D% CHO (g/100 mL)	Protein* (g/100 mL)	Cal/L	Na⁺ (mEq/L)	K⁺ (mEq/L)	Cl⁻ (mEq/L)	HCO₃⁻† (mEq/L)	Ca²⁺ (mEq/L)	mOsm/L
APPROXIMATE ELECTROLYTE COMPOSITION OF COMMONLY CONSUMED FLUIDS (NOT RECOMMENDED FOR ORAL REHYDRATION THERAPY)**									
Apple juice	11.9	—	—	0.4	26	—	—	—	700
Coca-Cola	10.9	—	—	4.3	0.1	—	13.4	—	656
Gatorade	5.9	—	—	21	2.5	17	—	—	377
G2	4.7	—	—	20	3.2	—	—	—	
Ginger ale	9	—	—	3.5	0.1	—	3.6	—	565
Milk	4.9	—	—	22	36	28	30	—	260
Orange juice	10.4	—	—	0.2	49	—	50	—	654
Powerade	5.8	—	—	18	2.7	—	—	—	264

*Protein or amino acid equivalent.

†Bicarbonate or equivalent (citrate, acetate, lactate).

‡Values are approximate; may vary from lot to lot.

**Values vary slightly depending on source.

CHO, Carbohydrate; HCO₃⁻, bicarbonate; NS, normal saline; WHO, World Health Organization.

TABLE 11-6

ELECTROLYTE COMPOSITION OF VARIOUS BODY FLUIDS

Fluid	Na^+ (mEq/L)	K^+ (mEq/L)	Cl^- (mEq/L)	Replacement Fluid
Gastric	20–80	5–20	100–150	½ NS
Pancreatic	120–140	5–15	90–120	NS
Small bowel	100–140	5–15	90–130	NS
Bile	120–140	5–15	80–120	NS
Ileostomy	45–135	3–15	20–115	1/2 NS or NS
Diarrhea	10–90	10–80	10–110	½ NS
Burns*	140	5	110	NS or LR
Sweat				
Normal	10–30	3–10	10–35	1/2 NS
Cystic fibrosis†	50–130	5–25	50–110	

*3–5 g/dL of protein may be lost in fluid from burn wounds.
†Replacement fluid dependent on sodium content.
LR, Lactated Ringer's; NS, normal saline.

1. **Parenteral fluid composition** (Table 11-5)
2. **Oral fluid composition** (Table 11-5)
   Oral rehydration therapy should be used in patients with mild to moderate dehydration without signs of shock, coma, acute abdomen, gastric distension, intractable vomiting, or excess stool losses
a. Method: Give 5–10 mL of oral rehydration solution (ORS) every 5–10 minutes, gradually increasing volume.
b. Deficit replacement:
   (1) Mild dehydration = 50 mL/kg over 4 hours
   (2) Moderate dehydration = 100 mL/kg over 4 hours
c. Maintenance: Infants should resume formula/breast milk by mouth (PO) ad lib. Children should continue with regular diet.
d. Ongoing losses: Regardless of the degree of dehydration, give additional 10 mL/kg of ORS for each additional diarrheal stool.

IV. ONGOING LOSSES

Represent continued losses of fluid and solute after initial presentation, as in persistent vomiting and/or diarrhea, high fever with diuresis, or nasogastric suction. Some of these losses can be measured directly and appropriately replaced based on known electrolyte concentrations (Table 11-6).[9]

V. SERUM ELECTROLYTE DISTURBANCES

A. Sodium

1. **Hyponatremia:**
a. Etiologies, diagnostic studies, and management (Table 11-7)
b. Factitious etiologies:
   (1) Hyperlipidemia: Na^+ decreased by $0.002 \times$ lipid (mg/dL)
   (2) Hyperproteinemia: Na^+ decreased by $0.25 \times$ [protein (g/dL) – 8]

TABLE 11-7

HYPONATREMIA*

Decreased Weight		Increased or Normal Weight
Renal Losses	**Extrarenal Losses**	**Increased or Normal Weight**
Na⁺-losing nephropathy	GI losses	Nephrotic syndrome
Diuretics	Skin losses	Congestive heart failure
Adrenal insufficiency	Third spacing	SIADH (see Chapter 10)
Cerebral salt-wasting syndrome	Cystic fibrosis	Acute/chronic renal failure
		Water intoxications
		Cirrhosis
		Excess salt-free infusions
LABORATORY DATA		
↑ Urine Na⁺	↓ Urine Na⁺	↓ Urine Na⁺†
↑ Urine volume	↓ Urine volume	↓ Urine volume
↓ Specific gravity	↑ Specific gravity	↑ Specific gravity
↓ Urine osmolality	↑ Urine osmolality	↑ Urine osmolality
MANAGEMENT (IN ADDITION TO TREATING UNDERLYING CAUSE)		
Replace losses	Replace losses	Restrict fluids

*Hyperglycemia and hyperlipidemia cause spurious hyponatremia.

†Urine Na⁺ may be appropriate for level of Na⁺ intake in patients with SIADH and water intoxication.

GI, Gastrointestinal; SIADH, syndrome of inappropriate antidiuretic hormone secretion.

    (3) Hyperglycemia: Na⁺ decreased 1.6 mEq/L for each 100-mg/dL rise in glucose

  c. Clinical manifestations: Nausea, headache, lethargy, seizure, coma

  2. **Hypernatremia:** Etiologies, diagnostic studies, and management (Table 11-8)

B. Potassium

  1. **Hypokalemia:**

  a. Etiologies and laboratory data (Table 11-9)

  b. Clinical manifestations: Skeletal muscle weakness or paralysis, ileus, cardiac arrhythmias.[12,13]Electrocardiogram (ECG) changes include delayed depolarization, with flat or absent T waves and, in extreme cases, U waves.

  c. Diagnostic studies:

    (1) Blood: Electrolytes, blood urea nitrogen/creatinine (BUN/Cr), creatine kinase (CK), glucose, renin, arterial blood gas (ABG)

    (2) Urine: Urinalysis, K⁺, Na⁺, Cl⁻, osmolality, 17-ketosteroids

    (3) Other: ECG, consider evaluation for Cushing syndrome (Chapter 10)

  d. Management: Rapidity of treatment should depend on symptom severity. See Formulary for dosage information:

    (1) Acute: Calculate deficit, and replace with potassium acetate or potassium chloride. Enteral replacement is safer when feasible, with less risk for iatrogenic hyperkalemia. Closely follow serum K⁺.

    (2) Chronic: Determine daily requirement, and replace with potassium chloride or potassium gluconate.

TABLE 11-8

HYPERNATREMIA

Decreased Weight		Increased Weight
Renal Losses	**Extrarenal Losses**	**Increased Weight**
Nephropathy	GI losses	Exogenous Na^+
Diuretic use	Skin losses	Mineralocorticoid excess
Diabetes insipidus	Respiratory*	Hyperaldosteronism
Postobstructive diuresis		
Diuretic phase of ATN		

LABORATORY DATA

↑ Urine Na^+	↓ Urine Na^+	Relative ↓ urine $Na^{+\dagger}$
↑ Urine volume	↓ Urine volume	Relative ↓ urine volume
↓ Specific gravity	↑ Specific gravity	Relative ↑ specific gravity

CLINICAL MANIFESTATIONS

Predominantly neurologic symptoms: lethargy, weakness, altered mental status, irritability, and seizures.[12,13] Additional symptoms may include muscle cramps, depressed deep tendon reflexes, and respiratory failure.

MANAGEMENT

Replace free water losses based on calculations in text and treat cause. Consider a natriuretic agent if there is increased weight.

*This cause of hypernatremia is usually secondary to free water loss, so the fractional excretion of sodium may be decreased or normal.

†Exogenous Na^+ administration will cause an increase in the fractional excretion of sodium.

ATN, Acute tubular necrosis; GI, gastrointestinal.

TABLE 11-9

CAUSES OF HYPOKALEMIA

	Decreased Stores		Normal Stores*
	Normal Blood Pressure		
Hypertension	**Renal**	**Extrarenal**	**Normal Stores***
Renovascular disease	RTA	Skin losses	Metabolic alkalosis
Excess renin	Fanconi syndrome	GI losses	Hyperinsulinemia
Excess mineralocorticoid	Bartter syndrome	High CHO diet	Leukemia
Cushing syndrome	DKA	Enema abuse	β_2-Catecholamines
	Antibiotics	Laxative abuse	Familial hypokalemic
	Diuretics	Anorexia nervosa	periodic paralysis
	Amphotericin B	Malnutrition	Familial

LABORATORY DATA

↑ Urine K^+	↑ Urine K^+	↓ Urine K^+	↑ Urine K^+

*Blood pressure may vary.

CHO, Carbohydrate; DKA, diabetic ketoacidosis; GI, gastrointestinal; RTA, renal tubular acidosis.

TABLE 11-10

CAUSES OF HYPERKALEMIA

Increased Stores		Normal Stores
Increased Urine K⁺	**Decreased Urine K⁺**	**Normal Stores**
Transfusion with aged blood	Renal failure	Tumor lysis syndrome
Exogenous K⁺ (e.g., salt substitutes)	Hypoaldosteronism	Leukocytosis (>100 K/µL)
Spitzer syndrome	Aldosterone insensitivity	Thrombocytosis (>750 K/µL)
	↓ Insulin	Metabolic acidosis*
	K⁺-sparing diuretics	Type IV RTA
	Congenital adrenal hyperplasia	Blood drawing (hemolyzed sample)
		Rhabdomyolysis/crush injury
		Malignant hyperthermia
		Theophylline intoxication

*For every 0.1-unit reduction in arterial pH, there is an approximately 0.2–0.4 mEq/L increase in plasma K⁺.
RTA, Renal tubular acidosis.

2. **Hyperkalemia:**
a. Etiologies (Table 11-10)
b. Clinical manifestations: Skeletal muscle weakness, paresthesias, and ECG changes. Typical ECG changes of hyperkalemia progress with increasing serum K⁺ values:
   (1) Peaked T waves
   (2) Loss of P waves with widening of QRS
   (3) ST-segment depression with further widening of QRS
   (4) Bradycardia, atrioventricular (AV) block, ventricular arrhythmias, torsades de pointes, and cardiac arrest
c. Management: Stop all IV infusions containing potassium; see algorithm in Fig. 11-3.

C. Calcium

1. **Hypocalcemia:**
a. Etiologies (Box 11-2)
b. Clinical manifestations: Tetany, neuromuscular irritability with weakness, paresthesias, fatigue, cramping, altered mental status, seizures, laryngospasm, cardiac arrhythmias[12,13]:
   (1) ECG changes (prolonged QT interval)
   (2) Trousseau sign (carpopedal spasm after arterial occlusion of an extremity for 3 minutes)
   (3) Chvostek sign (muscle twitching with percussion of facial nerve)
c. Diagnostic studies:
   (1) Blood: Total and ionized Ca^{2+}, phosphate, alkaline phosphatase, Mg^{2+}, total protein, BUN, creatinine, 25-OH vitamin D, parathyroid hormone (PTH):
      (a) Albumin: Δ of 1 g/dL changes total serum Ca^{2+} in the same direction by 0.8 mg/dL.
      (b) pH: Acidosis increases ionized calcium.

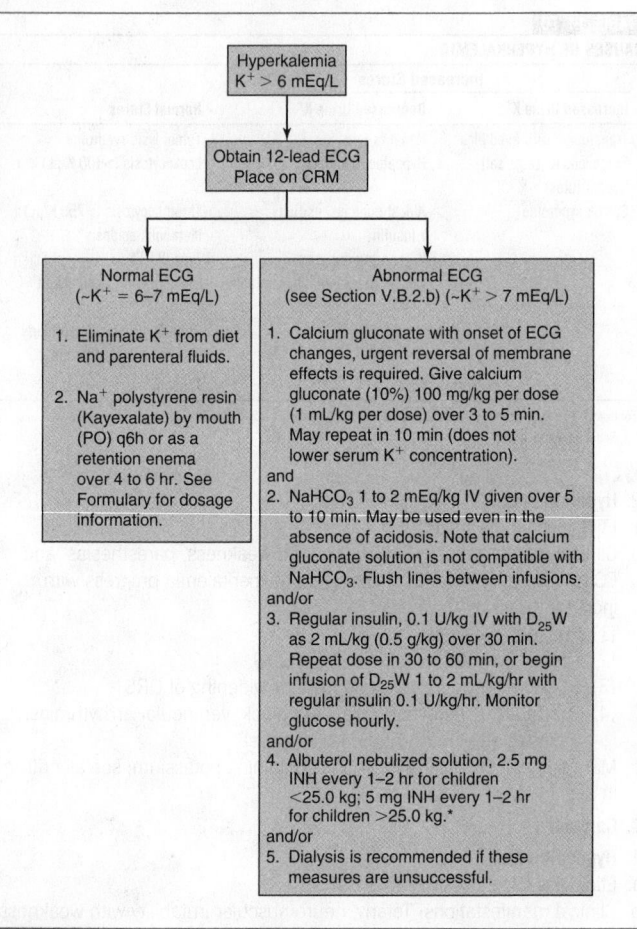

FIGURE 11-3

Algorithm for hyperkalemia. CRM, cardiorespiratory monitor; D25W, 25% dextrose in water; ECG, electrocardiogram; INH, inhaled; IV, intravenous. *Dosing for Albuterol. In: DRUG-DEX System (Internet database). Greenwood Village, Colo: Thomson Reuters (Healthcare). Updated periodically.

 (2) Urine: Ca^{2+}, phosphate, creatinine

 (3) Other: Chest x-ray (visualize thymus), ankle, and wrist films (assess for rickets), ECG (QT interval)

d. Management: See Formulary for dosing information:

 (1) Acute: Consider IV replacement (calcium gluconate, calcium gluceptate, or calcium chloride [cardiac arrest dose]).

 (2) Chronic: Consider use of oral supplements of calcium carbonate, calcium gluconate, calcium glubionate, or calcium lactate.

BOX 11-2	
ETIOLOGIES OF HYPOCALCEMIA AND HYPERCALCEMIA	
Hypocalcemia	**Hypercalcemia**
Hypoparathyroidism	Hyperparathyroidism
Vitamin D deficiency	Vitamin D intoxication
Hyperphosphatemia	Excessive exogenous calcium admin-
Pancreatitis	istration
Malabsorption states (malnutrition)	Malignancy
Drugs (anticonvulsants, cimetidine,	Prolonged immobilization
aminoglycosides, calcium	Thiazide diuretics
channel blockers)	Subcutaneous fat necrosis
Hypomagnesemia/hypermagnesemia	Williams syndrome
Maternal hyperparathyroidism (in	Granulomatous disease
neonates)	(e.g., sarcoidosis)
Ethylene glycol ingestion	Hyperthyroidism
Calcitriol (activated vitamin D)	Milk-alkali syndrome
insufficiency	
Tumor lysis syndrome	

e. Special considerations:
  (1) Symptoms of hypocalcemia refractory to Ca^{2+} supplementation may be caused by hypomagnesemia.
  (2) Significant hyperphosphatemia should be corrected before correction of hypocalcemia, because renal calculi or soft-tissue calcification may occur if total $[Ca^{2+}] \times [PO_4^{3-}] \geq 55$.

2. **Hypercalcemia:**
a. Etiologies (see Box 11-2)
b. Clinical manifestations: Weakness, irritability, lethargy, seizures, coma, abdominal cramping, anorexia, nausea, vomiting, polyuria, polydipsia, renal calculi, pancreatitis, ECG changes (shortened QT interval)
c. Diagnostic studies:
  (1) Blood: Total and ionized Ca^{2+}, phosphate, alkaline phosphatase, total protein, albumin, BUN, creatinine, PTH, 25-OH vitamin D
  (2) Urine: Ca^{2+}, phosphate, creatinine
  (3) Other: ECG (calculate QT interval), kidney, ureter, bladder (KUB) radiograph or renal ultrasound (assess for renal calculi)[14]
d. Management:
  (1) Treat the underlying disease.
  (2) Hydration: Increase urine output and Ca^{2+} excretion. If glomerular filtration rate and blood pressure are stable, give NS with maintenance K^+ at two to three times maintenance rate until Ca^{2+} is normalized.
  (3) Diuresis with furosemide.
  (4) Consider hemodialysis for severe or refractory cases.
  (5) Consider steroids in malignancy, granulomatous disease, and vitamin D toxicity to decrease vitamin D and Ca^{2+} absorption (in consultation with appropriate specialists).
  (6) Severe or persistently elevated Ca^{2+}: Consider calcitonin or bisphosphonate in consultation with endocrinologist.

> **BOX 11-3**
>
> **ETIOLOGIES OF HYPOMAGNESEMIA AND HYPERMAGNESEMIA**
>
> | Hypomagnesemia | Hypermagnesemia |
> |---|---|
> | **Increased Urinary Losses** | **Renal Failure** |
> | Diuretic use, renal tubular acidosis, hypercalcemia, chronic adrenergic stimulants, chemotherapy | **Excessive Administration** |
> | | Status asthmaticus, eclampsia/ preeclampsia, cathartics, enemas, phosphate binders |
> | **Increased Gastrointestinal Losses** | |
> | Malabsorption syndromes, severe malnutrition, diarrhea, vomiting, short bowel syndromes, enteric fistulas | |
> | **Endocrine Etiologies** | |
> | Diabetes mellitus, parathyroid hormone disorders, hyperaldosterone states | |
> | **Decreased Intake** | |
> | Prolonged parenteral fluid therapy with Mg^{2+}-free solutions | |

D. Magnesium

1. **Hypomagnesemia:**
a. Etiologies (Box 11-3)
b. Clinical manifestations: Anorexia, nausea, weakness, malaise, depression, nonspecific psychiatric symptoms, hyperreflexia, carpopedal spasm, clonus, tetany, ECG changes (atrial and ventricular ectopy; torsades de pointes)
c. Diagnostic studies:
   (1) Blood: Mg^{2+}, total and ionized Ca^{2+}
   (2) Other: Consider evaluation for renal/gastrointestinal losses or endocrine etiologies
d. Management: See Formulary for dosing and side effects:
   (1) Acute: Magnesium sulfate
   (2) Chronic: Magnesium oxide or magnesium sulfate

2. **Hypermagnesemia:**
a. Etiologies (see Box 11-3)
b. Clinical manifestations: Depressed deep tendon reflexes, lethargy, confusion, respiratory failure (in extreme cases)
   NOTE: Neonates born prematurely after tocolysis with magnesium sulfate are at high risk for respiratory sequelae, but serum magnesium levels tend to normalize within 72 hours.
c. Diagnostic studies: Mg^{2+}, total and ionized Ca^{2+}, BUN, creatinine
d. Management:
   (1) Stop supplemental Mg^{2+}
   (2) Diuresis
   (3) Ca^{2+} supplements such as calcium chloride (cardiac arrest doses), or calcium gluconate (see Formulary for dosing)
   (4) Dialysis if life-threatening levels are present

E. Phosphate

1. **Hypophosphatemia:**
a. Etiologies (Box 11-4)
b. Clinical manifestations: Symptomatic only at very low levels (<1 mg/dL), with irritability, paresthesias, confusion, seizures, myocardial depression, apnea in very low-birth-weight infants, and coma
c. Diagnostic studies
    (1) Blood: Phosphate, total and ionized Ca^{2+}, BUN, creatinine, Na, K, Mg^{2+}; consider PTH and vitamin D
    (2) Urine: Ca^{2+}, phosphate, creatinine, pH
d. Management:
    (1) Insidious onset of symptoms: PO potassium phosphate or sodium phosphate (see Formulary for dosing)
    (2) Acute onset of symptoms: IV potassium phosphate or sodium phosphate (see Formulary for dosing)

2. **Hyperphosphatemia:**
a. Etiologies (see Box 11-4)
b. Clinical manifestations: Symptoms of resulting hypocalcemia (see previous)
c. Diagnostic studies:
    (1) Blood: Phosphate, total and ionized Ca^{2+}, BUN, creatinine, Na, K, Mg^{2+}; consider PTH, vitamin D, complete blood cell count (CBC), arterial blood gas
    (2) Urine: Ca^{2+}, phosphate, creatinine, urinalysis
d. Management:
    (1) Restrict dietary phosphate.
    (2) Phosphate binders (calcium carbonate, aluminum hydroxide; use with caution in renal failure). See Formulary for dosing.
    (3) For cell lysis (with normal renal function), give an NS bolus and IV mannitol. See Chapter 22 for management of tumor lysis syndrome.
    (4) If patient has poor renal function, consider dialysis.

BOX 11-4	
ETIOLOGIES OF HYPOPHOSPHATEMIA AND HYPERPHOSPHATEMIA	
Hypophosphatemia	**Hyperphosphatemia**
Starvation	Hypoparathyroidism (rarely in the absence of renal insufficiency)
Protein-energy malnutrition	
Malabsorption syndromes	Excessive administration of phosphate (oral, intravenous, or enemas)
Intracellular shifts associated with respiratory or metabolic alkalosis	
Treatment of diabetic ketoacidosis	Tumor lysis syndrome
Corticosteroid administration	Reduction of glomerular filtration rate to <25% (may occur at smaller reductions in neonates)
Increased renal losses (e.g., renal tubular defects, diuretic use)	
Vitamin D–deficient and vitamin D–resistant rickets	
Very low-birth-weight infants when intake does not meet demand	

VI. ACID-BASE/OSMOLAR GAP DISTURBANCES

A. Definitions

1. **Serum osmolality:** Number of dissolved particles per kilogram. Can be calculated as follows:

$$2[\text{serum Na}^+] + \text{glucose (mg/dL)} /18 + \text{BUN (mg/dL)} /2.8$$

a. Normal range: 275–295 mOsm/kg

b. Serum osmolar gap = calculated serum osmolality − laboratory measured osmolality

   NOTE: May be elevated in some anion gap acidosis, but a markedly elevated osmolar gap in the setting of an anion gap acidosis is highly suggestive of acute methanol or ethylene glycol intoxication.

2. **Anion gap (AG):** Represents anions other than bicarbonate and chloride required to balance the positive charge of Na^+. (K^+ is considered negligible in AG calculations.)

$$AG = Na^+ - (Cl^- + HCO_3^-) \ (\text{Normal} : 12 \text{ mEq/L} \pm 2 \text{ mEq/L})$$

a. The majority of unmeasured anions contributing to the anion gap in normal individuals are albumin and phosphate. A decrease in either of these components will decrease the anion gap and could mask an increase in organic acids such as lactate. Correcting the anion gap for albumin concentration increases the utility of the traditional method. The following equation can be used; AG is measured in mEq/L and albumin is measured in g/dL[15]:

b. Corrected AG = Observed AG + 2.5 x (Normal albumin − Measured albumin)

3. **Acidosis (pH < 7.35):**

a. Respiratory acidosis: $Pco_2 > 45$ mmHg

b. Metabolic acidosis: Arterial bicarbonate < 22 mmol/L

4. **Alkalosis (pH > 7.45):**

a. Respiratory alkalosis: $Pco_2 < 35$ mmHg

b. Metabolic alkalosis: Arterial bicarbonate > 26 mmol/L

B. Rules for Determining Primary Acid-Base Disorders (see Table 24-3; Calculation of Expected Compensatory Response)[16]

1. **Determine the pH:** Body does not fully compensate for primary acid-base disorders, so the primary disturbance will shift the pH away from 7.40. Examine the Pco_2 and HCO_3^- to determine whether the primary disturbance is a metabolic acidosis/alkalosis or respiratory acidosis/alkalosis.

2. **Calculate the anion gap:** If anion gap is >20 mmol/L, there is a primary metabolic acidosis regardless of pH or serum bicarbonate concentration. (The body does not generate a large anion gap to compensate for a primary disorder.)

C. Etiology of Acid-Base Disturbances (Fig. 11-4)

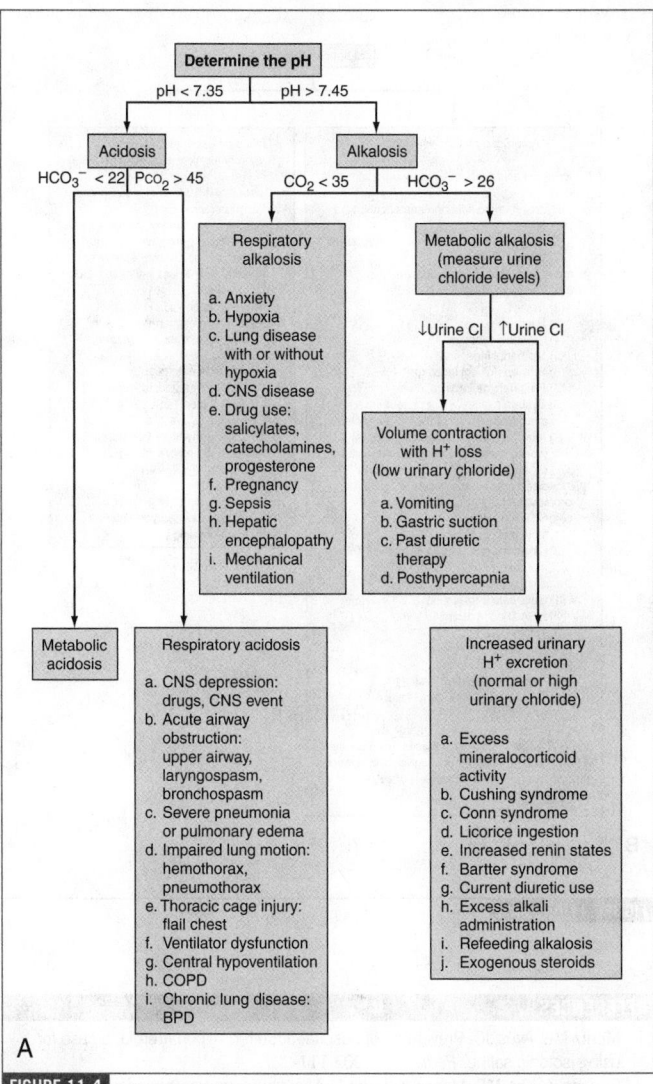

Determine the pH

pH < 7.35 — Acidosis
$HCO_3^- < 22$ $Pco_2 > 45$

pH > 7.45 — Alkalosis
$CO_2 < 35$ $HCO_3^- > 26$

Respiratory alkalosis

a. Anxiety
b. Hypoxia
c. Lung disease with or without hypoxia
d. CNS disease
e. Drug use: salicylates, catecholamines, progesterone
f. Pregnancy
g. Sepsis
h. Hepatic encephalopathy
i. Mechanical ventilation

Metabolic alkalosis (measure urine chloride levels)

↓Urine Cl   ↑Urine Cl

Volume contraction with H^+ loss (low urinary chloride)

a. Vomiting
b. Gastric suction
c. Past diuretic therapy
d. Posthypercapnia

Metabolic acidosis

Respiratory acidosis

a. CNS depression: drugs, CNS event
b. Acute airway obstruction: upper airway, laryngospasm, bronchospasm
c. Severe pneumonia or pulmonary edema
d. Impaired lung motion: hemothorax, pneumothorax
e. Thoracic cage injury: flail chest
f. Ventilator dysfunction
g. Central hypoventilation
h. COPD
i. Chronic lung disease: BPD

Increased urinary H^+ excretion (normal or high urinary chloride)

a. Excess mineralocorticoid activity
b. Cushing syndrome
c. Conn syndrome
d. Licorice ingestion
e. Increased renin states
f. Bartter syndrome
g. Current diuretic use
h. Excess alkali administration
i. Refeeding alkalosis
j. Exogenous steroids

A

FIGURE 11-4

A and B, Etiology of acid-base disturbances. BPD, bronchopulmonary dysplasia; CNS, central nervous system; COPD, chronic obstructive pulmonary disease; NSAID, nonsteroidal antiinflammatory drug.

Continued

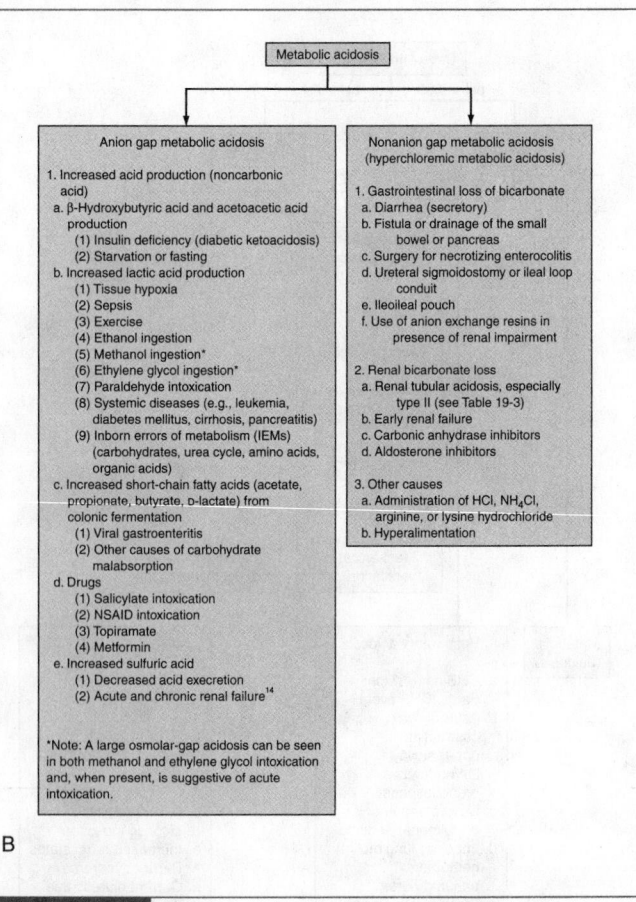

Metabolic acidosis

Anion gap metabolic acidosis

1. Increased acid production (noncarbonic acid)
   a. β-Hydroxybutyric acid and acetoacetic acid production
      (1) Insulin deficiency (diabetic ketoacidosis)
      (2) Starvation or fasting
   b. Increased lactic acid production
      (1) Tissue hypoxia
      (2) Sepsis
      (3) Exercise
      (4) Ethanol ingestion
      (5) Methanol ingestion*
      (6) Ethylene glycol ingestion*
      (7) Paraldehyde intoxication
      (8) Systemic diseases (e.g., leukemia, diabetes mellitus, cirrhosis, pancreatitis)
      (9) Inborn errors of metabolism (IEMs) (carbohydrates, urea cycle, amino acids, organic acids)
   c. Increased short-chain fatty acids (acetate, propionate, butyrate, D-lactate) from colonic fermentation
      (1) Viral gastroenteritis
      (2) Other causes of carbohydrate malabsorption
   d. Drugs
      (1) Salicylate intoxication
      (2) NSAID intoxication
      (3) Topiramate
      (4) Metformin
   e. Increased sulfuric acid
      (1) Decreased acid excecretion
      (2) Acute and chronic renal failure[14]

*Note: A large osmolar-gap acidosis can be seen in both methanol and ethylene glycol intoxication and, when present, is suggestive of acute intoxication.

Nonanion gap metabolic acidosis (hyperchloremic metabolic acidosis)

1. Gastrointestinal loss of bicarbonate
   a. Diarrhea (secretory)
   b. Fistula or drainage of the small bowel or pancreas
   c. Surgery for necrotizing enterocolitis
   d. Ureteral sigmoidostomy or ileal loop conduit
   e. Ileoileal pouch
   f. Use of anion exchange resins in presence of renal impairment

2. Renal bicarbonate loss
   a. Renal tubular acidosis, especially type II (see Table 19-3)
   b. Early renal failure
   c. Carbonic anhydrase inhibitors
   d. Aldosterone inhibitors

3. Other causes
   a. Administration of HCl, NH₄Cl, arginine, or lysine hydrochloride
   b. Hyperalimentation

B

FIGURE 11-4, cont'd

REFERENCES

1. Moritz ML, Ayus JC. Prevention of hospital-acquired hyponatremia: a case for using isotonic saline. *Pediatrics*. 2003:111-227.
2. Choong K, Kho ME, Menon K, Bohn D. Hypotonic versus isotonic saline in hospitalised children: a systematic review. *Arch Dis Child*. 2006;91:828.
3. Neville KA, Sandeman DJ, Rubinstein A. Prevention of hyponatremia during maintenance intravenous fluid administration: a prospective randomized study of fluid type versus fluid rate. *J Pediatr*. 2010;156:313-319.
4. Moritz ML, Ayus JC. Intravenous fluid management for the acutely ill child. *Curr Opin Pediatr*. 2011;23:186-193.

5. Roberts KB. Fluids and electrolytes: parenteral fluid therapy. *Pediatr Rev*. 2001;22:380-387.

6. Segar WE. Parenteral fluid therapy. *Curr Probl Pediatr*. 1972;3:23-40.

7. Finberg L, Kravath RE, Hellerstein S. *Water and Electrolytes in Pediatrics: Physiology, Pathology, and Treatment*. 2nd ed. Philadelphia: Saunders, 1993.

8. Hellerstein S. Fluids and electrolytes: clinical aspects. *Pediatr Rev*. 1993;14: 103-115.

9. Kliegman RM, Stanton B, St. Gene J, et al. *Nelson Textbook of Pediatrics*. 19th ed. Philadelphia: Saunders, 2011.

10. Oski FA. *Principles and Practice of Pediatrics*. 4th ed. Philadelphia: Saunders, 2006.

11. Nichols DG, Yaster M, Lappe DG, et al. *Golden Hour: The Handbook of Advanced Pediatric Life Support*. 3rd ed. St Louis: Mosby, 2011.

12. Barkin R. *Pediatric Emergency Medicine*. 2nd ed. St Louis: Mosby, 1997.

13. Feld LG, Kaskel FJ, Schoeneman MJ. The approach to fluid and electrolyte therapy in pediatrics. *Adv Pediatr*. 1988;35:497-535.

14. Fleisher G, Ludwig S, Henretig F. *Textbook of Pediatric Emergency Medicine*. Baltimore: Williams & Wilkins, 2010.

15. Figge J, Jabor A, Kazda A, Fencl V. Anion gap and hypoalbuminemia. *Crit Care Med*. 1998;26:1807-1810.

16. Haber RJ. A practical approach to acid-base disorders. *West J Med*. 1991;155:146-151.

Chapter 12

Gastroenterology

Tina Navidi, MD

⊙ See additional content on Expert Consult

I. WEBSITES

North American Society for Pediatric Gastroenterology, Hepatology, and Nutrition: www.naspghan.org
American College of Gastroenterology: www.acg.gi.org

II. GASTROINTESTINAL EMERGENCIES

A. Gastrointestinal Bleeding

1. **Presentation**—Blood loss from the gastrointestinal (GI) tract occurs in four ways: Hematemesis, hematochezia, melena, and occult bleeding.
2. **Differential diagnosis of GI bleeding:** Table 12-1.

TABLE 12-1

DIFFERENTIAL DIAGNOSIS OF GI BLEEDING

Age	Upper GI Tract	Lower GI Tract
Newborns (0–30 days)	Swallowed maternal blood Gastritis	Necrotizing enterocolitis Malrotation with midgut volvulus Anal fissure Hirschsprung disease
Infant (30 days–1 year)	Gastritis Esophagitis Peptic ulcer disease	Anal fissure Allergic proctocolitis Intussusception Meckel diverticulum Lymphonodular hyperplasia Intestinal duplication Infectious colitis
Preschool (1–5 years)	Gastritis Esophagitis Peptic ulcer disease Esophageal varices Epistaxis	Juvenile polyps Lymphonodular hyperplasia Meckel diverticulum Hemolytic-uremic syndrome Henoch-Schönlein purpura Infectious colitis Anal fissure
School age and adolescent	Esophageal varices Peptic ulcer disease Epistaxis Gastritis	Inflammatory bowel disease Infectious colitis Juvenile polyps Anal fissure Hemorrhoids

Modified from Pearl R. The approach to common abdominal diagnoses in infants and children. Part II. *Pediatr Clin North Am.* 1998;45:1287-1326.

3. **Initial evaluation and management**
a. Assess airway, breathing, circulation, and hemodynamic stability.
b. Perform physical examination, looking for evidence of bleeding.
c. Verify bleeding with rectal examination, testing of stool or emesis for occult blood, and/or gastric lavage.
d. Obtain baseline laboratory tests. Complete blood cell count (CBC), prothrombin time/partial thromboplastin time (PT/PTT), blood type and cross-match, reticulocyte count, blood smear, blood urea nitrogen (BUN)/creatinine, electrolytes, and a panel to assess for disseminated intravascular coagulation (D-dimer, fibrinogen).
e. Begin initial fluid resuscitation with normal saline or lactated Ringer solution. Consider transfusion if there is continued bleeding, symptomatic anemia, and/or a hematocrit level <20%. Initiate intravenous acid suppression therapy, preferably with a proton pump inhibitor (PPI).
f. Further evaluation and therapy based on assessment and site of bleeding:
   (1) + Gastric lavage: consider esophagogastroduodenoscopy (EGD) and testing for *H. Pylori*. Treatment may include histamine-2 (H2) blocker, PPI. (Use nasogastric tube with caution if esophageal varices are suspected.[1])
   (2) + Stool hemoccult: Abdominal film, upper GI study (± small bowel follow-through), air-contrast barium enema, colonoscopy, Meckel scan, tagged red cell scan. If signs/symptoms of infection exist, consider stool culture, stool ova and parasites, *Clostridium difficile* toxin.

B. Acute Abdominal Pain[2]

1. **Definition:** Severe abdominal pain (localized or generalized).[3] May require emergency surgical evaluation/intervention.
2. **Differential diagnosis:** Table 12-2
3. **Evaluation:**
a. History: Course and characterization of pain, diarrhea, emesis, melena, hematochezia, fever, last oral intake, emesis, menstrual history, vaginal symptoms, urinary symptoms, and respiratory symptoms. Assess GI history, travel history, and diet.
b. Physical examination: Vital signs, toxic appearing, rashes, arthritis, jaundice. Thorough general exam including: Abdominal tenderness on palpation, rebound/guarding, rigidity, masses, distention, change in bowel sounds. Rectal exam with stool Hemoccult test. Pelvic exam (discharge, masses, adnexal/cervical motion tenderness), genital exam.
c. Radiologic studies: Obtain plain abdominal radiographs to assess for obstruction, constipation, free air, gallstones, and kidney stones. Consider chest radiograph to evaluate for pneumonia, abdominal/pelvic ultrasonography, abdominal computed tomography (CT) with contrast (include rectal contrast for appendicitis evaluation).
d. Laboratory studies to consider: Electrolytes, chemistry panel, CBC, liver and kidney function tests, coagulation studies, blood type and screen/cross-match, urinalysis, amylase, lipase, gonorrhea/chlamydia cultures (or polymerase chain reaction probes), beta–human chorionic

---

TABLE 12-2

ACUTE ABDOMINAL PAIN

GI source	Appendicitis, pancreatitis, intussusception, malrotation with volvulus, inflammatory bowel disease, gastritis, bowel obstruction, mesenteric lymphadenitis, irritable bowel syndrome, abscess, hepatitis, perforated ulcer, Meckel diverticulitis, cholecystitis, choledocholithiasis, constipation, gastroenteritis
Renal source	Urinary tract infection, pyelonephritis, nephrolithiasis
Genitourinary (GU) source	Ectopic pregnancy, ovarian cyst/torsion, pelvic inflammatory disease, testicular torsion
Oncologic source	Wilms tumor, neuroblastoma, rhabdomyosarcoma, lymphoma
Other sources	Henoch-Schönlein purpura, pneumonia, sickle cell anemia, diabetic ketoacidosis, juvenile rheumatoid arthritis, incarcerated hernia

gonadotropin (β-hCG), erythrocyte sedimentation rate (ESR), C-reactive protein (CRP)

4. **Management:**
a. Immediate: Make the patient NPO (ensure that they have nothing by mouth). Begin rehydration. Consider nasogastric decompression, serial abdominal examinations, surgical/gynecologic/GI evaluation, pain control, and antibiotics as indicated.

III. CONDITIONS OF THE GI TRACT (ESOPHAGUS/STOMACH/BOWEL)

A. Vomiting

1. **Definition:** Forceful oral explusion of gastric contents, can be bilious (green or yellow) or nonbilious
2. **Diagnosis/evaluation:** Review feeding and medication history. Assess: bilious, hematemesis, acute vs. chronic. Consider: Electrolytes, CBC, UA, β-hCG, pancreatic enyzmes. Imaging: Plain abdominal film with upright view (rule out obstruction, free air), abdominal ultrasound, upper GI, neurologic evaluation and imaging. Nasogastric/orogastric tube decompression if GI obstruction suspected. Consider surgical consulltiation if bilious or hematemesis.
3. **Differential:** Table 12-3
4. **Management:** Hydration. Avoid antiemetic unless specific benign etiology is identified.

B. Diarrhea[4]

1. **Definition:** Usual stool output is 10 g/kg/day in children and 100 g/day in adults. Stool loss of >10 g/kg/day in infants and young children or >200 g/day in older children or adults is considered diarrhea.[5] Acute diarrhea is >3 loose or watery stools per day. Chronic diarrhea is diarrhea lasting more than 14 days.
2. **Diagnosis/evaluation:** History to assess acute vs. chronic, travel, recent antibiotic use, immune status. Consider laboratory evaluation: Electrolytes, CBC, stool Hemoccult, urine culture (young, febrile children), stool culture (febrile ± bloody stools), stool tests for leukocytes, *C. difficile*

TABLE 12-3

DIFFERENTIAL DIAGNOSIS OF VOMITING

Age	Typically Nonbilious	Typically bilious
Newborn & infant (0 days–1 year)	Overfeeding, physiologic reflux, milk protein sensitivity, pyloric stenosis, necrotizing enterocolitis, metabolic disorder, infection (GU, respiratory, GI), esophageal/gastric atresia/stenosis, Hirschsprung disease	Malrotation ± volvulus, intestinal atresia/stenosis, intussusception, pancreatitis
Preschool (1–5 years)	Cyclic vomiting, infectious (GI, GU), toxin ingestion, diabetic ketoacidosis (DKA), central nervous system (CNS) mass effect, eosinophilic esophagitis, posttussive, peptic disease, appendicitis	Malrotation, intussusception, incarcerated hernia, pancreatitis, intestinal dysmotility
School age & adolescent	Eating disorders, pregnancy, CNS mass effect, eosinophilic esophagitis, DKA, peptic disease, cyclic vomiting, toxins/drugs of abuse, infectious (GU, GI), appendicitis	Peritoneal adhesions, incarcerated hernia, pancreatitis, intestinal dysmotility

toxin, ova and parasites, viral antigens (e.g., rotavirus).

3. **Etiology:** Infectious or malabsorptive with osmotic or secretory mechanism

a. Osmotic diarrhea: Water is drawn into intestinal lumen by maldigested nutrients (e.g., celiac or pancreatic disease, lactose) or other osmotic compounds. Stool volume depends on diet and decreases with fasting (stool osmolar gap ≥100 mOsm/kg).

b. Secretory diarrhea: Water accompanies secreted or unabsorbed electrolytes into the intestinal lumen (e.g., excessive secretion of chloride ions caused by cholera toxin). Stool volume is increased and does not vary with diet (stool osmolar gap <100 mOsm/kg).

c. Stool osmolar gap = Stool Osm – (2 × [stool {Na}m Eq/L + stool {K} m Eq/L]). Stool Osm is infrequently measured: Standard value is 290 mOsm/kg.[6]

4. **Management**

a. Oral rehydration therapy (ORT): Mainstay of initial management regardless of etiology. Parenteral hydration is indicated in severe dehydration, hemodynamic instability, or failure of ORT. See Chapter 11 for oral rehydration solutions and calculation of deficit and maintenance fluid requirements.

b. Diet: Restart regular diet once patient is rehydrated, unless found to be the source of the diarrhea (e.g., gluten in celiac disease [CD]).

c. Other: Nonspecific antidiarrheal agents (e.g., adsorbents such as kaolin-pectin), antimotility agents (e.g., loperamide), antisecretory drugs, and toxin binders (e.g., cholestyramine) have limited data regarding efficacy and may adversely affect motility. If infectious, antimicrobial therapy may be indicated. If malabsorptive (e.g., CD, inflammatory bowel disease), therapy should be tailored to disease process.

d. Probiotics. Evidence supporting use of probiotics (live microorganisms in fermented foods that promote optimal health by establishing improved balance in intestinal microflora) is limited, but efficacy has been demonstrated in the following circumstances: antibiotic-associated diarrhea, mild to moderate acute diarrhea, *C. difficile* diarrhea (severe recurrent disease only), and prevention of atopic dermatitis. Probiotics are not regulated by the U.S. Food and Drug Administration (FDA), so there is no oversight of quality control (including potency).[7]

C. Constipation and Encopresis[8]

Normal stooling patterns by age: Infants 0–3 months, 2–3 bowel movements (BMs)/day; 6–12 months, 1.8/day; 1–3 years, 1.4/day; >3 years, 1/day

1. **Definitions:**
a. **Constipation:** Delay or difficulty in defecation for 2 or more weeks. Functional causes of constipation are most common.
   (1) Functional
   (2) Nonfunctional: See Table 12-4 for differential diagnosis.
   (3) **Diagnosis/evaluation:**
       (a) History: Timing of first meconium stool, family's definition of constipation, duration of condition and age of onset, toilet training experience, frequency/consistency/size of stools, pain or bleeding with defecation, presence of abdominal pain, soiling of underwear, stool withholding behavior, change in appetite, abdominal distention, anorexia, nausea, vomiting, weight loss, or poor weight gain, allergies, dietary history, medications, developmental history, psychosocial history, family history (constipation, thyroid disorders, cystic fibrosis).
       (b) Physical exam: External perineum, perianal exam, and digital anorectal exam. Stool occult blood test for all infants with constipation, any child with abdominal pain, failure to thrive, intermittent diarrhea, or family history of colon cancer or colonic polyps. Fecal impaction may be diagnosed with physical exam (hard mass within abdomen), digital exam (dilated rectal vault filled with stool), and/or abdominal radiography.
   (4) **Treatment of functional constipation:**
       (a) Disimpaction (2–5 days)
           (i) Oral/nasogastric approach: Polyethylene glycol electrolyte solutions effective for initial disimpaction. May also use magnesium hydroxide, magnesium citrate, lactulose, sorbitol, senna, or bisacodyl laxatives (avoid magnesium-containing products in infants owing to potential toxicity, beware of overdose in children).
           (ii) Rectal approach: Saline or mineral oil enemas. Avoid soapsuds, tap water, and magnesium enemas because of potential toxicity. Avoid enemas in infants; may use glycerin suppositories. Avoid phosphate-containing products owing

TABLE 12-4

DIFFERENTIAL DIAGNOSIS OF NON-FUNCTIONAL CONSTIPATION*

Anatomic malformations	Anal stenosis, anterior displaced anus, imperforate anus, pelvic mass (e.g., sacral teratoma)
Metabolic and GI	Cystic fibrosis, diabetes mellitus, gluten enteropathy, hypercalcemia, hypokalemia, hypothyroidism, multiple endocrine neoplasia type 2B
Neuropathic conditions	Neurofibromatosis, spinal cord abnormalities, spinal cord trauma, static encephalopathy, tethered cord
Intestinal nerve or muscle disorders	Hirschsprung disease, intestinal neuronal dysplasia, visceral myopathies, visceral neuropathies
Abnormal abdominal musculature	Down syndrome, gastroschisis, prune belly
Connective tissue disorders	Ehlers-Danlos syndrome, scleroderma, systemic lupus erythematosus
Drugs	Antacids, anticholinergics, antidepressants, antihypertensives, opiates, phenobarbital, sucralfate, sympathomimetics
Other	Botulism, cow's milk protein intolerance, heavy metal ingestion (lead), vitamin D intoxication

Modified from Constipation Guideline Committee of the North American Society for Pediatric Gastroenterology, Hepatology and Nutrition. Evaluation and treatment of constipation in infants and children. *J Pediatr Gastroenterol Nutr.* 2006;43:e1-e13.

*Note: Remember that functional constipation remains the most common cause.

to risk of acute phosphate nephropathy (reported with use of oral sodium phosphate products).
- (b) Maintenance therapy (usually 3–12 months): Goal is to prevent recurrence.
    - (i) Dietary changes: Increase intake of fluids and absorbable and nonabsorbable carbohydrates to soften stools. A balanced diet that includes whole grains, fruits, and vegetables is recommended. Data are too weak to support a definitive recommendation for fiber supplementation in the treatment of constipation in children.
    - (ii) Behavioral modifications: Regular toilet habits, positive reinforcement. Referral to mental health for help with motivational or behavioral concerns.
    - (iii) Medications: Polyethylene glycol (osmotic laxatives), lactulose, magnesium hydroxide, or sorbitol recommended. Avoid prolonged use of stimulant laxatives. Discontinue therapy gradually only after return of regular bowel movements with good evacuation.
- (5) **Special considerations in infants <1 year of age:** 2–4 oz of 100% fruit juice (e.g., prune, pear, apple) recommended in younger infants. Barley cereal, sorbitol-containing fruit purees, lactulose can be used in infants taking solid foods. Glycerin suppositories may be useful. Avoid mineral oil, stimulant laxatives, and phosphate enemas.

D. Inflammatory Bowel Disease (IBD)[9,10]

1. **Classification/types:**
a. **Crohn's disease:** Transmural inflammatory process affecting any segment of the GI tract. Abdominal pain in majority of cases. Other common symptoms include weight loss, diarrhea, lethargy, anorexia, fever, nausea, vomiting, growth retardation, malnutrition, delayed puberty, psychiatric symptoms, arthropathy, and erythema nodosum.[10]
b. **Ulcerative colitis (UC):** Chronic relapsing inflammatory disease of the colon and rectum. Symptoms (present for at least 2 weeks) include gross or occult rectal bleeding, diarrhea, abdominal pain with or around time of defecation. Exclusion of enteric pathogens (e.g., *Salmonella, Shigella, Yersinia, Campylobacter, Escherichia coli* 0157:H7, *C. difficile*) is necessary.[11] Weight loss, anorexia, lethargy are less common than in Crohn's disease.

2. **Evaluation:**
a. Complete history and physical exam, including family history, exposure to infectious agents or antibiotic treatment, assessment of hydration and nutritional status, signs of peritoneal inflammation, signs of systemic chronic disease. Stomatitis, perianal skin tags, fissures, fistulas are suggestive of Crohn's disease. Presence of fever, orthostasis, tachycardia, abdominal tenderness, distention, or masses suggests moderate to severe disease and need for hospitalization.
b. Laboratory assessment: CBC, ESR, CRP, serum urea and creatinine, serum albumin, liver function tests. IBD is associated with decreased hemoglobin and albumin, rise in platelet count, ESR, CRP (although children with UC may have normal hemoglobin, platelets, and ESR). Anti-neutrophil cytoplasmic antibodies (ANCA) may be elevated in UC. Diagnostic endoscopy is typically used to make diagnosis.

3. **Management:**
a. First-line therapy: Corticosteroids, 5-aminosalicylates, antibiotics
b. Second-line: Immunosuppression includes thiopurines, methotrexate, cyclosporine, tacrolimus, and anti-tumor necrosis factor (TNF) monoclonal antibodies.
c. Surgical intervention is indicated only after medical management has failed in both Crohn's and UC. In Crohn's, surgery is indicated for localized disease (strictures), abscess, or disease refractory to medical management.

E. Gastrointestinal Reflux Disease[12]

1. **Definitions:** Gastroesophageal reflux (GER) is passage of gastric contents into the esophagus, and gastroesophageal reflux disease (GERD) is defined as symptoms or complications of GER.

2. **Evaluation/diagnosis:**
a. History and physical examination: Usually sufficient to reliably diagnose GER, identify complications, and initiate management.
b. Esophageal pH monitoring: Valid and reliable method of measuring acid reflux.

c. Esophageal impedance monitoring: Combine with esophageal pH monitoring to detect both acid and nonacid reflux with greater sensitivity than pH monitoring alone.[13]

3. **Management:**

a. Diet: Milk protein sensitivity is one cause of unexplained vomiting in formula-fed infants; evidence supports a 2- to 4- week trial of extensively hydrolyzed protein formula. Milk-thickening agents decrease visible regurgitation but do not decrease GER. No evidence to support routine elimination of specific foods to treat GERD in older children.

b. Lifestyle: Prone or left-side sleeping position, elevation of head of bed may improve GER symptoms in adolescents. Infants up to 12 months should continue to sleep supine—sudden infant death syndrome (SIDS) risk far outweighs benefit of prone or lateral sleeping in GERD. (May consider prone positioning for infants while awake and monitored.) Obesity and large meal volume are associated with increased GER in adults.

c. Acid-suppressant therapy: Both PPIs and H_2 receptor antagonists (H_2RAs) are effective in relieving symptoms and promoting mucosal healing. PPIs are superior to H_2RAs. Smallest effective dose should be used for acid suppression.

d. Prokinetic therapy: Potential side effects of each currently available prokinetic agent outweigh potential benefits. There is insufficient evidence to support routine use of metoclopramide, erythromycin, bethanechol, or domperidone for GERD.

F. **Eosinophilic Esophagitis (EE)[14]**

1. **Definition:** Symptoms of esophageal dysfunction with ≥15 eosinophils/high-power field (hpf) on peripheral blood smear, and absence of pathologic GERD as evidenced by lack of responsiveness to high-dose PPI or normal pH monitoring of distal esophagus.

2. **Presentation:** Dysphagia, food impaction, chest pain, food refusal or intolerance, GER symptoms, emesis, abdominal pain, failure to thrive. High rate of atopy in children with EE.

3. **Diagnosis:** Endoscopy and esophageal biopsy, allergic evaluation for other atopic conditions.

4. **Management:** Dietary therapy (elemental formula or removal of specific foods identified by skin prick or atopy patch testing), PPI therapy (as co-treatment), may consider systemic steroids for emergencies (e.g., dysphagia leading to dehydration, weight loss), topical steroids for less severe symptoms (6- to 8- week course of fluticasone or budesonide metered-dose inhaler (MDI) administered orally *without* spacer). Data on use of steroids in EE are limited—recommendation based on expert opinion and current literature.

5. **Differential diagnosis** of esophageal eosinophilia: GERD, EE, eosinophilic gastroenteritis, Crohn's disease, connective tissue disease, hypereosinophilic syndrome, infection, drug hypersensitivity.

G. Celiac Disease[15]

1. **Definition:** An immune-mediated enteropathy caused by a permanent GI tract sensitivity to gluten in genetically susceptible individuals. Increased occurrence in children with type 1 diabetes mellitus, autoimmune thyroiditis, Down syndrome, Turner syndrome, Williams syndrome, selective immunoglobulin (Ig) A deficiency, and in first-degree relatives of those with celiac disease.

2. **Presentation:** Diarrhea, vomiting, abdominal pain, constipation, abdominal distention, failure to thrive. Non-GI symptoms include dermatitis herpetiformis, dental enamel hypoplasia of permanent teeth, osteoporosis, short stature, delayed puberty, and iron deficiency anemia resistant to oral iron.

3. **Diagnosis:** Measure IgA antibody to human recombinant tissue transglutaminase (TTG) and serum IgA (high prevalence of IgA deficiency in celiac disease). Endomysial antibody is subject to interpretation error and adds cost. If there is known selective IgA deficiency and symptoms are suggestive of celiac disease, testing with TTG IgG is recommended. Confirmation requires intestinal biopsy in all cases with findings of villous atrophy as a characteristic histopathologic feature.

4. **Management:** Lifetime gluten-free diet.

IV. CONDITIONS OF THE LIVER

A. Liver Function Studies: (Table 12-5)

1. **Synthetic function:** Albumin, prealbumin, PT, activated PTT, cholesterol. Elevated NH_3 is evidence of decreased ability to detoxify ammonia.

2. **Liver cell injury:** Elevation of aspartate aminotransferase, alanine aminotransferase, lactate dehydrogenase.

3. **Cholestasis:** Increased bilirubin, urobilinogen, γ-glutamyltransferase, alkaline phosphatase, 5'-nucleotidase, serum bile acids.

B. Acute Liver Failure (ALF)[16]

1. **Definition:** Biochemical evidence of liver injury with no history of known chronic liver disease, presence of coagulopathy not corrected by vitamin K administration, and international normalized ratio (INR) >1.5 if patient has encephalopathy or >2.0 if patient does not have encephalopathy. Causes of ALF vary in reversibility (with treatment or withdrawal of offending agent) and age of presentation.

2. **Etiologies** (incidence varies by age):

a. Infection: Herpesvirus, hepatitis A, hepatitis B, adenovirus, cytomegalovirus, Epstein-Barr virus, enterovirus, indeterminate

b. Vascular: Budd-Chiari syndrome, portal vein thrombosis, veno-occlusive disease, ischemic hepatitis

c. Immune dysregulation: Natural killer (NK) cell dysfunction (hemophagocytic lymphohistiocytosis), autoimmune

d. Inherited/metabolic: Wilson disease, mitochondrial, tyrosinemia, galactosemia, fatty acid oxidation defect, iron storage disease

TABLE 12-5

EVALUATION OF LIVER FUNCTION TESTS

Enzyme	Source	Increased	Decreased	Comments
AST/ALT	Liver, heart, skeletal muscle, pancreas, RBCs, kidney	Hepatocellular injury, rhabdomyolysis, muscular dystrophy, hemolysis, liver cancer	Vitamin B_6 deficiency, uremia	ALT more specific than AST for liver, AST > ALT in hemolysis, AST/ALT >2 in 90% of alcohol disorders in adults
Alkaline phosphatase	Osteoblasts, liver, small intestine, kidney, placenta	Hepatocellular injury, bone growth, disease, trauma, pregnancy, familial	Low phosphate, Wilson disease, zinc deficiency, hypothyroidism, pernicious anemia	Highest in cholestatic conditions; must be differentiated from bone source
GGT	Renal tubules, bile ducts, pancreas, small intestine, brain	Cholestasis, newborn period, induced by drugs	Estrogen therapy, artificially low in hyperbilirubinemia	Not found in bone, increased in 90% of primary liver disease, specific for hepatobiliary disease in nonpregnant patient
5'-NT	Intestine, liver cell membrane, brain, heart, pancreas	Cholestasis		Specific for hepatobiliary disease in nonpregnant patient
NH_3	Bowel flora, protein metabolism	Hepatic disease secondary to urea cycle dysfunction, hemodialysis, valproic acid therapy, urea cycle enzyme deficiency, organic acidemia and carnitine deficiency		Converted to urea in liver

AST/ALT, Aspartate aminotransferase/alanine aminotransferase; 5'-NT, 5'-nucleotidase; GGT, γ-glutamyl transpeptidase; RBCs, red blood cells.

e. Drugs/toxins: Acetaminophen, anticonvulsants
f. Other: Unknown, cancer/leukemia
3. **Presentation:** Prodrome of malaise, nausea, emesis, and anorexia. Jaundice and encephalopathy (hyperammonemia, cerebral edema) may be delayed by hours to weeks. Glucose instability with hypoglycemia, coagulopathy.
4. **Evaluation:**
a. Clinical: Neurologic status, signs of chronic liver disease, other chronic disease.

TABLE 12-6

INTERPRETATION OF THE SEROLOGIC MARKERS OF HEPATITIS B IN COMMON SITUATIONS

Serologic Marker				
HBsAg	Total HBcAb	IgM HBcAb	HBsAb	Interpretation
−	−	−	−	No prior infection, not immune
−	−	−	+	Immune after hepatitis B vaccination (if concentration ≥10 IU/mL or passive immunization from HBIG administration)
−	+	−	+	Immune after recovery from HBV infection
+	+	+	−	Acute HBV infection
+	+	−	−	Chronic HBV infection

HBsAg, Hepatitis B surface antigen; HBcAb, antibody to hepatitis B core antigen; HBsAb, antibody to hepatitis B surface antigen; HBIG, hepatitis B immune globulin.
From Davis AR, Rosenthal P. Hepatitis B in children. *Pediatr Rev.* 2008;29;111-120.

b. Laboratory: Electrolytes, BUN, creatinine, blood glucose, calcium, magnesium, phosphorous, blood gas, CBC with peripheral smear, reticulocyte count, liver function/production (albumin, aspartate aminotransferase [AST], alanine aminotransferase [ALT], alkaline phosphatase), INR, PT, PTT, ammonia, factors V, VII (depleted first in ALF), VIII, fibrinogen. Urine toxicology screen, serum acetaminophen level. Consider viral studies.
   NOTE: See Table 12-6 for interpretation of serologic markers of hepatitis B.
c. Imaging: Abdominal ultrasound with Doppler flows, head CT scan to exclude hemorrhage/edema, chest radiograph.
d. Studies to explore causation: Viral studies, immune function, metabolic studies, tissue biopsies.

C. Hyperbilirubinemia[17,18]

Bilirubin is the product of hemoglobin metabolism. There are two forms: Direct (conjugated) and indirect (unconjugated). Hyperbilirubinemia is usually the result of increased hemoglobin load, reduced hepatic uptake, reduced hepatic conjugation, or decreased excretion. Direct hyperbilirubinemia is defined as direct bilirubin >20% of total or direct bilirubin >2 mg/dL. See Table 12-7 for differential diagnosis of hyperbilirubinemia. Refer to Chapter 18 for evaluation and treatment of neonatal hyperbilirubinemia.

V. PANCREATITIS[19,20]

Inflammatory disease of the pancreas; falls into two major categories, acute and chronic.

A. Acute Pancreatitis

1. **Presentation:** Sudden onset of abdominal pain associated with rise of pancreatic digestive enzymes in serum or urine, with or without

TABLE 12-7

DIFFERENTIAL DIAGNOSIS OF HYPERBILIRUBINEMIA

INDIRECT HYPERBILIRUBINEMIA

Transient neonatal jaundice	Breast milk jaundice, physiologic jaundice Polycythemia, reabsorption of extravascular blood
Hemolytic disorders	Autoimmune disease, blood group incompatibility, hemoglobinopathies, microangiopathies, red cell enzyme deficiencies, red cell membrane disorders
Enterohepatic recirculation	Cystic fibrosis, Hirschsprung disease, ileal atresia, pyloric stenosis
Disorders of bilirubin metabolism	Acidosis, Crigler-Najjar syndrome, Gilbert syndrome, hypothyroidism, hypoxia
Miscellaneous	Dehydration, drugs, hypoalbuminemia, sepsis

DIRECT HYPERBILIRUBINEMIA

Biliary obstruction	Biliary atresia, choledochal cyst, fibrosing pancreatitis, gallstones or biliary sludge, inspissated bile syndrome, neoplasm, primary sclerosing cholangitis
Infection	Cholangitis, cytomegalovirus, Epstein-Barr virus, herpes simplex virus, histoplasmosis, HIV, leptospirosis, liver abscess, sepsis, syphilis, toxocariasis, toxoplasmosis, tuberculosis, urinary tract infection, varicella-zoster virus, viral hepatitis
Genetic/metabolic disorders	α_1-Antitrypsin deficiency, Alagille syndrome, Caroli disease, cystic fibrosis, Dubin-Johnson syndrome, galactokinase deficiency, galactosemia, glycogen storage disease, hereditary fructose intolerance, hypothyroidism, Niemann-Pick disease, rotor syndrome, tyrosinemia, Wilson disease
Chromosomal abnormalities	Trisomy 18, Trisomy 21, Turner syndrome
Drugs	Acetaminophen, aspirin, erythromycin, ethanol, iron, isoniazid, methotrexate, oxacillin, rifampin, steroids, sulfonamides, tetracycline, vitamin A
Miscellaneous	Neonatal hepatitis syndrome, parenteral alimentation, Reye syndrome

radiographic changes in the pancreas. Reversible process. Most common etiologies: Trauma, multisystem disease, drugs, infections, idiopathic, and congenital anomalies. See Table 12-8 for conditions associated with acute pancreatitis.

2. **Diagnosis/evaluation:**
a. Clinical signs/symptoms: Abdominal pain (sudden or gradual, most commonly epigastric), anorexia, nausea, vomiting, tachycardia, fever, hypotension, guarding/rebound tenderness/decreased bowel sounds, sonographic or radiologic evidence of pancreatic inflammation. Grey-Turner and Cullen signs are rare in children.
b. Laboratory findings:
   (1) Elevated lipase and amylase: ≥3 times above normal limit (but no correlation with disease severity). Lipase is more sensitive and specific for acute pancreatitis but normalizes more slowly, so it may be preferable to follow amylase after establishing diagnosis.[9]

TABLE 12-8

CONDITIONS ASSOCIATED WITH ACUTE PANCREATITIS

SYSTEMIC DISEASES

Infections	Coxsackie, CMV, cryptosporidium, EBV, hepatitis, influenza A or B, leptospirosis, mycoplasma, mumps, rubella, typhoid fever, varicella
Inflammatory and vasculitic disorders	Collagen vascular diseases, hemolytic uremic syndrome, Henoch-Schönlein purpura, IBD, Kawasaki disease
Sepsis/peritonitis/shock	
Transplantation	

IDIOPATHIC (UP TO 25% OF CASES)

MECHANICAL STRUCTURAL

Trauma	Blunt trauma, child abuse, ERCP
Perforation	
Anomalies	Annular pancreas, choledochal cyst, pancreatic divisum, stenosis, other
Obstruction	Parasites, stones, tumors

METABOLIC AND TOXIC FACTORS

Cystic fibrosis	
Diabetes mellitus	
Drugs/toxins	Salicylates, cytotoxic drugs (L-asparaginase), corticosteroids, chlorothiazides, furosemide, oral contraceptives (estrogen), tetracyclines, sulfonamides, valproic acid, azathioprine, 6-mercaptopurine
Hypercalcemia	
Hyperlipidemia	
Hypothermia	
Malnutrition	
Organic acidemia	
Renal disease	

CMV, Cytomegalovirus; EBV, Epstein-Barr virus; ERCP, endoscopic retrograde cholangiopancreatography.
Modified from Robertson MA. Pancreatitis. In: Walker WA et al, eds. *Pediatric Gastrointestinal Disease.* 3rd ed. New York: BC Decker, 2000:1321-1344; and Werlin SL. Pancreatitis. In: McMillan JA et al, eds. *Oski's Pediatrics.* Philadelphia: Lippincott Williams & Wilkins, 2006:2010-2012.

    (2) Additional findings: leukocytosis, hyperglycemia, glucosuria, hypocalcemia, hyperbilirubinemia.

3. **Management:**
a. Pancreatic rest: Nasogastric decompression, analgesia, intravenous fluid hydration, oral intake restriction. Enteral feeding via nasojejunal tube may be used for nutrition. (In adults, enteral nutrition is associated with lower incidence of infection, surgical intervention, and shorter hospital stay. Minimal pediatric evidence available.)
b. Antibiotics are reserved for only the most severe cases.

B. Chronic Pancreatitis

1. **Definition:** Progressive inflammatory process causing irreversible changes in the architecture and function of the pancreas. Common

complications include chronic abdominal pain, loss of exocrine function (malabsorption, malnutrition) and/or endocrine function (diabetes mellitus). Two major morphologic forms: calcific and obstructive (Table EC 12-A).

2. **Management:** (For acute exacerbations) same as management of acute pancreatitis. See Section V.A.3.

C. Miscellaneous Tests

For descriptions, see Expert Consult.

1. **Occult blood**

a. Purpose: To screen for presence of blood through detection of heme in stool

b. Method: Smear a small amount of stool on test areas of an occult blood test card and allow to air dry. Apply developer as directed.

c. Interpretation: Blue color resembling that of the control indicates presence of heme. Brisk transit of ingested red meat and inorganic iron may yield a false-positive result. Fruits and vegetables associated with false-positive results include cantaloupes, radishes, bean sprouts, cauliflower, broccoli, and grapes. Screening for presence of blood in gastric aspirates or vomitus should be performed using Gastroccult, not stool Hemoccult, cards.

2. **Quantitative fecal fat**

a. Purpose: To screen for fat malabsorption by quantitating fecal fat excretion.

b. Method: Patient should be on a normal diet (35% fat) with amount of calories and fat ingested recorded for 2 days before test and during the test itself. Collect and freeze all stools passed within 72 hours, send to laboratory for determination of total fecal fatty acid content.

c. Interpretation

(1) Total fecal fatty acid excretion of >5 g fat per 24 hours may suggest malabsorption. Results will vary with amount of fat ingested, and normal values have not been established for children <2 years of age.

(2) Coefficient of absorption (CA) is a more accurate indicator of fat malabsorption and does not vary with fat intake:

$$CA = (\text{Grams of fat ingested} - \text{Grams of fat excreted}) / (\text{Grams of fat ingested}) \times 100$$

Infants <6 months of age should absorb >85% of fat intake. By age 1 year, fat absorption should be at an adult level of >95%. Quantitative fecal fat is recommended over qualitative methods (e.g., staining with Sudan III), which depend on spot checks and are thus unreliable for diagnosing fat malabsorption.

REFERENCES

1. Koletzko S, Jones N, Goodman K, Gold B, et al. Evidence Based Guidelines from ESPGHAN and NASPGHAN for Helicobacter Pylori Infection in Children. Pediatric Gastroenterology, Hepatology and Nutrition. *J Pediatr Gastroenterol Nutr.* 2011;53:230-243

2. Moir CR. Abdominal pain in infants and children. *Mayo Clin Proc.* 1996;71(10):984-989.

3. World Health Organization. ICD-10. http://www.who.int/classifications/icd/en/2007. Available online; World Health Organization.

4. King CK, Glass R, Bresee JS, et al. Managing acute gastroenteritis among children: oral rehydration, maintenance, and nutritional therapy. *MMWR Recomm Rep.* 2003;52:1-16.

5. Vanderhoof JA. Chronic diarrhea. *Pediatr Rev.* 1998;19(12):418.

6. Thomas PD, Forbes A, Green J, et al. Guidelines for the investigation of chronic diarrhoea, 2nd ed. *Gut.* 2003;52(suppl 5):v1-15.

7. Clinical Practice Guideline. Clinical efficacy of probiotics: review of the evidence with focus on children. NASPGHAN Nutrition Committee Report. *J Pediatr Gastroenterol Nutr.* 2006;43:550-557.

8. Constipation Guideline Committee of the North American Society for Pediatric Gastroenterology, Hepatology and Nutrition. Evaluation and treatment of constipation in infants and children: recommendations of the North American Society for Pediatric Gastroenterology, Hepatology and Nutrition. *J Pediatr Gastroenterol Nutr.* 2006;43:e1-e13.

9. McMillan JA, Feigin RD, DeAngelis CD. *Oski's Pediatrics,* 4th ed. Philadelphia: Lippincott Williams & Wilkins; 2011.

10. Beattie RM, Croft NM, Fell JM, et al. Inflammatory bowel disease. *Arch Dis Child.* 2006;91:426-432.

11. Clinical Report: Differentiating ulcerative colitis from Crohn disease in children and young adults: report of a working group of the North American Society for Pediatric Gastroenterology, Hepatology, and Nutrition and the Crohn's and Colitis Foundation of America. *J Pediatr Gastroenterol Nutr.* 2007;44:653-674.

12. Vandenplas Y, Rudolph CD, DiLorenzo C, et al. Pediatric gastroesophageal reflux clinical practice guidelines: joint recommendations of the North American Society of Pediatric Gastroenterology, Hepatology, and Nutrition and the European Society of Pediatric Gastroenterology, Hepatology, and Nutrition. *J Pediatr Gastroenterol Nutr.* 2009;49:498-547.

13. Hirano I, Richter JE. Practice Parameters Committee of the American College of Gastroenterology. ACG practice guidelines: esophageal reflux testing. *Am J Gastroenterol.* 2007;102:668-685.

14. Furuta GT, Liacouras CA, Collins MH, et al. Eosinophilic esophagitis in children and adults: a systematic review and consensus recommendations for diagnosis and treatment. *Gastroenterology.* 2007;133:1342-1363.

15. Hill ID, Dirks MH, Liptak GS, et al. Guideline for the diagnosis and treatment of celiac disease in children: recommendations of the North American Society for Pediatric Gastroenterology, Hepatology and Nutrition. *J Pediatr Gastroenterol Nutr.* 2005;40:1-19.

16. Bucuvalas J, Yazigi N, Squires Jr RH. Acute liver failure in children. *Clin Liver Dis.* 2006;10:149-168.

17. Harb R, Thomas DW. Conjugated hyperbilirubinemia: screening and treatment in older infants and children. *Pediatr Rev.* 2007;28:83-91.

18. Moyer V, Freese DK, Whitington PF, et al. Guideline for the evaluation of cholestatic jaundice in infants: recommendations of the North American Society for Pediatric Gastroenterology, Hepatology and Nutrition. *J Pediatr Gastroenterol Nutr.* 2004;39:115-128.
19. Lowe ME. Pancreatitis in childhood. *Curr Gastroenterol Rep.* 2004;6:240-246.
20. Nydegger A, Couper RTL. Childhood pancreatitis. *J Gastroenterol Hepatol.* 2006;21(3):499-509.

Chapter 13

Genetics: Metabolism and Dysmorphology

Jessica Duis, MD

Continuous technologic advances make genetics a constantly evolving field. It is best discussed in separate sections entitled "Metabolism" and "Dysmorphology." When considering a particular diagnosis, a complete patient history should include details of the conception, pregnancy, prenatal ultrasound findings, delivery, postnatal growth, development, a three-generation family history in the form of a pedigree, and a comprehensive physical examination.

I. WEBSITES/DATABASES

Online Mendelian Inheritance in Man (OMIM): http://omim.org (includes a search engine for identifying genetic diseases based on clinical phenotype, gene, and OMIM number)

GeneReviews: www.genereviews.org; expert-authored and peer-reviewed descriptions of inherited disorders

National Newborn Screening and Genetics Resource Center: genes-r-us.uthscsa.edu/resources.htm

GeneTests: www.genetests.org (includes information on genetic diagnostic tests, genetic clinics in the United States and laboratories that perform genetic testing)

American College of Medical Genetics: www.acmg.net/resources/policies/ACT/condition-analyte-links.htm (includes ACT sheets and algorithm to help guide physicians after a positive newborn metabolic screen)

National Organization for Rare Disorders: www.rarediseases.org

II. METABOLISM

A. Newborn Metabolic Screening[1-3]

1. **Overview by state:** http://genes-r-us.uthscsa

2. **Timing:**

a. First screen should be performed within the first 48–72 hours of life (at least 24 hours after initiation of feeding).

b. Second screen (requested in some states) should be performed between 1 and 4 weeks of age (after 7 days).

c. Preterm infants: Perform initial screen at birth (to collect DNA before transfusions), another at 48–72 hours of age, a third at 7 days of age, and a final at 28 days or before discharge (whichever comes first).

3. **Abnormal results:**

a. Requires immediate follow-up and confirmatory testing; consult a geneticist.

b. ACT Sheets and Confirmatory Algorithms are available for more information on how to proceed with specific abnormalities: www.acmg.net/resources/policies/ACT/condition-analyte-links.htm.

B. Clinical Presentation[1,4,5] (Box 13-1)

1. **Neonatal:** After appearing well for a brief period of time, which can range from hours to a usual time frame of about 48–72 hours; illness often mistaken for sepsis develops and can progress to coma.

2. **Infancy:** Failure to thrive, poor feeding with vomiting, often presents at the time of intercurrent illness or when the infant begins fasting overnight (usually 7–12 months of age).

3. **Children and adults:** Often a presentation at the time of intercurrent illness; waxing and waning consciousness that may progress to coma.

C. Evaluation[1,5]

1. **Initial laboratory tests:** Complete metabolic panel (CMP), blood glucose, venous blood gas (VBG), ammonia, lactate, creatine kinase (CK), complete blood cell count (CBC) with differential, urine ketones (Box 13-2).

2. **If metabolic disease is suspected:** Consult a geneticist. General metabolic workup includes plasma amino acids (PAA), urine organic acids (UOA), acylcarnitine profile, quantitative plasma carnitine, lactate/pyruvate (refer to Table 13-1 for collection information).

3. **Special considerations:**[5-7]

a. Hyperammonemia: VBG, UOA, PAA, acylcarnitine profile, urine orotic acid (Fig. 13-1)

b. Hypoglycemia: During acute illness consider urine ketones, acylcarnitine profile, PAA, UOA, insulin, growth hormone, cortisol, C-peptide (Fig. 13-2)[8]

c. Metabolic acidosis: Ammonia, lactic acid, UOA, UA with urine pH, CMP (Fig. 13-3)

BOX 13-1

WHEN TO SUSPECT METABOLIC DISEASE[1,5]

Overwhelming illness in the neonatal period
Vomiting
Acute acidosis, anion gap
Massive ketosis
Hypoglycemia
Coagulopathy
Deep coma
Seizures, especially myoclonic
Hypotonia
Unusual odor of urine
Extensive dermatosis, especially monilial
Neutropenia, thrombocytopenia, or pancytopenia
Family history of siblings dying early

BOX 13-2

INITIAL LABORATORY INVESTIGATIONS[4,5]

BLOOD

Complete metabolic profile (special attention to bicarbonate and anion gap)
Blood glucose
Venous blood gas: pH, Pco_2, HCO_3, Po_2
Ammonia
Lactate
Creatine kinase
Complete blood cell count with differential
Plasma amino acids
Quantitative carnitine
Acylcarnitine profile

URINE

Ketones
Urinalysis
Reducing substances
Urine organic acids

TABLE 13-1

SAMPLE COLLECTION

Specimen Name	Volume (mL)	Tube	Handling Instructions
Chromosome microarray (SNP array)	2–5	Purple top	Do not freeze, may refrigerate.
Karyotype	2–5	Green top	Room temperature.
DNA-based testing	5–10	Purple top	Room temperature; ship in insulated container overnight.
Plasma ammonia	1–3	Purple top	Place on ice and transport immediately to laboratory.
Plasma amino acids	1–3	Green top	Take to laboratory immediately on ice; if must store, spin down and separate plasma and store at −20°C.
Quantitative carnitine (free and total carnitine)	1–3	Green top	Transport on ice.
Acylcarnitine profile	0.5–2.0	Green top	Transport on ice.
Lactate	2–3	Gray top	Immediately transport on ice.
Urine organic acids	3–5	Urine specimen container	Take immediately to laboratory on ice; if must store, store at −20°C.
Urine amino acids	1–5	Urine specimen container	Take immediately to laboratory on ice; if must store, store at −20°C.

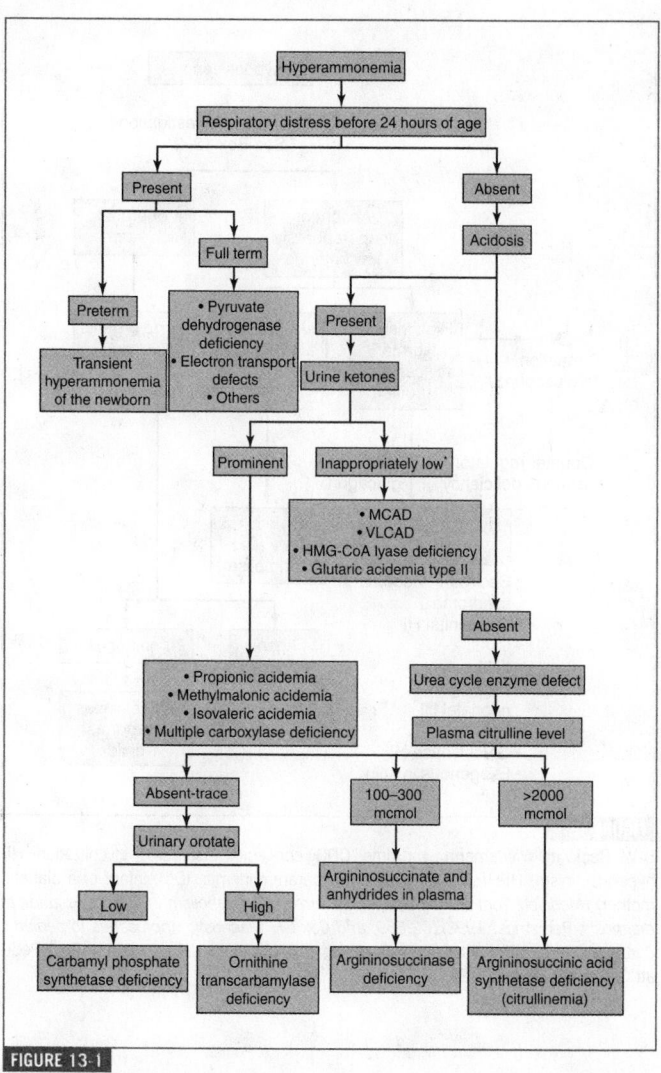

FIGURE 13-1

Differential diagnosis of hyperammonemia. *Indicates inappropriately low urinary ketones in the setting of symptomatic hypoglycemia. HMG-CoA, Hydroxymethylglutaryl-CoA; MCAD, medium-chain acyl-CoA dehydrogenase; SCAD, short-chain acyl-CoA dehydrogenase; VLCAD, very long-chain acyl-CoA dehydrogenase.[4,5]

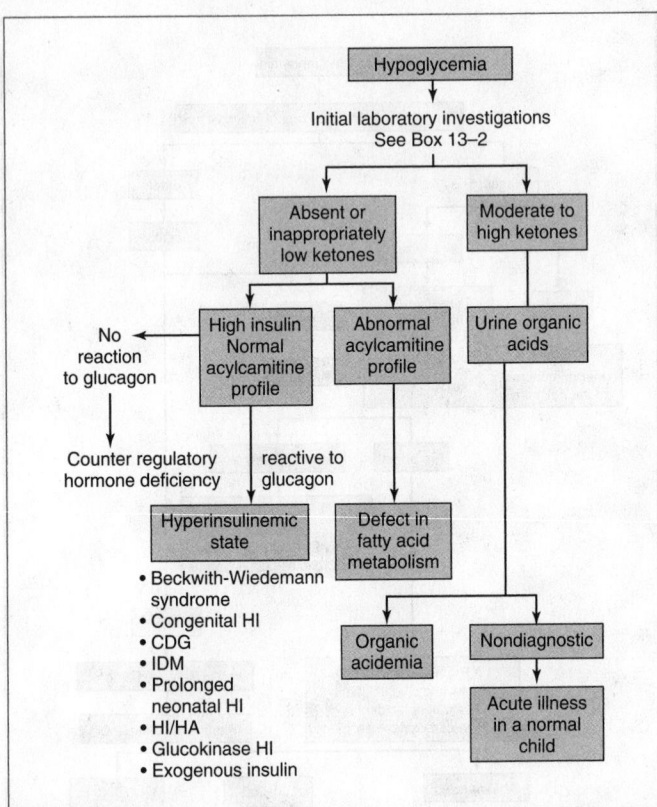

FIGURE 13-2

B-W, Beckwith-Wiedemann syndrome; CDG, congenital disorder of glycolization; HI, hyperinsulinism; HI/HA, hyperinsulinism/hyperammonemia; IDM, infant of a diabetic mother. *(Modified from Burton BK. Inborn errors of metabolism in infancy: a guide to diagnosis. Pediatrics. 1998;102:E69; and Cox GF. Diagnostic approaches to pediatric cardiomyopathy of metabolic genetic etiologies and their relation to therapy. Prog Pediatr Cardiol. 2007;24:15-25.)*

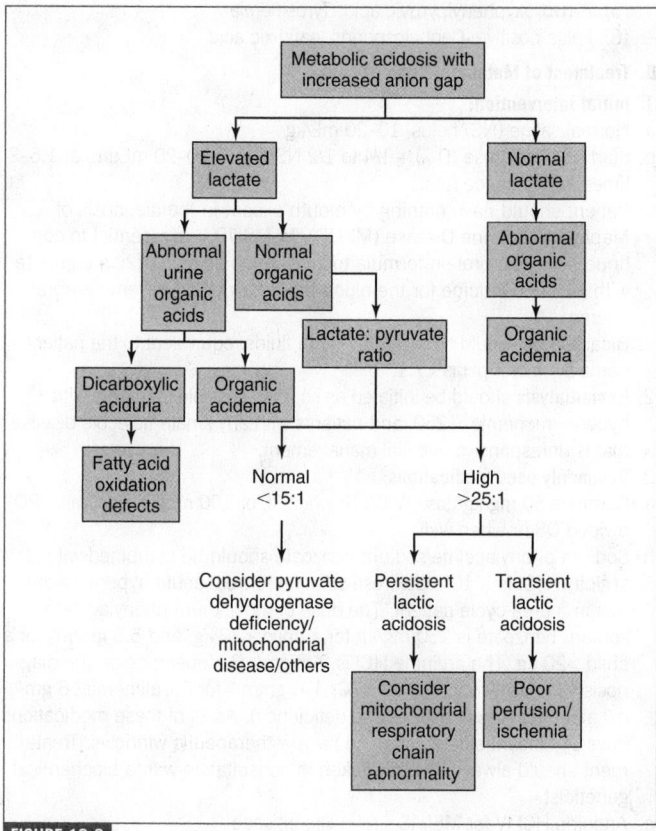

FIGURE 13-3

Metabolic acidosis with increased anion gap. (From Burton B. Inborn errors of metabolism in infancy: a guide to diagnosis. Pediatrics. 1998;102:E69.)

d. Neonatal seizures: CSF and plasma amino acids (done simultaneously to determine the glycine ratio to evaluate for nonketotic hyperglycinemia), CSF/serum glucose ratio, neurotransmitters, very long-chain fatty acids, organic acids, serum uric acid, urine sulfites. Consider trial of pyridoxine (100 mg intravenously [IV]), pyridoxal phosphate (30 mg/kg), and folinic acid (3 mg/kg) IV if uncontrollable.

e. Urine reducing substances (finding with differential):
   (1) Galactose: Galactosemia
   (2) Fructose: Hereditary fructose intolerance, fructosuria
   (3) Glucose: Diabetes mellitus, renal tubular defect
   (4) Xylose: Pentosuria

(5) P-hydroxyphenylpyruvic acid: Tyrosinemia

(6) False positive: Cephalosporins, nalidixic acid

D. Treatment of Metabolic Crisis[5-7]

1. Initial intervention:

a. Normal saline (NS) bolus, 10–20 mL/kg

b. Start 10% dextrose (D_{10}) + 1/4 to 1/2 NS + KCl (10–20 mEq/L) at 1.5–2 times maintenance rate.

c. Patient should have nothing by mouth except in the diagnosis of Maple Syrup Urine Disease (MSUD). In MSUD it is essential to continue synthetic protein formula to give amino acids that can compete with elevated leucine for the blood brain barrier to prevent cerebral edema.

d. Bicarbonate should be included in the fluids, equivalent to the patient's home dose or if pH is <7.1.

2. Hemodialysis should be initiated as soon as possible in infants with hyperammonemia > 250, and patients with any small-molecule disease that is unresponsive to initial management.

3. Commonly used medications:

a. Carnitine 50 mg/kg/dose IV Q6 hr when ill, or 100 mg/kg/day orally (PO) divided Q8 hr when well.

b. Sodium phenylacetate/sodium benzoate should be combined with arginine HCl in a 10% dextrose solution to treat acute hyperammonemia in a urea cycle patient. The dose of the sodium phenylacetate / sodium benzoate is 250 mg/kg for a child <20 kg, and 5.5 gm/m² for a child >20 kg. The arginine HCl is 2–6 gm/m², depending on the diagnosis (2 gm/m² for CPS and OTC; 4–6 gm/m² for Citrullinemia; 6 gm/m² alone for Argininosuccinase deficiency). As all of these medications have significant side effects and narrow therapeutic windows. Treatment should always be undertaken in consultation with a biochemical geneticist.

c. Arginine HCl IV for MELAS stroke-like episode.

d. Sodium benzoate for NKH

E. Some Common Metabolic Diseases in Brief[1,4-7]

1. Fatty acid oxidation (FAO) disorders:

a. Epidemiology: 1/10,000; autosomal recessive disorders:
   (1) Most common is medium-chain acyl-CoA dehydrogenase (MCAD).
   (2) Short-chain acyl-CoA dehydrogenase (SCAD) deficiency is picked up on newborn screen, but most patients have no problems even during intercurrent illness.

b. Presentation:
   (1) Hypoketotic hypoglycemia, lethargy, coma, vomiting
   (2) Disorders of long chains can present with rhabdomyolysis and/or cardiomyopathy

c. Diagnostic evaluation: Blood glucose, urine ketones, complete metabolic panel (CMP), VBG, creatine kinase (CK), ammonia, acylcarnitine profile, quantitative carnitine

d. Acute managment:
   (1) Bolus D_{10} 2 mL/kg in hypoglycemia and/or NS 20 mL/kg for volume repletion.
   (2) Start D_{10}+ 1/4 NS + KCl (based on serum level of K) and run at 1.5–2 times maintenance fluid rate.
   (3) Treat fever aggressively with antipyretics, and treat intercurrent infection.
e. Chronic management:
   (1) Carnitine supplementation for primary carnitine deficiencies and MCAD (avoid in very long-chain acyl-CoA dehydrogenase [VLCAD] and long-chain 3-hydroxyl-CoA dehydrogenase [LCHAD] disorders).
   (2) In disorders of very long-chain fatty acids, limit intake to low-fat foods and supplementation with medium-chain triglyceride oil.
   (3) In all FAO patients with mild intercurrent illness or decreased day-time intake, nighttime feeds Q4 hr are necessary.

2. **Organic acidemias:**
a. Epidemiology: All autosomal recessive:
   (1) 3-methylcrotonyl-CoA carboxylase deficiency (3-MCC): 1/15,000 (picked up on newborn screen, but most children are normal with-out problems during illness)
   (2) Glutaric acidemia type 1 (GA1): 1/30,000–40,000
   (3) Methylmalonic acidemia (MMA): 1/100,000
   (4) Propionic acidemia (PA): 1/150,000
   (5) Isovaleric acidemia: 1/150,000
   (6) Maple syrup urine disease (MSUD): 1/150,000
b. Presentation:
   (1) Neonatal: Well, full-term infant who develops lethargy, irritability, seizures, hypotonia, poor feeding, hypoglycemia, vomiting
   (2) Older infant/child: Failure to thrive, vomiting, global developmen-tal delays, choreoathetoid or dystonic movements secondary to metabolic stroke in the basal ganglia, bone marrow suppression, frequent infections, pancreatitis, cardiomyopathy
c. Diagnostic evaluation: Blood glucose, complete metabolic profile, urinalysis to look for infection and ketones, CBC with differential, VBG, ammonia, acylcarnitine profile, PAA, quantitative carnitine
d. Acute management:
   (1) Start infusion of D_{10}+ 1/4 NS + KCl at 1.5–2 times maintenance
   (2) May need bicarbonate, especially if on it daily at baseline
   (3) Stop all protein feeds (except in MSUD, where synthetic formula should be used at all times if possible)
   (4) Carnitine 50 mg/kg IV Q6 hr in MMA, PA
   (5) 10% glycine 500 mg/kg/day in isovaleric acidemia
e. Chronic Management: Formula that appropriately restricts amino acids; treatment with carnitine

3. **Urea cycle defects:**
a. Epidemiology: 1/30,000. Autosomal recessive, except for ornithine transcarbamylase (OTC) deficiency which is X-linked.

13

    (1) Most common is OTC deficiency.

    (2) OTC deficiency and carbamyl phosphate synthetase (CPS) deficiency are not picked up on newborn screening because it is difficult to distinguish between low and normal citrulline levels.

b. Presentation: Episodes of acute decompensation characterized by hyperammonemia, lethargy, seizures, coma, respiratory alkalosis, failure to thrive, poor appetite, vomiting, psychosis

c. Diagnostic evaluation: CMP, VBG, ammonia, PAA, urine orotic acid, urinalysis, CBC to determine if evidence for a bacterial infection.

d. Acute management:

    (1) Start IV fluids as per above, stop all protein intake, dialysis as indicated for ammonia > 250

    (2) Sodium benzoate/sodium phenylacetate and arginine IV

e. Chronic management: Sodium phenylbutyrate or glycerol phenylbutyrate, citrulline (for OTC deficiency and CPS deficiency), arginine (for citrullinemia and argininosuccinate lyase deficiency), protein-restricted diet

4. **Phenylketonuria (PKU):**

a. Epidemiology: Autosomal recessive, 1/10,000–15,000

b. Presentation: Intellectual disability if untreated

c. Diagnostic evaluation: Most infants diagnosed by newborn screening before clinical appearance; PAA to look at phenylalanine

d. Acute management: Phenylalanine-restricted diet

e. Chronic management: Phenylalanine-restricted diet; sapropterin effective in a subset of patients at a dose of 10–20 mg/kg/day

5. **Hereditary tyrosinemia (HT1):**

a. Epidemiology: Autosomal recessive, 1/100,000

b. Presentation: Severe liver failure, vomiting, bleeding, sepsis, hypoglycemia, renal tubulopathy (Fanconi syndrome). Chronic HT1 leads to cirrhosis, failure to thrive, rickets, neuropathy, tubulopathy, neurologic crises

c. Diagnostic evaluation: Complete metabolic panel, coagulation studies, CBC with differential, urine organic acids to quantitate succinylacetone, PAA

d. Acute management: Management of bleeding complications and providing replacement factors: 2-(2-nitro-4-trifluoromethyl-benzoyl)-1, 3-cyclohexanedione (NTBC), 1–2 mg/kg divided twice daily

e. Chronic management: Tyrosine- and phenylalanine-restricted diet, NTBC 1–2 mg/kg divided twice daily

6. **Mitochondrial diseases:**[6,9]

a. Epidemiology: 1/8500; can be caused by mutations in nuclear or mitochondrial DNA.

b. Presentation: Can involve any organ system; symptoms usually neurologic and myopathic. For in-depth discussion, access gene review at www.ncbi.nlm.nih.gov/books/NBK1224/.

c. Diagnostic evaluation: CMP, CK, VBG, CBC with differential, lactate/pyruvate, CSF levels of lactate/pyruvate, plasma and CSF amino acids, urine organic acids, urine amino acids, brain imaging, mitochondrial DNA testing. Muscle biopsy is no longer indicated except in the case of severe myopathy.

d. Acute management: ABCs, supportive therapy, encourage anaerobic metabolism.

e. Chronic management: Cocktail of antioxidants, vitamins, and cofactors.

7. **Lysosomal storage diseases:**[10]

a. Epidemiology:

(1) Mucopolysaccharidosis type I (Hurler syndrome, MPS I): 1/100,000; autosomal recessive

(2) Mucopolysaccharidosis type II (Hunter syndrome, MPS II): 1/140,000; X-linked recessive

(3) Mucopolysaccharidosis type III (Sanfilippo syndrome, MPS III): 1/100,000; autosomal recessive

(4) Mucopolysaccharidosis type IV (Morquio syndrome, MPS IV): 1/75,000-300,000; autosomal recessive

(5) Mucopolysaccharidosis type VI (Maroteaux-Lamy syndrome, MPS VI): 1/200,000-300,000; autosomal recessive

(6) Mucopolysaccharidosis type VII (Sly syndrome, MPS VII): Rare

b. Presentation:

(1) Infants normal at birth, except in Sly syndrome (MPS VII), where infants usually die from hydrops.

(2) Coarsening of facial features noted at about age 1 year. Progressive dysostosis multiplex, growth failure, hepatomegaly, deafness, psychomotor retardation, intellectual disability, hearing loss.

(3) Hurler syndrome (MPS I): Lethal by 10 years of age if not treated with bone marrow transplantation

(4) Sanfilippo syndrome (MPS III): Patients aggressive with extremely hyperkinetic behavior and tetraspasticity

(5) Morquio syndrome (MPS IV): Small stature with severe skeletal abnormalities

(6) Maroteaux-Lamy syndrome (MPS VI): Visceral involvement, normal intelligence

c. Diagnostic evaluation: CBC with differential, skeletal survey for dysostosis, specific enzyme activity

d. Acute management: Supportive therapy

e. Chronic management:

(1) Hurler syndrome (MPS I): Stem cell transplantation before 2 years of age may slow progression of cognitive decline but does not affect skeletal manifestations or corneal clouding

(2) Maroteaux-Lamy syndrome (MPS VI): Enzyme replacement

(3) Non-neuronopathic Hunter syndrome (MPS II): Enzyme replacement

8. **Disorders of carbohydrate metabolism—galactosemia:**

a. Epidemiology: Galactosemia, 1/30,000; autosomal recessive.

b. Presentation:

(1) Presents at 3–4 days of life with hypoglycemia, jaundice, diarrhea, hepatomegaly, hyperammonemia, poor feeding, vomiting. Other

presenting symptoms include failure to thrive, lethargy, seizures, cataracts, hepatic failure, and renal failure.

(2) Galactosemia should be considered in an infant with overwhelming *Escherichia coli* sepsis.

c. Diagnostic evaluation: Galactosemia often made on newborn screening. Obtain blood glucose, comprehensive metabolic panel, ammonia, co-agulation studies, urine for reducing substances, galactitol, erythrocyte galactose-1-phosphate, galactose-1-phosphate uridyltransferase (GALT) activity.

d. Acute management: ABCs, discontinue feeds, dextrose containing fluids.

e. Chronic management: Lactose-free and galactose-restricted diet for life.

9. **Glycogen storage disease (GSD):** For more information see GeneReviews at http://www.ncbi.nlm.nih.gov/books/NBK1312/ and http://www.ncbi.nlm.nih.gov/books/NBK26372/

a. Epidemiology: Autosomal recessive

(1) GSD type I: 1/100,000; GSD1a most common in persons of European descent

(2) GSD type III: 1/100,000

b. Presentation:

(1) GSD type I: Patients have hepatomegaly and renomegaly. They can present with severe hypoglycemia in the neonatal period, but more commonly present at age 3–4 months with hepatomegaly, lactic acidosis, hyperuricemia, hypoglycemia, and hyperlipidemia. They have doll-like facies and xanthomas. Progression of disease includes long-term growth retardation, short stature, osteoporosis, delayed puberty, hepatic adenomas, polycystic ovaries, renal disease, and pancreatitis. Unreated GSD1b is associated with recurrent bacterial infections and mucosal ulcers secondary to impaired neutrophil and monocyte function, along with chronic neutropenia.

(2) GSD type III: Patients have liver and muscle involvement. In infancy and early childhood, they present with ketotic hypoglycemia, hepatomegaly, hyperlipidemia, and elevated hepatic transaminases. GSD3a is associated with hypertophic cardiomyopathy and skeletal myopathy in the third to fourth decade.

c. Diagnosis:

(1) GSD type I: Blood glucose, lactate, uric acid, triglycerides, lipids, molecular genetic testing

(2) GSD type III: Ketotic hypoglycemia with fasting, transaminases, CK, molecular testing

d. Acute management: Prevent hypoglycemia, treat with dextrose-containing fluids.

e. Chronic management:

(1) GSD type I: Prevent hypoglycemia and may have to provide cornstarch or newly available Glycosade after consulting a geneticist.

Allopurinol to prevent gout. Lipid-lowering medications. Citrate supplementation to help prevent nephrolithiasis, nephrocalcinosis. Angiotensin-converting enzyme (ACE) inhibitors to treat microalbuminuria. Kidney transplant for end-stage renal disease. G-CSF for recurrent infections in GSD1b.

(2) GSD type III: High-protein diet and frequent feedings (Q3–4 hr) in infancy. Cornstarch or Glycosade to prevent hypoglycemia overnight.

F. Hypotonia[11,12]

1. **Definition:** Reduced resistance to passive range of motion in joints, characterized by an impaired ability to sustain postural control and movement against gravity.
2. **Central:** Depressed level of consciousness, predominantly axial weakness, normal strength with hypotonia, abnormalities of brain function, dysmorphic features, fisting of the hands, scissoring on vertical suspension, and other congenital malformations (Fig. 13-4A).
3. **Peripheral:** Alert, responds appropriately to surroundings, normal sleep/wake cycles, profound weakness, absent reflexes, feeding difficulties, decreased and/or lack of antigravity movement (see Fig. 13-4B).
4. **Combined hypotonia:** See Fig. 13-5

III. DYSMORPHOLOGY[1,2,13-15]

A. History

Pregnancy history, type of conception (natural vs. artificial reproductive technologies), perinatal history, developmental milestones, three-generation pedigree

B. Physical Examination[13]

1. **Major anomalies:** Create significant medical problems for the patient and may require specific surgical or medical management. Includes structural brain abnormalities, intellectual disability or developmental delays, failure to thrive, cleft lip and/or palate, congenital heart defects, skeletal dysplasia, severe limb abnormalities.
2. **Minor anomalies:** Features that vary in comparison to the normal population, with little serious medical or surgical consequences. Includes abnormally shaped ears or eyes, inverted nipples, birthmarks, abnormal structures of the hands and feet, abnormal skin folds or creases (e.g., single palmar crease).

C. Workup

1. **Imaging:**
a. Abdominal ultrasound, echocardiogram, brain imaging (head ultrasound or magnetic resonance imaging [MRI])
b. Genetic skeletal survey for patients with apparent short bones, short stature, visible external anomalies (asymmetry, proximal thumbs, skin dimpling)

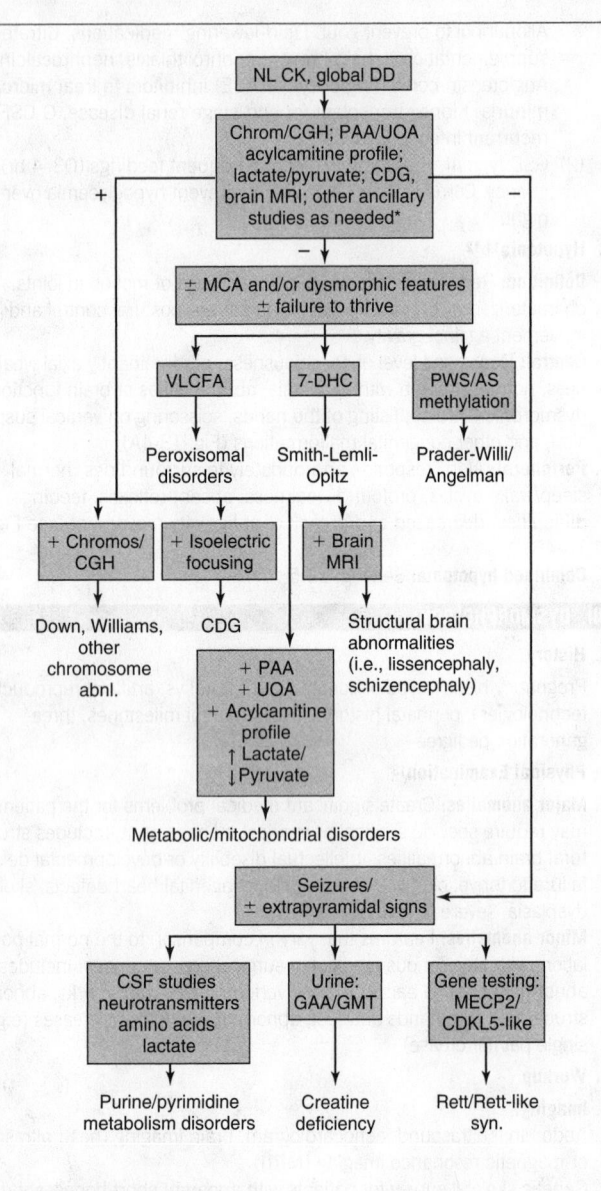

A (Central Hypotonia)

FIGURE 13-4, cont'd

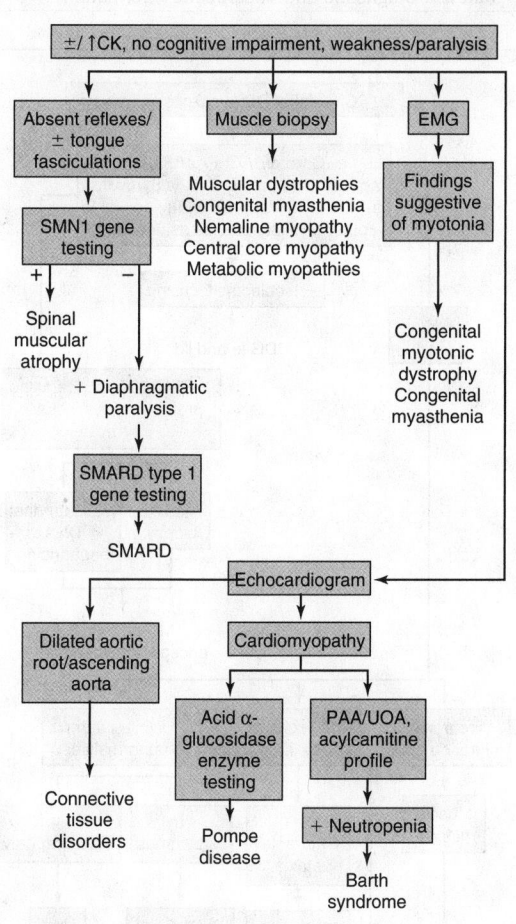

B (Peripheral Hypotonia)

FIGURE 13-4

Hypotonia. CDKL5, cyclin-dependent kinase-like 5; CK, creatine kinase; CPT II, carnitine palmitoyltransferase II; CSF, cerebrospinal fluid; DD, developmental delay; 7-DHC, 7-dehydrocholesterol; EMG, electromyography; GAA, guanidinoacetate; GMT, guanidinoacetate-N-methyltransferase; MCA, multiple congenital anomalies; MECP2, methyl CpG binding protein 2; NL CK, normal creatine kinase; PAA, plasma amino acids; PWS/AS, Prader-Willi syndrome/Angelman syndrome; SMARD, spinal muscular atrophy with respiratory distress; SMN1, survival of motor neuron 1; UAA, urine amino acids; UOA, urine organic acids; VLCFA, very long-chain fatty acids. *(From Lisi E, Cohn R. Genetic evaluation of the hypotonic pediatric patient: perspective from a hypotonia specialty clinic and review of the literature.* Dev Med Child Neurol. 2011;53:586-599.)

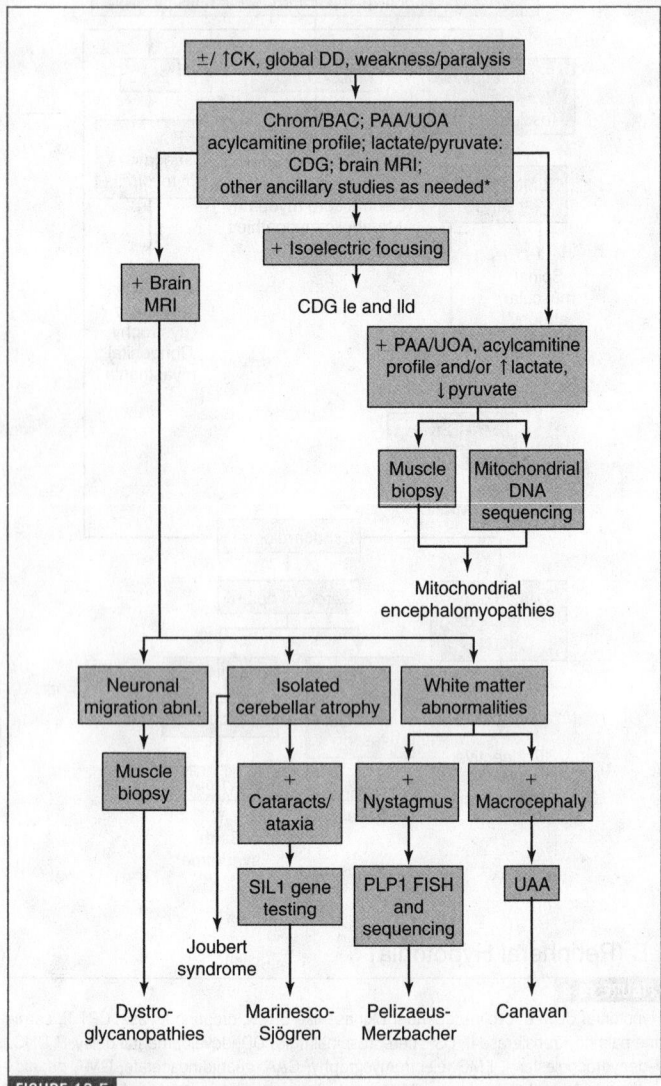

FIGURE 13-5

Combined hypotonia. FISH, fluorescence in situ hybridization; PLP1, proteolipid protein 1. *(From Lisi E, Cohn R. Genetic evaluation of the hypotonic pediatric patient: perspective from a hypotonia specialty clinic and review of the literature. Dev Med Child Neurol. 2011;53:586-599.)*

2. **Ophthalmologic examination**
3. **Hearing evaluation**
4. **Chromosome microarray:** Indicated when one major and two minor malformations are present; detects changes in copy number and genotype. This is first-line testing for chromosomal anomalies replacing the karyotype, except when specifically indicated (see below). This test may be done by single nucleotide polymorphism (SNP) array (which will also detect low-level mosaicism and consanguinity) or oligoarray. Both assays are equally sensitive at detecting copy number variation.
5. **Specific gene testing:** See www.genetests.org for reference.
6. **Whole-exome sequencing:** Consult a geneticist. This tests yields complex results well beyond the diagnosis and requires extensive pretest and posttest counseling.
7. **Karyotype:** Very rarely indicated anymore; indicated in suspected aneuploidy (e.g., trisomy 13, 18, 21, or monosomy X) and when assessing frequent miscarriages (to look for balanced translocation). Otherwise, first-line testing for chromosome abnormalities is a microarray.
8. **Fluorescence in situ hybridization (FISH):** Only rarely indicated.

D. Specific Syndromes

This section is not comprehensive; it covers a few common genetic syndromes. More complete information can be found in the following references: Jones[14], Hall and colleagues[13], http://omim.org, www.genereviews.org:

1. **Trisomy 21**[16]:
a. Epidemiology: Occurs in 1/700–1/1000 newborns (risk increases with advanced maternal age).
b. Most commonly due to maternal nondisjunction in 95%; few cases due to translocation (3%–4%).
c. Presentation: Hypotonia, small brachycephalic head, epicanthic folds, flat nasal bridge, upward-slanting palpebral fissures, Brushfield spots, small mouth, small ears, excessive skin at the nape of the neck, single transverse palmar (simian) crease, short fifth finger with clinodactyly, wide gap between the first and second toes, intellectual disability with a range from mild to severe, increased risk of congenital heart defects (50%), leukemia (<1%), hearing loss (75%), otitis media (50%–70%), Hirschsprung disease (<1%), gastrointestinal atresias (12%), eye disease (60%) including cataracts (15%) and severe refractive errors (50%), acquired hip dislocation (6%), obstructive sleep apnea (50%–75%), and thyroid disease (15%).
d. Diagnostic evaluation: First trimester screening with follow-up testing if increased risk; follow-up testing available includes noninvasive prenatal diagnosis with fetal circulating DNA in maternal serum; definitive results available through karyotype analysis at birth or prenatally by amniocentesis or chorionic villi sampling (CVS).
e. Health supervision: Guideline available at http://pediatrics.aappublications.org/content/107/2/442.full.html:

(1) Neonatal: Ophthalmologic evaluation for cataracts, hearing screen, echocardiogram, obtain complete blood count due to increased risk for leukemia vs. transient myeloproliferative disorder, consider ear-nose-throat (ENT) evaluation for any airway concerns, check thyroid studies or confirm normal on newborn screen (1% congenital hypothyroidism), early intervention services.

(2) Infancy: Risk of serous otitis media 50%–70%, may need referral to ENT if any concern for hearing loss, behavioral audiogram in all children at 1 year, evaluate vision at each visit, refer at 6 months for pediatric ophthalmology visit, thyroid studies at 6 and 12 months and then annually, early intervention services.

(3) Early childhood: Consider referral to ENT and audiology if concern for hearing loss, subjective evaluation of vision at each visit, referral to pediatric ophthalmology every 2 years, cervical spine roentgenogram at age 3 to 5 years to look for atlantoaxial instability or subluxation, thyroid screening annually, monitor for signs of obstructive sleep apnea.

(4) Late childhood: Audiologic and ophthalmologic exams annually, thyroid studies annually.

(5) Adolescence: Perform CBC and thyroid function tests, annual audiologic and ophthalmologic examinations.

2. **Trisomy 18**[14]:

a. Epidemiology: 1/5000 newborns (increased risk with advanced maternal age).

b. Most commonly due to maternal nondisjunction.

c. Features: Intrauterine growth restriction and polyhydramnios, small for gestational age at birth, clenched hands with overlapping fingers, hypoplastic nails, short sternum, prominent occiput, low-set and structurally abnormal ears, micrognathia, rocker-bottom feet, congenital heart disease, cystic and horseshoe kidneys, failure to thrive, seizures, hypertonia, significant developmental and cognitive impairments.

d. Diagnosis: First trimester screening with follow-up testing if increased risk; follow-up testing available includes noninvasive prenatal diagnosis with fetal circulating DNA in maternal serum; definitive results available through karyotype analysis at birth or prenatally by amniocentesis or chorionic villi sampling (CVS); approximately 90% will have abnormalities on ultrasound.

e. Previously thought to be invariably lethal in the neonatal period, now approximately 5%–10% make it to their first birthday.

3. **Trisomy 13**[14]:

a. Epidemiology: 1/5000 newborns (increased risk with advanced maternal age).

b. Features: Defects of forebrain development (holoprosencephaly), severe developmental disability, low-set malformed ears, cleft lip and palate, microphthalmia, scalp defects, aplasia cutis congenita, polydactyly (most frequently of the postaxial type), narrow hyperconvex nails, apneic spells, cryptorchidism, congenital heart defects.

c. Diagnosis: First-trimester screening with follow-up testing if increased risk. Available follow-up testing includes noninvasive prenatal diagnosis with fetal circulating DNA in maternal serum; definitive results available through karyotype analysis at birth or prenatally by amniocentesis or chorionic villi sampling (CVS); about 90% will have abnormalities on ultrasound.

d. Roughly 5% of pregnancies with trisomy 13 survive to birth, and only 5% of those survive the first 6 months of life.

4. **Turner syndrome (45,X)**[14,17]:

a. Epidemiology: 1/2000–5000 newborns (99% spontaneously abort).

b. Features: Slight intrauterine growth restriction, slow growth during infancy and childhood, gonadal dysgenesis and lack of a pubertal growth spurt. Intelligence is usually normal, but patients are at risk for cognitive, behavioral, and social impairments. Other features are lymphedema, micrognathia, dental crowding, deep-set and hyperconvex nails, broad chest with hypoplastic or inverted nipples, tibial exostosis, hearing loss, renal abnormalities, webbed neck, hypertension, congenital heart disease (most commony bicuspid aortic valve and coarctation of the aorta), and hypothyroidism.

c. Diagnosis: Karyotype

d. Health supervision: Guidelines available at http://pediatrics.aappublicati ons.org/content/111/3/692.full.html:

(1) Endocrine: Growth hormone usually initiated when height < 5th percentile (refer early to pediatric endocrinology), monitor for obesity and glucose intolerance, monitor for thyroid dysfunction.

(2) Cardiology: Baseline echocardiogram, close cardiac follow-up to monitor for aortic dilatation, monitor for hypertension and manage aggressively.

(3) HEENT: Hearing examination and audiology referral, monitor for strabismus.

(4) Renal: Evaluate for renal abnormalities (most commonly a horse-shoe kidney).

(5) Orthopedic: Hip examinations in infancy because of increased risk of congenital developmental hip dysplasia; evaluate for development of scoliosis.

(6) Provide psychosocial support.

5. **Connective tissue diseases**[14,18,19]:

a. Examples: Marfan, Loeys-Dietz, familial thoracic aortic aneurysm disease, bicuspid aortic valve and aneurysm syndromes, Ehlers-Danlos, Sphrintzen-Goldberg, cutis laxa syndromes, arterial tortuosity syndrome, Stickler syndrome (description of each of these is beyond the scope of this chapter).

b. Marfan: Prevalence 1/5000–10,000; autosomal dominant. Diagnostic criteria incorporate information from family history, medical history, physical examination, slit lamp examination, echocardiography.

13

(1) Features:
  (a) Myopia, displacement of the lens from the center of the pupil (60%), bone overgrowth and joint laxity, extremities disproportionately long for size of trunk, pectus carinatum or excavatum, scoliosis, dilatation of the aorta at level of sinuses of Valsalva, predisposition to aortic tear and rupture, mitral valve prolapsed, enlargement of proximal pulmonary artery, pneumothorax
  (b) Physical examination: Scoring of systemic features based on evaluation of the literature available at http://www.marfan.org/marfan/4470/Diagnostic-Criteria----Scoring-of-Systemic-Features/
(2) Diagnosis confirmed by molecular genetic testing of fibrillin-1 gene (FBN1).
(3) Surveillance: Annual ophthalmologic examination; annual echocardiography unless aortic root diameter exceeds ≈ 4.5 cm in adults (rates of aortic dilation exceed ≈ 0.5 cm/yr) and significant aortic regurgitation is present, then valve-sparing surgery to replace the aortic root; intermittent surveillance of the entire aorta with computed tomography (CT) or magnetic resonance angiography (MRA) scans beginning in young adulthood. Avoid contact sports, competitive sports, isometric exercise, and overstimulation of the cardiovascular system.
(4) Treatment with β-blocker (atenolol) is current standard of care, but a large-scale trial is underway to see whether angiotensin-II type 1 receptor blocker (losartan) may be more effective.

6. **Neurofibromatosis type I (NF1)**[14,20]:
a. Epidemiology: 1/4000; autosomal dominant
b. Diagnosis:
  (1) Two or more of the following: Six or more café au lait macules over 5 mm in greatest diameter in prepubertal individuals and over 15 mm greatest diameter in postpubertal individuals, two or more neurofibromas of any type or one plexiform neurofibroma, freckling in the axillary or inguinal regions, optic glioma, two or more Lisch nodules, a distinctive osseous lesion (e.g., sphenoid dysplasia, tibial pseudarthrosis), a first-degree relative (parent, sibling, offspring) with NF1 as defined by the above criteria
  (2) Other features: Short stature, macrocephaly, progressive scoliosis
  (3) Diagnostic evaluation: Molecular confirmation by NF1 gene testing
c. Surveillance: Annual genetics examination, annual ophthalmologic examination, developmental assessment of children, regular blood pressure monitoring, MRI for follow-up of clinically symptomatic tumors

7. **22q11 syndrome (velocardiofacial syndrome [VCFS], DiGeorge syndrome)**[15]:
a. Epidemiology: 1/4000–6000; autosomal dominant.
b. Features: Congenital heart disease (tetralogy of Fallot, interrupted aortic arch, ventricular septal defect, and truncus arteriosus most common), palatal abnormalities (velopharyngeal incompetence [VPI], cleft palate),

characteristic facial features, learning difficulties, immune deficiency (70%), hypocalcemia (50%), significant feeding problems (30%), renal anomalies (37%), hearing loss (both conductive and sensorineural), laryngotracheoesophageal anomalies, growth hormone deficiency, autoimmune disorders, seizures (without hypocalcemia), and skeletal abnormalities.

c. Diagnostic evaluation: SNP array is the gold standard; FISH is no longer recommended as first line. Assessments should include serum calcium, absolute lymphocyte count, B- and T-cell subsets, renal ultrasound, chest x-ray, cardiac examination, and echocardiogram.

8. **Fragile X syndrome**[21]:
a. Epidemiology: 1/4000 males and 1/8000 females; X-linked
b. Features:
   (1) Male: Mild to moderate intellectual disability, cluttered speech, autism, macrocephaly, large ears, prognathism, postpubertal macroorchidism, tall stature, seizures, tremor, ataxia
   (2) Female: A third are intellectually disabled; premature ovarian failure, tremor, ataxia
c. Diagnostic evaluation: Molecular genetic testing of the FMR1 gene; caused by expansion of the CGG nucleotide repeat in the FMR1 gene

REFERENCES

1. McMillan JA, Feigin RD, DeAngelis C. *Oski's Pediatrics: Principles and Practice.* 4th ed. Philadelphia: Lippincott Williams & Wilkins, 2006.
2. Seidel HM, Rosenstein B, Pathak A, et al. *Primary Care of the Newborn.* 4th ed. St Louis: Mosby, 2006.
3. Kaye CI. Committee on Genetics. Introduction to the newborn screening fact sheets. *Pediatrics.* 2006;118:1304-1312.
4. Burton BK. Inborn errors of metabolism in infancy: a guide to diagnosis. *Pediatrics.* 1998;102:E69.
5. Hoffman GF, Zschocke J, Nyhan W. *Inherited Metabolic Diseases: A Clinical Approach.* Heidelberg: Springer, 2010.
6. Saudubray JM, van den Berghe G, Walter JH. *Inborn Metabolic Diseases: Diagnosis and Treatment.* 5th ed. Heidelberg: Springer, 2012.
7. Scriver CR, Sly WS, Childs B, et al. *The Metabolic and Molecular Bases of Inherited Disease.* 8th ed New York: McGraw-Hill Professional, 2001.
8. Hoe FM. Hypoglycemia in infants and children. *Adv Pediatr.* 2008;55:367-384.
9. Chinnery PF. Mitochondrial Disease Overview; 2000. Last update 2010. GeneReviews Available at http://www.ncbi.nlm.nih.gov/books/NBK1224/.
10. Staretz-Chacham O, Lang TC. Lysosomal storage diseases in the newborn. *Pediatrics.* 2009;1:191-207.
11. Peredo DE, Hannibal MC. The floppy infant: evaluation of hypotonia. *Pediatr Rev.* 2009;30:e66-e76.
12. Lisi EC, Cohn RD. Genetic evaluation of the pediatric patient with hypotonia: perspective from a hypotonia specialty clinic and review of the literature. *Dev Med Child Neurol.* 2011;53:586-599.
13. Hall JG, Allanson J, Gripp K, et al. *Handbook of Physical Measurements.* 2nd ed. Oxford, UK: Oxford University Press, 2007.
14. Jones KL. *Smith's Recognizable Patterns of Human Malformation.* 6th ed. Philadelphia: Saunders, 2006.

13

15. Hennekam R, Allanson J, Krantz I. *Gorlin's Syndromes of the Head and Neck.* 5th ed. New York: Oxford University Press, 2010.

16. Bull Mj. Committee on Genetics. Health supervision for children with Down syndrome. *Pediatrics.* 2011;128:393-406.

17. Frias JL, Davenport ML. Committee on Genetics and Section on Endocrinology. Health supervision for children with Turner syndrome. *Pediatrics.* 2003;111: 692-702; reaffirmed 2009.

18. Loeys BL, Dietz HC, Braverman AC, et al. The revised Ghent nosology for the Marfan syndrome. *J Med Genet.* 2010;47:476-485. doi: 10.1136/jmg.2009.072785.

19. American Academy of Pediatrics, Committee on Genetics. Health supervision for children with Marfan syndrome. *Pediatrics.* 1996;98:978-982.

20. Hersh JH. Health supervision for children with neurofibromatosis. *Pediatrics.* 2008;121:633-642.

21. American Academy of Pediatrics, Committee on Genetics. Health supervision for children with Fragile X syndrome. *Pediatrics.* 2011;127:994-1006.

Chapter 14

Hematology

Radha Gajjar, MD, and Elizabeth Jalazo, MD

I. ANEMIA

A. General Evaluation

Anemia is defined as a reduction in hemoglobin (Hb) two standard deviations below the mean, based on age-specific norms (Table 14-1 and Fig. 14-1). Evaluation should include:

1. **Complete history,** including nutrition, menstruation, ethnicity, fatigue, pica, medication exposure, growth and development, blood loss, hyperbilirubinemia and family history of anemia, splenectomy, or cholecystectomy.

2. **Physical examination,** including evaluation of pallor, tachycardia, cardiac murmur, jaundice, hepatosplenomegaly, glossitis, tachypnea, koilonychia, angular cheilitis or signs of systemic illness.

3. **Initial laboratory tests** including complete blood cell count (CBC) with red blood cell (RBC) indices (mean corpuscular volume [MCV], mean corpuscular hemoglobin [MCH], red cell distribution width [RDW]), reticulocyte count, stool for occult blood, urinalysis, and serum bilirubin. Complete evaluation always includes a peripheral blood smear.

B. Diagnosis

Anemias may be categorized as macrocytic, microcytic, or normocytic. Table 14-2 gives an approach to diagnosis based on RBC production as measured by reticulocyte count and cell size. Note that normal ranges for Hb and MCV are age dependent.

C. Evaluation of Specific Causes of Anemia

1. **Iron-deficiency anemia:** Hypochromic/microcytic anemia with a low reticulocyte count and an elevated RDW.

a. Serum ferritin reflects total body iron stores after age 6 months and is the first value to fall in iron deficiency; may be falsely elevated with inflammation or infection.

b. Other indicators: Low serum iron, elevated total iron-binding capacity (TIBC), low mean corpuscular hemoglobin concentration (MCHC), elevated transferrin receptor level, and low reticulocyte Hb content.

c. Iron therapy should result in an increased reticulocyte count in 2–3 days and an increase in hematocrit (HCT) after 1–4 weeks of therapy. Iron stores are generally repleted after 3 months of therapy.

d. Mentzer index (MCV/RBC): Index >13.5 suggests iron deficiency; expect elevated RDW. Mentzer index <11.5 suggests thalassemia minor; expect low/normal RDW.

14

TABLE 14-1

AGE-SPECIFIC BLOOD CELL INDICES

Age	Hb (g/dL)*	HCT (%)*	MCV (fL)*	MCHC (g/dL RBC)*	Reticulocytes	WBCs (×10³/mL)†	Platelets (10³/mL)†
26–30 wk gestation‡	13.4 (11)	41.5 (34.9)	118.2 (106.7)	37.9 (30.6)	—	4.4 (2.7)	254 (180–327)
28 wk	14.5	45	120	31.0	(5–10)	—	275
32 wk	15.0	47	118	32.0	(3–10)	—	290
Term§ (cord)	16.5 (13.5)	51 (42)	108 (98)	33.0 (30.0)	(3–7)	18.1 (9–30)||	290
1–3 day	18.5 (14.5)	56 (45)	108 (95)	33.0 (29.0)	(1.8–4.6)	18.9 (9.4–34)	192
2 wk	16.6 (13.4)	53 (41)	105 (88)	31.4 (28.1)		11.4 (5–20)	252
1 mo	13.9 (10.7)	44 (33)	101 (91)	31.8 (28.1)	(0.1–1.7)	10.8 (4–19.5)	—
2 mo	11.2 (9.4)	35 (28)	95 (84)	31.8 (28.3)			—
6 mo	12.6 (11.1)	36 (31)	76 (68)	35.0 (32.7)	(0.7–2.3)	11.9 (6–17.5)	—
6 mo–2 yr	12.0 (10.5)	36 (33)	78 (70)	33.0 (30.0)		10.6 (6–17)	(150–350)
2–6 yr	12.5 (11.5)	37 (34)	81 (75)	34.0 (31.0)	(0.5–1.0)	8.5 (5–15.5)	(150–350)
6–12 yr	13.5 (11.5)	40 (35)	86 (77)	34.0 (31.0)	(0.5–1.0)	8.1 (4.5–13.5)	(150–350)
12–18 YR							
Male	14.5 (13)	43 (36)	88 (78)	34.0 (31.0)	(0.5–1.0)	7.8 (4.5–13.5)	(150–350)
Female	14.0 (12)	41 (37)	90 (78)	34.0 (31.0)	(0.5–1.0)	7.8 (4.5–13.5)	(150–350)
ADULT							
Male	15.5 (13.5)	47 (41)	90 (80)	34.0 (31.0)	(0.8–2.5)	7.4 (4.5–11)	(150–350)
Female	14.0 (12)	41 (36)	90 (80)	34.0 (31.0)	(0.8–4.1)	7.4 (4.5–11)	(150–350)

*Data are mean (− 2 SD).
†data are mean (± 2 SD).
‡Values are from fetal samplings.
§1 mo, capillary hemoglobin exceeds venous: 1 hr: 3.6-g difference; 5 day: 2.2-g difference; 3 wk: 1.1-g difference.
||Mean (95% confidence limits).

Hb, Hemoglobin; HCT, hematocrit; MCHC, mean cell hemoglobin concentration; MCV, mean corpuscular volume; RBC, red blood cell; WBC, white blood cell.

Data from Forestier F, Daffos F, Galacteros F, et al. Hematologic values between 18 and 30 normal fetuses between 18 and 30 weeks of gestation. *Pediatr Res.* 1986;20:342; Oski FA, Naiman JL. *Hematological Problems in the Newborn Infant.* Philadelphia: WB Saunders;1982; Nathan D, Oski FA. *Hematology of Infancy and Childhood.* Philadelphia: WB Saunders; 1998; Matoth Y, Zaizor K, Varsano I, et al. Postnatal changes in some red cell parameters. *Acta Paediar Scand.* 1971;60:317; and Wintrobe MM. *Clinical Hematology.* Baltimore: Williams & Wilkins; 1999.

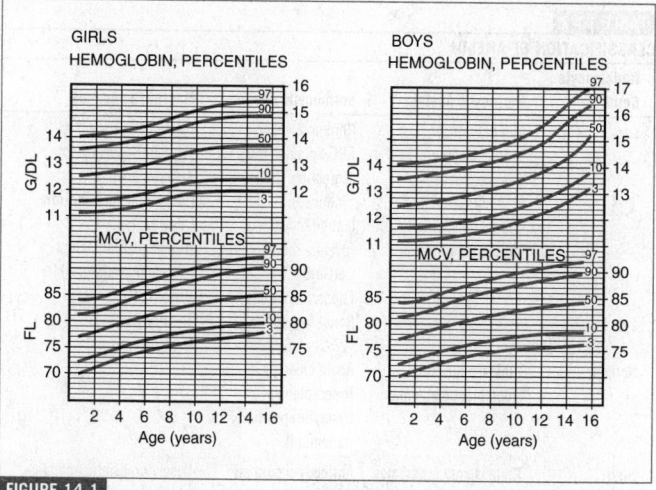

FIGURE 14-1

Hemoglobin and mean corpuscular volume (MCV) by age and gender. *(Data from Dallman PR, Siimes MA. Percentile curves for hemoglobin and red cell volume in infancy and childhood.* J Pediatr. *1979;94:26.)*

2. **Hemolytic anemia:** Rapid RBC turnover. Etiologies: Congenital membranopathies, hemoglobinopathies, enzymopathies, metabolic defects, and immune-mediated destruction. Useful studies include:
a. Reticulocyte count: Usually elevated; indicates increased production of RBCs to compensate for increased destruction. Corrected reticulocyte count (CRC) accounts for differences in HCT and is an indicator of erythropoietic activity. CRC >1.5 suggests increased RBC production secondary to hemolysis or blood loss.

$$CRC = \% \text{ Reticulocytes} \times \text{Patient HCT/Normal HCT}$$

b. Plasma aspartate aminotransferase (AST) and lactate dehydrogenase (LDH): Increased from release of intracellular enzymes. Serum LDH levels are significantly elevated in intravascular hemolysis and mildly elevated in extravascular hemolysis.
c. Haptoglobin: Binds free Hb; decreased with intravascular and extravascular hemolysis. Can also be decreased in patients with liver dysfunction secondary to decreased hepatic synthesis and in neonates.
d. Direct Coombs test: Tests for presence of antibody or complement on patient RBCs. May be falsely negative if affected cells have already been destroyed or antibody titer is low.
e. Indirect Coombs test: Tests for free autoantibody in patient's serum after RBC antibody binding sites are saturated. Positive indirect test with negative direct test is typical of alloimmune sensitization (e.g., transfusion reaction).

14

TABLE 14-2

CLASSIFICATION OF ANEMIA

Reticulocyte Count	Microcytic Anemia	Normocytic Anemia	Macrocytic Anemia
Low	Iron deficiency Lead poisoning Chronic disease Aluminum toxicity Copper deficiency Protein malnutrition	Chronic disease RBC aplasia (TEC, infection, drug induced) Malignancy Juvenile rheumatoid arthritis Endocrinopathies Renal failure	Folate deficiency Vitamin B_{12} deficiency Aplastic anemia Congenital bone marrow dysfunction (Diamond-Blackfan or Fanconi syndromes) Drug-induced Trisomy 21 Hypothyroidism
Normal	Thalassemia trait Sideroblastic anemia	Acute bleeding Hypersplenism Dyserythropoietic anemia II	—
High	Thalassemia syndromes Hemoglobin C disorders	Antibody-mediated hemolysis Hypersplenism Microangiopathy (HUS, TTP, DIC, Kasabach-Merritt) Membranopathies (spherocytosis, ellipto-cytosis) Enzyme disorders (G6PD, pyruvate kinase) Hemoglobinopathies	Dyserythropoietic anemia I, III Active hemolysis

DIC, Disseminated intravascular coagulation; G6PD, glucose-6–phosphate dehydrogenase; HUS, hemolytic-uremic syndrome; RBC, red blood cell; TEC, transient erythroblastopenia of childhood; TTP, thrombotic thrombocytopenic purpura.

Data from Nathan D, Oski FA. *Hematology of Infancy and Childhood*, 6th ed. Philadelphia: WB Saunders, 2003.

f. Osmotic fragility test: Useful in diagnosis of hereditary spherocytosis. Can also be positive in ABO incompatibility, autoimmune hemolytic anemia, or anytime spherocytes are present.

g. Glucose-6–phosphate dehydrogenase (G6PD) assay: Quantitative test to diagnose G6PD deficiency, an X-linked disorder affecting 10%–14% of African American males. May be normal immediately after a hemolytic episode because older, more enzyme-deficient cells have been lysed. For a comprehensive list of oxidizing drugs, go to: http://g6pddeficiency.org/index.php?cmd=contraindicated.

h. Heinz body preparation: detects precipitated Hb within RBCs; present in unstable hemoglobinopathies and enzymopathies during oxidative stress (e.g., G6PD deficiency).

3. **Red cell aplasia:** variable cell size, low reticulocyte count, variable platelet and white blood cell (WBC) counts. Bone marrow aspiration evaluates RBC precursors in the marrow to look for marrow dysfunction, neoplasm, or specific signs of infection.

a. Acquired aplasias:

   (1) Infectious causes: parvovirus in children with rapid RBC turnover (infects RBC precursors), Epstein-Barr virus (EBV), cytomegalovirus (CMV), human herpesvirus type 6, or human immunodeficiency virus (HIV).

   (2) Transient erythroblastopenia of childhood (TEC): Occurs from age 6 months to 4 years, with >80% of cases presenting after age 1 year with a normal or slightly low MCV and low reticulocyte count. Spontaneous recovery usually occurs within 4–8 weeks.

   (3) Exposures include radiation and various drugs and chemicals.

b. Congenital aplasias: Typically macrocytic anemias

   (1) Fanconi anemia: Autosomal recessive disorder, usually presents before 10 years of age; may present with pancytopenia. Patients may have thumb abnormalities, renal anomalies, microcephaly, or short stature. Chromosomal fragility studies can be diagnostic.

   (2) Diamond-Blackfan anemia: Autosomal recessive pure RBC aplasia; presents in the first year of life. Associated with congenital anomalies in 30%-47%[12] of cases, including triphalangeal thumb, short stature, and cleft lip.

c. Aplastic anemia: Idiopathic bone marrow failure, usually macrocytic.

4. **Physiologic anemia of infancy (physiologic nadir):** Decrease in Hb until oxygen needs exceed oxygen delivery, usually at Hb of 9–11 mg/dL. Normally occurs at age 8–12 weeks for full-term infants and age 3–6 weeks for preterm infants.

5. **Anemia of chronic inflammation:** usually normocytic with normal to low reticulocyte count. Iron studies reveal low iron, TIBC, and transferrin and elevated ferritin.

II. HEMOGLOBINOPATHIES

A. Hemoglobin Electrophoresis

Involves separation of Hb variants based on molecular charge and size. All positive sickle preparations and solubility tests for sickle Hb (e.g., Sickledex) should be confirmed with electrophoresis or isoelectric focusing (component of mandatory newborn screening in many states). Table 14-3 outlines neonatal Hb electrophoresis patterns.

B. Sickle Cell Anemia

Caused by a genetic defect in β-globin; 8% of African Americans are carriers; 1 in 500 African Americans have sickle cell anemia.

TABLE 14-3

NEONATAL HEMOGLOBIN (Hb) ELECTROPHORESIS PATTERNS*

FA	Fetal Hb and adult normal Hb; the normal newborn pattern
FAV	Indicates presence of both HbF and HbA, but an anomalous band (V) is present that does not appear to be any of the common Hb variants.
FAS	Indicates fetal Hb, adult normal HbA, and HbS, consistent with benign sickle cell trait
FS	Fetal and sickle HbS without detectable adult normal HbA. Consistent with clinically significant homozygous sickle Hb genotype (S/S) or sickle β-thalassemia, with manifestations of sickle cell anemia during childhood.
FC†	Designates presence of HbC without adult normal HbA. Consistent with clinically significant homozygous HbC genotype (C/C), resulting in a mild hematologic disorder presenting during childhood.
FSC	HbS and HbC present. This heterozygous condition could lead to manifestations of sickle cell disease during childhood.
FAC	HbC and adult normal HbA present, consistent with benign HbC trait
FSA	Heterozygous HbS/β-thalassemia, a clinically significant sickling disorder
F†	Fetal HbF is present without adult normal HbA. May indicate delayed appearance of HbA but is also consistent with homozygous β-thalassemia major or homozygous hereditary persistence of fetal HbF.
FV†	Fetal HbF and an anomalous Hb variant (V) are present.
AF	May indicate prior blood transfusion. Submit another filter paper blood specimen when infant is 4 mo of age, at which time the transfused blood cells should have been cleared.

*Hemoglobin variants are reported in order of decreasing abundance; for example, FA indicates more fetal than adult hemoglobin.
†Repeat blood specimen should be submitted to confirm original interpretation.
NOTE: HbA: $\alpha_2\beta_2$; HbF: $\alpha_2\gamma_2$; HbA$_2$: $\alpha_2\delta_2$.

1. **Diagnosis:** Often made on newborn screen with Hb electrophoresis. The sickle preparation and Sickledex are rapid tests that are positive in all sickle hemoglobinopathies. False-negative test results may be seen in neonates and other patients with a high percentage of fetal Hb.
2. **Complications** (Table 14-4): A hematologist should be consulted.
3. **Health maintenance**[1,2]: Ongoing consultation and clinical involvement with a pediatric hematologist and/or sickle cell program are essential (Table 14-5).
4. **Hemoglobin electrophoresis (outside neonatal period):** hemoglobin SF, SCF, SAF—other Hb combinations may sickle.

C. Thalassemias

Defects in α- or β-globin production. The predominant adult hemoglobin is HbA ($\alpha_2\beta_2$), a tetramer composed of two α and two β chains. The α-Globin production is dependent on four genes, and β-globin production is dependent on two genes. Imbalance in production of globin chains leads to precipitation of excess chains, causing ineffective erythropoiesis and shortened survival of mature RBCs.

1. **α-Thalassemias:**
a. Silent carriers (α–/αα): not anemic, childhood and adult hemoglobin electrophoresis usually normal.

TABLE 14-4

SICKLE CELL DISEASE COMPLICATIONS

Complication	Evaluation	Treatment
Fever (T ≥38.5°C)	History and physical CBC with differential Reticulocyte count Blood cultures Chest x-ray Other cultures as indicated	IV antibiotics (third-generation cephalosporin, other antibiotics as indicated, especially if penicillin-resistant pneumococcus suspected) Admit if ill appearing, <3 yr of age, concerning lab results, or complications. Some centers use antibiotics with a long half-life and reevaluate in 24 hr as an outpatient.
Vaso-occlusive crisis Children <2 yr, dactylitis Children >2 yr, unifocal or multifocal pain	History and physical CBC with differential Reticulocyte count Type and screen	Oral analgesics as an outpatient, as tolerated IV analgesics and IV fluids if outpatient therapy fails (parenteral narcotics in form of PCA and parenteral NSAIDs, usually in combination) Aggressive early treatment of pain is essential.
Acute chest syndrome New pulmonary infiltrate with fever, cough, chest pain, tachypnea, dyspnea, or hypoxia	History and physical CBC with differential Reticulocyte count Blood cultures Chest x-ray Type and screen	Admit O_2, incentive spirometry, bronchodilators IV antibiotics (third-generation cephalosporin and macrolide) Analgesia, IV fluids Simple transfusion or partial exchange for moderately severe illness; double the packed cell volume exchange transfusion for severe or rapidly progressing illness. High-dose dexamethasone controversial (risk of readmission for pain or other SCD-related issues)[7]
Splenic sequestration Acutely enlarged spleen and Hb level ≥2 g/dL below patient's baseline	History and physical CBC Reticulocyte count Type and hold	Serial abdominal exams IV fluids and fluid resuscitation as necessary RBC transfusion or, in severe cases, exchange transfusion for cardiovascular compromise and Hb <4.5 g/dL. (Autotransfusion may occur with recovery, leading to increased Hb and CHF. Transfuse cautiously.)

Continued

14

TABLE 14-4

SICKLE CELL DISEASE COMPLICATIONS (Continued)

Complication	Evaluation	Treatment
Aplastic crisis Acute illness with Hb below patient's baseline and low reticulocyte count May follow viral illnesses, especially parvovirus B19	History and physical CBC with differential Reticulocyte count Type and screen Parvovirus serology and polymerase chain reaction	Admit IV fluids PRBCs for symptomatic anemia Isolation to protect susceptible individuals and women of childbearing age until parvovirus excluded
Other complications Priapism, CVA, TIA, gallbladder disease, avascular necrosis, hyphema*		

*Hyphema in a patient with sickle cell trait is an ophthalmologic emergency

NOTE: CVA requires emergency transfusion guided by a hematologist and a neurologist experienced with sickle cell disease. Exchange transfusion preferable to simple transfusion if possible.[8]

Abbreviations: CBC, Complete blood cell count; CHF, congestive heart failure; CVA, cerebrovascular accident; Hb, hemoglobin; IV, intravenous; NSAIDs, nonsteroidal anti-inflammatory drugs; PCA, patient-controlled analgesia; PRBCs, packed red blood cells; RBC, red blood cells; SCD, sickle cell disease; T, temperature; TIA, transient ischemic attack.

TABLE 14-5

SICKLE CELL DISEASE HEALTH MAINTENANCE

IMMUNIZATIONS	Maintenance
Pneumococcal vaccine	Vaccinate with 13-valent conjugate vaccine as per routine childhood schedule, 23-valent polysaccharide vaccine at age 2, booster at age 5.
Meningococcal vaccine	Give at age 2 and every 5 yr thereafter.
Influenza vaccine	Vaccinate yearly beginning at age 6 mo.
MEDICATIONS	
PCN	Begin as soon as SCD diagnosis made (125 mg BID; increase dose to 250 mg BID at age 3*).
Folic acid	Consider supplementation, start by age 1.
Hydroxyurea	Consider with frequent crises or in severe disease.†
IMAGING	
Transcranial Doppler (TCD)	Perform annually from ages 2 to 16 to evaluate for increased risk of cerebrovascular accident (CVA).
OTHER	
Ophthalmology	Perform annually from age 10 to evaluate for sickle retinopathy.
Growth and development, school/social issues, counseling regarding fevers	Review closely at all visits.

*Prophylaxis may be discontinued by age 5 if patient has had no prior severe pneumococcal infections or splenectomy and has documented pneumococcal vaccinations, including second 23-valent vaccination. Practice patterns vary. Some continue penicillin indefinitely.

†Increases levels of fetal Hb and decreases HbS polymerization in cells. Has been shown to significantly decrease episodes of vaso-occlusive crises, dactylitis, acute chest syndrome, number of transfusions, and hospitalizations.[9,13] May decrease mortality in adults.

PCN, Penicillin; SCD, sickle cell disease.

b. α-Thalassemia trait (α–/α–) or (αα/––): Causes mild microcytic anemia, childhood and adult hemoglobin electrophoresis usually normal. Hb Barts can be seen in infancy (e.g., on state newborn screens) in patients with α-thalassemia trait.

c. HbH disease (β_4) (α–/––): Causes moderately severe anemia.

d. Hb Bart/hydrops fetalis (––/––): Hb Bart (γ_4) cannot deliver oxygen; usually fatal.

2. **β-Thalassemia:** Found throughout the Mediterranean, Middle East, India, and Southeast Asia. Ineffective erythropoiesis is more severe in β-thalassemia than α-thalassemia because excess α chains are more unstable than β chains. Adult hemoglobin electrophoresis with decreased hemoglobin A, increased hemoglobin A_2, and increased hemoglobin F.

a. Thalassemia trait/thalassemia minor (β/β+) or (β/β0): Usually asymptomatic, with microcytosis out of proportion to anemia, sometimes with erythrocytosis.

b. Thalassemia intermedia (β+/β+): Presents at about age 2 years with moderate compensated anemia that may become symptomatic, leading to heart failure, pulmonary hypertension, splenomegaly, and bony expansion, usually in second or third decade of life.

c. Thalassemia major/Cooley's anemia (β0/β0, β+/β0, or β+/β+): Presence of anemia within first 6 months of life, with hepatosplenomegaly and progressive bone marrow expansion that may lead to frontal bossing, maxillary hyperplasia, and other skeletal deformities. Regular transfusions required to avoid anemia.

III. NEUTROPENIA

An absolute neutrophil count (ANC) <1500/µL, although neutrophil counts vary with age (Table 14-6). Severe neutropenia is defined as an ANC <500/µL. Children with significant neutropenia are at risk for bacterial and fungal infections. Granulocyte colony-stimulating factor may be indicated. Transient neutropenia secondary to viral illness rarely causes significant morbidity. Autoimmune neutropenia is a common cause of neutropenia in children 6 mo–6 yr. Testing for antineutrophil antibodies is indicated in this age group and may obviate the need for more extensive workup. For management of fever and neutropenia in oncology patients, see Chapter 22, Figure 22-1. Box 14-1 lists causes.

IV. THROMBOCYTOPENIA

A. Definition

Platelet count <150,000/µL. Clinically significant bleeding is unlikely with platelet counts >20,000/µL in the absence of other complicating factors.

B. Causes of Thrombocytopenia

1. **Idiopathic thrombocytopenic purpura (ITP):** A diagnosis of exclusion; can be acute or chronic. WBC count, Hb levels, and peripheral blood smear are normal. Many require no therapy, and indications for treatment of patients without significant bleeding are not well established.

TABLE 14-6

AGE-SPECIFIC LEUKOCYTE DIFFERENTIAL

Age	Total Leukocytes* Mean (range)	Neutrophils† Mean (range)	%	Lymphocytes Mean (range)	%	Monocytes Mean	%	Eosinophils Mean	%
Birth	18.1 (9–30)	11 (6–26)	61	5.5 (2–11)	31	1.1	6	0.4	2
12 hr	22.8 (13–38)	15.5 (6–28)	68	5.5 (2–11)	24	1.2	5	0.5	2
24 hr	18.9 (9.4–34)	11.5 (5–21)	61	5.8 (2–11.5)	31	1.1	6	0.5	2
1 wk	12.2 (5–21)	5.5 (1.5–10)	45	5.0 (2–17)	41	1.1	9	0.5	4
2 wk	11.4 (5–20)	4.5 (1–9.5)	40	5.5 (2–17)	48	1.0	9	0.4	3
1 mo	10.8 (5–19.5)	3.8 (1–8.5)	35	6.0 (2.5–16.5)	56	0.7	7	0.3	3
6 mo	11.9 (6–17.5)	3.8 (1–8.5)	32	7.3 (4–13.5)	61	0.6	5	0.3	3
1 yr	11.4 (6–17.5)	3.5 (1.5–8.5)	31	7.0 (4–10.5)	61	0.6	5	0.3	3
2 yr	10.6 (6–17)	3.5 (1.5–8.5)	33	6.3 (3–9.5)	59	0.5	5	0.3	3
4 yr	9.1 (5.5–15.5)	3.8 (1.5–8.5)	42	4.5 (2–8)	50	0.5	5	0.3	3
6 yr	8.5 (5–14.5)	4.3 (1.5–8)	51	3.5 (1.5–7)	42	0.4	5	0.2	3
8 yr	8.3 (4.5–13.5)	4.4 (1.5–8)	53	3.3 (1.5–6.8)	39	0.4	4	0.2	2
10 yr	8.1 (4.5–13.5)	4.4 (1.5–8.5)	54	3.1 (1.5–6.5)	38	0.4	4	0.2	2
16 yr	7.8 (4.5–13.0)	4.4 (1.8–8)	57	2.8 (1.2–5.2)	35	0.4	5	0.2	3
21 yr	7.4 (4.5–11.0)	4.4 (1.8–7.7)	59	2.5 (1–4.8)	34	0.3	4	0.2	3

*Numbers of leukocytes are $\times 10^3/\mu L$; ranges are estimates of 95% confidence limits; percents refer to differential counts.
†Neutrophils include band cells at all ages and a small number of metamyelocytes and myelocytes in the first few days of life.
Adapted from Cairo MS, Brauho F. Blood and blood-forming tissues. In: Randolph AM, ed. *Pediatrics.* 21st ed. New York: McGraw-Hill, 2003.

BOX 14-1

DIFFERENTIAL DIAGNOSIS OF CHILDHOOD NEUTROPENIA

ACQUIRED	CONGENITAL
Infection	Cyclic neutropenia
Immune-mediated	Severe congenital neutropenia
Chronic benign neutropenia of childhood	(e.g., Kostmann syndrome)
	Shwachman-Diamond syndrome
Hypersplenism	Fanconi anemia
Vitamin B_{12}, folate, copper deficiency	Metabolic disorders (e.g., amino acidopa-thies, Barth syndrome, glycogen storage disorders)
Drugs or toxic substances	
Aplastic anemia	Osteopetrosis
Malignancies or preleukemic disorders	Neutropenia with pigmentation abnormalities (e.g., Chédiak-Higashi anomaly)
Ionizing radiation	

a. Treatment options:
   (1) Intravenous immune globulin (see Formulary for IVIG dosing)
   (2) Corticosteroids (i.e., prednisone 2 mg/kg/day or up to 30 mg/kg methylprednisolone for up to 3 days)
   (3) Anti-Rh (D) immune globulin (WinRho). Useful only in Rh-positive nonsplenectomized patients. Should not be used in patients with preexisting hemolysis or renal disease; monitor for signs of intravascular hemolysis after administration. Disseminated intravascular coagulation (DIC) has been reported. See package insert for blackbox warning and monitoring guidelines.
   (4) Consider rituximab in chronic cases.[3]
   (5) Splenectomy or chemotherapy may be considered in chronic cases. Platelet transfusions are not generally helpful but necessary in life-threatening bleeding.

2. **Neonatal thrombocytopenia:** May be caused by:
a. Decreased production: Results from aplastic disorders, congenital malignancy such as leukemia, and viral infections
b. Increased consumption: Usually result of DIC due to infection or asphyxia.
c. Immune mediated: Immunoglobulin (Ig)G or complement attach to platelets and cause destruction. Specific causes include preeclampsia, sepsis, maternal ITP, and platelet alloimmunization.

3. **Neonatal alloimmune thrombocytopenia (NAIT):** Transplacental maternal antibodies (usually against PLA-1 antigen/HPA-1a) cause fetal platelet destruction. If severe, a transfusion of maternal platelets will be more effective than random donor platelets in raising infant's platelet count.
a. Evaluation/diagnosis:
   (1) Check maternal platelet count and platelet-associated IgG. Mother's platelet count should be normal and platelet-associated IgG usually negative.
   (2) Absence of maternal PLA-1 antigen/HPA-1a or other specific antigens
   (3) Study of mother's or infant's plasma with a panel of known minor platelet antigens
   (4) Mixing study of maternal or neonatal plasma and paternal platelets.

4. **Causes of microangiopathic hemolytic anemia:** DIC, hemolytic-uremic syndrome/thrombotic thrombocytopenic purpura (HUS/TTP)
a. HUS/TTP: Characterized by the triad of microangiopathic hemolytic anemia, uremia, and thrombocytopenia. HUS is often triggered by bacterial enteritis, especially caused by *Escherichia coli* O157:H7, although there are a variety of causes. HUS does not typically include coagulation abnormalities like those seen in DIC. Avoid blood products in patients with HUS thought to be secondary to pneumococcal infection. TTP includes the triad of HUS in addition to fever and central nervous system (CNS) changes and is more common in older adolescents and adults.
b. DIC (see Box 14-5)

5. **Other causes of thrombocytopenia:** Infection causing marrow suppression, malignancy, HIV, drug-induced thrombocytopenia, marrow

infiltration, cavernous hemangiomas (Kasabach-Merritt syndrome), thrombocytopenia with absent radii syndrome (TAR), thrombosis, hypersplenism, and other rare inherited disorders (e.g., Wiskott-Aldrich, Paris-Trousseau, Noonan, and DiGeorge syndromes; myosin 9– associated megaplatelet disorders; chromosomal abnormalities).

V. COAGULATION (FIG. 14-2)

A. Tests of Coagulation

An incorrect anticoagulant-to-blood ratio will give inaccurate results. Table 14-7 lists normal hematologic values for coagulation testing.

1. **Activated partial thromboplastin time (aPTT):** Measures intrinsic system; requires factors V, VIII, IX, X, XI, XII, fibrinogen, and prothrombin. May be prolonged in heparin administration, hemophilia, von Willebrand disease (v WD), DIC, and in the presence of circulating inhibitors (e.g., lupus anticoagulants).

2. **Prothrombin time (PT):** Measures extrinsic pathway; requires factors V, VII, X, fibrinogen, and prothrombin. May be prolonged in warfarin

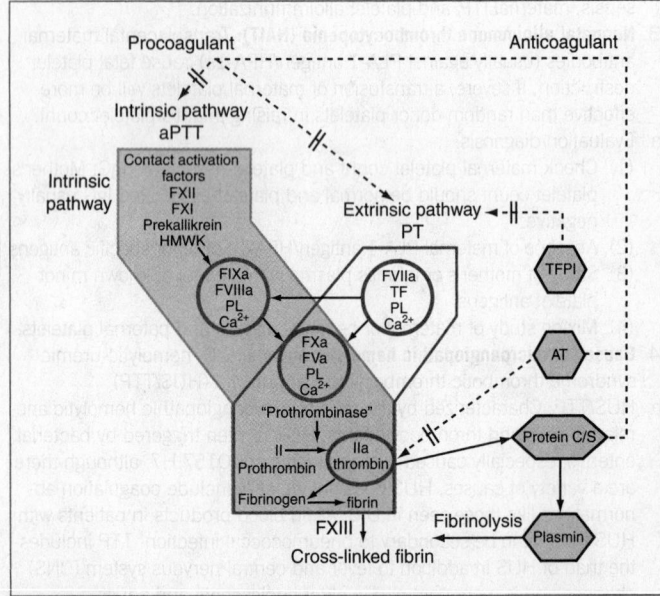

FIGURE 14-2

Coagulation cascade. AT, Antithrombin; F, factor; HMWK, high-molecular-weight kininogen; PL, phospholipid; TF, tissue factor; TFPI, tissue factor pathway inhibitor. (*Adaptation courtesy James Casella and Clifford Takemoto.*)

TABLE 14-7

AGE-SPECIFIC COAGULATION VALUES

Coagulation Test	Preterm Infant, (30–36 wk), Day of Life 1*	Term Infant, Day of Life 1	Day of Life 3	1 Month–1 yr	1–5 yr	6–10 yr	11–16 yr	Adult
PT (sec)	13.0 (10.6–16.2)	15.6 (14.4–16.4)	14.9 (13.5–16.4)	13.1 (11.5–15.3)	13.3 (12.1–14.5)	13.4 (11.7–15.1)	13.8 (12.7–16.1)	13.0 (11.5–14.5)
INR		1.26 (1.15–1.35)	1.20 (1.05–1.35)	1.00 (0.86–1.22)	1.03 (0.92–1.14)	1.04 (0.87–1.20)	1.08 (0.97–1.30)	1.00 (0.80–1.20)
aPTT (sec)†	53.6 (27.5–79.4)	38.7 (34.3–44.8)	36.3 (29.5–42.2)	39.3 (35.1–46.3)	37.7 (33.6–43.8)	37.3 (31.8–43.7)	39.5 (33.9–46.1)	33.2 (28.6–38.2)
Fibrinogen (g/L)	2.43 (1.50–3.73)	2.80 (1.92–3.74)	3.30 (2.83–4.01)	2.42 (0.82–3.83)	2.82 (1.62–4.01)	3.04 (1.99–4.09)	3.15 (2.12–4.33)	3.1 (1.9–4.3)
Bleeding time (min)*					6 (2.5–10)	7 (2.5–13)	5 (3–8)	4 (1–7)
Thrombin time (sec)	14 (11–17)	12 (10–16)*		17.1 (16.3–17.6)	17.5 (16.5–18.2)	17.1 (16.1–18.5)	16.9 (16.2–17.6)	16.6 (16.2–17.2)
Factor II (U/mL)	0.45 (0.20–0.77)	0.54 (0.41–0.69)	0.62 (0.50–0.73)	0.90 (0.62–1.03)	0.89 (0.70–1.09)	0.89 (0.67–1.10)	0.90 (0.61–1.07)	1.10 (0.78–1.38)
Factor V (U/mL)	0.88 (0.41–1.44)	0.81 (0.64–1.03)	1.22 (0.92–1.54)	1.13 (0.94–1.41)	0.97 (0.67–1.27)	0.99 (0.56–1.41)	0.89 (0.67–1.41)	1.18 (0.78–1.52)
Factor VII (U/mL)	0.67 (0.21–1.13)	0.70 (0.52–0.88)	0.86 (0.67–1.07)	1.28 (0.83–1.60)	1.11 (0.72–1.50)	1.13 (0.70–1.56)	1.18 (0.69–2.00)	1.29 (0.61–1.99)
Factor VIII (U/mL)	1.11 (0.50–2.13)	1.82 (1.05–3.29)	1.59 (0.83–2.74)	0.94 (0.54–1.45)	1.10 (0.36–1.85)	1.17 (0.52–1.82)	1.20 (0.59–2.00)	1.60 (0.52–2.90)
vWF (U/mL)*	1.36 (0.78–2.10)	1.53 (0.50–2.87)			0.82 (0.47–1.04)	0.95 (0.44–1.44)	1.00 (0.46–1.53)	0.92 (0.5–1.58)
Factor IX (U/mL)	0.35 (0.19–0.65)	0.48 (0.35–0.56)	0.72 (0.44–0.97)	0.71 (0.43–1.21)	0.85 (0.44–1.27)	0.96 (0.48–1.45)	1.11 (0.64–2.16)	1.30 (0.59–2.54)
Factor X (U/mL)	0.41 (0.11–0.71)	0.55 (0.46–0.67)	0.60 (0.46–0.75)	0.95 (0.77–1.22)	0.98 (0.72–1.25)	0.97 (0.68–1.25)	0.91 (0.53–1.22)	1.24 (0.96–1.71)
Factor XI (U/mL)	0.30 (0.08–0.52)	0.30 (0.07–0.41)	0.57 (0.24–0.79)	0.89 (0.62–1.25)	1.13 (0.65–1.62)	1.13 (0.65–1.62)	1.11 (0.65–1.39)	1.12 (0.67–1.96)
Factor XII (U/mL)	0.38 (0.10–0.66)	0.58 (0.43–0.80)	0.53 (0.14–0.80)	0.79 (0.20–1.35)	0.85 (0.36–1.35)	0.81 (0.26–1.37)	0.75 (0.14–1.17)	1.15 (0.35–2.07)
PK (U/mL)*	0.33 (0.09–0.57)	0.37 (0.18–0.69)			0.95 (0.65–1.30)	0.99 (0.66–1.31)	0.99 (0.53–1.45)	1.12 (0.62–1.62)
HMWK (U/mL)*	0.49 (0.09–0.89)	0.54 (0.06–1.02)			0.98 (0.64–1.32)	0.93 (0.60–1.30)	0.91 (0.63–1.19)	0.92 (0.50–1.36)
Factor XIIIa (U/mL)*	0.70 (0.32–1.08)	0.79 (0.27–1.31)			1.08 (0.72–1.43)	1.09 (0.65–1.51)	0.99 (0.57–1.40)	1.05 (0.55–1.55)
Factor XIIIs (U/mL)*	0.81 (0.35–1.27)	0.76 (0.30–1.22)			1.13 (0.69–1.56)	1.16 (0.77–1.54)	1.02 (0.60–1.43)	0.97 (0.57–1.37)
d-Dimer						0.26 (0.10–0.56)	0.27 (0.16–0.39)	0.18 (0.05–0.42)
FDPs*	1.47 (0.41–2.47)	1.34 (0.58–2.74)	0.22 (0.11–0.42)	0.25 (0.09–0.53)				Borderline titer = 1.25–1.50 Positive titer <1.50

Continued

14

TABLE 14-7

AGE-SPECIFIC COAGULATION VALUES (Continued)

Coagulation Test	Preterm Infant (30–36 wk), Day of Life 1*	Term Infant, Day of Life 1	Day of Life 3	1 Month–1 yr	1–5 yr	6–10 yr	11–16 yr	Adult
COAGULATION INHIBITORS								
ATIII (U/mL)*	0.38 (0.14–0.62)	0.63 (0.39–0.97)			1.11 (0.82–1.39)	1.11 (0.90–1.31)	1.05 (0.77–1.32)	1.0 (0.74–1.26)
α₂-M (U/mL)*	1.10 (0.56–1.82)	1.39 (0.95–1.83)			1.69 (1.14–2.23)	1.69 (1.28–2.09)	1.56 (0.98–2.12)	0.86 (0.52–1.20)
C1-Inh (U/mL)*	0.65 (0.31–0.99)	0.72 (0.36–1.08)			1.35 (0.85–1.83)	1.14 (0.88–1.54)	1.03 (0.68–1.50)	1.0 (0.71–1.31)
α₂-AT (U/mL)*	0.90 (0.36–1.44)	0.93 (0.49–1.37)			0.93 (0.39–1.47)	1.00 (0.69–1.30)	1.01 (0.65–1.37)	0.93 (0.55–1.30)
Protein C (U/mL)	0.28 (0.12–0.44)	0.32 (0.24–0.40)	0.33 (0.24–0.51)	0.77 (0.28–1.24)	0.94 (0.50–1.34)	0.94 (0.64–1.25)	0.88 (0.59–1.12)	1.03 (0.54–1.66)
Protein S (U/mL)	0.26 (0.14–0.38)	0.36 (0.28–0.47)	0.49 (0.33–0.67)	1.02 (0.29–1.62)	1.01 (0.67–1.36)	1.09 (0.64–1.54)	1.03 (0.65–1.40)	0.75 (0.54–1.03)
FIBRINOLYTIC SYSTEM*								
Plasminogen (U/mL)	1.70 (1.12–2.48)	1.95 (1.60–2.30)			0.98 (0.78–1.18)	0.92 (0.75–1.08)	0.86 (0.68–1.03)	0.99 (0.7–1.22)
TPA (ng/mL)					2.15 (1.0–4.5)	2.42 (1.0–5.0)	2.16 (1.0–4.0)	4.90 (1.40–8.40)
α₂-AP (U/mL)	0.78 (0.4–1.16)	0.85 (0.70–1.0)			1.05 (0.93–1.17)	0.99 (0.89–1.10)	0.98 (0.78–1.18)	1.02 (0.68–1.36)
PAI (U/mL)					5.42 (1.0–10.0)	6.79 (2.0–12.0)	6.07 (2.0–10.0)	3.60 (0–11.0)

*Data from Andrew M, Paes B, Milner R, et al. Development of the human anticoagulant system in the healthy premature infant. *Blood.* 1987;70:165–172; Andrew M, Paes B, Milner R, et al. Development of the human anticoagulant system in the healthy premature infant. *Blood.* 1988;72:1651–1657; and Andrew M, Vegh P, Johnston M, et al. Maturation of the hemostatic system during childhood. *Blood.* 1992;8:1998–2005.

†aPTT values may vary depending on reagent.

α₂-AP, α₂-Antiplasmin; α₂-AT, α₂-antitrypsin; α₂-M, α₂-macroglobulin; aPTT, activated partial thromboplastin time; ATIII, antithrombin III; FDPs, fibrin degradation products; HMWK, high-molecular-weight kininogen; INR, international normalized ratio; PAI, plasminogen activator inhibitor; Pk, prekallikrein; PT, prothrombin time; TPA, tissue plasminogen activator; VIII, factor VIII procoagulant; vWF, von Willebrand factor.

Adapted from Monagle P, Barnes C, Ignjatovic, V, et al. Developmental haemostasis. Impact for clinical haemostasis laboratories. *Thromb Haemost.* 2006;95:362–372.

administration, deficiencies of vitamin K–associated factors, malabsorption, liver disease, DIC, and the presence of circulating inhibitors.

3. **Platelet function testing:** Platelet aggregation and the Platelet Function Analyzer-100 (PFA-100) system are in vitro methods for measuring platelet function. Bleeding time (BT) evaluates clot formation, including platelet number and function and von Willebrand factor (vWF). Always assess the platelet number and history of ingestion of platelet inhibitors (e.g., nonsteroidal antiinflammatory drugs [NSAIDs]) before any platelet function testing.

B. Hypercoagulable States

Present clinically as venous or arterial thrombosis (Box 14-2)

1. **Laboratory evaluation**[4,5]:
a. Initial laboratory screening includes PT and high-sensitivity aPTT; if PT or aPTT are prolonged, a mixing study to look for circulating anticoagulants.
b. Extended workup for hypercoagulable states (Box 14-3): A hematologist should be consulted.

BOX 14-2

HYPERCOAGULABLE CONDITIONS

CONGENITAL	ACQUIRED
Protein C and S deficiency: Hereditary autosomal dominant disorder. Heterozygotes have three- to sixfold increased risk for venous thrombosis.	**Endothelial damage:** Causes include vascular catheters, smoking, diabetes, hypertension, surgery, hyperlipidemia.
Antithrombin III deficiency: Hereditary autosomal dominant disorder. Homozygotes die in infancy.	**Hyperviscosity:** Macroglobulinemia, polycythemia, sickle cell disease
Factor V Leiden (activated protein C resistance): 2%–5% of European whites are heterozygotes with two- to fourfold increased risk for venous thrombosis; 1 in 1000 are homozygotes, with 80- to 100-fold increased risk for venous thrombosis.	**Antiphospholipid antibodies:** Seen in patients with systemic lupus erythematosus or other autoimmune diseases; can occur with infections or idiopathically. Associated with venous and arterial thromboses and spontaneous abortions.
Homocystinemia: Increased levels of homocysteine associated with arterial and venous thromboses, often due to MTHFR abnormalities	**Platelet activation:** Caused by essential thrombocytosis, oral contraceptives, heparin-induced thrombocytopenia
Others: Prothrombin mutation (G20210A), plasminogen abnormalities, fibrinogen abnormalities	**Others:** Drugs, malignancy, liver disease, inflammatory disease such as inflammatory bowel disease, paroxysmal nocturnal hemoglobinuria, lipoprotein A

MTHFR, Methyltetrahydrofolate reductase.

c. Identification of one risk factor (e.g., indwelling vascular catheter) does not preclude the search for others, especially when accompanied by a family or personal history of thrombosis.

2. **Treatment of thromboses:**

a. Unfractionated heparin (UFH): Used for treatment or prevention of deep venous thrombosis (DVT) or pulmonary embolism (PE), atrial fibrilliation, mechanical heart valve, arterial thrombosis, cerebral sinovenous thrombosis, cardioembolic arterial ischemic stroke, homozygous purpura fulminans, and for bridge to warfarin therapy

(1) See Tables 14-8 to 14-11 for UFH bolus and drip adjustment guidelines for goal heparin anti-Xa level range of 0.3–0.7 U/mL or aPTT range 50–80 seconds.

(2) UFH may be reversed with protamine.

(3) UFH or low-molecular-weight-heparin (LMWH) therapy should continue for at least 5–7 days while initiating warfarin for treatment of venous thrombosis.

Contraindications: Patients with known hypersensitivity to heparin, major active bleeding, known or suspected heparin-induced thrombocytopenia (HIT), or concurrent epidural therapy

Precautions: Patients at high risk for bleeding (general bleeding precaution protocols must be implemented) or with platelet count

---

BOX 14-3

EXTENDED WORKUP FOR HYPERCOAGULABLE STATES*

Suggested tiered testing approach:

First Tier:

Antithrombin III activity (antithrombin III deficiency and dysfunction)

Activated protein C resistance assay (screening test for factor V Leiden)

Factor V Leiden (DNA-based assay for factor V Leiden)

Factor II 20210A (prothrombin mutation)

Homocysteine

Methyltetrahydrofolate reductase (MTHFR) genetic testing if homocysteine elevated

Dilute Russell viper venom test (antiphospholipid antibody syndrome)

Anticardiolipin screening enzyme-linked immunosorbent assay (ELISA; anticardiolipin antibodies)

Protein C activity (protein C deficiency and dysfunction)

Protein S activity (protein S deficiency and dysfunction)

Factor VIII, IX, XI

Second Tier (less common conditions):

Platelet neutralization procedure (lupus anticoagulant)

Plasminogen activity

Tissue plasminogen activator (TPA) antigen

Plasminogen activator inhibitor activity (PAI-1; measures activity of this TPA inhibitor)

α_2-Antiplasmin activity (measures activity of this plasmin inhibitor)

Lipoprotein (a) (Lp[a]) promotes decreased fibrinolysis

---

*Where necessary, abnormality tested for is listed in parentheses.

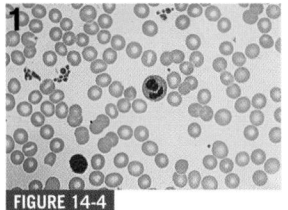

FIGURE 14-4

Normal smear. Round RBCs with central pallor about one third of the cell's diameter, scattered platelets, occasional white blood cells.

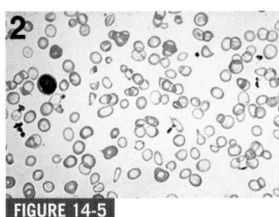

FIGURE 14-5

Iron deficiency. Hypochromic/microcytic RBCs, poikilocytosis, plentiful platelets, occasional ovalocytes and target cells.

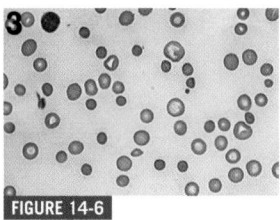

FIGURE 14-6

Spherocytosis. Microspherocytes a hallmark (densely stained RBCs with no central pallor).

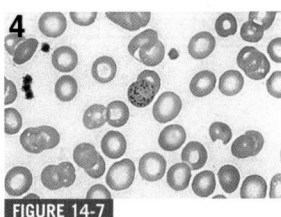

FIGURE 14-7

Basophilic stippling as a result of precipitated RNA throughout the cell; seen with heavy metal intoxication, thalassemia, iron deficiency, and other states of ineffective erythropoesis.

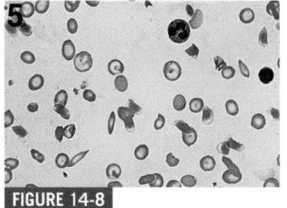

FIGURE 14-8

Hemoglobin SS disease. Sickled cells, target cells, hypochromia, poikilocytosis, Howell-Jolly bodies; nucleated RBCs common (not shown).

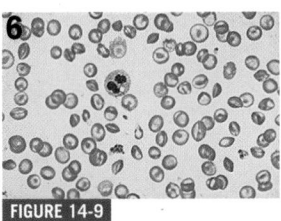

FIGURE 14-9

Hemoglobin SC disease. Target cells, oat cells, poikilocytosis; sickle forms rarely seen.

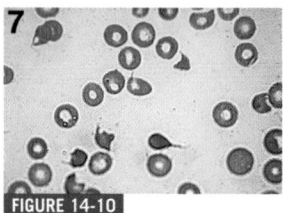

FIGURE 14-10

Microangiopathic hemolytic anemia. RBC fragments, anisocytosis, poly-chromasia, decreased platelets.

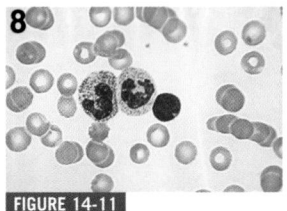

FIGURE 14-11

Toxic granulations. Prominent dark blue primary granules; commonly seen with infection and other toxic states (e.g., Kawasaki disease).

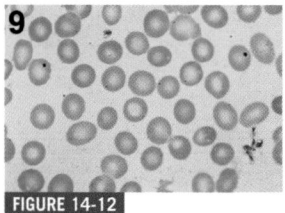

FIGURE 14-12

Howell-Jolly body. Small, dense nuclear remnant in an RBC; suggests splenic dysfunction or asplenia.

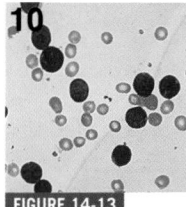

FIGURE 14-13

Leukemic blasts showing large nucleus-to-cyto-plasm ratio.

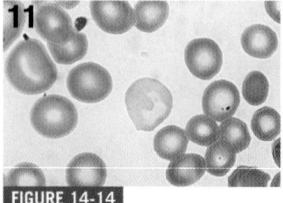

FIGURE 14-14

Polychromatophilia. Diffusely baso-philic because of RNA staining; seen with early release of reticulocytes from the marrow.

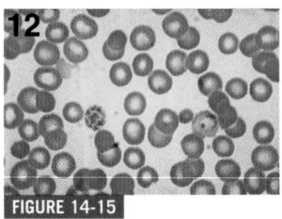

FIGURE 14-15

Malaria. Intraerythrocytic parasites.

TABLE 14-8

UNFRACTIONATED HEPARIN DOSE INITIATION GUIDELINES FOR GOAL aPTT RANGE OF 50–80 SECONDS*

Age	Loading Dose (No Loading Dose for Stroke Patients)	Initial Infusion Rate	Monitoring Parameters
Neonates and infants <1 yr	75 units/kg intravenously (IV)	28 units/kg/hr	Obtain aPTT 4 hr after loading dose.
Children ≥1 yr–16 yr	75 units/kg IV (max dose = 7700 units)	20 units/kg/hr (initial max rate = 1650 units/hr)	Obtain aPTT 4 hr after loading dose.
Patients >16 yr	70 units/kg (max dose = 7700 units)	15 units/kg/hr (initial max rate = 1650 units/hr)	Obtain aPTT 4 hr after loading dose.

*Reflects antifactor Xa level of 0.3–0.7 IU/mL with current activated partial thromboplastin time (aPTT) reagents at Johns Hopkins Hospital 2/3/11. Therapeutic aPTT range may vary with different aPTT reagents.

TABLE 14-9

UNFRACTIONATED HEPARIN DOSE ADJUSTMENT ALGORITHM FOR GOAL aPTT RANGE OF 50–80 SECONDS*

aPTT (seconds)	Bolus (units/kg)	Hold (minutes)	Rate Change	Repeat aPTT (hours)
≤39	50	0	Increase 20%	4 hr
40–49	0	0	Increase 10%	4 hr
50–80	0	0	0	4 hr, then next day once two consecutive values are in range
81–100	0	0	Decrease 10%	6 hr
101–125	0	30–60 min	Decrease 20%	6 hr
≥125†	0	60–120 min until aPTT <115 sec	Decrease 30%; restart when aPTT <115 sec	6 hr after infusion is restarted

*Reflects antifactor Xa level of 0.3–0.7 IU/mL with current activated partial thromboplastin (aPTT) reagents at Johns Hopkins Hospital 2/3/11. Therapeutic aPTT range may vary with different aPTT reagents.
†Confirm that specimen was not drawn from heparinized line or same extremity as site of heparin infusion.

TABLE 14-10

UNFRACTIONATED HEPARIN DOSE INITIATION GUIDELINES FOR GOAL ANTI-Xa ACTIVITY OF 0.3-0.7 UNITS/ML

Age	Loading Dose (No Bolus for Stroke Patients)	Initial Infusion Rate	Monitoring Parameters
Neonates and infants <1 year	75 units/kg IV	28 units/kg/hr	Obtain anti-Xa 4 hours after loading dose
Children ≥1 year–16 years	75 units/kg IV (max dose = 7700 units)	20 units/kg/hr (max rate = 1650 units/hour)	Obtain anti-Xa 4 hours after loading dose
Patients > 16 years	70 units/kg (max dose = 7700 units)	15 units/kg/hr (max rate = 1650 units/hr)	Obtain anti-Xa 4 hours after loading dose

---

TABLE 14-11

UNFRACTIONATED HEPARIN DOSE ADJUSTMENT ALGORITHM FOR GOAL ANTI-Xa ACTIVITY OF 0.3–0.7 UNITS/ML

Anti-Xa level	Bolus (units/kg)	Hold (minutes)	Rate Change	Repeat anti-Xa (hours)
≤0.1	50	0	Increase 20%	4 hr
0.2	0	0	Increase 10%	4 hr
0.3–0.7	0	0	0	4 hr, then next day once two consecutive values are in range
0.8–0.9	0	0	Decrease 10%	6 hr
1.0–1.1	0	30–60	Decrease 20%	6 hr
>1.2*	0	60–120 until anti-Xa <1.0	Decrease 30%; restart when anti-Xa activity <1.0	6 hr after infusion is restarted

*Confirm that specimen was not drawn from heparinized line or same extremity as site of heparin infusion.

<50,000/mm³. Avoid intramuscular injections and avoid other drugs that affect platelet function (e.g., NSAIDs, aspirin, clopidogrel). Baseline labs prior to institution of UFH therapy (to assess baseline coagulation state): aPTT, PT, BMP, Heme-8.

b. LMWH[4,5]: Administered subcutaneously, has a longer half-life, more predictable pharmacokinetics, and requires less monitoring. Also associated with lower risk for HIT.

(1) Dose depends on preparation. See Formulary for enoxaparin dosage information.

(2) Monitor LMWH therapy by following anti-Xa activity. Therapeutic range is 0.5–1.0 U/mL for thrombosis treatment and 0.1–0.3 U/mL for prophylactic dosing. Blood for anti-Xa activity should be drawn 4 hours after dose.

(3) LMWH-induced bleeding can be partially reversed with protamine. Consult hematologist for protamine reversal protocol.

c. Warfarin: Used for long-term anticoagulation. Patient should receive heparin (UFH or LMWH) while initiating warfarin therapy, owing to possibility of hypercoagulability from decreased protein C and S levels.

(1) Usually administered orally at an initiation dose for 1–2 days, followed by a daily dose sufficient to maintain the PT/INR in the desired range. Infants often require higher daily doses. Levels should be measured every 1–4 weeks. Table 14-12 lists dose adjustment guidelines, and Table 14-13 outlines management of excessive anticoagulation.

(2) Efficacy is greatly affected by dietary intake of vitamin K. Patients should receive appropriate dietary education.

(3) Box 14-4 lists medications that influence warfarin therapy.

d. Anticoagulant therapy alters many coagulation tests:

(1) Heparin prolongs aPTT, thrombin time, dilute Russell Viper Venom test (dRVVT), and mixing studies.

TABLE 14-12

ADJUSTMENT AND MONITORING OF WARFARIN TO MAINTAIN AN INTERNATIONAL NORMALIZED RATIO (INR) BETWEEN 2 AND 3*,[11]

I. DAY 1 INITIAL DOSING

1. Newborn: for age <3 mo, there are limited data for safety and efficacy of warfarin. Higher dose may be needed in neonates and infants.
2. Infants and children:
   - If baseline INR is 1–1.3, dose = 0.2 mg/kg/dose orally Q24 hr (max 7.5 mg/dose)‡
   - If baseline INR >1.3, liver dysfunction, postoperative cardiac Fontan procedure patients, NPO/poor nutrition, receiving broad-spectrum antibiotics, receiving medications causing significant drug/drug interactions, receiving medications with CYP2C9 enzyme inhibition (e.g., amiodarone, metronidazole, fluconazole, Bactrim), or slow metabolizer of warfarin, dose = 0.1 mg/kg/dose Q24 hr (max 5 mg/dose)

II. DAYS 2–4

Dose Adjustment for Goal INR of 2–3

Day 2		Day 3 and 4	
INR Level	**Action**	**INR Level**	**Action**
1.1–1.3	Repeat initial dose	1.1–1.3	Repeat initial dose*
1.4–1.9	50% of initial dose	1.4–1.9	50% of initial dose*
≥2	Hold dose for 24 hr, then restart at 50% of initial dose	2–3	50% of initial dose†
		3.1–3.5	25% of initial dose†
		>3.5	Hold dose until INR <3.5, then restart at 50% of previous dose†

III. DAY 5 AND MAINTENANCE

Maintenance Dosing

≥5 Days	
INR Level	**Action**
1.1–1.4	Increase weekly dose by 20%
1.5–1.9	Increase weekly dose by 10%
2–3	Continue current dose
3.1–3.5	Decrease weekly dose by 10%
>3.5	Hold dose, recheck INR daily until INR <3.5, then restart at 20% less than previous dose

*If INR is not >1.5 on day 4, patient should be reassessed, and dose/kg should be adjusted on an individual basis.
†Consult pediatric hematology for patient-specific recommendations on reduced dosing.
‡Reported average daily dose to maintain INR of 2–3 for infants is 0.33 mg/kg; for adolescents, 0.09 mg/kg; and for adults, from 0.04–0.08 mg/kg.
Adapted from The Johns Hopkins Hospital Children's Center pediatric policies, procedures, and protocols general care (Policy Number GEN069), Baltimore, 2010.

14

TABLE 14-13

MANAGEMENT OF EXCESSIVE WARFARIN ANTICOAGULATION

INR <5 without serious bleeding	Hold warfarin. Recheck INR daily. When INR approaches therapeutic range, resume warfarin at lower dose and follow INR daily.*
INR ≥5 but <8 without serious bleeding	Hold warfarin. Recheck INR every 12–24 hr. If high risk for bleeding, consider low dose of vitamin K oral or IV (30 mcg/kg for patients <40 kg in weight; 1–2.5 mg for patients >40 kg). When INR approaches therapeutic range, resume warfarin at a lower dose.*
INR ≥8 without serious bleeding	Hold warfarin. Recheck INR every 6–12 hr. Give vitamin K orally (PO) or IV (30 mcg/kg for patients <40 kg in weight; 1–2.5 mg for patients >40 kg). INR reduction expected to occur within 12–24 hours with IV or 24–48 hours with PO vitamin K. Repeat vitamin K as necessary. When INR approaches therapeutic range, resume warfarin at a lower dose.*
Serious bleeding at any INR elevation	Hold warfarin. Monitor INR every 6 hr. Give vitamin K IV (2.5–5 mg). Vitamin K may be repeated as needed. Consider use of FFP (10–15 mL/kg IV), recombinant factor VIIa (16 mcg/kg IV), prothrombinase complex concentrate, or rhFVIIa (Novoseven) IV. Restart warfarin when INR approaches therapeutic range and when clinically appropriate at a lower dose.*
Life-threatening bleeding at any INR	Hold warfarin. Monitor INR every 2–4 hr. Administer vitamin K IV at 5–10 mg. Repeat vitamin K as needed. Transfuse FFP (10–15 mL/kg IV), consider rhFVIIa (Novoseven) or prothrombinase complex concentrate. Restart warfarin when INR approaches therapeutic range and when clinically appropriate at a lower dose.*

*Refer to Table 14-12.
NOTE: Always evaluate for bleeding risks and potential drug interactions.
FFP, Fresh frozen plasma; INR, international normalized ratio; IV, intravenous; rhVIIa, activated recombinant human factor VII.
Adapted from The Johns Hopkins Hospital Children's Center pediatric policies, procedures, and protocols general care (Policy Number GEN069), Baltimore, 2010.

(2) Warfarin prolongs PT, aPTT, and dRVVT. Warfarin reduces the activity of vitamin K–dependent factors (II, VII, IX, X, protein C and S).
e. Thrombolytic therapy should be considered for life- or limb-threatening thrombosis. Consult a hematologist.
NOTE: Children receiving anticoagulation therapy should be protected from trauma. Subcutaneous injections should be used when possible, and caution should be used with intramuscular injections. The use of antiplatelet agents and arterial punctures should be avoided.

BOX 14-4

MEDICATIONS THAT INFLUENCE WARFARIN THERAPY*

SIGNIFICANT INCREASE IN INR	SIGNIFICANT DECREASE IN INR
Amiodarone	Amobarbital
Anabolic steroids	Aprepitant
Bactrim (TMP/SMZ)	Butabarbital
Chloramphenicol	Carbamazepine
Disulfiram	Dicloxacillin
Fluconazole	Griseofulvin
Isoniazid	Methimazole
Metronidazole	Phenobarbital
Miconazole	Phenytoin
Phenylbutazone	Primidone
Quinidine	Propylthiouracil
Sulfinpyrazone	Rifabutin
Sulfisoxazole	Rifampin
Tamoxifen	Secobarbital

MODERATE INCREASE IN INR	MODERATE DECREASE IN INR
Cimetidine	Atazanavir
Ciprofloxacin	Efavirenz
Clarithromycin	Nafcillin
Delavirdine	Ritonavir
Efavirenz	
Itraconazole	
Lovastatin	
Omeprazole	
Propafenone	
Ritonavir	

INR, International normalized ratio; TMP/SMZ, trimethoprim/sulfamethoxazole.
*Numerous medications not listed in this table can affect warfarin administration.

14

C. Bleeding Disorders (Fig. 14-3 and Box 14-5)

1. **Differential diagnosis of bleeding disorders** (Table 14-14 and Box 14-5)
2. **Desired factor replacement goals in hemophilia** (Table 14-15)

VI. BLOOD COMPONENT REPLACEMENT

A. Blood Volume

Requirements are age specific (Table 14-16).

B. Blood Product Components

1. **RBCs:** Decision to transfuse RBCs should be made with consideration of clinical symptoms and signs, degree of cardiorespiratory or CNS disease, cause and course of anemia, and options for alternative therapy, noting risks for transfusion-associated infections and reactions.

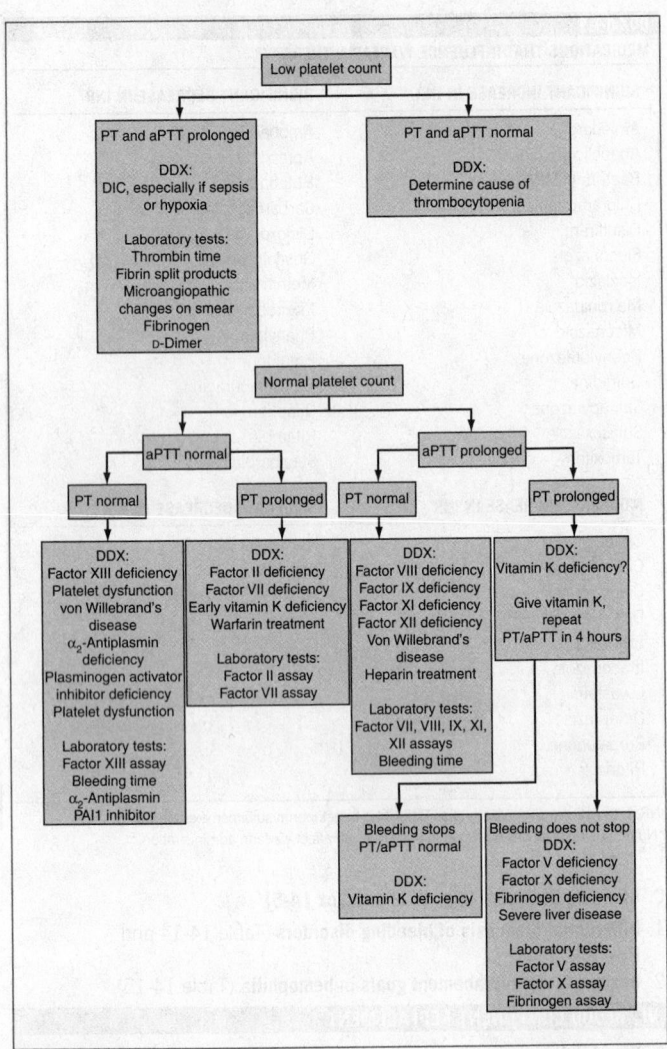

FIGURE 14-3

Differential diagnosis (DDX) of bleeding disorders. aPTT, Activated partial thromboplastin time; DIC, disseminated intravascular coagulation; PT, prothrombin time.

TABLE 14-14

COMMON COAGULATION DISORDERS

Factor VIII deficiency (hemophilia A)*	Characteristics: X-linked recessive, prolonged aPTT, reduced factor VIII activity, normal PT and BT Treatment: a. Treat with factor VIII concentrate, preferably recombinant factor VIII to reduce risk of infection. b. Factor level recovers by 2% per 1 unit of factor VIII per kg of body weight (refer to Table 14-15). c. First dose has shorter half-life, so if redosing needed, second dose should be given after 4–8 hr. Subsequent doses can be given every 12 hr. d. Continuous infusion often desirable—example, surgical patients or those requiring prolonged therapy usually need 50 U/kg loading dose, followed by 3–5 U/kg/hr. e. For suspected intracranial bleeding, replace to 100% **before** diagnostic procedure (e.g., computed tomography [CT] scan). f. Dose calculation: units of factor VIII needed = weight (kg) × desired % replacement × 0.5.
Factor IX deficiency (hemophilia B or Christmas disease)*	Characteristics: X-linked recessive, prolonged aPTT, reduced factor IX activity Treatment: a. Treat with factor IX concentrate, preferably recombinant to reduce risk of infection. b. Factor level usually recovers by 1% for each unit of factor IX concentrate per kg of body weight. c. Half-life of factor IX 18–24 hr. Similar to factor VIII, if second dose needed, it should be given at a shorter interval. d. Recombinant factor IX has a shorter half-life; consider evaluation of in vivo factor survival in patient. e. Replace to 100% **before** diagnostic procedure if intracranial bleeding is suspected. f. Dose calculation: units of factor IX needed = weight (kg) × desired % replacement (may be advisable to multiply by 1.2 for recombinant factor IX).

Continued

TABLE 14-14

COMMON COAGULATION DISORDERS (Continued)

von Willebrand disease	Characteristics: vWF binds platelets to subendothelial surfaces and carries and stabilizes factor VIII.
	Type 1: Decreased activity of vWF and proportionally decreased quantity of vWF. Mild to moderate bleeding. Prolonged BT, normal platelet count, platelet dysfunction on platelet function testing, aPTT normal in most cases but may be mildly prolonged.
	Type 2: Characterized by four subtypes, all with various functional abnormalities of vWF. Mild to moderate bleeding but in some cases can be severe.
	Type 3: Absence or near absence of vWF, with reduction of factor VIII and severe bleeding.
	Treatment:
	a. Majority of patients with type 1 vWD respond to DDAVP (desmopressin acetate) with increases in vWF activity from two- to threefold over baseline (DDAVP responsiveness should be established by prior testing). IV or intranasal DDAVP may be used for minor bleeding or surgical procedures.
	b. DDAVP may be contraindicated in the rare vWD type 2B, because it may exacerbate thrombocytopenia.
	c. For more severe disease or patients who do not respond to DDAVP, treatments of choice are purified plasma-derived products containing both vWF and factor VIII (HUMATE P, Alphanate, or Wilate). These concentrates are preferred because they are virally inactivated.
	d. Aminocaproic acid 100 mg/kg IV or PO every 4–6 hr (up to 30 g/day) may be useful for treatment of mucosal bleeding and as prophylaxis for dental extraction.

*All patients with hemophilia should be vaccinated with hepatitis A and B vaccines.

aPTT, Activated partial thromboplastin; BT, bleeding time; IV, intravenous; PO, per os; PT, prothrombin time; vWF, von Willebrand factor.

TABLE 14-15

DESIRED FACTOR REPLACEMENT IN HEMOPHILIA

Bleeding Site	Desired Level (%)
Minor soft tissue bleeding	20–30
Joint	40–70
Simple dental extraction	50
Major soft tissue bleeding	80–100
Serious oral bleeding	80–100
Head injury	100+
Major surgery (dental, orthopedic, other)	100+

NOTE: A hematologist should be consulted for all major bleeding and before surgery.

Round to the nearest vial; do not exceed 200%.

a. Packed RBC (PRBC) transfusion: Concentrated RBCs with HCT of 55%–70%. A typed and cross-matched blood product is preferred when possible; O-negative (or O-positive) blood may be used if transfusion cannot be delayed. O-negative is preferred for females of childbearing age to reduce risk for Rh sensitization.

(1) Unless rapid replacement is required for acute blood loss or shock, infuse no faster than 2–3 mL/kg/hr (generally 10–15 mL/kg aliquots over 4 hr) to avoid congestive heart failure.

(2) Rule of thumb in severe compensated anemia: Give an X mL/kg aliquot, where X = patient Hb (g/dL); for example, if Hb = 5 g/dL, transfuse 5 mL/kg over 4 hours.

(3) To calculate the volume of PRBC to achieve a desired HCT, use the following equation:

$$\text{Volume of PRBCs (mL)} = \text{EBV (mL)} \times \text{(desired HCT} - \text{actual HCT)}\ \text{HCT of PRBCs}$$

where EBV is the estimated blood volume (see Table 14-16 for age-specific EBV) and HCT of PRBCs is usually 55%–70%

(4) A unit of blood is 500 mL, but approximately 300 mL after processing without significant loss of red cells. This may vary with type of diluents used and time of storage, owing to red cell compaction.

b. Leukocyte-poor PRBCs:

(1) Filtered RBCs: 99.9% of WBCs removed from product; used for cytomegalovirus (CMV)-negative patients to reduce risk for CMV transmission. Also reduces likelihood of a nonhemolytic febrile transfusion reaction.

(2) Washed RBCs: 92%–95% of WBCs removed from product. Similar advantages to leukocyte-poor filtered RBCs. Although filtered leukocyte-poor blood is now more commonly used, washing may be helpful if a patient has preexisting antibodies to blood products (e.g., patients who have complete IgA deficiency or history of urticarial transfusion reactions).

TABLE 14-16

ESTIMATED BLOOD VOLUME (EBV)

Age	Total Blood Volume (mL/kg)
Preterm infants	90–105
Term newborns	78–86
1–12 mo	73–78
1–3 yr	74–82
4–6 yr	80–86
7–18 yr	83–90
Adults	68–88

Data from Nathan D, Oski FA. *Hematology of Infancy and Childhood.* Philadelphia: WB Saunders, 1998.

c. Irradiated blood products:
   (1) Many blood products (PRBCs, platelet preparations, leukocytes, FFP, and others) contain viable lymphocytes capable of proliferation and engraftment in the recipient, causing graft-versus-host disease (GVHD). Irradiation with 1500 cGy before transfusion may prevent GVHD but does not prevent antibody formation against donor white cells. Engraftment most likely in young infants, immunocompromised patients, and patients receiving blood from first-degree relatives.
   (2) Indications: Intensive chemotherapy, leukemia, lymphoma, bone marrow transplantation, solid organ transplantation, known or suspected immune deficiencies, intrauterine transfusions, and transfusions in neonates.
d. CMV-negative blood: Obtained from donors who test negative for CMV. May be given to neonates or other immunocompromised patients, including those awaiting organ or marrow transplant who are CMV negative.

2. **Platelets:** Indicated to treat severe or symptomatic thrombocytopenia. Should not be refrigerated because this promotes premature platelet activation and clumping. Bacteremia secondary to contamination more common than with refrigerated blood products.
a. Single-donor product: Preferred over pooled concentrate for patients with antiplatelet antibodies.
b. Leukocyte-poor: Use if there is a history of significant acute febrile platelet transfusion reactions.
c. Usually give $4 U/m^2$, or approximately 10 mL/kg of normally concentrated platelet product. Platelet count is raised by 10,000 to 15,000/μL by giving $1 U/m^2$. For infants and children, 10 mL/kg will increase platelet count by about 50,000/μL.
d. Hemorrhagic complications are rare with platelet counts >20,000/μL. A transfusion *trigger* of 10,000/μL is recommended by many in the absence of serious bleeding complications. Platelet count >50,000/μL is advisable for minor procedures; >100,000/μL is advisable for major surgery or intracranial operation.
e. Usually unit = 50 mL after processing, $\geq 5.5 \times 10^{11}$ plt/unit.

3. **FFP:** Contains all clotting factors except platelets. Used in severe clotting factor deficiencies with active bleeding or in combination with vitamin K to achieve rapid reversal of effects of warfarin. Also replaces anticoagulant factors (antithrombin III, protein C, protein S). Used in treatment of DIC, vitamin K deficiency with active bleeding, or TTP. One milliliter of FFP expected to provide 1 unit of activity of all factors except labile factor V and VIII, but individual units may vary. Usual amount is 10–15 mL/kg; repeat doses as needed. In acquired TTP, plasma exchange is the treatment of choice. Usually unit = 250–300 mL after processing.

4. **Cryoprecipitate:** Enriched for factor VIII (5–10 U/mL), vWF, and fibrinogen. Historically useful for children with factor VIII or vWF deficiency in the context of active bleeding, but concentrates or recombinant products now preferred because of lower risk for viral transmission. Useful for raising fibrinogen when small volumes are required. Usually unit = 10–15 mL after processing (80 units factor VIII and 250 mg fibrinogen).

5. **Monoclonal factor VIII:** Highly purified factor derived from pooled human blood using monoclonal antibodies.

6. **Recombinant factor VIII or IX:** Highly purified with less (theoretical) infectious risk than pooled human products. There is risk for inhibitor formation, as with other products.

C. PRBC Exchange Transfusion

1. **Partial PRBC exchange transfusion may be indicated** for sickle cell patients with acute chest syndrome, stroke, intractable pain crisis, or refractory priapism. Replace with Sickledex-negative cells. Follow HCT carefully during transfusion to avoid hyperviscosity, maintaining HCT <35%.

2. **Indications for double packed volume PRBC exchange transfusion** include severe acute chest and CVA. This is based on twice the patient's calculated packed cell volume. Goal is to reduce percentage of HbS to <30%. Expected reduction in percentage of circulating sickle cells is 60%–80%.

3. **To calculate the volume of PRBC needed for a double packed volume PRBC exchange, use the following equation:**

$$\text{Desired volume of exchange} = \text{EBV (mL)} \times \text{Patient HCT} \times 2/(\text{HCT of PRBC})$$

where EBV is the age-dependent estimated blood volume (see Table 14-16), and HCT of PRBC is 55%–70%.

D. Complications of Transfusions

1. **Acute transfusion reactions:**

a. Acute hemolytic reaction: most often the result of blood group incompatibility. Signs and symptoms include fever, chills, tachycardia, hypotension, and shock. Treatment includes immediate cessation of blood transfusion and institution of supportive measures. Laboratory findings include DIC, hemoglobinuria, and positive Coombs test.

b. Febrile nonhemolytic reaction: Usually the result of inflammatory cytokines; common in previously transfused patients. Symptoms include fever, chills, and diaphoresis. Stop transfusion and evaluate. Prevention includes premedication with antipyretics, antihistamines, corticosteroids, and if necessary, use of leukocyte-poor PRBCs.

c. Urticarial reaction: Reaction to donor plasma proteins. Stop transfusion immediately; treat with antihistamines, and epinephrine and steroids if there is respiratory compromise (see also treatment of anaphylaxis, Chapter 1). Use washed or filtered RBCs with the next transfusion.

   d. Evaluation of acute transfusion reaction:

     (1) Patient's urine: Test for hemoglobin.

     (2) Patient's blood: Confirm blood type, screen for antibodies, and repeat direct Coombs test (DCT) on pretransfusion and posttransfusion sera.

     (3) Donor blood: Culture for bacteria.

2. **Delayed transfusion reaction:** Usually due to minor blood group antigen incompatibility, with low or absent titer of antibodies at time of transfusion. Occurs 3–10 days after transfusion. Symptoms include fatigue, jaundice, and dark urine. Laboratory findings include anemia, positive Coombs test, new RBC antibodies, and hemoglobinuria. The need for acute intervention is much less likely than with acute reactions.

3. **Transmission of infectious diseases**[6,10]: Blood supply is tested for HIV types 1 and 2, HTLV types I and II, hepatitis B, hepatitis C, syphilis, and West Nile virus. Data from *2009 Red Book* estimate the risk for transmitting infection (estimated per unit) as follows: HIV (1 in 2,000,000); HTLV (1 in 641,000); hepatitis B (1 in 63,000–500,000); hepatitis C (1 in 100,000); parvovirus (1 in 10,000). CMV, hepatitis A, parasitic, tickborne, and prion diseases may also be transmitted by blood products.

4. **Sepsis:** Occurs with products contaminated with bacteria, particularly platelets, because they are stored at room temperature. Risk for transmitting bacteria in PRBCs is 1 in 5 million units, and in platelets is 1 in 100,000.

E. Reasons Not to Consider a Directed Donor

1. **Donors less likely to be truthful about risk**
2. **Increase risk of transfusion-related GVHD if from a relative**
3. **Can alloimmunize if potential bone marrow donor**

F. Reasons to Consider a Directed Donor

1. **Chronic transfusion programs** (e.g., thalassemia or sickle cell disease), where donors provide antigen-matched red cells repetitively for the same patient
2. **NAIT,** where maternal platelets lack causative antigens and represent optimal therapy

---

VII. INTERPRETING BLOOD SMEARS

See Figures 14-4 through 14-15 for examples of blood smears. Examine the blood smear in an area where the RBCs are nearly touching but do not overlap.

A. RBC

Examine size, shape, and color.

B. WBC

A rough estimate of the WBC count can be made by looking at the smear under high power (×100 magnification). Each one cell per high-power field correlates with approximately 500 WBC/mm³ (×20 magnification).

C. Platelets

A rough estimate of platelet count is one platelet per high-power field corresponds to 10,000–15,000/µL. Platelet clumps usually indicate >100,000 platelets/µL.

REFERENCES

1. American Academy of Pediatrics, Section on Hematology/Oncology Committee on Genetics. Health supervision in children with sickle cell disease. *Pediatrics.* 2002;109:526-535.
2. Driscoll MC. Sickle cell disease. *Pediatr Rev.* 2007;28:259-268.
3. Bennett CM, Rogers ZR, Kinnamon DD, et al. Prospective phase 1/2 study of rituximab in childhood and adolescent chronic immune thrombocytopenic purpura. *Blood.* 2006;107:2639-2642.
4. Streiff MB, Kickler TS. *The Johns Hopkins Hospital Hemostatic Testing and Antithrombotic Therapy Manual.* 3rd ed. Baltimore: Johns Hopkins Hospital, 2007.
5. *The Johns Hopkins Hospital Children's Center pediatric policies, procedures, and protocols general care.* Baltimore, 2010.
6. Red Book. *2009 Report of the Committee on Infectious Diseases.* 28th ed. Elk Grove Village, IL: American Academy of Pediatrics, 2009.
7. Strouse JJ, Takemoto CM, Keefer JR, et al. Corticosteroids and increased risk of readmission after acute chest syndrome in children with sickle cell disease. *Pediatr Blood Cancer.* 2008;50:1006-1012.
8. Hulbert ML, Scothorn DJ, Panepinto JA, et al. Exchange blood transfusion for first overt stroke is associated with a lower risk of subsequent stroke than simple transfusion: a retrospective cohort of 137 children with sickle cell anemia. *J Pediatr.* 2006;149:710-712.
9. Brawley OW, Cornelius LJ, Edwards LR, et al. National Institutes of Health Consensus Development Conference statement: hydroxyurea treatment for sickle cell disease. *Ann Intern Med.* 2008;148:932-938.
10. Red Cross Blood Testing. www.redcrossblood.org. Accessed December 10, 2010.
11. Monagle P, Chan AC, Goldenberg NA. Antithrombotic therapy in neonates and children. *Chest.* 2012:e737S-e801S.
12. Lipton JM, Ellis SR. Diamond-Blackfan anemia: diagnosis, treatment, and molecular pathogenesis. *Hematol Oncol Clin North Am.* 2009;23:261-282.
13. Wang WC, Ware RE, Miller ST. Hydroxycarbamide in very young children with sickle-cell anaemia: a multicentre, randomised, controlled trial (BABY-HUG). *Lancet.* 2011;377:1663-1672.

14

Chapter 15

Immunology and Allergy

Emily Braun, MD

I. ALLERGIC RHINITIS[1-4]

A. Epidemiology

1. **Most common chronic condition:** Affects 10%–30% of children
2. **Significant impact on quality of life,** including school performance and sleep patterns, as demonstrated in multiple studies
3. **Increases risk for** recurrent otitis media, asthma, acute and chronic sinusitis
4. **Risk factors:** Atopic family history, serum immunoglobulin (Ig) E >100 IU/mL before age 6 years, higher socioeconomic status, maternal smoke exposure in first year of life

B. Diagnosis

1. **History:**
a. Allergen-driven mucosal inflammation leading to cyclical exacerbations or persistent symptoms
b. Symptoms: Nasal (congestion, rhinorrhea, pruritus), ocular (pruritus, tearing), postnasal drip (sore throat, cough, pruritus)
c. Patterns: Seasonal (depending on local allergens) vs. perennial (with seasonal peaks)
d. Coexisting atopic diseases common (eczema, asthma, food allergy)
2. **Physical examination:**
a. Allergic facies with shiners, mouth breathing, transverse nasal crease ("allergic salute"), accentuated lines below lower eyelids (Dennie-Morgan lines)
b. Nasal mucosa may be normal to pink to pale gray, ± swollen turbinates.
c. Injected sclera with or without clear discharge, conjunctival cobblestoning
3. **Diagnostic studies:**
a. Diagnosis can be made on clinical grounds, but skin testing can be confirmatory.
b. Skin testing: Gold standard, determination of specific IgE involved
c. Total IgE: Nonspecific, limited value
d. Peripheral blood eosinophil count: Not sensitive enough to be diagnostic
e. Nasal smear for eosinophils: Quick, easy screen with good positive predictive value
f. Measurement of specific IgE: Identifies presence of serum IgE to selected antigens
g. Imaging studies: Not useful
h. Consider sleep study to evaluate for obstructive sleep apnea and pulmonary function tests (PFT) to evaluate for asthma.

C. Differential Diagnosis

1. **Vasomotor rhinitis:** Symptoms made worse by scents, alcohol, or changes in temperature or humidity
2. **Infectious rhinitis:** Viral vs. bacterial
3. **Episodic rhinitis:** Allergic nasal symptoms elicited by sporadic exposures to inhaled aeroallergens
4. **Adenoid hypertrophy**
5. **Rhinitis medicamentosa:** Rebound rhinitis from prolonged use of nasal vasoconstrictors
6. **Sinusitis:** Acute or chronic
7. **Nonallergic rhinitis with eosinophilia syndrome (NARES)**
8. **Nasal polyps**

D. Treatment

1. **Allergen avoidance:**
a. Relies on identification of triggers, most common of which are pollens, fungi, dust mites, insects, animals
b. Difficult to avoid ubiquitous airborne allergens
c. HEPA filter use may be of use when animal allergens are a concern
d. Thorough housecleaning and allergy-proof bed coverings can be useful

2. **Oral antihistamines** (diphenhydramine, cetirizine):
a. First-line treatment
b. Second-generation preparations preferable (loratadine, desloratadine, fexofenadine, cetirizine, levocetirizine)
c. Adverse effects: Sedation and anticholinergic side effects more prominent with first-generation agents

3. **Intranasal corticosteroids** (fluticasone, mometasone, budesonide, flunisolide, ciclesonide, triamcinolone):
a. Second-line treatment
b. Most effective maintenance therapy for nasal congestion
c. Potential benefit for ocular symptoms
d. No proven adverse effect on long-term growth
e. Adverse effects: nasal irritation, sneezing, bleeding
f. Recognize potential risk of adrenal suppression at high doses of inhaled or intranasal steroids

4. **Leukotriene inhibitors** (montelukast): Alone or in combination with antihistamines

5. **Mast cell stabilizers** (intranasal cromolyn):
a. Inexpensive and easily available
b. Most effective as prophylaxis
c. Few adverse effects

6. **Intranasal antihistamines** (azelastine, olopatadine):
a. Effective for acute symptoms
b. Not studied in children younger than 5 years
c. Adverse effects: Bitter taste, systemic absorption with sedation

7. **Anticholinergics** (ipratropium):
a. Useful for rhinorrhea only
b. Adverse effects: Drying of nasal mucosa
8. **Immunotherapy:**
a. Success rate is high when patients are chosen carefully and when performed by an allergy specialist.
b. Consider when drug side effects are limiting or triggering allergens are difficult to avoid.
c. Not recommended for patients with poor adherence to therapy or those with poorly-controlled asthma
d. Not well studied in children younger than 5 years
e. May reduce risk for future development of asthma, and treatment of allergic rhinitis may improve asthma control.
9. **Nasal rinsing with hypertonic saline:** Tolerable and inexpensive
10. **Ophthalmic agents:** Can be used to treat allergic conjunctivitis (Table 15-1). Up to 60% of patients with allergic rhinitis have concomitant conjunctivitis.

TABLE 15-1

EXAMPLES OF OPHTHALMIC AGENTS INDICATED FOR TREATMENT OF ALLERGIC CONJUNCTIVITIS

Brand Name	Ingredient	Dose
Alocril (≥3 yr) Sol: 5 mL	Nedocromil sodium 2% (mast cell stabilizer), benzalkonium chloride	1–2 drops several times a day; remove contact lenses during therapy
Patanol/Pataday (≥3 yr) Sol: 5 mL	Olopatadine 0.1% (H₁-antagonist and mast cell stabilizer)	1 drop once daily–BID
Zaditor (≥3 yr) Sol: 5 mL	Ketotifen fumarate 0.025% (H₁-antagonist and mast cell stabilizer)	1 drop Q8–12 hr

II. FOOD ALLERGY[5-9]

A. Epidemiology

1. **Prevalence is 6%–8% in pediatric population**
2. **Most common allergens in children:** Milk, eggs, peanuts, tree nuts (e.g., cashew, walnut), soy, wheat

B. Manifestations of Food Allergy:

1. **Often a combination of several syndromes;** symptoms can occur within minutes to hours of ingesting food.
2. **Diagnosis requires** both sensitization (demonstration of allergen-specific IgE) and clinical symptoms after exposure to allergen.
3. **Rarely presents with isolated respiratory symptoms.**
4. **Anaphylaxis:** see Chapter 1, Allergic Emergencies (Anaphylaxis)
5. **Skin syndromes:**
a. Urticaria/angioedema:
   (1) Chronic urticaria is rarely related to food allergy.
   (2) Acute urticaria due to food allergy predicts risk for future anaphylaxis.

b. Atopic dermatitis/eczema:
   (1) Food allergy is more common in patients with atopic dermatitis.
   (2) Even if not apparent by history, at least a third of children with moderate to severe atopic dermatitis have IgE-mediated food allergies.
   (3) Acute and chronic skin changes often coexist.

6. **Gastrointestinal syndromes:**

a. Oral allergy syndrome:
   (1) Pollen-associated food allergy caused by cross-reactivity of antibodies to pollens (e.g., apple or tree pollen)
   (2) Pruritus of oral mucosa after ingestion of certain fresh fruits and vegetables in patients with pollen allergies
   (3) Rarely results in edema of oral mucosa
   (4) Symptoms rarely progress beyond mouth
   (5) Inciting antigens are destroyed by cooking

b. Allergic eosinophilic gastroenteritis, esophagitis:
   (1) May cause abdominal pain, diarrhea, early satiety
   (2) May be confused with reflux
   (3) Characterized by eosinophilic infiltration of digestive tract

c. Food-induced enterocolitis:
   (1) Presents in infancy
   (2) Vomiting and diarrhea (may contain blood); when severe, may lead to lethargy, dehydration, hypotension, acidosis
   (3) Most commonly associated with milk, soy

d. Infantile proctocolitis:
   (1) Confined to distal colon and can present with diarrhea or blood-streaked and mucousy stools
   (2) Symptoms usually resolve within 72 hours of stopping offending agent; rarely leads to anemia.

7. **Respiratory syndromes:**

a. Rhinitis (see Section I)

b. Asthma (see Chapter 24)

C. **Diagnosis of Food Allergy (Fig. 15-1)**

1. **History and physical examination:**

a. Identify specific foods and whether fresh vs. cooked.

b. Establish timing and nature of reactions; patient should keep a food diary.

c. Mainstays of diagnosis, but skin testing needed to identify trigger foods.

2. **Skin testing:**

a. Skin prick test has poor positive predictive value but very good negative predictive value.

b. Patient must not be taking antihistamines.

c. Widespread skin conditions (e.g., dermatographism, urticaria, severe eczema) may decrease accuracy.

d. Intradermal tests have high false-positive rates and higher risk.

e. Atopy patch testing (APT): Under investigation; no guidelines for use at this time.

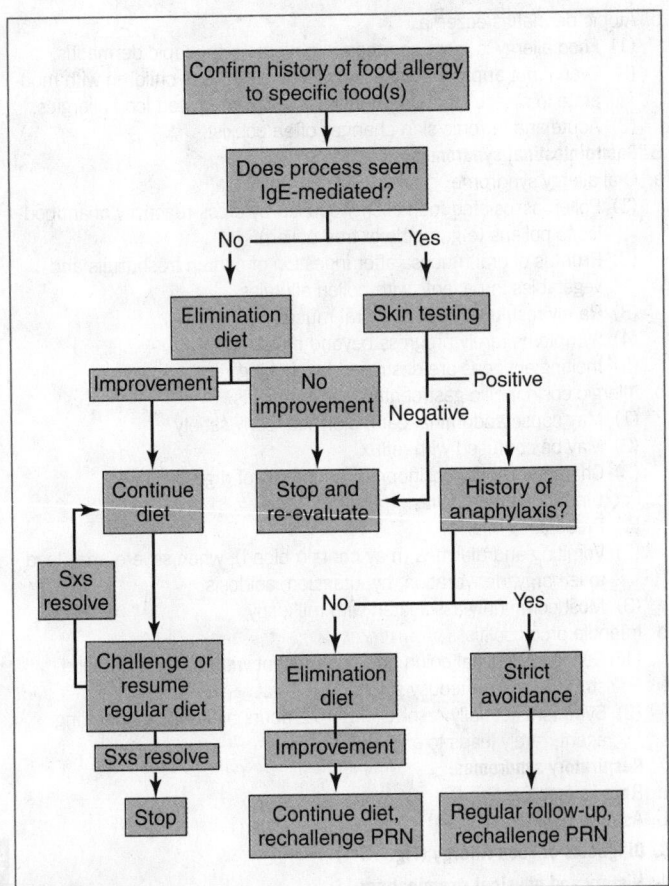

FIGURE 15-1

Evaluation and management of food allergy. Sxs, Symptoms. *(Data from Wood RA. The natural history of food allergy. Pediatrics. 2003;111:1631-1637; and Wood RA. Up to Date 2009. http://www.uptodate.com.)*

3. **Measurement of allergen-specific IgE:**
   a. Like skin tests, has poor positive predictive value, excellent negative predictive value
   b. Commonly used antigens include milk, eggs, peanuts, tree nuts (e.g., cashew, walnut), soy, wheat
   c. Levels above a certain range (different for different antigens) have increasing positive predictive value
   d. Useful in patients with dermatologic conditions that preclude skin testing

e. IgE binding to specific allergen components currently in clinical use, enzyme assays based on anti-IgE antibodies

f. IgG testing not useful

4. **Oral food challenges:**

a. Can verify clinical reactivity to a specific food allergen

b. Must be done under close medical supervision with emergency medications readily available

c. Patient must not be taking antihistamines

d. Most effective when double-blinded using graded doses of disguised food

5. **Trial elimination diet:**

a. Helpful if improvement with removal of food from diet

b. May be used prior to oral food challenge to clear food from system

D. Differential Diagnosis

1. **Food intolerance:** Nonimmunologic, based on toxins or other properties of foods leading to adverse effects

2. **Malabsorption syndromes:**

a. Cystic fibrosis, celiac disease (see Chapter 12), lactase deficiency

b. Gastrointestinal (GI) malformations

E. Treatment

1. **Allergen avoidance** is the most important intervention for all types of food allergy.

a. Patients must pay close attention to food ingredients.

b. Infants with milk, soy allergies may be placed on elemental formula.

c. Nutritional counseling and regular growth monitoring are recommended.

2. **For angioedema, urticaria:**

a. Epinephrine is first-line treatment

b. Antihistamines, corticosteroids

c. Broad differential.

3. **Atopic dermatitis:** Symptomatic control (see Chapter 8)

4. **Anaphylaxis:** Epinephrine, all at-risk patients should have an epinephrine auto-injector.

5. **Food-specific immunotherapy** is under investigation; used to induce clinical desensitization to specific allergens.

F. Natural History

1. **About one third of allergies** are lost in a 1- to 2-year period (peanut, tree nut, and shellfish allergies rarely outgrown, however).

2. **Patients with prior anaphylaxis** also usually outgrow their food allergies.

3. **Skin tests and radioallergosorbent testing (RAST)** may remain positive even though symptoms resolve.

III. DRUG ALLERGY[10-11]

A. Epidemiology

1. **Drug allergy:** Immunologically mediated response to an agent in a sensitized person.

15

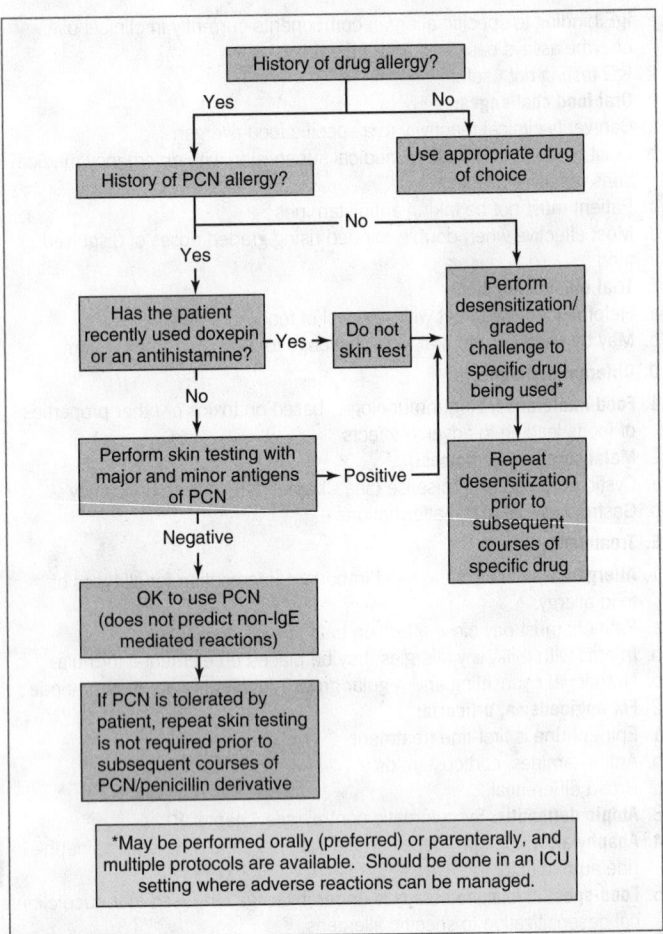

FIGURE 15-2

Evaluation and management of drug allergy. PCN, Penicillin. *(Adapted from Solensky R. Allergy to penicillins. Up to Date 2009. http://www.uptodate.com.)*

2. **Drug intolerance:** Undesirable pharmacologic effect.
3. **Although 10% of patients report penicillin allergy,** after evaluation, about 90% of individuals can tolerate penicillin.
B. **Diagnosis**
1. **History:** Cutaneous manifestations are the most common presentation for drug allergic reactions.

2. **Diagnostic studies:**
a. Penicillin is the only agent for which optimal negative predictive values for IgE-mediated reactions have been established.
b. Skin testing with major and minor antigens of penicillin.

C. **Management (Fig. 15-2)**

1. **Desensitization:** Immunologic IgE induction of tolerance, progressive administration of an allergenic substance to render effector cells less reactive
2. **Graded challenge:** Administration of progressively increasing doses of a drug until full dose is reached; does not modify a patient's response to the drug

IV. EVALUATION OF SUSPECTED IMMUNODEFICIENCY (TABLES 15-2 AND 15-3)[12-19]

V. IMMUNOGLOBULIN THERAPY[20-22]

A. **Intravenous Immunoglobulin (IVIG)**

1. **Indications:**
a. Replacement therapy for antibody-deficient disorders:
   (1) 400–500 mg/kg IV every 4 weeks to start.
   (2) Children with severe hypogammaglobulinemia (<100 mg/dL) may benefit from a total *loading* dose of 800 mg/kg given in two separate doses a few days apart, followed by 400–500 mg/kg every month.
   (3) Adjust dosing based on clinical response and to maintain trough IgG level of at least 500 mg/dL.
b. Immune thrombocytopenic purpura:
   (1) Initially 400–2000 mg/kg (up to 1000 mg/kg given on a single day or in divided doses over 2–5 consecutive days).
   (2) Maintenance dose: 400–1000 mg/kg/dose every 3–6 weeks based on clinical response and platelet count.
   (3) May also use Rho(D) immune globulin (Win Rho) in Rh-positive patients.
c. Kawasaki disease:
   (1) 2 g/kg × 1 dose over 8–12 hr.
   (2) If signs and symptoms persist, consider second dose of 2 g/kg.
   (3) Doses should be started within first 10 days of symptoms.
d. Pediatric human immunodeficiency virus (HIV) infection with antibody deficiency (IgG concentration <400 mg/dL, failure to form antibodies to common antigens, recurrent serious bacterial infections, or measles prophylaxis): Dosing same as for antibody-deficient disorders mentioned previously.
e. Bone marrow transplantation:
   (1) 400–500 mg/kg/dose to start; adjust dosing to maintain trough IgG level of at least 400 mg/dL
   (2) May decrease incidence of infection and death but not acute graft-versus-host disease
f. Other potential uses:
   (1) Guillain-Barré syndrome
   (2) Refractory dermatomyositis and polymyositis
   (3) Chronic inflammatory demyelinating polyneuropathy

15

TABLE 15-2

WHEN TO SUSPECT IMMUNODEFICIENCY

Recurrent Infections	Opportunistic Infections	Severe Infections	Other Conditions
6 or more new infections in 1 yr Recurrent tissue or organ abscesses 2 or more serious sinus infections in 1 yr 2 or more pneumonias in 1 yr	*Pneumocystis jiroveci* pneumonia *Pseudomonas* sepsis Invasive infection with *Neisseria* spp.	2 or more months of antibiotics with little effect Sepsis in the absence of a known risk (e.g., indwelling vascular catheter, neutropenia) Bacterial meningitis Pneumonia with empyema Resistant superficial or oral candidiasis	Failure to gain weight or grow normally Family history of immunodeficiency or unexplained early deaths Lymphopenia in infancy Complications from a live vaccine Part of a syndrome complex (e.g., Wiskott-Aldrich [with thrombocytopenia, eczema], DiGeorge syndrome [with facial dysmorphism, congenital cardiac disease, hypoparathyroidism])

Adapted from Stiehm ER. Approach to the child with recurrent infections. Up to Date 2009. http://www.uptodate.com.

TABLE 15-3

EVALUATION OF SUSPECTED IMMUNODEFICIENCY

Suspected Functional Abnormality	Clinical Findings	Initial Tests	More-Advanced Tests
Antibody (e.g., common variable immunodeficiency, X-linked agammaglobulinemia, IgA deficiency)	Sinopulmonary and systemic infections (pyogenic bacteria) Enteric infections (enterovirus, other viruses, *Giardia* spp.) Autoimmune diseases (immune thrombocytopenia, hemolytic anemia, inflammatory bowel disease)	Immunoglobulin levels (IgG, IgM, IgA) Antibody levels to T-cell–dependent protein antigens (e.g., tetanus or pneumococcal conjugate vaccines) Antibody levels to T-cell–independent polysaccharide antigens in a child ≥2 yr (e.g., pneumococcal polysaccharide vaccine such as Pneumovax)	B-cell enumeration Immunofixation electrophoresis
Cell-mediated immunity (e.g., severe combined immunodeficiency, DiGeorge syndrome)	Pneumonia (pyogenic bacteria, fungi, *Pneumocystis jiroveci*, viruses)	Total lymphocyte counts HIV ELISA/Western blot/PCR	T-cell enumeration (CD3, CD4, CD8) In vitro T-cell proliferation to mitogens, antigens, or allogeneic cells FISH 22q11 for DiGeorge deletion

TABLE 15-3

EVALUATION OF SUSPECTED IMMUNODEFICIENCY (Continued)

Suspected Functional Abnormality	Clinical Findings	Initial Tests	More-Advanced Tests
Phagocytosis (chronic granulomatous disease, leukocyte adhesion deficiency, Chédiak-Higashi syndrome)	Cutaneous infections, abscesses, lymphadenitis (staphylococci, enteric bacteria, fungi, mycobacteria), poor wound healing	WBC/neutrophil count and morphology	Nitroblue tetrazolium (NBT) test or dihydro-rhodamine (DHR) reduction test Chemotactic assay Phagocytic assay
Spleen	Bacteremia/hematogenous infection (pneumococcus, other streptococci, *Neisseria* spp.)	Peripheral blood smear for Howell-Jolly bodies Hemoglobin electrophoresis (HbSS)	Technetium-99 spleen scan or sonogram
Complement	Bacterial sepsis and other bloodborne infections (encapsulated bacteria, especially *Neisseria* spp.) Lupus, glomerulonephritis Angioedema	CH50 (total hemolytic complement)	Alternative pathway assay (AH50) Mannose-binding lectin level Individual complement component assays

ELISA, Enzyme-linked immunosorbent assay; FISH, fluorescent in situ hybridization; HIV, human immunodeficiency virus; PCR, polymerase chain reaction; WBC, white blood cell.

From Lederman HM. Clinical presentation of primary immunodeficiency diseases. In: McMillan J. *Oski's Pediatrics.* Philadelphia: Lippincott Williams & Wilkins; 2006:2441-2444.

2. **Precautions and adverse reactions:**
a. Severe systemic symptoms (hemodynamic changes, respiratory difficulty, anaphylaxis).
b. Less-severe systemic reactions (headache, myalgia, fever, chills, nausea, vomiting) may be alleviated by decreasing infusion rate or premedication with IV corticosteroids, antihistamines, and/or antipyretics.
c. Aseptic meningitis syndrome.
d. Acute renal failure (increased risk with preexisting renal insufficiency and with sucrose-containing IVIG).
e. Acute venous thrombosis (increased risk with sucrose-containing IVIG).
f. Use with caution in patients with undetectable IgA level due to trace amounts of IgA in IVIG (can lead to IgE-mediated anaphylaxis), although routine screening for IgA deficiency is not recommended in potential recipients.

B. **Intramuscular Immunoglobulin (IMIG)**

1. **Indications:**
a. Hepatitis A prophylaxis
b. Measles prophylaxis
c. Rubella prophylaxis

d. Rabies prophylaxis

e. Varicella-Zoster prophylaxis (independent of HIV status)

2. **Precautions and adverse reactions:**

a. Severe systemic symptoms (hemodynamic changes, anaphylaxis).

b. Local symptoms at injection site increase with repeated use; risk of local tissue injury.

c. High risk for anaphylactoid reactions if given intravenously.

d. Use with caution in patients with undetectable IgA levels, owing to trace amounts of IgA in IMIG.

3. **Dose of IMIG:**

a. Hepatitis A postexposure prophylaxis: 0.02 mL/kg given within 14 days of exposure. Immunoglobulin is not needed if at least one dose of hepatitis A vaccine was given at ≥1 month before exposure.

b. Measles prophylaxis: 0.25 mL/kg/dose (maximum dose 15 mL) given within 6 days of exposure in immunocompetent patient, and 0.5 mL/kg (maximum dose 15 mL) immediately following exposure in immunocompromised patients.

c. Rubella prophylaxis during pregnancy: 0.55 mL/kg/dose within 72 hours of exposure.

d. Rabies: 20 international units (IU)/kg single dose administered as soon as possible after exposure with the first dose of rabies vaccine.

e. Varicella-zoster postexposure prophylaxis (independent of HIV status): (GamaSTAN™ S/D): 0.6-1.2 mL/kg/dose as a single dose within 72 hours of exposure

4. **Administration:**

a. No more than 5 mL should be given at one site in an adult or large child.

b. Smaller amounts per site (1–3 mL) for smaller children and infants.

c. Administration of >15 mL at one time is essentially never warranted.

d. Peak serum levels achieved by 48 hours; immune effect lasts 3–4 weeks.

e. Intravenous or intradermal use of IMIG is absolutely contraindicated.

C. Subcutaneous Immunoglobulin

1. **Indication:** Replacement therapy for antibody deficiency.

2. **Dose:**

a. 100–125 mg/kg weekly (maximum rate: 20 mL/hour; doses >15 mL usually should be divided between sites, but it depends on the amount of subcutaneous tissue).

b. Larger doses can be given simultaneously in multiple sites or more frequently than once weekly.

c. Using the same areas for injections improves tolerability.

3. **Precautions and adverse reactions:** similar to IMIG and IVIG; fewer systemic reactions because more slowly absorbed into circulation.

4. **Considerations:** does not require venous access or special nursing (parents can administer) but may require multiple needlesticks in larger children because of volume restriction per site.

D. Specific Immunoglobulins

1. Hyperimmune globulins:

a. Prepared from donors with high titers of specific antibodies

b. Includes hepatitis B immune globulin (HBIG), varicella-zoster immuneglobulin (VZIG), cytomegalovirus immune globulin (CMV-IG), Rho(D) immune globulin, and others

2. Monoclonal antibody preparations (rituximab, palivizumab, and others)

VI. IMMUNOLOGIC REFERENCE VALUES

A. Serum IgG, IgM, IgA, and IgE Levels (Table 15-4)

B. Serum IgG, IgM, IgA, and IgE Levels for Low Birth Weight Preterm Infants (Table 15-5)

C. Serum IgG Subclass Levels (Table 15-6)

D. Lymphocyte Enumeration (Table 15-7)

E. Serum Complement Levels (Table 15-8)

TABLE 15-4

SERUM IMMUNOGLOBULIN LEVELS*

Age	IgG (mg/dL)	IgM (mg/dL)	IgA (mg/dL)	IgE (IU/ml)
Cord blood (term)	1121 (636–1606)	13 (6.3–25)	2.3 (1.4–3.6)	0.22 (0.04–1.28)
1 mo	503 (251–906)	45 (20–87)	13 (1.3–53)	
6 wk				0.69 (0.08–6.12)
2 mo	365 (206–601)	46 (17–105)	15 (2.8–47)	
3 mo	334 (176–581)	49 (24–89)	17 (4.6–46)	0.82 (0.18–3.76)
4 mo	343 (196–558)	55 (27–101)	23 (4.4–73)	
5 mo	403 (172–814)	62 (33–108)	31 (8.1–84)	
6 mo	407 (215–704)	62 (35–102)	25 (8.1–68)	2.68 (0.44–16.3)
7–9 mo	475 (217–904)	80 (34–126)	36 (11–90)	2.36 (0.76–7.31)
10–12 mo	594 (294–1069)	82 (41–149)	40 (16–84)	
1 yr	679 (345–1213)	93 (43–173)	44 (14–106)	3.49 (0.80–15.2)
2 yr	685 (424–1051)	95 (48–168)	47 (14–123)	3.03 (0.31–29.5)
3 yr	728 (441–1135)	104 (47–200)	66 (22–159)	1.80 (0.19–16.9)
4–5 yr	780 (463–1236)	99 (43–196)	68 (25–154)	8.58 (1.07–68.9)[†]
6–8 yr	915 (633–1280)	107 (48–207)	90 (33–202)	12.89 (1.03–161.3)[‡]
9–10 yr	1007 (608–1572)	121 (52–242)	113 (45–236)	23.6 (0.98–570.6)[§]
14 yr				20.07 (2.06–195.2)
Adult	994 (639–1349)	156 (56–352)	171 (70–312)	13.2 (1.53–114)

*Numbers in parentheses are the 95% confidence intervals (CIs).

[†]IgE data for 4 yr.

[‡]IgE data for 7 yr.

[§]IgE data for 10 yr.

From Kjellman NM, Johansson SG, Roth A. Serum IgE levels in healthy children quantified by a sandwich technique (PRIST). *Clin Allergy.* 1976;6:51-59; Jolliff CR, Cost KM, Stivrins PC, et al. Reference intervals for serum IgG, IgA, IgM, C3, and C4 as determined by rate nephelometry. *Clin Chem.* 1982;28:126-128; and Zetterström O, Johansson SG. IgE concentrations measured by PRIST in serum of healthy adults and in patients with respiratory allergy: a diagnostic approach. *Allergy.* 1981;36:537-547.

15

SERUM IMMUNOGLOBULIN LEVELS FOR LOW BIRTH WEIGHT PRETERM INFANTS

Age (mo)	Plasma IG Concentrations in 25- to 28-Wk Gestation Infants			Plasma IG Concentrations in 29- to 32-Wk Gestation Infants		
	IgG (mg/dL)*	IgM (mg/dL)*	IgA (mg/dL)*	IgG (mg/dL)*	IgM (mg/dL)*	IgA (mg/dL)*
0.25	251 (114–552)†	7.6 (1.3–43.3)	1.2 (0.07–20.8)	368 (186–728)†	9.1 (2.1–39.4)	0.6 (0.04–1.0)
0.5	202 (91–446)	14.1 (3.5–56.1)	3.1 (0.09–10.7)	275 (119–637)	13.9 (4.7–41)	0.9 (0.01–7.5)
1.0	158 (57–437)	12.7 (3.0–53.3)	4.5 (0.65–30.9)	209 (97–452)	14.4 (6.3–33)	1.9 (0.3–12.0)
1.5	134 (59–307)	16.2 (4.4–59.2)	4.3 (0.9–20.9)	156 (69–352)	15.4 (5.5–43.2)	2.2 (0.7–6.5)
2.0	89 (58–136)	16.0 (5.3–48.9)	4.1 (1.5–11.1)	123 (64–237)	15.2 (4.9–46.7)	3.0 (1.1–8.3)
3	60 (23–156)	13.8 (5.3–36.1)	3.0 (0.6–15.6)	104 (41–268)	16.3 (7.1–37.2)	3.6 (0.8–15.4)
4	82 (32–210)	22.2 (11.2–43.9)	6.8 (1.0–47.8)	128 (39–425)	26.5 (7.7–91.2)	9.8 (2.5–39.3)
6	159 (56–455)	41.3 (8.3–205)	9.7 (3.0–31.2)	179 (51–634)	29.3 (10.5–81.5)	12.3 (2.7–57.1)
8–10	273 (94–794)	41.8 (31.1–56.1)	9.5 (0.9–98.6)	280 (140–561)	34.7 (17–70.8)	20.9 (8.3–53)

*Geometric mean.
†Numbers in parentheses are ±2 SD.
From Ballow M, Cates KL, Rowe JC, et al. Development of the immune system in very low birth weight (less than 1500 g) premature infants: concentrations of plasma immunoglobulins and patterns of infections. *Pediatr Res.* 1986;9:899-904.

SERUM IgG SUBCLASS LEVELS*

Age (yr)	IgG1 (mg/dL)	IgG2 (mg/dL)	IgG3 (mg/dL)	IgG4 (mg/dL)
0.5–1	290 (140–620)	58 (41–130)	41 (11–85)	0.2 (0–0.8)
1–1.5	350 (170–650)	62 (40–140)	42 (12–87)	3 (0–26)
1.5–2	400 (220–720)	80 (50–180)	44 (14–91)	7 (0–41)
2–3	450 (240–780)	95 (55–200)	46 (15–93)	14 (0–69)
3–4	480 (270–810)	115 (65–220)	48 (16–96)	20 (1–94)
4–6	500 (300–840)	130 (70–250)	50 (17–97)	26 (2–116)
6–9	570 (350–910)	170 (85–330)	54 (20–100)	37 (3–158)
9–12	600 (370–930)	210 (10–400)	58 (22–109)	47 (4–190)
12–18	580 (370–910)	260 (110–480)	63 (24–116)	49 (5–196)
Adult	500 (280–800)	300 (115–570)	64 (24–120)	35 (5–125)

*Numbers in parentheses are the 95% confidence intervals (CIs).
From Schauer U, Stemberg F, Rieger CH, et al. IgG subclass concentrations in certified reference material 470 and reference values for children and adults determined with the binding site reagents. *Clin Chem.* 2003;49:1924-1929.

TABLE 15-7

T AND B LYMPHOCYTES IN PERIPHERAL BLOOD

Age	CD3 (Total T cell) Count*,† (%)†	CD4 count*,† (%)†	CD8 Count*,† (%)†	CD19 (B cell) Count*,† (%)†
0–3 mo	2.50–5.50 (53–84)	1.60–4.00 (35–64)	0.56–1.70 (12–28)	0.30–2.00 (6–32)
3–6 mo	2.50–5.60 (51–77)	1.80–4.00 (35–56)	0.59–1.60 (12–23)	0.43–3.00 (11–41)
6–12 mo	1.90–5.90 (49–76)	1.40–4.30 (31–56)	0.50–1.70 (12–24)	0.61–2.60 (14–37)
1–2 yr	2.10–6.20 (53–75)	1.30–3.40 (32–51)	0.62–2.00 (14–30)	0.72–2.60 (16–35)
2–6 yr	1.40–3.70 (56–75)	0.70–2.20 (28–47)	0.49–1.30 (16–30)	0.39–1.40 (14–33)
6–12 yr	1.20–2.60 (60–76)	0.65–1.50 (31–47)	0.37–1.10 (18–35)	0.27–0.86 (13–27)
12–18 yr	1.00–2.20 (56–84)	0.53–1.30 (31–52)	0.33–0.92 (18–35)	0.11–0.57 (6–23)
Adult‡	0.70–2.10 (55–83)	0.30–1.40 (28–57)	0.20–0.90 (10–39)	

*Absolute counts (number of cells per microliter $\times 10^{-3}$).

†Normal values (10th to 90th percentile).

‡From Comans-Bitter WM, de Groot R, van den Beemd R, et al. Immunotyping of blood lymphocytes in childhood. Reference values for lymphocyte subpopulations. *J Pediatr.* 1997;130:388-393.

From Shearer WT, Rosenblatt HM, Gelman RS, et al. Lymphocyte subsets in healthy children from birth through 18 years of age: the Pediatric AIDS Clinical Trials Group P1009 study. *J Allergy Clin Immunol.* 2003;112:973-980.

TABLE 15-8

SERUM COMPLEMENT LEVELS*

Age	C3 (mg/dL)	C4 (mg/dL)
Cord blood (term)	83 (57–116)	13 (6.6–23)
1 mo	83 (53–124)	14 (7.0–25)
2 mo	96 (59–149)	15 (7.4–28)
3 mo	94 (64–131)	16 (8.7–27)
4 mo	107 (62–175)	19 (8.3–38)
5 mo	107 (64–167)	18 (7.1–36)
6 mo	115 (74–171)	21 (8.6–42)
7–9 mo	113 (75–166)	20 (9.5–37)
10–12 mo	126 (73–180)	22 (12–39)
1 yr	129 (84–174)	23 (12–40)
2 yr	120 (81–170)	19 (9.2–34)
3 yr	117 (77–171)	20 (9.7–36)
4–5 yr	121 (86–166)	21 (13–32)
6–8 yr	118 (88–155)	20 (12–32)
9–10 yr	134 (89–195)	22 (10–40)
Adult	125 (83–177)	28 (15–45)

*Numbers in parentheses are the 95% confidence intervals (CIs).

Modified from Jolliff CR, Cost KM, Stivrins PC, et al. Reference intervals for serum IgG, IgA, IgM, C3, and C4 as determined by rate nephelometry. *Clin Chem.* 1982;28:126-128.

15

VII. COMPLEMENT PATHWAY (FIG. 15-3)

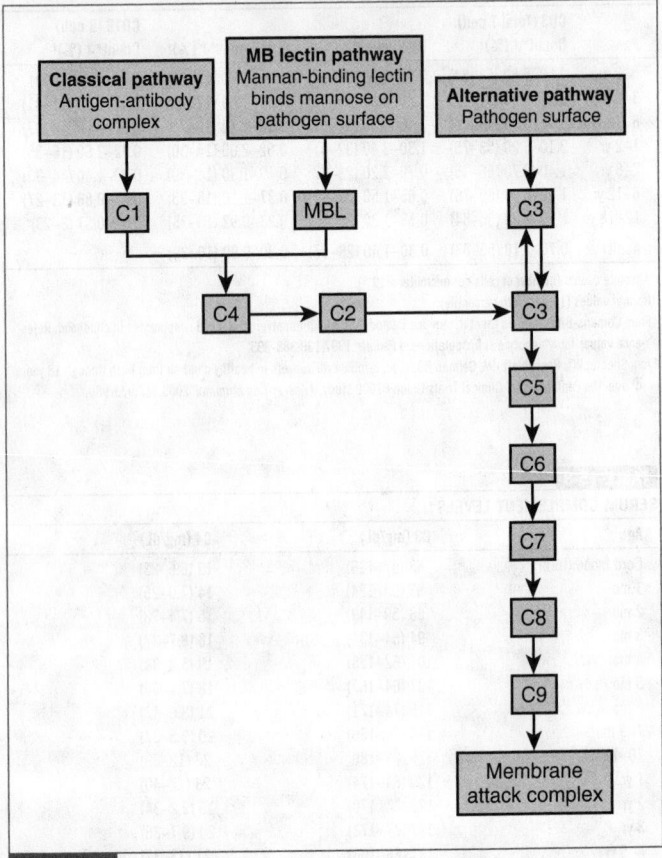

FIGURE 15-3

Complement pathway. MB, Mannan-binding; MBL, mannan-binding lectin.

REFERENCES

1. Blaiss MS. Antihistamines: treatment selection criteria for pediatric seasonal allergic rhinitis. *Allergy Asthma Proc*. 2005;26:95-102.
2. Garavello DW, DiBerardino F, Romagnoli M, et al. Nasal rinsing with hypertonic solution: an adjunctive treatment for pediatric seasonal allergic rhinoconjunctivitis. *Int Arch Allergy Immunol*. 2005;137:310-314.
3. Gelfand EW. Pediatric allergic rhinitis: factors affecting treatment choice. *Ear Nose Throat J*. 2005;84:163-168.

4. Wallace DV, Dykewicz MS, Bernstein DI, et al. The diagnosis and management of rhinitis: an updated practice parameter. *J Allergy Clin Immunol.* 2008;122 (suppl 2):S1-84.

5. Burks W. Diagnostic tools for food allergy. Up to Date 2009. Available at www.uptodate.com.

6. Chapman JA. Food allergy: a practice parameter. *Ann Allergy Asthma Immunol.* 2006;96(3 suppl 2):S1-68.

7. Lifschitz CH. Dietary protein-induced proctitis/colitis, enteropathy, and enterocolitis of infancy. Up to Date 2009. Available at www.uptodate.com.

8. Burks AW, Jones SM, Boyce JA, et al. NIAID-Sponsored 2010 Guidelines for Managing Food Allergy: applications in the pediatric population. *Pediatrics.* 2011;128:955-965.

9. Sicherer SH, Wood RA. Clinical report: allergy testing in childhood: using allergen-specific IgE testing. *Pediatrics.* 2012;129:193-197.

10. Solensky R. Allergy to penicillins. Up to Date 2009. Available at www.uptodate.com.

11. Solensky R, Khan DA. Drug allergy: an updated practice parameter. *Ann Allergy Asthma Immunol.* 2010;105:259-273.

12. Bonilla FA, Bernstein IL, Khan DA, et al. Practice parameter for the diagnosis and management of primary immunodeficiency. *Ann Allergy Asthma Immunol.* 2005;94:S1.

13. Bonilla FA, Geha RS. Primary immunodeficiency diseases. *J Allergy Clin Immunol.* 2003;111(suppl 2):S571-S581.

14. Bonilla FA, Geha RS. Update on primary immunodeficiency diseases. *J Allergy Clin Immunol.* 2006;117(suppl 2 Mini-Primer):S435-S441.

15. Fleisher TA. Back to basics: primary immune deficiencies: windows into the immune system. *Pediatr Rev.* 2006;27:363-372.

16. Geha RS, Notarangelo LD, Casanova JL, et al. International Union of Immunological Societies Primary Immunodeficiency Diseases Classification Committee. Primary immunodeficiency diseases: an update from the International Union of Immunological Societies Primary Immunodeficiency Diseases Classification Committee. *J Allergy Clin Immunol.* 2007;120:776-794.

17. Lederman HM. Clinical presentation of primary immunodeficiency diseases. In: McMillan J, ed. *Oski's Pediatrics.* Philadelphia:: Lippincott Williams & Wilkins; 2006:2441-2444.

18. Stiehm ER. Approach to the child with recurrent infections. Up to Date 2009. Available at www.uptodate.com.

19. Stiehm ER, Ochs HD, Winkelstein JA. Immunodeficiency disorders: general considerations. In: Stiehm ER, Ochs HD, Winkelstein JA, eds. *Immunologic disorders in infants and children.* 5th ed. Philadelphia: Elsevier/Saunders; 2004.

20. Garcia-Lloret M, McGhee S, Chatila TA, et al. Immunoglobulin replacement therapy in children. *Immunol Allergy Clin North Am.* 2008;28:833-849.

21. Moore ML, Quinn JM. Subcutaneous immunoglobulin replacement therapy for primary antibody deficiency: advancements into the 21st century. *Ann Allergy Asthma Immunol.* 2008;101:114-121.

22. Orange J, Hossny EM, Weiler CR, et al. Use of intravenous immunoglobulin in human disease: a review of evidence by members of the Primary Immunodeficiency Committee of the American Academy of Allergy, Asthma, and Immunology. *J Allergy Clin Immunol.* 2006;117:S525-S553.

Chapter 16

Immunoprophylaxis

Jennifer Albon, MD

⊗ See additional content on Expert Consult

I. WEBSITES

American Academy of Pediatrics: *Red Book: 2012 Report of the Committee on Infectious Diseases,* 29th ed. 2012: http://aapredbook.aappublications.org/

Food and Drug Administration: Vaccines Licensed for Immunization and Distribution in the US with Supporting Documents (including all package inserts): http://www.fda.gov/BiologicsBloodVaccines/Vaccines/ApprovedProducts/

Centers for Disease Control and Prevention: Vaccines and Immunization: Includes immunization schedules and *Morbidity and Mortality Weekly Reports* pertaining to vaccines: http://www.cdc.gov/vaccines/

Centers for Disease Control and Prevention: Travelers' Health: http://www.cdc.gov/travel/

Influenza vaccines A and B: www.cdc.gov/flu/professionals/antivirals/index.htm

Vaccine Adverse Event Reporting System: http://vaers.hhs.gov/index

World Health Organization: Vaccine, Blood, and Biologics: http://www.who.int/immunization/en/

II. IMMUNIZATION SCHEDULES

Recommended Childhood Immunization Schedule (Fig. 16-1) and Catch-up Immunization Schedules, with minimum age for initial vaccination, minumum intervals between doses (Fig. 16-2), and accompanying footnotes (Fig. 16-3)[1]

III. IMMUNIZATION GUIDELINES

A. Vaccine Informed Consent

Current forms for the vaccine information statement (VIS) can be obtained from the Centers for Disease Control and Prevention (CDC). The most recent VIS must be provided to the patient (non minor) or parent/guardian, with documentation of version date and date vaccine administered.

B. Vaccine Administration

1. **Preferred sites of administration of intramuscular (IM) and subcutaneous (SQ) vaccines:**
   a. <18 months old: Anterolateral thigh
   b. Toddlers: Anterolateral thigh or deltoid (deltoid preferred if large enough)
   c. Adolescents and young adults: Deltoid
2. **Route:**
   a. IM: Deep into muscle to avoid tissue damage from adjuvants, usually with a 22G–25G needle, ⅞ to 1 inch long in infants and toddlers, and 1 to 2 inches long in adolescents and young adults

Figure 1. Recommended immunization schedule for persons aged 0 through 18 years – United States, 2014.
(FOR THOSE WHO FALL BEHIND OR START LATE, SEE THE CATCH-UP SCHEDULE [FIGURE 2]).

These recommendations must be read with the footnotes that follow. For those who fall behind or start late, provide catch-up vaccination at the earliest opportunity as indicated by the green bars in Figure 1. To determine minimum intervals between doses, see the catch-up schedule (Figure 2). School entry and adolescent vaccine age groups are in bold.

Vaccine	Birth	1 mo	2 mos	4 mos	6 mos	9 mos	12 mos	15 mos	18 mos	19–23 mos	2-3 yrs	**4-6 yrs**	7-10 yrs	**11-12 yrs**	13–15 yrs	16–18 yrs
Hepatitis B[1] (HepB)	1st dose	←2nd dose→			←3rd dose→											
Rotavirus[2] (RV) RV1 (2-dose series); RV5 (3-dose series)			1st dose	2nd dose	See footnote 2											
Diphtheria, tetanus, & acellular pertussis[3] (DTaP: <7 yrs)			1st dose	2nd dose	3rd dose			←4th dose→				5th dose				
Tetanus, diphtheria, & acellular pertussis[4] (Tdap: ≥7 yrs)														(Tdap)		
Haemophilus influenzae type b[5] (Hib)			1st dose	2nd dose	See footnote 5		←3rd or 4th dose, See footnote 5→									
Pneumococcal conjugate[6] (PCV13)			1st dose	2nd dose	3rd dose		←4th dose→									
Pneumococcal polysaccharide[6] (PPSV23)																
Inactivated poliovirus[7] (IPV) (<18 yrs)			1st dose	2nd dose	←3rd dose→							4th dose				
Influenza[8] (IIV; LAIV) 2 doses for some: See footnote 8					Annual vaccination (IIV only)						Annual vaccination (IIV or LAIV)					
Measles, mumps, rubella[9] (MMR)							←1st dose→					2nd dose				
Varicella[10] (VAR)							←1st dose→					2nd dose				
Hepatitis A[11] (HepA)							←2-dose series, See footnote 11→									
Human papillomavirus[12] (HPV2: females only; HPV4: males and females)														(3-dose series)		
Meningococcal[13] (Hib-MenCY ≥ 6 weeks; MenACWY-D ≥9 mos; MenACWY-CRM ≥ 2 mos)			See footnote 13											1st dose		Booster

Range of recommended ages for all children | Range of recommended ages for catch-up immunization | Range of recommended ages for certain high-risk groups | Range of recommended ages during which catch-up is encouraged and for certain high-risk groups | Not routinely recommended

This schedule includes recommendations in effect as of January 1, 2014. Any dose not administered at the recommended age should be administered at a subsequent visit, when indicated and feasible. The use of a combination vaccine generally is preferred over separate injections of its equivalent component vaccines. Vaccination providers should consult the relevant Advisory Committee on Immunization Practices (ACIP) statement for detailed recommendations, available online at http://www.cdc.gov/vaccines/hcp/acip-recs/index.html. Clinically significant adverse events that follow vaccination should be reported to the Vaccine Adverse Event Reporting System(VAERS) online (http://www.vaers.hhs.gov) or by telephone (800-822-7967). Suspected cases of vaccine-preventable diseases should be reported to the state or local health department. Additional information, including precautions and contraindications for vaccination, is available from CDC online (http://www.cdc.gov/vaccines/recs/vac-admin/contraindications.htm) or by telephone (800-CDC-INFO [800-232-4636]). This schedule is approved by the Advisory Committee on Immunization Practices (http//www.cdc.gov/vaccines/acip), the American Academy of Pediatrics (http://www.aap.org), the American Academy of Family Physicians (http://www.aafp.org), and the American College of Obstetricians and Gynecologists (http://www.acog.org).

NOTE: The above recommendations must be read along with the footnotes of this schedule.

FIGURE 16-1

Recommended immunization schedule for persons aged 0–18 years—United States, 2013. *(From ACIP Childhood/Adolescent Immunization Work Group: Advisory Committee on Immunization Practices [ACIP] recommended immunization schedule for persons aged 0 through 18 years—United States, 2013.* MMWR Recomm Rep. *2013; 62:2-8. Available at www.cdc.gov.)*

FIGURE 2. Catch-up immunization schedule for persons aged 4 months through 18 years who start late or who are more than 1 month behind—**United States, 2014.**

The figure below provides catch-up schedules and minimum intervals between doses for children whose vaccinations have been delayed. A vaccine series does not need to be restarted, regardless of the time that has elapsed between doses. Use the section appropriate for the child's age. Always use this table in conjunction with Figure 1 and the footnotes that follow.

Vaccine	Minimum Age for Dose 1	Minimum Interval Between Doses			
		Dose 1 to dose 2	**Dose 2 to dose 3**	**Dose 3 to dose 4**	**Dose 4 to dose 5**
		Persons aged 4 months through 6 years			
Hepatitis B	Birth	4 weeks	8 weeks and at least 16 weeks after first dose; minimum age for the final dose is 24 weeks		
Rotavirus	6 weeks	4 weeks	4 weeks		
Diphtheria, tetanus, & acellular pertussis	6 weeks	4 weeks	4 weeks	6 months	6 months
Haemophilus influenzae type b	6 weeks	(see footnotes)	(see footnotes)	(see footnotes)	
Pneumococcal	6 weeks	(see footnotes)	(see footnotes)	(see footnotes)	
Inactivated poliovirus	6 weeks	4 weeks	4 weeks	6 months minimum age 4 years for final dose	
Meningococcal	6 weeks	8 weeks	See footnote 13	See footnote 13	
Measles, mumps, rubella	12 months	4 weeks			
Varicella	12 months	3 months			
Hepatitis A	12 months	6 months			
		Persons aged 7 through 18 years			
Tetanus, diphtheria, tetanus, diphtheria, & acellular pertussis	7 years	4 weeks	4 weeks if first dose of DTaP/DT administered at younger than 12 months; 6 months if first dose of DTaP/DT administered at age 12 months or older and no further doses needed for catch-up	6 months if first dose of DTaP/DT administered at younger than 12 months	
Human papillomavirus	9 years	Routine dosing intervals are recommended			
Hepatitis A	12 months	6 months			
Hepatitis B	Birth	4 weeks	8 weeks (and at least 16 weeks after first dose)		
Inactivated poliovirus	6 weeks	4 weeks	4 weeks	6 months	
Meningococcal	6 weeks	8 weeks	See footnote 13		
Measles, mumps, rubella	12 months	4 weeks			
Varicella	12 months	3 months if person is younger than age 13 years; 4 weeks if person is aged 13 years or older			

NOTE: The above recommendations must be read along with the footnotes of this schedule.

FIGURE 16-2

Catch-up immunization schedule for persons aged 4 months–18 years who start late or who are more than 1 month behind—United States, 2013. (From ACIP Childhood/Adolescent Immunization Work Group: Advisory Committee on Immunization Practices [ACIP] recommended immunization schedule for persons aged 0 through 18 years—United States, 2013. MMWR Recomm Rep. 2013;62:2–8. Available at www.cdc.gov.)

Footnotes — Recommended immunization schedule for persons aged 0 through 18 years—United States, 2014

For further guidance on the use of the vaccines mentioned below, see:
http://www.cdc.gov/vaccines/hcp/acip-recs/index.html.

For vaccine recommendations for persons 19 years of age and older, see the adult immunization schedule.

Additional information

- For contraindications and precautions to use of a vaccine and for additional information regarding that vaccine, vaccination providers should consult the relevant ACIP statement available online at http://www.cdc.gov/vaccines /acip-recs/index.html.
- For purposes of calculating intervals between doses, 4 weeks = 28 days. Intervals of 4 months or greater are determined by calendar months.
- Vaccine doses administered 4 days or less before the minimum interval are considered valid. Doses of any vaccine administered ≥5 days earlier than the minimum interval or minimum age should not be counted as valid doses and should be repeated as age-appropriate. The repeat dose should be spaced after the invalid dose by the recommended minimum interval. For further details, see *MMWR, General Recommendations on Immunization and Reports / Vol. 60 / No. 2; Table 1. Recommended and minimum ages and intervals between vaccine doses* available online at http://www.cdc.gov/mmwr/pdf/rr/rr6002.pdf.
- Information on travel vaccine requirements and recommendations is available at http://wwwnc.cdc.gov/travel/destinations/list.
- For vaccination of persons with primary and secondary immunodeficiencies, see Table 13, "*Vaccination of persons with primary and secondary immunodeficiencies*," in General Recommendations on Immunization (ACIP), available at http://www.cdc.gov/mmwr/pdf/rr/rr6002.pdf.; and American Academy of Pediatrics. Immunization in Special Clinical Ctrumstances, in Pickering LK, Baker CJ, Kimberlin DW, Long SS eds. *Red Book: 2012 report of the Committee on Infectious Diseases. 29th ed.* Elk Grove Village, IL: American Academy of Pediatrics.

1. **Hepatitis B (HepB) vaccine. (Minimum age: birth)**
   Routine vaccination:
   At birth:
   - Administer monovalent HepB vaccine to all newborns before hospital discharge.
   - For infants born to hepatitis B surface antigen (HBsAg)-positive mothers, administer HepB vaccine and 0.5 mL of hepatitis B immune globulin (HBIG) within 12 hours of birth. These infants should be tested for HBsAg and antibody to HBsAg (anti-HBs) 1 to 2 months after completion of the HepB series, at age 9 through 18 months (preferably at the next well-child visit).
   - If mother's HBsAg status is unknown, within 12 hours of birth administer HepB vaccine regardless of birth weight. For infants weighing less than 2,000 grams, administer HBIG in addition to HepB vaccine within 12 hours of birth. Determine mother's HBsAg status as soon as possible and, if mother is HBsAg-positive, also administer HBIG for infants weighing 2,000 grams or more as soon as possible, but no later than age 7 days.

   Doses following the birth dose:
   - The second dose should be administered at age 1 or 2 months. Monovalent HepB vaccine should be used for doses administered before age 6 weeks.
   - Infants who did not receive a birth dose should receive 3 doses of a HepB-containing vaccine on a schedule of 0, 1 to 2 months, and 6 months starting as soon as feasible. See Figure 2.
   - Administer the second dose 1 to 2 months after the first dose (minimum intervals of 4 weeks), administer the third dose at least 8 weeks after the second dose AND at least 16 weeks after the **first** dose. The final (third or fourth) dose in the HepB vaccine series should be administered no earlier than age 24 weeks.
   - Administration of a total of 4 doses of HepB vaccine is permitted when a combination vaccine containing HepB is administered after the birth dose.

   Catch-up vaccination:
   - Unvaccinated persons should complete a 3-dose series.
   - A 2-dose series (doses separated by at least 4 months) of adult formulation Recombivax HB is licensed for use in children aged 11 through 15 years.
   - For other catch-up guidance, see Figure 2.

2. **Rotavirus (RV) vaccines. (Minimum age: 6 weeks for both RV1 [Rotarix] and RV5 [RotaTeq])**
   Routine vaccination:
   Administer a series of RV vaccine to all infants as follows:
   1. If Rotarix is used, administer a 2-dose series at 2 and 4 months of age.
   2. If RotaTeq is used, administer a 3-dose series at ages 2, 4, and 6 months.
   3. If any dose in the series was RotaTeq or vaccine product is unknown for any dose in the series, a total of 3 doses of RV vaccine should be administered.

   Catch-up vaccination:
   - The maximum age for the first dose in the series is 14 weeks, 6 days; vaccination should not be initiated for infants aged 15 weeks, 0 days or older.
   - The maximum age for the final dose in the series is 8 months, 0 days.
   - For other catch-up guidance, see Figure 2.

FIGURE 16-3—cont'd

Continued

16

For further guidance on the use of the vaccines mentioned below, see:
http://www.cdc.gov/vaccines/hcp/acip-recs/index.html.

3. **Diphtheria and tetanus toxoids and acellular pertussis (DTaP)
    vaccine. (Minimum age: 6 weeks. Exception: DTaP-IPV [Kinrix]:4
    years)**
    Routine vaccination:
    - Administer a 5-dose series of DTaP vaccine at ages 2, 4, 6, 15 through 18 months, and 4
      through 6 years. The fourth dose may be administered as early as age 12 months, provided at
      least 6 months have elapsed since the third dose.

    Catch-up vaccination:
    - The fifth dose of DTaP vaccine is not necessary if the fourth dose was administered at age 4 years
      or older.
    - For other catch-up guidance, see Figure 2.

4. **Tetanus and diphtheria toxoids and acellular pertussis (Tdap)
    vaccine. (Minimum age: 10 years for Boostrix, 11 years for
    Adacel)**
    Routine vaccination:
    - Administer 1 dose of Tdap vaccine to all adolescents aged 11 through 12 years.
    - Tdap may be administered regardless of the interval since the last tetanus and diphtheria
      toxoid-containing vaccine.
    - Administer 1 dose of Tdap vaccine to pregnant adolescents during each pregnancy (preferred
      during 27 through 36 weeks gestation) regardless of time since prior Td or Tdap vaccination.

    Catch-up vaccination:
    - Persons aged 7 years and older who are not fully immunized with DTaP vaccine should
      receive Tdap vaccine as 1 (preferably the first dose in the catch-up series; additional doses are
      needed, use Td vaccine). For children 7 through 10 years who receive a dose of Tdap as part of
      the catch-up series, an adolescent Tdap vaccine dose at age 11 through 12 years should NOT
      be administered. Td should be administered instead 10 years after the Tdap dose.
    - Persons aged 11 through 18 years who have not received Tdap vaccine should receive a dose
      followed by tetanus and diphtheria toxoids (Td) booster doses every 10 years thereafter.
    - Inadvertent doses of DTaP vaccine:
      - If administered inadvertently to a child aged 7 through 10 years may count as part of the
        catch-up series. This dose may count as the adolescent Tdap dose, or the child can later
        receive a Tdap booster dose at age 11 through 12 years.
      - If administered inadvertently to an adolescent aged 11 through 18 years, the dose should be
        counted as the adolescent Tdap booster.
    - For other catch-up guidance, see Figure 2.

5. ***Haemophilus influenzae* type b (Hib) conjugate vaccine. (Minimum
    age: 6 weeks for PRP-T [ACTHIB, DTaP-IPV/Hib (Pentacel) and
    Hib-MenCY (MenHibrix)], PRP-OMP [PedvaxHIB or COMVAX], 12
    months for PRP-T [Hiberix])**
    Routine vaccination:
    - Administer a 2- or 3-dose Hib vaccine primary series and a booster dose (dose 3 or 4
      depending on vaccine used in primary series) at age 12 through 15 months to complete a full
      Hib vaccine series.
    - The primary series with ActHIB, MenHibrix, or Pentacel consists of 3 doses and should be
      administered at 2, 4, and 6 months of age. The primary series with PedvaxHib or COMVAX
      consists of 2 doses and should be administered at 2 and 4 months of age; a dose at age 6
      months is not indicated.
    - One booster dose (dose 3 or 4 depending on vaccine used in primary series) of any Hib
      vaccine should be administered at age 12 through 15 months. An exception is Hiberix vaccine.
      Hiberix should only

FIGURE 16-3—cont'd

For further guidance on the use of the vaccines mentioned below, see:
http://www.cdc.gov/vaccines/hcp/acip-recs/index.html.

5. *Haemophilus influenzae* type b (Hib) conjugate vaccine (cont'd)

- For recommendations on the use of MenHibrix in patients at increased risk for meningococcal disease, please refer to the meningococcal vaccine footnotes and also to *MMWR* March 22, 2013; 62(RR02);1-22, available at http://www.cdc.gov/mmwr/pdf/rr/rr6202.pdf.

Catch-up vaccination:

- If dose 1 was administered at ages 12 through 14 months, administer a second (final) dose at least 8 weeks after dose 1, regardless of Hib vaccine used in the primary series.
- If the first 2 doses were PRP-OMP (PedavaxHIB or COMVAX), and were administered at age 11 months or younger, the third (and final) dose should be administered at age 12 through 15 months and at least 8 weeks after the second dose.
- If the first dose was administered at age 7 through 11 months, administer the second dose at least 4 weeks later and a third (and final) dose at age 12 through 15 months or 8 weeks after second dose, whichever is later, regardless of Hib vaccine used for first dose.
- If first dose is administered at younger than 12 months of age and second dose is given between 12 through 14 months of age, a third (and final) dose should be given 8 weeks later.
- For unvaccinated children aged 15 months or older, administer only 1 dose.
- For other catch-up guidance, see Figure 2. For catch-up guidance related to MenHibrix, please see the meningococcal vaccine footnotes and also *MMWR* March 22, 2013; 62 (RR02);1-22, available at http://www.cdc.gov/mmwr/pdf/rr/rr6202.pdf.

Vaccination of persons with high-risk conditions:

- Children aged 12 through 59 months who are at increased risk for Hib disease, including chemotherapy recipients and those with anatomic or functional asplenia (including sickle cell disease), human immunodeficiency virus (HIV) infection, immunoglobulin deficiency, or early component complement deficiency, who have received either no doses or only 1 dose of Hib vaccine before 12 months of age, should receive 2 additional doses of Hib vaccine 8 weeks apart; children who received 2 or more doses of Hib vaccine before 12 months of age should receive 1 additional dose.
- For patients younger than 5 years of age undergoing chemotherapy or radiation treatment who received a Hib vaccine dose(s) within 14 days of starting therapy or during therapy, repeat the dose(s) at least 3 months following therapy completion.
- Recipients of hematopoietic stem cell transplant (HSCT) should be revaccinated with a 3-dose regimen of Hib vaccine starting 6 to 12 months after successful transplant, regardless of vaccination history; doses should be administered at least 4 weeks apart.
- A single dose of any Hib-containing vaccine should be administered to unimmunized* children and adolescents 15 months of age and older undergoing an elective splenectomy; if possible, vaccine should be administered at least 14 days before procedure.
- Hib vaccine is not routinely recommended for patients 5 years or older. However, 1 dose of Hib vaccine should be administered to unimmunized* persons aged 5 years or older who have anatomic or functional asplenia (including sickle cell disease) and unvaccinated persons 5 through 18 years of age with human immunodeficiency virus (HIV) infection
  * Patients who have not received a primary series and booster dose or at least 1 dose of Hib vaccine after 14 months of age are considered unimmunized.

6. **Pneumococcal vaccines. (Minimum age: 6 weeks for PCV13, 2 years for PPSV23)**

Routine vaccination with PCV13:

- Administer a 4-dose series of PCV13 vaccine at ages 2, 4, and 6 months and at age 12 through 15 months.
- For children aged 14 through 59 months who have received an age-appropriate series of 7-valent PCV (PCV7), administer a single supplemental dose of 13-valent PCV (PCV13).

Catch-up vaccination with PCV13:

- Administer 1 dose of PCV13 to all healthy children aged 24 through 59 months who are not completely vaccinated for their age.
- For other catch-up guidance, see Figure 2.

Vaccination of persons with high-risk conditions with PCV13 and PPSV23:

- All recommended PCV13 doses should be administered prior to PPSV23 vaccination if possible.
- For children 2 through 5 years of age with any of the following conditions: chronic heart disease (particularly cyanotic congenital heart disease and cardiac failure); chronic lung disease (including asthma if treated high-dose oral corticosteroid therapy); diabetes melitus;cerebrospinal fluid leak; cochlear implant; sickle cell disease and other hemoglobinopathies;anatomic or functional asplenia; HIV infection; chronic renal failure; nephrotic syndrome;diseases associated with treatment with immunosuppressive drugs or radiation therapy,including malignant neoplasms, leukemias, lymphomas, and Hodgkin disease; solid organtransplantation; or congenital immunodeficiency:
  1. Administer 1 dose of PCV13 if 3 doses of PCV (PCV7 and/or PCV13) were received previously.
  2. Administer 2 doses of PCV13 at least 8 weeks apart if fewer than 3 doses of PCV (PCV7 and/or PCV13) were received previously.

FIGURE 16-3—cont'd

16

Continued

For further guidance on the use of the vaccines mentioned below, see:
http://www.cdc.gov/vaccines/hcp/acip-recs/index.html.

6. **Pneumococcal vaccines (cont'd)**

   - 3. Administer 1 supplemental dose of PCV13 if 4 doses of PCV7 or other age-appropriate complete PCV7 series was received previously.
   - 4. The minimum interval between doses of PCV (PCV7 or PCV13) is 8 weeks.
   - 5. For children with no history of PPSV23 vaccination, administer PPSV23 at least 8 weeks after the most recent dose of PCV13.

   - For children aged through 18 years who have cerebrospinal fluid leak; cochlear implant; sickle cell disease and other hemoglobinopathies; anatomic or functional asplenia; congenital or acquired immunodeficiencies; HIV infection; chronic renal failure; nephrotic syndrome; diseases associated with treatment with immunosuppressive drugs or radiation therapy, including malignant neoplasms, leukemias, lymphomas, and Hodgkin disease; generalized malignancy; solid organ transplantation; or multiple myeloma.

     1. If neither PCV13 nor PPSV23 has been received previously, administer 1 dose of PCV13 now and 1 dose of PPSV23 at least 8 weeks later.
     2. If PCV13 has been received previously but PPSV23 has not, administer 1 dose of PPSV23 at least 8 weeks after the most recent dose of PCV13.
     3. If PPSV23 has been received but PCV13 has not, administer 1 dose of PCV13 at least 8 weeks after the most recent PPSV23 dose.

   - For children aged 6 through 18 years with chronic heart disease (particularly cyanotic congenital heart disease and cardiac failure), chronic lung disease (including asthma if treated with high-dose oral corticosteroid therapy), diabetes mellitus, alcoholism, or chronic liver disease, who have not received PPSV23, administer 1 dose of PPSV23. If PCV13 has been received previously, then PPSV23 should be administered at least 8 weeks after any prior PCV13 dose.

   - A single revaccination with PPSV23 should be administered 5 years the first dose to children with sickle cell disease or other hemoglobinopathies; anatomic or functional asplenia; congenital or acquired immunodeficiencies; HIV infection; chronic renal failure; nephrotic syndrome; diseases associated with treatment with immunosuppressive drugs or radiation therapy, including malignant neoplasms, leukemias, lymphomas, and Hodgkin disease; generalized malignancy; solid organ transplantation; or multiple myeloma.

7. **Inactivated poliovirus vaccine (IPV). (Minimum age: 6 weeks)**

   Routine vaccination:

   - Administer a 4-dose series of IPV at ages 2, 4, 6 through 18 months, and 4 through 6 years. The final dose in the series should be administered on or after the fourth birthday and at least 6 months after the previous dose.

   Catch-up vaccination:

   - In the first 6 months of life, minimum age and minimum intervals are only recommended if the person is at risk for imminent exposure to circulating poliovirus (i.e., travel to a polio-endemic region or during an outbreak).
   - If 4 or more doses are administered before age 4 years, an additional dose should be administered at age 4 through 6 years and at least 6 months after the previous dose.
   - A fourth dose is not necessary if the third dose was administered at age 4 years or older and at least 6 months after the previous dose.
   - If both OPV and IPV were administered as part of a series, a total of 4 doses should be administered, regardless of the child's current age. IPV is not routinely recommended for U.S. residents aged 18 years or older.
   - For other catch-up guidance, see Figure 2.

8. **Influenza vaccines. (Minimum age: 6 months for inactivated influenza vaccine [IIV], 2 years for live, attenuated influenza vaccine [LAIV])**

   Routine vaccination

   - Administer influenza vaccine annually to all children beginning at age 6 months. For most healthy, nonpregnant persons aged 2 through 49 years, either LAIV or IIV may be used. However, LAIV should NOT be administered to some persons, including 1) those with asthma, 2) children 2 through 4 years who NOT be administered to some persons, including 1) those with asthma, 2) children 2 through 4 years who had wheezing in the past 12 months, or 3) those who have any other underlying medical conditions that perdispose them to influenza complications. For all other contraindications to use of LAIV, see *MMWR* 2013; 62 (No. RR-7):1-43, available at http://www.cdc.gov/mmwr/pdf/rr/rr6207.pdf.

   For children aged 6 months through 8 years:

   - For the 2013–14 season, administer 2 doses (separated by at least 4 weeks) to children who are receiving influenza vaccine for the first time. Some children in this age group who have been vaccinated previously will also need 2 doses. For additional guidance, follow dosing guidelines in the 2013-14 ACIP influenza vaccine recommendations, *MMWR* 2013; 62 (No. RR-7):1-43, available at http://www.cdc.gov/mmwr/pdf/rr/rr6207.pdf.
   - For the 2014–15 season, follow dosing guidelines in the 2014 ACIP influenza vaccine recommendations.

   For persons aged 9 years and older:

   - Administer 1 dose.

FIGURE 16-3—cont'd

For further guidance on the use of the vaccines mentioned below, see:
http://www.cdc.gov/vaccines/hcp/acip-recs/index.html.

9. **Measles, mumps, and rubella (MMR) vaccine. (Minimum age: 12 months for routine vaccination)**
   Routine vaccination:
   - Administer a 2-dose series of MMR vaccine at ages12 through 15 months and 4 through 6 years. The second dose may be administered before age 4 years, provided at least 4 weeks have elapsed since the first dose.
   - Administer 1 dose of MMR vaccine to infants aged 6 through 11 months before departure from the United States for international travel. These children should be revaccinated with 2 doses of MMR vaccine, the first at age 12 through 15 months (12 months if the child remains in an area where disease risk is high), and the second dose at least 4 weeks later.
   - Administer 2 doses of MMR vaccine to children aged 12 months and older before departure from the United States for international travel. The first dose should be administered on or after age 12 months and the second dose at least 4 weeks later.

   Catch-up vaccination:
   - Ensure that all school-aged children and adolescents have had 2 doses of MMR vaccine; the minimum interval between the 2 doses is 4 weeks.

10. **Varicella (VAR) vaccine. (Minimum age: 12 months)**
    Routine vaccination:
    - Administer a 2-dose series of VAR vaccine at ages 12 through 15 months and 4 through 6 years. The second dose may be administered before age 4 years, provided at least 3 months have elapsed since the first dose. If the second dose was administered at least 4 weeks after the first dosr, it can be accepted as valid.

    Catch-up vaccination:
    - Ensure that all persons aged 7 through 18 years without evidence of immunity (see *MMWR* 2007; 56 [No. RR-4], available at http://www.cdc.gov/mmwr/pdf/rr/rr5604.pdf) have 2 doses of varicella vaccine. For children aged 7 through 12 years, the recommended minimum interval between doses is 3 months (if the second dose was administered at least 4 weeks after the first dose, it can be accepted as valid); for persons 13 years and older, the minimum interval between doses is 4 weeks.

11. **Hepatitis A (HepA) vaccine. (Minimum age: 12 months)**
    Routine vaccination:
    - Initiate the 2-dose HepA vaccine series at 12 through 23 months; separate the 2 doses by 6 to 18 months.
    - Children who have received 1 dose of HepA vaccine before age 24 months should receive a second dose 6 to 18 months after the first dose.
    - For any person aged 2 years and older who has not already received the HepA vaccine series, 2 doses of HepA vaccine separated by 6 to 18 months may be administered if immunity against hepatitis A virus infection is desired.

    Catch-up vaccination:
    - The minimum interval between the two doses is 6 months.

    Special populations:
    - Administer 2 doses of HepA vaccine at least 6 months apart to previously unvaccinated persons who live in areas where vaccination programs target older children, or who are at increased risk for infection. This includes persons traveling to or working in countries that have high or intermediate endemicity of infection; men having sex with men; users of injection and non-injection illicit drugs; persons who work with HAV-infected primates or with HAV in a research laboratory; persons with clotting-factor disorders; persons with chronic liver disease; and persons who anticipate close, personal contact (e.g., household or regular babysitting) with an international adoptee during the first 60 days after arrival in the United States from a country with high or intermediate endemicity. The first dose should be administered as soon as the adoption is planned, ideally 2 or more weeks before the arrival of the adoptee.

12. **Human papillomavirus (HPV) vaccines. (Minimum age: 9 years for HPV2 [Cervarix] and HPV4 [Gardasil])**
    Routine vaccination:
    - Administer a 3-dose series of HPV vaccine on a schedule of 0, 1-2, and 6 months to all adolescents aged 11 through 12 years. Either HPV4 or HPV2 may be used for females, and only HPV4 may be used for males.
    - The vaccine series may be started at age 9 years.
    - Administer the second dose 1 to 2 months after the first dose (minimum interval of 4 weeks), administer the third dose 24 weeks after the first dose and 16 weeks after the second dose (minimum interval of 12 weeks).

    Catch-up vaccination:
    - Administer the vaccine series to females (either HPV2 or HPV4) and males (HPV4) at age 13 through 18 years if not previously vaccinated.
    - Use recommended routine dosing intervals (see above) for vaccine series catch-up.

16

FIGURE 16-3—cont'd

Continued

For further guidance on the use of the vaccines mentioned below, see: http://www.cdc.gov/vaccines/hcp/acip-recs/index.html.

13. **Meningococcal conjugate vaccines. (Minimum age: 6 weeks for Hib-MenCY [MenHibrix], 9 months for MenACWY-D [Menactra], 2 months for MenACWY-CRM [Menveo])**
    Routine vaccination:
    - Administer a single dose of Menactra or Menveo vaccine at age 11 through 12 years, with a booster dose at age 16 years.
    - Adolescents aged 11 through 18 years with human immunodeficiency virus (HIV) infection should receive a 2-dose primary series of Menactra or Menveo with at least 8 weeks between doses.
    - For children aged 2 months through 18 years with high-risk conditions, see below.

    Catch-up vaccination:
    - Administer Menactra or Menveo vaccine at age 13 through 18 years if not previously vaccinated.
    - If the first dose is administered at age 13 through 15 years, a booster dose should be administered at age 16 through 18 years with a minimum interval of at least 8 weeks between doses.
    - If the first dose is administered at age 16 years or older, a booster dose is not needed.
    - For other catch-up guidance, see Figure 2.

    Vaccination of persons with high-risk conditions and other persons at increased risk of disease:
    - Children with anatomic or functional asplenia (including sickle cell disease):
      1. For children younger than 19 months of age, administer a 4-dose infant series of MenHibrix or Menveo at 2, 4, 6, and 12 through 15 months of age.
      2. For children aged 19 through 23 months who have not completed a series of MenHibrix or Menveo, administer 2 primary doses of Menveo at least 3 months apart.
      3. For children aged 24 months and older who have not received a complete series of MenHibrix or Menveo or Menactra, administer 2 primary doses of either Menactra or Menveo at least 2 months apart. If Menactra is administered to a child with asplenia (including sickle cell disease), do not administer Menactra until 2 years of age and at least 4 weeks after the completion of all PCV13 doses.
    - Children with persistent complement component deficiency
      1. For children younger than 19 months of age, administer a 4-dose infant series of either MenHibrix or Menveo at 2, 4, 6, and 12 through 15 months of age.
      2. For children 7 through 23 months who have not initiated vaccination, two options exist depending on age and vaccine brand:
         a. For children who initiate vaccination with Menveo at 7 months through 23 months of age, a 2-dose series should be administered with the second dose after 12 months of age and at least 3 months after the first dose.
         b. For children who initiate vaccination with Menactra at 9 months through 23 months of age, a 2-dose series of Menactra should be administered at least 3 months apart.
         c. For children aged 24 months and older who have not received a complete series of MenHibrix, Menveo, or Menactra, administer 2 primary doses of either Menactra or Menveo at least 2 months apart.
    - For children who travel to or reside in countries in which meningococcal disease is hyperendemic or epidemic, including countries in the African meningitis belt or the Hajj, administer an age-appropriate formulation and series of Menactra or Menveo for protection against serogroups A and W meningococcal disease. Prior receipt of MenHibrix is not sufficient for children traveling to the meningitis belt or the Hajj because it does not contain serogroups A or W.
    - For children at risk during a community outbreak attributable to a vaccine serogroup, administer or complete the age- and formulation-appropriate series of MenHibrix, Menactra, or Menveo.
    - For booster doses among persons with high-risk conditions, refer to *MMWR* 2013; 62 (RR02);1-22, available at http://www.cdc.gov/mmwr/preview/mmwrhtml/rr6202a1.htm.

    Catch-up recommendations for persons with high-risk conditions:
    1. If MenHibrix is administered to achieve protection against meningococcal disease, a complete age-appropriate series of MenHibrix should be administered.
    2. If the first dose of MenHibrix is given at or after 12 months of age, a total of 2 doses should be given at least 8 weeks apart to ensure protection against serogroups C and Y meningococcal disease.
    3. For children who initiate vaccination with Menveo at 7 months through 9 months of age, a 2-dose series should be administered with the second dose after 12 months of age and at least 3 months after the first dose.
    4. For other catch-up recommendations for these persons, refer to *MMWR* 2013; 62 (RR02);1-22, available at http://www.cdc.gov/mmwr/preview/mmwrhtml/rr6202a1.htm.
    For complete information on use of meningococcal vaccines, including guidance related to vaccination of persons at increased risk of infection, see *MMWR* March 22, 2013; 62 (RR02);1-22, available at http://www.cdc.gov/mmwr/pdf/rr/rr6202.pdf.

FIGURE 16-3

Footnotes: Recommended immunization schedule for persons aged 0 through 18 years—United States, 2013. *(From ACIP Childhood/Adolescent Immunization Work Group: Advisory Committee on Immunization Practices [ACIP] recommended immunization schedule for persons aged 0 through 18 years—United States, 2013.* MMWR Recomm Rep. *2013;62:2-8. Available at www.cdc.gov.)*

b. SQ: Into pinched skin fold with a 23G–25G, ⅝- to ¾-inch needle

3. **Simultaneous administration:**

a. Routine childhood vaccines are safe and effective when administered simultaneously at different sites, generally 1–2 inches apart. This includes inactivated and live vaccines.

b. If live vaccines are not given at the same visit, an interval of 28 days should be allotted between them.

C. Vaccine Types

1. **Live vaccines:** Influenza (intranasal); measles, mumps, and rubella (MMR); polio (oral); rotavirus; tuberculosis (BCG); typhoid (oral); varicella; yellow fever

2. **Nonlive vaccines:** Diphtheria, tetanus, pertussis combination vaccines (DTaP/DT/Td/Tdap), hepatitis A (HepA), hepatitis B (HepB), *Haemophilus influenzae* type b (Hib), human papillomavirus (HPV), influenza (injectable), Japanese encephalitis, meningococcal, pneumococcal, rabies, typhoid (injectable)

D. Misconceptions

1. Misconceptions about the need for and safety of recommended immunizations have been associated with underimmunization and/or delay in immunization.

2. The CDC and American Academy of Pediatrics (AAP) publish Provider Resources for Vaccine Conversations with Parents, available athttp://www.cdc.gov/vaccines/hcp/patient-ed/conversations/index.html, for up-to-date vaccine information and resources to effectively communicate with parents regarding vaccines.

E. General Indications and Precautions for All Vaccines

This information is based on the Advisory Committee on Immunization Practices (ACIP) and the Committee on Infectious Diseases from the AAP and may vary from those listed on the manufacturers' inserts[2]:

1. **Contraindications** (vaccines should not be given):

a. Anaphylactic reaction to a vaccine or a vaccine constituent contraindicates further doses of that vaccine or vaccines containing that substance (e.g., streptomycin and neomycin).

2. **Precautions:** If risks are believed to outweigh benefits, immunization should be withheld; if benefits are believed to outweigh risks (e.g., to complete primary series, during an outbreak, or foreign travel, immunization should be given)

a. Moderate or severe illnesses with or without a fever

b. Anaphylactic latex allergy (vaccines supplied in vials or syringes that contain natural rubber, a list is available from the CDC at http://www.cdc.gov/vaccines/pubs/pinkbook/downloads/appendices/B/latex-table.pdf)

3. **Misconceptions:** Vaccines should be given in the circumstances below, as well as those listed in the specific vaccine sections:

a. Mild to moderate local reaction (soreness, redness, swelling) after a dose of an injectable antigen; low-grade or moderate fever after a previous vaccine dose

b. Nonanaphylactic latex allergies (e.g., contact allergy to latex gloves)

c. Mild acute illness with or without low-grade fever, current antimicrobial therapy, or convalescent phase of illnesses

d. Malnutrition

e. Family history of adverse event to immunization

f. History of penicillin or other nonspecific allergies

g. Unimmunized or immunodeficient household contact (exception is live attenuated influenza virus [LAIV], which should not be administered to close contacts of persons with severe immunosuppression)

h. Pregnancy of mother or household contact

i. Breast-feeding (nursing infant *OR* lactating mother). Exception: yellow fever vaccine, which is a precaution.

IV. IMMUNOPROPHYLAXIS GUIDELINES FOR SPECIAL HOSTS

A. Children at High Risk for Pneumococcal Disease

1. **Definition:**

a. Immunocompetent children: Those with chronic heart disease, chronic lung disease, diabetes mellitus, cerebrospinal fluid (CSF) leaks, cochlear implants

b. Immunocompromised children: Those with asplenia (functional or anatomic), human immunodeficiency virus (HIV), chronic renal failure or nephrotic syndrome, malignancy, immunosuppressive therapy, congenital immunodeficiency

2. **For those <6 years of age,** complete primary series with PCV13 (pneumococcal conjugate vaccine).

3. **For those >6 years of age** and not fully immunized, give 1 dose of PCV13, no matter how many prior doses previously received.

4. Give 1 dose of 23PS (23-valent pneumococcal polysaccharide vaccine) ≥8 weeks after last dose of PCV13 if ≥2 years of age.

5. **For Immunocompromised children:** A single booster of 23PS is indicated after 5 years of age but should not be repeated.[3]

B. Children at High Risk for Meningococcal Disease

1. **Definition:** Those with asplenia (functional or anatomic) or persistent complement deficiency.

2. **If <19 months,** give Hib MenCY or MenACWY-CRM vaccine series.

3. **If 9–23 months** and have persistent complement deficiency, can alternatively give meningococcal conjugate vaccine MenACWY-D series.

4. **When ≥2 years,** give either MenACWY series. Boosters of MenACWY should be given every 5 years in this group. For travelers to countries in the "meningitis belt" or the Hajj, children should receive protection against groups A and W-135 with MCV4 doses if ≥age 9 months, and receive boosters every 3 years (children aged 2–6 years) or 5 years (children >age 6).

C. Children at High Risk for Hib Disease

1. **Definition:** Those with immunocompromising conditions including cancers, anatomic or functional asplenia, and HIV.

2. **If <12 months,** give primary series.

3. **If 12–59 months** and have received only 1 dose, should receive 2 additional doses separated by 8 weeks. If 2 doses received before 12 months, should receive a third dose.
4. **If >5 years** and unimmunized, should receive 1 dose.

D. Functional or Anatomic Asplenia (Including Sickle Cell Disease)

1. **Penicillin prophylaxis:** See Chapter 14.
2. **Pneumococcal vaccines:** See Section IV.A.
3. **Meningococcal vaccines:** See Section IV.B.
4. **Hib vaccines:** See Section IV.C.
5. **Children ≥2 years** undergoing elective splenectomy should ideally receive pneumococcal and MCV vaccines at least 2 weeks before surgery for optimal immune response and may also benefit from another dose of Hib

E. Congenital Immunodeficiency Disorders

1. **Live vaccines are generally contraindicated.** See Table 1.16 in the *AAP Red Book*[2] for details regarding individual immunodeficiencies.
2. **Inactivated vaccines should be given** according to the routine schedule. Immune response may vary and may be inadequate; titers can be used to assess response.
3. **Immunoglobulin (Ig) therapy** may be indicated.
4. **Household contacts:** Immunize according to routine immunization schedule.

F. Known or Suspected HIV Disease

1. **Inactivated vaccines should be given** according to the routine immunization schedule. Influenza vaccine should be given yearly.
a. Pneumococcal vaccines: See Section IV.A
b. Meningococcal vaccines: Administer 2 doses at least 8 weeks apart starting at age 11 years
c. Hib vaccines: See Section IV.C
2. **Live vaccines:**
a. MMR and varicella vaccines should be given to asymptomatic or mildly symptomatic patients with CD4 cell count of 15% or greater.[4] Do not administer the measles, mumps, rubella, and varicella (MMRV) combination vaccine.
b. Do not administer LAIV. Oral (live attenuated) poliovirus (OPV) and BCG vaccine are generally not given except in areas where risk of disease is thought to outweigh possibility of vaccine-associated disease.
3. **Passive immunoprophylaxis or chemoprophylaxis should be considered** after exposures.

G. Oncology Patients

(See Table 16-1 for general guidelines.)

1. **During active chemotherapy,** immune response to vaccines may be less than ideal. Titers may be useful to assess response.
2. **All live vaccines** should be delayed at least 3 months after immunosuppressive therapy has been discontinued.
3. **Hematopoietic stem cell transplant recipients:** Will need reimmunization against vaccine-preventable illnesses after their transplantation. See

TABLE 16-1

IMMUNIZATION FOR GENERAL ONCOLOGY PATIENTS

Vaccine	Indications and Comments
DTaP/Tdap, Hib, HBV, IPV	Indicated for incompletely immunized children
PCV13, 23PS	Indicated for incompletely immunized children (see Section IV.A)
Meningococcal	Consider in asplenic patients (see Section IV.B)
Influenza	Defer in active chemotherapy; may give as early as 3–4 wk after remission and off chemotherapy if during influenza season; peripheral granulocyte and lymphocyte counts should be >1000/µL; should be given to household contacts
MMR	Contraindicated until child is in remission and finished with all chemotherapy for 3–6 mo; may need reimmunization after chemotherapy if titers have fallen below protective levels
Varicella	Consider immunizing children who have remained in remission and have finished chemotherapy for >1 yr; with absolute lymphocyte count of >700/µL and platelet count of >1000,000/µL within 24 hr of immunization; check titers of previously immunized children to verify protective levels of antibodies

Data from American Academy of Pediatrics. *Red Book: 2012 Report of the Committee on Infectious Diseases*. 29th ed. Elk Grove Village, Ill: AAP, 2012.

Table EC 16-A for guidelines regarding when vaccination can be reinitiated after transplantation.

H. Patients with Solid Organ Transplants

Administer live vaccines at least a month before tranplant. Ensure all other vaccines are up to date. Safety and efficacy of inactivated vaccines after transplant are still unclear; they are generally given as scheduled after 6 months post transplant, when immunosuppression is less intense.

I. Patients on Corticosteroids

Only live vaccines are potentially contraindicated (see Table 16-2 for details).

TABLE 16-2

LIVE VACCINE IMMUNIZATION FOR PATIENTS RECEIVING CORTICOSTEROID THERAPY

Steroid Dose	Recommended Guidelines
Topical, inhaled, or local injection of steroids	Live vaccines can generally be given; if there is clinical evidence of immunosuppression, wait 1 mo after cessation of therapy.
Low-dose steroids (<2 mg/kg/day or <20 mg/day of prednisone equivalent), including physiologic doses	Live vaccines may be given.
High-dose steroids (≥2 mg/kg/day or ≥20 mg/day of prednisone equivalent)	
Duration of therapy < 14 days	May give live vaccines immediately after cessation of therapy (but consider 2-wk delay in administration).
Duration of therapy ≥ 14 days	Do not give live vaccines until therapy has been discontinued for 1 mo.

Modified from American Academy of Pediatrics. *Red Book: 2012 Report of the Committee on Infectious Diseases*. 29th ed. Elk Grove Village, Ill: AAP, 2012.

J. Patients on Biological Response Modifier Therapy (Cytokine Inhibitors)

Administer live vaccines a minimum of 4 weeks before initiating therapy. Ensure all other vaccines are up to date. Vaccine efficacy unclear while on therapy.

K. Pregnancy

1. **Give Tdap during each pregnancy** (preferred during 27th–36th wk of gestation), regardless of prior immunization status. Generally inactivated influenza vaccine is also strongly recommended.
2. Other inactivated vaccines are considered precautionary and generally deferred until after the pregnancy.
3. **Live vaccines** are generally contraindicated during pregnancy. The only exception is yellow fever, which is precautionary and should be given if the risk of yellow fever is high when travelling.

L. Preterm and Low-Birth-Weight Infants

1. **Immunize according to chronologic age, using regular vaccine dosage.**
2. **HepB:** Initiation of HepB vaccine may be delayed for infants of hepatitis B surface antigen (HBsAg)-negative mothers until the child is >2 kg or age 2 months, whichever is earlier. See Fig. 16-4 for management of preterm infant born to mother with HepB.

M. Patients Treated with Immunoglobulin or Other Blood Products

See Table EC 16-B for suggested intervals between any immunoglobulin or blood product administration (including packed red blood cells [pRBCs]) and MMR or varicella immunization. This time allows decrease in passive antibodies so children will have an adequate response to the vaccine, but they should not be considered adequately protected after product administrations. Blood products and immunogloblin are not thought to interfere with non-measles or varicella vaccines.

N. Travelers to Foreign Countries

See CDC's Travel Health page on vaccinations (available at http://www.cdc.gov/travel/page/vaccinations.htm) for specific recommendations. on vaccines by destination. If assistance in obtaining appropriate vaccines for a patient/referral to a travel clinic is indicated, authorized U.S. yellow fever vaccination clinics are generally good options (searchable at http://www.cdc.gov/travel/yellow-fever-vaccination-clinics/search.htm).

V. IMMUNOPROPHYLAXIS GUIDELINES FOR SPECIFIC DISEASES

A. Diphtheria/Tetanus/Pertussis Vaccines and Tetanus Immunoprophylaxis

1. **Description:**
a. DTaP: Diphtheria and tetanus toxoids combined with acellular pertussis vaccine; preferred formulation for children <7 years of age.
b. DT: Diphtheria and tetanus toxoids without pertussis vaccine; use in children <7 years of age in whom pertussis vaccine is contraindicated.
c. Td: Tetanus toxoid with one third to one sixth the dose of diphtheria toxoid of other preparations; use in individuals ≥age 7 years in whom pertussis vaccine is contraindicated.

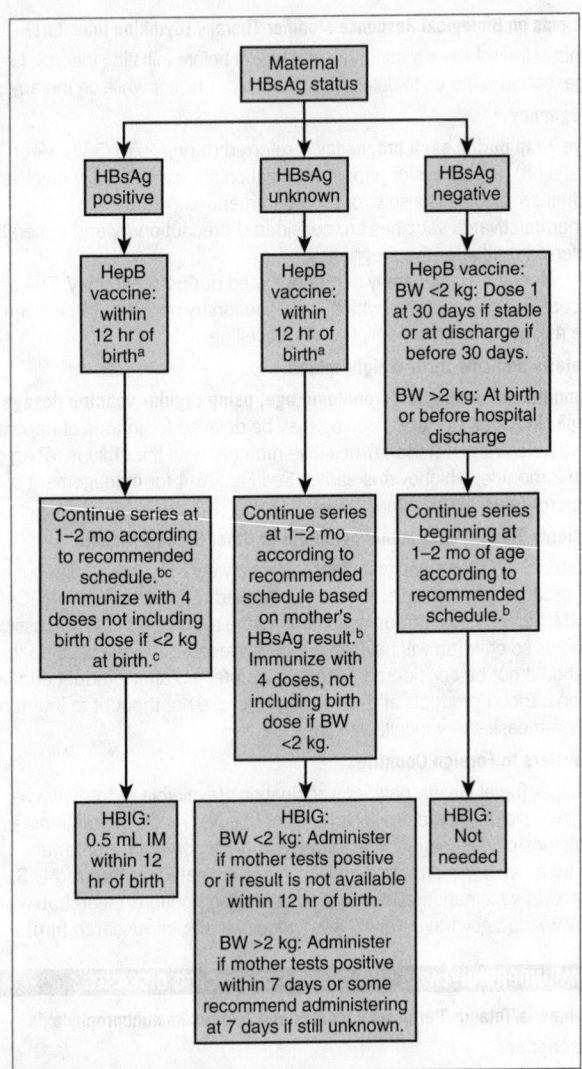

```
                    ┌──────────────────┐
                    │  Maternal        │
                    │  HBsAg status    │
                    └──────────────────┘
```

HBsAg positive

HepB vaccine: within 12 hr of birth[a]

Continue series at 1–2 mo according to recommended schedule.[b,c] Immunize with 4 doses not including birth dose if <2 kg at birth.[c]

HBIG: 0.5 mL IM within 12 hr of birth

HBsAg unknown

HepB vaccine: within 12 hr of birth[a]

Continue series at 1–2 mo according to recommended schedule based on mother's HBsAg result.[b] Immunize with 4 doses, not including birth dose if BW <2 kg.

HBIG: BW <2 kg: Administer if mother tests positive or if result is not available within 12 hr of birth.

BW >2 kg: Administer if mother tests positive within 7 days or some recommend administering at 7 days if still unknown.

HBsAg negative

HepB vaccine: BW <2 kg: Dose 1 at 30 days if stable or at discharge if before 30 days.

BW >2 kg: At birth or before hospital discharge

Continue series beginning at 1–2 mo of age according to recommended schedule.[b]

HBIG: Not needed

FIGURE 16-4

Management of neonates born to mothers with unknown or positive hepatitis B surface antigen (HbsAg) status. BW, Birth weight; HBIG, hepatitis B immune globulin; HepB, hepatitis B virus. [a]Only single antigen vaccine should be used. [b]A fourth vaccine dose is required if using combination vaccines. [c]Reimmunization may be required based on anti-HBs. Test at 9–18 mo of age. (*Data from American Academy of Pediatrics. Red Book: 2012 Report of the Committee on Infectious Diseases. 29th ed. Elk Grove Village, Ill: AAP, 2012.*)

d. Tdap (Boostrix and Adacel): Tetanus and diphtheria toxoids combined with acellular pertussis vaccine. Boostrix can be given at age 10 years, Adacel at age 11 years.

2. **Contraindications:**

a. Encephalopathy within 7 days of administration of previous dose of DTaP.

b. Progressive neurologic disorder may merit permanent deferral of pertussis immunization. Reconsider pertussis immunization at each visit. Use DT or Td if pertussis vaccine is permanently deferred in children ≥age 1 year (children <1 year should not receive DT; risk for diphtheria and tetanus is low in first year of life). After first birthday, initiate either DT or DTaP immunization, as clinically indicated.

c. **Precautions:**

(1) Seizure disorder or seizures within 3 days of receiving a previous dose of DTaP:

(a) Poorly controlled or new-onset seizures: Defer pertussis immunization until seizure disorder is well controlled and progressive neurologic disorder is excluded; then give DTaP and antipyretics around the clock for 24 hours after immunization.

(b) Personal or family history of febrile seizures: Give DTaP and antipyretics around the clock for 24 hours after immunization.

(2) Temperature of 40.5°C (104.8°F) within 48 hours after immunization with a previous dose of DTaP

(3) Collapse or shock-like state (hypotonic-hyporesponsive episode) within 48 hours of receiving a previous dose of DTaP

(4) Persistent inconsolable crying lasting 3 hours within 48 hours of receiving a previous dose of DTaP

(5) Guillain-Barré syndrome (GBS) within 6 weeks after a prior dose (however, completion of the primary series in children is usually justified)

d. **Misconceptions (vaccines should be given):** Family history of seizures (see above) or family history of sudden infant death syndrome

3. **Side effects:** Substantially decreased with DTaP compared to DTP. Local tenderness (8%–11%), fever ≥ 38.0°C (8%–24%, more common in subsequent doses), anorexia (8%–11%), drowsiness (19%–33%), vomiting (4%–7%), crying ≥ 1 hour (1%–2%). Severe side effects of allergic reactions, persistent crying > 3 hours, hypotonic-hyporesponsive episode, seizures, and body temperature > 40.5°C that were more common with DTP vaccine are very rare with DTaP.[5]

4. **Administration:**

a. DTaP, DT, Td, or TdaP: Dose is 0.5 mL IM

b. Tetanus Ig (TIG): Dose is 10 mL/kg IM

5. **Special considerations:**

a. Tetanus prophylaxis in wound management (Table 16-3)

b. Pertussis exposure:

(1) Immunize all unimmunized or partially immunized close contacts <age 7 years and >age 10 years, according to the recommended

TABLE 16-3

INDICATIONS FOR TETANUS PROPHYLAXIS

Prior Tetanus Toxoid Doses	Clean, Minor Wounds		All Other Wounds	
	Tetanus Vaccine*	TIG	Tetanus Vaccine*	TIG
Unknown or < 3	Yes	No	Yes	Yes
≥3, last < 5 yr ago	No	No	No	No†
≥3, last 5–10 yr ago	No	No	Yes	No†
≥3, last > 10 yr ago	Yes	No	Yes	No†

*Vaccine choice for child <age 7 yr is DTaP, and Tdap if >age 7 years (DT or Td if pertussis is contraindicated).

†Any child with HIV infection or who is within the first year after bone marrow transplantation should receive TIG for any tetanus-prone wound, regardless of vaccination status.

Modified from American Academy of Pediatrics. *Red Book: 2012 Report of the Committee on Infectious Diseases.* 29th ed. Elk Grove Village, Ill: AAP, 2012.

schedule. Give fourth dose of DTaP if third dose was given >6 months prior. Give booster dose of DTaP if last dose was given >3 years prior and child is <age 7 years.

(2) Postexposure chemoprophylaxis with azithromycin, erythromycin or clarithromycin. Alternatives include trimethoprim-sulfamethoxazole (see Table 3.44 of the 2012 *Red Book* for more details[2]).

B. *Haemophilus influenzae* Type B Immunoprophylaxis

1. **Description:** The three licensed vaccines consist of a capsular polysaccharide antigen (PRP) conjugated to a carrier protein. It is not necessary to use the same formulation for the entire series.

a. PRP-OMP (PedvaxHIB): Conjugated to outer membrane protein of *Neisseria meningitidis;* requires only two doses in primary series (2 and 4 months) plus booster at 12–15 months. If PRP-OMP is used only for part of the immunization series, the recommended number of doses to complete the series is based on the other Hib vaccine used. Children without prior DTaP vaccine may respond better to PRP-OMP than to other formulations.

b. PRP-T (ActHIB): Conjugated to tetanus toxoid. Approved for ages 2–18 months.

c. PRP-T (Hiberix): Conjugated to tetanus toxoid. Approved as a booster dose in ages 15 months to 4 years.

2. **Contraindications:** None

3. **Side effects:** Local pain, redness, and swelling in 25% of recipients (mild, lasting <24 hours)

4. **Administration:** Dose is 0.5 mL IM

5. **Special considerations:**

a. See Section IV.C.

b. Children with invasive Hib disease at age <24 months: Begin Hib immunization 1 month after acute illness and continue as if previously unimmunized. Vaccination is not required if invasive disease develops after age 24 months. Consider immunologic workup for any child with invasive Hib disease after completing the immunization series.

c. Post exposure: Generally rifampin is recommended for unvaccinated household or daycare contacts <4 years of age.

C. Hepatitis A Virus Immunoprophylaxis

1. **Description:** Two brands of HepA vaccine are available—Havrix and Vaqta (both preservative-free), which are licensed only for children ≥age 12 months.
2. **Contraindications:** Anaphylactic reaction to aluminum hydroxyphosphate sulfate, aluminum hydroxide, or neomycin.
3. **Side effects:** Local reactions are typically mild and include injection site tenderness (21%), redness, swelling and warmth (4%), rash (1%), fever (11%), and headache (<9%). No serious adverse events have been reported.[6,7]
4. **Administration:**
   a. HepA vaccine: Dose is 0.5 mL IM for ages 1–18 years and 1 mL IM for ≥ age 19 years
   b. HepA Ig: Dose is 0.02 mL/kg (max dose, 5 mL) IM
5. **Special considerations:**
   a. Preexposure immunoprophylaxis for travelers
      (1) HepA vaccine is preferred for travelers ≥12 months old; a single dose usually provides adequate immunity if time does not allow a second dose before travel.
      (2) HepA Ig is protective for up to 5 months and can be given without vaccine to children <age 12 months before travel.
   b. Postexposure immunoprophylaxis: If exposed in the last 2 weeks and <12 months old, should receive HepA Ig. If ≥age 12 months, should receive HepA vaccine. If it has been >2 weeks since exposure, no prophylaxis is indicated if <age 12 months, but HepA vaccine might be considered if ≥age 12 months and exposure could be ongoing.

D. Hepatitis B Virus Immunoprophylaxis

1. **Description:**
   a. HepB vaccine: Adsorbed HBsAg produced recombinantly. Different recombinant vaccines may be used interchangeably.
   b. HBIG: Prepared from plasma containing high-titer anti-HBsAg antibodies and negative for antibodies to HIV and HCV.
2. **Contraindications:** Anaphylactic reaction to yeast
3. **Side effects:** Pain at injection site (3%–29%) or fever >37.7°C (1%–6%); immediate hypersensitivity reaction is very rare
4. **Administration:**
   a. Recombivax: Dose is 5 mcg IM (0.5 mL pediatric formulation) for patients <age 20 years, 10 mcg IM (1 mL adult formulation) ≥age 20 years, and 40 mcg IM (1 mL dialysis formulation) for dialysis patients.
   b. Energix-B: Dose is 10 mcg IM (0.5 mL) for patients <age 20 years, 20 mcg IM (1 mL) ≥age 20 years, and 40 mcg IM (2 mL) for dialysis patients.
   c. HBIG: Dose for infants is 0.5 mL IM; for older children, 0.06 mL/kg IM.

16

5. **Special considerations:**
a. Infants of mothers who are HBsAg positive or unknown will have a different schedule (Fig. 16-4).
b. See Table 16-4 for HepB prophylaxis after percutaneous exposure to blood.

E. Human Papillomavirus Immunoprophylaxis

1. **Description:** Two approved vaccines:
a. HPV4 (Gardasil) vaccine protects against HPV types 6, 11, 16, and 18; administered to both females and males. Has efficacy against cervical, vulvar, and vaginal cancers caused by types 16 and 18; against genital warts, in females and males, caused by types 6 and 11.[8]
b. HPV2 (Cervarix) has been approved for females and protects against HPV types 16 and 18.
2. **Contraindications:** Anaphylaxis to yeast.
3. **Side effects:** Pain, swelling, and erythema at injection site (83%, 25%, and 25%, respectively), fever (10%), nausea (6%), dizziness (4%), syncope. Recommend observation for syncope for 15 minutes after administration.[8]
4. **Administration:** Dose is 0.5 mL IM. First dose can be given at ≥age 9 years but recommended at age 11–12 years.
5. **Special considerations:** Females or males with evidence of current HPV infection, such as cervical dysplasia or warts of a positive HPV DNA test, should still be immunized.

F. Influenza Immunoprophylaxis

Influenza strains can change year to year, particularly in time of pandemic flu; please refer to the CDC for up-to-date guidelines at www.cdc.gov/flu/professionals/antivirals/index.htm.

TABLE 16-4

HEPATITIS B VIRUS PROPHYLAXIS AFTER PERCUTANEOUS EXPOSURE TO BLOOD

Exposed Person	Positive	HBsAg Status of Source of Blood	
		Negative	Unknown
Unimmunized	HBIG and HBV series	HBV series	HBV series
Previously immunized			
Known responder	No treatment	No treatment	No treatment
Known nonresponder	HBIG and HBV series	No treatment	Treat as if positive if known high risk source *OR* give HBIG × 2 (1 mo apart)*
Response unknown	Test exposed person for anti-HBsAg and HBV booster dose	No treatment	Test exposed person for anti-HBs: If inadequate, HBV booster dose If adequate (>10 mIU/mL), no treatment

*Preferred if already received two vaccine series with failure to respond.
Modified from American Academy of Pediatrics. *Red Book: 2012 Report of the Committee on Infectious Diseases.* 29th ed. Elk Grove Village, Ill: AAP, 2012.

1. **Description:** Activated and inactivated influenza vaccines are produced in embryonated eggs. Vaccines contain multiple viral strains (including both type A and type B strains) based on expected prevalent influenza strains for the upcoming winter:
   a. Inactivated influenza vaccines: Split-virus vaccines with subvirion or purified surface antigen vaccines available; given IM to children ≥age 6 months
   b. LAIV: Given intranasally to healthy children >age 2 years
2. **Contraindications:** Anaphylaxis to eggs is a contraindication to both IM and intranasal influenza vaccines; anaphylaxis to gelatin (which is in some influenza vaccines [look at package insert]). Contraindications specific to LAIV are pregnancy, asthma, children <age 5 years with wheezing in the past 12 months, immunocompromised, or on aspirin treatment:
   a. **Precautions:** GBS within 6 weeks after a previous influenza vaccine dose
   b. **Misconceptions (vaccines should be given):** Less severe or local manifestations of allergy to egg and pregnancy (give inactivated vaccine to pregnant patients)
3. **Side effects:** Fever 6–24 hours after immunization in children <age 2 years (10%–35%); rare in children >age 2 years. Local reactions are uncommon in children <13 years of age; 10% in children ≥13 years. There are no statistically significant differences observed between placebo and LAIV recipients for fever, rhinitis, or nasal congestion. If there is an association between the influenza vaccine and GBS, the risk is rare and ≤1–2 cases per million doses.
4. **Administration:** Give annually during the fall in preparation for winter influenza season:
   a. Inactivated: Dose is 0.25 mL IM for ages 6–35 months and 0.5 mL IM for ≥age 3 years.
   b. LAIV: Dose is 0.2 mL intranasally.
5. **Special considerations:**
   a. **Chemoprophylaxis for influenza A and B:** High rates of resistance of influenza A and B to amantadine and rimantadine and of influenza A to oseltamivir cause recommendations to vary by season and location. Please refer to www.cdc.gov/flu/professionals/antivirals/index.htm:
      (1) Chemoprophylaxis against influenza A and B: Oseltamivir (≥2 weeks) and zanamivir (≥5 years)
      (2) Chemoprophylaxis against influenza A only: Amantadine or rimantadine (≥1 year)
      (3) Indications for chemoprophylaxis:
         (a) Unimmunized high-risk children, including those for whom the vaccine is contraindicated or children immunized <2 weeks before influenza outbreak.
         (b) Unimmunized individuals in close contact with or providing care to high-risk individuals
         (c) Immunodeficient individuals unlikely to have protective response to vaccine

16

    (d) Control of outbreaks in a closed setting

    (e) Immunized high-risk individuals if vaccine strain different from circulating strain

  (4) Chemoprophylaxis is not a substitute for immunization and does not interfere with the immune response to the inactivated virus vaccine. LAIV should not be administered until >48 hours after completing antiviral therapy for influenza.[9] Do not administer chemoprophylaxis until at least 2 weeks after administration of LAIV.

b. Infants <age 6 months cannot be immunized. Close contacts should receive the vaccine.

G. Japanese Encephalitis (JE) Immunoprophylaxis

See Expert Consult for more information.

H. Measles/Mumps/Rubella Immunoprophylaxis

1. **Description:**

a. MMR: Combination vaccine composed of live attenuated viruses. Measles and mumps vaccines are grown in chick embryo cell culture; rubella vaccine is prepared in human diploid cell culture.

b. Measles Ig: IM and IV immunoglobulin preparations contain similar concentration of measles antibody.

c. Rubella Ig: Data showing decreased clinical infection, viral shedding, and rates of viremia are limited.[2]

2. **Contraindications:** Anaphylactic reaction to neomycin or gelatin or immunocompromise

a. **Precautions:**

  (1) Recent (within 3–11 months, depending on product and dose) blood product administration (see Section IV.M).

  (2) Thrombocytopenia or history of thrombocytopenic purpura. In most instances, benefits of immunization will be much greater than potential risks, particularly because there is a higher risk of thrombocytopenia after measles or rubella disease.

  (3) Tuberculosis or positive purified protein derivative (PPD) tuberculin test. A theoretical basis exists for concern that measles vaccine might exacerbate tuberculosis. Before administering MMR to people with untreated active tuberculosis, initiating antituberculosis therapy is advisable.

b. **Misconceptions (vaccines should be given):** PPD testing may be done on the day of immunization (otherwise, postpone PPD 4–6 weeks because of suppression of response), breast-feeding, pregnancy of mother of recipient, immunodeficiency in a family member or household contact, HIV infection, nonanaphylactic reactions to gelatin or neomycin, anaphylactic reaction to eggs (consider observing patient for 90 minutes after vaccine administration; skin testing is not predictive of hypersensitivity reaction and therefore is not recommended), history of seizures

3. **Side effects:** Fever to 39.4°C or higher develops in 5%–15% of immunized persons, usually between 6 and 12 days after immunization and

can last up to 5 days; febrile seizures are rare and occur 8–14 days after the first dose (fevers should be treated with antipyretics in those with a history of seizures); transient rash (5%); transient thrombocytopenia (1 in 25,000 to 1 in 2 million) 2–3 weeks after immunization; encephalitis and encephalopathy (<1 in 1 million).[2]

4. **Administration:**
a. MMR vaccine: Dose is 0.5 mL SQ.
b. Measles Ig dose: Standard-dose Ig for children and pregnant women: 0.25 mL/kg (maximum dose, 15 mL) IM. High-dose Ig for immunocompromised children (including those with HIV infection): 0.5 mL/kg (maximum dose, 15 mL) IM. Not required if IVIG received within 3 weeks before exposure.

5. **Special considerations:**
a. Measles postexposure immunoprophylaxis:
   (1) Vaccine prevents or modifies disease if given within 72 hours of exposure; it is the intervention of choice for measles outbreak.
   (2) Measles Ig prevents or modifies disease if given within 6 days of exposure. It is indicated in susceptible household contacts, pregnant women, children <age 1 year, and immunocompromised individuals (including HIV-infected children), regardless of immunization status. It is not indicated for non immunocompromised contacts who have received one dose of the vaccine at ≥age 12 months.
b. Rubella postexposure immunoprophylaxis:
   (1) Rubella Ig can be considered in rubella-susceptible women exposed to confirmed rubella early in pregnancy if termination of the pregnancy is refused.

I. Meningococcal Immunoprophylaxis

1. **Description:** Meningococcal vaccines are available against groups A, C, Y, and W-135 for children. No vaccine is available for group B because of poor immunogenicity:
a. Hib MenCY (Men Hibrix): Conjugate vaccine against Hib and meningococcus groups C and Y; for patients 6 weeks–18 months of age
b. MenACWY-D (Menactra): A tetravalent conjugate vaccine against groups A, C, Y, and W-135; for patients ≥9 months of age
c. MenACWY-CRM (Menveo): A tetravalent conjugate vaccine against groups A, C, Y, and W-135; for patients ≥2 years of age
d. MPSV4: A quadrivalent serogroup-specific vaccine against groups A, C, Y, and W-135; made from purified capsular polysaccharide antigen; for patients >5 years of age

2. **Contraindications:** Anaphalaxis to tetanus toxoid, diphtheria toxoid, or any natural rubber latex.
a. **Precaution:** History of GBS

3. **Side effects:**
a. MenACWY: Mild localized erythema and pain lasting 1–2 days (occurs infrequently), fever (2%–5%), headache, irritability, fatigue

16

b. Hib MenCY: Similar to Hib vaccine alone, with local injection-site pain, redness, and swelling common (15%–46%), as is irritability (62%–71%), drowsiness (49%–63%), loss of appetite (30%–34%), and fever (11%–26%)[10]

4. **Administration:** Dose is 0.5 mL IM for MenACWY and Hib MenCY, and 0.5 mL SQ for MPSV4.

5. **Special considerations:**

a. See Sections IV.B and IV.F.

b. Postexposure immunoprophylaxis:

   (1) Indications: Contact with the index case within 7 days before the onset of illness, including household, child care, and nursery school contacts; direct exposure to the index case's secretions, including mouth-to-mouth and unprotected endotracheal intubation, those who frequently slept in the home of the index case, and passengers next to the index case during airline flights longer than 8 hours.

   (2) Treatment should be given within 24 hours of primary case diagnosis. Rifampin is the drug of choice with single dose ciprofloxacin or ceftriaxone as alternatives.

c. Hib MenCY or MCV4 can be given for outbreak control.

J. Pneumococcal Immunoprophylaxis

1. **Description:**

a. PCV13: Pneumococcal conjugate vaccine includes 13 purified capsular polysaccharides of *Streptococcus pneumoniae,* each coupled to a variant of diphtheria toxin. PCV7 had serotypes 4, 6B, 9V, 14, 18C, 19F, and 23F, and serotypes 1, 3, 5, 6A, 7F, and 19A were added to PCV13.[3]

b. 23PS: Purified capsular polysaccharide includes antigen from 23 serotypes (1, 2, 3, 4, 5, 6B, 7F, 8, 9N, 9V, 10A, 11A, 12F, 14, 15B, 17F, 18C, 19A, 19F, 20, 22F, 23F, and 33F[3]) of *S. pneumoniae.* Approved for children aged 2 years and older with certain underlying medical conditions.

2. **Contraindications:** None.

3. **Side effects:** Pain or erythema at injection site (>50%, with <10% interfering with limb movement); irritability (14%–86%), decreased appetite (16%–51%), decreased sleep (7%–47%), increased sleep (3%–72%), less commonly fever within 1–2 days after administration (1%–37%).[11]

4. **Administration:** Dose for both PCV13 and 23PS is 0.5 mL given IM. Concurrent administration of PCV13 and 23PS vaccines is not recommended.

5. **Special considerations:**

a. See Section IV.A.

b. For children <age 60 months who received PCV7 for their primary series, they should complete the series with PCV13. If they have already received their full four-dose series of PCV7, they should receive one dose of PCV13 if <age 60 months (or older with a condition at special risk for pneumococcal disease).

K. Poliomyelitis Immunoprophylaxis

1. **Description:**
a. IPV: Inactivated injectable vaccine; contains three types of poliovirus grown in Vero cells and inactivated in formaldehyde.[12]
b. OPV: Live viral oral vaccine; no longer available in the United States. Children who have received the appropriate number of doses of OPV in other countries should be considered adequately immunized.
2. **Administration:** Dose is 0.5 mL IM or SQ.
3. **Contraindications:** Anaphylactic reactions to neomycin, streptomycin, polymyxin B, 2-phenoxyethanol, and formaldehyde. OPV should generally not be given to immunocompromised children.
4. **Side effects:** 0%–29% local reactions, 0%–4% fever[13]; no serious side effects have been associated with use of IPV.

L. Rabies Immunoprophylaxis

1. **Description:**
a. Three rabies vaccines are available for prophylaxis: Human diploid cell vaccine (HDCV), rabies vaccine adsorbed (RVA), and purified chicken embryo cell vaccine (PCECV).
b. Human rabies immune globulin (RIG): Antirabies Ig prepared from plasma of donors hyperimmunized with rabies vaccine.
2. **Contraindications:** Anaphylaxis to gelatin (present in some vaccines [look at package insert]). PCECV can be used if there is a serious allergic reaction to HDCV.
3. **Side effects:** Uncommon in children. In adults, local reactions in 15%–25%, mild systemic reactions (e.g.,headache, abdominal pain, nausea, muscle aches, dizziness) in 10%–20%, and neurologic illness similar to GBS or focal central nervous system disorder (reported with HDCV but not believed to be causally related). Immune complex–like reaction (urticaria, arthralgia, angioedema, vomiting, fever, malaise) 2–21 days after immunization with HDCV is rare in primary series, but 6% after booster dose.
4. **Administration:**
a. Rabies vaccines: Dose is 1 mL IM. Do not administer in same part of body or in same syringe as RIG.
b. RIG: Dose is 20 IU/kg. Infiltrate around the wound and give remainder IM.
5. **Special considerations:**
a. Preexposure prophylaxis: Indicated for high-risk groups, including veterinarians, animal handlers, laboratory workers, children living in high-risk environments, those traveling to high-risk areas, and spelunkers:
   (1) Three injections of HDCV or PCEC vaccine on days 0, 7, and 21 or 28.
   (2) Rabies serum antibody titers should be followed at 6-month intervals for those at continuous risk and at 2-year intervals for those with risk for frequent exposure; give booster doses only if titers are nonprotective.

16

TABLE 16-5

RABIES POSTEXPOSURE PROPHYLAXIS

Animal Type	Evaluation and Disposition of Animal	Postexposure Prophylaxis Recommendations
Dogs, cats, ferrets	Healthy and available for 10 days' observation.	Do not begin prophylaxis unless animal develops signs of rabies.
	Rabid or suspected rabid; euthanize animal and test brain.	Provide immediate immunization and RIG.
	Unknown (escaped).	Consult public health officials.
Skunk, raccoon, bat,* fox, woodchuck, most other carnivores	Regard as rabid unless geographic area is known to be free of rabies or until animal is euthanized and proven negative by testing.	Provide immediate immunization and RIG.†
Livestock, rodents, rabbit, other mammals	Consider individually.	Consult public health officials; these bites rarely require treatment.

*In the case of direct contact between a human and a bat, consider prophylaxis even if a bite, scratch, or mucous membrane exposure is not apparent.

†Treatment may be discontinued if animal fluorescent antibody is negative.

Modified from American Academy of Pediatrics. *Red Book: 2012 Report of the Committee on Infectious Diseases.* 29th ed. Elk Grove Village, Ill: AAP, 2012.

b. Postexposure prophylaxis (Table 16-5):
  (1) General wound management: Clean immediately with soap and water and flush thoroughly. Avoid suturing wound unless indicated for functional reasons. Consider tetanus prophylaxis and antibiotics if indicated. Report all patients suspected of rabies infection to public health authorities.
  (2) Indications: Infectious exposures include bites, scratches, or contamination of open wound or mucous membrane with infectious material of a rabid animal or human.
  (3) Vaccine for postexposure prophylaxis:
    (a) Unimmunized: 1 mL IM on days 0, 3, 7, and 14. The fifth dose is only necessary for children who are immunosuppressed and should be given on day 28.
    (b) Previously immunized (including preexposure and postexposure): 1 mL IM on days 0 and 3. Do not give RIG.
  (4) Vaccine and RIG should be given jointly except in previously immunized patients (no RIG required). If vaccine is not immediately available, give RIG alone and vaccinate later. If RIG is unavailable, give vaccine alone. RIG may be given within 7 days after initiating immunization.

M. Respiratory Syncytial Virus (RSV) Immunoprophylaxis

1. **Description:** Palivizumab (monoclonal RSV-Ig) is a humanized mouse monoclonal IgG to RSV.
2. **Contraindications:** None.
3. **Side effects:** Comparable to placebo; upper respiratory tract infection, otitis media, fever, rhinitis, and liver function test elevation occurred 1%–3% more commonly than with placebo.

4. **Administration:** Dose is 15 mg/kg IM. Give palivizumab at onset of RSV season (November 1 for most of the United States, July 1 for southeast Florida, September 15 for north central and southwest Florida) and then monthly as indicated.
5. **Special considerations:**
a. Indications[13]:
   (1) Infants and children <age 2 years with chronic lung disease (CLD) who have required medical therapy (oxygen, bronchodilators, diuretics, or corticosteroids) within the 6 months before the RSV season. These children should receive a maximum of five doses. Data are limited, but these patients may also benefit from prophylaxis during a second RSV season.
   (2) Infants <32 weeks' estimated gestational age (EGA) at birth who do not have CLD may benefit from prophylaxis with palivizumab. These children should receive a maximum of five doses:
      (a) EGA < 29 weeks: If <12 months at the start of RSV season
      (b) EGA 29 to <32 weeks: If <6 months at the start of RSV season
   (3) Infants 32 weeks to <35 weeks EGA who are <age 3 months at the start of the RSV season and who are likely to have increased RSV exposure (child care attendance or siblings < 5 years of age). These children should receive a maximum of three doses, none being after 3 months of age.
   (4) Infants with congenital abnormalities of the airway or neuromuscular disease and should receive a maximum of five doses during the first year of life.
   (5) Infants with hemodynamically significant cyanotic or acyanotic congenital heart disease who are ≤24 months of age should be considered for prophylaxis. This includes children who:
      (a) Are receiving medication for treatment of congestive heart failure.
      (b) Have moderate to severe pulmonary hypertension.
      (c) Have a cyanotic heart lesion. Children who have undergone a surgical procedure where bypass was used should receive a postoperative dose of palivizumab as soon as clinically stable.
   (6) There are no specific recommendations for severely immunocompromised children, but they may benefit from prophylaxis.

N. Rotavirus Immunoprophylaxis

1. **Description:** Two vaccines available
a. RotaTeq (RV5): Pentavalent live viral vaccine containing five reassortant human and bovine rotavirus strains in the form of an oral solution given in three doses
b. Rotarix (RV1): Live human attenuated rotavirus in the form of an oral solution given in two doses
2. **Contraindications:** Severe allergic reaction to latex (RV1 only)
a. **Precautions:** Preexisting chronic gastrointestinal disease, history of intussusception, spina bifida, or bladder exstrophy

16

b. **Misconceptions (vaccines should be given):** Breast-feeding or immuno-deficient family member/contact

3. **Side effects:** Diarrhea (24%), vomiting (15%), otitis media (14.5%), nasopharyngitis (7%), and bronchospasm (1%). Adverse events among Rotarix and placebo occurred at similar rates.[15,16]

4. **Administration:**

a. RotaTeq: Dose is 2 mL orally (PO). Vaccine is packaged in single-dose tubes to be administered without dilution. Do not readminister if infant spits out or vomits dose. Given in three doses, typically at 2, 4, and 6 months of age.

b. Rotarix: Dose is 1 mL PO. Vaccine is packaged to be reconstituted only with the accompanying diluent. If the infant spits out or vomits a dose, a single replacement dose at the same visit may be considered. Given in two doses, typically at 2 and 4 months of age.

5. **Special considerations:**

a. Premature infants can begin the series at 6 weeks of chronologic age if clinically stable.

b. Infants who received antibody-containing products can receive the first dose 42 days after the product was given.

O. Tuberculosis Immunoprophylaxis

See Expert Consult for more information.

P. Typhoid Fever Immunoprophylaxis

1. **Description:** Two typhoid vaccines are available and induce a protective response in 50%–80% of recipients:

a. Vi capsular polysaccharide vaccine (ViCPS) administered IM for children ≥age 2 years

b. Oral live attenuated vaccine (Ty21a) for ≥age 6 years

2. **Contraindications:** Immunocompromised (for Ty21a only)

a. **Other precautions:** Taking antibiotics that would be active against *Salmonella typhi* (for Ty21a only)

3. **Side effects:** For children receiving ViCPS, local soreness/pain (13%–14%), erythema (7%), induration (3%), impaired limb use not found, subjective fever (3%), and decreased activity (2%)[17]

4. **Administration:**

a. ViCPS: Dose is 0.5 mL IM for children ≥age 2 weeks before potential exposure. Booster dose every 2 years.

b. Ty21a: Four capsules that must be swallowed whole (one taken every other day) and finished ≥1 week before potential exposure. Booster series every 5 years.

5. **Special considerations:** Indicated for travelers to endemic areas

Q. Varicella Immunoprophylaxis

1. **Description:**

a. Vaccine: Cell-free live attenuated varicella virus vaccine

b. Varicella-zoster immune globulin (VariZIG): Prepared from plasma containing high-titer antivaricella antibodies

2. **Contraindications:** Anaphylactic reaction to neomycin or gelatin, or immunocompromised:
a. **Other precautions:** Recent (within 3–11 months, depending on product and dose) blood product administration (see Section IV.M)
b. **Misconceptions (vaccines should be given):** Pregnancy of mother of recipient, immunodeficiency in a household contact (including HIV infection)
3. **Side effects:** Injection site reactions (20%), fever (15%), mild varicelliform rash within 5–26 days of vaccine administration (3%–5%), although most thought to be due to wild-type VZV infection. Vaccine rash often very mild, but patient may be infectious; reversion to wild-type virus has not been reported.[18]
4. **Administration:**
a. Varicella vaccine: Dose is 0.5 mL SQ.
b. VariZIG: Dose is 12.5 units/kg IM (maximum dose, 625 U; minimum dose, 125 U). If VariZIG is unavailable, can give IVIG 400 mg/kg IV.
5. **Special considerations:**
a. Do not give vaccine for 5 months after VariZIG; do not give concurrently with VariZIG. Avoid salicylates for 6 weeks after vaccine administration if possible. Avoid antiviral treatment for 21 days after vaccination.
b. Consider vaccine in household contacts of immunocompromised hosts. If a rash develops in the immunized person, avoid direct contact if possible.
c. Postexposure prophylaxis:
    (1) Candidates for VariZIG or acyclovir who have had significant exposure include immunocompromised individuals without a history of varicella or varicella immunization, susceptible pregnant women, newborn infants, hospitalized preterm infants
        (a) Significant exposures: Household contact, face-to-face indoor play, onset of varicella in the mother of a newborn from 5 days before to 2 days after delivery (even if mother received VariZIG during pregnancy), hospital exposures (roommate, face-to-face contact with infectious individual, visit by contagious individual, or intimate contact with person with active zoster lesions)
    (2) Potential interventions for people without evidence of immunity include:
        (a) Varicella vaccine ideally administered within 3 days but up to 5 days after exposure for immunocompetent children.
        (b) VariZIG given as one dose up to 96 hours after exposure (give as soon as possible). IVIG can be used if VariZIG is unavailable.
        (c) Oral acyclovir can also be given beginning 7 days after exposure.

R. Yellow Fever Immunoprophylaxis
1. **Description:** Live attenuated virus vaccine approved for children ≥age 6 months but recommended for children ≥age 9 months
2. **Contraindications:** Anaphylaxis to eggs or gelatin. Skin testing with yellow fever vaccine is recommended before administration in children with a

history of immediate hypersensitivity reaction (e.g., anaphylaxis or generalized urticaria) to eggs. Immunocompromised individuals also at risk:

a. **Precautions:** Age 6–8 months (see below), pregnancy, breast-feeding, or asymptomatic HIV infection

3. **Side effects:** Yellow fever vaccine rarely found to be associated with risk of viscerotropic disease (multiple-organ system failure) and neurotropic disease (postvaccine encephalitis). Increased risk of adverse events in persons of any age with thymic dysfunction and an increased risk of postvaccine encephalitis in younger children (<9 months).

4. **Administration:** Dose is 0.5 mL IM. Booster necessary every 10 years.

5. **Special considerations:**

a. Yellow fever is endemic in areas of sub-Saharan Africa and South America. Vaccine is required by some countries as a condition of entry.

b. Vaccine is available in the United States only in designated centers. A list of centers that provide yellow fever vaccine (and usually other travel vaccines) can be found at http://wwwnc.cdc.gov/travel/yellow-fever-vaccination-clinics/search.htm.

S. Combination Vaccines

1. **Comvax = PRP-OMP (Hib)/HepB:** 6 weeks–71 months of age

2. **Kinrix = DTaP-IPV:** Given commonly as fifth dose of DTaP and fourth dose of IPV at age 4–6 years

3. **Pediarix = DTaP/HepB/IPV:** 6 weeks–7 years of age; minimum interval is 6 weeks

a. Higher rates of fever are reported with combination vaccine than the vaccines administered separately.

4. **Pentacel = DTaP-IPV/PRP-T (Hib):** 6 weeks–4 years of age

5. **Proquad = measles/mumps/rubella/varicella[17]:** 12 months–12 years of age:

a. Unless caregiver prefers MMRV vaccine, CDC recommends that MMR and varicella vaccines be administered separately for the first dose in 12- to 47-month child, owing to studies showing increased risk for febrile seizure with combination vaccine in this age group. Combination MMRV vaccine can be used for second dose or as first dose for children >age 48 months.

6. **TriHIBit = DTaP/PRP-T (Hib):** Fourth dose of Hib and DTaP series between 15–18 months

7. **Twinrix = HepA/HepB:** ≥18 years of age. Administered in a three-dose schedule given at 0, 1 month, and 6 months; dose is 1 mL

8. **MenHibrix = Hib / MenCY:** 6 weeks to 23 months of age

REFERENCES

1. Centers for Disease Control and Prevention. Available at www.cdc.org
2. American Academy of Pediatrics. Red Book: 2012 Report of the Committee on Infectious Diseases. 29th ed Elk Grove Village, Ill: AAP, 2012.
3. Nuorti JP, Whitney CG, Centers for Disease Control and Prevention. Prevention of pneumococcal disease among infants and children–use of 13-valent pneumococcal conjugate vaccine and 23-valent pneumococcal polysaccharide vaccine—recommendations of the Advisory Committee on Immunization Practices (ACIP). *MMWR Recomm Rep.* 2010;59(RR-11):1-18.

4. Pickering LK, Baker CJ, Freed GL, et al. Immunization programs for infants, children, adolescents, and adults: clinical practice guidelines by the Infectious Diseases Society of America. *Clin Infect Dis.* 2009;49:817-840.
5. Sanofi Pasteur package insert for Daptacel.
6. GlaxoSmithKline package insert for Havrix (hepatitis A vaccine).
7. Merck package insert for Vaqta (hepatitis A vaccine).
8. Merck package insert for Gardasil.
9. Centers for Disease Control and Prevention. Prevention and control of seasonal influenza with vaccines: recommendations of the Advisory Committee on Immunization Practices (ACIP). *MMWR Recomm Rep.* 2009;58:1-52.
10. GlaxoSmithKline package insert for MenHibRix.
11. Wyeth package insert for Prevnar 13.
12. Centers for Disease Control and Prevention. Updated recommendations of the Advisory Committee on Immunization Practices (ACIP) regarding routine poliovirus vaccination. *MMWR Recomm Rep.* 2009;58:829-830.
13. Sanofi Pasteur package insert for IPOL (poliovirus vaccine inactivated).
14. Meissner HC, Bocchini JA. Reducing RSV hospitalizations: AAP modifies recommendations for use of palivizumab in high-risk infants, young children. *AAP News.* 2009;30:1.
15. GlaxoSmithKline package insert for Rotarix (rotavirus vaccine).
16. Merck package insert for RotaTeq (rotavirus vaccine).
17. Sanofi Pasteur package insert for Typhoid Vi Polysaccharide Vaccine.
18. Merck package insert for Varivax.
19. Merck package insert for ProQuad (measles, mumps, rubella, and varicella live virus vaccine).

16

Chapter 17

Microbiology and Infectious Disease

Edith Dietz, MD, and Courtney Mangus, MD

💬 See additional content on Expert Consult

I. MICROBIOLOGY

A. Collection of Specimens for Blood Culture

1. **Preparation:** To minimize contamination, clean venipuncture site with 70% isopropyl ethyl alcohol. Apply tincture of iodine or 10% povidone-iodine and allow to dry for at least 1 minute, or scrub site with 2% chlorhexidine for 30 seconds and allow to dry for 30 seconds. Clean blood culture bottle injection site with alcohol only.
2. **Collection:** Two sets of cultures of equal blood volume should be obtained for each febrile episode, based on patient weight: <8 kg, 1–3 mL each; 8–13 kg, 4–5 mL; 14–25 kg, 10–15 mL each; >25 kg, 20–30 mL each (modified from Kaditis et al. 1996[1]). Total blood volume drawn should not exceed more than 1% of patient's total blood volume.

B. Rapid Microbiologic Identification of Common Aerobic Bacteria (Fig. 17-1)

C. Choosing Appropriate Antibiotic Based on Sensitivities

1. **Minimum inhibitory concentration (MIC):** Lowest concentration of an antimicrobial agent that prevents visible growth; MICs are unique to each agent. Antibiotic selection should be based on whether agent is "susceptible" rather than MIC.
2. **See Tables 17-1 through 17-6 for spectrum of activity of commonly used antibiotics.**[2,3]
   Note: Antibiotic sensitivities can vary greatly with local resistance patterns. Follow published institutional guidelines and culture results for individual patients and infections. When possible, always use agent with narrowest spectrum of activity particularly when organism susceptibilities are known.

II. INFECTIOUS DISEASE

A. Fever Without Localizing Source: Evaluation and Management Guidelines

1. **Age < 28 days:** Hospitalize for full evaluation (Fig. 17-2). Owing to the greater risk of serious bacterial infections in young infants with fever, a conservative approach is warranted.
2. **Age 29–90 days:** Well-appearing infants who meet low-risk criteria may potentially be managed as outpatients if reliable follow-up and monitoring is ensured.

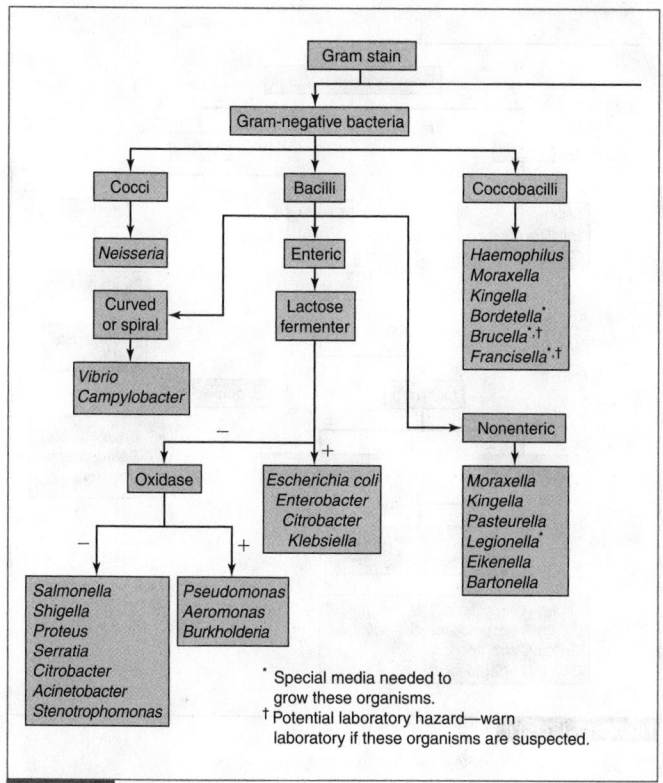

FIGURE 17-1

Algorithm demonstrating identification of aerobic bacteria.

3. **Age > 90 days:** Traditionally, similar risk-stratification strategies were advocated and used to aid evaluation and management of febrile children >90 days of age. However, the marked decline in invasive infections due to *Haemophilus influenzae* type b and *Streptococcus pneumoniae*, since introduction of conjugate vaccines, has significantly reduced the likelihood of serious bacterial infection in a well-appearing child within this age group:

a. If ill-appearing without source of infection identified, consider admission and empirical antimicrobial therapy.

b. If source of infection identified, treat accordingly.

c. If well-appearing and without foci of infection, many experts now advocate urinalysis + urine culture as the only routine diagnostic test if reliable

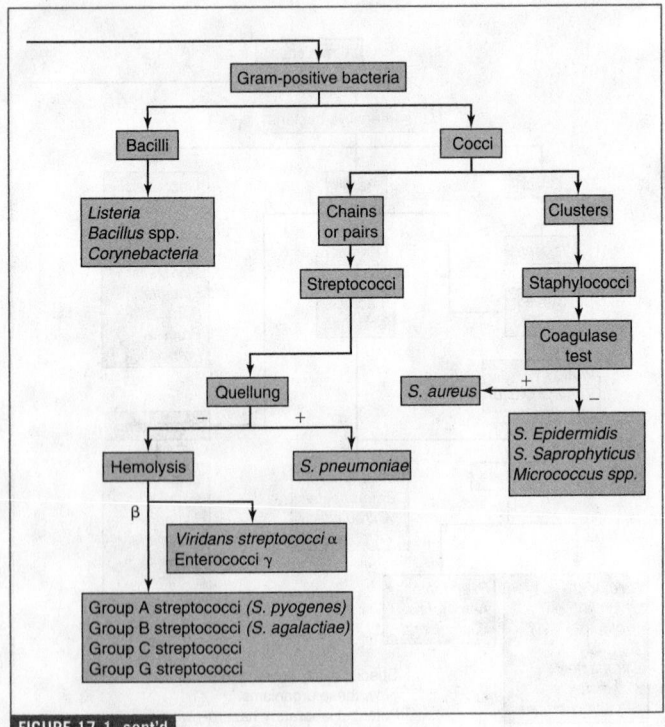

FIGURE 17-1, cont'd

follow-up and monitoring is ensured, including all females and uncircumcised males <age 2 years, all circumcised males <age 6 months, and all children with known genitourinary tract abnormalities.[4,5]

B. Intrauterine and Perinatal Infections

1. **Intrauterine (congenital) infections:** The acronym TORCH (toxoplasmosis, other, rubella, cytomegalovirus [CMV], herpes symplex virus [HSV]) is used to describe a group of infections (including a large number that fall under "other") outlined individually in Table 17-7. These infections often present in the neonate with overlapping findings: intrauterine growth retardation (IUGR), hematologic insult, ocular abnormalities, central nervous system (CNS) signs, and other organ system involvement (e.g., pneumonitis, myocarditis, nephritis, hepatitis).[6-8] Workup and management of these infections is detailed in Table 17-7.

TABLE 17-1

β-LACTAMS

	Gram-Positive Organisms	Gram-Negative Organisms	Anaerobes	Spirochetes
PENICILLINS				
Natural penicillins (Pen G or Pen V)	*Streptococcus pyogenes, Streptococcus agalactiae, Streptococcus pneumoniae* (with about 10%–20% resistance), *Listeria*	*Neisseria meningitidis*	Oral but not all gut anaerobes (gut organisms can make β-lactamases)	Syphilis Leptospirosis
Nafcillin, oxacillin, dicloxacillin	MSSA, CoNS (high levels of resistance)			
Amoxicillin, ampicillin	*S. pyogenes, S. agalactiae, S. pneumoniae, Viridans streptococcus, Listeria, Enterococcus fecalis*	Non–β-lactamase-producing *Escherichia coli, Haemophilus influenzae, Proteus*	Oral but not all gut anaerobes (gut organisms can make β-lactamases)	*Borrelia burgdorferi* (Lyme disease)
Amoxicillin/clavulanic acid (Augmentin), ampicillin/ sulbactam (Unasyn)	Amoxicillin coverage plus MSSA	β-Lactamase-producing Gram-negative organisms (>95% of *E. coli, H. influenzae*)	Oral and gut anaerobes	
Piperacillin/tazobactam (Zosyn), ticarcillin/clavulanate (Timentin)	*E. fecalis*, MSSA, *S. pyogenes, S. agalactiae*	β-Lactamase-producing Gram-negative organisms (majority of *E. coli, H. influenzae*) as well as *Pseudomonas, Serratia, Citrobacter* (varies based on local epidemiology)	Oral and gut anaerobes	
CEPHALOSPORINS				
Do not cover LAME (*Listeria*, Atypicals such as *Mycoplasma* and *Chlamydia*, MRSA [except for ceftaroline], and Enterococci)				
First-generation: cephalexin, cefazolin	MSSA, *S. pyogenes, S. agalactiae*	Very good coverage of enteric Gram-negative organisms (e.g., *E. coli, Klebsiella*, etc.), *Moraxella catarrhalis*		

Continued

TABLE 17-1

β-LACTAMS (Continued)

	Gram-Positive Organisms	Gram-Negative Organisms	Anaerobes	Spirochetes
Second-generation: cefuroxime ("true," same as first-generation "derived")	True, same as first-generation Derived, little activity	β-Lactamase–producing Gram-negative organisms (E. coli, H. influenzae, Klebsiella spp., Proteus spp., M. catarrhalis, etc.), Enterobacter, some Neisseria spp.	Derived have moderate activity (poor coverage of gut anaerobes)	
Third-generation: ceftriaxone, cefotaxime, ceftazidime IV (oral: Suprax = cefixime, Vantin = cefpodoxime, Omnicef = cefdinir) *Good CNS penetration*	*S. pneumoniae* (majority), *S. pyogenes, S. agalactiae, Viridans streptococci*, other streptococci	Ceftriaxone/cefotaxime and orals: β-lactamase–producing Gram-negatives (E. coli, H. influenzae, M. catarrhalis, Klebsiella, Proteus, Neisseria, etc.) Ceftazidime: β-lactamase–producing Gram-negatives, Pseudomonas	None	*B. burgdorferi*
Fourth-generation: cefepime *Good CNS penetration*	Same as third-generation plus MSSA	β-Lactamase–producing Gram-negatives, Pseudomonas		
CARBAPENEMS				
Meropenem, imipenem	MSSA, S. pneumoniae, S. pyogenes, S. agalactiae, Enterococcus	β-Lactamase–producing Gram-negatives, including some very resistant Pseudomonas spp., Acinetobacter spp., Serratia spp., Klebsiella spp., E. coli	Oral and gut (not Clostridium difficile)	
Ertapenem	MSSA	β-Lactamase–producing Gram-negatives (less active against Pseudomonas and Acinetobacter than other carbapenems)	All oral and gut (not C. difficile)	
MONOBACTAMS				
Aztreonam		Covers most aerobic Gram-negative bacilli, including about 2/3 of Pseudomonas spp.		

CNS, Central nervous system; CoNS, coagulase-negative staphylococci; MRSA, methicillin-resistant *Staphylococcus aureus*; MSSA, methicillin-sensitive *Staphylococcus aureus*.

TABLE 17-2

FLUOROQUINOLONES

	Gram-Positive Organisms	Gram-Negative Organisms	Anaerobes	Other
Ciprofloxacin	*Bacillus* spp., including *Bacillus anthracis*	Broad coverage, including *Pseudomonas*; emerging *Neisseria* resistance		*Mycobacterium, Bartonella, Rickettsia*
Levofloxacin	Excellent *Streptococcus pneumoniae* coverage; some MSSA and *S. epidermidis* coverage	Almost same coverage as ciprofloxacin		Great atypical coverage
Moxifloxacin	Same as levofloxacin	Good enteric coverage; poor *Pseudomonas* coverage	Best anaerobic coverage of quinolones	Good for MTB and MAI

MAI, *Mycobacterium avium* subsp. *intracellulare*; MSSA, methicillin-sensitive *Staphylococcus aureus*; MTB, *Mycobacterium tuberculosis*.

TABLE 17-3

MACROLIDES

	Gram positive organisms	Atypicals	Others
Clarithromycin	Reasonably good against *Streptococcus pneumonia* (~50-70%)	*Mycoplasma, Chlamydia pneumoniae, Legionella*	*Bartonella henslae, Bordetella pertussis, Campylobacter,* and *H. flu*
Erythromycin	Same as clarithromycin	Above and *Chlamydia trachomatis*	Diptheria, Entamoeba histolytica
Azithromycin	Same as clarithromycin	Above plus *Toxoplasmosis* (with pyrimethamine)	*N. gonorrhea, Treponema pallidum* (Syphilis), *Haemophilus ducreyi* (chancre)

TABLE 17-4

TETRACYCLINES

	Gram-Positive Organisms	Atypicals	Others
Doxycycline and tetracycline	Some streptococci, pneumococci, MSSA, MRSA, *Propionibacterium acnes*	*Mycoplasma, Chlamydia, Legionella*	*Haemophilus influenzae*, some anaerobic activity, *Borrelia burgdorferi, Rickettsia, Francisella tularensis* (tularemia), *Vibrio, Helicobacter pylori*

MRSA, Methicillin-resistant *Staphylococcus aureus*; MSSA, methicillin-sensitive *Staphylococcus aureus*.

TABLE 17-5

AMINOGLYCOSIDES

	Gram-Negative Organisms
Gentamicin and streptomycin	Almost all Gram-negative organisms; synergy with ampicillin for *Enterococcus*
Tobramycin and amikacin	Almost all Gram-negative organisms

17

TABLE 17-6

SINGLE DRUG CLASS

	Gram-Positive Organisms	Gram-Negative Organisms	Other
Clindamycin	Broad Gram-positive coverage: MRSA, MSSA, *Streptococcus pyogenes*, *Streptococcus agalactiae*	Second-line agent for *Campylobacter jejuni* and *Gardnerella vaginalis*	Oral anaerobes; some *Chlamydia trachomatis* and *Mycoplasma* spp. coverage; and *Gardnerella vaginalis*
Metronidazole	Anaerobic Gram-positive organisms: *Clostridium* spp., *Peptostreptococcus*	*Helicobacter pylori* and gram-negative anaerobes: *Bacteroides* spp., *Prevotella*, *Fusobacterium*	*Entamoeba histolytica, Giardia lambia, Trichomonas vaginalis*, and *G. vaginalis*
Linezolid	MRSA, MSSA, *Enterococcus* (including VRE), CoNS, *S. pyogenes S. agalactiae*, *Streptococcus pneumoniae*, *S. viridans*	None	*Mycobacterium* spp., *Nocardia*
Vancomycin	MRSA, MSSA, *Enterococcus* (except VRE), CoNS, *S. pyogenes* and *agalactiae*, *S. pneumoniae, C. difficile* (orally)	None	
Trimethoprim + Sulfamethoxazole	MRSA, MSSA, *Listeria* (second choice if PCN allergy)	Many Gram-negative bacilli, including *Stenotrophomonas*	PCP (*Pneumocystis jiroveci*), *Toxoplasma gondii, Nocardia*

CoNS, Coagulase-negative staphylococci; MRSA, methicillin-resistant *Staphylococcus aureus*; MSSA, methicillin-sensitive *Staphylococcus aureus*; PCN, penicillin; PCP, *Pneumocystis* pneumonia; VRE, vancomycin-resistant *Enterococcus*.

2. **Perinatal viral infections:** Perinatal varicella-zoster virus (VZV), HSV, enterovirus, and CMV infections can be severe, with profound morbidity and mortality. Although VZV, HSV, hepatitis B, and hepatitis C can all cause intrauterine (congenital) infection, perinatal infection around the time of birth is more common. It can be difficult to clinically distinguish neonatal VZV and HSV lesions.[9] Workup and management of these infections is detailed in Table 17-8.

3. **Group B streptococcal (GBS) infection:**

a. Adequate maternal intrapartum prophylaxis is intravenous (IV) penicillin, ampicillin, or cefazolin ≥4 hours before delivery.[9] Fig. 17-3 shows an algorithm for secondary prevention of early-onset GBS disease in newborns.

b. Late-onset GBS: See Table 17-9.

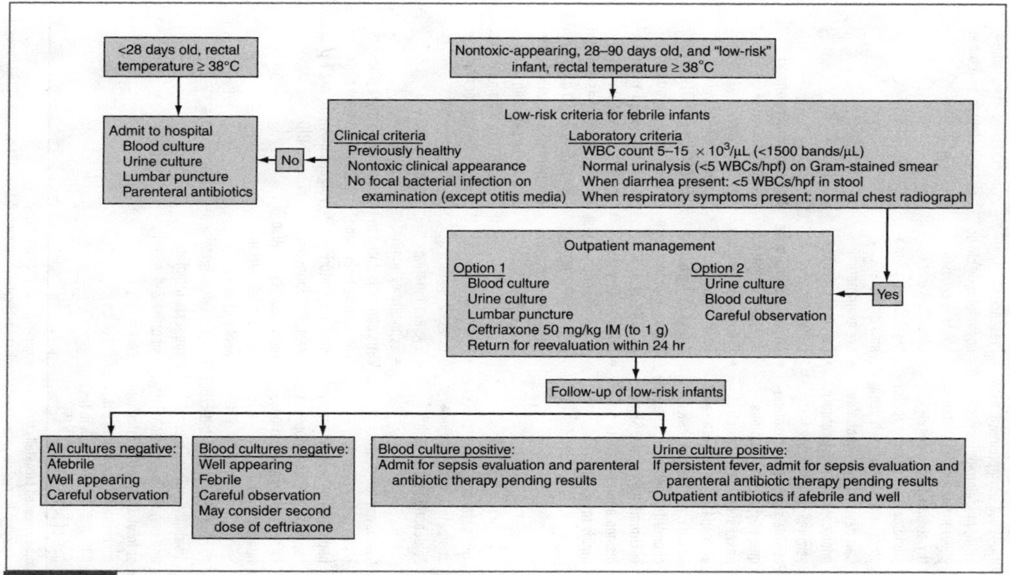

<28 days old, rectal temperature ≥ 38°C
Admit to hospital
Blood culture
Urine culture
Lumbar puncture
Parenteral antibiotics
No
Nontoxic-appearing, 28–90 days old, and "low-risk" infant, rectal temperature ≥ 38°C
Low-risk criteria for febrile infants
Clinical criteria
Previously healthy
Nontoxic clinical appearance
No focal bacterial infection on examination (except otitis media)
Laboratory criteria
WBC count 5–15 × 10³/µL (<1500 bands/µL)
Normal urinalysis (<5 WBCs/hpf) on Gram-stained smear
When diarrhea present: <5 WBCs/hpf in stool
When respiratory symptoms present: normal chest radiograph
Yes
Outpatient management
Option 1
Blood culture
Urine culture
Lumbar puncture
Ceftriaxone 50 mg/kg IM (to 1 g)
Return for reevaluation within 24 hr
Option 2
Urine culture
Blood culture
Careful observation
Follow-up of low-risk infants
All cultures negative:
Afebrile
Well appearing
Careful observation
Blood cultures negative:
Well appearing
Febrile
Careful observation
May consider second dose of ceftriaxone
Blood culture positive:
Admit for sepsis evaluation and parenteral antibiotic therapy pending results
Urine culture positive:
If persistent fever, admit for sepsis evaluation and parenteral antibiotic therapy pending results
Outpatient antibiotics if afebrile and well

FIGURE 17-2

Algorithm for management of a previously healthy infant ≤90 days of age with a fever without localizing signs. This algorithm is a suggested but not exhaustive approach. hpf, High-power field. *(Modified from Baraff LJ. Management of fever without source in infants and children.* Ann Emerg Med. *2000;36:602-614; and Baraff LJ. Management of infants and young children with fever without source.* Pediatr Ann. *2008;37:673-679.)*

TABLE 17-7

CONGENITAL INFECTIONS

Infective Agent	Clinical Findings	Diagnostic Testing	Therapy
Toxoplasmosis	70%–90% asymptomatic at birth; maculopapular rash, generalized lymphadenopathy, hepatosplenomegaly, jaundice, pneumonitis, petechiae, and thrombocytopenia. Can develop hydrocephalus, microcephaly, chorioretinitis, seizures, and hearing loss	• Presence of immunoglobulin (Ig) M or IgA is diagnostic; persistence of IgG beyond age 12 mo also diagnostic • Eye examination • Cerebral calcifications best seen on CT	Pyrimethamine + sulfadiazine with folinic acid for at least 12 months
Syphilis*	Possible signs: hepatosplenomegaly, snuffles (copious nasal secretions), lymphadenopathy, mucocutaneous lesions, pneumonia, osteochondritis, hemolytic anemia, or thrombocytopenia. Skin lesions and secretions are highly infectious	• All women should be screened prenatally • If maternal serology positive, screen infant using nontreponemal test such as VDRL or RPR • Confirmatory test using treponemal test such as FTA-ABS or MHA-TP.† See Table EC 17-A	**For abnormal neonatal testing/physical examination:** aqueous penicillin G, 50,000 U/kg IV Q12 hr (age 1 week or younger) or Q8 hr (>age 1 week); *or* procaine penicillin G, 50,000 U/kg IM as a single daily dose for 10 days **For normal neonatal tests:** benzathine penicillin G, 50,000 U/kg IM, single dose
Rubella*	IUGR, cataracts, cardiac anomalies, deafness, "blueberry muffin rash"	• IgM positive at birth–3 months • Eye examination • Echocardiogram	Supportive care for newborn Ensure mother is immunized
Cytomegalovirus (CMV)	90% asymptomatic at birth: IUGR, jaundice, hepatosplenomegaly, microcephaly, thrombocytopenia, intracranial calcifications, hearing loss	Virus can be isolated in cell culture from urine, stool, respiratory tract, CSF, peripheral blood leukocytes. Also can test IgM within 3 weeks of birth	Ganciclovir 6 mg/kg/dose IV Q12 hr for 6 weeks Valganciclovir 16 mg/kg/dose PO BID
Parvovirus B19	Fetal hydrops, IUGR, intellectual disability, isolated pleural and pericardial effusions; risk of fetal death when infection occurs during pregnancy is 2%–6%, greatest risk in first half of pregnancy	Positive serum IgM suggests infection occurred 2–4 months earlier	Supportive care

*All mothers should be screened prenatally for rubella immune status and syphilis.

†Link to diagnostic algorithm for syphilis: http://aapredbook.aappublications.org/content/1/SEC131/SEC268/F2192.large.jpg.

‡See 2012 American Academy of Pediatrics *Red Book* for isolation recommendations.

BID, Twice daily; CSF, cerebrospinal fluid; CT, computed tomography; IM, intramuscular; IUGR, intrauterine growth retardation; IV, intravenous; FTA-ABS, fluorescent treponemal antibody absorption test; MHA-TP, microhemagglutination assay for *Treponema pallidum* antibodies; PO, oral; RPR, rapid plasma reagin; VDRL, Venereal Disease Research Laboratory test.

TABLE 17-8

PERINATAL INFECTIONS

Infective Agent	Clinical Findings	Diagnostic Testing	Therapy
Herpes simplex virus (HSV)	HSV can present any time within the first 1–3 weeks of life as: 1. Disease localized to SEM. 2. Localized CNS infection. 3. Disseminated disease with severe pneumonitis and hepatitis. Disseminated disease often presents in the first to second week of life; CNS disease presents later, often in the second to third week of life.	• Surface culture: conjunctiva, nasopharynx, mouth, rectum, blood, CSF, skin vesicles • PCR: blood, CSF • Ancillary: CMP looking for elevated transaminase; CXR looking for pneumonitis	Acyclovir 20 mg/kg/dose IV Q8 hr • 14 days for skin, eye, and mouth disease • 21 days with up to 6 months prophylaxis for disseminated disease
Varicella[10]	Maternal infection from 5 days prior or 2 days after delivery can result in severe neonatal infection in first 2 weeks. Can include pneumonitis, encephalitis, purpura fulminans, bleeding, death. Maternal infection >5 days before delivery and GA >28 weeks causes milder disease.	• DFA of vesicle scraping • PCR from vesicle or CSF	Infant: VariZIG and/or acylovir if mother developed primary varicella (not zoster) between 5 days before and 2 days after delivery, and hospitalized preterm infants < 28 weeks or ≥ 28 weeks if mother lacks historical or serologic evidence of protection.
Enterovirus	Neonates can develop severe infection: hepatitis, myocarditis, meningitis, encephalitis, pneumonitis, DIC.	RNA PCR from throat, stool, rectal swab, urine, blood, or CSF	IVIG
Hepatitis B virus (HBV)[11]	In utero transmission accounts for <2% of perinatal infections. If mother is both HBsAg positive and HBeAg positive, risk for development of chronic HBV infection is 70%–90% by age 6 months unless postexposure immunoprophylaxis is given. Risk is 5%–20% when mother is HBsAb positive and HBeAg negative. Appropriate prophylaxis is highly effective.	ALT is usually normal at birth, with detectable HBeAg and high HBV DNA concentrations (≥20,000 IU/mL). Testing for HBsAg and anti-HBs should be done at 9 and 18 months in infants with HBsAg-positive mothers	Newborns of HBsAg-positive or unknown mothers should receive HBV vaccine and HBIG 0.5 mL IM within 12 hours of life. (See FIGURE 16-4. Management of neonates born to mothers with unknown or positive HBsAg status.) Breast-feeding not contraindicated

Continued

17

TABLE 17-8
PERINATAL INFECTIONS (Continued)

Infective Agent	Clinical Findings	Diagnostic Testing	Therapy
Hepatitis C virus (HCV)	Risk of perinatal transmission is 5% and occurs only from women who are HCV RNA positive at time of delivery. Maternal co-infection with HIV is associated with increased risk of perinatal transmission.	HCV RNA can be detected in serum or plasma within 1–2 weeks after exposure and weeks before onset of liver enzyme abnormalities. Maternal anti-HCV antibodies can persist up to 18 months.	No therapy until HCV status ascertained. Nonpegylated interferon-α-2b plus ribavirin approved in children aged 3–17 years, but no data for neonates. Refer to pediatric hepatitis specialist. Breast-feeding not contraindicated.
Human immunodeficiency virus (HIV)*	Most mother-to-child transmission occurs perinatally, with lower rates of transmission occurring in utero and postnatally through breast-feeding. Risk factors for transmission: 1. Greater viral exposure, especially maternal viral load. 2. Risk increases with longer duration of ruptured membranes, more months of breast-feeding, vaginal delivery, or laboring before cesarean section.	• If high risk of acquiring infection (i.e., high maternal VL), HIV DNA PCR at 48–72 hours of life • If lower risk, test at 2 weeks of life	See Table 17-12 Breastfeeding contraindicated

ALT, Alanine aminotransferase; CMP, comprehensive metabolic panel; CNS, central nervous system; CSF, cerebrospinal fluid; CXR, chest x-ray; DFA, direct fluorescent antibody; DIC, disseminated intravascular coagulation; GA, gestational age; HBIG, hepatitis B immune globulin; IM, intramuscular; IV, intravenous; IVIG, intravenous immunoglobulin; PCR, polymerase chain reaction; sAb, surface antibody; sAg, surface antigen; SEM, skin, eyes, mouth; VL, viral load; VZIG, varicella-zoster immune globulin.

*From Panel on Treatment of HIV-Infected Pregnant Women and Prevention of Perinatal Transmission. Recommendations for use of antiretroviral drugs in pregnant HIV-1-infected women for maternal health and interventions to reduce perinatal HIV transmission in the United States. Available at http://aidsinfo.nih.gov/contentfiles/lvguidelines/PerinatalGL.pdf. Tables 8 and 9. Accessed December 11, 2012.

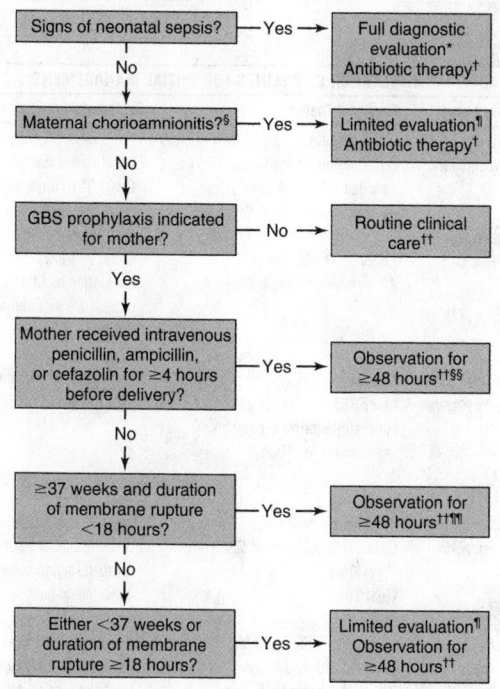

Signs of neonatal sepsis? —Yes→ Full diagnostic evaluation* Antibiotic therapy†

No ↓

Maternal chorioamnionitis?§ —Yes→ Limited evaluation¶ Antibiotic therapy†

No ↓

GBS prophylaxis indicated for mother? —No→ Routine clinical care††

Yes ↓

Mother received intravenous penicillin, ampicillin, or cefazolin for ≥4 hours before delivery? —Yes→ Observation for ≥48 hours††§§

No ↓

≥37 weeks and duration of membrane rupture <18 hours? —Yes→ Observation for ≥48 hours††¶¶

No ↓

Either <37 weeks or duration of membrane rupture ≥18 hours? —Yes→ Limited evaluation¶ Observation for ≥48 hours††

* Full diagnostic evaluation includes a blood culture, a complete blood count (CBC), including white blood cell differential and platelet counts, chest radiograph (if respiratory abnormalities are present), and lumbar puncture (if patient is stable enough to tolerate procedure and sepsis is suspected).

† Antibiotic therapy should be directed toward the most common causes of neonatal sepsis, including intravenous ampicillin for GBS and coverage for other organisms (including *Escherichia coli* and other gram-negative pathogens) and should take into account local antibiotic resistance patterns.

§ Consultation with obstetric providers is important to determine the level of clinical suspicion for chorioamnionitis. Chorioamnionitis is diagnosed clinically and some of the signs are nonspecific.

¶ Limited evaluation includes blood culture (at birth) and CBC with differential and platelets (at birth and/or at 6-12 hours of life).

†† If signs of sepsis develop, a full diagnostic evaluation should be conducted and antibiotic therapy initiated.

§§ If ≥37 weeks' gestation, observation may occur at home after 24 hours if other discharge criteria have been met, access to medical care is readily available, and a person who is able to comply fully with instructions for home observation will be present. If any of these conditions is not met, the infant should be observed in the hospital for at least 48 hours and until discharge criteria are achieved.

¶¶ Some experts recommend a CBC with differential and platelets at age 6-12 hours.

FIGURE 17-3

Algorithm for secondary prevention of early-onset group B streptococcal (GBS) disease among newborns. (From Verani JR, McGee L, Schrag SJ; Division of Bacterial Diseases, National Center for Immunization and Respiratory Diseases, Centers for Disease Control and Prevention [CDC]. Prevention of perinatal group B streptococcal disease—revised guidelines from CDC, 2010. MMWR Recomm Rep. 2010;59:1-36.)

TABLE 17-9		
NEONATAL BACTERIAL INFECTIONS: GUIDELINES FOR INITIAL MANAGEMENT		
Infectious Syndrome	**Empirical Therapy**	**Comments**
Conjunctivitis	Saline irrigation regardless of etiology	
Chlamydia trachomatis	Erythromycin 50 mg/kg/day PO/IV divided QID for 14 days *Alt: azithromycin for 5 days*	Exudative conjunctivitis. Onset 3–10 days. Topical treatment ineffective
Neisseria gonorrheae	Ceftriaxone 25–50 mg/kg IV/IM, single dose (max 125 mg) *Alt: cefotaxime, single dose*	Exudative conjunctivitis. Onset 2–4 days. Admit for evaluation and treatment of possible disseminated disease
Meningitis		
GBS, *Escherichia coli*, *Listeria monocytogenes*	Ampicillin + cefotaxime. Treat 14 days for GBS infection, 21 days for *Listeria* For gram-negative organisms: cefotaxime for 21 days	Gentamicin not recommended; poor CSF penetration
Pneumonia		
GBS, *Staphylococcus aureus*, *L. monocyto-genes*	Ampicillin + gentamicin Consider vancomycin if MRSA prevalent Treat 10–21 days, depending on severity	Blood cultures indicated Effusions should be drained; Gram stain and culture collected on fluid
C. trachomatis	Erythromycin 50 mg/kg/day PO/IV divided QID for 14 days *Alt: azithromycin for 5 days*	Presents at 2–19 weeks of life with staccato cough, tachypnea, rales, bilateral infiltrates, and hyperinflation on CXR; usually afebrile
Septic arthritis		
S. aureus, GBS, gram-negative bacilli	(Cefotaxime or gentamicin) + (nafcillin or oxacillin if *S. aureus* suspected)	Drainage necessary
Sepsis	Ampicillin + (gentamicin or cefotaxime)	

First antibiotic listed indicates treatment of choice. Alternative regimens are listed in italics. Cultures should be obtained when clinically appropriate; antibiotic coverage should be narrowed when organism and suscebility information is available.

Alt., Alternative; CSF, cerebrospinal fluid; CXR, chest x-ray; GBS, group B streptococcal; IM, intramuscular; IV, intravenous; MRSA, methicillin-resistant *Staphylococcus aureus*; PO, oral; QID, four times daily.

C. Common Neonatal Bacterial Infections and Pediatric Infections: Guidelines for Initial Management (Table 17-9 and Table 17-10)

D. Sexually Transmitted and Genitourinary Infections

1. **Common sexually transmitted infections (Table 17-11)**
2. **Pelvic inflammatory disease:**
a. Differential diagnosis is broad and includes endometriosis, tubo-ovarian abscess, ovarian cyst, ectopic pregnancy, acute surgical abdomen, irritable bowel disease (IBD), pyelonephritis, dysmenorrhea, septic/threatened abortion.

TABLE 17-10

COMMON PEDIATRIC INFECTIONS: GUIDELINES FOR INITIAL MANAGEMENT

Infectious Syndrome	Usual Etiology	Suggested Empirical Therapy	Suggested Length of Therapy/Comments
Bites			
Human	*Streptococcus* spp., *Staphylococcus aureus*, oral anaerobes, *Eikenella corrodens*, *Haemophilus* spp.	**PO:** amoxicillin/clavulanate Alt: *clindamycin + (third-generation cephalosporin or TMP/SMX)* **IV:** ampicillin/sulbactam Alt: *TMP/SMX + clindamycin*	For all bites, cleaning, irrigation, and débridement are critical. Human: 5–7 days. Assess immunization status (tetanus, hepatitis B) and HIV risk.
Dog/cat	Add *Pasteurella multocida*, *Streptococcus* spp., *Capnocytophaga*, oral anaerobes	Same	Animal: 7–10 days Assess tetanus immunization status, risk of rabies.
Catheter-related bloodstream infections	*S. aureus*, CoNS, enteric Gram-negative bacilli including Pseudomonas, Candida spp.	Immunocompetent: vancomycin + third-generation cephalosporin Immunocompromised: vancomycin + (cefepime or piperacillin/tazobactam)	Consider catheter removal and fungal coverage as clinically indicated.
Cellulitis	GAS, *S. aureus* (MSSA or MRSA)	**PO:** cephalexin; *clindamycin if MRSA prevalence high* **IV:** oxacillin; *clindamycin or vancomycin if MRSA prevalence high* TMP/SMX is not active against GAS	5 days Incision and drainage alone may be adequate and should be performed when indicated; obtain cultures for susceptibility. Hospitalize for severe infections, limb-threatening infections, immunocompromised status.
Conjunctivitis (suppurative, non-neonatal)	*Streptococcus pneumoniae*, *Haemophilus influenzae* (nontypeable), *Moraxella*, viral *Neisseria gonorrhoeae*	Ophthalmic erythromycin, bacitracin/polymyxin B, or polymyxin B/TMP Ceftriaxone IM	5 days Ointments preferred for infants or young children. Single dose. Consider *Chlamydia* treatment as clinically indicated.
Dacrocystitis	*S. pneumoniae*, *H. influenzae*, *S. aureus*, *Streptococcus pyogenes*, *Pseudomonas aeruginosa*	Initial management: warm compresses **PO:** oxacillin or cephalexin	Consider ophthalmologic evaluation to relieve obstruction.

Continued

17

TABLE 17-10

COMMON PEDIATRIC INFECTIONS: GUIDELINES FOR INITIAL MANAGEMENT (Continued)

Infectious Syndrome	Usual Etiology	Suggested Empirical Therapy	Suggested Length of Therapy/Comments
Dental abscesses	Oral flora, including anaerobes	Clindamycin or amoxicillin/clavulanic acid	Consider dental evaluation for surgical drainage.
Gastroenteritis (Bacterial)	*Escherichia coli*	Antibiotics strongly discouraged because of possible increased risk of HUS occurring in patients with *E. coli* 0157:H7 treated with antibiotics[12] Azithromycin or ciprofloxacin for traveler's diarrhea	
	Salmonella spp.	Ceftriaxone *Alt: azithromycin, ampicillin, amoxicillin, or TMP/SMX for susceptible strains*	10–14 days for infants <age 3 months, bacteremia, toxic appearance, hemoglobinopathy, or immunosuppressed. Antibiotics generally not indicated otherwise.
	Shigella spp.	Ceftriaxone, azithromycin, or fluoroquinolone	5 days for dysentery, immunosuppressed, or to prevent spread in mild disease. Oral cephalosporins not useful. High rates resistance with amoxicillin or TMP/SMX.
	Yersinia spp.	TMP/SMX, aminoglycosides, cefotaxime, flouroquinolone, or tetracycline	Usually no antibiotic therapy is recommended except with bacteremia, extraintestinal infections, or immunocompromised hosts.
	Campylobacter spp.	Azithromycin or erythromycin	5–7 days; shortens duration of fecal shedding
	Clostridium difficile	Metronidazole Oral vancomycin for severe infection	10 days Stop the precipitating antibiotic therapy
Influenza	Influenza A and B	Recommendations vary yearly based on characteristics and resistance patterns	See http://www.cdc.gov/flu/ for most up-to-date recommendations.

TABLE 17-10

COMMON PEDIATRIC INFECTIONS: GUIDELINES FOR INITIAL MANAGEMENT (Continued)

Infectious Syndrome	Usual Etiology	Suggested Empirical Therapy	Suggested Length of Therapy/Comments
Intraabdominal infections	E. coli, Enterococcus, Bacteroides spp., Clostridium spp., Peptostreptococcus, P. aeruginosa, S. aureus, other Gram-negative bacilli	**Single agent:** piperacillin-tazobactam, ticarcillin-clavulanate **Combo:** (ceftriaxone or cefepime) + metronidazole	4–7 days For patients with health care–associated infection, consider MRSA coverage.
Lymphadenitis	Viruses, GAS, S. aureus, anaerobes, atypical mycobacteria, Actinomyces, Bartonella henselae (cat scratch disease), Mycobacterium tuberculosis	**PO:** amoxicillin/clavulanate; clindamycin if MRSA prevalent **Alt:** cephalexin or dicloxacillin **IV:** oxacillin or cefazolin; clindamycin if MRSA prevalent	Surgical excision with M. tuberculosis, atypical mycobacteria. Needle aspiration with B. henselae. If allergic to PCN: cefdinir, cefuroxime, or vancomycin
Mastoiditis (acute)	S. pneumoniae, S. pyogenes, S. aureus, H. influenzae (nontypeable)	Third-generation cephalosporin	4 weeks Surgical management required; definitive therapy should be guided by culture obtained at surgery.
Meningitis (non-neonatal) age > 1 month	S. pneumoniae, Neisseria meningitidis, H. influenzae	Ceftriaxone + vancomycin For severe PCN allergy, consider chloramphenicol + vancomycin or levofloxacin	Duration depends on organism. See Red Book, 2012 for chemoprophylaxis recommendations for contacts of meningococcal and Hib disease. Dexamethasone use, except for with H. influenzae, is controversial.
Orbital cellulitis	S. pneumoniae, H. influenzae (nontypeable), Moraxella catarrhalis, S. aureus, GAS	Ampicillin/sulbactam; OR (cefotaxime or ceftriaxone) AND (clindamycin or vancomycin or oxacillin)	10 days Recommend ophthalmologic consultation; CT to evaluate intracranial extension.

Continued

17

TABLE 17-10

COMMON PEDIATRIC INFECTIONS: GUIDELINES FOR INITIAL MANAGEMENT (Continued)

Infectious Syndrome	Usual Etiology	Suggested Empirical Therapy	Suggested Length of Therapy/Comments
Osteomyelitis			
Uncomplicated	*S. aureus*, GAS, *Streptococcus* spp., *Kingella kingae* (≤4 years)	Oxacillin, nafcillin, or clindamycin *Alt: TMP-SMX*	4–6 weeks Clindamycin ineffective as monotherapy for *Kingella.*
Foot puncture	Add *P. aeruginosa* coverage	Add ceftazidime or antipseudomonal PCN	
Sickle cell disease	Add *Salmonella* spp. coverage	Add ceftriaxone	
Otitis media (acute)[13]	*S. pneumoniae*, *H. influenzae* (nontypeable), *M. catarrhalis*	High dose Amoxicillin 80–90 mg/kg/day If child has received Amoxicillin within the past 30 days or has concurrent purulent conjunctivitis, Amoxicillin-Clavulanate is recommended *Alt/PCN Allergy: Cefdinir, Cefpodoxime, Ceftriaxone* For treatment failure (persistent symptoms 48-72 hours after initial treatment): Amoxicillin-Clavulanate or Ceftriaxone (IM daily x 3 days) *Alt: Clindamycin + 3rd generation cephalosporin*	10 days for children age < 2 years and all children with severe symptoms 7 days for children ages 2-5 years with mild-moderate symptoms 5-7 days days for children > age 6 years with mild-moderate symptoms Consider watchful waiting in patients 6-23 months with unilateral, nonsevere symptoms or in patients > 2 years with nonsevere symptoms Consider tympanocentesis and specialist consultations
Otitis externa (uncomplicated)	*Pseudomonas*	Eardrops: ciprofloxacin	7–10 days Analgesics for pain
Parotitis	*S. aureus* most common; also oral flora, gram-negative rods, viruses (including mumps, HIV, EBV), or noninfectious causes	PO: clindamycin or nafcillin/oxacillin or amoxicillin/clavulanic acid	Sialogogues, local heat, gentle massage of gland from posterior to anterior, and hydration provide symptomatic relief. Surgical drainage may be required. Consider HIV test if chronic parotitis.

TABLE 17-10

COMMON PEDIATRIC INFECTIONS: GUIDELINES FOR INITIAL MANAGEMENT (Continued)

Infectious Syndrome	Usual Etiology	Suggested Empirical Therapy	Suggested Length of Therapy/Comments
Periorbital cellulitis (preseptal)	GAS and Streptococcus spp., S. aureus, H. influenzae (nontypeable), M. catarrhalis	Ampicillin/sulbactam or amoxicillin/clavulate or third-generation cephalosporin Consider adding vancomycin, TMP/SMX, or clindamycin if concern for MRSA	10–14 days If secondary to local trauma and not associated with sinusitis, treat as staph/strep cellulitis.
Pertussis	Bordetella pertussis	Azithromycin, erythromycin Azithromycin for age < 1 month	5 days for Azithromycin. 10 days for Erythromycin Chemoprophylaxis for close contacts
Pharyngitis	GAS, group C and G streptococci, Arcanobacterium haemolyticum, viruses (including coxsackievirus, other enteroviruses, EBV)	PCN V or amoxicillin Benzathine PCN G × 1 for GAS Alt: clindamycin, macrolide, or cephalexin	10 days (to prevent acute rheumatic fever in GAS infection). Supportive treatment only for viral pharyngitis.
Pneumonia (non-neonatal)			
Age < 5 years	S. pneumoniae, Mycoplasma, Chlamydia pneumoniae, GAS, S. aureus, viruses, influenza	**Outpatient:** amoxicillin (high-dose), ± azithromycin (atypical coverage) Alt: clindamycin **Inpatient:** ampicillin ± azithromycin Alt: ceftriaxone + azithromycin	10 days Atypical organisms (Mycoplasma, Chlamydia) are more likely in children >age 5 years. Add vancomycin or clindamycin if severe illness or features suggestive of S. aureus (pleural effusion, cavitation).
Age > 5 years (and immunized)	S. pneumoniae, Mycoplasma, C. pneumoniae, GAS, S. aureus, viruses, influenza	**Outpatient:** azithromycin ± amoxicillin (high dose) Alt: azithromycin ± clindamycin **Inpatient:** ampicillin + azithromycin Alt: ceftriaxone or cefotaxime + azithromycin	7–10 days Vancomycin or clindamycin if severe illness or features suggestive of S. aureus (pleural effusion, cavitation).

Continued

17

TABLE 17-10

COMMON PEDIATRIC INFECTIONS: GUIDELINES FOR INITIAL MANAGEMENT (Continued)

Infectious Syndrome	Usual Etiology	Suggested Empirical Therapy	Suggested Length of Therapy/Comments
Nonimmunized child (for *H. influenzae*, *S. pneumoniae*)	See above	Ceftriaxone or cefotaxime ± azithromycin	Consider vancomycin or clindamycin for MRSA coverage.
Spinal fusion infections	*Staphylococcus*, *Streptococcus* spp.; enteric or genitourinary Gram-negative organisms	Vancomycin + piperacillin/tazobactam	Greater than 3 months Consider washout of wound initially. Deep tissue culture of wound may direct treatment. Removal of instrumentation may be necessary.
Septic arthritis (non-neonatal)			
Age < 5 years	*S. aureus*, GAS, *S. pneumoniae*, *Kingella kingae* (≤4 years)	Clindamycin or oxacillin. Add amoxicillin for *Kingella*	3 weeks (IV) Aspiration of affected joint recommended. May switch to PO after response.
Age > 5 years	*S. aureus*, GAS, *Streptococcus* spp.	Nafcillin, oxacillin, or clindamycin Alt: *vancomycin*	
Adolescent	Add *N. gonorrhoeae*	Add ceftriaxone	
Sinusitis[20]			
Acute	*S. pneumoniae*, *H. influenzae*, *M. catarrhalis*	Amoxicillin/clavulanate Alt: *cefpodoxime or cefixime* If PCN allergy: levofloxacin If no improvement in 3–5 days, broaden coverage	10 days If severe/fails to respond, consider imaging and/or drainage.
Chronic	Add *S. aureus*, anaerobes	Amoxicillin/clavulanic acid, cefpodoxime, cefuroxime, or cefdinir Alt: *fluoroquinolone*	7 days after resolution of symptoms.
Seriously ill or immuno-compromised	Add *Pseudomonas*, gram-negative bacilli, *Mucor*, *Rhizopus*, *Aspergillus*	Cefepime or piperacillin/tazobactam ± amphotericin B	Surgical intervention needed.

TABLE 17-10

COMMON PEDIATRIC INFECTIONS: GUIDELINES FOR INITIAL MANAGEMENT (Continued)

Infectious Syndrome	Usual Etiology	Suggested Empirical Therapy	Suggested Length of Therapy/Comments
Tracheitis	*S. aureus, S. pneumoniae*, GAS, *M. catarrhalis, H. influenzae*, *Pseudomonas*	Ceftriaxone + clindamycin if community-acquired Cefepime or piperacillin-tazobactam if ventilator or tracheostomy dependent	5 days
UTI			
Cystitis	*E. coli*, Enterobacteriaceae, *Proteus* spp., *Staphylococcus saprophyticus*, *Enterococcus* spp.	**PO:** TMP/SMX, cefixime **IV:** cefotaxime or ceftriaxone OR ampicillin and gentamicin Alt: nitrofurantoin or ciprofloxacin	7–14 days Consider phenazopyridine for comfort (urine and other secretions may turn red). For severe PCN allergy or resistant organisms.
Pyelonephritis	*E. coli*, Enterobacteriaceae, *Proteus* spp., *Enterococcus* spp.	Ceftriaxone OR ampicillin + gentamicin Alt: cefixime or ciprofloxacin	7–14 days Outpatient treatment if well appearing. Consider initial dose of parenteral therapy.
Abnormal host/urinary tract	Add *Pseudomonas*, resistant gram-negative organisms	Piperacillin/tazobactam or cefepime	7–14 days
Ventriculoperitoneal shunt, infected	*S. epidermidis, S. aureus*, Enterobacteriaceae, *Propionibacterium acnes*	Vancomycin + cefepime	10–21 days, depending on organism and response. Shunt removal or revision is often required for successful treatment.

First antibiotics listed indicate treatment of choice. *Alternative treatment regimens are listed in italics.* Cultures should be obtained when clinically appropriate; antibiotic coverage should be narrowed once organism and susceptibility information is available.

CoNS, Coagulase-negative staphylococci; CT, computed tomography; CXR, chest x-ray; EBV, Epstein-Barr virus; FDA, U.S. Food and Drug Administration; GAS, group A streptococcus; GBS, group B streptococcus; Hib, *Haemophilus influenzae* type b; HIV, human immunodeficiency virus; IM, intramuscular; IV, intravenous; MRSA, methicillin-resistant *Staphylococcus aureus*; MSSA, methicillin-sensitive *Staphylococcus aureus*; PCN, penicillin; PO, by mouth; TMP/SMX, trimethoprim/sulfamethoxazole; UTI, urinary tract infection.

Recommendations modified from American Academy of Pediatrics. Pickering LK, Baker CJ, Kimberlin DW, Long SS, eds. *Red Book: 2012 Report of the Committee on Infectious Diseases.* 29th ed. Elk Grove Village, Ill: AAP, 2012; and McMillan JA, Siberry GK, Dick JD, et al. *The Harriet Lane Handbook of Pediatric Antimicrobial Therapy.* Philadelphia: Mosby Elsevier, 2009.

TABLE 17-11

SEXUALLY TRANSMITTED AND GENITOURINARY INFECTIONS: GUIDELINES FOR MANAGEMENT

Infection	Clinical Diagnosis	Empirical Therapy	Comments
Bacterial vaginosis		Metronidazole 500 mg PO BID OR Metronidazole Gel 0.75% (5 g) intravaginally daily OR Clindamycin Cream 2% 5 g intravaginally	7 days 5 days 7 days
Chlamydia **infections**	Uncomplicated urethritis, endocervicitis, or proctitis	Azithromycin 1 g PO once *OR* Doxycycline 100 mg PO BID for 7 days *Alt: erythromycin PO QID or fluoroquinolone for 7 days*	Consider empirical treatment for gonorrhea secondary to common co-infection. See below for instructions for therapy for sexual partners.
	Chlamydia infection in pregnancy	Azithromycin 1 g PO once Amoxicillin 500 mg PO TID for 7 days Erythromycin PO QID for 7 days	Repeat testing (3 weeks posttreatment) to document chlamydial eradication is in all pregnant patients.
Gonorrhea infections	Uncomplicated infection of the cervix, urethra, rectum, or pharynx	Ceftriaxone 250 mg IM once, ***PLUS*** Azithromycin 1 g PO once	Dual treatment is recommended for gonorrhea secondary to organism resistance.
	Epididymitis	Ceftriaxone 250 mg IM once, ***PLUS*** Doxycycline 100 mg PO BID for 10 days	For MSM, add a fluoroquinolone for 10 days.
	Disseminated gonococcal infections	Ceftriaxone 1 g IV/IM daily *Alt: cefotaxime 1g IV q8 hours*	Can switch to cefixime 400 mg PO BID 24–48 hours after clinical improvement. Total therapy course: 7 days.
Pelvic inflammatory disease	See Chapter 17 Section II.D.2.C	**Outpatient:** ceftriaxone 250 mg IM once, ***PLUS*** Doxycycline 100 mg PO BID for 14 days ± metronidazole 500 mg PO BID x 14 days	
		Inpatient: regimen A (2g Cefotetan IV Q12 hr OR 2g Cefoxitin IV Q6 hr) plus doxycycline 100 mg IV Q12 hr **Regimen B:** clindamycin 900 mg IV Q8 hr plus gentamicin 2 mg/kg loading dose, then 1.5 mg/kg IV Q8 hr maintenance (or single daily dosing)	Switch to oral therapy 24 hours after clinical improvement to complete 14 days of treatment with doxycycline BID or clindamycin QID.
Syphilis	Primary, secondary, or early latent syphilis (<1 year duration)	Benzathine PCN G 50,000 U/kg (max 2.4 million units) IM (single dose) *Alt: doxycycline 100 mg PO BID for 14 days **OR** tetracycline 500 mg PO QID for 14 days*	Data is limited for penicillin alternatives

TABLE 17-11

SEXUALLY TRANSMITTED INFECTIONS: GUIDELINES FOR MANAGEMENT (Continued)

Infection	Clinical Diagnosis	Empirical Therapy	Comments
	Late syphilis (>1 year duration); tertiary syphilis	Benzathine PCN G 50,000 U/kg (max 2.4 million units) IM Q1 week for 3 weeks *Alt: doxycycline 100 mg PO BID for 28 days OR tetracycline 500 mg PO QID for 28 days*	
	Neurosyphilis	See formulary for dosing	
Trichomonas		Metronidazole 2 g PO once	Refer partner for testing and treatment.
Herpes (genital, non-neonatal)		Acyclovir or Valacyclovir	See formulary for treatment for initial infection and recurrence
Candidiasis (Vulvovaginal)		Fluconazole PO OR intravaginal cream	See formulary

PCN G, penicillin G.

Patients should be instructed to refer their partners for diagnosis, testing, and treatment. For dosing for children ≤8 years of age or <45 kg or for additional alternative regimens, please refer to the CDC Treatment Guidelines, 2010: http://www.cdc.gov/std/treatment/2010/.

b. Workup: Pelvic and bimanual examination, gonorrhea/chlamydia (GC/CT) testing, HIV, human chorionic gonadotropin (hCG), wet preparation, erythrocyte sedimentation rate (ESR), C-reactive protein (CRP), and urinalysis/urine culture (UA/UCx) if clinically indicated. Consider a complete blood cell count (CBC) with differential and pelvic ultrasound if the patient is ill-appearing, has an adnexal mass on bimanual examination, or is not improving after antibiotics.

c. Minimum diagnostic criteria: Uterine, adnexal, or cervical motion tenderness without other identifiable causes. One or more of the following additional criteria enhances specificity: fever (>38.3°C), mucopurulent vaginal or cervical discharge, leukocytes on saline microscopy, increased ESR or CRP, laboratory documentation of chlamydial or gonorrhea infection.

d. Treatment: Empirical treatment is indicated for all sexually active females if minimum diagnostic criteria are met and no other cause for symptoms is identified. See Table 17-11 and the Centers for Disease Control and Prevention (CDC) STD Treatment Guidelines for most up-to-date information (http://www.cdc.gov/std/treatment/2010/pid.htm).

e. Admission criteria: Cannot exclude acute surgical abdomen, presence of tubo-ovarian abscess, pregnancy, immunodeficiency, severe illness (nausea, vomiting, anorexia), inability to tolerate or follow outpatient oral regimen, failure to respond to appropriate outpatient therapy, follow-up cannot be ensured.

E. Human Immunodeficiency Virus and Acquired Immunodeficiency Syndrome

Recommendations provided are current at the time of publication. Please see the CDC guidelines on the diagnosis and management of children with HIV infection at www.aidsinfo.nih.gov/ for the most up-to-date recommendations.

1. **Counseling and testing:** Legal requirements for consent vary by state. Counseling includes informed consent for testing, implications of positive test results, and prevention of transmission:

a. Prenatal testing:
   (1) CDC guidelines state that HIV screening should be included in the routine panel of prenatal tests for all pregnant women, on an opt-out basis, after notifying the patient that testing will be conducted.[14]
   (2) CDC also recommends that repeat HIV antibody testing occur in the third trimester, preferably before 36 weeks of gestation.[14]

b. Perinatal and newborn testing:
   (1) For women in labor with undocumented HIV infection status during pregnancy or for infants born to mothers with unknown HIV status, a rapid HIV test should be performed on the mother on an opt-out basis.
   (2) If an HIV rapid antibody test is positive, confirmatory testing (e.g., Western blot) should be pursued. If confirmatory testing is positive, virologic testing (HIV DNA polymerase chain reaction (PCR) or HIV RNA assay) should be completed.

c. Adolescent testing: CDC recommends HIV screening with opt-out consent as part of routine clinical care in all healthcare settings for patients, beginning at age 13 years. Repeat HIV-1 antibody testing should be performed on a regular basis for adolescents who remain at risk of HIV-1 infection. When there is suspicion for recent exposure, virologic testing should be pursued.

2. **Management of perinatal HIV exposure[14,15]:** Recommendations provided are current at the time of publication; check the recent recommendations for most current therapy at www.aidsinfo.nih.gov/:

a. Prevention of mother-to-child transmission[16]: Three interventions are recommended to reduce transmission, including use of antiretroviral therapy during pregnancy, during delivery, and in the newborn; elective cesarean section for women with viral load >1000 copies/mL; and use of breast-feeding alternatives where they are found to be affordable, feasible, acceptable, sustainable, and safe. Healthcare professionals who are treating HIV-infected pregnant women and their newborn infants should report all instances of prenatal exposure to antiretroviral drugs (ARVs) to the Antiretroviral Pregnancy Registry (1-800-258-4263 or www.apregistry.com):
   (1) Pregnancy: Current guidelines recommend use of three-drug regimens during pregnancy and labor for all pregnant women with HIV infection. Zidovudine (ZDV) should be included in the pregnant woman's regimen (initiated at 14–34 weeks' gestation), because it has been shown to significantly reduce vertical transmission of HIV in combination with postnatal ZDV to the infant (Table 17-12). Elective cesarean section is recommended if possible at 38 weeks for all HIV-infected pregnant women with viral load >1000 copies/mL at time of delivery or who have unknown viral load. In the United

TABLE 17-12
DIAGNOSIS AND MANAGEMENT FOR INFANTS WITH IN UTERO HIV EXPOSURE

Age	Laboratory Tests to Obtain*	Management	Comments
Newborn	(1) HIV DNA PCR if maternal status unknown and preliminary testing positive. Umbilical cord blood should not be used, owing to possible contamination with maternal blood. (2) Baseline CBC with differential.	(1) Start ZDV 4 mg/kg/dose PO BID, or 3 mg/kg IV Q12 hr within 12 hours of delivery. (2) Nevirapine if no maternal ARV: three doses at 12 mg/dose; first dose within 48 hours of birth, second dose 48 hours after first dose, third dose 96 hours after second dose.	Lower dose of ZDV for premature (<35 weeks GA) infants. Lower dose of nevirapine for infants <2 kg; concern for bone marrow suppression.
2–3 weeks	(1) HIV DNA PCR (or RNA assay)—consent signed if no prior consent for testing on chart (2) CBC with differential.	Check ZDV dosing and administration. Assess psychosocial needs, consider case management referral.	HIV antibody testing is not routine—only if lacking evidence of maternal HIV status (otherwise, antibody is expected to be positive in HIV-exposed infants).
4–6 weeks	(1) HIV DNA PCR (or RNA assay)—consent signed if no prior consent for testing on chart. (2) CBC with differential (use discretion, based on results of previous CBC).	(1) Discontinue ZDV regardless of PCR result (ZDV monotherapy is used during first 6 weeks for prophylaxis only). (2) Presumptively exclude HIV infection if results of ≥2. weeks PCR and ≥4 weeks PCR both negative. No TMP-SMX needed. (3) If PCR results not yet known, begin TMP-SMX at 75 mg/m²/dose BID for 3 consecutive days of week.	(1) If TMP-SMX is not tolerated, alternatives are aerosolized pentamidine, dapsone, or atovaquone (see Table EC 17-Bon Expert Consult for dosing guidelines). (2) TMP-SMX can be discontinued as soon as results of both ≥2 weeks PCR and ≥4 weeks PCR are negative. (3) **NOTE:** One single HIV-1 DNA PCR test has a sensitivity of 95% and a specificity of 97% for samples collected from infected infants 1 to 36 months of age.
2 months		(1) Check TMP-SMX dosing and administration if still needed. (2) Discontinue TMP-SMX if meets criteria above for negative testing.	Routine well-child check and immunizations.

Continued

17

TABLE 17-12

DIAGNOSIS AND MANAGEMENT FOR INFANTS WITH IN UTERO HIV EXPOSURE (Continued)

Age	Laboratory Tests to Obtain*	Management	Comments
4 months	HIV DNA PCR (or RNA assay).	Definitively exclude HIV infection: two negative PCRs (one ≥1 month, one ≥4 months) as long as no signs/symptoms of HIV infection.	(1) HIV is diagnosed (infected child) if any two separate DNA PCR assay results are positive. (2) If HIV infection is definitively excluded, infant needs only routine comprehensive well-child care, including all routine immunizations.
12, 15, 18 months	HIV antibody optional (to document clearance of maternal antibody—usually by 12 months but may persist to 18 months).		(1) Routine TB risk assessment, especially if HIV-infected household contacts, to determine need for PPD. (2) Routine well-child care and immunizations including MMR and varicella.

*Any abnormal result requires prompt pediatric HIV specialist consultation.
ARV, Antiretroviral drug; CBC, complete blood cell count; GA, gestational age; MMR, measles/mumps/rubella; PCR, polymerase chain reaction; PPD, purified protein derivative; TB, tuberculosis; TMP-SMX, trimethoprim-sulfamethoxazole; ZDV, zidovudine.
Modified from Department of Health and Human Services guidelines for pediatric and perinatal HIV infection (see www.aidsinfo.nih.gov for more detailed information). Accessed January 24, 2013.

States, current recommendations are that HIV-infected women should not breast feed.

(2) Labor: For women with undetermined HIV status who are found to be positive on HIV rapid antibody test, antiretroviral prophylaxis should be administered to both mother and newborn without waiting for results of confirmatory HIV testing. If confirmatory test results are negative, prophylaxis may be discontinued and breast-feeding initiated.

(3) Newborn: Oral administration of ZDV at 4 mg/kg/dose BID, beginning as soon as possible after birth and continuing for the first 6 weeks of life. If the mother received no prenatal ARVs, the infant should also be treated with nevirapine (three doses) in the first week of life (see Table 17-8 or Table 17-12). If infant prophylaxis with antiretrovirals in addition to ZDV is being considered, choice of drugs should be determined in consultation with an expert in pediatric HIV infection. Monitor ZDV toxicity with periodic CBC with differential count. Main toxicities are anemia and neutropenia. Consultation with an expert in pediatric HIV infection is advised if discontinuation of antiretrovirals is considered because of toxicity.

Exclusion of HIV infection is based on two negative antibody tests on different specimens after 6 months of age, or two negative virologic tests, one after 1 month of age and another after 4 months of age.

3. **Diagnosis and management of HIV-exposed infants** (Table 17-12)[17]
4. **Opportunistic infections:**
a. *Pneumocystis jiroveci* pneumonia (PCP) is the most common of the opportunistic infections. Trimethoprim-sulfamethoxazole (TMP-SMX) is recommended for all HIV-exposed infants until HIV infection is reasonably excluded, for all HIV-infected infants until age 12 months and for HIV-infected children and adolescents older than 1 year whose CD4 values fall into the severe immune suppression category (CD4 percentage < 15% or CD4 count < 200 cells/mm³)[17]
b. For more detailed information, see Table EC 17-B on Expert Consult. Drug regimens for prevention and treatment of opportunistic infection in HIV infected children are given.
5. **Management of HIV-infected infants and children**
Treatment guidelines change frequently; it is important to reference the most up-to-date guidelines at http://www.aidsinfo.nih.gov/:
a. Criteria for initiation of antiretroviral therapy (ART)[8]:
   (1) <12 months: All HIV-infected infants <age 12 months, regardless of immunologic, virologic, or clinical status should receive antiretroviral therapy.
   (2) >12 months–3 years: Asymptomatic patients with CD4 cell count <1000 cells/mm³ or CD4 percentage <25% should initiate ART.
   (3) >3 years–5 years: Asymptomatic patients with CD4 cell count <750 cells/mm³ or CD4 percentage <25% should initiate ART.
   (4) 5 years and up: Asymptomatic patients with CD4 cell count <500 cells/mm³ or CD4 percentage <25%.

(5) ART initiation should be considered in asymptomatic patients >12 months of age with plasma HIV RNA levels >100,000 copies/mL and in all patients who develop symptoms.

b. Revised pediatric HIV classification system.

c. Antiretroviral regimen: If an infant is identified as HIV infected while receiving ZDV prophylaxis, therapy should be changed to a three-drug regimen. For drug choices, refer to http://www.aidsinfo.nih.gov/.

d. Clinical and laboratory monitoring in HIV-infected children: Immune status (CD4 count or percentage), viral load, and evidence of HIV progression (plasma HIV RNA) should be monitored at diagnosis and every 3–4 months. Other testing to perform at diagnosis includes HIV genotype, CBC with differential, serum chemistry with liver and renal function, lipid profile, and urinalysis. Drug toxicity should also be monitored on a regular basis. Careful attention to routine aspects of pediatric care (e.g., growth, development, vaccines) is essential. Screening for hepatitis B and C infection, as well as for tuberculosis, is also recommended for all HIV-infected patients.[17]

e. Immunizations in HIV-infected or HIV-exposed infants and children: Perinatally exposed infants should receive all scheduled infant immunizations. Live vaccines, measles/mumps/rubella (MMR) and varicella vaccine should be given to asymptomatic HIV-infected children and adolescents (see Chapter 16). HIV-infected children should receive pneumococcal conjugated vaccine 23 (PCV23) at age 2 and 5 years. Influenza vaccine should be given annually in the fall to all infected children ≥age 6 months and to children ≥age 6 months who have HIV-infected household contacts.

F. Tuberculosis (TB)

1. Types of testing[8]:

a. **IGRA** (immunologic-based testing with interferon gamma release assay): Measures interferon-gamma (IFN-γ) production from T lymphocytes in response to stimulation with antigens that are fairly specific to *Mycobacterium tuberculosis* complex. Similar sensitivity to tuberculin skin test (TST) but higher specificity (because antigens used are not found in bacillus Calmette-Guérin (BCG) or most pathogenic nontuberculous mycobacteria):

(1) Testing of immune-competent children 5 years of age or older in place of a TST

(2) May be useful to determine whether a BCG-immunized child with a reactive TST more likely has latent TB infection or has a false-positive TST reaction caused by the BCG

b. **TST:**

(1) Most common method for diagnosing latent TB infection in asymptomatic persons. BCG immunization is not a contraindication.

(2) Inject 5 tuberculin units (5 TU) of purified protein derivative (0.1 mL) intradermally with a 27-gauge needle on the volar aspect of the forearm to form a 6- to 10-mm wheal. Results of skin testing should be read 48–72 hours later.

(3) Definition of positive Mantoux test (regardless of whether BCG has been previously administered): Box 17-1.

BOX 17-1

DEFINITIONS OF POSITIVE TUBERCULIN SKIN TESTING[9]

INDURATION ≥ 5 MM

Children in close contact with known or suspected contagious cases of tuberculosis
Children suspected to have tuberculosis based on clinical or radiographic findings
Children on immunosuppressive therapy or with immunosuppressive conditions
(including HIV infection)

INDURATION ≥ 10 MM

Children at increased risk for dissemination based on young age (<4 yr) or with other
medical conditions (cancer, diabetes mellitus, chronic renal failure, or malnutrition)
Children with increased exposure: those born in or whose parents were born
in endemic countries; those with travel to endemic countries; those exposed to
HIV-infected adults, homeless persons, illicit drug users, nursing home residents,
incarcerated or institutionalized persons, migrant farm workers

INDURATION ≥ 15 MM

Children ≥4 yr without any risk factors

---

   c. The incubation period from TB infection to a positive TST or IGRA is
approximately 2–10 weeks.

2. **Who to test:**

a. Contacts of people with confirmed or suspected infectious TB (contact
investigation)

b. Children with clinical or radiographic findings of TB

c. Children immigrating from or with history of travel to TB-endemic areas,
including international adoptees; children with close contacts from TB-
endemic areas (if the child is well, TST should be delayed for up to 10
weeks after return)

d. Children who will be starting T-cell suppressive immunomodulatory
therapy

e. Annual testing for HIV-Infected children starting at age 3–12 months
(TST only; IGRA not recommended)

f. Incarcerated adolescents

3. **Drug therapy:**

a. Treatment of latent TB infection:

   (1) Indications:

      (a) Children with positive tuberculin tests but no evidence of clinical
disease

      (b) Recent contacts, especially HIV-infected children, of people
with infectious TB, even if tuberculin test and clinical evidence
are not indicative of disease

   (2) Recommendations (see Formulary for specific doses and
Table EC 17-C):

      (a) Isoniazid-susceptible: 9 months isoniazid daily (if daily therapy
not possible, alternative is DOT [directly observed therapy] twice
weekly for 9 months)

(b) Isoniazid-resistant: 6 months of rifampin daily (alternative is DOT twice weekly for 6 months)

(c) If resistant to isoniazid and rifampin, consult infectious disease specialist

b. Treatment for active TB infection[8]: consultation with infectious disease specialist recommended. See Table EC 17-C. (For details, see 2012 American Academy of Pediatrics *Red Book*.)

G. Selected Tickborne Illnesses[9]

For all of the following illnesses, infection typically occurs between spring and fall seasons.

1. Lyme disease:

a. Geographic distribution: New England and Middle Atlantic, Upper Midwest, and Pacific Northwest.

b. Presentation:

(1) *Early localized disease:* 3–32 days after tick bite. Erythema migrans (annular rash at site of bite, target lesion with clear or necrotic center), fever, headache, myalgia, malaise

(2) *Early disseminated disease:* 3–10 weeks after the tick bite. Secondary erythema migrans with multiple smaller target lesions, cranioneuropathy (especially facial nerve palsy), systemic symptoms as previously listed, and lymphadenopathy; 1% may develop carditis with heart block or aseptic meningitis

(3) *Late disease:* Intermittent recurrent symptoms occur 2–12 months from initial tick bite. Pauciarticular arthritis affecting large joints (7% of those untreated), peripheral neuropathy, encephalopathy

c. Transmission: Spirochete *Borrelia burgdorferi.* Inoculation occurs by the bite of a deer tick, *Ixodes scapularis* or *Ixodes pacificus;* disseminates systemically through blood and lymphatics. Transmission of *B. burgdorferi* requires 24–48 hours of tick attachment.

d. Diagnosis:

(1) Early disease, clinical diagnosis: During first 4 weeks of infection, diagnostic tests are insensitive and generally not recommended.

(2) Early disseminated and late disease: Combination of clinical findings and serologic tests. A stepwise approach should be taken:

(a) First, perform a quantitative test for serum antibodies using EIA (enzyme immunoassay) or IFA (immunofluorescent assay). IgM will become detectable at 3–4 weeks and peak at 6–8 weeks. IgG is only used to confirm late diagnosis. Of note, false-positive results of these assays occur as result of cross-reactivity with viral infections, other spirochetal infections, and autoimmune diseases.

(b) If immunoassay is positive, Western blot should be used to confirm diagnosis. (If immunoassay is negative, no further testing indicated.)

(c) Lumbar puncture as clinically indicated. Lyme-disease–specific antibodies can be isolated from the cerebrospinal fluid (CSF) in patients with CNS inovlvement.

e. Treatment: Antibiotic prophylaxis not routinely recommended for ticks attached <24–48 hours.
   (1) Early localized disease: Doxycycline 4 mg/kg (max 100 mg/dose) PO BID for 14–21 days is treatment of choice for patients ≥ 8 years. Amoxicillin or cefuroxime for 14–21 days recommended for younger children.
   (2) Early disseminated and late-onset disease manifestations are treated by the same oral regimen as early disease, with the following durations: Multiple erythema migrans (21 days), isolated facial palsy (14–21 days), and arthritis (28 days). Persistent or recurrent arthritis (>2 months), carditis, meningitis, or encephalitis may be treated with ceftriaxone or parenteral penicillin (14–28 days).

2. **Rocky Mountain spotted fever**[8]:
a. Geographic distribution: Widespread. Most common in south Atlantic, southeastern, and south central United States.
b. Presentation: Incubation period is ≈1 week (range 2–14 days):
   (1) Symptoms: Fever, headache, myalgia, nausea, anorexia, abdominal pain, diarrhea. Severe disease may manifest in CNS, cardiac, pulmonary, gastrointestinal tract, renal involvement, disseminated intravascular involvement, and shock leading to death.
   (2) Rash: Usually appears by day 6; initially erythematous and macular; progresses to maculopapular and petechial due to vasculitis. Rash usually appears on wrists and ankles and spreads proximally. Palms and soles are often involved.
   (3) Laboratory manifestations: Thrombocytopenia, hyponatremia, and anemia. White blood cell count usually normal.
c. Transmission: *Rickettsia rickettsii,* an obligate intracellular pathogen transmitted to humans by a tick bite.
d. Diagnosis: By rickettsial group-specific serologic tests, which may be negative early in the illness. A fourfold or greater change between acute- and convalescent-phase serum specimens is diagnostic. Probable diagnosis can be established by a single serum titer of 1:64 or greater by IFA assay. Culture of *R. rickettsii* is generally not attempted because of danger of transmission to laboratory personnel. *R. rickettsii* can be obtained by immunohistochemical staining of tissue specimens obtained before initiation of antimicrobial therapy. This method is highly specific but not sensitive.
e. Treatment: Doxycycline is recommended drug for children of any age and should be started as soon as the diagnosis is suspected. Duration: 7–10 days and is continued until patient is afebrile for ≥3 days and has demonstrated clinical improvement.
f. For discussion of other rickettsial spotted fever infections that are clinically similar but epidemiologically distinct, see 2012 *Red Book* (Section 3).

3. **Ehrlichiosis**[8]:
a. Geographic distribution: Southeastern, south central, and midwestern United States.

b. Presentation: Systemic febrile illness with headache, chills, rigors, malaise, myalgia, arthralgia, nausea, vomiting, anorexia, or acute weight loss. Rash is variable in location and appearance:

  (1) Laboratory manifestations: Leukopenia, anemia, and transaminitis are common. CSF studies with lymphocytic pleocytosis or elevated protein are also common.

  (2) More severe disease: Pulmonary infiltrates, bone marrow hypoplasia, respiratory failure, encephalopathy, meningitis, disseminated intravascular coagulation (DIC), spontaneous hemorrhage, and renal failure.

c. Transmission: *Ehrlichia chaffeensis* (human monocytic ehrlichiosis [HME]) and *Ehrlichia ewingii* associated with the bite of a Lone Star tick *(Amblyomma americanum),* although other tick species may be vectors. Mammalian reservoirs include white-tailed deer and white-footed mice.

d. Diagnosis: Confirmed by isolation of *Ehrlichia* organisms from blood or CSF, a fourfold or greater change in IgG-specific antibody titer by IFA assay between acute and convalescent serum specimens, PCR assay amplification of ehrlichial DNA from a clinical specimen, or detection of an intraleukocytoplasmic cluster of bacteria in conjunction with a single IFA titer ≥64. PCR from acute-phase peripheral blood of patients with ehrlichiosis seems sensitive, specific, and promising for early diagnosis.

e. Treatment: Doxycycline 4 mg/kg/day BID IV or PO (max 100 mg/dose). Ehrlichiosis may be severe or fatal in untreated patients; initiate treatment early. Failure to respond within first 3 days should suggest infection with an agent other than *Ehrlichia.* Treatment should be continued for at least 3 days after defervescence, for a minimum total course of 7 days.

4. **Anaplasmosis:** Though clinically very similar, ehrlichiosis and anaplasmosis are now described separately. The previous information on clinical presentation and treatment is the same for anaplasmosis. Differences from ehrlichiosis are as follows: caused by *Anaplasma phagocytophilum* (human granulocytotrophic anaplasmosis [HGA]), transmitted by the deer tick *(Ixodes scapularis)* or western black-legged tick *(Ixodes pacificus),* diagnosis via *Anaplasma* organisms using techniques as described previously. Most cases are reported from the north central and northeastern United States, and from northern California.

H. Fungal and Yeast Infections

1. Diagnosis:

a. Place specimen (nail or skin scrapings, biopsy specimens, fluids from tissues or lesions) in 10% potassium hydroxide (KOH) on glass slide to look for hyphae, pseudohyphae.

b. Germ tube screen of yeast (3 hours) for *Candida albicans:* All germ tube–positive yeast are *C. albicans,* but not all *C. albicans* are germ tube positive.

2. **Common community-acquired fungal infections, etiology, and treatment** (Table 17-13)

TABLE 17-13

COMMON COMMUNITY-ACQUIRED FUNGAL INFECTIONS

Disease	Usual Etiology	Suggested Therapy	Suggested Length of Therapy
Tinea capitis (ringworm of scalp)	*Trichophyton tonsurans, Microsporum canis*	Oral griseofulvin (ultramicro) give with fatty foods. Fungal shedding decreased with 1%–2.5% selenium sulfide shampoo *Alt:* terbinafine, itraconazole (total 2–4 weeks), or fluconazole (once weekly)	4–8 wk or 2 wk after clinical resolution
Tinea corporis/pedis/ cruris (ringworm of body/feet/genital region)	*Epidermophyton floccosum, Trichophyton rubrum, Trichophyton mentagrophytes, Microsporum canis*	Topical antifungal (miconazole, clotrimazole) once daily or BID; terbinafine BID	1–4 wks for either therapy
Oral candidiasis (thrush) in immuno-competent patients	*Candida albicans, Candida tropicalis*	Nystatin suspension or clotrimazole troche (only nystatin for infants)	7–10 days, then continue 3 days after clinical resolution
Candidal skin infections (intertriginous)	*C. albicans*	Topical nystatin, miconazole, clotrimazole	3 days after clinical resolution
Tinea unguium (ringworm of nails)	*T. mentagrophytes, T. rubrum, E. floccosum*	Oral griseofulvin *Alt:* oral terbinafine, itraconazole, fluconazole	6–12 mo 4–6 mo for alternatives (once weekly for fluconazole)

Modified from McMillan JA, Lee CKK, Siberry G, Dick J. *The Harriet Lane Handbook of Pediatric Antimicrobial Therapy.* Philadelphia: Mosby, 2009. See Table 1-5 for further details regarding treatment of fungal infections.

I. Exposures to Bloodborne Pathogens and Postexposure Prophylaxis (PEP)

1. **HIV[8,18,19]:** Updated guidelines may be found at aidsinfo.nih.gov:
a. Occupational exposure, risk for occupational transmission of HIV:
   (1) Needlesticks: Three infections for every 1000 exposures (0.3%). Risk is greater when exposure involves a larger volume of blood and/or higher titer of HIV, as in a deep injury, visible blood on the device causing the injury, a device previously used in the source patient's vein or artery, or a source patient in the late stages of HIV infection.
   (2) Mucous membrane exposure: One infection for every 1000 exposures (0.1%). Risk may be higher with larger volume of blood and a higher titer of HIV, prolonged skin contact, extensive surface area of exposure, or skin integrity that is visibly compromised.
b. Nonoccupational HIV exposure in children and adolescents[19]:
   (1) Injury from needles of discarded syringes: No confirmed reports of HIV acquisition from percutaneous injury by a needle found in the

community. If needle or syringe is found to have visible blood and source is known to be HIV infected, PEP should be considered. Testing the syringe for HIV is not practical or reliable.

(2) Repeated sexual encounters or a single episode of sexual abuse: Risk is highest with unprotected receptive anal intercourse (5 per 1,000 exposures), intermediate with receptive vaginal intercourse (1 per 1,000 exposures), and even lower with insertive vaginal intercourse. If exposure source has genital ulcer disease or another sexually transmitted infection, or if there was tissue damage, risk for HIV transmission is higher, increasing the benefit of PEP relative to burden and risk for drug toxicity.

(3) Human milk[14]: PEP is not warranted for a single exposure to human breast milk.

(4) Human bites: Transmission is extremely rare even when saliva is contaminated with blood. Saliva inhibits HIV infectivity; HIV is rarely isolated from saliva, and concentrations of HIV in saliva of HIV-infected persons is low even in the presence of periodontal disease.

c. Prophylaxis:

(1) Optimally, PEP should be initiated as soon as possible, preferably within 1–3 hours of exposure but no later than 72 hours. The usual duration of PEP, if tolerated, is 28 days. The benefits of PEP are greatest when risk of infection is high, intervention is prompt, and adherence is likely.

(2) A clinician with experience in treating individuals with HIV infection should be consulted whenever possible (without causing PEP initiation delay) before initiating therapy. Decision about need for PEP is based on HIV status of source, type and severity of potential exposure, and individual risk tolerance. PEP generally comprises two-drug or three-drug regimens, frequently available in fixed-dose combination pills for older children and adults. No clear evidence of superior efficacy of a three-drug regimen over a two-drug regimen in preventing HIV infection after exposure, but many experts prefer to use three drugs; this practice must be balanced against the increased toxicity potential when additional drugs are used. Typical regimens include two nucleoside reverse-transcriptase inhibitors (NRTIs) (e.g., ZDV + lamivudine or, in adolescent/adults, tenofovir + emtricitabine), two NRTIs plus a protease inhibitor (PI) (e.g., lopinavir/ritonavir) or two NRTIs plus a non-nucleoside reverse-transcriptase inhibitor (NNRTI) (e.g., efavirenz). Full descriptions of potential regimens can be found in CDC and American Academy of Pediatrics (AAP) guidelines.

(3) Use of ZDV alone as PEP is no longer recommended. For most recent recommendations, refer to CDC and AAP guidelines. The CDC's PEP hotline (open 24 hours daily) is 888-448-4911.

2. **Hepatitis B:** Most readily transmitted of the bloodborne pathogens. Recommendations for hepatitis B prophylaxis in nonimmune person after percutaneous exposure to blood that contains (or might contain)

hepatitis B surface antigen (HBsAg) include hepatitis B immune globulin and initiation of hepatitis B vaccine series. For details, see Chapter 16.

3. **Hepatitis C:** No preventive therapy available. Serologic testing and follow-up are important to document if infection occurs. Infections become chronic in the majority of patients.

J. Infectious Diseases in Internationally Adopted Children

For more information, see American Academy of Pediatrics. Medical evaluation of internationally adopted children for infectious diseases. In: Pickering LK, Baker CJ, Kimberlin DW, et al, eds. *Red Book: 2012 Report of the Committee on Infectious Diseases.* 29th ed. Elk Grove Village, Ill: AAP, 2012.[8]

REFERENCES

1. Kaditis A, O'Marcaigh A, Rhodes K, et al. Yield of positive blood cultures in pediatric oncology patients by a new method of blood culture collection. *Pediatr Infect Dis J.* 1996;15:615-620.
2. Cosgrove SE, Avdic E, et al. The Johns Hopkins Hospital Antimicrobial Stewardship Program Antibiotic Guidelines. 2012; 1-160.
3. McMillan JA, Siberry GK, et al. The Harriet Lane Handbook of Pediatric Antimicrobial Therapy. Philadelphia: Mosby Elsevier, 2009.
4. Shapiro ED. Fever without localizing signs. In: Long SS, Pickering LK, Prober CG, eds. *Principles and Practice of Pediatric Infectious Disease.* 3rd ed: PA, Philadelphia, Churchill Livingstone, 2008.
5. Barraff L. Management of infants and young children with fever without a source. *Pediatr Ann.* 2008;27:673-679.
6. Kliegman RE, Stanton B, St Geme J, et al. *Nelson Textbook of Pediatrics.* 19th ed. Philadelphia: Elsevier, 2010.
7. Del Pizzo J. Focus on diagnosis: congenital infections (TORCH). *Pediatr Rev.* 2011;32:537-542.
8. American Academy of Pediatrics, In: Pickering LK, Baker CJ, Kimberlin DW, et al, eds. *Red Book: 2012 Report of the Committee on Infectious Diseases.* 29th ed. Elk Grove Village, Ill: AAP, 2012.
9. Verani JR, McGee L, Schrag SJ; Division of Bacterial Diseases, National Center for Immunization and Respiratory Diseases, Centers for Disease Control and Prevention (CDC). Prevention of perinatal group B streptococcal disease—revised guidelines from CDC, 2010. *MMWR Recomm Rep.* 2010;59(RR-10):1-36.
10. Centers for Disease Control and Prevention. A new product (VariZIG) for postexposure prophylaxis of varicella available under an investigational new drug application expanded access protocol. *MMWR Morb Mortal Wkly Rep.* 2006;55:209-210.
11. Wong VC, Reesink HW, Lelie PN, et al. Prevention of the HBsAg carrier state in newborn infants of mothers who are chronic carriers of HBsAG and HBeAg by administration of hepatitis-B vaccine and hepatitis-B immunoglobulin: double-blind randomized placebo-controlled study. *Lancet.* 1984;1:921-926.
12. Wong CS, Jelacic S, Habeeb RL, et al. The risk of hemolytic-uremic syndrome after antibiotic treatment of *Escherichia coli* O157:H7 infections. *N Engl J Med.* 2000;342:1930-1936.
13. Lieberthal AS, et al. The diagnosis and management of acute otitis media. *Pediatrics.* 2013;131:e964-e999.

14. AAP Committee on Pediatric AIDS. HIV testing and prophylaxis to prevent mother-to-child transmission in the United States. *Pediatrics*. 2008;122:1127-1134.

15. Perinatal HIV Guidelines Working Group. *Public Health Service Task Force Recommendations for Use of Antiretroviral Drugs in Pregnant HIV-1-Infected Women for Maternal Health and Interventions to Reduce Perinatal HIV-1 Transmission in the United States*. Rockville, Md: National Institutes of Health, 2009.

16. Panel on Treatment of HIV-Infected Pregnant Women and Prevention of Perinatal Transmission. Recommendations for Use of Antiretroviral Drugs in Pregnant HIV-1-Infected Women for Maternal Health and Interventions to Reduce Perinatal HIV Transmission in the United States. Available at http://aidsinfo.nih.gov/contentfiles/lvguidelines/PerinatalGL.pdf. Accessed January 24, 2013.

17. Simpkins EP, Siberry GK, Hutton N. Thinking about HIV infection. *Pediatr Rev*. 2009;30:337-349.

18. Centers for Disease Control and Prevention. Updated U.S. Public Health Service guidelines for the management of occupational exposures to HIV and recommendations for postexposure prophylaxis. *MMWR Recomm Rep*. 2005;54(RR-09): 1-17.

19. Havens P, American Academy of Pediatrics Committee on Pediatric AIDS. Postexposure prophylaxis in children and adolescents for nonoccupational exposure to human immunodeficiency virus. *Pediatrics*. 2003;11:1475-1489.

20. Wald ER, et al. Clinical practice guideline for the diagnosis and management of acute bacterial sinusitis in children aged 1 to 18 years. *Pediatrics*. 2013. Jul; 132(1): e262-e280.

Chapter 18

Neonatology

Lauren Beard, MD

See additional content on Expert Consult

I. WEBSITES

www.nicuniversity.org

Outcomes calculator: http://www.nichd.nih.gov/about/org/der/branches/ppb/programs/epbo/pages/epbo_case.aspx

Neonatal dermatology: http://www.adhb.govt.nz/newborn/TeachingResources/Dermatology/Dermatology.htm

III. NEWBORN RESUSCITATION

A. Neonatal Advanced Life Support (NALS) Algorithm for Neonatal Resuscitation (Fig. 18-1)

For infants with meconium in the amniotic fluid, routine intrapartum oropharyngeal and nasopharyngeal **suctioning is not recommended**. If the infant is not vigorous, endotracheal intubation should be performed immediately after birth, and suction should be applied to the endotracheal tube as it is withdrawn.[1]

B. Endotracheal Tube Size and Depth of Insertion (see Table 18-1)

C. Ventilatory Support (See Chapter 4)

D. Vascular Access (See Chapter 3 for Umbilical Venous Catheter and Umbilical Artery Catheter Placement)

NOTE: During initial resuscitation, umbilical venous catheter (UVC) should be inserted just far enough to obtain blood return; no measurement or verified placement necessary initially.

IV. NEWBORN ASSESSMENT

A. Vital Signs and Birth Weight

1. **Normal vital signs:** HR 120–160 bpm, respiratory rate (RR) 40–60 breaths/min, rectal temperature 36.5°–37.5°C
2. **Arterial blood pressure:** Related to birth weight, gestational age (see Chapter 7).
3. **See Chapter 21 for growth charts for the premature infant.**
4. **Weight:** Extremely low birth weight (ELBW) < 1000 g, very low birth weight (VLBW) < 1500 g, low birth weight (LBW) < 2500 g, small for gestational age (SGA) < 10% for gestational age, large for gestational age (LGA) > 90% for gestational age

B. Apgar Scores (Table 18-2)

Assess at 1 and 5 minutes. Repeat at 5-minute intervals if 5-minute score is <7.[2]

TABLE 18-1

PREDICTED ENDOTRACHEAL TUBE SIZE AND DEPTH BY BIRTH WEIGHT AND GESTATIONAL AGE

Gestational Age (wk)	Weight (g)	ETT Size (mm)	ETT Depth of Insertion (cm from Upper Lip)
23–24	500–600	2.5	5.5
25–26	700–800	2.5	6
27–29	900–1000	2.5	6.5
30–32	1100–1400	2.5–3.0	7
33–34	1500–1800	3.0	7.5
35–37	1900–2400	3.0–3.5	8
38–40	2500–3100	3.5	8.5

NOTE: Based on Tochen's 1979 study, the "7-8-9-10" rule recommended that 1-, 2-, 3-, or 4-kg babies were to be intubated at a "tip to lip" distance of 7, 8, 9, or 10 cm, respectively. However, recent literature suggests these guidelines may better represent appropriate endotracheal tube (ETT) depth of insertion.

Data from Peterson J, Johnson N, Deakins K, et al. Accuracy of the 7-8-9 rule for endotracheal tube placement in the neonate. *J Perinatol.* 2006;26:333–336.

C. New Ballard Gestational Age Estimation

The Ballard score is most accurate when performed between age 12 and 20 hours.[3] Approximate gestational age is calculated based on the sum of the neuromuscular and physical maturity ratings (Fig. 18-2).

1. **Neuromuscular maturity:**
a. Posture: Observe infant quiet and supine. Score 0 for arms, legs extended; 1 for starting to flex hips and knees, arms extended; 2 for stronger flexion of legs, arms extended; 3 for arms slightly flexed, legs flexed and abducted; and 4 for full flexion of arms and legs.
b. Square window: Flex hand on forearm enough to obtain fullest possible flexion without wrist rotation. Measure angle between hypothenar eminence and ventral aspect of forearm.
c. Arm recoil: With infant supine, flex forearms for 5 seconds, fully extend by pulling on hands, then release. Measure the angle of elbow flexion to which arms recoil.
d. Popliteal angle: Hold infant supine with pelvis flat, thigh held in knee-chest position. Extend leg by gentle pressure and measure popliteal angle.
e. Scarf sign: With baby supine, pull infant's hand across the neck toward opposite shoulder. Determine how far elbow will reach across. Score 0 if elbow reaches opposite axillary line, 1 if past midaxillary line, 2 if past midline, and 3 if elbow unable to reach midline.
f. Heel-to-ear maneuver: With baby supine, draw foot as near to head as possible without forcing it. Observe distance between foot and head and degree of extension at knee.
2. **Physical maturity:** Based on developmental stage of eyes, ears, breasts, genitalia, skin, lanugo, and plantar creases (see Fig. 18-2)

D. Birth Trauma

1. **Extradural fluid collections** (Table 18-3, Fig. 18-3):

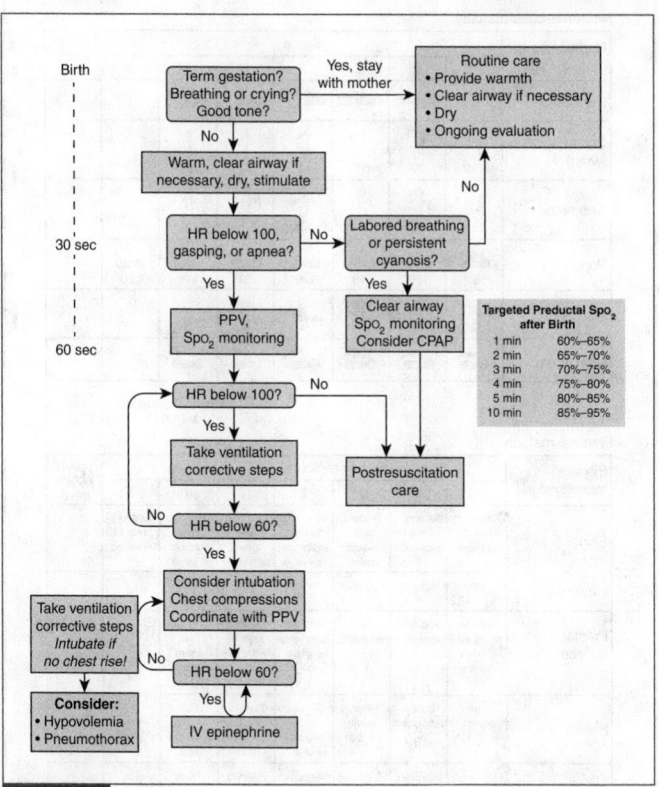

FIGURE 18-1

Overview of resuscitation in the delivery room. CPAP, Continuous positive airway pressure; HR, heart rate; IV, intravenous; PPV, positive pressure ventilations; Spo_2, oxygen saturation by pulse oximetry. *(From Kattwinkel J, Perlman JM, Aziz K, et al. 2010 American Heart Association guidelines for cardiopulmonary resuscitation and emergency cardiovascular care. Part 15: Neonatal resuscitation. Circulation. 2010;122:S909–S919.)*

Text within figure:

Birth

Term gestation? Breathing or crying? Good tone? — Yes, stay with mother → Routine care
- Provide warmth
- Clear airway if necessary
- Dry
- Ongoing evaluation

No ↓

Warm, clear airway if necessary, dry, stimulate

30 sec

HR below 100, gasping, or apnea? — No → Labored breathing or persistent cyanosis? — No → (Routine care)

Yes ↓   Yes ↓

PPV, Spo_2 monitoring   Clear airway Spo_2 monitoring Consider CPAP

60 sec

Targeted Preductal Spo_2 after Birth

1 min	60%–65%
2 min	65%–70%
3 min	70%–75%
4 min	75%–80%
5 min	80%–85%
10 min	85%–95%

HR below 100? — No → Postresuscitation care

Yes ↓

Take ventilation corrective steps

HR below 60? — No

Yes ↓

Consider intubation Chest compressions Coordinate with PPV

Take ventilation corrective steps *Intubate if no chest rise!* — No ← HR below 60?

Consider:
- Hypovolemia
- Pneumothorax

Yes ↓

IV epinephrine

TABLE 18-2
APGAR SCORES

Score	0	1	2
Heart rate	Absent	<100 bpm	>100 bpm
Respiratory effort	Absent, irregular	Slow, crying	Good
Muscle tone	Limp	Some flexion of extremities	Active motion
Reflex irritability (nose suction)	No response	Grimace	Cough or sneeze
Color	Blue, pale	Acrocyanosis	Completely pink

Data from Apgar V. Proposal for a new method of evaluation of the newborn infant. *Anesth Analg.* 1953;32:260.

18

Neuromuscular maturity

Neuromuscular maturity sign	Score							Record score here
	−1	0	1	2	3	4	5	
Posture								
Square window (wrist)	> 90°	90°	60°	45°	30°	0°		
Arm recoil		180°	140–180°	110–140°	90–110°	< 90°		
Popliteal angle	180°	160°	140°	120°	100°	90°	< 90°	
Scarf sign								
Heel to ear								

TOTAL NEUROMUSCULAR MATURITY SCORE

Physical maturity

Physical maturity sign	Score							Record score here
	−1	0	1	2	3	4	5	
Skin	Sticky, friable, transparent	Gelatinous, red, translucent	Smooth, pink, visible veins	Superficial peeling and/or rash, few veins	Cracking, pale areas, rare veins	Parchment, deep cracking, no vessels	Leathery, cracked, wrinkled	
Lanugo	None	Sparse	Abundant	Thinning	Bald areas	Mostly bald		
Plantar surface	Heel-toe: 40–50 mm: −1 <40 mm: −2	>50 mm, no crease	Faint red marks	Anterior transverse crease only	Creases anterior two thirds	Creases over entire sole		
Breast	Imperceptible	Barely perceptible	Flat areola, no bud	Stippled areola, 1–2 mm bud	Raised areola, 3–4 mm bud	Full areola, 5–10 mm bud		
Eye/ear	Lids fused: loosely: −1 tightly: −2	Lids open, pinna flat, stays folded	Sl. curved pinna, soft, slow recoil	Well-curved pinna, soft but ready recoil	Formed and firm, instant recoil	Thick cartilage, ear stiff		
Genitals (male)	Scrotum flat, smooth	Scrotum empty, faint rugae	Testes in upper canal, rare rugae	Testes descending, few rugae	Testes down, good rugae	Testes pendulous, deep rugae		
Genitals (female)	Clitoris prominent and labia flat	Prominent clitoris and small labia minora	Prominent clitoris and enlarging minora	Majora and minora equally prominent	Majora large, minora small	Majora cover clitoris and minora		

TOTAL PHYSICAL MATURITY SCORE

Score	Maturity rating														Gestational age (weeks)
Neuromuscular_____ Physical_____ Total_____	Score	−10	−5	0	5	10	15	20	25	30	35	40	45	50	By dates_____ By ultrasound_____ By exam_____
	Weeks	20	22	24	26	28	30	32	34	36	38	40	42	44	

FIGURE 18-2

Neuromuscular and physical maturity (New Ballard Score). *(Modified from Ballard JL et al. New Ballard Score, expanded to include extremely premature infants.* J Pediatr. *1991;119:417–423.)*

2. **Fractured clavicle:** Possible crepitus/deformity on day 1 ± swelling/ discomfort on day 2
3. **Brachialplexus injuries:** Erb palsy (C5-6) most common, but also possible to have Klumpke (C8-T1; least common) and total brachial plexus palsy (C5-T1). See Section XII.

E. Neonatal Hypoxic-Ischemic Encephalopathy (HIE): Initial Management[4]

1. **Hypothermia protocol:** Infants with evidence of HIE shortly after birth who are > 36 weeks' gestation should be considered for hypothermia. Protocol should be initiated within 6 hours of delivery.
2. **Criteria for hypothermia vary by center but typically include one or more of the following:**
a. Cord gas or blood gas in the first hour of life with a pH <7.0 or base deficit of >16. For infants with a pH of 7.01–7.15 or base deficit of 10–15.9, additional criteria should be met (e.g., significant perinatal event).

TABLE 18-3

BIRTH-RELATED EXTRADURAL FLUID COLLECTIONS

	Caput Succedaneum	Cephalohematoma	Subgaleal Hemorrhage
Location	At point of contact; can extend across sutures	Usually over parietal bones; does not cross sutures	Beneath epicranial aponeurosis; may extend to orbits or nape of neck
Findings	Vaguely demarcated; pitting edema, shifts with gravity	Distinct margins; initially firm, more fluctuant after 48 hr	Firm to fluctuant, ill-defined borders; may have crepitus or fluid waves
Timing	Maximal size/firmness at birth; resolves in 48–72 hrs	Increases after birth for 12–24 hr; resolution over weeks	Progressive after birth; resolution over weeks
Size	Minimal	Rarely severe	May be severe, especially in the setting of associated coagulopathy

Data from DJ Davis. Neonatal subgaleal hemorrhage: diagnosis and management. *CMAJ.* 2001;164:1452.

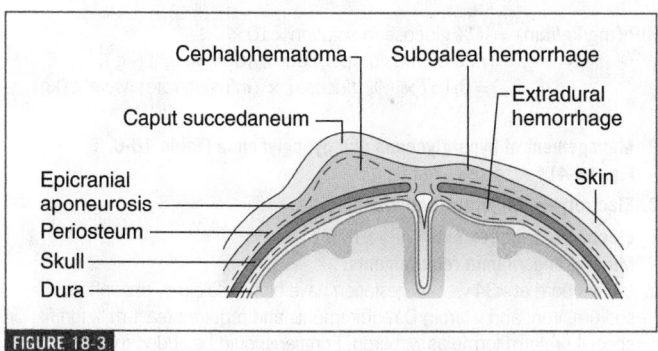

FIGURE 18-3

Types of extradural fluid collections seen in newborn infants.

b. 10-minute APGAR ≤ 5

c. Evidence of moderate to severe encephalopathy

d. Need for assisted ventilation at birth for at least 10 minutes

F. Selected Anomalies, Syndromes, and Malformations (See Chapter 13 for Common Syndromes/Genetic Disorders)

1. **VATER association:** **V**ertebral anomalies, **A**nal anomalies and anal atresia, **T**racheoesophageal fistula, **E**sophageal atresia, and **R**adial and/or **R**enal defects. May also include vascular (cardiac) defects.

2. **CHARGE syndrome** (associated with mutations in gene *CHD7* on chromosome 8q12): **C**oloboma, **H**eart disease, choanal **A**tresia, **R**etarded growth and development (may include central nervous system [CNS] anomalies), **G**enital anomalies (may include hypogonadism), **E**ar abnormalities or deafness.

3. **Infant of a diabetic mother:** Sacral agenesis, femoral hypoplasia, heart defects, and cleft palate. May also include preaxial radial defects, microtia, cleft lip, microphthalmos, holoprosencephaly, microcephaly, anencephaly, spina bifida, hemivertebra, urinary tract defects, and polydactyly.

4. **Fetal alcohol syndrome:** SGA, short palpebral fissures, epicanthal folds, flat nasal bridge, long philtrum, thin upper lip, small hypoplastic nails. May be associated with cardiac defects.

V. FLUIDS, ELECTROLYTES, AND NUTRITION

A. Fluids

1. **Insensible water loss in preterm infants (Table 18-4).**

2. **Water requirements of newborns (Table 18-5).**

B. Glucose

1. **Requirements:** Preterm neonates require about 5–6 mg/kg/min of glucose (40–100 mg/dL).[5] Term neonates require about 3–5 mg/kg/min of glucose. The formula to calculate glucose infusion rate (GIR) is as follows:

$$\text{GIR (mg/kg/min)} = [(\%\,\text{glucose in solution} \times 10 \times \\ (\text{rate of infusion per hour})]/[60 \times \text{weight (kg)}]$$
$$= 0.167 \times (\%\,\text{glucose}) \times (\text{infusion rate})/\text{weight (kg)}$$

2. **Management of hyperglycemia and hypoglycemia (Table 18-6, Fig. 18-4).[6]** Also see Chapter 10.

C. Electrolytes, Minerals, and Vitamins

1. **Electrolyte requirements (**Table 18-7)

2. **Mineral and vitamin requirements:**

a. Infants born at <34 weeks' gestation have higher calcium, phosphorus, sodium, iron, and vitamin D requirements and require breast-milk fortifier or special preterm formulas with iron. Fortifier should be added to breast milk only after the second week of life.

TABLE 18-4

INSENSIBLE WATER LOSS IN PRETERM INFANTS*

Body Weight (g)	Insensible Water Loss (mL/kg/day)
<1000	60–70
1000–1250	60–65
1251–1500	30–45
1501–1750	15–30
1751–2000	15–20

*Estimates of insensible water loss at different body weights during the first few days of life.
Data from Veille JC. Management of preterm premature rupture of membranes. *Clin Perinatol.* 1988;15:851-862.

TABLE 18-5

WATER REQUIREMENTS OF NEWBORNS

Birth Weight (g)	Water Requirements (mL/kg/24 hr) by Age		
	1–2 days	3–7 days	7–30 days
<750	100–250	150–300	120–180
750–1000	80–150	100–150	120–180
1000–1500	60–100	80–150	120–180
>1500	60–80	100–150	120–180

Data from Taeusch HW, Ballard RA, eds. *Schaeffer and Avery's Diseases of the Newborn.* 7th ed. Philadelphia: WB Saunders, 1998.

TABLE 18-6

MANAGEMENT OF HYPERGLYCEMIA AND HYPOGLYCEMIA[6]

	Hypoglycemia	Hyperglycemia
Definition	Serum glucose < 40 mg/dL in term and late preterm infants	Serum glucose > 125 mg/dL in term infants, >150 mg/dL in preterm infants
Differential diagnosis	Insufficient glucose delivery Decreased glycogen stores Increased circulating insulin (infant of a diabetic mother, maternal drugs, Beckwith-Wiedemann syndrome, tumors) Endocrine and metabolic disorders Sepsis or shock Hypothermia, polycythemia, or asphyxia	Excess glucose administration Sepsis Hypoxia Hyperosmolar formula Neonatal diabetes mellitus Medications
Evaluation	Assess for symptoms and calculate glucose delivery to infant. Laboratory evaluation: serum glucose (bedside); complete blood cell count with differential; electrolytes; blood, urine, ± cerebrospinal fluid (CSF) cultures; urinalysis; insulin and C-peptide levels if warranted.	
Management	(See Fig. 18-4.) If glucose < 40 and symptomatic, treat with intravenous glucose (dose = 200 mg/kg, which is equivalent to dextrose 10% at 2 mL/kg). Change dextrose infusion rates gradually. Generally, no more than 2 mg/kg/min in a 2-hr interval. (See Chapter 10 for further guidelines.) Monitor glucose levels every 30–60 min until normal.	Gradually decrease glucose infusion rate if receiving >5 mg/kg/min. Monitor glucosuria. Consider insulin infusion for persistent hyperglycemia.

18

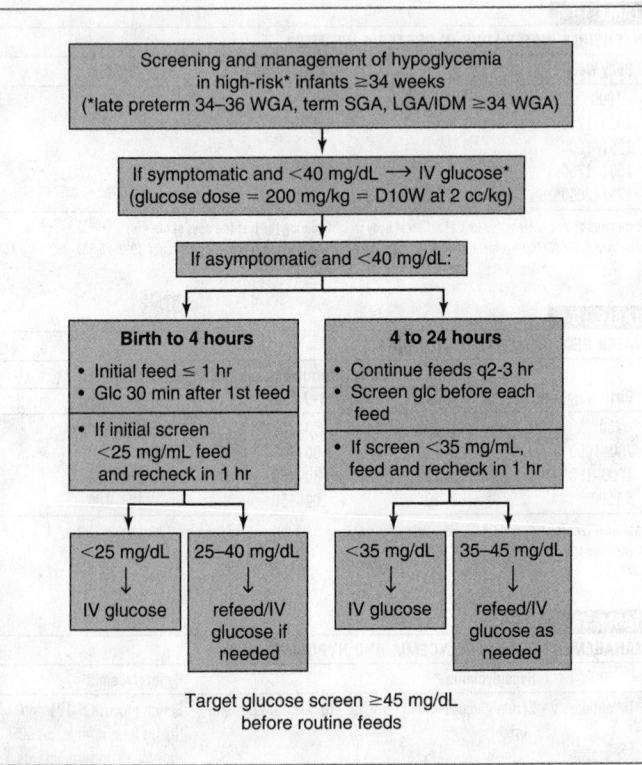

FIGURE 18-4

Screening for and management of postnatal glucose homeostasis in late-preterm (34–36 6/7 weeks) and term small-for-gestational-age and large-for-gestational-age infants of diabetic mothers. D1OW, 10% dextrose in water; glc, glucose; IDM, infant of diabetic mother; IV, intravenous; LGA, large for gestational age; SGA, small for gestational age; WGA, weeks gestational age. (*Modified from Adamkin DH, Committee on Fetus and Newborn. Postnatal glucose homeostasis in late-preterm and term infants.* Pediatrics. *2011;127:575–579*).

TABLE 18-7		
ELECTROLYTE REQUIREMENTS		
	Before 48 Hours of Life	**After 48–72 Hours of Life**
Sodium	None unless serum sodium < 135 mEq/L, without evidence of volume overload	Term infants: 2–3 mEq/kg/day Preterm infants: 3–5 mEq/kg/day
Potassium	None	1–2.5 mEq/kg/day if adequate urine output is established and serum level < 4.5 mEq/L

b. Iron: Enterally fed preterm infants require elemental iron supplementation of 2 mg/kg/day after age 4–8 weeks.

D. Nutrition

1. Growth and caloric requirements:

a. Preterm infants (healthy and thermoneutral environments):

    (1) Caloric requirements: 115–130 kcal/kg/day (up to 150 kcal/kg/day for very low-birth-weight infants)

    (2) Growth (after 10 days of life): 15–20 g/kg/day

b. Term infants:

    (1) Caloric requirements: 100–120 kcal/kg/day

    (2) Growth (after 10 days of life): 10 g/kg/day

2. Total parenteral nutrition (see Chapter 21)

VI. CYANOSIS IN THE NEWBORN

A. Differential Diagnosis

1. **General:** Hypothermia, hypoglycemia, sepsis, shock

2. **Neurologic:** Central apnea, central hypoventilation, intraventricular hemorrhage (IVH), meningitis

3. **Respiratory:** Persistent pulmonary hypertension of the newborn (PPHN), diaphragmatic hernia, pulmonary hypoplasia, choanal atresia, pneumothorax, respiratory distress syndrome (RDS), transient tachypnea of the newborn (TTN), pneumonia, meconium aspiration

4. **Cardiac:** Congestive heart failure, congenital cyanotic heart disease

5. **Hematologic:** Polycythemia, methemoglobinemia

6. **Medications:** Respiratory depression from maternal medications (e.g., magnesium sulfate, narcotics)

B. Evaluation

1. **Physical examination:** Note central vs. peripheral and persistent vs. intermittent cyanosis, respiratory effort, single vs. split S_2, presence of heart murmur. Acrocyanosis is often a normal finding in newborns.

2. **Clinical tests:** Oxygen challenge test (see Chapter 7), preductal/postductal arterial blood gases or pulse oximetry to assess for right-to-left shunt, and transillumination of chest for possible pneumothorax.

3. **Other data:** Complete blood cell count (CBC) with differential, serum glucose, chest radiograph, electrocardiogram (ECG), echocardiography. Consider blood, urine, and cerebrospinal fluid (CSF) cultures if sepsis is suspected, and methemoglobin level if cyanosis is out of proportion to hypoxemia.

VII. RESPIRATORY DISEASES

A. General Respiratory Considerations

1. Exogenous surfactant therapy:

a. Indications: RDS in preterm infants, meconium aspiration, pneumonia, persistent pulmonary hypertension.

b. Administration: If infant is ≤26 weeks' gestation, first dose is typically given in delivery room or as soon as stabilized; repeat dosing may follow at 6-hour intervals.

c. Complications: Pneumothorax, pulmonary hemorrhage.

2. **Supplemental O₂:** Adjust inspired oxygen to maintain O_2 saturation between 85% and 94% until retina is fully vascularized, between 94% and 98% if retinas are mature (see Section XIII), and >97% in cases of pulmonary hypertension.

B. Respiratory Distress Syndrome

1. **Definition:** Deficiency of pulmonary surfactant (a phospholipid protein mixture that decreases surface tension and prevents alveolar collapse). Surfactant is produced by type II alveolar cells in increasing quantities from 32 weeks' gestation:

a. Maternal administration of steroids antenatally has been shown to decrease neonatal morbidity and mortality. Risk for RDS is decreased in babies born >24 hours and <7 days after maternal steroid administration.

b. Other factors that accelerate lung maturity: Maternal hypertension, sickle cell disease, narcotic addiction, intrauterine growth retardation, prolonged rupture of membranes, and fetal stress

2. **Incidence:**

a. <30 weeks' gestation: 60% without antenatal steroids, 35% in those who received antenatal steroids

b. 30–34 weeks' gestation: 25% without antenatal steroids, 10% in those who received antenatal steroids

c. >34 weeks' gestation: 5%

3. **Risk factors:** Prematurity, maternal diabetes, cesarean section without antecedent labor, perinatal asphyxia, second twin, previous infant with RDS.

4. **Clinical presentation:** Respiratory distress worsens during first few hours of life, progresses over 48–72 hours, and subsequently improves:

a. Recovery is accompanied by brisk diuresis.

b. Chest x-ray findings: *Reticulogranular* pattern to lung fields; may obscure heart borders.

5. **Management:**

a. Support ventilation and oxygenation

b. Surfactant therapy

C. Persistent Pulmonary Hypertension of the Newborn (PPHN)

1. **Etiology:** Idiopathic or secondary to conditions leading to increased pulmonary vascular resistance. Most commonly seen in term or postterm infants, infants born by cesarean section, and infants with a history of fetal distress and low Apgar scores. Usually presents within 12–24 hours of birth:

a. Vasoconstriction secondary to hypoxemia and acidosis (e.g., neonatal sepsis)

b. Interstitial pulmonary disease (meconium aspiration syndrome, pneumonia)

c. Hyperviscosity syndrome (polycythemia)

d. Pulmonary hypoplasia, either primary or secondary to congenital diaphragmatic hernia or renal agenesis

2. **Diagnostic features:**

a. Severe hypoxemia (Pa_{O_2} < 35–45 mm Hg in 100% O_2) disproportionate to radiologic changes

b. Structurally normal heart with right-to-left shunt at foramen ovale and/or ductus arteriosus; decreased postductal oxygenation compared with preductal (difference of at least 7–15 mm Hg between preductal and postductal Pa_{O_2} is significant)

c. Must be distinguished from cyanotic heart disease. Infants with heart disease will have an abnormal cardiac examination and show little to no improvement in oxygenation with increased fraction of inspired O_2 (Fi_{O_2}) and hyperventilation. See Chapter 7 for interpretation of oxygen challenge test.

3. **Principles of therapy:**

a. **Improve oxygenation:** Supplemental oxygen (Fi_{O_2}) to improve alveolar oxygenation. Optimize oxygen-carrying capacity with blood transfusions as needed.

b. **Minimize pulmonary vasoconstriction:**

   (1) Minimal handling of infant and limited invasive procedures. Sedation and occasionally paralysis of intubated neonates may be necessary.

   (2) Alkalosis (pH 7.45–7.55): Metabolic or respiratory (Pco_2 in low 30s); may improve oxygenation, although not noted to affect outcome. Avoid severe hypocarbia (Pco_2 < 30), which can be associated with myocardial ischemia and decreased cerebral blood flow. Hyperventilation may result in barotrauma, predisposing to chronic lung disease, so should be minimized if possible. Consider high-frequency ventilation.

c. **Maintenance of systemic blood pressure and perfusion:** Reversal of right-to-left shunt through volume expanders and/or inotropes.

d. **Consider pulmonary vasodilator therapy:**

   (1) Inhaled nitric oxide (NO): Reduces pulmonary vascular resistance (PVR). Blended with ventilatory gases and titrated to effect. Typical starting dose is 20 parts per million (ppm). Unlikely to be efficacious >40 ppm. Complications include methemoglobinemia (reduce NO dose for methemoglobin >4%), NO_2 poisoning (reduce NO dose for NO_2 concentration >1–2 ppm).

   (2) Prostaglandin I_2 (prostacyclin): A complex molecule made from arachidonic acid; major endogenous pulmonary vasodilator. Normally produced by lung when lung vessels are constricted.

e. **Broad-spectrum antibiotics:** Sepsis is a common underlying cause of PPHN.

f. **Consider extracorporeal membrane oxygenation (ECMO):** Reserved for cases of severe cardiovascular instability, oxygenation index (OI) > 40 for >3 hour, or alveolar-arterial gradient (A-a$_{O_2}$) ≥ 610 for 8 hours (see Chapter 4 for calculation of OI and A-a$_{O_2}$. Pa_{O_2} should be postductal).

18

Patients typically need to be >2000 g and >34 weeks' gestation; should have head ultrasound and echocardiogram before initiating ECMO.

4. **Mortality depends on underlying diagnosis:** Mortality rates generally lower for RDS and meconium aspiration but higher in sepsis and diaphragmatic hernia.

D. Spontaneous Pneumothorax

1. Seen in 1%–2% of normal newborns.
2. Associated with use of high inspiratory pressures and underlying diseases such as RDS, meconium aspiration, and pneumonia.
3. Patient should be monitored in a neonatal intensive care unit (NICU) setting.

VIII. APNEA AND BRADYCARDIA

A. Apnea[7]

1. **Definition:** Respiratory pause > 20 seconds, or a shorter pause associated with cyanosis, pallor, hypotonia, or bradycardia < 100 bpm. In preterm infants, apnea may be central (no diaphragmatic activity), obstructive (upper airway obstruction), or mixed central and obstructive. Common causes of apnea in the newborn are listed in Figure 18-5.

2. **Incidence:** Apnea of prematurity occurs in most infants born at <28 weeks' gestation, ≈50% of infants born at 30–32 weeks' gestation, and <7% of infants born at 34–35 weeks' gestation. Usually resolves by 34–36 weeks' postconceptual age but may persist after term in infants born at <25 weeks' gestation.

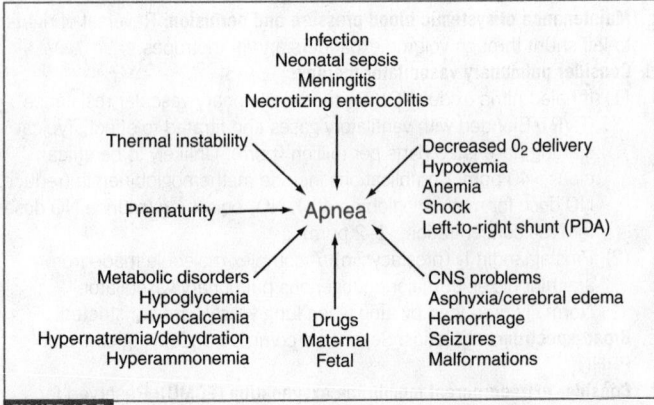

FIGURE 18-5

Causes of apnea in the newborn. CNS, Central nervous system; PDA, patent ductus arteriosus. (*From Klaus MH, Fanaroff AA. Care of the High-Risk Neonate. 5th ed. Philadelphia: WB Saunders, 2001:268.*)

3. **Management:**
a. Consider pathologic causes for apnea.
b. Pharmacotherapy with caffeine or other stimulants.
c. Continuous positive airway pressure or mechanical ventilation (see Chapter 4 for details).

B. Bradycardia Without Central Apnea
Etiologies include obstructive apnea, mechanical airway obstruction, gastroesophageal reflux, increased intracranial pressure (ICP), increased vagal tone (defecation, yawning, rectal stimulation, placement of nasogastric [NG] tube), electrolyte abnormalities, heart block.

IX. CARDIAC DISEASES

A. Patent Ductus Arteriosus (PDA)
1. **Definition:** Failure of ductus arteriosus to close in first few days of life, or reopening after functional closure. Typically results in left-to-right shunting of blood once PVR has decreased. If PVR remains high, blood may be shunted right to left, resulting in hypoxemia (see Section VII.C).
2. **Incidence:** Up to 60% in preterm infants weighing <1500 g, higher in those <1000 g. Female-to-male ratio is 2:1. Obligatory PDA is found in 10% of infants with congenital heart disease.
3. **Risk factors:** Most often related to hypoxia and immaturity. Term infants with PDA usually have structural defects in ductal vessel walls.
4. **Diagnosis:**
a. Examination: Systolic murmur that may be continuous, best heard at left upper sternal border or left infraclavicular area. May have apical diastolic rumble due to increased blood flow across mitral valve in diastole. Bounding peripheral pulses with widened pulse pressure if large shunt. Hyperactive precordium and palmar pulses may be present.
b. ECG: Normal or left ventricular hypertrophy in small to moderate PDA. Biventricular hypertrophy in large PDA.
c. Chest radiograph: May have cardiomegaly and increased pulmonary vascular markings, depending on size of shunt.
d. Echocardiogram.
5. **Management:**
a. Ongoing controversy over indications for treatment, timing of intervention, and best management strategy
b. Indomethacin: Prostaglandin synthetase inhibitor; 80% closure rate in preterm infants:
   (1) For dosage information and contraindications, see Formulary.
   (2) Complications: Transient decrease in glomerular filtration rate and decreased urine output, transient gastrointestinal bleeding (not associated with increased incidence of necrotizing enterocolitis [NEC]), prolonged bleeding time and disturbed platelet function for 7–9 days independent of platelet number (not associated with increased incidence of intracranial hemorrhage). Spontaneous

isolated intestinal perforations are seen with indomethacin use. Rates are higher with concomitant hydrocortisone use.

c. Ibuprofen[7,8]: As effective as indomethacin but fewer renal adverse effects

d. Surgical ligation of the duct

B. Cyanotic Heart Disease

See Chapter 7.

X. HEMATOLOGIC DISEASES

A. Unconjugated Hyperbilirubinemia in the Newborn[9]

1. **Overview:** During first 3–4 days of life, serum bilirubin increases from 1.5 mg/dL (cord blood) to 6.5 ± 2.5 mg/dL:

a. Maximum rate of bilirubin increase for normal infants with nonhemolytic hyperbilirubinemia: 5 mg/dL/24 hr, or 0.2 mg/dL/hr

b. Consider pathologic cause: Visible jaundice or total bilirubin concentration > 5 mg/dL on first day of life

c. Risk factors: Birth weight < 2500 g, breast-feeding, prematurity

2. **Evaluation:**

a. Maternal prenatal testing: ABO and Rh (D) typing and serum screen for isoimmune antibodies

b. Infant or cord blood: Blood smear, direct Coombs test, blood and Rh typing (if maternal blood type is O, Rh negative, or prenatal blood typing was not performed)

3. **Management:**

a. Phototherapy: Ideally, intensive phototherapy should produce a decline of total serum bilirubin (TSB) level of 1–2 mg/dL within 4–6 hours, with further decline subsequently:
   (1) Preterm newborn (Table 18-8)
   (2) Term newborn (Fig. 18-6)

b. Intravenous immune globulin (IVIG) (>35 weeks' gestational age): In isoimmune hemolytic disease, IVIG administration (0.5–1 g/kg over 2 hours) is recommended if TSB is rising despite intensive phototherapy, or TSB level is within 2–3 mg/dL of exchange level. Repeat in 12 hours if needed.

c. Neonatal double-volume exchange transfusion (see Table 18-8 and Fig. 18-7):
   (1) Volume: 160 mL/kg for full-term infant, 160–200 mL/kg for preterm infant.

TABLE 18-8

GUIDELINES FOR USE OF PHOTOTHERAPY IN PRETERM INFANTS <1 WEEK OF AGE

Weight (g)	Phototherapy (mg/dL)	Consider Exchange Transfusion (mg/dL)
500–1000	5–7	12–15
1000–1500	7–10	15–18
1500–2500	10–15	18–20
>2500	>15	>20

(2) Route: During exchange, blood is removed through umbilical arterial catheter (UAC) and an equal volume is infused through umbilical venous catheter (UVC). If UAC is unavailable, use a single venous catheter.

(3) Rate: Exchange in 15-mL increments for vigorous full-term infants. Exchange at 2–3 mL/kg/min in premature/less stable infants to avoid trauma to red blood cells.

(4) Complications: Emboli, thromboses, hemodynamic instability, electrolyte disturbances, coagulopathy, infection, death.

NOTE: CBC, reticulocyte count, peripheral smear, bilirubin, Ca^{2+}, glucose, total protein, infant blood type, Coombs test, and newborn screen should be performed on a *preexchange sample* of blood; they are of no diagnostic value on postexchange blood. If indicated, save preexchange blood for serologic or chromosome studies.

B. Conjugated Hyperbilirubinemia

1. **Definition:** Direct bilirubin > 2.0 mg/dL and > 10% of TSB

2. **Etiology:** Biliary obstruction/atresia, choledochal cyst, hyperalimentation, α_1-antitrypsin deficiency, hepatitis, sepsis, infections (especially urinary tract infections), hypothyroidism, inborn errors of metabolism, cystic fibrosis, red blood cell abnormalities

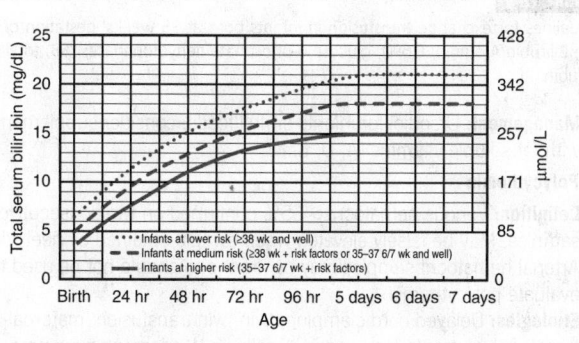

- Use total bilirubin. Do not subtract direct reacting or conjugated bilirubin.
- Risk factors: Isoimmune hemolytic disease, G6PD deficiency, asphyxia, significant lethargy, temperature instability, sepsis, acidosis, or albumin < 3.0 g/dL (if measured).
- For well infants 35–37 6/7 wk can adjust TSB levels for intervention around the medium risk line. It is an option to intervene at lower TSB levels for infants closer to 35 wk and at higher TSB levels for those closer to 37 6/7 wk.
- It is an option to provide conventional phototherapy in hospital or at home at TSB levels 2–3 mg/dL (35–50 mmol/L) below those shown, but home phototherapy should not be used in any infant with risk factors.

FIGURE 18-6

Guidelines for phototherapy in infants born at 35 weeks' gestation or more. G6PD, Glucose-6-phosphate dehydrogenase; TSB, total serum bilirubin.

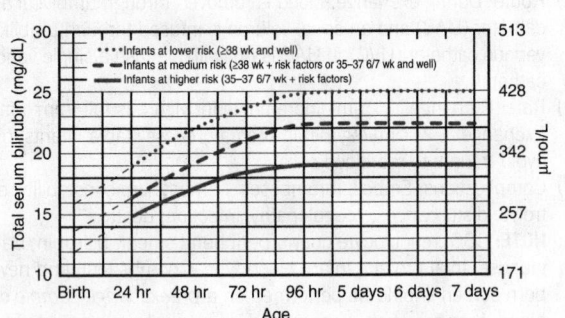

- The dashed lines for the first 24 hours indicate uncertainty due to a wide range of clinical circumstances and a range of responses to phototherapy.
- Immediate exchange transfusion is recommended if infant shows signs of acute bilirubin encephalopathy (hypertonia, arching, retrocollis, opisthotonos, fever, high-pitched cry) or if TBS is ≥5 mg/dL (85 μmol/L) above these lines.
- Risk factors: Isoimmune hemolytic disease, G6PD deficiency, asphyxia, significant lethargy, temperature instability, sepsis, acidosis.
- Measure serum albumin and calculate B/A ratio.
- Use total bilirubin. Do not subtract direct reacting or conjugated bilirubin.
- If infant is well and 35–37 6/7 wk (median risk) can individualize TSB levels for exchange based on actual gestational age.

FIGURE 18-7

Guidelines for exchange transfusion in infants born at 35 weeks' gestation or more. B/A, Bilirubin/Albumin; G6PD, glucose-6-phosphate dehydrogenase; TSB, total serum bilirubin.

3. **Management:** Ursodiol for infants on full feeds; consider supplementation with fat-soluble vitamins (A, D, E, K)

C. Polycythemia

1. **Definition:** Venous hematocrit > 65% confirmed on two consecutive samples. May be falsely elevated when sample obtained by heel stick. Arterial hematocrit samples may be lower and should not be used to evaluate polycythemia.

2. **Etiologies:** Delayed cord clamping, twin-twin transfusion, maternal-fetal transfusion, intrauterine hypoxia, Beckwith-Wiedemann syndrome, maternal gestational diabetes, neonatal thyrotoxicosis, congenital adrenal hyperplasia, trisomy 13, 18, or 21.

3. **Clinical findings:** Plethora, respiratory distress, cardiac failure, tachypnea, hypoglycemia, irritability, lethargy, seizures, apnea, jitteriness, poor feeding, thrombocytopenia, hyperbilirubinemia.

4. **Complications:** Hyperviscosity predisposes to venous thrombosis and CNS injury. Hypoglycemia may result from increased erythrocyte utilization of glucose.

5. **Management:** Partial exchange transfusion for symptomatic infants, with isovolemic replacement of blood with isotonic fluid. Blood is exchanged

in 10- to 20-mL increments to reduce hematocrit to <55. (See Chapter 14 to calculate amount of blood to be exchanged. Use birth weight (kg) × 90 mL/kg for estimated blood volume in mL.)

XI. GASTROINTESTINAL DISEASES

A. Necrotizing Enterocolitis

1. **Definition:** Serious intestinal inflammation and injury thought to be secondary to bowel ischemia, immaturity, and infection.
2. **Incidence:** More common in preterm (3%–4% of infants <2000 g) and African-American infants. Occurs principally in infants who have been fed.
3. **Risk factors:** Prematurity, asphyxia, hypotension, polycythemia-hyperviscosity syndrome, umbilical vessel catheterization, exchange transfusion, bacterial and viral pathogens, enteral feeds, PDA, congestive heart failure, cyanotic heart disease, RDS, intrauterine cocaine exposure.
4. **See Table EC 18-B:**
a. Systemic: Temperature instability, apnea, bradycardia, metabolic acidosis, hypotension, disseminated intravascular coagulopathy (DIC).
b. Intestinal: Elevated pregavage residuals with abdominal distention, blood in stool, absent bowel sounds, and/or abdominal tenderness or mass. Elevated pregavage residuals in the absence of other clinical symptoms rarely raise suspicion of NEC.
c. Radiologic: Ileus, intestinal pneumatosis, portal vein gas, ascites, pneumoperitoneum.
5. **Management:** Nothing by mouth, nasogastric tube decompression, maintain adequate hydration and perfusion, antibiotics for 7–14 days, surgical consultation. Surgery is performed for signs of perforation or necrotic bowel.

B. Bilious Emesis Differential

See Table EC 18-C.
See Chapter 12.

1. **Mechanical:** Annular pancreas, intestinal atresia/duplication/malrotation/obstruction (including adjacent organomegaly), meconium plug or ileus, Hirschsprung, imperforate anus.
2. **Functional (i.e., poor motility):** NEC, electrolyte abnormalities, sepsis
NOTE: Must eliminate malrotation as an etiology because its complication (volvulus) is a surgical emergency.

C. Abdominal Wall Defects

See Table EC 18-D.

XII. NEUROLOGIC DISEASES

A. Intraventricular Hemorrhage (IVH)

1. **Definition:** Intracranial hemorrhage usually arising in the germinal matrix and periventricular regions of the brain.

2. **Incidence:**
a. 30%–40% of infants <1500 g; 50%–60% of infants <1000 g
b. Highest incidence in first 72 hours of life: 60% within 24 hours, 85% within 72 hours, <5% after 1 week of age
3. **Diagnosis and classification:** Ultrasonography; grade is based on maximum amount of hemorrhage seen by age 2 weeks:
a. Grade I: Hemorrhage in germinal matrix only
b. Grade II: IVH without ventricular dilation
c. Grade III: IVH with ventricular dilation (30%–45% incidence of motor and cognitive impairment)
d. Grade IV: IVH with periventricular hemorrhagic infarct (60%–80% incidence of motor and cognitive impairment)
4. **Screening:** Indicated in infants <32 weeks' gestational age within first week of life; repeat in second week.
5. **Prophylaxis:** Maintain acid-base balance and avoid fluctuations in blood pressure. Indomethacin is considered for IVH prophylaxis in some newborns (<28 weeks' gestation, birth weight <1250 g) and is most efficacious if given in first 6 hours of life, but has not been shown to impact long-term outcome.[10]
6. **Outcome:** Infants with grade III and IV hemorrhages have a higher incidence of neurodevelopmental disabilities and an increased risk for posthemorrhagic hydrocephalus.

B. **Periventricular Leukomalacia**

1. **Definition and ultrasound findings:** Ischemic necrosis of periventricular white matter, characterized by CNS depression within first week and ultrasound findings of cysts with or without ventricular enlargement caused by cerebral atrophy
2. **Incidence:** More common in preterm infants but also occurs in term infants; 3.2% in infants <1500 g
3. **Etiology:** Primarily ischemia-reperfusion injury, hypoxia, acidosis, hypoglycemia, acute hypotension, low cerebral blood flow
4. **Outcome:** Commonly associated with cerebral palsy with or without sensory and cognitive deficit

C. **Neonatal Seizures (See Chapter 20)**

D. **Neonatal Abstinence Syndrome**

Onset of symptoms usually occurs within first 24–72 hours of life (methadone may delay symptoms until 96 hours or later). Symptoms may last weeks to months. Box 18-1 shows signs and symptoms of opiate withdrawal.

E. **Peripheral Nerve Injuries**

1. **Etiology:** Result from lateral traction on shoulder (vertex deliveries) or head (breech deliveries).
2. **Clinical features (see Table 18-9).**
3. **Management:** Evaluate for associated trauma (clavicular and humeral fractures, shoulder dislocation, facial nerve injury, cord injuries). Full recovery is seen in 85%–95% of cases in first year of life.

BOX 18-1

OPIATE WITHDRAWAL

Signs and Symptoms of Opiate Withdrawal

W	Wakefulness
I	Irritability, insomnia
T	Tremors, temperature variation, tachypnea, twitching (jitteriness)
H	Hyperactivity, high-pitched cry, hiccoughs, hyperreflexia, hypertonia
D	Diarrhea (explosive), diaphoresis, disorganized suck
R	Rub marks, respiratory distress, rhinorrhea, regurgitation
A	Apnea, autonomic dysfunction
W	Weight loss
A	Alkalosis (respiratory)
L	Lacrimation (photophobia), lethargy
S	Seizures, sneezing, stuffy nose, sweating, sucking (nonproductive)

TABLE 18-9

PLEXUS INJURIES

Plexus Injury	Spinal Level Involved	Clinical Features
Erb-Duchenne palsy (90% of cases)	C5–C6 Occasionally involves C4	Adduction and internal rotation of arm. Forearm is pronated; wrist is flexed. Diaphragm paralysis may occur if C4 is involved.
Total palsy (8%–9% of cases)	C5–T1 Occasionally involves C4	Upper arm, lower arm, and hand involved. Horner syndrome (ptosis, anhydrosis, and miosis) exists if T1 is involved.
Klumpke paralysis (<2% of cases)	C7–T1	Hand flaccid with little control. Horner syndrome if T1 is involved.

XIII. RETINOPATHY OF PREMATURITY (ROP)[11]

A. Definition

Interruption of normal progression of retinal vascularization.

B. Etiology

Exposure of the immature retina to high oxygen concentrations can result in vasoconstriction and obliteration of the retinal capillary network, followed by vasoproliferation. Risk is greatest in the most immature infants.

C. Diagnosis—Dilated Funduscopic Examination

Dilated funduscopic examination should be performed in the following patients:

1. All infants born ≤30 weeks' gestation
2. Infants born >30 weeks' gestation with unstable clinical course, including those requiring cardiorespiratory support
3. Any infant with a birth weight ≤1500 grams

D. Timing[12]

1. For all infants ≤27 weeks' gestation at birth, initial ROP screening examination should be performed at 31 weeks' postmenstrual age.

2. For all infants ≥28 weeks' gestation at birth, initial ROP screening examination should be performed at 4 weeks chronologic age.

3. For infants born before 25 weeks' gestation, consider earlier screening at 6 weeks chronologic age (even if before 31 weeks' postmenstrual age) on the basis of severity of comorbidities. This may enable earlier detection and treatment of aggressive posterior ROP, which is a severe form of rapidly progressive ROP.

E. Classification

1. Stage:

a. Stage 1: Demarcation line separates avascular from vascularized retina

b. Stage 2: Ridge forms along demarcation line

c. Stage 3: Extraretinal fibrovascular proliferation tissue forms on ridge

d. Stage 4: Partial retinal detachment

e. Stage 5: Total retinal detachment

2. **Zone** (Fig. 18-8)

3. **Plus disease:** Abnormal dilation and tortuosity of posterior retinal blood vessels in two or more quadrants of retina; may be present at any stage

4. **Number of clock hours or 30-degree sectors involved**

F. Management[11]

1. **Type 1 ROP:** Peripheral retinal ablation should be considered. Type 1 ROP classified as:

a. Zone I: Any stage ROP with plus disease

b. Zone I: Stage 3 ROP without plus disease

c. Zone II: Stage 2 or 3 ROP with plus disease

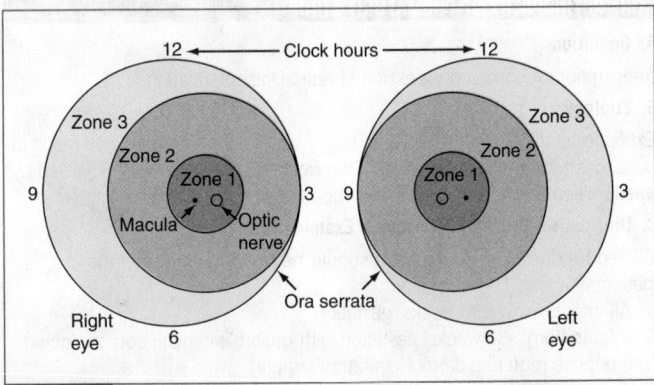

FIGURE 18-8

Zones of the retina. (*From American Academy of Pediatrics. Screening examination of premature infants for retinopathy of prematurity, AAP policy statement. Pediatrics. 2013;131:189–195.*)

2. **Type 2 ROP:** Serial examinations rather than retinal ablation should be considered. Type 2 ROP classified as:
a. Zone I: Stage 1 or 2 ROP without plus disease
b. Zone II: Stage 3 ROP without plus disease
3. **Follow-up** (Table 18-10)

TABLE 18-10

SUGGESTED SCHEDULE FOR FOLLOW-UP OPHTHALMOLOGIC EXAMINATION IN RETINOPATHY OF PREMATURITY (ROP)

≤1 Week	1–2 Weeks	2 Weeks	2–3 Weeks
Stage 1 or 2 ROP: zone I Stage 3 ROP: zone II	Stage 2 ROP: zone II Immature vascularization: posterior zone II	Stage 1 ROP: zone II	Stage 1 or 2 ROP: zone III
Immature vascularization: zone I, no ROP	Immature vascularization: posterior zone II	Immature vascularization: zone II, no ROP	Regressing ROP: zone III
Immature retina extends into posterior zone II near boundary of zone I	Unequivocally regressing ROP: zone I	Unequivocally regressing ROP: zone II	

NOTE: The presence of plus disease in zone I or II indicates that peripheral ablation rather than observation is appropriate.

From American Academy of Pediatrics. Screening examination of premature infants for retinopathy of prematurity, AAP policy statement. *Pediatrics*. 2013;131:189-195.

XIV. CONGENITAL INFECTIONS

See Chapter 17.

XV. COMMONLY USED MEDICATIONS IN THE NEONATAL INTENSIVE CARE UNIT (TABLE 18-11)

For neonatal specific drug dosing, refer to formulary or the Neofax.

TABLE 18-11

DOSING OF COMMONLY USED ANTIBIOTICS IN THE NEONATAL INTENSIVE CARE UNIT, BASED ON POSTMATERNAL AND POSTNATAL AGE

AMPICILLIN (GBS bacteremia = 150–200 mg/kg/day; GBS meningitis = 300–400 mg/kg/day) **CEFOTAXIME** 50 mg/kg/dose (gonococcal infections = 25 mg/kg/dose) (GC ophthalmia Ppx if maternal GC infection is present = 100 mg/kg × 1 dose) **OXACILLIN** 25–50 mg/kg/dose	**VANCOMYCIN** (bacteremia = 10 mg/kg/dose; meningitis = 15 mg/mg/dose)	**METRONIDAZOLE**† (loading = 15 mg/kg/dose; maintenance = 7.5 mg/kg/dose)

18

Continued

TABLE 18-11

DOSING OF COMMONLY USED ANTIBIOTICS IN THE NEONATAL INTENSIVE CARE UNIT, BASED ON POSTMATERNAL AND POSTNATAL AGE—cont'd

Dosing Interval Chart			Dosing Interval Chart			Dosing Interval Chart		
PMA (weeks)	Postnatal (days)	Interval (hours)	PMA (weeks)	Postnatal (days)	Interval (hours)	PMA (weeks)	Postnatal (days)	Interval (hours)
≤29	0–28	12	≤29	0–14	18	≤29	0–28	48
	>28	8		>14	12		>28	24
30–36	0–14	12	30–36	0–14	12	30–36	0–14	24
	>14	8		>14	8		>14	12
37–44	0–7	12	37–44	0–7	12	37–44	0–7	24
	>7	8		>7	8		>7	12
≥45	All	6	≥45	All	6	≥45	All	8

GENTAMICIN

FLUCONAZOLE†

(Invasive candidiasis: loading = 12–25 mg/kg/dose; maintenance = 6–12 mg/kg/dose)

Dosing Chart				Dosing Interval Chart		
PMA (weeks)	Postnatal (days)	Dose (mg/kg)	Interval (hours)	Gest. Age (weeks)	Postnatal (days)	Interval (hours)
≤29*	0–7	5	48	≤29	0–14	48
	8–28	4	36		>14	24
	≥29	4	24	30 and older	0–7	48
30–34	0–7	4.5	36		>7	24
	≥8	4	24			
≥35	All	4	24			

*Or significant asphyxia, PDA, or treatment with indomethacin.

†Thrush = 6 mg/kg/dose on day 1, then 3 mg/kg/dose orally (PO) Q24 hr, regardless of gestational or postnatal age.

GBS, Group B *Streptococcus;* GC, gonococcus; Gest., gestational; PDA, patent ductus arteriosus; PMA, postmaternal age; Ppx, prophylaxis.

Online Neofax: http://neofax.thomsonhc.com/neofax/index.php. 2010. Thomson Reuters Inc. • Application Version: 3.0.0.4 • User Manual Version: 200901.

REFERENCES

1. Wiswell TE, Gannon CM, Jacob J, et al. Delivery room management of the apparently vigorous meconium-stained neonate: results of the multicenter, international collaborative trial. *Pediatrics*. 2000;105:1-7.
2. Apgar V. A proposal for new method of evaluation of the newborn infant. *Anesth Analg*. 1953;32:260-267.
3. Ballard JL, Khoury JC, Wedig K, et al. New Ballard Score, expanded to include extremely premature infants. *J Pediatr*. 1991;119:417-423.
4. Tagin MA, Woolcott CG, Vincer MJ, et al. Hypothermia for neonatal hypoxic ischemic encephalopathy: an updated systemic review and meta-analysis. *Arch Pediatr Adolesc Med*. 2012;166:558-566.
5. Cornblath M. Neonatal hypoglycemia. In: Donn SM, Fisher CW, eds. *Risk Management Techniques in Perinatal and Neonatal Practice*. Armonk, NY: Futura, 1996.
6. American Academy of Pediatrics. Clinical practice guideline. *Pediatrics*. 2004; 114:297-316.
7. Klaus MH, Fanaroff AA. *Care of the High-Risk Neonate*. 5th ed. Philadelphia: Saunders, 2001.
8. Ohlsson A, Walia R, Shah SS. Ibuprofen for the treatment of patent ductus arteriosus in preterm and/or LBW infants. *Cochrane Database Syst Rev*. 2008;1. CD003481.
9. American Academy of Pediatrics: Subcommittee on Hyperbilirubinemia: Management of hyperbilirubinemia in the newborn infant 35 or more weeks of gestation. *Pediatrics*. 2004;114(1):297-316. Erratum in Pediatrics 2004;114(4):1138.
10. Schmidt B, Davis P, Moddemann D, et al. Long-term effects of indomethacin prophylaxis in ELBW infants. *N Engl J Med*. 2001;344:1966-1972.
11. Good WV. Early Treatment for Retinopathy of Prematurity Cooperative Group. Revised indications for the treatment of retinopathy of prematurity: results of the early treatment for retinopathy of prematurity randomized trial. *Arch Ophthalmol*. 2003;121:1684-1694.
12. Fierson WM. American Academy of Pediatrics Section on Ophthalmology, American Academy of Ophthalmology; American Association for Pediatric Ophthalmology and Strabismus; American Association of Certified Orthoptists. Screening examination of premature infants for retinopathy of prematurity. *Pediatrics*. 2013;131:189-195.

Chapter 19

Nephrology

Katie Shaw, MD

I. WEBSITES

The International Pediatric Hypertension Association:
www.pediatrichypertension.org
American Academy of Pediatrics (AAP) Urinary Tract Infection (UTI)
Practice Guidelines for Children 2–24 months: UTI Guidelines 2011
National Kidney Disease Education Program: NKDEP Website
National Kidney Foundation: www.kidney.org

II. URINALYSIS, URINE DIPSTICK, AND MICROSCOPY[1]

Urinalysis (UA) components are useful in clinical evaluation but rarely
diagnositic in isolation. The clinican should be mindful of the possibility of
false-positive and false-negative results, particularly with the dipstick, owing
to a variety of factors.

Best if urine specimen is evaluated within 1 hour after voiding. Annual
screening UAs are no longer recommended by the AAP.

A. Color

Normal urine varies in color from almost colorless to amber.

B. Turbidity

Cloudy urine can be normal; is most often the result of crystal formation at
room temperature. Uric acid crystals form in acidic urine, and phosphate
crystals form in alkaline urine. Cellular material and bacteria can also cause
turbidity.

C. Specific Gravity

1. **Purpose:** Used as a measurement of a kidney's ability to concentrate
   urine. Easily determined surrogate of osmolality.
2. **Normal findings:** Between 1.003 and 1.030.
3. **Special circumstances:**
   a. Isosthenuria: Excretion of urine with osmolality equal to plasma (neither
      concentrated or diluted). Typically a specific gravity of 1.010.
   b. Disease states affecting the kidney's ability to concentrate urine may
      have a urine specific gravity fixed at 1.010 (i.e., chronic kidney disease).
   c. Glucose, abundant protein, and iodine-containing contrast materials can
      give falsely high readings.

D. pH

1. **Purpose:** Used in determining the renal tubules' ability to maintain
   normal hydrogen ion concentration.
2. **Findings:** Normal ranges from 4.5–8, with an average range of 5–6.

E. Protein

1. **Purpose:** Used for screening and monitoring proteinuria. Should be quantified more precisely when needed for diagnostic purposes (see Section VII and related figures).
2. **Findings:** Dipstick provides readings of negative, trace, 1+ (~30 mg/dL), 2+ (~100 mg/dL), 3+ (~300 mg/dL), and 4+ (>1000 mg/dL).

F. Sugars

1. **Purpose:** Used to detect sugar in urine; glucosuria is always abnormal.
2. **Findings:** Glucosuria is suggestive but not diagnostic of diabetes mellitus or proximal renal tubular disease (see Section VIII). Blood level of glucose at which kidney tubular reabsorption is exceeded is typically between 160 and 180 mg/dL.
3. **Special circumstances:** Different tests are available to detect glucose/sugars. Reduction tests (e.g., Clinitest) will detect other sugars such as galactose, lactose, fructose, pentoses, and glucose. Enzyme tests (e.g., Clinistix) are specific for glucose only.

G. Ketones

1. **Purpose:** Used to detect altered metabolism by detecting breakdown of fatty acids and fats. Useful in patients with diabetes and altered carbohydrate metabolism.
2. **Findings:** Except for trace amounts, ketonuria suggest ketoacidosis, usually due to diabetes mellitus or catabolism induced by inadequate intake. Neonatal ketoacidosis may occur with metabolic defects (e.g., propionic acidemia, methylmalonic aciduria, glycogen storage disease).

H. Nitrite

See Section III.E.1.a

I. Leukocyte Esterase

See Section III.E.1.b

J. Hemoglobin, Myoglobin

1. **Purpose:** Used to detect glomerular or urologic injury.
2. **Findings:** Dipstick reads positive with intact red blood cells (as few as 3–4 red blood cells [RBCs]/high-powered field [hpf]), hemoglobin, or myoglobin. Hemoglobinuria is seen with intravascular hemolysis or in a hematuric urine that has been standing for an extended period. Myoglobinuria is seen in crush injuries, vigorous exercise, major motor seizures, fever, malignant hyperthermia, electrocution, snake bites, and ischemia.

K. Bilirubin, Urobilinogen (Table 19-1)

Dipstick measures each individually.

1. **Urine bilirubin:** Positive with conjugated hyperbilirubinemia; in this form, bilirubin is water soluble and excreted by the kidney.
2. **Urobilinogen:** Increased in all cases of hyperbilirubinemia where there is no obstruction to enterohepatic circulation.

TABLE 19-1

URINALYSIS FOR BILIRUBIN/UROBILINOGEN

	Normal	Hemolytic Disease	Hepatic Disease	Biliary Obstruction
Urine urobilinogen	Normal	Increased	Increased	Decreased
Urine bilirubin	Negative	Negative	±	Positive

L. Red Blood Cells (RBC)

1. **Purpose:** Used to differentiate the presence of hemoglobinuria/myoglobinuria from intact RBCs.
2. **Findings:** Centrifuged urine normally contains <5 RBCs/hpf. Examination of RBC morphology may help localize the source of bleeding; dysmorphic RBCs suggest a glomerular origin, whereas normal RBCs suggest lower tract bleeding. See Section VI for further definitions and evaluation of persistent hematuria.

M. White Blood Cells (WBC)

1. **Purpose:** Used to detect infection or inflammation anywhere in the genitourinary tract.
2. **Findings:** ≥5 white blood cells (WBCs)/hpf of a properly spun urine specimen is suggestive of urinary tract infection (UTI). Relative to UTI, sterile pyuria is much less common in the pediatric population. If sterile pyuria is present, it is usually transient and accompanies systemic infectious or inflammatory disorders (e.g., Kawasaki disease).

N. Epithelial Cells

1. **Purpose:** Sqaumous epithelial cells are used as an index of possible contamination by vaginal secretions in females or by foreskin in uncircumcised males.
2. **Findings:** Any amount indicates possible contamination.

O. Sediment

Using light microscopy, unstained centrifuged urine can be examined for formed elements, including casts, cells, and crystals.

P. Urine Gram Stain

Gram stain is used to screen for UTIs. One organism per high-power field in uncentrifuged urine represents at least 10^5 colonies/mL.

III. EVALUATION AND MANAGEMENT OF URINARY TRACT INFECTIONS[3]

A. History

Obtain voiding history (stool, urine), stream characteristics in toilet-trained children, sexual intercourse, sexual abuse, circumcision, masturbation, pinworms, prolonged baths, bubble baths, evaluation of growth curve, recent antibiotic use, and family history of vesicoureteral reflux (VUR), recurrent UTIs, or chronic kidney disease.

B. Physical Examination

Vital signs, especially blood pressure, abdominal examination for flank masses, bowel distention, evidence of impaction, meatal stenosis or circumcision in males, vulvovaginitis or labial adhesions in females, neurologic examination of lower extremities, perineal sensation and reflexes, and rectal and sacral examination (for anteriorly placed anus).

C. Risk Factors

Recent AAP guidelines for children 2–24 months provide resources to help clinicians stratify the risk of UTI in the absence of another source of infection in a febrile child.
1. **Females are at higher risk for UTI than males.**
2. **Uncircumcised males are at higher risk.**
3. **Other risk factors include nonblack race, fever ≥39°C, and fever >1-2 days.**

D. Method of Obtaining Urine Sample

1. **If a child is 2 months to 2 years of age, has a fever, and appears sufficiently ill to warrant immediate antibiotics,** obtain urinalysis and urine culture by transurethral catheterization.
2. **If a child is 2 months to 2 years of age, has a fever, and does not appear ill enough to warrent immediate antibiotics,** obtain urine by catheterization or the most convenient method available. If UA does not suggest UTI, it is reasonable to avoid antimicrobial therapy. If UA does suggest UTI, urine culture should be obtained by catheterization.

E. Diagnosis

1. **To establish the diagnosis of UTI,** both urinalysis results suggestive of infection and positive urine culture are recommended.
a. Nitrite test:
   (1) Purpose: Used to detect nitrites produced by reduction of dietary nitrates by urinary gram-negative bacteria (especially *Escherichia coli, Klebsiella,* and *Proteus*).
   (2) Findings: Positive test is strongly suggestive of a UTI because of high specificity. Nitrite sensitivity is 15%-82% and specificity is 90%-100%.
   (3) Special circumstances: False-negative (low sensitivity) results commonly occur with insufficient time for conversion of urinary nitrates to nitrites (age-dependent voiding frequency) and inability of bacteria to reduce nitrates to nitrites (many gram-positive organisms such as *Enterococcus, Mycobacterium* spp., and fungi).
b. Leukocyte esterase test:
   (1) Purpose: Used to detect esterases released from broken-down leukocytes. An indirect test for WBCs.
   (2) Findings: Positive test is more sensitive (67%-84%) than specific (64%-92%) for a UTI.
c. Pyuria: Defined at a threshold of 5 WBCs/hpf. Absence of pyuria is rare if a true UTI is present.

d. Urine culture:
   (1) Suprapubic aspiration: >50,000 colony-forming units (CFUs) neces-
       sary to diagnose a UTI. Some resources do consider <50,000 CFUs
       diagnostic of a UTI. Recommend clinical correlation.
   (2) Transurethral catheterization: >50,000 CFUs necessary to diagnose
       a UTI.
   (3) Clean catch: >100,000 CFUs necessary to diagnose a UTI.
   (4) Bagged specimen: Positive culture cannot be used to document a
       UTI.
   (5) Catheter Associated (indwelling urethral or suprapubic): No specific
       data for pediatric patients. Adult IDSA guidelines define as presence
       of symptoms and signs compatible with UTI and > 1000 CFU/mL of
       1 or more bacterial species in a single catheter urine specimen or
       in a midstream voided urine specimen from patient whose catheter
       has been removed within previous 48 hours.[2]

F. Culture-Positive UTI

Treatment: Based on urine culture and sensitivities if possible; for empirical
therapy, see Chapter 17.

1. **Upper versus lower UTI:** Fever, systemic symptoms, and costoverte-
   bral angle tenderness suggest pyelonephritis (upper UTI) rather than
   cystitis (lower UTI). Fever that persists for >48 hours after initiating
   appropriate antibiotics is also suggestive of pyelonephritis. Although a
   99mTc-dimercaptosuccinic acid (DMSA) scan is the gold standard to
   diagnose pyelonephritis, infants with febrile UTI are assumed to have
   pyelonephritis and are treated as such.
2. **Organisms:** *E. coli* is the most common cause of pediatric UTI. Other
   common pathogens include *Klebsiella, Proteus* spp., *Staphylococcus
   saprophyticus*, and *Staphylococcus aureus*. Group B streptococci and
   other bloodborne pathogens are important in neonatal UTIs, whereas
   Enterococcus and *Pseudomonas* are more prevalent in abnormal hosts
   (e.g., recurrent UTI, abnormal anatomy, neurogenic bladder, hospitalized
   patients, or those with frequent bladder catheterizations).
3. **Treatment considerations:**
a. Hospitalize all febrile children age <4 weeks, and treat with intravenous
   (IV) antibiotics, owing to risk for bacteremia and meningitis.
b. Parenteral antibiotics for children who are toxic, dehydrated, or unable
   to tolerate oral medication due to vomiting or noncompliance. Studies
   comparing duration are inconclusive, but experts traditionally recommend 7–10 days for uncomplicated cases and 14 days for toxic children
   and those with pyelonephritis. Some recent studies have shown that 2–4
   days of oral antibiotics in uncomplicated lower tract UTIs are as effective
   as 7–10 days of oral treatment.[4]
4. **Inadequate response to therapy:** Repeat urine culture in children with
   expected response is controversial but generally thought to be unnecessary. Repeat culture, as well as renal ultrasound to rule out an abscess
   or urinary obstruction, is indicated in children with poor response to

Grade I	Grade II	Grade III	Grade IV	Grade V
Ureter only	Ureter, pelvis, calyces; no dilatation, normal calyceal fornices	Mild or moderate dilatation and/or tortuosity of ureter; mild or moderate dilatation of the pelvis, but no or slight blunting of the fornices	Moderate dilatation and/or tortuosity of the ureter; mild dilatation of renal pelvis and calyces; complete obliteration of sharp angle of fornices, but maintenance of papillary impressions in majority of calyces	Gross dilatation and tortuosity of ureter; gross dilatation of renal pelvis and calyces; papillary impressions are no longer visible in majority of calyces

FIGURE 19-1

International classification of vesicoureteral reflux. *(Modified from Rushton H. Urinary tract infections in children: epidemiology, evaluation, and management.* Pediatr Clin North Am. *1997;44:5; and International Reflux Committee. Medical vs. surgical treatment of primary vesicoureteral reflux: report of the International Reflux Study Committee.* Pediatrics. *1981;67:392.)*

therapy. Repeat cultures should also be considered in patients with recurrent UTIs to rule out persistent bacteriuria.

5. **Imaging studies** (Fig. 19-1):
a. Anatomic evaluation: New guidelines for children aged 2–24 months continue to recommend obtaining an ultrasound of the kidneys and bladder after the first UTI is diagnosed. In a change from prior recommendations, a voiding cystourethrogram (VCUG) is recommended after a second UTI is diagnosed or as indicated by an abnormal kidney and bladder ultrasound (hydronephrosis, scarring, or other findings to suggest either high-grade vesicoureteral reflux [VUR] or obstructive uropathy).[3]
    (1) Kidney and Bladder Ultrasonography: To evaluate for gross structural defects, obstructive lesions, positional abnormalities, and kidney

size and growth. Should be done at the earliest convenient time unless the child fails to demonstrate expected clinical response, which should prompt a more immediate kidney sonogram.

(2) VCUG: To evaluate bladder anatomy, emptying, and VUR. May be substituted with radionuclide cystogram (RNC), which has 1/100 the radiation exposure of VCUG and increased sensitivity for transient reflux. RNC does not visualize urethral anatomy, is not sensitive for low-grade reflux, and cannot grade reflux.

b. Abdominal radiograph: If indicated, to evaluate stool pattern and for spinal dysraphism.

c. Dimercaptosuccinic acid (DMSA): ^{99m}Tc-DMSA scan can detect areas of decreased uptake that may represent acute pyelonephritis or chronic kidney scarring; does not differentiate between the two. Routine use not recommended; may be indicated in patients with an abnormal VCUG or kidney sonography, in patients with history of asymptomatic bacteriuria and fever. Repeat in 3–6 months if initial study is positive to evaluate for persistent infection and kidney scarring if clincally indicated.

d. Diethylenetriamine pentaacetic acid (DTPA)/mercaptoacetyl triglycine (MAG-3): In the setting of hydronephrosis, can be used to assess drainage of the urinary collecting system to characterize possible upper urologic tract obstructions at ureteropelvic or ureterovesico junction. May also be used for indications given above for DMSA.

6. **Managment of VUR:**

a. Antibiotic prophylaxis: Conventionally, low-dose antibiotic prophylaxis has been recommended in all children with VUR and obstructive disease. New guidelines call into question the efficacy of antibiotic prophylaxis in preventing UTI and subsequent kidney disease in the setting of VUR; studies are ongoing to determine its role.[5-7] The Randomized Intervention for the Management of Vesicoureteral Reflux (RIVUR) Study is a randomized double-blinded controlled clinical trial (only in the United States) aiming to answer the question of antibiotic prophylaxis necessity and results are anticipated in 2014 after the publication of this edition.

b. Surgical intervention: Persistence/grade of VUR is typically monitored yearly, often in consultation with a pediatric urologist. Higher-grade VUR that persists as the child grows may ultimately require surgical intervention, the timing of which may be affected by factors such as presence of bilateral VUR, kidney/scarring, other underlying urologic disease, recurrent kidney infections, and/or ease of family follow-up. No model predicting the resolution of VUR has been verified.

7. **Asymptomatic bacteriuria:** Defined as bacteria in urine on microscopy and Gram stain in an afebrile, asymptomatic patient without pyuria. Antibiotics not necessary if voiding habits and urinary tract are normal. DMSA may be helpful in differentiating pyelonephritis from fever and coincidental bacteriuria.

8. **Referral to pediatric urology:** Consider in children with abnormal voiding patterns based on history or imaging, neurogenic bladder, abnormal anatomy, recurrent UTI, or poor response to appropriate antibiotics.

TABLE 19-2

NORMAL VALUES OF GLOMERULAR FILTRATION RATE

Age	GFR (Mean) (mL/min/1.73 m²)	Range (mL/min/1.73 m²)
Neonates <34 wk gestational age		
2–8 days	11	11–15
4–28 days	20	15–28
30–90 days	50	40–65
Neonates >34 wk gestational age		
2–8 days	39	17–60
4–28 days	47	26–68
30–90 days	58	30–86
1–6 mo	77	39–114
6–12 mo	103	49–157
12–19 mo	127	62–191
2 yr–adult	127	89–165

From Holliday MA, Barratt TM. *Pediatric Nephrology*. Baltimore: Williams & Wilkins, 1994:1306.

IV. KIDNEY FUNCTION TESTS

A. Tests of Glomerular Function

1. **Glomerulogenesis is complete at 36 weeks' gestation.** Glomerular filtration rate (GFR) increases over the first few years of life related to glomerular maturation.
2. **Normal GFR values as measured by inulin clearance (gold standard)** are shown in Table 19-2.
3. **Creatinine clearance (CCr):**
   Timed urine specimen: Standard measure of GFR; closely approximates inulin clearance in the normal range of GFR. When GFR is low, CCr overestimates GFR. Usually inaccurate in children with obstructive uropathy or problems with bladder emptying.

$$CCr \ (mL/min/1.73 \ m^2) = (U \times [V/P]) \times 1.73/BSA,$$

   where U (mg/dL) = urinary creatinine concentration; V (mL/min) = total urine volume (mL) divided by the duration of the collection (min) (24 hours = 1440 min); P (mg/dL) = serum creatinine concentration (may average two levels); and BSA (m²) = body surface area.
4. **Estimated GFR (eGFR) from plasma creatinine:** Convenient estimate of kidney function in clinical venue as challenging to determine if creatinine is normal, given variation related to body size/muscle mass. If body habitus is markedly abnormal or precise measurement of GFR is needed, consider determining GFR by methods other than estimation. Creatinine must be in steady state to estimate GFR; use caution in the setting of acute kidney injury. Two equations to calculate estimated GFR:
   a. Bedside Chronic Kidney Disease in Children (CKiD) cohort: Newly developed equation based on current laboratory methodologies to determine creatinine. Recommended for eGFR determination in children aged 1–16 years. Estimated GFRs of ≥75 mL/min/1.73 m² determined by this

PROPORTIONALITY CONSTANT FOR CALCULATING GLOMERULAR FILTRATION RATE

Age	k Values
Low birth weight during first year of life	0.33
Term AGA during first year of life	0.45
Children and adolescent girls	0.55
Adolescent boys	0.70

AGA, Appropriate for gestational age.

Data from Schwartz GJ, Brion LP, Spitzer A. The use of plasma creatinine concentration for estimating glomerular filtration rate in infants, children, and adolescents. *Pediatr Clin North Am.* 1987;34:571.

equation likely represent normal kidney function; clinical correlation is recommended as always with GFR estimation.[8]

$$\text{eGFR (mL/min/1.73 m}^2) = 0.413 \times (L/Pcr),$$

where *0.413* is proportionality constant, L = height (cm), and Pcr = plasma creatinine (mg/dL).

b. Schwartz equation: Traditional equation for eGFR. However, given changes in laboratory assays used to determine creatinine, this equation systemically overestimates GFR and should be considered when applying clinically:

$$\text{eGFR (mL/min/1.73 m}^2) = kL/Pcr,$$

where k = proportionality constant; L = height (cm); and Pcr = plasma creatinine (mg/dL) (Table 19-3).

c. Modification of Diet in Renal Disease (MDRD) and Chronic Kidney Disease Epidemiology Collaboration (CKD-EPI): Used to calculate GFR in those > 18 years old. (See NKDEP website.)

5. **Other measurements of GFR:** May be used when more precise determination of GFR is needed (e.g., dosing of chemotherapy). These methods include iothalamate, DTPA, and iohexol.

B. Tests of Kidney Tubular Function

1. **Proximal tubule:**

a. Proximal tubule reabsorption: Proximal tubule is responsible for reabsorption of electrolytes, glucose, and amino acids. Studies to evaluate proximal tubular function compare urine and blood levels of specific compounds, arriving at a percentage of tubular reabsorption (Tx):

$$Tx = 1 - [(Ux/Px)/(UCr/PCr)] \times 100\%,$$

where Ux = concentration of compound in urine; Px = concentration of compound in plasma; Ucr = concentration of creatinine in urine; and Pcr = concentration of creatinine in plasma. This formula can be used for amino acids, electrolytes, calcium, and phosphorus. For example, in the setting of hypophosphatemia, tubular reabsorption of phosphorus near 100% would be expected in a kidney with preserved proximal tubular function.

b. Calculation of fractional excretion of sodium (FENa) is derived from the equation[9]:

$$FENa = [(UNa/PNa)/(UCr)/(PCr)] \times 100\%.$$

FENa is usually <1% in prerenal azotemia or glomerulonephritis and >1% (usually >3%) in acute tubular necrosis (ATN) or postrenal azotemia. Infants have diminished ability to reabsorb sodium; FENa in volume-depleted infants is <3%. Recent diuretic use may give inaccurate results. A fractional excretion of urea (FEurea) may be useful in certain clincal scenarios:

$$FEurea = [(Uurea/Purea)/(UCr/PCr)] \times 100\%$$

FEurea is usually <35% in prerenal azotemia and >50% in ATN.[9]

c. Glucose reabsorption: Glucosuria must be interpreted in relation to simultaneously determined plasma glucose concentration. If plasma glucose concentration is <160 mg/dL and glucose is present in urine, this implies abnormal tubular reabsorption of glucose and proximal renal tubular disease (see Section II.F).

d. Bicarbonate reabsorption: Majority occurs in proximal tubule. Abnormalities in reabsorption lead to type 2 renal tubular acidosis (RTA; see Table 19-9).

2. **Distal tubule:**

a. Urine acidification: A urine acidification defect (distal RTA) should be suspected when random urine pH values are >6 in the presence of moderate systemic metabolic acidosis. Confirm acidification defects by simultaneous venous or arterial pH, plasma bicarbonate concentration, and determination of the pH of fresh urine.

b. Urine concentration occurs in the distal tubule: Urine osmolality, ideally on a first morning urine specimen, can be used to evaluate capacity to concentrate urine. (For more formal testing, see the water deprivation test in Chapter 10.)

c. Urine calcium: Hypercalciuria may be seen with distal RTA, vitamin D intoxication, hyperparathyroidism, immobilization, excessive calcium intake, use of steroids or loop diuretics, or idiopathic. Diagnosis is as follows:

   (1) 24-hour urine: Calcium > 4 mg/kg/24 hr (gold standard)
   (2) Spot urine: Determine calcium/creatinine (Ca/Cr) ratio. Normal urine Ca/Cr ratio does not rule out hypercalciuria. Correlate clinically and follow elevated spot urine Ca/Cr ratio with a 24-hr urine calcium determination if indicated (Table 19-4).[10]

TABLE 19-4

AGE-ADJUSTED CALCIUM/CREATININE RATIOS

Age	Ca^{2+}/Cr Ratio (mg/mg) (95th Percentile for Age)
<7 mo	0.86
7–18 mo	0.60
19 mo–6 yr	0.42
Adults	0.22

From Sargent JD, Stukel TA, Kresel J, et al. Normal values for random urinary calcium-to-creatinine ratios in infancy. *J Pediatr.* 1993;123:393.

V. ACUTE KIDNEY INJURY[11,12]

A. Definition

Sudden decline in kidney function, clinically represented by rising creatinine, with or without changes in urine output.

B. Etiology (Table 19-5)

Causes are generally subdivided into three categories:

1. **Prerenal:** Impaired perfusion of kidneys, the most common cause of acute kidney injury (AKI) in children. Volume depletion is a common cause of prerenal AKI.
2. **Renal:**
a. Parenchymal disease due to vascular or glomerular lesions
b. ATN: Typically a diagnosis of exclusion when no evidence of renal parenchymal disease is present and prerenal and postrenal causes have been eliminated if possible
3. **Postrenal:** Obstruction of the urinary tract, commonly due to inherited anatomic abnormalities

TABLE 19-5

ETIOLOGIES OF ACUTE KIDNEY INJURY

Prerenal	**Decreased true intravascular volume:** e.g., hemorrhage, volume depletion, sepsis, burns
	Decreased effective intravascular volume: e.g., congestive heart failure, hepatorenal syndrome
	Altered glomerular hemodynamics: e.g., NSAIDs, ACE inhibitors (when renal perfusion is already low)
Intrinsic renal	**Acute tubular necrosis:** *Hypoxic/ischemic insults* *Drug-induced*—aminoglycosides, amphotericin B, acyclovir, chemotherapeutic agents (ifosfomide, cisplatin) *Toxin-mediated*—endogenous toxins (myoglobin, hemoglobin); exogenous toxins (ethylene glycol, methanol)
	Interstitial nephritis: *Drug-induced*—ß-lactams, NSAIDs (may be associated with high-grade protein-uria), sulfonamides, PPIs *Idiopathic*
	Uric acid nephropathy (tumor lysis syndrome)
	Glomerulonephritis: In most severe degree, presents as rapidly progressive glomerulonephritis (RPGN)
	Vascular lesions: Renal artery thrombosis, renal vein thrombosis, cortical necrosis, hemolytic uremic syndrome
	Hypoplasia/dysplasia: idiopathic or exposure to nephrotoxic drug in utero
Postrenal	**Obstruction in a solitary kidney** **Bilateral ureteral obstruction** **Urethral obstruction** **Bladder dysfunction**

ACE, Angiotensin-converting enzyme; NSAIDs, nonsteroidal antiinflammatory drugs; PPIs, proton pump inhibitors.
Data from Andreoli SP. Acute kidney injury in children. *Pediatr Nephrol.* 2009;24:253-263.

C. Clinical Presentation

Pallor, decreased urine output, edema, hypertension, vomiting, and lethargy. The hallmark of early kidney failure is often oliguria.

1. **Oliguria:** Urine output <300 mL/m²/24 hr, or <0.5 mL/kg/hr in children and <1.0 mL/kg/hr in infants. May be an appropriate physiologic response to water depletion (prerenal state) or a reflection of intrinsic or obstructive kidney disease.

a. Blood urea nitrogen/creatinine (BUN/Cr) ratio (both in mg/dL): Interpret ratios with caution in small children with low serum creatinines
   (1) 10-20 (normal ratio): Suggests intrinsic renal disease in the setting of oliguria
   (2) >20: Suggests volume depletion, prerenal azotemia, or gastrointestinal bleeding
   (3) <5: Suggests liver disease, starvation, inborn error of metabolism

b. Laboratory differentiation of oliguria (Table 19-6)

D. Acute Tubular Necrosis

Clinically defined by three phases:

1. **Oliguric phase:** Period of severe oliguria that may last days. If oliguria or anuria persists for longer than 3–6 weeks, kidney recovery from ATN is less likely.
2. **High urine output phase:** Begins with increased urine output and progresses to passage of large volumes of isosthenuric urine containing sodium levels of 80–150 mEq/L.
3. **Recovery phase:** Signs and symptoms usually resolve rapidly, but polyuria may persist for days to weeks.

E. Treatment Considerations

1. **Placement of indwelling catheter to monitor urine output.**
2. **Prerenal and postrenal factors** should be excluded and intravascular volume maintained with appropriate fluids in consultation with a pediatric nephrologist.

F. Complications

Often dependent on clinical severity; usually includes fluid overload (hypertension, congestive heart failure [CHF], pulmonary edema), electrolyte disturbances (hyperkalemia), metabolic acidosis, hyperphosphatemia, and uremia.

TABLE 19-6		
LABORATORY DIFFERENTIATION OF OLIGURIA		
Test	Prerenal	Renal
FENa	≤1%	>3%
BUN/Cr ratio	>20:1	<10:1
Urine specific gravity	>1.015	<1.010

G. Acute Dialysis

1. **Indications:**

When metabolic or fluid derangements are not controlled by aggressive medical management alone. Generally accepted criteria include the following, although a nephrologist should always be consulted:

a. **Acidosis:** Intractable metabolic acidosis.

b. Electrolyte abnormalities: Hyperkalemia >6.5 mEq/L despite restriction of delivery and medical management. Calcium and phosphorus imbalance (e.g., hypocalcemia with tetany, seizures in the presence of a very high serum phosphate level). Derangements implicated in neurologic abnormalities.

c. Ingestions or accumulation of dialyzable toxin or poison: Lithium, ammonia, alcohol, barbiturates, ethylene glycol, isopropanol, methanol, salicylates, theophylline. When available, poison control centers can provide guidance and expertise.

d. Volume overload: Evidence of pulmonary edema or hypertension.

e. Uremia: BUN >150 mg/dL (lower if rising rapidly), uremic pericardial effusion, neurologic symptoms.

2. **Techniques:**

a. Peritoneal dialysis: Requires catheter to access peritoneal cavity, as well as adequate peritoneal perfusion. May be used acutely or chronically.

b. Intermittent hemodialysis: Requires placement of special vascular access catheters. May be method of choice for certain toxins (e.g., ammonia, uric acid, poisons) or when there are contraindications to peritoneal dialysis.

c. Continuous arteriovenous hemofiltration/hemodialysis (CAVH/D) and continuous venovenous hemofiltration/hemodialysis (CVVH/D):

(1) Requires special vascular access catheter.

(2) Lower efficiency of solute removal compared with intermittent hemodialysis, but higher efficiency is not necessary because of the continuous nature of this form of dialysis.

(3) Sustained nature of dialysis allows for more gradual removal of volume/solutes, which is ideal for patients with hemodynamic or respiratory instability.

VI. HEMATURIA AND ASSOCIATED DISORDERS[13,14]

A. Definitions

1. **Gross hematuria:** Blood in urine visible to the naked eye.

2. **Microscopic hematuria:** Blood not visible to naked eye, but ≥5 red blood cells per high-power field (RBCs/hpf).

3. **Red urine that is not hematuria:** Hemoglobinuria, myoglobinuria, brick dust urine (precipitated urates in typically acidic urine of neonates).

4. **Persistent hematuria:** Three positive urinalyses, based on dipstick and microscopic examination over at least a 2- to 3-week period, warranting further evaluation.

5. **Extraglomerular hematuria:** No RBC casts, minimal if any proteinuria.

TABLE 19-7

CAUSES OF HEMATURIA IN CHILDREN

Kidney-related disease	Isolated glomerular disease	IgA nephropathy, Alport syndrome, thin glomerular basement membrane nephropathy, postinfectious/poststreptococcal glomerulonephritis, membranous nephropathy, membrano-proliferative glomerulonephritis, focal segmental glomerulo-sclerosis, antiglomerular basement membrane disease
	Multisystem disease involving glomerulus	Systemic lupus erythematosus nephritis, Henoch-Schönlein purpura nephritis, granulomatosis with polyangiitis, poly-arteritis nodosa, Goodpasture syndrome, hemolytic-uremic syndrome, sickle cell glomerulopathy, HIV nephropathy
	Tubulointersti-tial disease	Pyelonephritis, interstitial nephritis, papillary necrosis, acute tubular necrosis
	Vascular	Arterial or venous thrombosis, malformations (aneurysms, hemangiomas), nutcracker syndrome, hemoglobinopathy (sickle cell trait/disease)
	Anatomic	Hydronephrosis, cystic kidney disease, polycystic kidney disease, multicystic dysplasia, tumor, trauma
Urinary tract disease		Inflammation (cystitis, urethritis)
		Urolithiasis
		Trauma
		Coagulopathy
		Arteriovenous malformations (AVMs)
		Bladder tumor
		Factitious syndrome

Data from Kliegman RM, Stanton BF, St. Geme JW, et al. *Nelson Textbook of Pediatrics*. 19th ed. Philadelphia: Saunders; 2011:1779.

6. **Glomerular hematuria:** Most often tea-colored urine but may be red/pink, RBC casts, dysmorphic RBCs, associated with proteinuria.
7. **Acute nephritic syndrome:** Classically tea-colored urine, facial or body edema, hypertension, and oliguria.

B. Etiologies (Table 19-7)

C. Evaluation (Fig. 19-2)

1. **Differentiate glomerular and extraglomerular hematuria:** Examine urine sediment looking for RBC casts and protein.
  a. Glomerular hematuria
    (1) Determine whether isolated kidney disease or multisystem disease: Complete blood cell count (CBC) with differential and smear, serum electrolytes with Ca, BUN/Cr, serum protein/albumin, and other testing driven by history and exam, including ANA, hepatitis B and C serologies, HIV, family history, audiology screen if indicated.
    (2) Consider other studies to determine underlying diagnosis: C3/C4, antineutrophil antibody (c- and p-ANCA), anti–double-stranded DNA

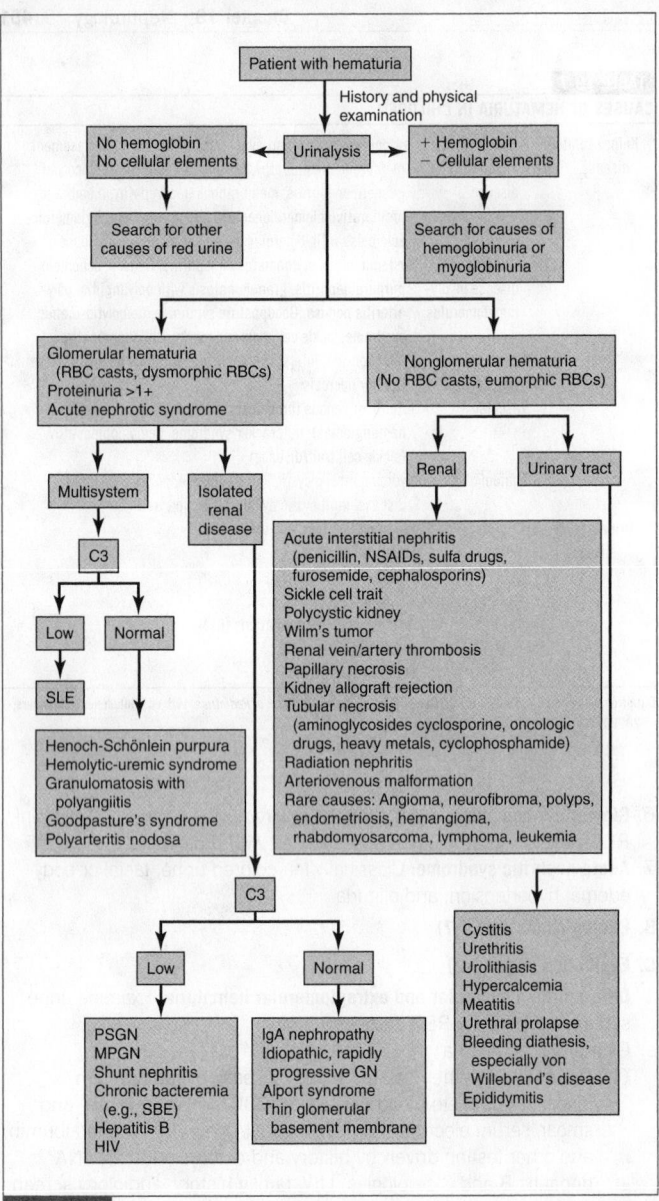

FIGURE 19-2

Diagnostic strategy for hematuria. GN, Glomerulonephritis; HIV, human immunodeficiency virus; MPGN, membranoproliferative glomerulonephritis; NSAIDS, nonsteroidal antiinflammatory drugs; PSGN, poststreptococcal glomerulonephritis; RBC, red blood cell; SBE, subacute bacterial endocarditis; SLE, systemic lupus erythematosus.

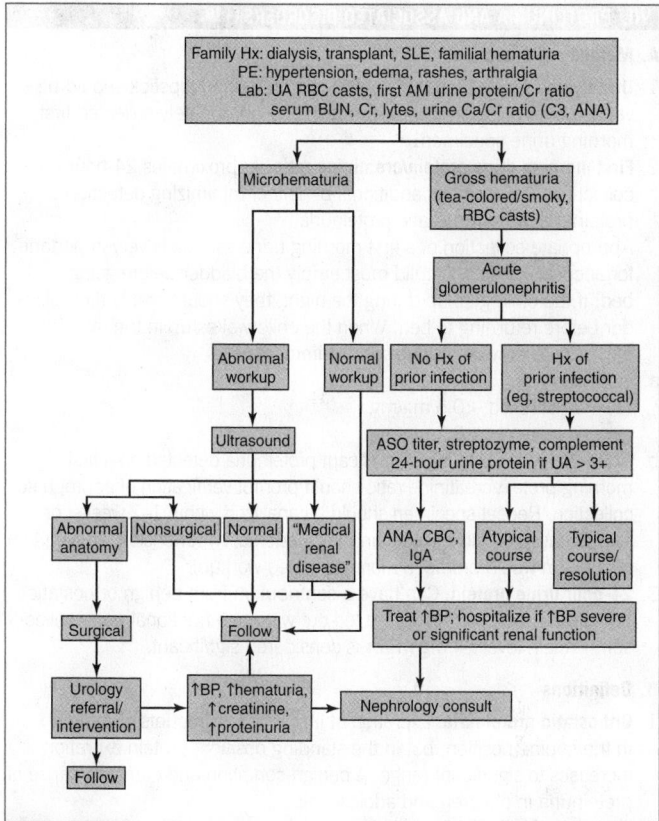

FIGURE 19-3

Management algorithm for hematuria. *(Data from Hay WM, Levin MJ, Deterding RR, Azbug MJ, Sondheimer JM. CURRENT Diagnosis & Treatment Pediatrics. 21st edition. Available at www.accessmedicine.com, Figure 24-1.*

b. Extraglomerular hematuria
   (1) Rule out infection: Urine culture, gonorrhea, chlamydia
   (2) Rule out trauma: History, consider imaging of abdomen/pelvis
   (3) Investigate other potential causes: urine Ca/Cr ratio or 24-hour urine for kidney stone risk analysis, sickle cell screen, kidney/bladder ultrasound. Consider serum electrolytes with Ca, consider prothrombin time/partial thromboplastin time (PT/PTT).

D. Management (Fig. 19-3)

VII. PROTEINURIA AND ASSOCIATED DISORDERS[14,15]

A. Methods of Detection

1. **Urinalysis:** See Section II.E. Proteinuria on a urine dipstick should be verified by a protein/creatinine ratio in an appropriately collected first morning urine specimen.

2. **First morning urine protein/creatinine ratio:** Approximates 24-hour urine collections well and has additional benefit of minimizing detection of proteinuria from orthostatic proteinuria.

   Appropriate collection of a first morning urine sample is very important for accurate results. A child must empty the bladder before going to bed. If the child gets up during the night, they should empty their bladder before returning to bed. When the child wakes up in the morning, they should provide a urine sample immediately.

   a. Normal ratios:
      (1) <2 years old: <0.5 mg/mg
      (2) >2 years old: <0.2 mg/mg
   b. Abnormal ratios (mg/mg): Significant proteinuria detected on a first morning protein/creatinine ratio should prompt verification of appropriate collection. Repeat specimen should be analyzed within 1–2 weeks, or sooner based on clinical scenario (e.g., edema, hypertension, or symptom of concern would prompt a more expedited workup).

3. **24-hour urine protein:** Can have a contribution from benign orthostatic proteinuria, which cannot be ruled out without a fractional urine collection. Protein level >4 mg/m^2/hr is considered significant.

B. Definitions

1. **Orthostatic proteinuria:** Excretion of insignificant amounts of protein in the supine position, but in the standing position, protein excretion increases to significant range. A benign condition and common cause of proteinuria in children and adolescents.

2. **Fixed proteinuria:** Proteinuria found on first morning urine void over several consecutive days. Suggestive of kidney disease.

3. **Microalbuminuria:** Presence of albumin in urine below detectable range of dipsticks. In adults, defined as 30–300 mg/g creatinine. Most often used in screening for kidney disease secondary to diabetes.

4. **Significant proteinuria:** UPr:UCr ratio 0.2–2.0 mg/mg or 4–40 mg/m^2/hr in a 24-hour collection.

5. **Nephrotic-range proteinuria:** UPr:UCr ratio >2 mg/mg or >40 mg/m^2/hr in a 24-hour collection. In adults, 24-hour urine protein excretion of 3000 mg/24 hr.

6. **Nephrotic syndrome:** Nephrotic-range proteinuria, hypoalbuminemia, and edema. Also associated with hyperlipidemia (cholesterol >200 mg/dL).

C. Etiologies (Box 19-1)

See Section VII.E for information about nephrotic syndrome.

BOX 19-1

CAUSES OF PROTEINURIA

Transient proteinuria: Caused by fever, exercise, dehydration, cold exposure, seizure, stress

Orthostatic proteinuria

Glomerular diseases with isolated proteinuria: Idiopathic (minimal change disease) nephrotic syndrome, focal segmental glomerulosclerosis, mesangial proliferative glomerulonephritis, membranous nephropathy, membranoproliferative glomerulonephritis, amyloidosis, diabetic nephropathy, sickle cell nephropathy

Glomerular diseases with proteinuria as a prominent feature: Acute postinfectious glomerulonephritis, immunoglobulin (Ig) A nephropathy

Tubular disease: Cystinosis, Wilson disease, acute tubular necrosis, tubulointerstitial nephritis, polycystic kidney disease, renal dysplasia

Data from Kliegman RM, Stanton BF, St. Geme JW, et al. *Nelson Textbook of Pediatrics*. 19th ed. Philadelphia: Saunders, 2011:1801.

BOX 19-2

BASIC EVALUATION OF SIGNIFICANT (NEPHROTIC AND NON-NEPHROTIC) PROTEINURIA

Complete metabolic panel with phosphorus

C3 and C4

Antinuclear antibody, anti–double-stranded DNA

Hepatitis B, C, and HIV in high-risk populations

Antineutrophil antibodies (c- and p-ANCA)

Kidney and bladder ultrasonography

Referral to nephrologist

D. Evaluation[16]

Further evaluation is necessary if proteinuria is significant and not secondary to orthostatic proteinuria (Box 19-2).

E. Nephrotic Syndrome[17]

Manifestation of a glomerular disorder secondary to primary kidney disease, a systemic disorder resulting in glomerular injury, or rarely certain drugs

1. **Clinical manifestations**

Hypoalbuminemia and decrease in oncotic pressure results in generalized edema. Initial swelling commonly occurs on the face (especially periorbital), as well as in the pretibial area. Eye swelling is often mistaken for allergic reactions or seasonal allergies.

2. **Etiologies** (Table 19-8 and Box 19-3)

3. **Management of minimal change nephrotic syndrome (MCNS):** empirical corticosteroid treatment without kidney biopsy is recommended for children without atypical features. Hospitalization recommended for children with overwhelming edema or infection.

a. Steroid-responsive: Roughly 95% of patients with MCNS and 20% with focal segmental glomerulosclerosis (FSGS) achieve remission within 4–8 weeks of starting prednisone. Prednisone starts with 60 mg/m² or 2 mg/kg/day (maximum dose, 60 mg/day) for 6 weeks, followed by

TABLE 19-8

ETIOLOGIES OF NEPHROTIC SYNDROME

Primary Causes (90%)	Secondary Causes (10%)
Minimal change nephrotic syndrome (MCNS): 85% of idiopathic causes in children	Infections (HIV, hepatitis B, hepatitis C)
Focal segmental glomerulosclerosis (FSGS)	Systemic lupus erythematosus
Membranous nephropathy	Diabetes mellitus
IgA nephropathy	Drugs
Genetic disorders involving the slit diaphragm	Malignancy (leukemias, lymphomas)

BOX 19-3

FACTORS SUGGESTING DIAGNOSIS OTHER THAN IDIOPATHIC MINIMAL CHANGE NEPHROTIC SYNDROME

Age <1 year or >10 years
Family history of kidney disease
Extrarenal disease (arthritis, rash, anemia)
Chronic disease of another organ or systemic disease
Symptoms due to intravascular volume expansion (hypertension, pulmonary edema)
Kidney failure
Active urine sediment (red blood cell casts)

40 mg/m^2 or 1.5 mg/kg on alternate days for 6 weeks, followed by a prednisone taper. Response is the best prognostic indicator, including the likelihood of underlying MCNS.

b. Frequently relapsing: Defined as two or more relapses within 6 months of initial response, or four or more relapses in any 12-month period.

c. Steroid-dependent: Defined as two consecutive relapses during tapering or within 14 days of cessation of steroids. Some patients can be managed with low-dose steroids given daily or on alternate days, but many still relapse. Second-line treatments for frequently relapsing and steroid-dependent nephrotic syndrome: Cyclophosphamide, mycophenolate mofetil (MMF), calcineurin inhibitors, or levamisole.

d. Steroid-resistant: Lack of remission or partial remission after 8 weeks of corticosteroids. Second-line agents, including calcineurin inhibitors or MMF, are often introduced once steroid resistance is confirmed.

e. Further evaluation: Biopsy recommended for macroscopic hematuria, persistent creatinine elevation, low complement levels, and persistent proteinuria after 4–8 weeks of adequate steroid treatment.

f. Complications: AKI, thromboembolic disease, infection, and side effects of systemic steroids.

VIII. TUBULAR DISORDERS

A. Renal Tubular Acidosis (Table 19-9)[9,18]

A group of transport defects resulting in abnormal urine acidification; due to deficiencies of reabsorption of bicarbonate (HCO_3^-), excretion of

TABLE 19-9

BIOCHEMICAL AND CLINICAL CHARACTERISTICS OF VARIOUS TYPES OF RENAL TUBULAR ACIDOSIS

	Type 1 (Distal)	Type 2 (Proximal)	Type 4 (Hypoaldosteronism)
Mechanism	Impaired distal acidification	Impaired bicarbonate absorption	Decreased aldosterone secretion or aldosterone effect
Etiology	Hereditary Sickle cell Toxins/drugs Cirrhosis Obstructive uropathy Connective tissue disorder	Hereditary Metabolic disease Fanconi syndrome Prematurity Toxins/heavy metals Amyloidosis PNH	Absolute mineralocorticoid deficiency Adrenal failure CAH DM Pseudohypoaldosteronism Interstitial nephritis
Minimal urine pH	>5.5	<5.5 (urine pH can be >5.5 with a bicarbonate load)	<5.5
Fractional excretion of bicarbonate (FeHCO₃)	↓ (<5%)	↑ (>15%)	↓ (<5%)
Plasma K+ concentration	Normal or ↓	Usually ↓	↑
Urine anion gap	Positive	Positive or negative	Positive
Nephrocalcinosis/ nephrolithiasis	Common	Rare	Rare
Treatment	1–3 mEq/kg/day of HCO₃ (5–10 mEq/kg/day if bicarb wasting)	5–20 mEq/kg/day of HCO₃	1–5 mEq/kg/day of HCO₃ May add Fludrocortisone and potassium binders

CAH, Congenital adrenal hyperplasia; DM, diabetes mellitus.; PNH, paroxysmal nocturnal hemoglobinuria.

Adapted from Holiday MA et al. *Pediatric Nephrology*. Baltimore: Williams & Wilkins, 1994:650.

hydrogen ions (H+), or both. Results in a persistent nonanion-gap metabolic acidosis accompanied by hyperchloremia. Renal tubular acidosis (RTA) syndromes often do not progress to kidney failure but are instead characterized by a normal GFR. Clinical presentation may be characterized by failure to thrive, polyuria, constipation, vomiting, and dehydration.

1. **Fractional excretion of bicarbonate (FeHCO₃) should be checked after a HCO₃ load.** Can help differentiate the types of RTA. Equation is based on the same concept found in Section IV.B.1:

$$FeHCO_3 = ([UHCO_3/PHCO_3]/[UCr/PCr]) \times 100\%$$

2. **Urine anion gap (UAG) is useful in differentiating types of RTA,** but it should not be used when a patient is volume depleted or has an anion-gap metabolic acidosis.

$$UAG = UNa + UK - UCl$$

B. Type 3 (Combined Proximal and Distal) RTA

Infants with mild type 1 and mild type 2 defects were previously classified as type 3 RTA. Studies have shown that this is not a genetic entity itself, which has resulted in reclassification as a subtype of type 1 RTA that occurs primarily in premature infants.

C. Fanconi Syndrome

Generalized dysfunction of the proximal tubule resulting not only in bicarbonate loss but also in variable wasting of phosphate, glucose, and amino acids. May be hereditary, as in cystinosis and galactosemia, or acquired through toxin injury and other immunologic factors. Clinically characterized by rickets and impaired growth.

D. Nephrogenic Diabetes Insipidus

1. **Water conservation is dependent on antidiuretic hormone (ADH) and its effects on the distal renal tubules.** Polyuria, a hallmark of nephrogenic diabetes insipidus (NDI), is due to diminished or lack of response of the ADH receptor in the distal renal tubules. Hereditary defects of ADH receptor or acquired insults (e.g., interstitial nephritis, sickle cell disease, lithium toxicity, chronic kidney disease [CKD]) may underlie NDI.
2. **Must be differentiated from other causes of polyuria:**
   a. Central diabetes insipidus: ADH deficiency that may be idiopathic or acquired (through infection or pituitary trauma)
   b. Diabetes mellitus
   c. Psychogenic polydipsia
   d. Cerebral salt wasting

IX. CHRONIC KIDNEY DISEASE[19]

Kidney damage for >3 months, as defined by structural or functional abnormalities, with or without decreased GFR. Classified as:

Stage I: Kidney injury with normal or increased GFR
Stage II: GFR 60–89 mL/min/1.73 m^2
Stage III: GFR 30–59 mL/min/1.73 m^2
Stage IV: GFR 15–29 mL/min/1.73 m^2
Stage V: GFR <15 mL/min/1.73 m^2 or dialysis

A. Etiology

There is a close association with age when kidney failure is first detected. CKD in children <5 years is most commonly due to congenital abnormalities (e.g., kidney hypoplasia/dysplasia, urologic malformations), whereas older children more commonly have acquired glomerular diseases (e.g., glomerulonephritis, FSGS) or hereditary disorders (e.g., Alport syndrome).

B. Clinical Manifestations (Table 19-10)

1. **Edema:**
   Secondary to excessive accumulation of both Na^+ and water. Causes of generalized edema include:

TABLE 19-10

CLINICAL MANIFESTATIONS OF CHRONIC KIDNEY DISEASE

Manifestation	Mechanisms
Uremia	Decline in GFR
Acidosis	Urinary bicarbonate wasting
	Decreased excretion of NH_4 and acid
Sodium wasting	Solute diuresis, tubular damage
	Aldosterone resistance
Sodium retention	Nephrotic syndrome
	CHF
	Reduced GFR
Urinary concentrating defect	Solute diuresis, tubular damage
	ADH resistance
Hyperkalemia	Decline in GFR, acidosis
	Aldosterone resistance
Renal osteodystrophy	Impaired production of 1,25 (OH) vitamin D
	Decreased intestinal calcium absorption
	Impaired phosphorus excretion
	Secondary hyperparathyroidism
Growth retardation	Protein-calorie deficiency
	Renal osteodystrophy
	Acidosis
	Anemia
	Inhibitors of insulin-like growth factors
Anemia	Decreased erythropoietin production
	Low-grade hemolysis
	Bleeding, iron deficiency
	Decreased erythrocyte survival
	Inadequate folic acid intake
	Inhibitors of erythropoiesis
Bleeding tendency	Thrombocytopenia
	Defective platelet function
Infection	Defective granulocyte function
	Glomerular loss of immunoglobulin/opsonins
Neurologic complaints	Uremic factors
Gastrointestinal ulceration	Gastric acid hypersecretion/gastritis
	Reflux
	Decreased motility
Hypertension	Sodium and water overload
	Excessive renin production
Hypertriglyceridemia	Diminished plasma lipoprotein lipase activity
Pericarditis and cardiomyopathy	Unknown
Glucose intolerance	Tissue insulin resistance

ADH, Anti-diuretic hormone; CHF, congestive heart failure; GFR, glomerular filtration rate; NH_4, ammonium.
Adapted from Brenner BM. *Brenner and Rector's The Kidney.* 6th ed. Philadelphia: WB Saunders, 2000.

a. Inability to excrete Na^+ with or without water (e.g., glomerular diseases resulting in decreased GFR)
b. Decreased oncotic pressure (e.g., nephrotic syndrome, protein-losing enteropathy, hepatic failure, CHF)
c. Reduced cardiac output (e.g., CHF, pericardial disease)
d. Mineralcorticoid excess (e.g., hyperreninemia, hyperaldosteronism)
2. **Other manifestations below in Table 19-10**

X. CHRONIC HYPERTENSION[20-22]

NOTE: For management of acute hypertension and normal BP parameters, see Chapters 4 and 7.

A. Definition

1. **Normal blood pressure (BP):** Systolic and diastolic BP <90th percentile for age, gender, and height. See Tables 7-1 and 7-2.
2. **High-normal BP (prehypertension):** Systolic and/or diastolic BP between 90th and 95th percentiles for age, gender, and height, or if BP exceeds 120/80 (even if <90th precentile for age, gender, and height).
3. **Hypertension:** Systolic and/or diastolic BPs >95th percentile for age, gender, and height on three separate occasions.
4. **Measurement of BP in children:**
a. Children ≥3 years should have BP measured at all routine and emergency visits. Children <3 years with risk factors (e.g.,history of prematurity/low birth weight, congenital heart disease, kidney disease or family history of kidney disease, history of malignancy, solid organ or bone marrow transplant) should have BP measured.
b. BP should be measured in a seated position 5 minutes after resting quietly; auscultation is preferred.
c. Appropriate cuff size has a bladder width at least 40% of upper arm circumference at midway point. Bladder length should cover 80%–100% of arm circumference. Cuffs that are too small may result in falsely elevated BPs. Choose a larger-sized cuff if there is a choice between two.

B. Etiologies of Hypertension in Neonates, Infants, and Children (Table 19-11)

C. Evaluation of Chronic Hypertension

1. **Rule out factitious causes of hypertension** (improper cuff size or measurement technique [e.g., manual vs. oscillometric]), nonpathologic causes of hypertension (e.g., fever, pain, anxiety, muscle spasm), and iatrogenic mechanisms (e.g., medications, excessive fluid administration).
2. **History:** Headache, blurred vision, dyspnea on exertion, edema, obstructive sleep apnea (OSA) symptoms, endocrine symptoms (diaphoresis, flushing, constipation, weakness, etc.), history of neonatal intensive care unit (NICU) stay, rule out pregnancy, history of UTIs, history of medications and supplements, illicit drug use, or any family history of kidney dysfunction or hypertension.

TABLE 19-11

CAUSES OF HYPERTENSION BY AGE GROUP

Age	Most Common	Less Common
Neonates/infants	Renal artery thrombosis after umbilical artery catheterization Coarctation of aorta Renal artery stenosis	Bronchopulmonary dysplasia Medications Patent ductus arteriosus Intraventricular hemorrhage
1–10 yr	Renal parenchymal disease Coarctation of aorta	Renal artery stenosis Hypercalcemia Neurofibromatosis Neurogenic tumors Pheochromocytoma Mineralocorticoid excess Hyperthyroidism Transient hypertension Immobilization-induced Sleep apnea Essential hypertension Medications
11 yr–adolescence	Renal parenchymal disease Essential hypertension	All diagnoses listed in this table

Modified from Sinaiko A. Hypertension in children. *N Engl J Med.* 1996;335:26.

3. **Physical examination:** Four-extremity pulses and BPs, endocrine disease stigmata, edema, hypertrophied tonsils, skin lesions, abdominal mass, or abdominal bruit.

4. **Clinical evaluation of confirmed hypertension:**

a. Laboratory studies: UA with microscopic evaluation, urine culture, serum electrolytes, CBC, Cr, BUN, fasting glucose, and lipid panel.

b. Imaging: Kidney and bladder ultrasonography and echocardiography. Consider renovascular imaging as indicated.

c. Consider (as indicated) thyroid function tests, urine catecholamines, plasma and urinary steroids, plasma renin, aldosterone, and toxicology screen. Consider polysomnography and retinal examination.

5. **Consider referral to specialist in hypertension.**

D. **Treatment of Hypertension**

1. **Nonpharmacologic:** Aerobic exercise, sodium restriction, smoking cessation, and weight loss indicated in all patients with hypertension. Reevaluate BP after lifestyle interventions, and begin pharmacologic therapy if hypertension persists.

2. **Pharmacologic:** Indications include secondary hypertension, symptomatic hypertension, target-organ damage, diabetes mellitus, and persistent hypertension despite nonpharmacologic measures.

E. **Classification of Hypertension in Children and Adolescents, with Measurement Frequency and Therapy Recommendations (Table 19-12)**

TABLE 19-12

CLASSIFICATION OF HYPERTENSION IN CHILDREN AND ADOLESCENTS AND THERAPY RECOMMENDATIONS

	SBP or DBP Percentile	Frequency of BP Measurement	Pharmacologic Therapy (in Addition to Lifestyle Modifications)
Normal	<90th percentile	Recheck at next physical examination	None
Prehypertension	90th to <95th percentile or if BP exceeds 120/80 mm Hg even if <90th percentile	Recheck in 6 months	None unless compelling indications: CKD, DM, heart failure, or LVH
Stage 1 hypertension	95th–99th percentile plus 5 mm Hg	Recheck in 1–2 weeks, sooner if patient is symptomatic; if persistently elevated on 2 additional occasions, evaluate or refer	Initiate therapy based on symptoms, secondary hypertension, end-organ damage, diabetes, persistent hypertension despite nonpharmacologic measures
Stage 2 hypertension	>99th percentile plus 5 mm Hg	Evaluate or refer within 1 week or immediately if the patient is symptomatic	Initiate therapy

CKD, Chronic kidney disease; DBP, diastolic blood pressure; DM, diabetes mellitus; LVH, left ventricular hypertrophy; SBP, systolic blood pressure.

Modified from National High Blood Pressure Education Program Working Group on High Blood Pressure in Children and Adolescents: The fourth report on the diagnosis, evaluation and treatment of high blood pressure in children and adolescents. *Pediatrics.* 2004;114:555-576.

F. Antihypertensive Drugs for Outpatient Management of Hypertension in Children 1–17 Years of Age (Table 19-13)

XI. NEPHROLITHIASIS[23,24]

A. Epidemiology

Lower incidence than adults but increasingly recognized.

B. Risk Factors

Congenital and structural urologic abnormalities (urinary stasis), hypercalciuria, hyperoxaluria/oxalosis, hypocitraturia, other metabolic abnormalities.

C. Presentation

Microscopic hematuria (90%), flank/abdominal pain (50%–75%), gross hematuria (30%–55%), concomitant UTI in up to 20%. Have higher likelihood than adults of having asymptomatic stones, especially younger children.

D. Diagnosis

Ultrasonography is an effective and preferred modality, particularly at centers with expertise, given benefit of avoiding radiation exposure. In certain scenarios (radiolucent stones such as uric acid stones, ureteral stones,

TABLE 19-13

ANTIHYPERTENSIVE DRUGS FOR OUTPATIENT MANAGEMENT OF HYPERTENSION IN CHILDREN 1–17 YEARS OF AGE

Class	Drug	Comments
Angiotensin-converting enzyme (ACE) inhibitor	Benazepril Captopril Enalapril Fosinopril Lisinopril Quinapril	Blocks angiotensin I to angiotensin II Decreases proteinuria while preserving renal function Contraindicated in pregnancy, compromised renal perfusion Check serum potassium and creatinine periodically to monitor for hyperkalemia and uremia Monitor for cough and angioedema
Angiotensin-II receptor blocker (ARB)	Irbesartan Losartan	Contraindicated in pregnancy Check serum potassium and creatinine periodically to monitor for hyperkalemia and uremia
α- and β-Blockers	Labetalol Carvedilol	Causes decreased peripheral resistance and decreased heart rate Contraindications: asthma, heart failure, insulin-dependent diabetes Heart rate is dose-limiting May impair athletic performance
β-Blocker	Atenolol Metoprolol Propranolol	Decreases heart rate, cardiac output, and renin release. Noncardioselective agents (e.g., propranolol) are contraindicated in asthma and heart failure Metoprolol and atenolol are β_1 selective Heart rate is dose-limiting May impair athletic performance Should not be used in insulin-dependent diabetics
Calcium channel blocker	Amlodipine Felodipine Isradipine	Acts on vascular smooth muscles Renal perfusion/function is minimally affected; generally few side effects Amlodipine and isradipine can be compounded into suspensions
	Extended-release nifedipine	May cause tachycardia
Central α-agonist	Clonidine	Stimulates brainstem α_2 receptors and decreases peripheral adrenergic drive May cause dry mouth and/or sedation (↓ opiate withdrawal) Transdermal preparation also available Sudden cessation of therapy can lead to severe rebound hypertension

TABLE 19-13

ANTIHYPERTENSIVE DRUGS FOR OUTPATIENT MANAGEMENT OF HYPERTENSION IN CHILDREN 1–17 YEARS OF AGE (Continued)

Class	Drug	Comments
Diuretic	Furosemide Bumetanide	Side effects are hyponatremia, hypokalemia, and ototoxicity
	Hydrochlorothia- zide (HCTZ) Chlorthalidone	Side effects are hypokalemia, hypercalcemia, hyperuricemia, and hyperlipidemia
	Spironolactone Triamterene Amiloride	Useful as add-on therapy in patients being treated with drugs from other drug classes Potassium-sparing diuretics are modest antihypertensives. They may cause severe hyperkalemia, especially if given with ACE inhibitor or ARB
Peripheral α-antagonist	Doxazosin Prazosin Terazosin	May cause hypotension and syncope, especially after first dose
Vasodilator	Hydralazine	Hydralazine can cause a lupus-like syndrome Directly acts on vascular smooth muscle and is very potent Tachycardia, Na retention, and water retention are common side effects
	Minoxidil	Used in combination with diuretics or β-blockers Minoxidil is usually reserved for patients with hypertension resistant to multiple drugs

Modified from National High Blood Pressure Education Program Working Group on High Blood Pressure in Children and Adolescents. The fourth report on the diagnosis, evaluation, and treatment of high blood pressure in children and adolescents. *Pediatrics.* 2004;114:568-569; Hospital for Sick Children. *The HSC Handbook of Pediatrics.* 9th ed. St. Louis: Mosby, 1997; Sinaiko A. Treatment of hypertension in children. *Pediatr Nephrol.* 1994;8:603-609; and Khattak S et al. Efficacy of amlodipine in pediatric bone marrow transplant patients. *Clin Pediatr.* 1998;37:31-35.

and lack of ultrasonographic expertise), noncontrast helical CT may be preferred to improve diagnostic sensitivity.

E. Management:

1. **Pain control, urine culture, hydration.** Some centers initiate α-blockers to facilitate stone passage, although evidence of benefit in children is equivocal.

2. **Urologic intervention** (extracorporeal shock wave lithotripsy, ureteroscopy, and percutaneous nephrolithostomy). May be necessary in setting of unremitting pain or urinary obstruction, especially in the setting of AKI or at-risk patient (e.g., solitary kidney, etc.).

3. **Collect and analyze stone composition to aid in prevention of future stones.**

F. Workup

Up to 75% of children with a kidney stone will have a metabolic abnormality (e.g., hypercalciuria, hyperoxaluria, hyperuricosuria, cystinuria). Workup should include analysis of the stone (if possible), urinalysis, basic metabolic panel, and phosphate, magnesium, and uric acid levels.

If evidence of elevated calcium or phosphate, obtain parathyroid hormone (PTH) level and consider checking 25- and 1,25(OH) vitamin D levels. A 24-hour urine collection should be obtained several weeks after the stone has passed, and urine sodium, calcium, urate, oxalate, citrate, creatinine, and cystine should be evaluated.

G. Prevention

1. **Recurrence of a kidney stone in children is common.**
2. **All children with history of stones should increase fluid intake** (e.g., at least 2 L/day in those >10 years old).
3. **Targeted interventions of any identified metabolic abnormalities** (e.g., low-sodium diet in those with hypercalciuria). Pharmacologic interventions are also available in certain scenarios (e.g., citrate supplementation).

REFERENCES

1. Fischbach FT, Dunning MB. *A Manual of Laboratory and Diagnostic Tests.* 8th ed. Philadelphia: Lippincott Williams & Wilkins, 2008.
2. Hooton T, et al. Diagnosis, Prevention, and Treatment of Catheter-Associated Urinary Tract Infections in Adults: 2009 International Clinical Practice Guidelines from the Infectious Disease Society of America. *Clinical Infectious Diseases.* 2010;50:625-663.
3. Subcommittee on Urinary Tract Infection, Steering Committee on Quality Improvement and Management. Urinary tract infection: clinical practice guideline for the diagnosis and management of the initial UTI in febrile infants and children 2 to 24 months. *Pediatrics.* 2001;128:595-610.
4. Michael M, Hodson EM, Craig JC, et al. Short versus standard duration oral antibiotic therapy for acute urinary tract infection in children. *Cochrane Database Syst Rev.* 2003; (Issue 1). Art. No.: CD003966. doi: 10.1002/14651858. CD003966.
5. Elder JS, Peters CA, Arant BS Jr, et al. Pediatric Vesicoureteral Reflux Guidelines Panel summary report on the management of primary vesicoureteral reflux in children. *J Urol.* 1997;157:1846-1851.
6. Conway PH, Cnaan A, Zaoutis T, et al. Recurrent urinary tract infections in children: risk factors and association with prophylactic antimicrobials. *JAMA.* 2007;298:179-186.
7. Craig JC, Irwig LM, Knight JF, et al. Does treatment of vesicoureteric reflux in childhood prevent end-stage renal disease attributable to reflux nephropathy? *Pediatrics.* 2000;105:1236-1241.
8. Schwartz GJ, Munoz A, Schneider MF. New equations to estimate GFR in children with CKD. *J Am Soc Nephrol.* 2009;20:629-637.
9. Carmody JB. Focus on diagnosis: urine electrolytes. *Pediatr Rev..* 2011;32:65-68.
10. Sargent JD, Stukel TA, Kresel J, et al. Normal values for random urinary calcium to creatinine ratios in infancy. *J Pediatr.* 1993;123:393.
11. Whyte DA, Fine RN. Acute renal failure in children. *Pediatr Rev.* 2008;29:299-306.
12. Andreoli SP. Acute kidney injury in children. *Pediatr Nephrol.* 2009;24:253-263.
13. Massengill SF. Hematuria. *Pediatr Rev.* 2008;29:342-348.
14. Kliegman RM, Stanton BF. *Nelson Textbook of Pediatrics.* 19th ed. Philadelphia: Saunders, 2011.

15. Cruz C, Spitzer A. When you find protein or blood in urine. *Contemp Pediatr.* 1998;15:89.
16. Gipson DS, Massengill SF, Yao L, et al. Management of childhood-onset nephrotic syndrome. *Pediatrics.* 2009;124:747-757.
17. Gordillo R, Spitzer A. The nephrotic syndrome. *Pediatr Rev..* 2009;30:94-104.
18. Soriano JR. Renal tubular acidosis: the clinical entity. *J Am Soc Nephrol.* 2002;13:2160-2170.
19. Whyte DA, Fine RN. Chronic kidney disease in children. *Pediatr Rev.* 2008;29:335-341.
20. Sinaiko A. Hypertension in children. *N Engl J Med.* 1996;335:26.
21. National High Blood Pressure Education Program Working Group on High Blood Pressure in Children and Adolescents. The fourth report on the diagnosis, evaluation and treatment of high blood pressure in children and adolescents. *Pediatrics.* 2004;114:555-576.
22. Brady TM, Solomon B, Siberry G. Pediatric hypertension: a review of proper screening, diagnosis, evaluation and treatment. *Contemp Pediatr.* 2008;25:46-56.
23. Tanaka ST, Pope JC. 4th. Pediatric stone disease. *Curr Urol Rep.* 2009;10:138-143.
24. McKay CP. Renal stone disease. *Pediatr Rev.* 2010;31:179-188.

⊘ See additional content on Expert Consult

I. WEBSITES

Child Neurology Society: www.childneurologysociety.org
American Academy of Neurology Practice Guidelines: aan.com/practice/guideline
American Heart Association Statement on Management of Stroke in Infants and Children: stroke.ahajournals.org

II. NEUROLOGIC EXAMINATION

A. Mental Status

Evaluate alertness and orientation to time, person, place, and current situation. Assess attentiveness and behavior in infants. Play interests are a window into development.

B. Cranial Nerves (Table 20-1)

C. Motor

1. **Muscle bulk.**
2. **Tone:** Infants with low tone will slip when held under their arms.
   a. Passive movements: Resting resistance to examiner's movement
   b. Active movements: Regulation of power with defined movements (e.g., posture, gait, pull to stand)
3. **Power/strength:** Assess and quantify activity (e.g., rising from floor, distance of standing broad jump, time to run 30 feet or climb 10 stairs [Box 20-1])

D. Sensory (Fig. 20-1, Table 20-2)

1. **Spinal cord level:** Best assessed with pinprick and temperature. If concerned about spinal cord impairment, ask about continence. Compare lower with upper, check both anterior and posterior trunk.
2. **Intraspinal lesions:**
   a. Anterior pathways: Pinprick and temperature
   b. Posterior pathways: Vibratory and joint position sense
3. **Root/plexus/nerve impairment:** Pin sensibility, consult dermatomal/nerve maps (see Fig. 20-1)
4. **Polyneuropathy:** Large fiber (vibration and position sense) versus small fiber (pinprick and temperature). Compare distal with proximal sites in a limb, and lower with upper extremities.

E. Tendon Reflexes

This assessment is most helpful in localizing other abnormalities, especially in the presence of weakness or asymmetry. Compare right with

TABLE 20-1

CRANIAL NERVES

Function/Region	Cranial Nerve	Test/Observation
Olfactory	I	Smell (e.g., coffee, vanilla, peppermint)
Vision	II	Acuity, fields, fundus
Pupils	II, III	Sympathetics, size, reaction to light, accommodation
Eye movements and eyelids	III, IV, VI	Range and quality of eye movements, saccades, pursuits, nystagmus, ptosis
Sensation	V	Corneal reflexes, facial sensation
Muscles of mastication	V	Clench teeth
Facial strength	VII	Degree of expression of emotions; strength of eye closure, smile, and puffing out cheeks; facial symmetry
Hearing	VIII	Localize sound, attend to finger rub, audiologic testing
Mouth, pharynx	IX, X	Swallowing, speech quality, symmetrical palatal elevation, gag reflex
Head control	XI	Lateral head movement, shoulder shrug
Tongue movement	XII	Tongue protrusion

BOX 20-1

STRENGTH RATING SCALE

0/5: No movement (i.e., no palpable tension at tendon)
1/5: Flicker of movement
2/5: Movement in a gravity-neutral plane
3/5: Movement against gravity, but not resistance
4/5: Subnormal strength against resistance
5/5: Normal strength against resistance

left sides, upper with lower extremities, and distal with proximal reflexes (Box 20-2 and Table EC 20-A on Expert Consult).

1. **Isolated abnormality of reflexes:** Little significance in the setting of normal strength and coordination
2. **Brisk reflexes combined with weakness:** Indicate upper motor neuron disorder
3. **Absent reflexes:**
a. Muscle disease: Reflexes usually diminished commensurate with power
b. Selective reflex dropout: Spinal cord, root, or nerve lesion
F. Coordination and Movement
1. **Evaluate general coordination while watching activities** (e.g., throwing a ball, dressing, writing, drawing)
2. **Test for cerebellar function:** Rapid alternating movements, finger-to-nose, heel-to-shin, walking, running
3. **Extra movements:** Quality and conditions under which they are enhanced or suppressed (tremor, dystonia, chorea, athetosis, tics, myoclonus)

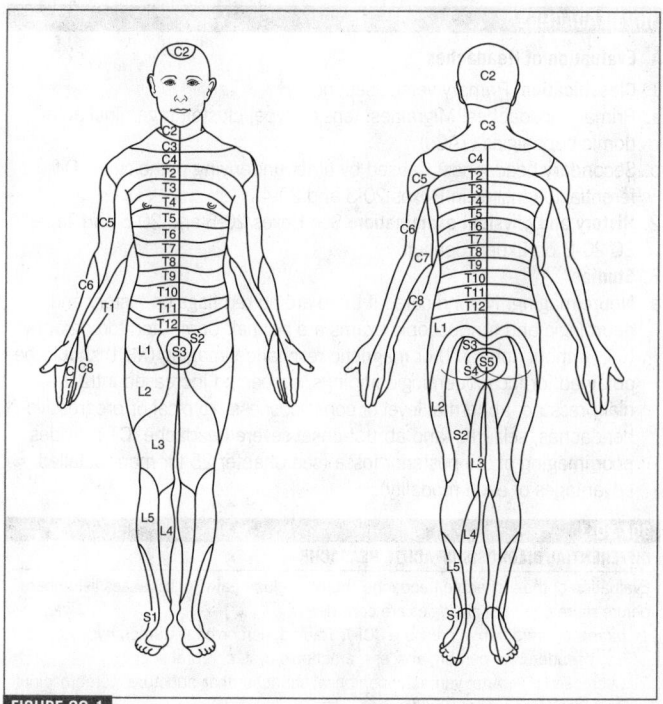

TABLE 20-2

UPPER AND LOWER MOTOR NEURON FINDINGS

On Exam	Upper	Lower
Power	Decreased	Decreased
Reflexes	Increased	Decreased
Tone	Increased	Normal or decreased
Babinski	Upgoing (present)	Downgoing (normal)
Fasciculations	Absent	Present
Muscle wasting	Absent	Present

BOX 20-2

REFLEX RATING SCALE

0: None
1+: Diminished (need use of clasped hands/gritting teeth to engage reflex)
2+: Normal
3+: Increased (reflexes cross neighboring joint or cross to other side)
4+: Hyperactive with clonus

III. HEADACHES[1-3]

A. Evaluation of Headaches

1. **Classification:** Primary versus secondary[4]
a. Primary headaches: Migraines, tension-type, cluster, trigeminal autonomic cephalgias (TACs)
b. Secondary headaches: Caused by other underlying pathologies. Differential diagnoses in Boxes 20-3 and 20-4.
2. **History and physical examination:** See Boxes 20-5 and 20-6 and Table EC 20-B on Expert Consult.
3. **Studies**[2]
a. Neuroimaging: Not indicated if there are no red flags on history and neurologic and funduscopic exams are normal. Computed tomography (CT [without contrast]) or magnetic resonance imaging (MRI) should be obtained for focal neurologic findings, suspected increased intracranial pressure, abnormal level of consciousness, atypical or progressive headaches, seizures, and abrupt-onset severe headache. CT provides poor imaging of the posterior fossa (see Chapter 25 for more detailed advantages of each modality).

BOX 20-3

DIFFERENTIAL DIAGNOSIS OF ACUTE HEADACHE

Evaluation of the first acute headache should exclude pathologic causes listed here before more common etiologies are considered.

1. Increased intracranial pressure (ICP): Trauma, hemorrhage, tumor, hydrocephalus, pseudotumor cerebri, abscess, arachnoid cyst, cerebral edema
2. Decreased ICP: After ventriculoperitoneal shunt, lumbar puncture, cerebrospinal fluid leak from basilar skull fracture
3. Meningeal inflammation: Meningitis, leukemia, subarachnoid or subdural hemorrhage
4. Vascular: Vasculitis, arteriovenous malformation, hypertension, cerebrovascular accident
5. Bone, soft tissue: Referred pain from scalp, eyes, ears, sinuses, nose, teeth, pharynx, cervical spine, temporomandibular joint
6. Infection: Systemic infection, encephalitis, sinusitis, etc.
7. First migraine

BOX 20-4

DIFFERENTIAL DIAGNOSIS OF RECURRENT OR CHRONIC HEADACHES

1. Migraine (with or without aura)
2. Tension
3. Analgesic rebound
4. Caffeine withdrawal
5. Sleep deprivation (e.g., in children with sleep apnea) or chronic hypoxia
6. Tumor
7. Psychogenic: conversion disorder, malingering, depression, acute stress, mood disorder
8. Cluster headache
9. Chronic daily headache

BOX 20-5

HEADACHE WARNING SIGNS ON HISTORY

1. Pain that awakens child from sleep
2. Age <3 years
3. Pain made worse with straining or Valsalva
4. Explosive onset
5. Focal deficits
6. Headache associated with emesis
7. Changes in chronic pattern or steady worsening of headaches
8. Altered mental status: Changes in mood, personality, school performance
9. Concurrent fever

BOX 20-6

IMPORTANT HISTORICAL INFORMATION IN EVALUATING HEADACHE

1. Age at onset
2. Associated trauma
3. Presence or absence of aura
4. Change in weight or other constitutional symptoms
5. Change in vision or any other neurologic symptoms
6. Frequency, severity, and duration of headaches (ask about school absences)
7. Quality, site, and radiation of pain (focal occipital pain is concerning for secondary headaches)
8. Associated symptoms such as weakness, tingling, photophobia, phonophobia
9. Triggers and alleviating/exacerbating factors
10. Family history of migraine
11. Changes and new stressors in school or at home

BOX 20-7

LUMBAR PUNCTURE[5]

- Indications: Fever, infection, concern for pseudotumor cerebri or other causes of increased intracranial pressure after negative imaging.
- Contraindications: Elevated intracranial pressure or mass effect, owing to concern for herniation. Obtain a head CT before lumbar puncture if this is a concern.
- Standard tests: Cell counts + differential, Gram stain, cerebrospinal fluid (CSF) culture, protein, glucose. Consider viral studies (HSV, enterovirus, etc.).
- Special tests: Manometer for opening pressure if concern for pseudotumor cerebri. Performed in a lateral decubitus position with legs extended.
- Correction for white blood cells (WBCs): Expected CSF WBC count = (red blood cells [RBCs] CSF/RBCs serum) × WBCs serum.
- Xanthochromia: Yellow or pink discoloration of CSF due to breakdown of hemoglobin. If CSF is xanthochromic, suspect subarachnoid hemorrhage.

---

b. Laboratory studies: Not routinely indicated if no red flags
c. Lumbar puncture: Not routinely indicated if no red flags (Box 20-7)
d. Electroencephalogram (EEG): Not routinely indicated if no red flags

B. Migraine Headache

1. Box 20-8 **lists diagnostic criteria.** Migraines are typically throbbing, pulsatile, or pressure-like in children. They are usually bifrontal in children

---

BOX 20-8

DIAGNOSTIC CRITERIA FOR PEDIATRIC MIGRAINE WITHOUT AURA[4,6]

At least five attacks fulfilling the following criteria and not attributable to another disorder:

1. Headache lasts 1–72 hours (untreated or unsucessfully treated)
2. At least two of the following characteristics:
   a. Unilateral or bilateral
   b. Pulsating quality
   c. Moderate to severe in intensity
   d. Aggravated by or causing avoidance of routine physical activities
3. At least one of the following occur during the headache:
   a. Nausea and/or vomiting
   b. Photophobia and phonophobia (which may be inferred from behavior)

---

and unilateral in adolescents and adults. There are many potential triggers (e.g., stress, caffeine, menses, sleep disruption).

2. **Classification**[4]:

a. Classic: With aura. *Aura* is any neurologic symptom that occurs prior to onset of a migraine (e.g., visual aberrations, paresthesias, numbness, dysphasia).

b. Common: Without aura

3. **Precursors to migraines and close associations include** cyclic vomiting, abdominal migraines, recurrent abdominal pain, paroxysmal vertigo of childhood, paroxysmal torticollis of infancy, and motion sickness.

4. **Treatment**[7,8]: Includes reassurance and education regarding lifestyle modification (sleep, hygiene, exercise, stress reduction, fluids, not missing meals). Refer any child with focal neurologic deficits to a pediatric neurologist.

a. Acute symptomatic: Avoid medication overuse (>2-3 doses/week); it can lead to rebound headache.

   (1) Dark, quiet room and sleep.
   (2) Nonsteroidal antiinflammatory drugs (NSAIDs [e.g., naproxen, ibuprofen, ketorolac]).
   (3) Acetaminophen.
   (4) Caffeine (e.g., Excedrin).
   (5) Triptans (Table 20-3). Objective data support nasal sumatriptan, which has been studied in children as young as 5 years of age. In 2009, the U.S. Food and Drug Administration (FDA) approved almotriptan for migraine treatment in adolescents aged 12–17.
   (6) Antiemetics (e.g., metoclopramide, prochlorperazine, promethazine) if nausea is a factor.
   (7) Steroids (e.g., methylprednisolone) may be useful in intractable cases, although evidence is lacking.
   (8) Magnesium may be useful in intractable cases, although evidence is lacking.
   (9) Sodium valproate.

TABLE 20-3

ABORTIVE TRIPTANS FOR MIGRAINE (SEE FORMULARY FOR SPECIFIC DOSING)

Medication	Dose (Preparation*)	Duration†
Sumatriptan (Imitrex)	6 mg (SQ); 5, 20 mg (NS); 25, 50, 100 mg (T)	Short
Rizatriptan (Maxalt)	5, 10 mg (T); 5, 10 mg (D)	Short
Zolmitriptan (Zomig)	2.5, 5 mg (T); 2.5, 5 mg (D); 5 mg (NS)	Short
Almotriptan (Axert)	6.25, 12.5 mg (T)	Short
Eletriptan (Relpax)	20, 40 mg (T)	Short
Naratriptan (Amerge)	1, 2.5 mg (T)	Long
Frovatriptan (Frova)	2.5 mg (T)	Long

*D, Dissolvable tablet; NS, nasal spray; SQ, subcutaneous; T, tablet.
†Short (4-hr half-life); long (12- to 24-hr half-life).

TABLE 20-4

PREVENTIVE THERAPIES FOR MIGRAINE (SEE FORMULARY FOR DOSING)

Medications	Adverse Effects	Consider in Patients with the Following Comorbidities
ANTICONVULSANT MEDICATIONS		
Divalproex sodium (Depakote)	Dizziness, drowsiness, weight gain, gastrointestinal upset, teratogenicity, potential liver injury	Bipolar, epilepsy, underweight
Topiramate (Topamax)	Cognitive changes, weight loss, sensory changes, paresthesias, kidney stones	Obesity, epilepsy
ANTIDEPRESSANT MEDICATIONS		
Amitriptyline (Elavil)	Sedation, dry mouth, constipation	Depression, insomnia
Nortriptyline	Sedation, dry mouth, constipation	Depression, insomnia
ANTIHISTAMINE MEDICATION		
Cyproheptadine (Periactin)	Sedation, increased appetite	Seasonal allergies, poor appetite, insomnia
β-BLOCKER		
Propranolol (Inderal)	Hypotension, exacerbates exercise-induced asthma, masks hypoglycemia	Hypertension
CALCIUM CHANNEL BLOCKER		
Flunarizine	Drowsiness, weight gain	Hypertension

b. Chronic treatment (if >3 per month and if migraines interfere with daily functioning or school):
   (1) Avoid triggers and stress. Balanced diet restrictive of certain migraine-causing foods (especially caffeine). Headache journal to help identify potential triggers. Encourage aerobic exercise and regular sleep. Keep hydrated.
   (2) Offer counseling when appropriate; also consider biofeedback, acupuncture, yoga, and massage therapy if parents are interested.
   (3) Consider medications (Table 20-4)

IV. PAROXYSMAL EVENTS

A. Differential Diagnosis of Recurrent Events That Mimic Epilepsy in Childhood (Table 20-5)

B. Seizures: First and Recurrent[9,10]

1. **Seizure:** Paroxysmal synchronized discharge of cortical neurons resulting in alteration of function (motor, sensory, cognitive)
2. **Causes of seizures**
a. Diffuse brain dysfunction: Fever, metabolic compromise, toxin or drugs, hypertension

---

TABLE 20-5

DIFFERENTIAL DIAGNOSIS OF RECURRENT EVENTS THAT MIMIC EPILEPSY IN CHILDHOOD[9]

Event	Differentiation from Epilepsy
Pseudoseizure (psychogenic seizure)	No EEG changes except movement artifact during event; movements thrashing rather than clonic; brief/absent postictal period; most likely to occur in patient with epilepsy
Paroxysmal vertigo (toddler)	Patient frightened and crying; no loss of awareness; staggers and falls, vomiting, dysarthria
GER in infancy, childhood	Paroxysmal dystonic posturing associated with meals (Sandifer syndrome)
Breath-holding spells (18 mo–3 yr)	Loss of consciousness and generalized convulsions, always provoked by an event that makes child cry
Syncope	Loss of consciousness with onset of dizziness and clouded or tunnel vision; slow collapse to floor; triggered by postural change, heat, emotion, etc.
Cardiogenic syncope	Abnormal ECG/Holter monitor finding (e.g., prolonged QT, atrioventricular block, other arrhythmias); exercise a possible trigger; episodic loss of consciousness without consistent convulsive movement
Cough syncope	Prolonged cough spasm during sleep in asthmatic, leading to loss of consciousness, often with urinary incontinence
Paroxysmal dyskinesias	May be precipitated by sudden movement or startle; not accompanied by change in alertness
Shuddering attacks	Brief shivering spells with continued awareness
Night terrors (4–6 yr)	Brief nocturnal episodes of terror without typical convulsive movements
Rages (6–12 yr)	Provoked and goal-directed anger
Tics/habit spasms	Involuntary, nonrhythmic, repetitive movements not associated with impaired consciousness; suppressible
Narcolepsy	Sudden loss of tone secondary to cataplexy; emotional trigger; no postictal state or loss of consciousness; EEG with recurrent REM sleep attacks
Migraine (confusional)	Headache or visual changes that may precede attack; family history of migraine; autonomic or sensory changes that can mimic focal seizure; EEG with regional area of slowing during attack
Myoclonus	Involuntary muscle jerking or twitch

ECG, Electrocardiography; EEG, electroencephalography; GER, gastroesophageal reflux; REM, rapid eye movement.

b. Focal brain dysfunction: Stroke, neoplasm, focal cortical dysgenesis, trauma

3. **Febrile illness**–associated seizures[11]

a. Definitions:

   (1) Simple febrile seizure: Primary generalized seizure associated with fever in a child 6–60 months of age that is non-focal, lasts <15 minutes and does not recur in a 24-hour period

   (2) Complex febrile seizure: Seizure associated with a fever in a child 6–60 months of age that is focal, lasts >15 minutes, or recurs within a 24-hour period

b. No further workup is necessary for a simple febrile seizure in a neurologically intact child who appears well, has a normal neurologic exam, is fully immunized, and has no meningeal signs.

c. Neuroimaging, blood work, and EEG are not routinely recommended in previously healthy children who have a simple febrile seizure. Further studies should be directed toward ascertaining the source of the fever.

d. Perform a lumbar puncture in any child with seizures and meningeal signs or symptoms (e.g., nuchal rigidity, Kernig and/or Brudzinski signs, etc.).

e. Consider lumbar puncture in these circumstances:

   (1) Infant 6–12 months of age if incomplete or unknown *Haemophilus influenzae* or *Streptococcus pneumoniae* immunizations.

   (2) Febrile seizure in a child pretreated with antibiotics. Antibiotics can mask signs and symptoms of meningitis.

4. **Evaluation of nonfebrile seizures**

a. If clinically indicated, check glucose, Na, K, Ca, Phos, blood urea nitrogen (BUN), creatinine (Cr), complete blood cell count (CBC), tox screen.

b. Blood pressure (BP): Supine and upright.

c. EEG: Recommended in all children with first nonfebrile seizure to evaluate for an epilepsy syndrome.[12] Routine interictal EEGs are frequently normal. Repeat EEGs, prolonged EEG monitoring with video, or studies done with sleep deprivation or photic stimulation may be more informative.

d. If this is not the first seizure and patient is receiving antiepileptic therapy, a change in seizure pattern should prompt a drug level (see Table 20-7 for therapeutic drug levels).

e. Imaging: Although not required for diagnosis, MRI and CT can detect focal brain abnormalities that may predispose to focal seizures.

   (1) Head ultrasound may be used in early infancy and requires open fontanelles.

   (2) Head CT without contrast: Can detect mass lesions, acute hemorrhage, hydrocephalus, and calcifications secondary to congenital disease such as cytomegalovirus infection. Obtain a head CT only when concerned about a mass or bleed or in an emergency situation.

   (3) Brain MRI with contrast: Obtain in infants with epilepsy and children with recurrent partial seizures, focal neurologic deficits, or developmental delay. Not routinely indicated when evaluating a first-time seizure.

5. **Seizure disorders (epilepsy):** Assess seizure type (Table 20-6), epilepsy classification (Box 20-9), and severity of disorder

TABLE 20-6

SPECIAL SEIZURE SYNDROMES[9,13,14]

Syndrome	Etiology	Evaluation	Treatment	Comment
Neonatal seizures	Brain malformation, hypoxic-ischemic-encephalopathy, intracranial hemorrhage, inborn errors of metabolism, CNS infection, cerebral infarction, hypoglycemia, hypocalcemia, hypomagnesemia	Screen for electrolyte and metabolic abnormalities and pyridoxine deficiency; workup for sepsis, LP, head ultrasound, CT or MRI; EEG	Treat underlying abnormality, consider pyridoxine ± EEG, phenobarbital (± additional agents).	Occurs within first 28 days of life; may be myoclonic, tonic, clonic, or subtle; presents as blinking, chewing, bicycling, or apnea; distinguished from jitteriness by vital sign changes and inability to provoke or inhibit
Infantile spasms	Symptomatic—67%. May be secondary to CNS malformation, acquired infantile brain injury, tuberous sclerosis, inborn errors of metabolism Cryptogenic—33%	EEG (shows hypsarrhythmia), MRI	High-dose steroids, vigabatrin, topiramate, ketogenic diet	Usual onset after age 2 mo, peak onset 4–6 mo; initiate treatment as soon as possible. Presents as sudden flexion or extension of the trunk and extremities, often in clusters
Absence seizures	Unknown	EEG (sudden generalized 3-Hz spike and slow-wave discharges)	Ethosuximide, valproic acid	Age of onset 4–8 years; provoked by hyperventilation: staring spells ± automatisms (eye blinking, mouth movements); often resolves spontaneously by puberty; good neurologic outcome
Benign rolandic epilepsy/BECTS (benign epilepsy of childhood with centrotemporal spikes)	Unknown	EEG (characteristic pattern of centrotemporal spikes)	No treatment necessary; avoid sleep deprivation; if seizures are frequent, may use carbamazepine or levetiracetam.	Age of onset 2–13 years; seizures are nocturnal and consist of hemisensory or motor phenomena of the face, motor findings in limbs; most patients outgrow by age 16–18.

Juvenile myoclonic epilepsy	Unknown genetic predisposition	Clinical history, sleep-deprived EEG (reveals generalized spike and wave discharges with normal background activity)	Levetiracetam, other meds for generalized seizure	Adolescent onset; morning myoclonus; 75%–95% have GTC seizures; good intellectual outcome, no progressive deterioration
Panayiotopoulos syndrome	Benign age-related focal seizure disorder; Prolonged seizure with predominately autonomic symptoms	EEG (shifting and/or multiple foci, often occipital spikes)	Often not treated owing to benign nature of condition	Syndrome specific to childhood; symptoms include vomiting, pallor, eye deviation, sweating, ± convulsions
Lennox-Gastaut syndrome	Cryptogenic or symptomatic	Interictal EEG (reveals slow spike and wave discharges)	Pharmacologic and nonpharmacologic treatments have varying degrees of effectiveness.	Age of onset 1–9 years; multiple seizure types, often intractable; intellectual disability

CNS, Central nervous system; CT, computed tomography; EEG, electroencephalography; GTC, generalized tonic-clonic; LP, lumbar puncture; MRI, magnetic resonance imaging.

BOX 20-9

INTERNATIONAL CLASSIFICATION OF EPILEPTIC SEIZURES[10]

I. Partial seizures (seizures with focal onset)
   1. Simple partial seizures (consciousness unimpaired)
      a. With motor signs
      b. With somatosensory or special sensory symptoms
      c. With autonomic symptoms or signs
      d. With psychic symptoms (higher cerebral functions)
   2. Complex partial seizures (consciousness impaired)
      a. Starting as simple partial seizures
         (a) Without automatisms
         (b) With automatisms (e.g., lip smacking, drooling, dazed-eyes look)
      b. With impairment of consciousness at onset
         (a) Without automatisms
         (b) With automatisms
   3. Partial seizures evolving into secondarily generalized seizures
II. Generalized seizures
   1. Absence seizures: Brief lapse in awareness without postictal impairment
      (atypical absence seizures may have mild clonic, atonic, tonic, automatism, or
      autonomic components)
   2. Myoclonic seizures: Brief, repetitive, symmetric muscle contractions
   3. Clonic seizures: Rhythmic jerking, flexor spasm of extremities
   4. Tonic seizures: Sustained muscle contraction
   5. Tonic-clonic seizures
   6. Atonic seizures: Abrupt loss of muscle tone
III. Unclassified epileptic seizures

---

6. **Status epilepticus**[15]: Traditionally defined as continuous or recurrent
   seizures lasting ≥30 minutes without the patient regaining consciousness. For treatment purposes, status epilepticus can be diagnosed after
   5 minutes of continuous seizure or at least two discrete seizures without
   complete recovery of consciousness between them. See Chapter 1 for
   treatment guidelines.

7. **Treatment**[12,16]:

a. If patient's first seizure, seizure was nonfocal, and patient has returned
   to baseline: No antiepileptic medication indicated. Overall recurrence of
   seizure varies from 14%–65% in the first year. Most recurrences occur
   within 1–2 years after the initial event. Epileptiform abnormalities on
   EEG indicate a higher chance of recurrence.

b. Educate parents and patient (as age appropriate) regarding epilepsy
   basics.[17] Review seizure first aid. Recommend supervision during
   bathing or swimming. Know driver's license laws in the state. Advocate
   teacher and school awareness.

c. Pharmacotherapy (Table 20-7): Weigh risk of future seizures without
   therapy against risk for treatment side effects plus residual seizures
   despite therapy. Reserve pharmacotherapy for recurrent afebrile
   seizures. Monotherapy may reduce complications; polytherapy increases
   risk of complications and side effects more than efficacy.

TABLE 20-7

COMMONLY USED ANTICONVULSANTS

Anticonvulsant (Trade Name)	Standard Therapeutic Levels (mg/dL)	Efficacy (Generalized/Partial)	IV Preparation Available?	Side Effects
Carbamazepine (Tegretol/Carbatrol)	8–12	P	No	Sedation, ataxia, diplopia, Stevens-Johnson syndrome, blood dyscrasias, hepatotoxicity, may worsen generalized seizures
Clobazam (Onfi)	n/a	G/P	No	Sedation, dizziness
Clonazepam (Klonopin)	n/a	G/P	No	Sedation, drooling, dependence
Ethosuximide (Zarontin)	40–100	G (absence)	No	Gastrointestinal upset
Felbamate (Felbatol)	40–100	G/P	No	Weight loss, hepatotoxicity, sleep disturbances, aplastic anemia (1:7900)
Gabapentin (Neurontin)	3–18	P	No	Weight gain, leg edema, dizziness
Lacosamide (Vimpat)	n/a	P	Yes	Sedation, reduced benefit with sodium channel drugs
Lamotrigine (Lamictal)	3–18	G/P	No	Rash (increased risk in combination with valproate)
Levetiracetam (Keppra)	n/a	G/P	Yes	Behavioral changes, irritability, rare psychosis
Oxcarbazepine (Trileptal)	MHD level (5–40)	P	No	Hyponatremia
Phenobarbital (Luminal)	15–40	G/P	Yes	Altered cognition, sedation
Phenytoin (Dilantin)	10–20	P	Yes	Hirsutism, gingival hyperplasia, teratogenicity, rash, purple-glove syndrome with infusion
Pregabalin (Lyrica)	n/a	P	No	Peripheral edema, weight gain, constipation, dizziness, ataxia, sedation
Rufinamide (Banzel)	n/a	G (Lennox-Gastaut)	No	Shortened QT interval, nausea, dizziness, sedation, headache
Tiagabine (Gabitril)	n/a	P	No	Can worsen generalized seizures
Topiramate (Topamax)	2–20	G/P	No	Cognitive side effects, weight loss, renal stones, acidosis, glaucoma
Valproic acid (Depakote, Depakene)	75–100	G/P	Yes	Weight gain, alopecia, hepatotoxicity, pancreatitis, PCOS, teratogenicity
Vigabatrin (Sabril)	n/a	G (infantile spasms)	No	Rash, weight gain, irritability, dizziness, sedation, visual field defects (requires ophthalmology evaluations)
Zonisamide (Zonegran)	20–40	G/P	No	Renal stones, weight loss; rare: Stevens-Johnson syndrome, aplastic anemia

G, Generalized; MHD, 10-Monohydroxy metabolite; n/a, not available; P, partial; PCOS, polycystic ovarian syndrome.
Based on personal communication with Eric Kossoff, MD, Johns Hopkins Pediatric Neurology.

20

d. Ketogenic diet[18]: High-fat, low-carbohydrate therapy typically used for intractable seizures. Especially effective for infantile spasms, GLUT1 deficiency, Doose syndrome, pyruvate dehydrogenase deficiency. Urine ketones can be monitored to assess compliance. Side effects include acidosis with bicarbonate value as low as 10–15 mEq/L, kidney stones, growth disturbance, and constipation. Typically used for 2 years, but can be maintained for longer.

C. Special Seizure Syndromes[13,17]

See Table 20-6 for seizure types, etiologies, evaluation, and treatment of many common seizure syndromes.

V. HYDROCEPHALUS[19]

A. Diagnosis[19]

Assess increasing head circumference, misshapen skull, frontal bossing, bulging large anterior fontanelle, increased ICP (setting-sun eye sign due to upward gaze paresis, increased tone/reflexes, vomiting, irritability, papilledema), and developmental delay. Obtain neuroimaging if increase in head circumference crosses more than two percentile lines or if patient is symptomatic. Differentiate hydrocephalus from megalencephaly or hydrocephalus *ex vacuo*.

B. Treatment

1. **Medical:**
a. Emergently manage acute increase of ICP (see Chapter 4).
b. Slowly progressive hydrocephalus: Acetazolamide and furosemide may provide temporary relief by decreasing the rate of CSF production(see Formulary for dosing).
2. **Surgical:** CSF shunting
a. Shunts: Ventriculoperitoneal (VP) shunts used most commonly.
   (1) Shunt dysfunction may be caused by infection, obstruction (clogging or kinking), disconnection, and migration of proximal and distal tips. Patient will develop signs of increased ICP with shunt malfunction.
   (2) Evaluation of shunt integrity: Obtain head CT to evaluate shunt position, ventricular size, and evidence of increased ICP. Obtain shunt series (skull, neck, chest, and abdominal radiographs) to look for kinking or disconnection. Referral to a neurosurgeon is then warranted to test shunt function and for possible percutaneous shunt drainage.
b. Endoscopic third ventriculostomy (ETV) may be used to avoid ventricular shunting.

VI. ATAXIA[20,21]

A. Ataxia definition: impaired coordination of movement and balance

B. Differential Diagnosis of Acute Ataxia (Box 20-10)

C. Evaluation (Box 20-11)

BOX 20-10

DIFFERENTIAL DIAGNOSIS OF ACUTE ATAXIA

1. Drug ingestion (e.g., phenytoin, carbamazepine, sedatives, hypnotics, phency-clidine) or intoxication (e.g., alcohol, ethylene glycol, hydrocarbon fumes, lead, mercury, thallium)
2. Postinfectious (cerebellitis [e.g., varicella], acute disseminated encephalomy-elitis)
3. Head trauma (cerebellar contusion or hemorrhage, posterior fossa hematoma, vertebrobasilar dissection, postconcussive syndrome)
4. Basilar migraine
5. Benign paroxysmal vertigo (migraine equivalent)
6. Intracranial mass lesion (tumor, abscess, vascular malformation)
7. Opsoclonus-myoclonus: Chaotic eye movement combined with ataxia and myoclonus of either postinfectious or paraneoplastic (neuroblastoma or other neural crest tumors) etiology
8. Hydrocephalus
9. Infection (e.g., labyrinthitis)
10. Seizure (ictal or postictal)
11. Vascular events (e.g., cerebellar hemorrhage or stroke)
12. Guillain-Barré syndrome or Miller-Fisher variant (ataxia, ophthalmoplegia, and areflexia). Warning: If bulbar signs present, patient may lose ability to protect airway.
13. Rare inherited paroxysmal ataxias
14. Inborn errors of metabolism (e.g., mitochondrial disorders, aminoacidopathies, urea cycle defects) (See Chapter 13 for workup.)
15. Multiple sclerosis
16. Somatoform disorders (conversion)

BOX 20-11

EVALUATION OF ACUTE ATAXIA (BASED ON CLINICAL SCENARIO)

1. Complete blood cell count (CBC), electrolytes, urine and serum toxicology
2. Imaging (computed tomography [CT] and/or magnetic resonance imaging [MRI])
3. Lumbar puncture (LP)
4. Electroencephalography (EEG)
5. If neuroblastoma is suspected (opsoclonus-myoclonus), obtain urine vanillylman-delic acid and homovanillic acid and imaging of chest and abdomen.

VII. STROKE[22-25]

A. Etiology

Risk factors for childhood stroke: Congenital heart disease, cerebral arteriopathies, hematologic disorders (sickle cell disease, prothrombotic state), serious systemic infection (meningitis, sepsis), head or neck trauma causing arterial dissection, and drugs

---

BOX 20-12

DIFFERENTIAL DIAGNOSIS OF ACUTE-ONSET FOCAL NEUROLOGIC DEFICIT

1. Hemiplegic migraine
2. Focal seizure
3. Postictal (Todd) paralysis
4. Cervical spinal cord injury (deficits spare face)
5. Ischemic stroke
6. Hemorrhagic stroke

BOX 20-13

INITIAL WORKUP OF ACUTE STROKE

1. Imaging: STAT noncontrast head computed tomography. Subsequently can obtain magnetic resonance imaging (diffusion-weighted) and magnetic resonance angiography of head and neck.
2. Initial laboratory studies: Complete blood cell count, comprehensive metabolic panel, erythrocyte sedimentation rate, prothrombin time, partial thromboplastin time, international normalized ratio, type and screen, urine toxicology screen
3. Echocardiogram
4. Hypercoagulability workup
5. Other studies to consider on a case-by-case basis: Fasting lipid panel, rheumatologic and metabolic studies, hemoglobin electrophoresis, and HIV testing

---

B. Differential Diagnosis (Box 20-12)

Stroke should be considered in the differential diagnosis for any child who presents with acute-onset focal neurologic deficit, focal seizures with prolonged postictal paralysis, new-onset refractory focal status epilepticus, altered mental status, or unexplained encephalopathy.

C. Initial Workup (Box 20-13)

D. Management[24]

1. **Supportive care is critical** and should proceed rapidly and parallel with initial workup. Ensure airway patency, provide supplemental oxygen to maintain $Sao_2 > 94\%$, and start maintenance intravenous (IV) fluids.
2. **Optimize cerebral perfusion pressure:** Ensure adequate fluid volume and maintenance of median BP for age. Treatment of hypertension is controversial. Unless BP is extremely elevated, *do not* use acute antihypertensive therapy, because hypertension may be a compensatory reaction to maintain cerebral perfusion.
3. **Monitoring:** Assess neurologic status frequently. Aim for normoglycemia (blood glucose 60–120 mg/dL). Treat fevers, with goal core temperature <37°C. Treat seizures aggressively. Correct dehydration and anemia.
4. **Deep venous thrombosis (DVT) prophylaxis for immobilized patients.**
5. **Antiplatelet and anticoagulation therapy:** If no evidence of hemorrhage, aspirin is typically recommended (1–5 mg/kg/day). Long-term anticoagulation with low-molecular-weight heparin or warfarin may be considered by a specialist on a case-by-case basis in children with substantial risk

of recurrent cardiac embolism and cerebral venous sinus thrombosis, and in selected hypercoagulable states.

6. **Children with sickle cell disease:** Hydration and urgent exchange transfusion to reduce sickle hemoglobin to <30% is recommended. Consult hematology.

7. **Urgent neurology consultation,** along with transfer to a tertiary care center with expertise in childhood stroke.

8. **Thrombolytic therapy not recommended for children** (American Heart Association [AHA] guidelines).

REFERENCES

1. Forsyth R, Farrell K. Headache in childhood. *Pediatr Rev.* 1999;20:39-45.
2. Lewis DW, Ashwal S, Dahl G, et al. Practice parameter: evaluation of children and adolescents with recurrent headaches. *Neurology.* 2002;59:490-498.
3. Brenner M, Oakley C, Lewis D. The evaluation of children and adolescents with headache. *Curr Pain Headache Rep.* 2008;12:361-366;Oct;12(5).
4. Headache Classification Subcommittee of the International Headache Society. The International Classification of Headache Disorders, 2nd ed. *Cephalalgia.* 2004;24 Suppl 1:9-160.
5. Fishman RA. *Cerebrospinal Fluid in Diseases of the Nervous System.* 2nd ed. Philadelphia: Saunders, 1992:190.
6. Blume HK. Pediatric headache: a review. *Pediatr Rev.* 2012;33:562-576.
7. Lewis D, Ashwal S, Hershey A, et al. Practice parameter: pharmacological treatment of migraine headache in children and adolescents. *Neurology.* 2004;63:2215-2224.
8. Hershey AD, Kabbouche MA, Powers SW. Treatment of pediatric and adolescent migraine. *Pediatr Ann.* 2010;39:416-423.
9. Murphy JV, Dehkharghani F. Diagnosis of childhood seizure disorders. *Epilepsia.* 1994;35(Suppl 2):S7-S17.
10. Committee on Classification and Terminology of the International League against Epilepsy. Classification of epilepsia: its applicability and practical value of different diagnostic categories. *Epilepsia.* 1996;38:1051-1059.
11. Subcommittee on Febrile Seizures, American Academy of Pediatrics. Neurodiagnostic evaluation of the child with a simple febrile seizure. *Pediatrics.* 2011;127:389-394.
12. Hirtz D, Berg A, Bettis D, et al. Practice parameter: treatment of the child with a first unprovoked seizure. *Neurology.* 2003;60:166-175.
13. Scher MS. Seizures in the newborn infant: diagnosis, treatment and outcomes. *Clin Perinatol.* 1997;24:735-772.
14. Singer HS, Kossoff EH. In: *Treatment of Pediatric Neurological Disorders.* Boca Raton, FL: Taylor & Francis Group, 2005.
15. Lowenstein DH, Bleck T, Macdonald RL. It's time to revise the definition of status epilepticus. *Epilepsia.* 1999;40:120-122.
16. Baumann RJ, Duffner PK. Treatment of children with simple febrile seizures: the AAP practice parameter. *Pediatr Neurol.* 2000;23:11-17.
17. Freeman JM, Vining EPG, Pillas DJ. *Seizures and Epilepsy in Childhood: A Guide.* 3rd ed. Baltimore: Johns Hopkins Press, 2002.
18. Kossoff EH, Hartman AL. Ketogenic diets: new advances for metabolism-based therapies. *Curr Opin Neurol.* 2012;25:173-178.

19. Kliegman RM, Stanton BF. In: Kliegman RM, et al, eds. *Nelson textbook of pediatrics.* 19th ed Philadelphia: Saunders; 2011.

20. Dinolfo EA. Evaluation of ataxia. *Pediatr Rev.* 2001;22:177-178.

21. Ryan M. Acute ataxia in childhood. *J Child Neurol.* 2003;18:309-316.

22. Ichord R. Treatment of pediatric neurologic disorders. In: Singer H, Kossoff EH, Hartman AL, et al, ed. *Treatment of Pediatric Neurologic Disorders.* Boca Raton, FL: Taylor & Francis Group, 2005.

23. Monagle P, Chalmers E, Chan AK, et al. Antithrombotic therapy in neonates and children: ACCP evidence-based clinical practice guidelines, 8th ed. *Chest.* 2008;1336(6 Suppl):887S-968S.

24. Roach ES, Golomb M, Adams R, et al. Guidelines on management of stroke in infants and children. *Stroke.* 2008;39:2644-2691.

25. Royal College of Physicians of London. Paediatric Stroke Working Group. *Stroke in Childhood: Clinical Guidelines for Diagnosis, Management and Rehabilitation.* London: Royal College of Physicians, 2004.

Chapter 21
Nutrition and Growth
Michael Koldobskiy, MD, PhD, and Jenifer Thompson, MS, RD, CSP

🔗 See additional content on Expert Consult

I. WEBSITES

A. Professional and Government Organizations:

1. Growth Charts and Nutrition Information: http://www.cdc.gov
2. AAP Children's Health Topics: http://www.healthychildren.org
3. Academy of Nutrition and Dietetics: http://www.eatright.org
4. American Society for Parenteral and Enteral Nutrition: http://www.clinnutr.org
5. National Institute of Child Health and Human Development: Breastfeeding: http://www.nichd.nih.gov/health/topics/breastfeeding.cfm
6. U.S. Department of Agriculture healthy eating guidelines: http://www.cnpp.usda.gov/dietaryguidelines.htm and http://www.choosemyplate.gov

B. Infant and Pediatric Formula Company Websites for Obtaining Complete and Up-to-Date Product Information. Information regarding more specialized and metabolic formulas can be found using these websites:

1. Enfamil, Enfacare, Nutramigen, and Pregestimil: http://www.meadjohnson.com
2. Carnation, Good Start, Nutren, Peptamen, Vivonex, Boost, and Resource: http://www.nestle-nutrition.com and http://www.nestleinfantnutrition.com
3. Alimentum, Elecare, Ensure, Neosure, Pediasure, Pedialyte, and Similac: http://www.abbottnutrition.com
4. America's Store Brand and Bright Beginnings: http://www.pbmproducts.com
5. Ketocal, Neocate, and Pepdite: http://www.shsna.com

II. ASSESSMENT OF NUTRITIONAL STATUS

A. Elements of Nutritional Assessment

1. **Anthropometric measurements** (weight, length/height, head circumference, body mass index [BMI], skin folds): Data plotted on growth charts according to age and compared with a reference population
2. **Clinical assessment** (general appearance [e.g., hair, skin, oral mucosa] and gastrointestinal symptoms of nutritional deficiencies)
3. **Dietary evaluation** (feeding history, current intake)
4. **Physical activity and exercise**
5. **Laboratory findings** (comparison with age-based norms)

B. **Indicators of Nutritional Status[1] (Growth Charts) (Figs. 21-1 to 21-9; Figures EC 21-A to 21-G on Expert Consult)**

1. **Growth:** Ideally, should be evaluated over time, but one measurement can be used for screening. Height (or length), weight, and weight for height should be plotted on a growth chart for every patient.

2. **BMI:** Defined as an index of healthy weight and a predictor of morbidity and mortality risk. Used to classify underweight and overweight individuals.[2] BMI should be determined and plotted for children ≥2 years. Use this formula to calculate BMI:

$$BMI = wt\ (kg)\ /[height\ (m)^2]$$

or

$$BMI = wt\ (lb)/[height\ (in)^2] \times 703$$

NOTE: Height indicates height measured by stadiometer, not recumbent length.

3. **BMI percentile:** BMI percentile is plotted on the Centers for Disease Control and Prevention (CDC) growth charts for children ≥2 years. Although not a direct measure of body fat, it is a reliable indicator of body fatness in most children and adolescents[2]:

4. **Interpretation of growth charts:**
a. Stunting: Length or height for age <5th percentile
b. Underweight:
   (1) Children <3 years: weight for length <5th percentile
   (2) Children ≥2 years: BMI for age <5th percentile
c. Healthy weight: BMI for age 5th percentile to <85th percentile
d. Overweight: Children >2 years: BMI for age 85th to <95th percentile
e. Obese:
   (1) Children <3 years: Weight for length >95th percentile
   (2) Children ≥2 years: BMI for age ≥95th percentile

5. **Recommendations for management of overweight and obese children** (also see Figure EC 21-H on Expert Consult)[3,4]
a. Management is three-tiered focused on identification, assessment, and prevention:
   (1) Identification: Calculate BMI at each well-child visit
   (2) Assessment: Medical risk, behavior risk, and attitude
   (3) Prevention: Targeted at behaviors and treatment interventions based on BMI stratification
b. Based on expert committee opinions, the Childhood Obesity Action Network has also developed an implementation guide for assessment and management of childhood obesity.[5]

6. **Growth charts:** For boys and girls, including weight, height, head circumference, BMI, and height velocity (see Figs. 21-1 to 21-9 and Figures EC 21-A to 21-G on Expert Consult). CDC recommends that clinicians in the United States use the 2006 WHO international growth charts rather than

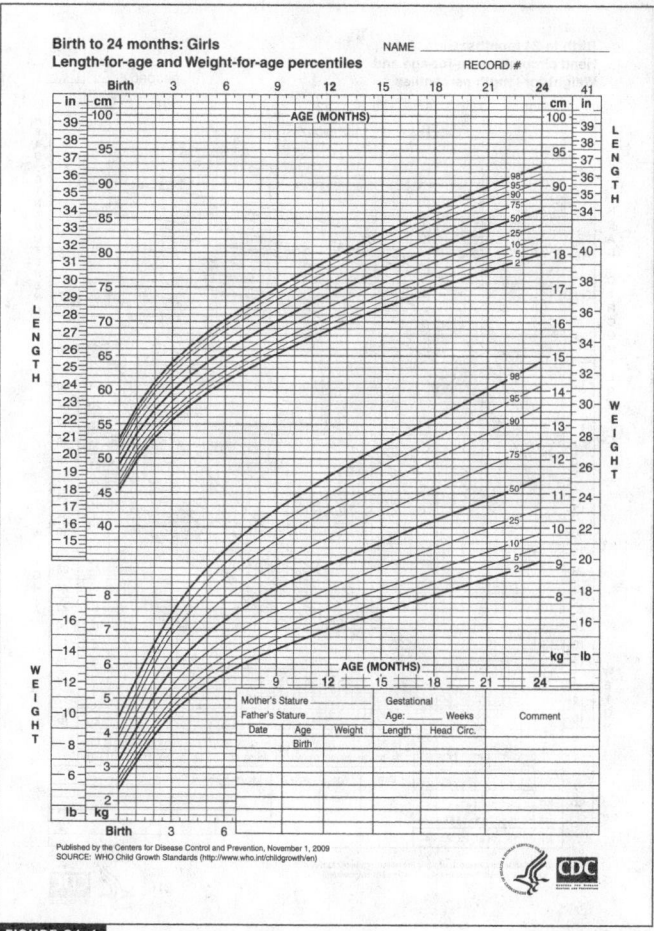

21

FIGURE 21-1

Length and weight for girls, birth to age 24 months. *(Published by the Centers for Disease Control and Prevention, November 1, 2009. SOURCE: WHO Child Growth Standards* [http://www.who.int/childgrowth/en].*)*

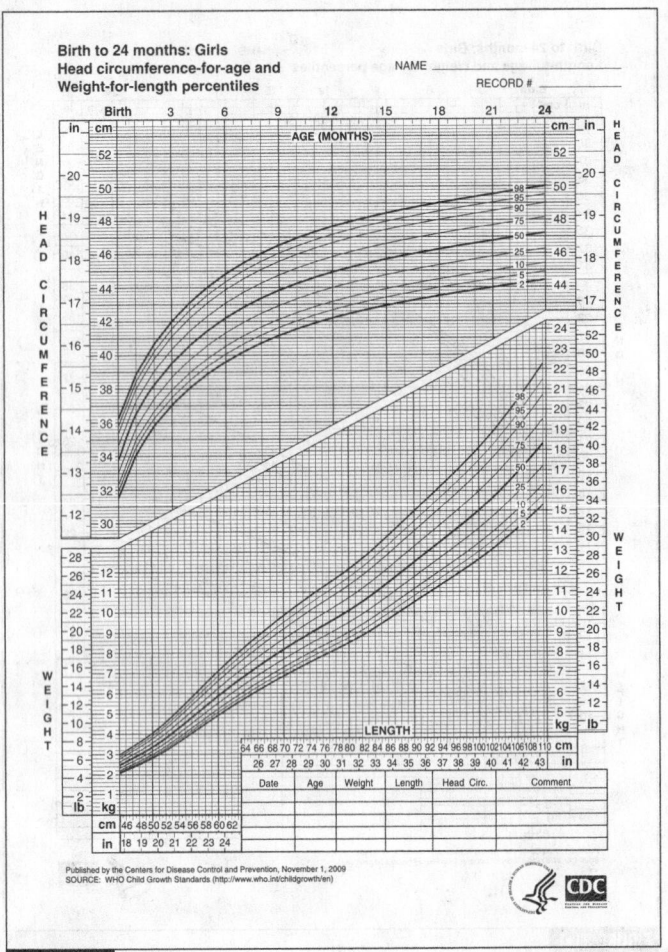

FIGURE 21-2

Head circumference and length-to-weight ratio for girls, birth to age 24 months. *(Published by the Centers for Disease Control and Prevention, November 1, 2009. SOURCE: WHO Child Growth Standards [http://www.who.int/childgrowth/en].)*

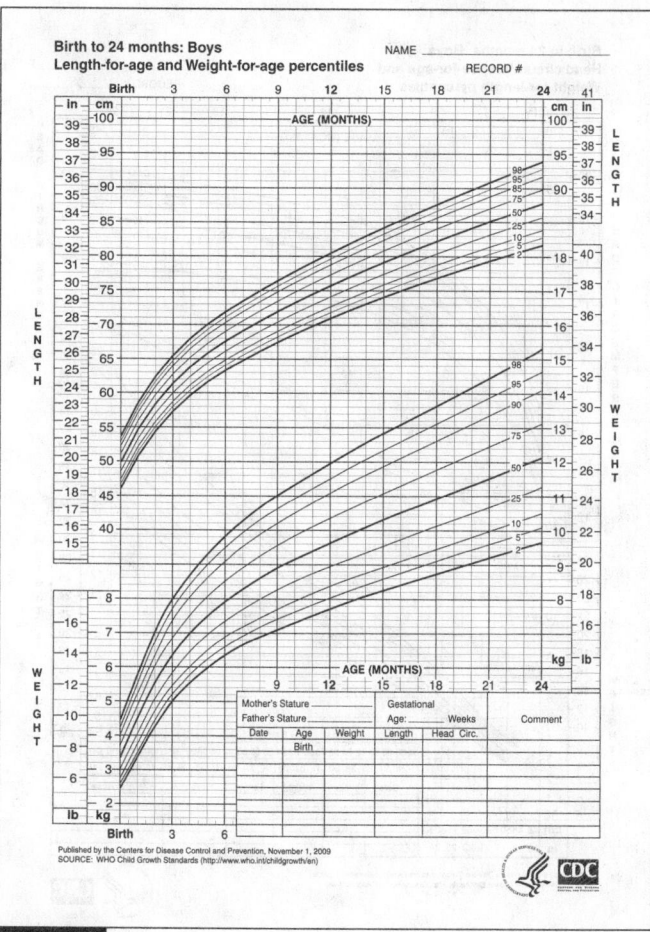

FIGURE 21-3

Length and weight for boys, birth to age 24 months. *(Published by the Centers for Disease Control and Prevention, November 1, 2009. SOURCE: WHO Child Growth Standards* [http://www.who.int/childgrowth/en].*)*

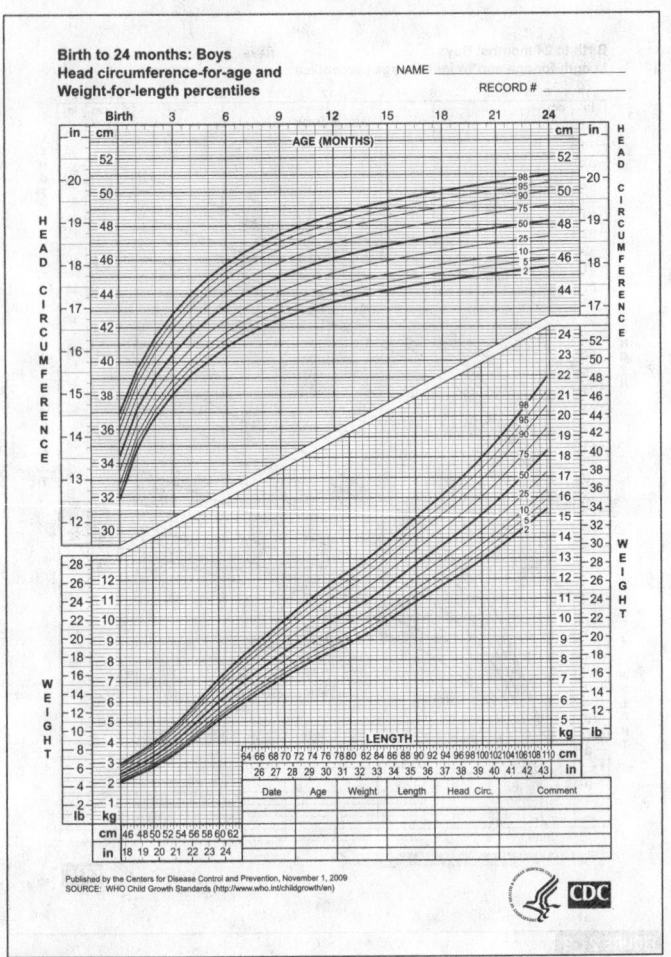

FIGURE 21-4

Head circumference and length-to-weight ratio for boys, birth to age 24 months. *(Published by the Centers for Disease Control and Prevention, November 1, 2009. SOURCE: WHO Child Growth Standards* [http://www.who.int/childgrowth/en].)

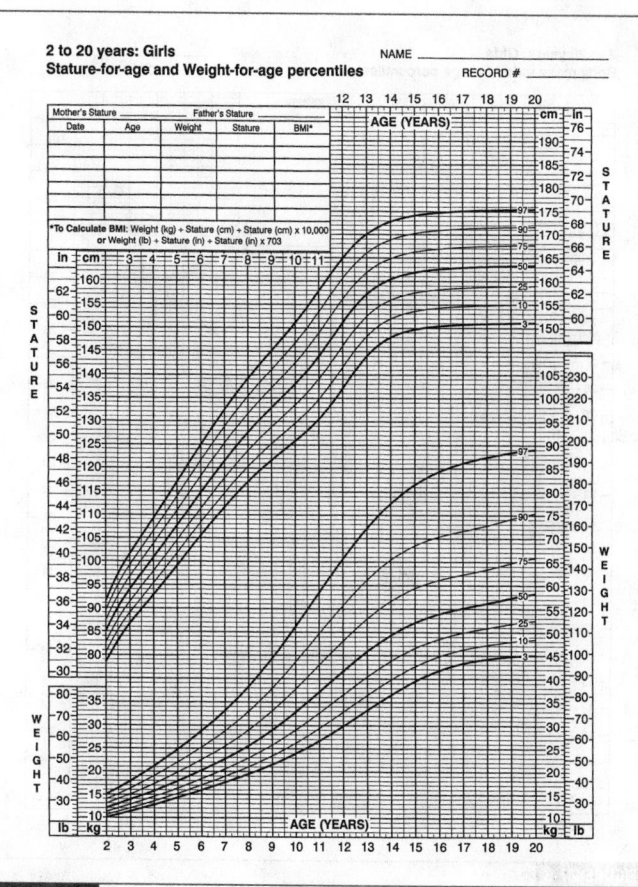

FIGURE 21-5

Stature and weight for girls ages 2–20 years. *(Developed by the National Center for Health Statistics in collaboration with the National Center for Chronic Disease Prevention and Health Promotion, 2000.)*

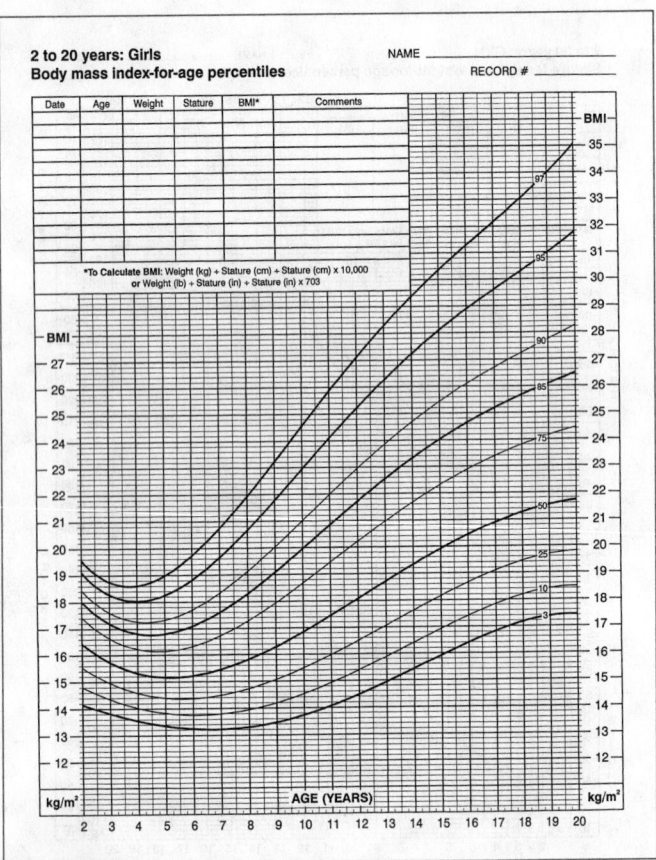

FIGURE 21-6

Body mass index for girls ages 2–20 years. (*Developed by the National Center for Health Statistics in collaboration with the National Center for Chronic Disease Prevention and Health Promotion, 2000.*)

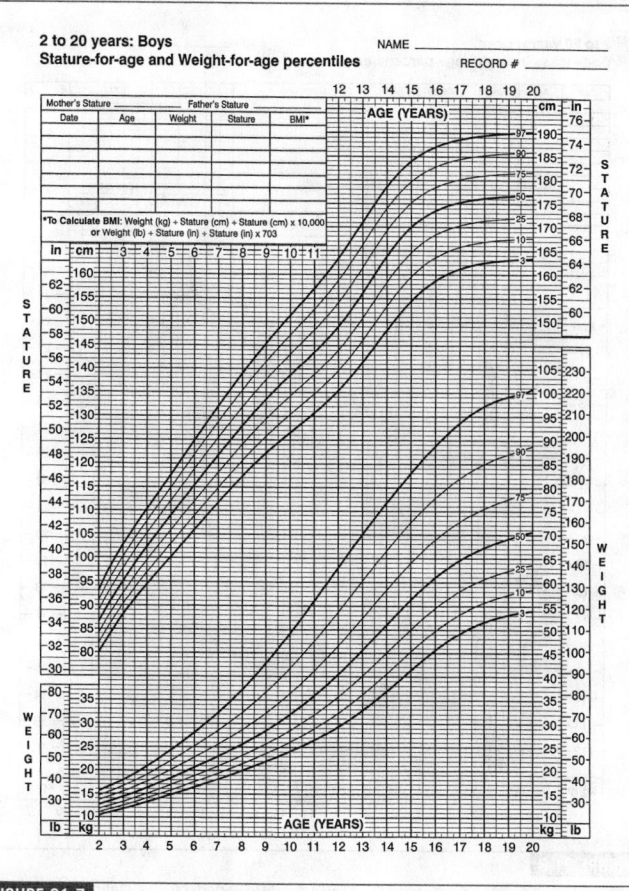

FIGURE 21-7

Stature and weight for boys ages 2–20 years. *(Developed by the National Center for Health Statistics in collaboration with the National Center for Chronic Disease Prevention and Health Promotion, 2000.)*

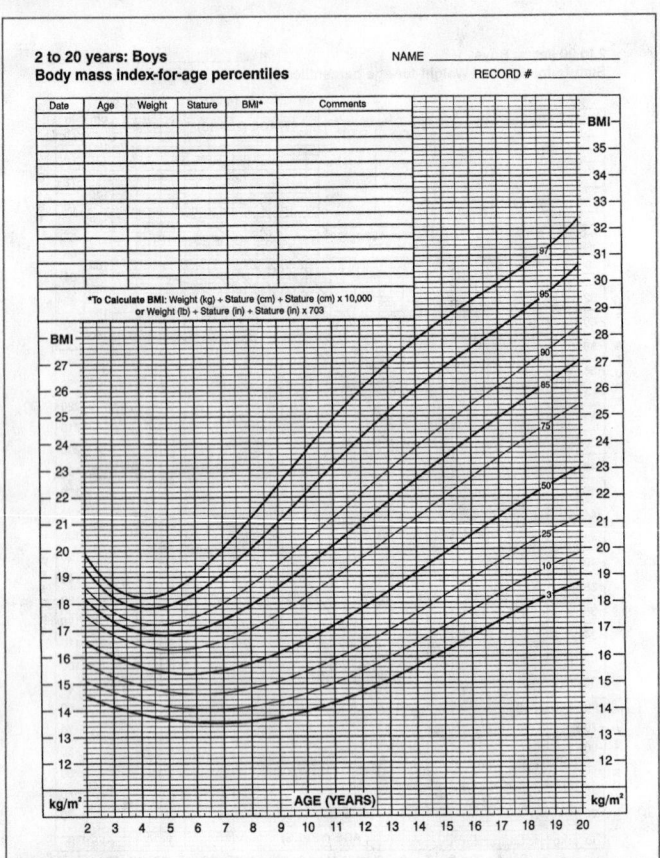

FIGURE 21-8

Body mass index for boys ages 2–20 years. *(Developed by the National Center for Health Statistics in collaboration with the National Center for Chronic Disease Prevention and Health Promotion, 2000.)*

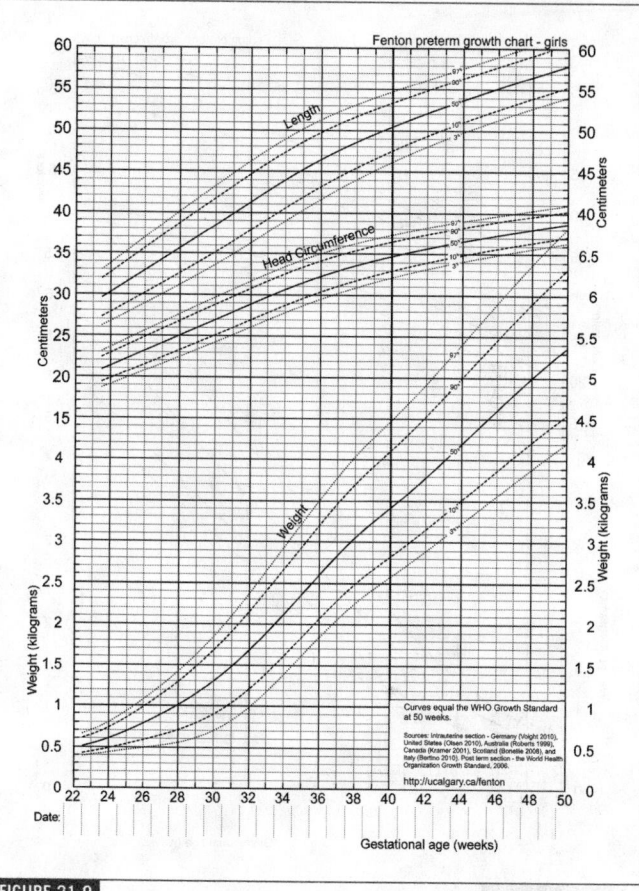

FIGURE 21-9

Length, weight, and head circumference for preterm infants. *(From Fenton RT, Kim HJ. A systematic review and meta-analysis to revise the Fenton growth chart for preterm infants.* BMC Pediatrics. *2013, 13:59.)*

Continued

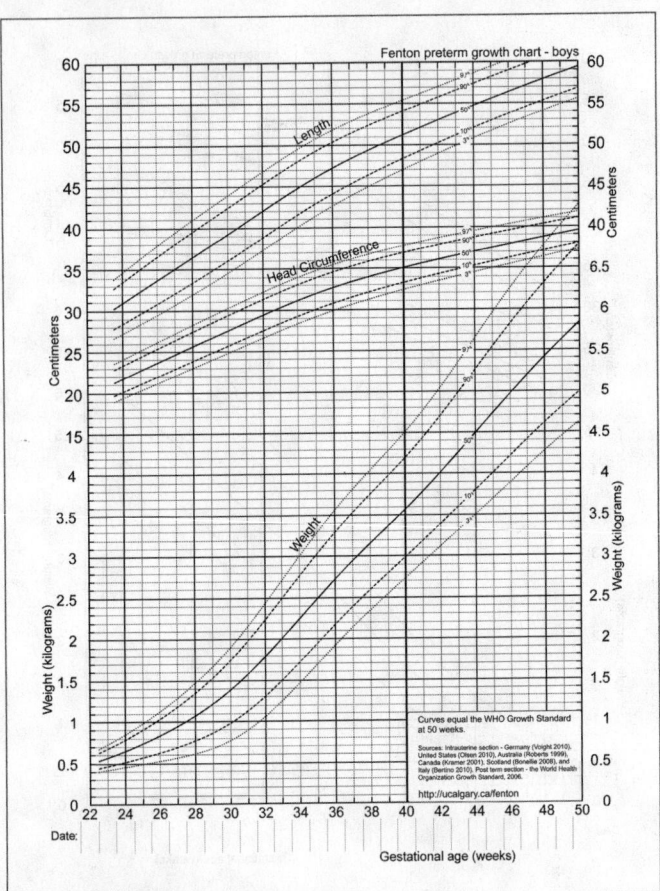

FIGURE 21-9, cont'd

the CDC growth charts for children aged <24 months. Growth charts for children ages 0–20 years, including 2000 CDC growth charts for ages 0–36 months and 2006 WHO growth charts for ages 0–24 months, can be downloaded from http://www.cdc.gov/growthcharts/

7. **Growth charts for special populations:**
a. Down syndrome: http://www.ndss.org; follow links to health care and growth charts (also see Figures EC 21-D to 21-G on Expert Consult)
b. Turner syndrome: http://aappolicy.aappublications.org/cgi/content/full/pediatrics;111/3/692/F1
c. Achondroplasia: http://aappolicy.aappublications.org/cgi/content/full/pediatrics;116/3/771

8. **Waist circumference and waist/height ratio:** Both waist circumference (WC) and waist/height ratio are indicators of visceral fat or abdominal obesity in children and adolescents aged 2–19 years. Increased visceral adiposity measured by WC increases the risk of obesity-related morbidity and mortality. WC should be measured at the high point of the iliac crest when the individual is standing and at minimal respiration. Waist/height ratio is calculated as a ratio of waist circumference (cm) and height (cm).[6] See CDC waist circumference tables for individuals ages 2–19 years: http://www.cdc.gov/nchs/data/nhsr/nhsr010.pdf, Table 18

III. ESTIMATING ENERGY NEEDS

A. Definitions of Energy Needs[2]

1. **Basal metabolic rate (BMR):** Rate of energy expenditure after an overnight fast, resting comfortably, supine, awake, and motionless in a thermoneutral environment.
2. **Basal energy expenditure (BEE):** BMR over 24 hours.
3. **Thermic effect of food (TEF):** Increase in energy expenditure elicited by food consumption.
4. **Energy deposition:** Energy requirement for growth.
5. **Total energy expenditure (TEE):** Sum of BEE, TEF, physical activity, thermoregulation, and energy expended in depositing new tissues and/or producing milk.
6. **Physical activity level (PAL):** Ratio of total to basal daily energy expenditure (TEE/BEE). Describes and accounts for physical activity habits.
7. **Physical activity coefficient (PA):** The physical activity coefficient that correlates with PAL (Table 21-1) can be used to calculate estimated energy requirements (EER [see Section III.B]).

B. Estimated Energy Requirements[2]

1. **EER:** Dietary energy intake predicted to maintain energy balance in a healthy individual. In children, EER includes the needs associated with growth. For most healthy infants and children, the equations here can be used to determine energy needs.
a. For infants, children, and adolescents, EER (kcal/day) = TEE + energy deposition

TABLE 21-1

PHYSICAL ACTIVITY COEFFICIENTS

	Sedentary Activity (Physical Activity Levels Required for Independent Living)	Low Active (30–45 min Sustained Daily Activity)	Active (60 min Sustained Daily Activity)	Very Active (≥90 min Sustained Daily Activity)
PAL	≥1.0 but <1.4	≥1.4 but <1.6	≥1.6 but <1.9	≥1.9 but <2.5
PA (boys ages 3–18)	1.00	1.13	1.26	1.42
PA (girls ages 3–18)	1.00	1.16	1.31	1.56

PA, Physical activity coefficient; PAL, physical activity level.

b. For most hospitalized patients, it can be assumed PAL = sedentary, PA = 1

2. **EER equations (calculate calories/day):**

a. **Infants and young children:**
   (1) 0–3 months: EER = (89 × weight [kg] − 100) + 175
   (2) 4–6 months: EER = (89 × weight [kg] − 100) + 56
   (3) 7–12 months: EER = (89 × weight [kg] − 100) + 22
   (4) 13–35 months: EER = (89 × weight [kg] − 100) + 20

b. **Boys ages 3–18:**
   (1) 3–8 years: EER = 88.5 − (61.9 × age [yr]) + (PA × 26.7 × weight [kg]) + (903 × height [m]) + 20
   (2) 9–18 years: EER = 88.5 − (61.9 × age [yr]) + (PA × 26.7 × weight [kg]) + (903 × height [m]) + 25

c. **Girls ages 3–18:**
   (1) 3–8 years: EER = 135.3 − (30.8 × age [yr]) + (PA × 10 × weight [kg]) + (934 × height [m]) + 20
   (2) 9–18 years: EER = 135.3 − (30.8 × age [yr]) + (PA × 10 × weight [kg]) + (934 × height [m]) + 25

d. **Pregnancy (14–18 years):** EER = adolescent EER + pregnancy energy deposition:
   (1) First trimester = adolescent EER + 0 kcal
   (2) Second trimester = adolescent EER + 340 kcal
   (3) Third trimester = adolescent EER + 452 kcal

e. **Lactation (14–18 years):** EER = adolescent EER + milk energy output − weight loss:
   (1) First 6 months = adolescent EER + 500 − 170
   (2) Second 6 months = adolescent EER + 400 − 0

3. Table 21-2[2] contains the estimated EER for healthy boys and girls of median weight (weight for age at 50th percentile) at both sedentary and active PAL levels.

C. EER Under Stressed Conditions[7]

Calculation of BEE: In many cases, there is little need to provide critically ill patients with more than their BEE. Ideally, energy expenditure should

TABLE 21-2

SAMPLE ESTIMATED ENERGY REQUIREMENTS FOR HEALTHY BOYS AND GIRLS OF MEDIAN WEIGHT AND HEIGHT*

Age	Boys EER (kcal/kg/day)	Girls EER (kcal/kg/day)
0–2 mo	107	104
3 mo	95	95
4–35 mo	82	82

	Boys			Girls		
	Median Weight, Boys (kg)	Sedentary† (kcal/kg/d)	Active† (kcal/kg/d)	Median Weight, Girls (kg)	Sedentary† (kcal/kg/d)	Active† (kcal/kg/d)
3 yr	14.3	80	104	13.9	76	100
4 yr	16.2	74	97	15.8	70	93
5 yr	18.4	68	90	17.9	65	87
6 yr	20.7	63	84	20.2	61	81
7 yr	23.1	59	80	22.8	56	75
8 yr	25.6	56	75	25.6	52	71
9 yr	28.6	53	71	29.0	48	65
10 yr	31.9	49	67	32.9	44	60
11 yr	35.9	46	63	37.2	41	56
12 yr	40.5	44	60	41.6	38	52
13 yr	45.6	42	57	45.8	36	50
14 yr	51.0	40	55	49.4	34	47
15 yr	56.3	39	54	52.0	33	45
16 yr	60.9	38	52	53.9	32	44
17 yr	64.6	36	50	55.1	31	43
18 yr	67.2	35	49	56.2	30	42

*Weight and height for age at 50th percentile.
†See definition of sedentary and active PAL for further information.
EER, Estimated energy requirements.
From Otten JJ, Hellwig JP, Meyers LD, eds. *Dietary Reference Intakes: The Essential Guide to Nutrient Requirements.* Washington, DC: National Academies Press, 2006.

be measured in critically ill patients, but this requires expensive equipment and may not always be practical. Numerous prediction equations are available, and the following is from the *Dietary Reference Intakes*[7]:

For boys: BEE (kcal/d) = 68 − (43.3 × age [yr]) + (712 × height [m]) + (19.2 × weight [kg])

For girls: BEE (kcal/d) = 189 − (17.6 × age [yr]) + (625 × height [m]) + (7.9 × weight [kg])

Appropriate changes should be made as indicated by real (not fluid) weight gain and signs and symptoms of overfeeding.

D. Catch-up Growth Requirement for Malnourished Infants and Children (<3 years)[8,9]

1. **Growth failure** (also known as *failure to thrive*): Condition of undernutrition generally identified in the first 3 years of life. Can be described by

---

BOX 21-1

DETERMINING CATCH-UP GROWTH REQUIREMENTS

1. Plot the child's height and weight on CDC growth charts.
2. Determine recommended calories needed for age (recommended dietary allowances [RDA]).
3. Determine the ideal weight (50th percentile) for child's height.*
4. Multiply the RDA calories by ideal body weight for height (kg).
5. Divide this value by the child's actual weight (kg).
   For example, for a 12-month-old boy whose weight is 7 kg and length is 72 cm, RDA for age would be 98 kcal/kg/day, and ideal body weight for height is 9 kg (50th percentile weight for height). Thus his catch-up growth requirement would be as follows:

$$98 \text{ kcal/kg/day} \times (9 \text{ kg/7kg}) = 126 \text{ kcal/kg/day}.$$

---

*Ideal weight can be 10th–85th percentile weight for height, depending on past growth trends; clinical judgment should be used.

the following growth scenarios: Weight for age <5th percentile on the CDC growth charts, weight for length (or height) <5th percentile, or decreased growth velocity resulting in weight falling >2 major percentiles over 3–6 months (**NOTE:** WHO growth charts have been recently recommended by the CDC for children <24 months, and one may consider using these charts to define growth failure.)

2. **Catch-up growth:** Time period of accelerated growth as a result of caloric provision in excess of the recommended dietary allowances (RDAs). Approximately 20%–30% more energy may be required to achieve catch-up growth in children. Protein needs also increase. This should continue until the previous growth percentiles are regained. Catch-up in linear growth may lag several months behind that in weight. Box 21-1 lists the steps for determining catch-up growth requirements

   NOTE: Aggressive refeeding in the severely malnourished child can result in metabolic alterations, vomiting, diarrhea, and circulatory decompensation known as *refeeding syndrome* (hypophosphatemia, hypokalemia, hypomagnesemia, and glucose and/or fluid intolerance).[10]

IV. DIETARY REFERENCE INTAKES FOR INDIVIDUALS[7]

A. Dietary Reference Intakes

Dietary reference intakes (DRIs) are reference values based on quantitative estimates of nutrient intakes and measured in several ways:

1. **Estimated average requirement (EAR):** Daily nutrient intake level estimated to meet the requirement of half the healthy individuals in a particular life stage and gender group.
2. **Recommended dietary allowance (RDA):** EAR ± 2 standard deviations. The daily nutrient intake level estimated to meet the requirement of 97%–98% of healthy individuals in a particular life stage and gender group.
3. **Adequate intake (AI):** Observed range of intakes in a healthy population; used when data are insufficient to calculate EAR and RDA.

4. **Tolerable upper intake level (UL):** Highest daily nutrient intake level likely to pose no risk for adverse health effects to almost all individuals in the general population.

B. Protein Requirements (Table 21-3)[7]

C. Fat Requirements (Table 21-4)[7]

D. Vitamin Requirements (Table 21-5)[7]

1. **Vitamin D supplementation**
a. Breast-fed and partially breast-fed infants: Should be supplemented with 400 IU/day of vitamin D beginning in the first few days of life.

TABLE 21-3

PROTEIN REQUIREMENTS

Age	RDA (g/kg/day)
0–6 mo	1.52 (AI)*
7–12 mo	1.2
1–3 yr	1.05
4–8 yr	0.95
9–13 yr	0.95
14–18 yr	0.85
Pregnancy (first half)	Unchanged
Pregnancy (second half)	1.1
Lactation	1.3

*If sufficient scientific evidence is not available to establish RDA (recommended dietary allowance), an AI (adequate intake) is usually developed. For healthy breast-fed infants, the AI is the mean intake.

From Otten JJ, Hellwig JP, Meyers LD, eds. *Dietary Reference Intakes: The Essential Guide to Nutrient Requirements.* Washington, DC: National Academies Press, 2006.

TABLE 21-4

FAT REQUIREMENTS: ADEQUATE INTAKE (AI)*

Age	Total Fat (g/day)	Linoleic Acid (g/day)	α-Linolenic Acid (g/day)
0–6 mo	31	4.4 (n-6 PUFA)	0.5 (n-3 PUFA)
7–12 mo	30	4.6 (n-6 PUFA)	0.5 (n-3 PUFA)
1–3 yr	†	7	0.7
4–8 yr	†	10	0.9
9–13 yr, boys	†	12	1.2
9–13 yr, girls	†	10	1.0
14–18 yr, boys	†	16	1.6
14–18 yr, girls	†	11	1.1
Pregnancy	†	13	1.4
Lactation	†	13	1.3

*If sufficient scientific evidence is not available to establish RDA (recommended dietary allowance), an AI (adequate intake) is usually developed. For healthy breast-fed infants, the AI is the mean intake. The AI for other life stage and gender groups is believed to cover the needs of all healthy individuals in the group, but a lack of data or uncertainty in the data prevents being able to specify with confidence the percentage of individuals covered by this intake.
†No AI, estimated average requirement (EAR), or RDA established.
PUFA, Polyunsaturated fatty acid.

From Otten JJ, Hellwig JP, Meyers LD, eds. *Dietary Reference Intakes: The Essential Guide to Nutrient Requirements.* Washington, DC: National Academies Press, 2006.

TABLE 21-5

DIETARY REFERENCE INTAKES: RECOMMENDED INTAKES FOR INDIVIDUALS—VITAMINS

Life Stage	Vit. A[a] (IU)	Vit. C (mg/day)	Vit. D[b,c] (IU)	Vit. E[d] (IU)	Vit. K (mcg/day)	Thiamin (mg/day)	Riboflavin (mg/day)	Niacin[e] (mg/day)	Vit. B6 (mg/day)	Folate[f] (mcg/day)	Vit. B12 (mcg/day)	Pantothenic Acid (mg/day)	Biotin (mcg/day)	Choline[g] (mg/day)
INFANTS														
0–6 mo	1333	40*	400	4*	2.0*	0.2*	0.3*	2*	0.1*	65*	0.4*	1.7*	5*	125*
7–12 mo	1666	50*	400	5*	2.5*	0.3*	0.4*	4*	0.3*	80*	0.5*	1.8*	6*	150*
CHILDREN														
1–3 yr	1000	15	600	6	30*	0.5	0.5	6	0.5	150	0.9	2*	8*	200*
4–8 yr	1333	25	600	7	55*	0.6	0.6	8	0.6	200	1.2	3*	12*	25*
MALES														
9–13 yr	2000	45	600	11	60*	0.9	0.9	12	1.0	300	1.8	4*	20*	375*
14–18 yr	3000	75	600	15	75*	1.2	1.3	16	1.3	400	2.4	5*	25*	550*
19–30 yr	3000	90	600	15	120*	1.2	1.3	16	1.3	400	2.4	5*	30*	550*
FEMALES														
9–13 yr	2000	45	600	11	60*	0.9	0.9	12	1.0	300	1.8	4*	20*	375*
14–18 yr	2333	65	600	15	75*	1.0	1.0	14	1.2	400	2.4	5*	25*	400*
19–30 yr	2333	75	600	15	90*	1.1	1.1	14	1.3	400	2.4	5*	30*	425*

PREGNANCY

<18 yr	2500	80	600	15	75*	1.4	1.4	18	1.9	600	2.6	6*	30*	450*
19–30 yr	2567	85	600	15	90*	1.4	1.4	18	1.9	600	2.6	6*	30*	450*

LACTATION

<18 yr	4000	115	600	19	75*	1.4	1.6	17	2.0	500	2.8	7*	35*	550*
19–30 yr	4333	120	600	19	90*	1.4	1.6	17	2.0	500	2.8	7*	35*	550*

aOne International Unit (IU) = 0.3 mcg retinol equivalent.

bOne mcg cholecalciferol = 40 IU vitamin D.

cIn the absence of adequate exposure to sunlight.

dOne IU = 1 mg vitamin E.

eAs niacin equivalents (NE). 1 mg of niacin = 60 mg of tryptophan; 0–6 months = preformed niacin (not NE).

fAs dietary folate equivalents (DFE). 1 DFE = 1 mcg food folate = 0.6 mcg of folic acid from fortified food or as a supplement consumed with food = 0.5 mcg of a supplement taken on an empty stomach. In view of evidence linking folate intake with neural tube defects in the fetus, it is recommended that all women capable of becoming pregnant consume 400 mcg from supplements or fortified foods in addition to intake of food folate from a varied diet. It is assumed that women will continue consuming 400 mcg from supplements or fortified food until their pregnancy is confirmed and they enter prenatal care, which ordinarily occurs after the end of the periconceptual period—the critical time for formation of the neural tube.

gAlthough AIs have been set for choline, there are few data to assess whether a dietary supply of choline is needed at all life stages, and it may be that the choline requirement can be met by endogenous synthesis at some of these stages.

NOTE: This table (taken from the DRI reports; see www.nap.edu) presents recommended dietary allowances (RDAs) in **bold type** and adequate intakes (AIs) in regular type followed by an asterisk (*). RDAs and AIs may both be used as goals for individual intake. RDAs are set to meet the needs of almost all (97%–98%) individuals in a group. For healthy breast-fed infants, the AI is the mean intake. The AI for other life stage and gender groups is believed to cover needs of all individuals in the group, but lack of data or uncertainty in the data prevent being able to specify with confidence the percentage of individuals covered by this intake.

Modified from Otten JJ, Hellwig JP, Meyers LD, eds. *Dietary Reference Intakes: The Essential Guide to Nutrient Requirements.* Washington, DC: National Academies Press, 2006.

Supplementation should be continued unless the infant is taking 1000 mL/day of vitamin D–fortified formula.
b. Infants not breast-fed and older children: If ingesting <1000 mL/day of vitamin D–fortified formula, fortified foods, or milk, should receive supplementation of 400 IU/day
c. Adolescents: If not obtaining 600 IU of vitamin D through fortified milk (100 IU per 8-oz serving) and fortified food (fortified cereals, egg yolks), should be supplemented with 600 IU/day

2. **Examples of multivitamins for infants and children** (Tables 21-6 and 21-7)

E. Mineral Requirements (Table 21-8)[7]

1. **Iron supplementation**
a. Breast-fed term infants: Should receive 1 mg/kg of an oral iron supplement beggining at 4 months of age, preferably from iron-fortified cereal or, alternatively, elemental iron
b. Breast-fed preterm infants: Should receive 2 mg/kg/day by 1 month of age, which should be continued until the infant is weaned to iron-fortified formula or begins eating complementary foods
c. Formula-fed term infants: Receive adequate iron from fortified formula (4–12 mg/L) from birth to age 12 months
d. Formula-fed preterm infants: Need an additional supplementation of 1 mg/kg/day to get total daily dose of 2 mg/kg/day

2. **Fluoride supplementation**
a. Supplementation not needed during the first 6 months of life. Thereafter, 0.5 mg/day is recommended for exclusively breast-fed infants.

TABLE 21-6

INFANT MULTIVITAMIN DROPS ANALYSIS (PER ML)*

Nutrient	Poly-Vi-Sol [w/iron], Multivitamin [with iron]	Tri-Vi-Sol [w/iron]	AquADEKs†‡	D Vi-Sol	Fer-In-Sol
Vitamin A (IU)	1500	1500	5751	—	—
Vitamin D (IU)	400	400	400	400	—
Vitamin E (IU)	5	—	50	—	—
Vitamin C (mg)	35	35	45	—	—
Thiamin (mg)	0.5	—	0.6	—	—
Riboflavin (mg)	0.6	—	0.6	—	—
Niacin (mg)	8	—	6	—	—
Vitamin B$_6$ (mg)	0.4	—	0.6	—	—
Vitamin B$_{12}$ (mcg)	2	—	—	—	—
Vitamin K (mcg)	—	—	400	—	—
Iron (mg)	[10]	[10]	—	—	15
Fluoride (mg)	—	—	—	—	—
Zinc (mg)	—	—	5	—	—

*Standard dose = 1 mL.
†Also contains biotin 15 mcg; pantothenic acid 3 mg; 87% vitamin A as β-carotene; coenzyme Q$_{10}$ 2 mg; selenium 10 mcg.
‡Recommended for use in infants with fat malabsorption, such as cystic fibrosis, liver disease.

TABLE 21-7
MULTIVITAMIN TABLETS (ANALYSIS/TABLET)

	Flintstones Sour Gummies	Centrum Kids Complete	Flintstones Complete	Centrum Tablet*	AquADEKs (Softgel)	Source CF (Chewable)	Vitamax (Chewable)	Phlexy-Vits (7-g Packet)	Nano-VM 1–3 yrs. (2 Scoops)	Nano-VM 4–8 yrs. (2 Scoops)
Vitamin A (IU)	1000	3500	3000	3500	18,167	16,000a	5000b	2664	1000	1332
Vitamin D (IU)	100	400	400	400	800	1,000	400	400	400	400
Vitamin E (IU)	10	30	30	30	150	200	200	13.5	9	10
Vitamin K (mcg)	—	10	—	25	700	200	200	70	30	55
Vitamin C (mg)	15	60	60	60	75	800	60	50	15	25
Thiamin (mg)	—	1.5	1.5	1.5	1.5	1.5	1.5	1.2	0.5	0.6
Riboflavin (mg)	—	1.7	1.7	1.7	1.7	1.7	1.7	1.4	0.5	0.6
Niacin (mg)	—	20	15	20	20	10	20	20	6	8
Vitamin B$_6$ (mg)	0.5	2	2	2	1.9	1.9	2	1.6	0.5	0.6
Folate (mcg)	100	400	400	400	200	200	200	700	150	200
Vitamin B$_{12}$ (mcg)	2.5	6	6	6	12	6	6	5	0.9	1.2
Biotin (mcg)	38	45	40	30	100	100	300	150	8	12
Pantothenic acid (mg)	2.5	10	10	10	12	12	10	5	2	3
Calcium (mg)	—	108	100	200	—	—	—	1,000	500	800
Phosphorus (mg)	—	50	100	20	—	—	—	775	460	500
Iron (mg)	—	18	18	18	—	—	—	15.1	7	10

Continued

TABLE 21-7
MULTIVITAMIN TABLETS (ANALYSIS/TABLET) (Continued)

	Flintstones Sour Gummies	Centrum Kids Complete	Flintstones Complete	Centrum Tablet*	AquADEKs (Softgel)	Source CF (Chewable)	Vitamax (Chewable)	Phlexy-Vits (7-g Packet)	Nano-VM 1–3 yrs. (2 Scoops)	Nano-VM 4–8 yrs. (2 Scoops)
Iodine (mcg)	20	150	150	150	—	—	—	150	90	90
Magnesium (mg)	—	40	20	50	—	—	—	300	65	110
Zinc (mg)	1.2	15	12	11	10	15	7.5	11.1	3	5
Copper (mg)	—	2	2	0.5	—	—	—	1.5	0.34	0.44
Manganese (mg)	—	1	—	2.3	—	—	—	1.5	1.2	1.5
Chromium (mcg)	—	20	—	35	—	—	—	30	11	15
Molybdenum (mcg)	—	20	—	45	—	—	—	70	17	22
Selenium (mcg)	—	—	—	55	75	—	—	75	20	30
Fluoride (mg)	—	—	—	—	—	—	—	—	—	—
Choline (mg)	38	—	38	—	—	—	—	8.8	0	0
Sodium (mg)	—	—	10	—	—	—	—	<1.4	575	775
Potassium (mg)	—	—	—	80	—	—	—	—	0	0
Chloride	—	—	—	72	—	—	—	<0.35	0	0

*Contains boron, nickel, silicon, tin.
[a] Vitamin A: 88% β-carotene, 12% palmitate.
[b] Vitamin A as acetate and 50% β-carotene.

TABLE 21-8

DIETARY REFERENCE INTAKES: RECOMMENDED INTAKES—ELEMENTS

Life Stage	Calcium (mg/day)	Chromium (mcg/day)	Copper (mcg/day)	Fluoride (mg/day)	Iodine (mcg/day)	Iron (mg/day)	Magnesium (mg/day)	Manganese (mg/day)	Molybdenum (mcg/day)	Phosphorus (mg/day)	Selenium (mcg/day)	Zinc (mg/day)
INFANTS												
0–6 mo	200*	0.2*	200*	0.01*	110*	0.27*	30*	0.003*	2*	100*	15*	2*
7–12 mo	260*	5.5*	220*	0.5*	130*	11	75*	0.6*	3*	275*	20*	3
CHILDREN												
1–3 yr	700	11*	340	0.7*	90	7	80	1.2*	17	460	20	3
4–8 yr	1000	15*	440	1.0*	90	10	130	1.5*	22	500	30	5
MALES												
9–13 yr	1300	25*	700	2*	120	8	240	1.9*	34	1250	40	8
14–18 yr	1300	35*	890	3*	150	11	410	2.2*	43	1250	55	11
19–30 yr	1000	35*	900	4*	150	8	400	2.3*	45	700	55	11

Continued

TABLE 21-8

DIETARY REFERENCE INTAKES: RECOMMENDED INTAKES—ELEMENTS (Continued)

Life Stage	Calcium (mg/day)	Chromium (mcg/day)	Copper (mcg/day)	Fluoride (mg/day)	Iodine (mcg/day)	Iron (mg/day)	Magnesium (mg/day)	Manganese (mg/day)	Molybdenum (mcg/day)	Phosphorus (mg/day)	Selenium (mcg/day)	Zinc (mg/day)
FEMALES												
9–13 yr	1300	21*	700	2*	120	8	240	1.6*	34	1250	40	8
14–18 yr	1300	24*	890	3*	150	15	360	1.6*	43	1250	55	9
19–30 yr	1000	25*	900	3*	150	18	310	1.8*	45	700	55	8
PREGNANCY												
<18 yr	1300	29*	1000	3*	220	27	400	2.0*	50	1250	60	13
19–30 yr	1000	30*	1000	3*	220	27	350	2.0*	50	700	60	11
LACTATION												
<18 yr	1300	44*	1300	3*	290	10	360	2.6*	50	1250	70	14
19–30 yr	1000	45*	1300	3*	290	9	310	2.6*	50	700	70	12

NOTE: This table presents recommended dietary allowances (RDAs) in **bold type** and adequate intakes (AIs) in ordinary type followed by an asterisk (*). RDAs and AIs may both be used as goals for individual intake. RDAs are set to meet the needs of almost all (97%–98%) individuals in a group. For healthy breast-fed infants, the AI is the mean intake. The AI for other life stage and gender groups is believed to cover needs of all individuals in the group, but lack of data or uncertainty in the data prevent being able to specify with confidence the percentage of individuals covered by this intake.

Modified from Otten JJ, Hellwig JP, Meyers LD, eds. *Dietary Reference Intakes: The Essential Guide to Nutrient Requirements.* Washington, DC: National Academies Press; 2006. Includes updates from. Ross AC, Taylor CL, Yaktine AL, Del Valle HB, eds. *Dietary Reference Intakes for Calcium and Vitamin D.* Washington, DC: National Academies Press, 2011.

TABLE 21-9

FIBER REQUIREMENTS: ADEQUATE INTAKE*

Age	Total Fiber (g/day)
0–12 mo	Not determined
1–3 yr	19
4–8 yr	25
9–13 yr, boys	31
9–13 yr, girls	26
14–18 yr, boys	38
14–18 yr, girls	26
Pregnancy	28
Lactation	29

*Adequate intake (AI). If sufficient scientific evidence unavailable to establish recommended dietary allowance (RDA), an AI is usually developed. For healthy breast-fed infants, the AI is the mean intake. AI for other life stage and gender groups is believed to cover the needs of all healthy individuals in the group, but a lack of data or uncertainty in the data prevents being able to specify with confidence the percentage of individuals covered by this intake.

Modified from Otten JJ, Hellwig JP, Meyers LD, eds. *Dietary Reference Intakes: The Essential Guide to Nutrient Requirements.* Washington, DC: National Academies Press, 2006.

b. Consider fluoride supplementation for those patients who use bottled water and home filtration systems. Most bottled water does not contain adequate amounts of fluoride. Some home water treatment systems can reduce fluoride levels.

c. To avoid fluorosis, children should not use fluoridated toothpaste until age 2 years, and then only a small pea-sized amount up to age 6 years. See Formulary for complete fluoride recommendations (i.e., in areas where water is not fluoridated).

F. Fiber Requirements (Table 21-9)[7]

V. ENTERAL NUTRITION

A. Mixing Instructions for Full-Term Standard and Soy-Based Infant Formulas (Table 21-10)

B. Common Caloric Modulars

For the child who needs additional protein, carbohydrate, fat, or a combination (Table 21-11)

C. Enteral Formulas, Including Their Main Nutrient Components (Table 21-12)

A comprehensive (but not complete) list. Most of these formulas are cow's milk–based and designed for normal digestive tracts.

D. Clinical Conditions Requiring Special Diets, and Suggested Formula(s) (Table 21-13)

A comprehensive (but not complete) list of special clinical conditions (e.g., cow's milk allergy or intolerance) and the growing number of formulas designed for these conditions.

E. Common Oral Rehydration Solutions (Table 21-14)

TABLE 21-10

PREPARATION OF INFANT FORMULAS FOR FULL-TERM STANDARD AND SOY FORMULAS*

Formula Type	Caloric Concentration (kcal/oz)	Amount of Formula	Water (oz)
Liquid concentrates	20	13 oz	13 oz
(40 kcal/oz)	24	13 oz	8.5 oz
	27	13 oz	6.3 oz
	30	13 oz	4.3 oz
Powder (44 kcal/scoop)	20	1 scoop	2 oz
	24	3 scoops	5 oz
	27	3 scoops	4.25 oz
	30	3 scoops	4 oz

*Does not apply to Enfacare, Neocate Infant, Neosure. Enfamil AR should not be concentrated greater than 24 kcal/oz. Use a packed measure for Nutramigen LIPIL and Pregestimil LIPIL; all others unpacked powder.

TABLE 21-11

COMMON CALORIC MODULARS*

Component	Calories
PROTEIN	
Beneprotein (powder)	25 kcal/scoop (6 g protein)
Prosource protein powder	30 kcal/scoop (6 g protein)
Complete Amino Acid Mix	3.28 kcal/g (0.82 g protein)
Liquid Protein Fortifier	0.67 kcal/mL (0.167 g protein/mL)
CARBOHYDRATE	
Polycose	Powder: 3.8 kcal/g
SolCarb	3.75 kcal/g; 15 kcal/tablespoon
FAT	
MCT oil†	7.7 kcal/mL
Vegetable oil	8.3 kcal/mL
Microlipid	4.5 kcal/mL
Liquigen (emulsified MCT)	4.5 kcal/mL
FAT AND CARBOHYDRATE	
Duocal	42 kcal/15 mL; 25 kcal/scoop (59% Carb, 41% Fat, 35% fat as MCT)

*Use these caloric supplements when you want to increase protein or when you have reached the maximum concentration tolerated and wish to further increase caloric density.
†Medium-chain triglyceride (MCT) oil is unnecessary unless there is fat malabsorption.

TABLE 21-12

ENTERAL NUTRITION COMPONENTS (PER LITER)

A. INFANT FORMULAS

	Kcal/oz	Protein (g)	Fat (g)	Carbs (g)	Na (mEq)	K (mEq)	Ca (mg)	P (mg)	Fe (mg)	Osmolality
HUMAN MILK										
Term	20	11	39	72	8	14	279	143	0.3	286
Preterm	20	14	39	66	11	15	248	128	1.2	290
HUMAN MILK AND FORTIFIERS ANALYSIS										
Enfamil HMF Liquid + Preterm Human Milk (5 mL + 25 mL breastmilk)	24	32	48	65	20	20	1100	640	15	322
Similac HMF + Preterm Human Milk (1 pkt/25 mL)	24	23	41	82	17	30	1381	777	4.6	N/A
PRETERM FORMULAS										
Enfamil Enfacare	22	21	39	77	11	20	890	490	13.3	260
Enfamil Premature 20	20	20	34	74	17	17	1100	553	3.4	240
Enfamil Premature 24 High Protein	24	28	41	85	20	21	1340	670	15	300
Enfamil Premature 30	30	30	52	112	26	28	1670	840	18	300
Gerber Good Start Premature 20	20	20	35	71	16	21	1110	570	12	229
Gerber Good Start Premature 24 High Protein	24	29	42	78	19	25	1310	680	14	299
Gerber Good Start Premature 30	30	30	53	107	24	31	1660	860	18	341
Gerber Good Start Nourish	22	21	38	76	12	20	880	470	13	275
Similac Neosure	22	21	41	75	11	27	781	461	13.4	250
Similac Special Care 20	20	20	37	70	13	22	1217	676	12.2	235
Similac Special Care 24 High Protein	24	27	44	81	15	27	1461	811	14.6	280
Similac Special Care 30	30	30	67	78	19	34	1826	1014	18.3	325

Continued

21

TABLE 21-12

ENTERAL NUTRITION COMPONENTS (PER LITER) (Continued)

A. INFANT FORMULAS (Continued)

	Kcal/oz	Protein (g)	Fat (g)	Carbs (g)	Na (mEq)	K (mEq)	Ca (mg)	P (mg)	Fe (mg)	Osmolality
COW'S MILK–BASED FORMULAS										
Enfamil Infant	20	14	36	74	8	19	520	287	12	300
Enfamil Newborn	20	14	36	73	8	19	520	287	12	300
Enfamil A.R.	20	17	34	74	12	19	520	353	12	230 (240*)
Enfamil LactoFree	20	14	36	73	9	19	547	307	12	200
Enfagrow Toddler Transitions	20	18	36	70	10	23	1300	867	13.4	270
Evap. Milk (13 oz + 19 oz water + 30 mL corn syrup)	20	27	31	72	21	32	1066	832	0.8	N/A
Organic Milk–Based Infant Formula	20	15	36	71	7	15	420	280	12	294
Parent's Choice Premium Infant Formula	20	14	36	72	8	19	520	287	12	295
Similac Advance	20	14	37	76	7	18	528	284	12	310
Similac Go and Grow Milk-Based Formula	20	14	37	72	7	18	1014	548	13.5	300
Similac Sensitive	20	14	37	72	9	19	568	379	12.2	200
Similac Advance Organic	20	14	37	71	7	18	528	284	12.2	225
Similac PM 60/40	20	15	38	69	7	14	379	189	4.7	280
Similac for Spitup	20	14	37	72	9	19	568	379	12.2	180
SOY-BASED										
America's Store Brand Soy (also w/ARA/DHA)	20	17	36	68	11	21	700	460	12	164
Enfamil Prosobee	20	17	36	71	11	21	700	460	12	170
Enfagrow Soy Next Step	20	22	30	79	11	21	1300	867	13.3	230
Gerber Good Start Soy	20	17	34	75	12	20	704	422	12.1	180
Gerber Good Start 2 Soy	20	19	34	73	12	20	1273	710	13.4	175

21

Similac Soy Isomil	20	17	37	70	13	19	710	507	12.2	200
Similac for Diarrhea	20	18	37	68	13	19	710	507	12.2	240
Similac Go and Grow Soy-Based Formula	20	17	37	70	13	19	1014	676	13.5	200
CASEIN, EXTENSIVELY HYDROLYZED										
Alimentum	20	19	37	69	13	20	710	507	12.2	370
Nutramigen	20	19	36	69	14	19	627	347	12	300 (320*)
Nutramigen with Enflora LGG	20	19	36	69	14	19	627	347	12	300
Pregestimil	20	19	38	69	14	19	640	350	12.2	250
WHEY, PARTIALLY HYDROLYZED										
Gerber Good Start Gentle	20	15	34	78	8	19	449	255	10.1	250
Gerber Good Start Protect	20	15	34	75	8	19	449	255	10.1	250
Gerber Good Start 2 Gentle	20	15	34	78	8	19	1273	710	13.4	180
Gerber Good Start 2 Protect	20	15	34	75	8	19	1273	710	13.4	180
Gerber Good Start Soothe	20	15	34	75	8	19	480	270	10	195
WHEY AND CASEIN, PARTIALLY HYDROLYZED										
Enfamil Gentlease	20	15	36	72	10	19	547	307	12	230
AMINO ACID–BASED										
Elecare Infant	20	20	32	72	13	26	780	568	10	350
Neocate Infant	20	21	30	78	11	27	830	624	12.4	375
PurAmino	20	19	36	69	14	19	627	347	12	350
SPECIALIZED										
3232A	20	19	28	89	13	19	627	420	12.5	250
RCF	20	20	36	68	13	19	710	507	12.2	168
Enfaport	30	35	54	102	13	29	940	520	18	280

Continued

TABLE 21-12

ENTERAL NUTRITION COMPONENTS (PER LITER) (Continued)

B. TODDLER AND YOUNG CHILD 1–10 YEARS (Continued)

B. TODDLER AND YOUNG CHILD 1–10 YEARS

COW'S MILK–BASED FORMULAS

	Kcal/oz	Protein (g)	Fat (g)	Carbs (g)	Na (mEq)	K (mEq)	Ca (mg)	P (mg)	Fe (mg)	Osmolality
Boost Kid Essentials	30	30	38	135	24	30	1181	886	14	550/600/570
Boost Kid Essentials 1.5 (w/fiber)	45	42	75	165	30	33	1300	990	14	390 (405)
Carnation Instant Breakfast Essentials	24	43	16	105	24	27	1539	1539	13.8	N/A
Compleat Pediatric	30	38	39	132	33	42	1440	1000	14	380
Cow's Milk, 2%	15	35	20	50	22	41	1258	979	0.5	N/A
Cow's Milk, whole	19	34	34	48	22	40	1226	956	0.5	285
KetoCal 3:1	30	22	97	10	18	35	1140	801	16	180
KetoCal 4:1	43	30	144	6	26	55	1600	1300	22	197
Monogen	30	27	28	163	21	22	617	480	10.1	370
Nutren Junior (also w/fiber)	30	30	50	110	20	34	1000	800	14	350
Pediasure Enteral (also w/fiber)	30	30	40	133	17	34	972	845	14	335 (345)
Pediasure 1.5 (also w/fiber)	45	59	67	160 (165)	17	42	1476	1054	11	370 (390)
Pediasure Sidekicks	19	30	21	89	17	42	1055	844	11	420
Pediasure Sidekicks, Clear	18	30	0	120	8	4	175	750	9	325
Pediasure Vanilla	30	30	38	131	17	34	972	845	14	480
Pediasure with Fiber, Vanilla	30	30	38	135	17	34	972	845	14	480
Portagen	30	32	44	104	22	29	850	642	17	350

SOY-BASED

Bright Beginnings Soy Pediatric Drink	30	30	50	109	17	40	970	800	14	350

SEMI-ELEMENTAL, HYDROLYZED

	Kcal/oz	Protein (g)	Fat (g)	Carbs (g)	Na (mEq)	K (mEq)	Ca (mg)	P (mg)	Fe (mg)	Osmolality
Peptamen Junior Fiber	30	30	39	137	20	34	1000	800	14	390
Peptamen Junior with Prebio	30	30	39	137	20	34	1000	800	14	365
Peptamen Junior, unflavored (w/fiber, vanilla flavored)	30	30	39	138	20	34	1000	800	14	260 (390)
Peptamen Junior 1.5	45	45	68	180	30	51	1652	1352	20.8	450
Pediasure Peptide (also flavored)	30	30	41	134	31	35	1060	844	14	250 (390)
Pediasure Peptide 1.5	45	45	61	201	47	52	1580	1265	21	450
SOY AND PORK, HYDROLYZED										
Peptide Junior, Unflavored	30	31	50	106	18	35	1130	940	14	430
AMINO ACID–BASED										
Elecare Jr, Unflavored and Vanilla	30	31	49	109	20	39	1172	852	15	560
E028 Splash	30	25	35	146	9	24	620	620	7.7	820
Neocate Junior Flavored	30	35	47	110	19	36	1200	738	16	690
Neocate Junior Unflavored	30	33	50	104	18	35	1130	697	15	590
Vivonex Pediatric	24	24	24	130	17	31	970	800	10	360

C. OLDER CHILDREN AND ADULT STANDARD FORMULAS

	Kcal/oz	Protein (g)	Fat (g)	Carbs (g)	Na (mEq)	K (mEq)	Ca (mg)	P (mg)	Fe (mg)	Osmolality
COW'S MILK–BASED FORMULAS										
Boost	30	40	17	171	24	43	1250	1250	19	625
Boost Glucose Control	32	59	50	84	48	29	1160	928	15	400
Boost High Protein	30	63	25	138	31	41	1459	1250	19	650
Boost Plus	45	59	59	188	31	41	1,459	1250	19	670
Compleat	32	48	40	128	43	44	760	760	14	340
Ensure Clear	30	35	0	215	8	0	0	0	9	700
Ensure Immune Health	32	38	25	177	37	40	1266	1055	19	620

Continued

21

TABLE 21-12

ENTERAL NUTRITION COMPONENTS (PER LITER) (Continued)

C. OLDER CHILDREN AND ADULT STANDARD FORMULAS (Continued)

	Kcal/oz	Protein (g)	Fat (g)	Carbs (g)	Na (mEq)	K (mEq)	Ca (mg)	P (mg)	Fe (mg)	Osmolality
Ensure Plus	45	55	212	47	41	45	1266	1266	19	680
Glucerna 1.0 Cal	30	42	54	96	41	40	705	705	13	355
Jevity 1 Cal	32	44	35	155	40	40	910	760	14	300
Jevity 1.2 Cal	36	56	39	169	59	47	1200	1200	18	450
Jevity 1.5 Cal	45	64	50	216	61	55	1200	1200	18	525
Nepro	54	81	96	167	46	27	1060	700	19	585
Novasource Renal	60	74	100	200	39	21	1300	650	18	700/960
Nutren 1.0, vanilla (w/fiber)	30	40	38	127	38	32	668	668	12	370 (410)
Nutren 1.5, unflavored	45	60	68	169	51	48	1000	1000	18	430
Nutren 2.0	60	80	104	196	57	49	1340	1340	24	745
Optimental	30	51	28	139	49	44	1055	1055	13	585
Osmolite 1 Cal	32	44	35	144	40	40	760	760	14	300
Osmolite 1.2 Cal	36	56	39	158	58	46	1200	1200	18	360
Osmolite 1.5 Cal	45	63	49	204	61	46	1000	1000	18	525
Promote (w/fiber)	30	63	26	130	44	51	1200	1200	18	340 (380)
Pulmocare	45	63	93	106	57	50	1060	1060	19	475
Renalcal	60	35	83	291	0	0	0	0	0	600
Replete, unflavored	30	63	34	113	39	39	1000	1000	18	300/350
Resource 2.0	60	84	88	217	35	39	1042	1042	18.8	790
Resource Breeze	32	38	0	230	15	1	42	633	11	750
Suplena	54	45	96	205	35	29	1055	717	19	600
TwoCal HN	60	84	91	219	64	63	1050	1050	19	725

SOY-BASED										
Fibersource HN	36	53	39	160	52	51	1000	1000	17	490
Isosource 1.5 CAL	45	68	65	170	56	58	1070	1070	19	650/585
Isosource HN	36	53	39	160	48	49	1200	1200	15	490
SEMI-ELEMENTAL HYDROLYZED										
Peptamen, unflavored	30	40	39	127	25	39	800	700	18	270
Peptamen with Prebio	30	40	39	127	25	39	800	700	18	300
Peptamen 1.5, unflavored	45	68	56	188	45	48	1000	1000	27	550
Peptamen AF	36	76	55	107	35	41	800	800	14.4	390
Peptamen Bariatric	30	93	38	78	29	34	670	670	12	345
Perative	39	67	37	180	45	44	870	870	16	460
Pivot 1.5	45	94	51	172	61	51	1000	1000	18	595
Vital 1.0 Cal	30	40	38	130	46	36	705	705	13	390
Vital HN	30	42	11	185	25	36	667	667	12	500
AMINO ACID–BASED										
Tolerex	30	21	1.5	230	20	30	560	560	10	550
Vivonex RTF	30	50	12	175	29	31	670	670	12	630
Vivonex Plus	30	45	7	190	27	27	560	560	10	650
Vivonex T.E.N.	30	38	3	210	26	24	500	500	9	630

*Liquid formulation.

TABLE 21-13

FORMULAS FOR SPECIAL CLINICAL CIRCUMSTANCES

A. INFANTS

Preterm	
Pre-discharge	Enfamil Premature 20, 24 HP, 30
	Similac Special Care Advance 20, 24 HP, 30
	Gerber Good Start Premature 20, 24 HP, 30
Post-discharge (through 12 mo)	Enfamil Enfacare
	Similac Neosure
	Gerber Good Start Nourish
Lactose intolerance	Enfamil LactoFree
	Similac Sensitive
	Similac for Diarrhea
Vegetarian, lactose intolerance, or galacto-semia	America's Store Brand Soy Infant Formula
	Gerber Good Start Soy
	Gerber Good Start Soy 2
	Similac Go and Grow Soy-Based Formula (9–24 mo)
	Similac Soy Isomil
	Enfagrow Soy NEXT STEP (9–24 mo)
	Enfamil Prosobee
Protein (e.g., cow's milk) allergy/intolerance and/or fat malabsorption	Alimentum
	Elecare
	Neocate Infant (and w/DHA and ARA)
	Nutramigen
	PurAmino
	Pregestimil
Severe carbohydrate intolerance	3232A
	RCF
Requiring lower calcium and phosphorus	Similac PM 60/40

B. TODDLERS AND YOUNG CHILDREN AGES 1–10 YR

Vegetarian, lactose intolerance, or milk protein intolerance	Bright Beginnings Soy Pediatric Drink
Protein allergy/intolerance and/or fat malabsorption	Pediasure Peptide (and 1.5)
	Pepdite Jr
	Peptamen Jr (with and without Prebio)
	Vivonex Pediatric
	Elecare Jr
	Neocate Junior (Unflavored and Flavored)
	EO28 Splash
Fat malabsorption, intestinal lymphatic obstruction, chylothorax	Portagen
	Monogen
	Enfaport
Increased caloric needs	Boost Kids Essentials
	Carnation Instant Breakfast Essentials
	Nutren Junior (also with fiber)
	Pediasure (also with fiber)
Requiring clear liquid diet	Resource Breeze
	Ensure Clear
	Pediasure Sidekicks Clear

TABLE 21-13

FORMULAS FOR SPECIAL CLINICAL CIRCUMSTANCES (Continued)

Intractable epilepsy	KetoCal (3:1 and 4:1)

C. OLDER CHILDREN AND ADULTS

Tube feeding	
For malabsorption of protein and/or fat	Peptamen, Peptamen w/ Prebio, Peptamen 1.5
	Perative
	Tolerex
	Vital HN
	Vital 1.0 Cal
	Vivonex Plus and Vivonex T.E.N
For critically ill and/or malabsorption	Optimental
	Pulmocare
	Pivot 1.5
	Perative
For impaired glucose tolerance	Glucerna
	Glytrol
	Store Brand Diabetic Nutritional Drink
For dialysis patients	Magnacal Renal
	Nepro
	NutriRenal
For patients with acute renal failure not on dialysis	Renalcal
	Suplena
Increased caloric needs (oral)	
With a normal gastrointestinal (GI) tract	Boost, Boost with fiber
	Boost Plus, Boost High Protein
	Carnation Instant Breakfast Essentials with whole milk
	Ensure
	NUTRA Shake
For clear liquid diet	Resource Breeze
	Ensure Clear
	Pediasure Sidekicks Clear
For patients with cystic fibrosis (CF)	Scandishake with whole milk

TABLE 21-14

ORAL REHYDRATION SOLUTIONS

Solution	Kcal/mL (kcal/oz)	Carbohydrate (g/L)	Na (mEq/L)	K (mEq/L)	Osmolality (mOsm/kg H$_2$O)
CeraLyte-70	0.16 (4.9)	Rice digest (40)	70	20	N/A
CeraLyte-50	0.16 (4.9)	Rice digest (40)	50	20	N/A
CeraLyte-90	0.16 (4.9)	Rice digest (40)	90	20	N/A
Enfalyte	0.12 (3.7)	Rice syrup solids (30)	50	25	170
Oral Rehydration Salts (WHO)	0.06 (2)	Dextrose (20)	90	20	330
Pedialyte (unflavored)	0.1 (3)	Dextrose (25)	45	20	250

VI. PARENTERAL NUTRITION[12]

Necessary to adequately support the pediatric patient with insufficient enteral intake.

A. Situations Where Parenteral Nutrition(PN) is Suggested

1. **Inability to feed enterally** (e.g., extreme prematurity, tracheoesophageal fistulas)
2. **When alimentation via gastrointestinal tract has to be restricted for >5 days** (e.g., chylothorax/chylous ascites, bowel pseudo-obstruction)
3. **Gastrointestinal (GI) dysfunction and/or malabsorption** (e.g., short gut syndrome, intestinal atresias, enteric fistulas, gastroschisis)
4. **Increased losses or requirements** (e.g., severe diarrhea, intractable vomiting, persistent or severe failure to thrive)

B. Suggested Formulations for Initiation and Advancement of PN (Table 21-15)

Suggested glucose, protein, and fat during initiation, as well as recommendations for advancement and maximum allowable amounts

C. Recommended Parenteral Formulations (Table 21-16)

Based on age groups; includes recommendations for electrolytes, elements, and minerals

D. Suggested Monitoring Schedule for Patients Receiving Parenteral Nutrition (Table 21-17)

Important to monitor growth parameters, as well as laboratory studies for these patients on periodic basis

---

TABLE 21-15

INITIATION AND ADVANCEMENT OF PARENTERAL NUTRITION*

Nutrient	Initial Dose	Advancement	Maximum
Glucose	5%–10%	2.5%–5%/day	12.5% peripheral 18 mg/kg/min (maximum rate of infusion)
Protein	1–1.5 g/kg/day	0.5–1 g/kg/day	3–4 g/kg/day 10%–16% of calories
Fat†	0.5–1 g/kg/day	1 g/kg/day	4 g/kg/day 0.17 g/kg/hr (maximum rate of infusion)

*Acceptable osmolarity of parenteral nutrition through a peripheral line varies between 900 and 1050 osm/L by institution. An estimate of the osmolarity of parenteral nutrition can be obtained with the following formula: Estimated osmolarity = (dextrose concentration × 50) + (amino acid concentration × 100) + (mEq of electrolytes × 2). Consult individual pharmacy for hospital limitations.

†Essential fatty acid deficiency (EFAD) may occur in fat-free parenteral nutrition within 2–4 weeks in infants and children and as early as 2–14 days in neonates. A minimum of 2%–4% of total caloric intake as linoleic acid and 0.25%–0.5% as linolenic acid is necessary to meet essential fatty acid requirements.

Modified from Baker RD, Baker SS, Davis AM. *Pediatric Parenteral Nutrition.* New York: Chapman and Hall, 1997; and Cox JH, Melbardis IM. Parenteral nutrition. In: Samour PQ, King K, eds. *Handbook of Pediatric Nutrition.* 3rd ed. Boston: Jones and Bartlett Publishers, 2005.

TABLE 21-16

PARENTERAL NUTRITION FORMULATION RECOMMENDATIONS

Component	Preterm	Term Infants	1–3 yr	4–6 yr	7–10 yr	11–18 yr
Energy (kcal/kg/day)	85–105	90–108	75–90	65–80	55–70	30–55
Protein (g/kg/day)	2.5–4	2.5–3.5	1.5–2.5	1.5–2.5	1.5–2.5	0.8–2
Sodium (mEq/kg/day)	2–4	2–4	2–4	2–4	2–4	60–150 mEq/day
Potassium (mEq/kg/day)	2–4	2–4	2–4	2–4	2–4	70–180 mEq/day
Calcium (mg/kg/day)	50–60	20–40	10–20	10–20	10–20	200–800 mg/day
Phosphorus (mg/kg/day)	30–45	30–45	15–40	15–40	15–40	280–900 mg/day
Magnesium (mEq/kg/day)	0.5–1	0.25–1	0.25–0.5	0.25–0.5	0.25–0.5	8–24 mEq/day
Zinc (mcg/kg/day)	325–400	100–250	100	100	50	2–5 mg/day
Copper (mcg/kg/day)*	20	20	20	20	5–20	200–300 mcg/day
Manganese (mcg/kg/day)*	1	1	1	1	1	40–50 mcg/day
Selenium (mcg/kg/day)	2	2	2	2	1–2	40–60 mcg/day

*Copper and manganese needs may be lowered in cholestasis.

Modified from Baker RD, Baker SS, Davis AM. *Pediatric Parenteral Nutrition.* New York: Chapman and Hall, 1997; Cox JH, Melbardis IM. Parenteral nutrition. In: Samour PQ, King K, eds. *Handbook of Pediatric Nutrition.* 3rd ed. Boston: Jones and Bartlett Publishers, 2005; and American Society for Parenteral and Enteral Nutrition (ASPEN). Safe practices for parenteral nutrition. *JPEN J Parenter Enteral Nutr.* 2004;28(6):S39–S70.

TABLE 21-17

MONITORING SCHEDULE FOR PATIENTS RECEIVING PARENTERAL NUTRITION*

Variable	Initial Period†	Later Period‡
GROWTH		
Weight	Daily	2 times/wk
Height	Weekly (infants)	
	Monthly (children)	Monthly
Head circumference (infants)	Weekly	Monthly§
LABORATORY STUDIES		
Electrolytes and glucose	Daily until stable	Weekly
BUN/creatinine	Twice weekly	Weekly
Albumin or prealbumin	Weekly	Weekly
Ca^{2+}, Mg^{2+}, P	Twice weekly	Weekly
ALT, AST, ALP	Weekly	Weekly
Total and direct bilirubin	Weekly	Weekly
CBC	Weekly	Weekly
Triglycerides	With each increase	Weekly
Vitamins	—	As indicated
Trace minerals	—	As indicated

*For patients on long-term parenteral nutrition, monitoring every 2–4 weeks is adequate in most cases.

†The period before nutritional goals are reached or during any period of instability.

‡When stability is reached, no changes in nutrient composition.

§Weekly in preterm infants.

ALP, Alkaline phosphatase; ALT, alanine transaminase; AST, aspartate transaminase; BUN, blood urea nitrogen; CBC, complete blood cell count.

REFERENCES

1. Centers for Disease Control and Prevention (CDC). http://www.cdc.gov/growthcharts/.
2. Centers for Disease Control and Prevention (CDC). http://www.cdc.gov/healthyweight/assessing/bmi/index.html.
3. Barlow SE, Dietz WH. Obesity evaluation and treatment: Expert Committee recommendations. *Pediatrics*. 1998;102(3):e29.
4. Barlow S. Expert Committee. Expert Committee recommendations regarding the prevention, assessment, and treatment of child and adolescent overweight and obesity: summary report. *Pediatrics*. 2007;120:S164-S192.
5. The Childhood Obesity Action Network Expert Committee recommendation implementation guide. http://www.nichq.org/documents/coan-papers-and-publications/COANImplementationGuide62607FINAL.pdf.
6. Li C, Ford ES, Mokdad AH, et al. Recent trends in waist circumference and waist-height ratio among US children and adolescents. *Pediatrics*. 2006;118:e1390-e1398.
7. Otten JJ, Hellwig JP, Meyers LD, eds. *Dietary Reference Intakes: The Essential Guide to Nutrient Requirements*. Washington, DC: National Academies Press, 2006.
8. Ross AC, Manson JE, Abrams SA. The 2011 Report on dietary reference intakes for calcium and vitamin D from the Institute of Medicine: what clinicians need to know. *J Clin Endocrinol Metab*. Nov 29 2010. [Epub ahead of print].
9. Corrales KM, Utter SL. Growth failure. In: Samour PQ, King K, eds. *Handbook of Pediatric Nutrition*. Boston: Jones and Bartlett Publishers, 2005:391-406.
10. Solomon SM, Kirby DF. The refeeding syndrome: a review. *JPENJ Parenter Enteral Nutr*. 1990;14:90-96.
11. American Academy of Pediatrics Committee on Nutrition, Kleinman RE, ed. *Pediatric Nutrition Handbook*. 6th ed. Chicago: American Academy of Pediatrics, 2009.
12. American Society for Parenteral and Enteral Nutrition (ASPEN). Safe practices for parenteral nutrition. *JPEN J Parenter Enteral Nutr*. 2004;28(6):S39-S70. http://www.ashp.org/DocLibrary/BestPractices/2004ASPEN.aspx.

Chapter 22
Oncology
M. Eric Kohler, MD, PhD

⊗ See additional content on Expert Consult

I. WEBSITES

National Cancer Institute (NCI): http://www.cancer.gov/cancertopics/pdq/
pediatrictreatment

SEER (Surveillance, Epidemiology, and End Results) data from the NCI:
http://seer.cancer.gov/

Long-term follow-up guidelines for survivors of pediatric cancer: http://
www.survivorshipguidelines.org/

National Cancer Institute Clinical Trial Database:
www.cancer.gov/clinicaltrials

II. PRESENTING SIGNS AND SYMPTOMS OF PEDIATRIC MALIGNANCIES (TABLE 22-1)

NOTE: Common presenting signs and symptoms of many malignancies
include weight loss, failure to thrive, anorexia, malaise, fever, pallor, and
lymphadenopathy.

TABLE 22-1

PRESENTING SIGNS AND SYMPTOMS OF PEDIATRIC MALIGNANCIES[1,2]

Malignancy	Signs and Symptoms	Initial Workup*	Incidence by Age
ALL	Anorexia, fatigue, malaise, irritability, low-grade fevers, bone pain/limp ± bone tendernesss, bruising/bleeding, petechiae, hepatosplenomegaly, lymphadenopathy, painless testicular enlargement/mass	CBC with differential, peripheral blood smear, LDH, uric acid, electrolytes, including Ca and Phos	Peaks at age 2–5 years
AML	Similar to ALL; may also have subcutaneous nodules, gingival hyperplasia, chloromas (masses)	Same initial workup as ALL plus DIC testing	Peaks in first year of life, declines until age 4
Lymphoma	Painless lymphadenopathy, hepatosplenomegaly, stridor, cough, fever, weight loss, night sweats, fatigue, anorexia, pruritus, intussusception, focal neurologic symptoms, alcohol-induced pain	CBC with differential, peripheral smear, electrolytes including Ca and Phos, LFTs, ESR, ferritin, uric acid, LDH, CXR	HD peaks between 15 and 35 years of age; NHL peaks from age 5–19
Brain tumor	Headache, irritability, emesis, gait changes, focal neurologic symptoms, cranial nerve palsies, changes in vision, personality changes, diabetes insipidus, precocious puberty	MRI of brain and spine, ophthalmology examination, endocrine workup if pituitary dysfunction is suspected	Higher incidence in children <5 years

Continued

TABLE 22-1

PRESENTING SIGNS AND SYMPTOMS OF PEDIATRIC MALIGNANCIES (Continued)

Malignancy	Signs and Symptoms	Initial Workup*	Incidence by Age
Neuroblastoma	Abdominal mass, hepatomegaly, fever, irritability, bone pain, limp, subcutaneous nodules, SVC syndrome, Horner syndrome, periorbital ecchymoses, opsoclonus-myoclonus, secretory diarrhea	Abdominal ultrasound, CT chest/abdomen/pelvis, urine HVA and VMA	Peaks at <2 years of age
Wilms tumor	Abdominal mass, abdominal pain, hypertension, hematuria	Abdominal ultrasound, abdominal CT or MRI, urinalysis, CBC	Peaks at age 2–5
Bone sarcoma	Long-bone pain not relieved with conservative treatment; limp, swelling, fracture	X-ray of primary site, CT of chest	Peaks at age 10–20
Rhabdomyo-sarcoma	Localized symptoms based on location of tumor; painful or painless mass, proptosis, hearing loss, urinary obstruction, hematuria	CT or MRI of primary site	Peaks at <6 years of age and in adolescence
Retinoblas-toma	Leukocoria, strabismus, hyphema, irregular pupil(s)	Ophthalmology referral	Peaks at age 2
Hepatoblas-toma	Abdominal mass, anorexia, emesis, abdominal pain, fever	CBC, LFTs, AFP, hepatitis B and C titers, abdominal ultrasound	Peaks at <3 years of age
Histiocytic disease	Scaly papular rash, fever, weight loss, gingival hyperplasia, diarrhea, pituitary dysfunction, precocious puberty, polydipsia, polyuria, long-bone pain	Skeletal survey, CXR, CBC, LFTs, LDH, ferritin, uric acid, triglycerides, urine osmolality, skin biopsy	Variable
Gonadal tumor	Testicular masses, scrotal swelling. Ovarian tumors are typically asymptomatic until quite large	Ultrasound, CT or MRI, AFP, β-hCG, LDH	Peaks in adolescence

*Laboratory test and imaging suggestions are meant as a guide for evaluation of a potential malignancy. Patients warranting definitive testing should be referred to an oncologist.

AFP, α-Fetoprotein; ALL, acute lymphocytic leukemia; AML, acute myeloid leukemia; β-hCG, beta human chorionic gonadotropin; Ca, calcium; CBC, complete blood cell count; CT, computed tomography; CXR, chest x-ray; DIC, disseminated intravascular coagulation; ESR, erythrocyte sedimentation rate; HD, Hodgkin disease; HVA/VMA, homovanillic acid/vanillylmandelic acid (urine catecholamines); LDH, lactate dehydrogenase; LFTs, liver function tests; MRI, magnetic resonance imaging; NHL, non-Hodgkin lymphoma; Phos, phosphorus; SVC, superior vena cava.

III. EVALUATION OF LYMPHADENOPATHY[2,3]

A. Etiology

1. **Reactive lymph node (LN):** Majority of lymphadenopathy
2. **Direct infection of LN:** Suppurative lymphadenitis (typically due to *Staphylococcus* or *Streptococcus*) or indolent lymphadenitis (e.g., *Bartonella*, atypical *Mycobacterium* [tuberculosis])

3. **Malignancy:** Can be seen in leukemias, lymphomas, and some solid tumors. Less common than infectious causes
4. **Other causes:** Autoimmune disorders, drug reactions, serum sickness, hypothyroidism, and sarcoidosis

B. Physical Findings

1. **Size:** Cervical and axillary LN are typically <1 cm in size. Inguinal LN are typically <1.5 cm in size. Cervical LN >2 cm or palpable supraclavicular LN are associated with higher risk for malignancy.
2. **Palpation:** Tenderness is more common with reactive or infected LN but does not exclude malignancy. Fluctuance, warmth, and/or overlying erythema are more common in lymphadenitis. Hard, rubbery, fixed, or matted LN are suspicious for malignancy and require further investigation.

C. Initial Workup

1. **If reactive lymphadenopathy is suspected,** consider observation, with expected decrease in size over 4–6 weeks and resolution in 8–12 weeks.
2. **If lymphadenitis is suspected,** consider a 10–14 day trial of antibiotics with streptococcal and staphylococcal coverage.
3. **Laboratory studies:** Complete blood cell count (CBC) with differential, erythrocyte sedimentation rate (ESR), lactate dehydrogenase (LDH), specific serologies based on exposures and symptoms (*Bartonella*, Epstein-Barr virus [EBV], human immunodeficiency virus [HIV]), tuberculin skin testing, chest x-ray.

IV. COMMONLY USED CHEMOTHERAPEUTIC DRUGS AND ASSOCIATED ACUTE TOXICITIES (TABLE 22-2)

TABLE 22-2

CHARACTERISTICS OF CHEMOTHERAPEUTIC AGENTS

Drug Name (Drug Class)	Toxicity*
Asparaginase (L-Asp, PEG-Asp, Elspar, *Erwinia*) (*Enzyme*)	DLT: pancreatitis, seizures, hypersensitivity reactions (both acute and delayed; less with PEG-modified), encephalopathy Other: nausea, pancreatitis, hyperglycemia, azotemia, fever, coagulopathy, sagittal sinus thrombosis and other venous thromboses, hyperammonemia Long-term: stroke
Bevacizumab (Avastin) (*VEGF inhibitor*)	DLT: wound healing, hemorrhage, thromboembolic events, CHF Other: abdominal pain, constipation, mucositis, dizziness, headache, dyspnea, epistaxis
Bleomycin (Blenoxane) (*DNA strand breaker*)	DLT: anaphylaxis, pneumonitis Other: pain, fever, chills, mucositis, skin reactions Long-term: pulmonary fibrosis
Busulfan (Myleran) (*Alkylator*)	DLT: myelosuppression, mucositis, seizures, veno-occlusive disease Other: hyperpigmentation, hypotension Long-term: infertility, endocardial fibrosis, secondary malignancy

Continued

TABLE 22-2

CHARACTERISTICS OF CHEMOTHERAPEUTIC AGENTS (Continued)

Drug Name *(Drug Class)*	Toxicity*
Carboplatin (CBDCA, Paraplatin) *(DNA cross-linker)*	DLT: thrombocytopenia, nephrotoxicity Other: severe emesis, ototoxicity, peripheral neuropathy, optic neuritis (rare) Long-term: renal insufficiency, hearing loss
Carmustine (bischloroni-trosourea, BCNU, BiCNU) *(Alkylator)*	DLT: myelosuppression (prolonged cumulative) Other: vesicant; brownish discoloration of skin, hepatic and renal toxicity, severe emesis Long-term: pulmonary fibrosis, infertility, secondary malignancy
Cisplatin (*cis*-platinum, CDDP, Platinol) *(DNA cross-linker)*	DLT: tubular and glomerular nephrotoxicity (related to cumulative dose), peripheral neuropathy, severe emesis Other: myelosuppression, ototoxicity, SIADH (rare), papilledema and retrobulbar neuritis (rare) Long-term: renal insufficiency, hearing loss, peripheral neuropathy
Cladribine (2-CdA, Leustatin) *(Nucleotide analog)*	Myelosuppression, nausea and vomiting, headache, fever, chills, fatigue
Clofarabine (Clolar) *(Purine analog)*	Capillary leak syndrome, veno-occlusive disease, increased creatinine, hyperbilirubinemia
Cyclophosphamide (CTX, Cytoxan) *(Alkylator prodrug)*	DLT: leukopenia, cardiomyopathy Other: hemorrhagic cystitis (improved by mesna), emesis, direct ADH effect, SIADH Long-term: infertility, cardiomyopathy, secondary malignancy, leukoenceophalopathy
Cytarabine (Ara-C) *(Nucleotide analog)*	DLT: myelosuppression, cerebellar toxicity Other: rash, fever, conjunctivitis, nausea and vomiting, anorexia, diarrhea, metallic taste, severe GI ulceration, lethargy, ataxia, nystagmus, slurred speech, respiratory distress rapidly progressing to pulmonary edema, influenza-like syndrome
Dacarbazine (DIC, DTIC, imidazole carboxamide, DTIC-Dome) *(Alkylator)*	DLT: myelosuppression Other: severe emesis, transaminitis, facial paresthesias (rare), rash Long-term: infertility
Dactinomycin (actinomycin D) *(Antibiotic)*	DLT: myelosuppression, severe diarrhea Other: vesicant; nausea, acne, erythema, radiation recall, veno-occlusive disease Long-term: secondary malignancy
Daunorubicin (daunomycin) *(Anthracycline)*	DLT: leukopenia, arrhythmia, congestive heart failure (related to cumulative dose) Other: stomatitis, emesis, vesicant, red urine, radiation recall Long-term: cardiomyopathy
Doxorubicin (Adriamycin) *(Anthracycline)*	Refer to daunorubicin
Etoposide (VP-16, VePesid) *(Topoisomerase inhibitor)*	DLT: leukopenia, anaphylaxis (rare), transient cortical blindness Other: hyperbilirubinemia, transaminitis, peripheral neuropathy (rare), hypotension Long-term: secondary malignancy (AML)
Fludarabine (Fludara) *(Nucleotide analog)*	Myelosuppression, anorexia, increased AST, somnolence, fatigue Long-term: peripheral neuropathy, immunosuppression

TABLE 22-2

CHARACTERISTICS OF CHEMOTHERAPEUTIC AGENTS (Continued)

Drug Name (Drug Class)	Toxicity*
Fluorouracil (5-FU, Adrucil) (Nucleotide analog)	DLT: myelosuppression, mucositis, severe diarrhea
	Other: hand-foot syndrome, tear duct stenosis, hyperpigmentation, loss of nails, cerebellar syndrome (rare), anaphylaxis
Gemcitabine (Pyrimidine analog)	Peripheral edema, rash, nausea, vomiting, constipation, transaminase elevation, myalgias, neuropathy, HUS, pulmonary edema
Hydroxyurea (Hydrea) (Ribonucleotide reductase inhibitor)	DLT: leukopenia, pulmonary edema (rare)
	Other: megaloblastic erythropoiesis, hyperpigmentation, azotemia, transaminitis, radiation recall
Idarubicin (idamycin) (Anthracycline)	DLT: arrhythmia, cardiomyopathy (cumulative)
	Other: vesicant; diarrhea, mucositis, enterocolitis
	Long-term: cardiomyopathy
Ifosfamide (isophosphamide, Ifex) (Alkylator prodrug)	DLT: myelosuppression, mental status changes, dizziness, encephalopathy (rarely progressing to death), renal tubular damage
	Other: emesis, hemorrhagic cystitis (improved with mesna), direct ADH effect, SIADH, Fanconi syndrome
	Long-term: secondary malignancy, infertility
Irinotecan (Camptosar, IRN) (Topoisomerase I inhibitor)	DLT: diarrhea
	Other: nausea and vomiting, asthenia, hyperbilirubinemia, dizziness, cough, dyspnea
Imatinib (Gleevec) (Tyrosine kinase inhibitor)	CHF, edema, pelural effusion, rash, night sweats, weight gain, myalgias, fever
Lomustine (CCNU) (Alkylating agent)	Myelosuppression, nausea and vomiting, disorientation, fatigue
	Long-term: secondary malignancy (leukemia)
Mechlorethamine (nitrogen mustard, HN₂ [mustine], Mustargen) (Alkylator)	DLT: leukopenia, thrombocytopenia
	Other: severe emesis; vesicant; peptic ulcer (rare)
	Long-term: secondary malignancy, infertility
Melphalan (L-PAM, Alkeran) (Alkylator)	DLT: prolonged leukopenia, mucositis, diarrhea
	Other: pruritus, emesis
	Long-term: pulmonary fibrosis, secondary malignancy, infertility, cataracts
Mercaptopurine (6-MP) (Nucleotide analog)	DLT: hepatic necrosis and encephalopathy
	Other: headache, diarrhea, nausea
	Long-term: cirrhosis
Methotrexate (MTX, amethopterin, Folex, Mexate) (Folate antagonist)	DLT: mucositis, diarrhea, renal dysfunction, encephalopathy, cortical blindness, ventriculitis (intrathecal)
	Other: photosensitivity, erythema, excessive lacrimation, transaminitis, pleuritis
	Long-term: leukoencephalopathy, cirrhosis, pulmonary fibrosis, aseptic necrosis of bone, osteoporosis
Mitoxantrone (dihydroxyanthra-cenedione dihydrochloride, Novantrone) (DNA intercalator)	DLT: myelosuppression, cardiomyopathy
	Other: mucositis, blue-green urine
	Long-term: cardiomyopathy
Paclitaxel (Taxol) (Tubulin inhibitor)	DLT: neutropenia, anaphylaxis, ventricular tachycardia and myocardial infarction (rare)
	Other: mucositis, peripheral neuopathy, bradycardia, hypertriglyceridemia

Continued

22

TABLE 22-2

CHARACTERISTICS OF CHEMOTHERAPEUTIC AGENTS (Continued)

Drug Name *(Drug Class)*	Toxicity*
Procarbazine (Matulane) *(Alkylating agent)*	DLT: encephalopathy; pancytopenia, especially thrombocytopenia Other: emesis, paresthesias, dizziness, ataxia, hypotension; adverse effects with tyramine-rich foods, ethanol, MAOIs, meperidine, and many other drugs Long-term: secondary malignancy, infertility
Temozolomide (Temodar) *(Alkylating agent)*	DLT: myelosuppression Other: constipation, headache, nausea, seizures
Teniposide (VM-26) *(Topoisomerase inhibitor)*	DLT: leukopenia, anaphylaxis (rare) Other: hyperbilirubinemia, transaminitis Long-term: secondary malignancy (AML)
Thioguanine (6-TG, 6-thioguanine) *(Nucleotide analog)*	DLT: myelosuppression, mucositis, diarrhea Other: hyperbilirubinemia, transaminitis, decreased vibratory sensation, ataxia, dermatitis
Thiotepa *(Alkylating agent)*	DLT: cognitive impairment, leukopenia Other: increased AST, headache, dizziness, rash, desquamation Long-term: secondary malignancy (leukemia), impaired fertility, lower extremity weakness
Topotecan (Hycamptin) *(Topoisomerase inhibitor)*	DLT: leukopenia, peripheral neuropathy (rare), Horner syndrome Other: nausea, diarrhea, transaminitis, headache
Vinblastine (BVL, vincaleuko-blastine, Velban) *(Microtubule inhibitor)*	DLT: leukopenia Other: vesicant; constipation, bone pain (especially in the jaw), peripheral and autonomic neuropathy, SIADH (rare)
Vincristine (VCR, Oncovin) *(Microtubule inhibitor)*	DLT: peripheral and autonomic neuropathy, constipation, jaw pain, encephalopathy, foot drop, ptosis Other: vesicant; bone pain, hoarseness, SIADH (rare), hyperbilirubinemia
Vinorelbine (Navelbine) *(Microtubule inhibitor)*	Peripheral neuropathy, asthenia, hyperbilirubinemia, constipation, diarrhea, nausea, emesis
CHEMOTHERAPY ADJUNCTS	
Amifostine	Indication: reduces toxicity of radiation Side effects: hypotension (62%), nausea and vomiting, flushing, chills, dizziness, somnolence, hiccups, sneezing, hypocalcemia in susceptible patients (<1%), rigors (<1%), mild skin rash
Dexrazoxane	Indication: protective agent for anthracycline-induced cardiotoxicity Side effects: myelosuppression
Leucovorin	Indication: reduces methotrexate toxicity Side effects: allergic sensitization (rare)
Mesna	Indication: reduces risk of hemorrhagic cystitis Side effects: headache, limb pain, abdominal pain, diarrhea, rash

*The dose-limiting toxicity (DLT) is the toxicity most likely to require adjustment or withholding of drug.

ADH, Antidiuretic hormone; AML, acute myeloid leukemia; AST, aspartate transaminase; CHF, congestive heart failure; GI, gastrointestinal; HUS, hemolytic uremic syndrome; MAOI, monoamine oxidase inhibitor; PEG, polyethylene glycol; SIADH, syndrome of inappropriate antidiuretic hormone; VEGF, vascular endothelial growth factor.

Modified from *Physician's Desk Reference.* 64th ed. Montvale, NJ: Medical Economics, 2010; Taketomo CK, Hodding JH, Kraus DM. *American Pharmaceutical Association Pediatric Dosage Handbook.* 16th ed. Hudson OH: Lexi-Comp, 2009; and Micromedex 2.0: http://www.thomsonhc.com/micromedex2/librarian.

V. ONCOLOGIC EMERGENCIES[1,4,5]

A. Hyperleukocytosis/Leukostasis

1. **Etiology:** Elevated white blood cell (WBC) count (WBC > 100,000/μL) in leukemia patients, leading to leukostasis in the microcirculation and diminished tissue perfusion (notably in central nervous system [CNS] and lungs). This occurs more commonly and at lower WBC counts (>100,000/μL) in acute myeloid leukemia (AML [especially M4 and M5]) than in acute lymphocytic leukemia (ALL [typically requiring a WBC count >300,000/μL]). Leukostasis is very common in chronic myeloid leukemia (CML) but at WBC counts >300,000/μL.
2. **Presentation:** Hypoxia, tachypnea, and dyspnea from pulmonary leukostasis. Mental status changes, headaches, seizures, papilledema from cerebral leukostasis. Occasionally, gastrointestinal (GI) bleeding, abdominal pain, renal insufficiency, priapism, and intracranial hemorrhage. Leukostasis may be asymptomatic.
3. **Management:**
a. Transfuse platelets as needed to keep count above 20,000/μL.
b. Avoid red blood cell (RBC) transfusions because they will raise viscosity (keep hemoglobin ≤10 g/dL). If RBCs are required, consider partial exchange transfusion.
c. Hydration, alkalinization, and allopurinol should be initiated (as discussed in Section V.B).
d. Administer fresh frozen plasma (FFP) and vitamin K for coagulopathy.
e. Before cytotoxic therapy, consider leukapheresis or exchange transfusion to lower WBC count if CNS or pulmonary symptoms exist.
f. Start disease treatment as soon as patient is clinically stable.

B. Tumor Lysis Syndrome

1. **Etiology:** Lysis of tumor cells before or during early stages of chemotherapy (especially Burkitt lymphoma/leukemia, T-cell ALL).
2. **Presentation:** Hyperuricemia, hypocalcemia, hyperkalemia, hyperphosphatemia. Can lead to acute kidney injury due to precipitation of uric acid crystals and/or calcium phosphate crystals in renal tubules and micovasculature, respectively.
3. **Prevention and management:**
a. Hydration: Dextrose 5% (D_5) 1/4 normal saline (NS) ± 40 mEq/L $NaHCO_3$ (without K) at two times maintenance rate. Keep urine specific gravity <1.010 and urine output >100mL/m²/hr.
b. Hyperuricemia: Allopurinol inhibits formation of uric acid and can be given orally (PO) or intravenously (IV) (see Formulary for dosing). Rasburicase converts uric acid to the more soluble allantoin. Use in higher-risk patients, especially those with uric acid >7.5 mg/dL.
c. Monitor K^+, Ca^{2+}, phosphate, uric acid, and urinalysis closely (up to Q2 hr for high-risk patients). There is an increased risk of calcium phosphate precipitation when Ca × Phos > 60.
d. Manage abnormal electrolytes as described in Chapter 11. See Chapter 19 for dialysis indications.

e. Consider stopping alkalinization after uric acid levels return to normal to facilitate calcium phosphate excretion.

C. Spinal Cord Compression

1. **Etiology:** Intrinsic or extrinsic compression of spinal cord; occurs most commonly with brain tumors, sarcomas, leukemia with lymphomatous involvement, lymphoma, and neuroblastoma.
2. **Presentation:** Back pain (localized or radicular), weakness, sensory loss, change in bowel or bladder function. Prognosis for recovery based on duration and level of disability at presentation.
3. **Diagnosis:** Magnetic resonance imaging (MRI [preferred]) or computed tomography (CT) scan of spine. A plain film of spine has good specificity but detects only two thirds of abnormalities.
4. **Management:** (**Note:** Steroids may prevent acurate diagnosis of leukemia/lymphoma; plan diagnostic procedure as soon as possible)
a. In the presence of neurologic abnormalities, strong history, and rapid progression of symptoms, immediately start bolus dexamethasone 1–2 mg/kg/day IV and obtain an emergent MRI of the spine.
b. With back pain but less acute symptoms and no anatomic level of dysfunction, consider lower dose of dexamethasone, 0.25–0.5 mg/kg/day PO, divided Q6 hr. Perform MRI of spine within 24 hours.
c. If cause of tumor is known, emergent radiotherapy or chemotherapy is indicated for sensitive tumors; otherwise, emergent neurosurgery consultation is warranted.
d. If cause of tumor is unknown or debulking may remove most or all of tumor, surgery is indicated to decompress the spine.

D. Increased Intracranial Pressure

1. **Etiology:** Ventricular obstruction or impaired cerebrospinal fluid (CSF) flow.
2. **Presentation:** Headaches, irritability, lethargy, emesis (especially if projectile).
3. **Diagnosis:** Evaluate for vital sign changes (i.e., Cushing triad [↓ heart rate, ↑ systolic blood pressure, irregular respirations]). Funduscopic evaluation for papilledema. Obtain CT or MRI of the head (MRI more sensitive for diagnosis of posterior fossa tumors).
4. **Management:**
a. See Chapter 4 for basic intracranial pressure (ICP) management.
b. If tumor is the cause, start IV dexamethasone: 1–2 mg/kg as first dose, then 0.5 mg/kg Q6 hr.
c. Obtain emergent neurosurgical consultation.
d. Consider manitol for altered mental status and/or cardiovascular instability.

E. Cerebrovascular Accident

1. **Etiology:** Hyperleukocytosis, coagulopathy, thrombocytopenia, radiation (fibrosis) or chemotherapy-related (e.g., L-asparaginase–induced hemorrhage or thrombosis, methotrexate). Most common in patients with leukemia.

2. **Diagnosis and management:**

a. Platelet transfusions (and likely increase threshold for transfusion), FFP as needed to replace factors (e.g., if depleted by L-asparaginase)

b. Brain CT with contrast, MRI, magnetic resonance angiography (MRA), or magnetic resonance venography (MRV) if venous thrombosis is suspected

c. Administer heparin acutely, followed by warfarin, for thromboses (if no venous hemorrhage observed on MRI)

d. Avoid L-asparaginase.

e. Leukapheresis for hyperleukocytosis

F. Respiratory Distress and Superior Vena Cava Syndrome

1. **Etiology:** Mediastinal mass, edema, or thrombosis; typically seen with Hodgkin disease, non-Hodgkin lymphoma (e.g., lymphoblastic lymphoma), ALL (T-lineage), germ cell tumors

2. **Presentation:** Orthopnea, headaches, facial swelling, dizziness, plethora, acute respiratory distress or failure

3. **Diagnosis:** Chest radiograph. Consider CT or MRI to assess airway. Attempt diagnosis of malignancy (if not known) by least invasive method possible. Avoid sedation or general anesthesia if unstable, high risk.

4. **Management:**

a. Control airway

b. Biopsy (e.g., bone marrow, pleurocentesis, lymphnode biopsy) before therapy if patient can tolerate sedation or general anesthesia

c. Empiric therapy: radiotherapy, steroids, chemotherapy

G. Typhilitis (Neutropenic Enterocolitis)

1. **Etiology:** Inflammation of bowel wall, usually localized to cecum. Occurs most often in association with prolonged neutropenia.

2. **Presentation:** Right lower quadrant abdominal pain, nausea, diarrhea, fever (fever may be absent early in course; neutropenic patient with abdominal pain warrants evaluation for typhlitis and empirical antibacterial coverage). Risk for perforation.

3. **Diagnosis:**

a. Careful serial abdominal examinations

b. X-ray may show pneumatosis intestinalis, bowel wall edema

c. CT (IV and PO contrast) most sensitive imaging; may reveal bowel wall thickening, pneumatosis intestinalis

4. **Management:**

a. Nothing by mouth (NPO), IV fluids; consider nasogastric decompression.

b. Broad anaerobic and gram-negative antibiotic coverage (consider coverage for *Clostridium difficile*).

c. Follow closely with surgery consult.

H. Fever and Neutropenia

1. **Etiology:** Presumed infection (bacterial, viral, or fungal) in a neutropenic host. Bacterial infection is the most common documented infection. Occassionally, fevers may be due to medications.

2. **Presentation:** Fever, fatigue, chills, rigors, listlessness, lethargy, tachypnea, tachycardia, localized pain.
3. **Diagnosis:** Fever (temperature [T] > 38.3°C or T > 38.0°C for >1 hour) in the setting of neutropenia (ANC < 500 cells/μL, or < 1000 cells/μL but expected to drop to <500 in the next 48 hours).
4. **Management:** See Fig. 22-1.

VI. HEMATOPOIETIC STEM CELL TRANSPLANTATION (HSCT)[1,6]

A. Goal

Administer healthy functioning hematopoietic stem cells from the bone marrow, peripheral blood, or umbilical cord blood to a patient whose bone marrow is diseased (from hematologic malignancy) or depleted (after treatment with myeloablative chemotherapy). HSCT is also used for some congenital and acquired hematologic, immunologic, and metabolic disorders.

B. Types

1. **Allogeneic:**
a. Recipient is transfused with donor stem cells after a myeloablative preparative regimen that includes chemotherapy and often also radiation. Donors are screened for human leukocyte antigen (HLA) subtype matching to recipient. Possible donors include HLA-matched sibling, matched unrelated donors, umbilical cord stem cells, and haploidentical (half-matched) related donors.
b. Increased level of mismatch between donor and recipient increases graft-versus-tumor effect, but also increases risk for graft-versus-host complications and graft rejection.
c. Used commonly for AML, ALL (high risk/relapse), myelodysplastic syndrome, juvenile myelomonocytic leukemia (JMML), hemophagocytic lymphohistiocytosis, and a number of nonmalignant hematologic, immunologic, and metabolic disorders.

2. **Autologous:**
a. Donor is recipient. After several cycles of conventional chemotherapy, stem cells from patient are harvested (often with assistance of growth factors such as granulocyte colony-stimulating factor [GCSF] to mobilize), stored, and given back (rescue) after the patient has received what are myeloablative doses of chemotherapy and radiation.
b. Avoids the complication of graft-versus-host disease (GVHD).
c. Used for high-risk neuroblastoma, lymphoma, and various high-risk solid tumors.

C. Engraftment

1. Recipient's bone marrow is repopulated with donor stem cells that proliferate and mature.
2. Usually starts within 2–4 weeks of transplant and presents with an inflammatory response but can be significantly delayed with certain conditions, medications, or infection.

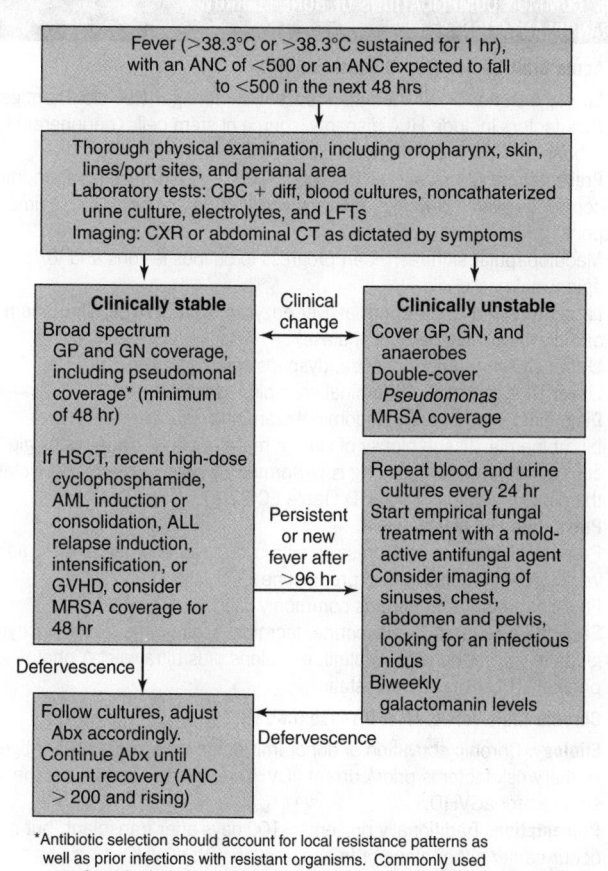

Fever (>38.3°C or >38.3°C sustained for 1 hr), with an ANC of <500 or an ANC expected to fall to <500 in the next 48 hrs

Thorough physical examination, including oropharynx, skin, lines/port sites, and perianal area
Laboratory tests: CBC + diff, blood cultures, noncathaterized urine culture, electrolytes, and LFTs
Imaging: CXR or abdominal CT as dictated by symptoms

Clinically stable
Broad spectrum GP and GN coverage, including pseudomonal coverage* (minimum of 48 hr)

If HSCT, recent high-dose cyclophosphamide, AML induction or consolidation, ALL relapse induction, intensification, or GVHD, consider MRSA coverage for 48 hr

Clinical change

Clinically unstable
Cover GP, GN, and anaerobes
Double-cover *Pseudomonas*
MRSA coverage

Persistent or new fever after >96 hr

Repeat blood and urine cultures every 24 hr
Start empirical fungal treatment with a mold-active antifungal agent
Consider imaging of sinuses, chest, abdomen and pelvis, looking for an infectious nidus
Biweekly galactomanin levels

Defervescence

Follow cultures, adjust Abx accordingly. Continue Abx until count recovery (ANC > 200 and rising)

Defervescence

*Antibiotic selection should account for local resistance patterns as well as prior infections with resistant organisms. Commonly used monotherapies include antipseudomonal β-lactams and fourth-generation cephalosporins or carbapenems.

FIGURE 22-1

Guideline for management of fever and neutropenia in children with cancer and/or undergoing hematopoietic stem cell transplantation. Abx, Antibiotics; ALL, acute lymphocytic leukemia; AML, acute myeloid leukemia; ANC, absolute neutrophil count; CBC, complete blood count; CT, computed tomography; CXR, chest x-ray; diff, differential; GN, gram-negative; GP, gram-positive; GVHD, graft-versus-host disease; HSCT, hemopoietic stem cell transplantation; LFTs, liver function tests; MRSA, methicillin-resistant Staphylococcus aureus. (Data from Lehrnbecher T, Phillips R, Alexander S, et al. Guideline for the management of fever and neutropenia in children with cancer and/or undergoing hematopoietic stem-cell transplantation. J Clin Oncol. 2012;30:4427-4438; Freifeld AG, Bow EJ, Sepkowitz KA, et al. Clinical practice guideline for the use of antimicrobial agents in neutropenic patients with cancer: 2010 update by the Infectious Diseases Society of America. Clin Infect Dis. 2011;52:e56-e93.)

VII. COMMON COMPLICATIONS OF BONE MARROW TRANSPLANTATION[1,6]

A. Acute Graft-Versus-Host Disease (aGVHD)

1. **Etiology:** Donor T-cell–mediated reaction to "foreign" (recipient) antigens. Risk factors include HLA disparity, source of stem cells (peripheral blood > bone marrow > umbilical cord blood).
2. **Presentation:** Classically occurs within 100 days of transplantation, most commonly within 6 weeks, but may occur or persist beyond this time point
   a. Maculopapular skin rash: Can progress to bullous lesions and toxic epidermal necrolysis
   b. Laboratory findings: Abnormal liver enzymes (direct hyperbilirubinemia and elevated alkaline phosphatase)
   c. Upper GI symptoms: Anorexia, dyspepsia, nausea, vomiting
   d. Lower GI symptoms: Abdominal cramping, diarrhea
3. **Diagnosis:** Triad of rash, abdominal cramping with diarrhea, hyperbilirubinemia. Tissue biopsy of skin or mucosa can provide histologic confirmation. Clinical staging is performed by organ system and dictates the clinical grading of aGVHD (Table EC 22-A).
4. **Prevention and management:**
   a. Prophylaxis: Immunosuppression with cyclosporine or tacrolimus; adjuvants are methotrexate and prednisone
   b. First-line treatment: Steroids commonly used
   c. Second-line agents: Cyclosporine, tacrolimus, sirolimus, antithymocyte globulin, mycophenolate mofetil, psoralens plus ultraviolet A photopheresis (PUVA) and pentostatin

B. Chronic Graft-Versus-Host Disease (cGVHD)

1. **Etiology:** Chronic activation of donor immune cells against host antigens. Primary risk factor is prior/current aGVHD. Other risk factors are the same as for aGVHD.
2. **Presentation:** Traditionally presents >100 days after transplant, but may occur earlier either alone or in conjunction with aGVHD:
   a. Skin is most commonly affected organ, with lichenoid changes on the face, palms, and soles and scleroderma-like changes, predominantly on extremities.
   b. Cholestasis and hepatitis can be seen with elevated alkaline phosphatase, bilirubin, aspartate aminotransferase, and alanine aminotransferase (AST/ALT).
   c. GI involvment results in lichenoid changes of oral mucosa, with painful ulcerations that may result in dysphagia. Esophageal strictures, chronic diarrhea, and malabsorption may also be seen.
   d. Dyspnea and cough may indicate lung involvement, with inflamation and fibrosis that can culminate in bronchiolitis obliterans.
   e. Xerophthalmia with chronically dry eyes, keratoconjunctivitis, and uveitis.

3. **Diagnosis:** Clinically diagnosed by classic findings in skin and GI system, as well as evidence of cholestasis. Skin and/or oral mucosa biopsies may be obtained for confirmation. Liver biopsy may be necessary in patients with suspected hepatic cGVHD.
4. **Prevention and management:**
a. Treatment should be targeted to affected tissues if cGVHD is limited to a single organ system.
b. Steroids continue to be first-line treatment.
c. Second-line agents are similar to those used in aGVHD.
d. Patients with cGVHD are functionally asplenic and immunosuppressed. They should receive four doses of pneumococcal conjugate vaccine 13 (PCV13) after transplant.

C. **Veno-occlusive Disease (Sinusoidal Obstruction Syndrome)**
1. **Etiology:** Occlusive fibrosis of terminal intrahepatic venules and sinusoids; occurs as a consequence of hematopoietic cell transplantation, hepatotoxic chemotherapy, and/or high-dose liver radiation. Typically occurs within 3 weeks of the insult, most common at the end of the first week after transplant.
2. **Presentation:** Tender hepatomegaly, jaundice, edema, ascites, and sudden weight gain.
3. **Diagnosis:**
a. Liver ultrasound with Doppler or MRI showing reversal of portal venous flow
b. Elevated bilirubin and ALT/AST
c. Prolongation of prothrombin time, decreased factor VII levels (in more severe disease)
d. Portal-hepatic venous gradient of >10 mmHg (invasive but sensitive)
4. **Prevention and management:**
a. Fluid and sodium restriction.
b. Defibrotide has been shown to be succesful in 35%–60% of patients with veno-occlusive disease (VOD).

D. **Thrombotic Microangiopathy: Thrombotic Thrombocytopenic Purpura (TTP) or Hemolytic Uremic Syndrome (HUS)**
1. **Etiology:** Post-HSCT, associated with immunosuppressants (cyclosporine, tacrolimus).
2. **Presentation:** Both TTP and HUS present with microangiopathic hemolytic anemia and thrombocytopenia. HUS completes the triad with renal insufficiency/failure, whereas TTP can be associated with neurologic symptoms.
3. **Diagnosis:** Anemia and thrombocytopenia on CBC, schistocytes on peripheral blood smear, hematuria, proteinuria, casts on urinalysis, elevated LDH, decreased haptoglobin, impaired renal function, elevated D-dimer on coagulation panel.
4. **Prevention and treatment:** Urgent plasma exchange if TTP is suspected; blood products, fluid management, dialysis.

E. Hemorrhagic Cystitis

1. **Etiology:** Pretransplant conditioning regimens (specifically those that include cyclophosphamide, pelvic, or total body irradiation) or viral (adenovirus, BK virus).
2. **Presentation:** Hematuria, dysuria, difficulty voiding.
3. **Diagnosis:** Urine viral polymerase chain reaction (PCR) assay, bacterial cultures, bladder ultrasound, CBC, coagulation studies.
4. **Prevention and management:** Hydration and mesna with preparative regimen. Treatment with aggressive hydration, blood products as indicated, cystoscopy, bladder irrigation, clot evacuation.

F. Mucositis

1. **Etiology:** Damage to endothelial cells of the GI tract from conditioning regimen, leading to breakdown of the mucosa. Typically peaks in the first 1–2 weeks after transplant.
2. **Presentation:** Oropharyngeal pain, abdominal pain, nausea, vomiting, diarrhea, intolerance of PO intake.
3. **Diagnosis:** Diagnosis is clinical.
4. **Prevention and management:** Supportive care aimed at pain control and nutrition. Local pain control with lidocaine-containing mouthwashes and bicarbonate rinses. Systemic pain control usually requires patient-controlled analgesia (PCA) infusion. Total parenteral nutrition (TPN) is commonly required.

VIII. HEMATOLOGIC CARE AND COMPLICATIONS[1]

NOTE: Transfuse only irradiated and leukoreduced packed red blood cells (PRBCs) and single-donor platelets, cytomegalovirus (CMV)-negative or leukofiltered PRBCs/platelets for CMV-negative patients. Use leukofiltered PRBCs/platelets for those who may undergo bone marrow transplantation (BMT) in the future, to prevent alloimmunization, or for those who have had nonhemolytic febrile transfusion reactions. Many oncology patients have nonhemolytic reactions (temperature elevation, rash, hypotension, respiratory distress) to PRBCs and/or platelet transfusion and will subsequently be premedicated with diphenhydramine and/or acetaminophen for future transfusions.

A. Anemia

1. **Etiology:** Blood loss, chemotherapy, marrow infiltration, hemolysis
2. **Management:**
a. See Chapter 14 for specific details on PRBC transfusions.
b. Hematocrit thresholds for PRBC transfusions in cancer patients are based on clinical status and symptoms and are not uncommonly <30 g/dL.

B. Thrombocytopenia

1. **Etiology:** Chemotherapy, marrow infiltration, consumptive coagulopathy, medications

2. **Management:**
a. See Chapter 14 for specific details on platelet transfusions.
b. In general maintain platelet count above 10,000 μL unless patient is actively bleeding or febrile, or before selected procedures (e.g., intramuscular [IM] injection). Consider maintaining platelet counts at higher levels for patients who have brain tumors, recent brain surgery, or history of stroke.

C. **Neutropenia**
1. **Etiology:** Chemotherapy, marrow infiltration, radiation
2. **Management:**
a. Broad-spectrum antibiotics with concomitant fever (see Fig. 22-1).
b. GCSF to assist in recovery of neutrophils.
c. Granulocyte transfusion can be performed in settings of infection or declining clinical status.

IX. NAUSEA TREATMENT IN CANCER PATIENTS[1]

A. **Etiology**

Usual cause is chemotherapy treatment. Also suspect opiate therapy, GI and CNS radiotherapy, obstructive abdominal process, elevated ICP, certain antibiotics, or hypercalcemia.

B. **Presentation**
1. **Acute:** Emesis within 24 hours of starting chemotherapy; occurs in one third of patients despite treatment.
2. **Delayed:** Emesis occurring >24 hours after chemotherapy. Risk factors include female gender, prior acute emesis, highly emetogenic agents (e.g., cisplatin).
3. **Anticipatory:** Emesis before chemotherapy administration.

C. **Therapy**

Hydration plus one or more antinausea medications (see Formulary for dosing)
1. **Serotonin (5-HT$_3$) antagonists:** Ondansetron, dolasetron, granisetron, or palonosetron. Usually a first-line therapy. Best for acute emesis. Risk of QT prolongation, widening of QRS.
2. **Histamine-1 antagonist:** Diphenhydramine; also cyproheptadine (with anticholinergic side effect of appetite stimulation).
3. **Steroids:** Dexamethasone; especially helpful in patients with brain tumor and as prophylaxis for delayed symptoms; synergy with 5-HT$_3$ antagonists.
4. **Benzodiazepines:** Lorazepam; used as an adjunct antiemetic agent.
5. **Metoclopramide:** Use diphenhydramine to reduce risk of extrapyramidal symptoms (EPS).
6. **Phenothiazines:** Promethazine, chlorpromazine; use diphenhydramine to reduce risk of EPS.
7. **Cannabinoids:** Dronabinol; can be helpful in resistant cases, especially in patients with large tumor burden. May also be used as an appetite stimulant in malnourished patients.
8. **Substance P and neurokinin-1 receptor antagonist:** Aprepitant; avoid with certain chemotherapy drugs (e.g., ifosfamide, etoposide).

X. ANTIMICROBIAL PROPHYLAXIS IN ONCOLOGY PATIENTS (TABLE 22-3)

NOTE: Treatment length and dosage may vary per protocol.

TABLE 22-3

ANTIMICROBIAL PROPHYLAXIS IN ONCOLOGY PATIENTS

Organism	Medication	Indication
Pneumocystis jiroveci	TMP-SMX, atovaquone, dapsone, or pentamidine	Chemotherapy and BMT per protocol (usually at least 6 mo after chemotherapy, 12 mo after BMT)
HSV	Acyclovir (dosing is different for zoster, varicella, and mucocutaneous HSV)	After BMT if patient or donor is HSV or CMV positive; recurrent zoster
Candida albicans	Fluconazole or voriconazole	After BMT (usually at least 28 days)
Gram-positive organisms	Penicillin	After BMT (usually at least 1 mo)

BMT, Bone marrow transplantation; CMV, cytomegalovirus; HSV, herpes simplex virus; TMP-SMX, trimethoprim-sulfamethoxazole.

XI. BEYOND CHILDHOOD CANCER: TREATING A CANCER SURVIVOR[1,7,8]

A. Understand the Treatment Regimen

1. **Identify all components of therapy received:** Comprehensive treatment summary from oncologist, summarizing:
a. Diagnosis: Site/stage, date, relapse
b. Chemotherapy: Cumulative doses, high dose vs. low dose for methotrexate and cytarabine
c. Radiation: Locations, cumulative dose
d. Surgeries: Dates, sites, resection
e. BMT: Preparation regimen, source of donor cells (including degree of HLA mismatch), GVHD, complications
f. Investigational treatments
g. Adverse drug reactions or allergies
2. **Follow up with any investigational treatments used.**
3. **Determine any potential problems by organ system,** and devise plan for routine evaluation.

B. Common Late Effects[1,2,7,NaN] (See Table EC 22-B)

Also see http://www.survivorshipguidelines.org/.

REFERENCES

1. Poplack D, Pizzo P. *Principles and Practice of Pediatric Oncology.* 6th ed. Philadelphia: Lippincott, Williams & Wilkins, 2011.
2. Kliegman RM, Behrman RE, Stanton BF, et al. *Nelson Textbook of Pediatrics.* 19th ed. Philadelphia: Saunders, 2011.
3. Friedmann AM. Evaluation and management of lymphadenopathy in children. *Pediatr Rev.* 2008;29:53-60.
4. Lehrnbecher T, Phillips R, Alexander S, et al. Guideline for the management of fever and neutropenia in children with cancer and/or undergoing hematopoietic stem-cell transplantation. *J Clin Oncol.* 2012;30:4427-4438.
5. Freifeld AG, Bow EJ, Sepkowitz KA, et al. Clinical practice guideline for the use of antimicrobial agents in neutropenic patients with cancer: 2010 update by the Infectious Diseases Society of America. *Clin Infect Dis.* 2011;52:e56-e93.
6. Bishop MR, ed. *Hematopoietic Stem Cell Transplantation.* New York: Springer, 2009.
7. Meck MM, Leary M, Sills RH. Late effects in survivors of childhood cancer. *Pediatr Rev.* 2006;27:257-262.
8. Pickering LK; American Academy of Pediatrics. *Red Book: 2012 Report of the Committee on Infectious Diseases.* 29th ed. Elk Grove Village, Ill: AAP, 2012.

22

Chapter 23

Palliative Care

Jessica Knight-Perry, MD

I. PALLIATIVE CARE

A. Website

For additional information please refer to American Academy of Hospice and Palliative Medicine at www.aahpm.org

B. Definition[1,2]

Palliative care is the active total care of the child's body, mind, and spirit with the intent to prevent and relieve suffering. It supports the best quality of life for the child and family beginning at diagnosis of a life-limiting condition and continuing regardless of whether the child receives treatment. Hospice care is a form of palliative care that focuses on the end of life and bereavement. Effective palliative care requires an interdisciplinary approach that works with child and family to determine goals of care. This is best accomplished when the palliative care team is involved as early in the child's course of illness as possible (Fig. 23-1).

C. Palliative Care Team Composition

1. **Child and family**
2. **Physician:** Primary care physician, specialist attending physician, fellow, resident, intern
3. **Nurses:** Primary nurse, charge nurse, home care nurse, hospice nurse
4. **Pain specialist and hospice palliative care specialist**
5. **Social worker**
6. **Child life specialist**

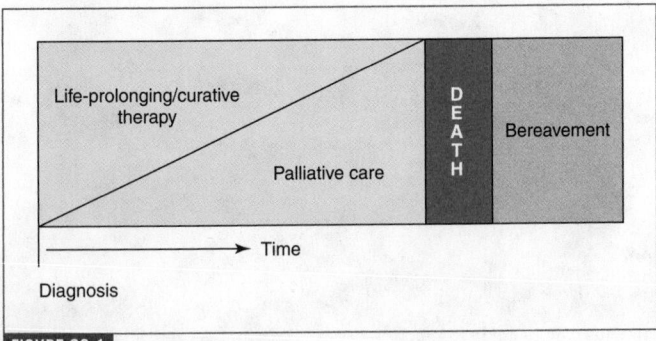

FIGURE 23-1

Current accepted model for palliative care.

7. **Pastoral care**
8. **Patient care coordinator and case manager**
9. **Bereavement coordinator**
10. **Community resources:** School, faith community, hospice program

II. COMMUNICATION AND DECISION MAKING

A. Decision-Making Tools (DMT)[3]

1. **Provides consistent, reliable format for discussion and formulation of plan of care.** Patients, families, and health care providers all participate in the process.

2. **Four domains of DMT should be updated regularly,** especially during "non-crisis" periods.

a. Medical indications: Diagnosis, symptoms, risk/benefits of treatment, cure/relapse rate, complications

b. Patient and family preferences: Information, decision making, desire for autonomy and privacy

c. Quality of life: Important activities of child, important relationships, emotional/spiritual well-being

d. Contextual issues: Identifying family unit, home environment, financial barriers, legal issues, cultural and spiritual beliefs

B. Family Meetings[4]

1. **Prepare the people and the messages.**
a. Why are you having the meeting?
b. Do you have all the information you need?
c. Are all clinicians in agreement about the patient's condition and the recommendations?
d. Are there decisions to be made?
e. Who should attend? Patient, parents, other important individuals? Which clinicians?
f. Who will take the lead role as the facilitator?

2. **Choose a private location with minimal distraction.**

3. **Begin by introducing all participants and the purpose of the meeting.**
a. Check whether any additional issues for discussion have arisen.

4. **Assess what the family knows and expects.**
a. What is their current understanding of the patient's condition?
b. What have they already been told?

5. **Describe the clinical situation.**
a. A brief, clear overview first. What is the big picture?
b. Then ask if the family wants and is ready for more details.
c. Periodically ask whether what you are saying is clear and makes sense.

6. **Encourage each member of the family to express concerns and questions.** Ask until there are no more questions.

7. **Explore the patient's and family's values and how they should influence decision making.**
a. Has there been any prior experience with serious medical decisions for this patient or another family member?

23

b. How does the family decide what is best?

c. Are there guides or principles that help the family decide?

8. **Propose goals for the patient's care that reflect the stated values.**

a. Begin with what treatments or interventions you recommend as beneficial and that support the goals of care.

b. If there are treatments you would not recommend because they do not support the overall goals of care, mention them later with your reason for not recommending.

c. Be prepared to listen compassionately and negotiate.

9. **Provide a concrete follow-up plan.**

a. Summarize the plan for care.

b. Agree on when to talk or meet again.

C. **Child Participation**

1. **Development of death concepts in children**[5-8] (Table 23-1).

2. **Child's capacity to participate in health care decisions.** Minor children can participate meaningfully in decision making if they demonstrate all of the following:

a. Communicate understanding of the medical information

b. State his or her preference

c. Communicate understanding of the consequences of decisions

D. **Advance Directive**

1. **Adolescents 18 years of age and older** can name another adult to make health care decisions if they are unable to speak for themselves.

2. **Health care team can help patients voice preferences** for future health care decisions.

TABLE 23-1

CONCEPTUALIZATION OF DEATH IN CHILDREN

Age Range	Characteristics	Concepts of Death	Interventions
0–2 yr	Achieve object permanence May sense something is wrong	None	Provide maximal comfort with familiar persons and favorite toys.
2–6 yr	Magical thoughts	Believes death is temporary Does not personalize death Believes death can be caused by thoughts	Minimize separation from parents; correct perceptions that the illness is punishment.
6–12 yr	Concrete thoughts	Understands death can be personal Interested in details of death	Be truthful, evaluate fears, provide concrete details if requested, allow participation in decision making.
12–18 yr	Reality becomes objective Capable of self-reflection	Searches for meaning, hope, purpose, and value of life	Be truthful, allow expression of strong feelings, allow participation in decision making.

III. LEGACY AND MEMORY MAKING

A. Memory Making

1. **Provide opportunities for the family to participate in memory making** (e.g., create memory boxes/packets, lock of hair, foot/hand molds or prints, videos, photographs).
2. **Older children may have specific wishes for funeral, memorial, or distribution of personal belongings.**

B. Rituals

Allow for culturally important rituals to be performed by the family (e.g., baptism, bathing, music, faith ceremonies or prayer).

C. Being at Home

For many children and families, the opportunity to be at home together, especially as a child approaches the end of life, is a top priority. Be sure to ask families about this early, before it is too late to transfer the patient and assess what preparations have to be made.

IV. DECISIONS TO LIMIT INTERVENTIONS

A. Do Not Attempt Resuscitation (DNAR)

1. **In the event of cardiorespiratory arrest,** cardiopulmonary resuscitation (CPR) is automatically initiated in hospitals by health care teams and in community settings by first responders. For patients with life-threatening conditions, CPR may not prolong or enhance quality of life, making it inconsistent with goals of care. The health care team should offer patients and families the option of forgoing CPR and other resuscitative interventions as part of an overall care plan that emphasizes comfort and quality of living (Box 23-1).
2. **If this option is desired,** physician must write a specific order *not* to attempt CPR (e.g., "In the event of cardiopulmonary arrest, do not attempt

---

BOX 23-1

SAMPLE FROM STATE OF MARYLAND EMS/DNAR FORMS AND BRACELET AUTHORIZATION FORM

The physician must sign the *Physician Certification and Order* and initial ONLY ONE of the two options on the form.

Option A:
    Maximum Efforts to Prevent Cardiac/Respiratory Arrest
    DNAR if Arrest Occurs—No CPR

Option B:
    Supportive Care Prior to Cardiac/Respiratory Arrest
    DNAR if Arrest Occurs—No CPR

NOTE: If a valid EMS/DNAR Order is located after resuscitation has begun, EMS personnel may withdraw resuscitation.

NOTE: Ambulance personnel cannot honor specific instructions in advance directives that do not conform to the care selections in the *Physician Certification and Order* (e.g., wants intubation but no CPR).

resuscitation."). Orders must follow local emergency medical services (EMS) policies for patients at home.

B. Do Not Escalate Treatment

When escalation of treatment no longer supports the goals of care, offer patients and families the option to forgo treatment changes even as the patient's condition worsens. Because death is expected, DNAR must also be discussed. Examples of such requests include:

1. **Do not increase the dose of current medications** (e.g., vasopressors).
2. **Do not add new medications** (e.g., antibiotics).
3. **Do not initiate new interventions** (e.g., dialysis, mechanical ventilation).
4. **Initiate and increase interventions** to treat pain and reduce suffering.

C. Discontinuing Current Interventions

When death is expected regardless of intervention, especially if current interventions are prolonging the dying process, patients and families can be offered the option of discontinuing these interventions (e.g., "Discontinue blood products, monitors, mechanical ventilation, medically provided hydration or nutrition."). Because death is expected, DNAR must also be discussed.

D. State Forms

MOLST (Medical Orders for Life-Sustaining Treatment) and POLST (Physician Orders for Life-Sustaining Treatment) Forms

1. **These are portable and enduring medical order forms** completed by patients or their authorized decision makers and signed by a physician. They contain orders regarding CPR and other life-sustaining treatments.
2. **If a state offers one of these forms,** the orders are valid for EMS providers as well as all health care providers and facilities within that state.
3. **A copy must be provided to the patient or authorized decision maker** within 48 hours of completion, or sooner if the patient is to be transferred.
4. **Please refer to your state's laws prior to completion of any documentation.** Additional information can be found at www.polst.org.

V. BODY, MIND, AND SPIRIT CHANGES AS DEATH APPROACHES[9]

A. Physical Changes

1. **Cardiac:** Blood pressure decreases, heart rate increases, and pulse becomes weaker.
2. **Circulation:** Cool extremities; cyanosis of fingers, nails, lips; mottling of skin
3. **Gastrointestinal:** Metabolism slows and appetite gradually decreases. Liquids are preferred to solids. The body will become naturally dehydrated, and fevers may occur as death approaches. Provide relief with ice chips, moist mouth swabs, antipyretic per rectum.

4. **Respiratory:** Variable pattern of breathing (tachypnea followed by periods of apnea); congestion secondary to secretion build-up; provide relief as follows:
   a. Turn patient every few hours, elevate head of bed, provide frequent mouth care, hyoscyamine as needed.
   b. Relief of air hunger: Morphine and lorazepam as needed, oxygen for comfort.
   c. **NOTE:** Deep suctioning is not helpful.
5. **Sensation changes:** Senses become overactive. Bright lights, noise, or television may be upsetting. Hearing is typically the last sense to diminish. Provide relief by dimming lights, reducing noise, and providing soft background music.
6. **Sleep:** Need for sleep increases as death approaches. Occasionally the child exhibits a surge of energy to play, eat, or socialize.

B. Emotional Changes

Detachment from the outside world: Reduced need to socialize leads to pulling inward of thoughts, emotions, and fears. Listen and reassure family about decreased interactions.

C. Mental Changes

Mental status: Confusion, restlessness, agitation, delirium. Provide relief by keeping child oriented to surroundings, surrounding him/her with family as a way to reinforce safety, and speaking in calm tones. Use lorazepam and haloperidol as needed.

D. Spiritual Changes

Spiritual: Child may call out or reach out for loved ones who are not physically present. Reassure the family that this is not unusual during the dying process.

VI. LAST HOURS: MEDICATION AND MANAGEMENT[10] (TABLE 23-2)

VII. DEATH PRONOUNCEMENT[11]

Residents may be called to pronounce the death of a patient in the hospital. This important task should be carried out with competence, compassion, and respect.

A. Preparation
1. **Know the child's name and gender.**
2. **Be prepared to answer simple pertinent questions** from family and friends.
3. **Consult with nursing staff for relevant information:** recent events, family response, family dynamics.
4. **Determine the need and call for interdisciplinary support:** social work, child life, pastoral care, bereavement coordinator.

B. Entering the Room
1. **Enter quietly and respectfully** along with the primary nurse.

TABLE 23-2

COMMON MEDICATIONS USED FOR SYMPTOMATIC RELIEF IN PALLIATIVE CARE

Indication	Medication	Initial Regimen
Pain	Morphine	0.3 mg/kg/dose PO, SL, PR Q2–4 hr* 0.1–0.2 mg/kg/dose IV Q2–4 hr* **NOTE:** Morphine should be titrated to symptomatic relief.
Dyspnea	Morphine	0.1–0.25 mg/kg/dose PO, SL, PR Q2–4 hr 0.05–0.1 mg/kg/dose IV Q2–4 hr 2.5–5 mg/3 mL normal saline nebulizer Q4hr **NOTE:** Nebulized morphine can cause severe broncho- spasm and worsen dyspnea. Nebulized fentanyl may be preferred.
Agitation	Lorazepam	0.05 mg/kg/dose PO, IV, SL, PR Q4–8 hr
	Haloperidol	0.01–0.02 mg/kg/dose PO, SL, PR Q8–12 hr
Pruritus	Diphenhydramine	0.5–1 mg/kg/dose PO, IV Q6–8 hr
Nausea and vomiting	Prochlorperazine	0.1–0.15 mg/kg/dose PO, PR Q6–8 hr
	Ondansetron	0.15 mg/kg/dose PO, IV Q6–8 hr
Seizures	Diazepam	0.3–0.5 mg/kg/dose PR Q2–4 hr
	Lorazepam	0.05–0.1 mg/kg/dose IV Q2–4 hr
Secretions	Hyoscyamine	0.03–0.06 mg/dose PO, SL Q4hr (if <2 yr) 0.06–0.12 mg/dose PO, SL Q4hr (if 2–12 yr) 0.12–0.25 mg/dose PO, SL Q4hr (if >12 yr)

*Infants <6 mo should receive one third to one half the dose.

IV, Intravenous; PO, oral; PR, rectal; SL, sublingual.

Adapted from Himelstein BP, Hilden JM, Boldt AM, et al. Pediatric palliative care. *N Engl J Med.* 2004;350:1752-1762.

2. **Introduce yourself and identify your role:**
a. "I am Dr. _____, the doctor on call."
b. Determine the relationships of those in the room.
c. Inform the family of the purpose of your visit ("I am here to examine your child"), and invite them to remain in the room.

C. Procedure for Pronouncement

1. **Check ID bracelet and pulse.**
2. **Respectfully check response to tactile stimuli.**
3. **Check for spontaneous respirations.**
4. **Check for heart sounds.**
5. **Record the time of death.**
6. **Inform the family of death.**
7. **Offer to contact other family members.**
8. **Remember to convey sympathy:** "I am so sorry for your loss."

D. Document Death in the Chart

1. **Write date, time of death, and the provider pronouncing the death.**
2. **Document absence of pulse, respirations, and heart sounds.**
3. **Identify family members who were present and informed of death.**
4. **Document notification of attending physician.**

E. Death Certificate

1. **Locate a copy of a sample death certificate for reference.**
2. **Use BLACK INK only and complete *Physician sections*.**
a. **NOTE:** Do *NOT* use abbreviations (e.g., spell out the month: January 31 and not 1/31).
b. **NOTE:** Do *NOT* cross out or use white out; must begin again if mistakes are made.
c. **NOTE:** Cardiopulmonary or respiratory arrest is *NOT* an acceptable primary cause of death.

F. Autopsy Consent

1. **Obtain family consent if indicated.**
2. **Plan follow-up to contact and review autopsy results.**

VIII. AFTER DEATH—BEREAVEMENT[11]

A. Etiquette

Families want to know that their children are not forgotten. Sending condolence cards, attending funerals, and contacting the family weeks to months later are all appropriate physician activities that are deeply valued by bereaved families. Respectful listening to families and sharing memories of the child help provide support during bereavement.

B. Available Services[12]

Be familiar with available services: pastoral care, social work, bereavement coordinator, community support groups, counseling services, bereavement follow-up programs.

REFERENCES

1. Sepulveda C. Palliative care: World Health Organization's global perspective. *J Pain Symptom Manage.* 2002;24:91-96.
2. Nelson R. Palliative care for children: policy statement. *Pediatrics.* 2007;119: 351-357.
3. Hays RM, Valentine J, Haynes G, et al. The Seattle Pediatric Palliative Care Project: effects on family satisfaction and health-related quality of life. *J Palliat Med.* 2006;9:716-728.
4. Back A, Arnold R, Tulsky J. *Mastering Communication with Seriously Ill Patients: Balancing Honesty with Empathy and Hope.* Cambridge University Press: New York, 2009:85-88.
5. Sourkes BM. *Armfuls of Time: The Psychological Experience of Children with Life-Threatening Illnesses.* Pittsburgh: University of Pittsburgh Press, 1995.
6. Corr CA. Children's understanding of death: striving to understand death. In: Doka KJ, ed. *Children mourning, mourning children.* Washington, DC: Hospice Foundation of America, 1995:8-10.
7. Corr CABalk DE, eds. *Handbook of Adolescent Death and Bereavement.* New York: Springer, 1996.
8. Faulkner K. Children's understanding of death. In: Armstrong-Dailey A, Zarbock S, eds. *Hospice Care for Children.* 2nd ed. New York: Oxford University Press, 2001:9-22.

9. Sigrist D. *Journey's End: A Guide to Understanding the Final Stages of the Dying Process*. Rochester, NY: Hospice of Rochester and Hospice of Wayne and Seneca Counties, Genesee Region Home Care, 1995.

10. Himelstein BP, Hilden JM, Boldt AM, et al. Pediatric palliative care. *N Engl J Med*. 2004;350:1752-1762.

11. Bailey A. *The Palliative Response*. Birmingham, AL: Menasha Ridge Press, 2003.

12. AAP Policy Statement. Committee on Bioethics and Committee on Hospital Care: Palliative care for children. *Pediatrics*. 2000;106(2 Pt 1):351-357.

Chapter 24

Pulmonology

Margaret Grala, MD

See additional content on Expert Consult

I. WEBSITES

American Lung Association: http://www.lung.org

Cystic Fibrosis Foundation: http://www.cff.org

American Academy of Allergy, Asthma and Immunology:
http://www.aaaai.org

National Heart Lung and Blood Institute: National Asthma Education and
Prevention Program: http://www.nhlbi.nih.gov

American Thoracic Society: http://www.thoracic.org

II. RESPIRATORY PHYSICAL EXAMINATION

A. Normal Respiratory Rates in Children (Table 24-1)

B. Inspection

Evaluate for chest wall abnormalities (barrel chest, pectus excavatum, or
pectus carinatum), symmetry, accessory muscle use, cyanosis of lips, skin,
or nails, or digital clubbing.

C. Palpation and Percussion

D. Auscultation (Table 24-2)

III. EVALUATION OF PULMONARY GAS EXCHANGE

A. Pulse Oximetry[1-5]

1. **Pulse oximetry** (Spo_2) is an indirect measurement of arterial O_2 saturation
   (Sao_2) estimated by light absorption characteristics of oxygenated and
   deoxygenated hemoglobin through the skin in peripheral blood.

TABLE 24-1

NORMAL RESPIRATORY RATES IN CHILDREN

Age (yr)	Respiratory Rate (breaths/min)
0–1*	24–38
1–3	22–30
4–6	20–24
7–9	18–24
10–14	16–22
14–18	14–20

*Slightly higher respiratory rates (i.e., 40–50 breaths/min) in the neonatal period may be normal in the absence of other signs and symptoms.

Data from Bardella IJ. Pediatric advanced life support: a review of the AHA recommendations. *Am Fam Phys.* 1999;60:1743-1750.

TABLE 24-2

RESPIRATORY AUSCULTATION

Sound	Description	Possible Causes
Crackles (rales)	Intermittent scratchy, bubbly noises Heard predominantly on inspiration Produced by reopening of airways closed on previous expiration	Bronchiolitis, pulmonary edema, pneumonia, asthma
Wheezes	Continuous, high-pitched, musical sound predominantly on expiration	Asthma, bronchiolitis, foreign body
Rhonchi	Continuous, low-pitched, nonmusical sound	Pneumonia, cystic fibrosis
Stridor	High-pitched, harsh, blowing sound Heard predominantly on inspiration	Croup, laryngomalacia, subglottic stenosis, allergic reaction, vocal cord dysfunction

2. **Important uses:**
a. Rapid and continuous assessment of oxygenation in acutely ill patients or patients requiring oxygen therapy
b. Assessment of oxygen requirements during feeding, sleep, exercise, or sedation
c. Monitoring of physiologic effects of apnea and bradycardia

3. **Limitations:**
a. Measures oxygen saturation, not O_2 delivery to tissues. A marginally low saturation in an anemic patient may be more significant because of their reduced O_2-carrying capacity.
b. Insensitive to hyperoxia because of the sigmoid shape of the oxyhemoglobin curve (Fig. 24-1).
c. Artificially increased: Carboxyhemoglobin levels >1%–2% (e.g., in chronic smokers or with smoke inhalation).
d. Artificially decreased: Patient motion, intravenous dyes (methylene blue, indocyanine green), opaque nail polish, and methemoglobin levels >1%.
e. Unreliable when pulse signal is poor: Hypothermia, hypovolemia, shock, edema, or movement artifact.
f. Spo_2 reading often does not correlate with Pao_2 in sickle cell disease.[6]

4. **Oxyhemoglobin dissociation curve** (see Fig. 24-1)

B. **Capnography**

1. **Measures CO_2 concentration of expired gas** by infrared spectroscopy or mass spectroscopy.

2. **End-tidal CO_2 ($ETco_2$) correlates with $Paco_2$** (usually within 5 mm Hg in healthy subjects).

3. **Can be used for demonstrating proper placement of an endotracheal tube,** continuous monitoring of CO_2 trends in ventilated patients, and monitoring ventilation during polysomnography.

C. **Blood Gases**

1. **Arterial blood gas (ABG):** Most accurate way to assess oxygenation (Pao_2), ventilation ($Paco_2$), and acid-base status (pH and HCO_3^-). See Chapter 27 for normal mean values.

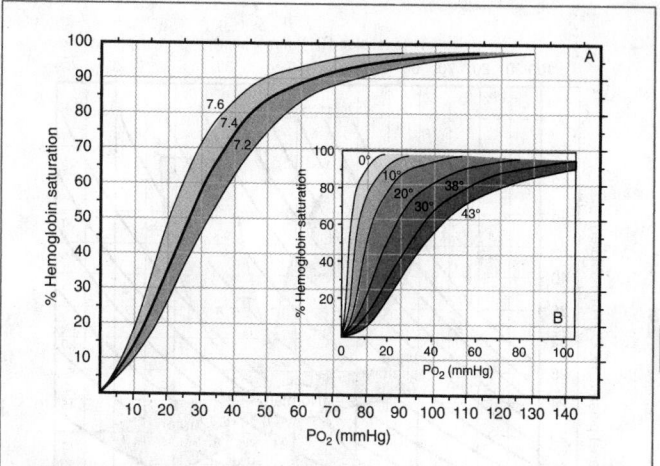

FIGURE 24-1

Oxyhemoglobin dissociation curve. **A,** Curve shifts to the left as pH increases. **B,** Curve shifts to the left as temperature decreases. *(Data from Lanbertsten CJ. Transport of oxygen, CO_2, and inert gases by the blood. In: Mountcastle VB, ed. Medical Physiology. 14th ed. St Louis: Mosby, 1980.)*

2. **Venous blood gas (VBG):** Pv_{CO_2} averages 6–8 mmHg higher than Pa_{CO_2}, and venous pH is slightly lower than arterial pH. Measurement is strongly affected by the local circulatory and metabolic environment.

3. **Capillary blood gas (CBG):** Correlation with ABG generally best for pH, moderate for P_{CO_2}, and worst for P_{O_2}.

D. Analysis of Acid-Base Disturbances[7-9]

1. **Determine primary disturbance,** then assess for mixed disorder by calculating expected compensatory response (Fig. 24-2 and Table 24-3).

IV. PULMONARY FUNCTION TESTS

Provide objective and reproducible measurements of airway function and lung volumes. Used to characterize disease, assess severity, and follow response to therapy.

A. Peak Expiratory Flow Rate (PEFR)

Maximal flow rate generated during a forced expiratory maneuver.

1. **Often used to follow the course of asthma and response to therapy** by comparing a patient's PEFR with the previous "personal best" and the normal predicted value

a. Limitations: Normal predicted values vary across different racial groups. Measurement is effort dependent and cannot be done reliably by many young children, and PEFR is insensitive to small airway function.

2. **Normal predicted PEFR values for children** (Table 24-4)

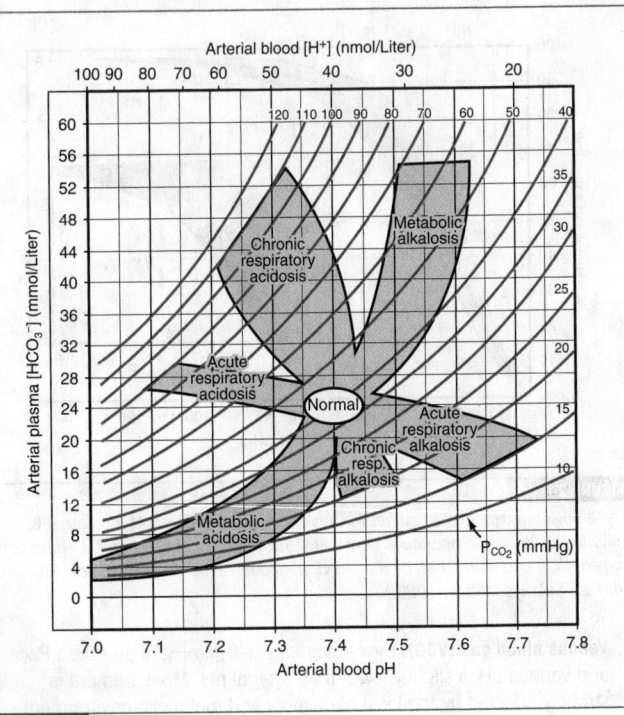

FIGURE 24-2

Interpretation of arterial blood gases. *(Modified from Siggaard-Anderson O. The Acid-Base Status of the Blood. 4th ed. Copenhagen: Munksgaard, 1976.)*

TABLE 24-3
CALCULATION OF EXPECTED COMPENSATORY RESPONSE

Disturbance	Primary Change	pH*	Expected Compensatory Response
Acute respiratory acidosis	↑$Paco_2$	↓pH	↑HCO_3^- by 1 mEq/L for each 10 mmHg rise in $Paco_2$
Acute respiratory alkalosis	↓$Paco_2$	↑pH	↓HCO_3^- by 1–3 mEq/L for each 10 mmHg fall in $Paco_2$
Chronic respiratory acidosis	↑$Paco_2$	↓pH	↑HCO_3^- by 4 mEq/L for each 10 mmHg rise in $Paco_2$
Chronic respiratory alkalosis	↓$Paco_2$	↑pH	↓HCO_3^- by 2–5 mEq/L for each 10 mmHg fall in $Paco_2$
Metabolic acidosis	↓HCO_3^-	↓pH	↓$Paco_2$ by 1–1.5 times fall in HCO_3^-
Metabolic alkalosis	↑HCO_3^-	↑pH	↑$Paco_2$ by 0.25–1 times rise in HCO_3^-

*Pure respiratory acidosis (or alkalosis): 10-mm Hg rise (fall) in $Paco_2$ results in an average 0.08 fall (rise) in pH. Pure metabolic acidosis (or alkalosis): 10-mEq/L fall (rise) in HCO_3^- results in an average 0.15 fall (rise) in pH.
Data from Schrier RW. *Renal and Electrolyte Disorders.* 3rd ed. Boston: Little, Brown, 1986.

TABLE 24-4

PREDICTED AVERAGE PEAK EXPIRATORY FLOW RATES FOR NORMAL CHILDREN

Height Inches (cm)	PEFR (L/min)	Height Inches (cm)	PEFR (L/min)
43 (109)	147	56 (142)	320
44 (112)	160	57 (145)	334
45 (114)	173	58 (147)	347
46 (117)	187	59 (150)	360
47 (119)	200	60 (152)	373
48 (122)	214	61 (155)	387
49 (124)	227	62 (157)	400
50 (127)	240	63 (160)	413
51 (130)	254	64 (163)	427
52 (132)	267	65 (165)	440
53 (135)	280	66 (168)	454
54 (137)	293	67 (170)	467
55 (140)	307		

PEFR, Peak expiratory flow rate.

Data from Voter KZ. Diagnostic tests of lung function. *Pediatr Rev.* 1996;17:53-63.

B. Maximal Inspiratory and Expiratory Pressures[10,11]

Maximal pressure generated during inhalation and exhalation against a fixed obstruction.

1. **Used as a measure of respiratory muscle strength.**
2. **Maximal inspiratory pressure (MIP)** is in the range of 80–120 cm H_2O at all ages. Maximum expiratory pressure (MEP) increases with age and is greater in males.
3. **A low MIP may be an indication for ventilatory support, and a low MEP correlates with decreased effectiveness of coughing.**

C. Spirometry (for Children ≥6 Years)

Plot of airflow versus time during rapid, forceful, and complete expiration from total lung capacity (TLC) to residual volume (RV). Useful to characterize different patterns of airway obstruction (Fig. 24-3). Usually performed before and after bronchodilation to assess response to therapy or after bronchial challenge to assess airway hyperreactivity.

1. **Important definitions** (Fig. 24-4)
a. Forced vital capacity (FVC): Maximum volume of air exhaled from the lungs after a maximum inspiration. Bedside measurement of vital capacity with a handheld spirometer can be useful in confirming or predicting hypoventilation associated with muscle weakness.
b. Forced expiratory volume in 1 second (FEV_1): Volume exhaled during the first second of the FVC maneuver.
c. Forced expiratory flow (FEF_{25-75}): Mean rate of airflow over the middle half of the FVC between 25% and 75% of FVC. Sensitive to medium and small airway obstruction.
2. **Interpretation of spirometry and lung volume readings** (Table 24-5).

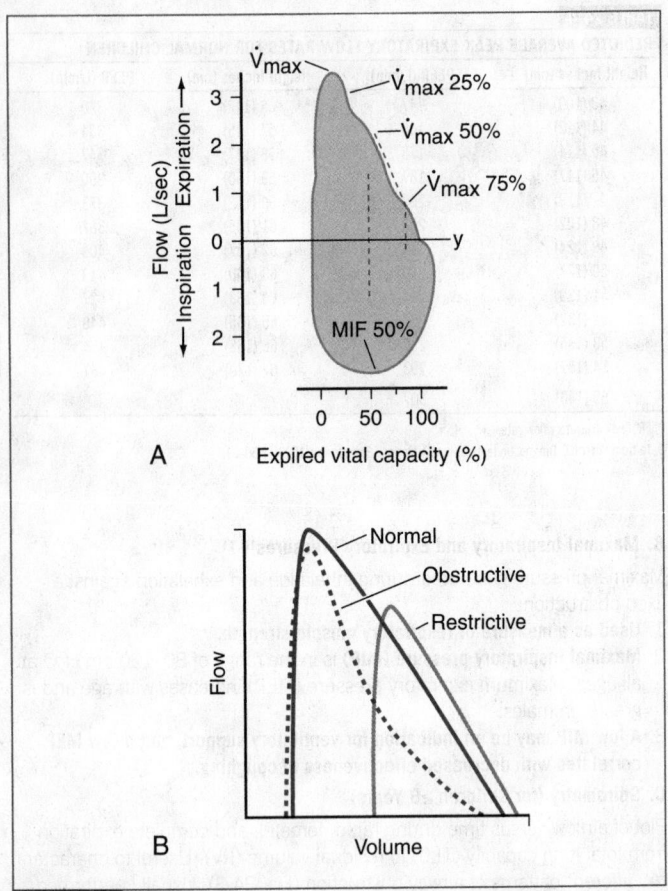

FIGURE 24-3

A, Normal flow-volume curve. **B,** Worsening intrathoracic airway obstruction as in asthma or cystic fibrosis. (**B,** *Data from Baum GL, Wolinsky E. Textbook of Pulmonary Diseases. 5th ed. Boston: Little, Brown, 1994.*)

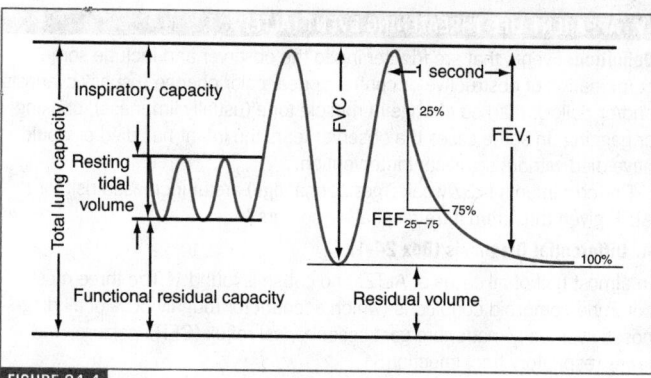

FIGURE 24-4

Lung volumes. FEF$_{25-75}$, Forced expiratory flow between 25% and 75% of FVC; FEV$_1$, forced expiratory volume in 1 second; FVC, forced vital capacity.

TABLE 24-5

INTERPRETATION OF SPIROMETRY AND LUNG VOLUME READINGS

	Obstructive Disease (Asthma, Cystic Fibrosis)	Restrictive Disease (Interstitial Fibrosis, Scoliosis, Neuromuscular Disease)
SPIROMETRY		
FVC*	Normal or reduced	Reduced
FEV$_1$*	Reduced	Reduced§
FEV$_1$/FVC†	Reduced	Normal
FEF$_{25-75}$	Reduced	Normal or reduced§
PEFR*	Normal or reduced	Normal or reduced§
LUNG VOLUMES		
TLC*	Normal or increased	Reduced
RV*	Increased	Reduced
RV/TLC‡	Increased	Unchanged
FRC	Increased	Reduced

*Normal range: ± 20% of predicted.
†Normal range: >85%.
‡Normal range: 20 ± 10%.
§Reduced proportional to FVC.

FEF$_{25-75}$, Forced expiratory flow between 25% and 75% of FVC; FEV$_1$, forced expiratory volume in 1 second; FRC, functional residual capacity; FVC, forced vital capacity; PEFR, peak expiratory flow rate; RV, residual volume; TLC, total lung capacity.

V. APPARENT LIFE-THREATENING EVENT (ALTE)[12,13]

Definition: Events that are frightening to the observer and include some combination of obstructive or central apnea, color change (usually cyanosis and/or pallor), marked change in muscle tone (usually limpness), choking, or gagging. In some cases the observer fears the infant has died or would have died without significant intervention.

Preterm infants (<37 weeks' gestational age) are at increased risk for ALTE given their immature respiratory centers.[14]

A. Differential Diagnosis (Box 24-1)

In almost half of all cases of ALTEs, no cause is found.[14] The three most common comorbid conditions (which account for roughly 50% of all diagnoses eventually made) are gastroesophageal reflux (GER), seizure, and lower respiratory tract infection.[14]

BOX 24-1

DIFFERENTIAL DIAGNOSIS OF APPARENT LIFE-THREATENING EVENT

I. Gastroenterologic

Gastroesophageal reflux disease
Gastroenteritis
Esophageal dysfunction
Surgical abdomen
Dysphagia

II. Neurologic

Seizure
Central apnea/hypoventilation
Meningitis/encephalitis
Hydrocephalus
Brain tumor
Neuromuscular disorders
Vasovagal reaction

III. Respiratory

Respiratory syncytial virus
Pertussis
Aspiration
Respiratory tract infection
Reactive airway disease
Foreign body

IV. Otolaryngologic

Laryngomalacia
Subglottic and/or laryngeal stenosis
Obstructive sleep apnea

V. Cardiovascular
Congenital heart disease
Cardiomyopathy
Cardiac arrhythmias/prolonged QT syndrome
Myocarditis
VI. Metabolic/Endocrine
Inborn error of metabolism
Hypoglycemia
Electrolyte disturbance
VII. Infectious
Sepsis
Urinary tract infection
VIII. Other Diagnosis
Child maltreatment
Shaken baby syndrome
Breath-holding spell
Choking
Drug or toxin reaction
Anemia
Periodic breathing
Factitious disorder imposed by another (Munchausen syndrome by proxy)

Modified from DeWolfe CC. Apparent life-threatening event: a review. *Pediatr Clin North Am.* 2005;52:4.

B. Workup

The clinical history and physical exam guide the workup. Treatment should be tailored to diagnosis and prevention of further events.

1. **If history and physical suggest a significant event took place,** consider obtaining a complete blood cell count (signs of infection or anemia), C-reactive protein, urinalysis, arterial blood gas (acid-base status and oxygenation), blood glucose (hypoglycemia), electrocardiogram (ECG [QT interval]), electrolytes, and potentially pertussis, respiratory syncytial virus (RSV), or other viral studies, depending on prevalence.[14]
2. **Further evaluations should be dictated by clinical picture, but some common studies are:**
a. Chest radiograph: Pneumonia, bronchiolitis, screen for cardiac disease
b. Cardiopulmonary monitoring and/or polysomnography: Continuous assessment of oxygenation and ventilation (especially for recurrent events or unusual apnea), rule out obstructive apnea
c. Barium swallow ± pH probe: Dysfunctional swallow, GER
d. Electroencephalography (EEG): Seizure disorder
e. Evaluation for non-accidental trauma, including head computed tomography (CT) if the history and physical raise concern
f. Urine toxicology: If suspicious of ingestion

VI. ASTHMA[15]

A chronic inflammatory disorder of the airways resulting in recurrent episodes of wheezing, breathlessness, chest tightness, and cough, particularly at night and in the early morning. These episodes are usually associated with obstruction of airflow in the lower airway and are reversible either spontaneously or with therapy. The inflammation causes increased airway hyperreactivity to a variety of stimuli: Viral infections, cold air, exercise, emotions, and environmental allergens and pollutants.

A. Clinical Manifestations

1. **Cough,** increased work of breathing (tachypnea, retractions, or accessory muscle use), wheezing, hypoxia, and hypoventilation. Crackles may also be present with asthma exacerbations.
2. **No audible wheezing** may indicate very poor air movement and severe bronchospasm.
3. **Chest radiographs** often show peribronchial thickening, hyperinflation, and patchy atelectasis.
   a. If persistent radiographic abnormalities, consider right middle lobe syndrome.

B. Management

1. **Acute management and status asthmaticus;** see Chapter 1
2. **Initial classification and initiation of treatment** for ages 0–4, 5–11, and ≥12 years: Figures 24-5, 24-6, and 24-7
3. **Stepwise approach to continued management** for ages 0–4, 5–11, and ≥12 years: Figures 24-8, 24-9, and 24-10

C. Prevention of Exacerbations

1. **Ensure up-to-date immunizations,** including influenza.
2. **Create an asthma action plan**
   (http://www.nhlbi.nih.gov/health/public/lung/index.htm#asthma or http://fha.maryland.gov/pdf/mch/Asthma_Action_Plan.pdf).
3. **Identify and minimize asthma triggers and environmental exposures,** including tobacco smoke, mold, pollen, dust mites, etc.
4. **Assess** symptom control, inhaler technique, and medication adherence with regular clinical evaluations.
   a. Consider specialist referral for formal pulmonary function test (PFT), monitoring, and allergy testing.
   b. For dosing guidelines on inhaled corticosteroids, please see Table EC 24-A on Expert Consult.

CLASSIFYING ASTHMA SEVERITY AND INITIATING TREATMENT IN CHILDREN 0–4 YEARS OF AGE

Assessing severity and initiating therapy in children who are not currently taking long-term control medication

Components of severity		Classification of asthma severity (0–4 years of age)			
				Persistent	
		Intermittent	Mild	Moderate	Severe
Impairment	Symptoms	≤2 days/week	>2 days/week but not daily	Daily	Throughout the day
	Nighttime awakenings	0	1–2×/month	3–4×/month	>1×/week
	Short-acting beta₂-agonist use for symptom control (not prevention of EIB)	≤2 days/week	>2 days/week but not daily	Daily	Several times per day
	Interference with normal activity	None	Minor limitation	Some limitation	Extremely limited
Risk	Exacerbations requiring oral systemic corticosteroids	0–1/year	≥2 exacerbations in 6 months requiring oral systemic corticosteroids, or ≥4 wheezing episodes/1 year lasting >1 day AND risk factors for persistent asthma		
		Consider severity and interval since last exacerbation. Frequency and severity may fluctuate over time. Exacerbations of any severity may occur in patients in any severity category.			
Recommended step for initiating therapy (See Fig. 24-8 for treatment steps.)		Step 1	Step 2	Step 3 and consider short course of oral systemic corticosteroids	
		In 2–6 weeks, depending on severity, evaluate level of asthma control that is achieved. If no clear benefit is observed in 4–6 weeks, consider adjusting therapy or alternative diagnoses.			

Key: EIB, exercise-induced bronchospasm

Notes
- The stepwise approach is meant to assist, not replace, the clinical decision making required to meet individual patient needs.
- Level of severity is determined by both impairment and risk. Assess impairment domain by patient's/caregiver's recall of previous 2–4 weeks. Symptom assessment for longer periods should reflect a global assessment such as inquiring whether the patient's asthma is better or worse since the last visit. Assign severity to the most severe category in which any feature occurs.
- At present, there are inadequate data to correspond frequencies of exacerbations with different levels of asthma severity. For treatment purposes, patients who had ≥2 exacerbations requiring oral systemic corticosteroids in the past 6 months, or ≥4 wheezing episodes in the past year, and who have risk factors for persistent asthma may be considered the same as patients who have persistent asthma, even in the absence of impairment levels consistent with persistent asthma.

FIGURE 24-5

Guidelines for classifying asthma severity and initiating treatment in infants and young children (0–4 years of age). (Adapted from NAEPP—Expert Panel Report 3. Guidelines for the Diagnosis and Management of Asthma, August 2007. http://www.nhlbi.nih.gov/guidelines/asthma/asthgdln.htm.)

CLASSIFYING ASTHMA SEVERITY AND INITIATING TREATMENT IN CHILDREN 5–11 YEARS OF AGE

Assessing severity and initiating therapy in children who are not currently taking long-term control medication

Components of severity		Classification of asthma severity (5–11 years of age)			
			Persistent		
		Intermittent	Mild	Moderate	Severe
Impairment	Symptoms	≤2 days/week	>2 days/week but not daily	Daily	Throughout the day
	Nighttime awakenings	≤2×/month	3–4×/month	>1×/week but not nightly	Often 7×/week
	Short-acting beta₂-agonist use for symptom control (not prevention of EIB)	≤2 days/week	>2 days/week but not daily	Daily	Several times per day
	Interference with normal activity	None	Minor limitation	Some limitation	Extremely limited
	Lung function	• Normal FEV$_1$ between exacerbations • FEV$_1$ >80% predicted • FEV$_1$/FVC >85%	• FEV$_1$ = >80% predicted • FEV$_1$/FVC >80%	• FEV$_1$ = 60%–80% predicted • FEV$_1$/FVC = 75%–80%	• FEV$_1$ <60% predicted • FEV$_1$/FVC <75%
Risk	Exacerbations requiring oral systemic corticosteroids	0–1/year (see note)	≥2/year (see note) →→→		
		Consider severity and interval since last exacerbation. ←— Frequency and severity may fluctuate over time —→ for patients in any severity category.			
		Relative annual risk of exacerbations may be related to FEV$_1$.			
Recommended step for initiating therapy		Step 1	Step 2	Step 3, medium-dose ICS option	Step 3, medium-dose ICS option, or step 4
					and consider short course of oral systemic corticosteroids
(See Fig. 24-9 for treatment steps.)		In 2–6 weeks, evaluate level of asthma control that is achieved, and adjust therapy accordingly.			

Key: EIB, exercise-induced bronchospasm; FEV$_1$, forced expiratory volume in 1 second; FVC, forced vital capacity; ICS, inhaled corticosteroids

Notes
• The stepwise approach is meant to assist, not replace, the clinical decision making required to meet individual patient needs.
• Level of severity is determined by both impairment and risk. Assess impairment domain by patient's/caregiver's recall of previous 2–4 weeks and spirometry. Assign severity to the most severe category in which any feature occurs.
• At present, there are inadequate data to correspond frequencies of exacerbations with different levels of asthma severity. In general, more frequent and intense exacerbations (e.g., requiring urgent, unscheduled care, hospitalization, or ICU admission) indicate greater underlying disease severity. For treatment purposes, patients who had ≥2 exacerbations requiring oral systemic corticosteroids in the past year may be considered the same as patients who have persistent asthma, even in the absence of impairment levels consistent with persistent asthma.

FIGURE 24-6

Guidelines for classifying asthma severity and initiating treatment in children 5–11 years of age. (*Adapted from NAEPP—Expert Panel Report 3. Guidelines for the Diagnosis and Management of Asthma, August 2007.* http://www.nhlbi.nih.gov/guidelines/asthma/asthgdln.htm.)

CLASSIFYING ASTHMA SEVERITY AND INITIATING TREATMENT IN YOUTHS≥12 YEARS OF AGE

Assessing severity and initiating treatment for patients who are not currently taking long-term control medications

Components of severity		Classification of asthma severity ≥12 years of age			
			Persistent		
		Intermittent	Mild	Moderate	Severe
Impairment Normal FEV$_1$/FVC: 8–19 yr 85% 20–39 yr 80% 40–59 yr 75% 60–80 yr 70%	Symptoms	≤2 days/week	>2 days/week but not daily	Daily	Throughout the day
	Nighttime awakenings	≤2×/month	3–4×/month	>1×/week but not nightly	Often 7×/week
	Short-acting beta$_2$-agonist use for symptom control (not prevention of EIB)	≤2 days/week	>2 days/week but not daily, and not more than 1 time on any day	Daily	Several times per day
	Interference with normal activity	None	Minor limitation	Some limitation	Extremely limited
	Lung function	• Normal FEV$_1$ between exacerbations • FEV$_1$ >80% predicted • FEV$_1$/FVC normal	• FEV$_1$ >80% predicted • FEV$_1$/FVC normal	• FEV$_1$ >60% but <80% predicted • FEV$_1$/FVC reduced 5%	• FEV$_1$ <60% predicted • FEV$_1$/FVC reduced >5%
Risk	Exacerbations requiring oral systemic corticosteroids	0–1/year (see note)	≥2/year (see note)		
		Consider severity and interval since last exacerbation. ◄— Frequency and severity may fluctuate over time —► for patients in any severity category.			
		Relative annual risk of exacerbations may be related to FEV$_1$.			
Recommended step for initiating treatment (See Fig. 24-10 for treatment steps.)		Step 1	Step 2	Step 3 and consider short course of oral systemic corticosteroids	Step 4 or 5
		In 2–6 weeks, evaluate level of asthma control that is achieved and adjust therapy accordingly.			

Key: FEV$_1$, forced expiratory volume in 1 second; FVC, forced vital capacity; ICU, intensive care unit

Notes
- The stepwise approach is meant to assist, not replace, the clinical decision making required to meet individual patient needs.
- Level of severity is determined by both impairment and risk. Assess impairment domain by patient's/caregiver's recall of previous 2–4 weeks and spirometry. Assign severity to the most severe category in which any feature occurs.
- At present, there are inadequate data to correspond frequencies of exacerbations with different levels of asthma severity. In general, more frequent and intense exacerbations (e.g., requiring urgent, unscheduled care, hospitalization, or ICU admission) indicate greater underlying disease severity. For treatment purposes, patients who had ≥2 exacerbations requiring oral systemic corticosteroids in the past year may be considered the same as patients who have persistent asthma, even in the absence of impairment levels consistent with persistent asthma.

FIGURE 24-7

Guidelines for classifying asthma severity and initiating treatment in youth 12 and older. (*Adapted from NAEPP—Expert Panel Report 3. Guidelines for the Diagnosis and Management of Asthma, August 2007.* http://www.nhlbi.nih.gov/guidelines/asthma/asthgdln.htm.)

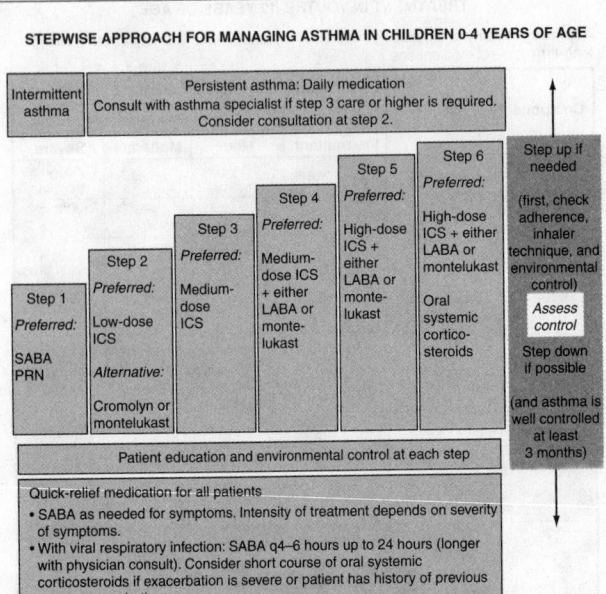

STEPWISE APPROACH FOR MANAGING ASTHMA IN CHILDREN 0-4 YEARS OF AGE

Intermittent asthma

Persistent asthma: Daily medication
Consult with asthma specialist if step 3 care or higher is required.
Consider consultation at step 2.

Step 1
Preferred:
SABA PRN

Step 2
Preferred:
Low-dose ICS
Alternative:
Cromolyn or montelukast

Step 3
Preferred:
Medium-dose ICS

Step 4
Preferred:
Medium-dose ICS + either LABA or montelukast

Step 5
Preferred:
High-dose ICS + either LABA or montelukast

Step 6
Preferred:
High-dose ICS + either LABA or montelukast
Oral systemic corticosteroids

Step up if needed
(first, check adherence, inhaler technique, and environmental control)

Assess control

Step down if possible
(and asthma is well controlled at least 3 months)

Patient education and environmental control at each step

Quick-relief medication for all patients
• SABA as needed for symptoms. Intensity of treatment depends on severity of symptoms.
• With viral respiratory infection: SABA q4–6 hours up to 24 hours (longer with physician consult). Consider short course of oral systemic corticosteroids if exacerbation is severe or patient has history of previous severe exacerbations.
• Caution: Frequent use of SABA may indicate the need to step up treatment. See text for recommendations on initiating daily long-term-control therapy.

Key: Alphabetical order is used when more than one treatment option is listed within either preferred or alternative therapy. ICS, inhaled corticosteroid; LABA, long-acting inhaled beta$_2$-agonist; SABA, short-acting inhaled beta$_2$-agonist

Notes:
• The stepwise approach is meant to assist, not replace, the clinical decision making required to meet individual patient needs.aaaa

• If alternative treatment is used and response is inadequate, discontinue it and use the preferred treatment before stepping up.

• If clear benefit is not observed within 4–6 weeks and patient/family medication technique and adherence are satisfactory, consider adjusting therapy or alternative diagnosis.

• Studies on children 0–4 years of age are limited. Step 2 preferred therapy is based on Evidence A. All other recommendations are based on expert opinion and extrapolation from studies in older children.

FIGURE 24-8

Stepwise approach for managing asthma in infants and young children (0–4 years of age). *(Adapted from NAEPP—Expert Panel Report 3. Guidelines for the Diagnosis and Management of Asthma, August 2007.* http://www.nhlbi.nih.gov/guidelines/asthma/ast hgdln.htm.*)*

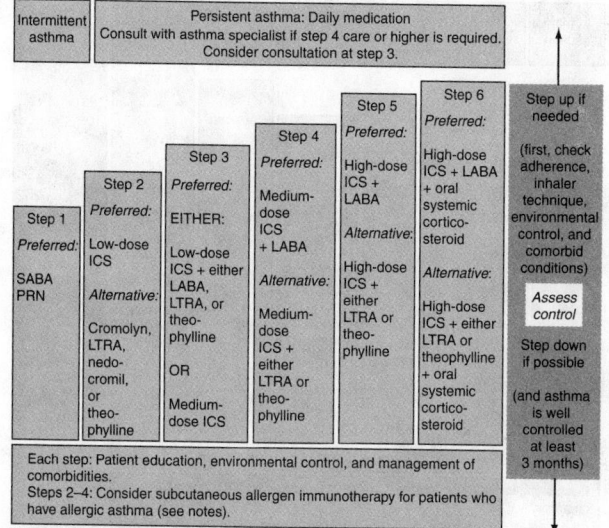

STEPWISE APPROACH FOR MANAGING ASTHMA IN CHILDREN 5–11 YEARS OF AGE

Intermittent asthma	Persistent asthma: Daily medication Consult with asthma specialist if step 4 care or higher is required. Consider consultation at step 3.

Step 1
Preferred:
SABA PRN

Step 2
Preferred:
Low-dose ICS
Alternative:
Cromolyn, LTRA, nedocromil, or theophylline

Step 3
Preferred:
EITHER:
Low-dose ICS + either LABA, LTRA, or theophylline
OR
Medium-dose ICS

Step 4
Preferred:
Medium-dose ICS + LABA
Alternative:
Medium-dose ICS + either LTRA or theophylline

Step 5
Preferred:
High-dose ICS + LABA
Alternative:
High-dose ICS + either LTRA or theophylline

Step 6
Preferred:
High-dose ICS + LABA + oral systemic corticosteroid
Alternative:
High-dose ICS + either LTRA or theophylline + oral systemic corticosteroid

Step up if needed
(first, check adherence, inhaler technique, environmental control, and comorbid conditions)
Assess control
Step down if possible
(and asthma is well controlled at least 3 months)

Each step: Patient education, environmental control, and management of comorbidities.
Steps 2–4: Consider subcutaneous allergen immunotherapy for patients who have allergic asthma (see notes).

Quick-relief medication for all patients
• SABA as needed for symptoms. Intensity of treatment depends on severity of symptoms: up to 3 treatments at 20-minute intervals as needed. Short course of oral systemic corticosteroids may be needed.
• Caution: Increasing use of SABA or use >2 days a week for symptom relief (not prevention of EIB) generally indicates inadequate control and the need to step up treatment.

Key: **Alphabetical order is used when more than one treatment option is listed within either preferred or alternative therapy.** ICS, inhaled corticosteroid; LABA, long-acting inhaled beta$_2$-agonist; LTRA, leukotriene receptor antagonist; SABA, short-acting inhaled beta$_2$-agonist

Notes:
• The stepwise approach is meant to assist, not replace, the clinical decision making required to meet individual patient needs.
• If alternative treatment is used and response is inadequate, discontinue it and use the preferred treatment before stepping up.
• Theophylline is a less desirable alternative due to the need to monitor serum concentration levels.
• Step 1 and step 2 medications are based on Evidence A. Step 3 ICS + adjunctive therapy and ICS are based on Evidence B for efficacy of each treatment and extrapolation from comparator trials in older children and adults—comparator trials are not available for this age group; steps 4–6 are based on expert opinion and extrapolation from studies in older children and adults.
• Immunotherapy for steps 2–4 is based on Evidence B for house-dust mites, animal danders, and pollens; evidence is weak or lacking for molds and cockroaches. Evidence is strongest for immunotherapy with single allergens. The role of allergy in asthma is greater in children than in adults. Clinicians who administer immunotherapy should be prepared and equipped to identify and treat anaphylaxis that may occur.

FIGURE 24-9

Stepwise approach for managing asthma in children 5–11. (*Adapted from NAEPP—Expert Panel Report 3. Guidelines for the Diagnosis and Management of Asthma, August 2007.* http://www.nhlbi.nih.gov/guidelines/asthma/asthgdln.htm.)

STEPWISE APPROACH FOR MANAGING ASTHMA IN YOUTH ≥12 YEARS OF AGE AND ADULTS

Intermittent asthma	Persistent asthma: Daily medication
	Consult with asthma specialist if step 4 care or higher is required. Consider consultation at step 3.

Step 1
Preferred:
SABA PRN

Step 2
Preferred:
Low-dose ICS
Alternative:
Cromolyn, LTRA, nedocromil, or theophylline

Step 3
Preferred:
Low-dose ICS + either LABA, OR Medium-dose ICS
Alternative:
Low-dose ICS + either LTRA, Theophylline, or zileuton

Step 4
Preferred:
Medium-dose ICS + LABA
Alternative:
Medium-dose ICS + either LTRA, theophylline, or zileuton

Step 5
Preferred:
High-dose ICS + LABA
AND
Consider omalizumab for patients who have allergies

Step 6
Preferred:
High-dose ICS + LABA + oral corticosteroid
AND
Consider omalizumab for patients who have allergies

Step up if needed
(first, check adherence, environmental control, and comorbid conditions)

Assess control

Step down if possible
(and asthma is well controlled at least 3 months)

Each step: Patient education, environmental control, and management of comorbidities.

Steps 2–4: Consider subcutaneous allergen immunotherapy for patients who have allergic asthma (see notes).

Quick-relief medication for all patients

- SABA as needed for symptoms. Intensity of treatment depends on severity of symptoms: up to 3 treatments at 20-minute intervals as needed. Short course of oral systemic corticosteroids may be needed.
- Use of SABA >2 days a week for symptom relief (not prevention of EIB) generally indicates inadequate control and the need to step up treatment.

Key: Alphabetical order is used when more than one treatment option is listed within either preferred or alternative therapy. EIB, exercise-induced bronchospasm; ICS, inhaled corticosteroid; LABA, long-acting inhaled β_2-agonist; LTRA, leukotriene receptor antagonist; PRN, as needed; SABA, shortacting inhaled β_2-agonist

Notes:
- The stepwise approach is meant to assist, not replace, the clinical decision making required to meet individual patient needs.
- If alternative treatment is used and response is inadequate, discontinue it and use the preferred treatment before stepping up.
- Zileuton is a less-desirable alternative due to limited studies as adjunctive therapy and the need to monitor liver function. Theophylline requires monitoring of serum concentration levels.
- In step 6, before oral systemic corticosteroids are introduced, a trial of high-dose ICS + LABA + either LTRA, theophylline, or zileuton may be considered, although this approach has not been studied in clinical trials.
- Step 1, 2, and 3 preferred therapies are based on Evidence A; step 3 alternative therapy is based on Evidence A for LTRA, Evidence B for theophylline, and Evidence D for zileuton. Step 4 preferred therapy is based on Evidence B, and alternative therapy is based on Evidence B for LTRA and theophylline and Evidence D for zileuton. Step 5 preferred therapy is based on Evidence B. Step 6 preferred therapy is based on Expert Panel Report 2 (1997) and Evidence B for omalizumab.
- Immunotherapy for steps 2–4 is based on Evidence B for house-dust mites, animal danders, and pollens; evidence is weak or lacking for molds and cockroaches. Evidence is strongest for immunotherapy with single allergens. The role of allergy in asthma is greater in children than in adults.
- Clinicians who administer immunotherapy or omalizumab should be prepared and equipped to identify and treat anaphylaxis that may occur.

FIGURE 24-10

Stepwise approach for managing asthma in youth 12 and older. *(Adapted from NAEPP—Expert Panel Report 3. Guidelines for the Diagnosis and Management of Asthma, August 2007.* http://www.nhlbi.nih.gov/guidelines/asthma/asthgdln.htm.*)*

VII. BRONCHIOLITIS[16]

Bronchiolitis is a lower respiratory tract infection common in infants and children 2 years of age and younger. It is characterized by acute inflammation, edema, and necrosis of airway epithelium, leading to increased mucus production and bronchospasm. It is most commonly caused by RSV, but can also be seen with other viruses including: parainfluenza, adenovirus, mycoplasma, and human metapneumovirus.

A. Clinical Manifestations

1. **Variable and dynamic course** ranging from transient apnea and mucus plugging to progressive lower airway disease
   a. Initial symptoms: Clear rhinorrhea, diminished appetite, fever, cough
   b. Later symptoms: Tachypnea, wheezing, dyspnea, irritability
2. **Radiographic findings:** Hyperinflation and patchy atelectasis

B. Treatment

Mainstay is supportive care.

1. **Consider hospitalization** based on clinical presentation, need for supplemental oxygen, or inability to feed. Should be strongly considered for patients <12 weeks, history of prematurity, underlying cardiopulmonary disease, or immunodeficiency.
2. **Supplemental oxygen therapy** for consistently low oxygen saturation (Sp_{O_2}).
   a. Consider maintaining higher Sp_{O_2} for those with fever, acidosis, or hemoglobinopathies due to oxyhemoglobin desaturation curve, or for increased work of breathing.
3. **A trial of bronchodilators is an option** but should be continued only if there is documented improved clinical response.
4. **Corticosteroids and antibiotics** should not be used routinely in bronchiolitis (unless signs of bacterial con-infection).
5. **Fluid support is often needed** owing to increased losses from tachypnea, fever, and poor oral intake.
   a. Hold oral feedings in hospitalized infants who are very tachypneic to minimize risk of aspiration.
6. **Consider hypertonic saline nebulizer treatments** in previously healthy infants while they are hospitalized.
   a. Albuterol is often given with hypertonic saline nebulizer treatments to reduce the bronchospasm induced by hypertonic saline.

C. Clinical Pearls

1. **In infants younger than 3 months with RSV,** there is an appreciable incidence of co-infection with urinary tract infection (UTI) and/or acute otitis media, but pneumonia is uncommon.[16]
2. **Infants hospitalized for bronchiolitis** are more likely to have recurrent wheezing.
3. **Ensure RSV immunoprophylaxis** for high-risk infants. See Chapter 16.

24

VIII. BRONCHOPULMONARY DYSPLASIA(BPD)[17-19]

Also known as chronic lung disease of prematurity or chronic lung disease of infancy, BPD is a chronic pulmonary condition that usually evolves after premature birth, characterized by the need for oxygen supplementation >21% for at least 28 days after birth. Thought to be a result of airway inflammation, damage from hyperoxia, hypoxia, or mechanical ventilation; results in interference with normal lung alveolar, airway, and vascular development.

A. Diagnostic Criteria

1. **Severity based on oxygen requirement** at time of assessment and characterized as mild if on room air, moderate if requiring <30% oxygen, or severe if requiring >30% oxygen and/or positive pressure.
a. If gestational age at birth was <32 weeks: Assess infant at 36 weeks' postmenstrual age or at discharge to home, whichever comes first.
b. If gestational age at birth >32 weeks: Assess infant at 28–56 days postnatal age or at discharge to home, whichever comes first.

B. Clinical Manifestations and Management of Established BPD

1. **Children with BPD** may have persistent respiratory symptoms, airway hyperreactivity, and supplemental oxygen requirements, especially during intercurrent illness. These children often require some combination of the following for their lung disease:
a. Bronchodilators.
b. Antiinflammatory agents.
c. Supplemental oxygen therapy.
d. Diuretics.
e. Severe cases may require tracheostomy and prolonged mechanical ventilation.
f. Remember RSV and flu prophylaxis.
2. **Need close monitoring for complications,** which can affect multiple organ systems besides lungs: Pulmonary or systemic hypertension, electrolyte abnormalities, nephrocalcinosis (from chronic diuretics), neurodevelopmental or growth delay, aspiration from dysphagia and/or GER, and more severe superinfections with RSV or flu.

IX. CYSTIC FIBROSIS (CF)[20-22]

An autosomal recessive disorder in which mutations of the cystic fibrosis transmembrane conductance regulator (*CFTR*) gene reduce the function of a chloride channel that usually resides within mucosal epithelial cells in the airways, pancreatic ducts, biliary tree, intestine, vas deferens, and sweat glands. Most patients have chronic progressive obstructive pulmonary disease, pancreatic exocrine insufficiency with protein and fat malabsorption, and abnormally high sweat electrolyte concentrations.

A. Clinical Manifestations (Table 24-6)

B. Diagnosis

Over half of patients are diagnosed by 6 months of age, three fourths by 2 years.

TABLE 24-6

MAJOR CLINICAL MANIFESTATIONS OF CYSTIC FIBROSIS BY ORGAN SYSTEM

Respiratory	Chronic productive cough, hemoptysis
	Bronchiectasis, bronchitis, pneumonia
	Sinusitis
	Nasal polyposis
Gastrointestinal	Meconium ileus
	Rectal prolapse
	Pancreatic insufficiency
	Distal intestinal obstruction syndrome (DIOS)
	Fat-soluble vitamin deficiency (A, D, E, K)
	Liver disease including cirrhosis
Genitourinary	Infertility (male) and decreased fertility (female)
	Absence of vas deferens
Miscellaneous	Increased sweat electrolytes
	Hypokalemic alkalosis
	Digital clubbing
	Pulmonary hypertrophic osteoarthropathy
	Failure to thrive

1. **Quantitative pilocarpine ionoelectrophoresis (sweat chloride) test:** Gold standard for diagnosis.
   a. Positive for CF: >60 mEq/L (mEq/L = mmol/L)
   b. Indeterminant:
      (1) Infants <6 months: Indeterminant if 30–60 mEq/L
      (2) Children >6 months: Indeterminant if 40–60 mEq/L
   c. Normal:
      (1) Infants <6 months: Normal if <30 mEq/L
      (2) Children >6 months: Normal if <40 mEq/L
2. **DNA testing is becoming increasingly important in diagnosis.** Over 1800 mutations have been described, most common is F508del (present in 70% of those with CF).
3. **Many states have adopted universal newborn screening (NBS)** by measuring infants' immunoreactive trypsinogen (IRT) levels and/or DNA testing for most common mutations. A confirmatory sweat chloride test should be performed promptly in those patients who have a positive NBS result.
4. **Clinical pearl:** Elevated sweat chloride levels can be from other disorders, including untreated adrenal insufficiency, glycogen storage disease type 1, fucosidosis, hypothyroidism, nephrogenic diabetes insipidus, ectodermal dysplasia, malnutrition, mucopolysaccharidosis, panhypopituitarism, or poor testing technique.

C. Pulmonary Therapies

1. **Airway clearance therapy (ACT)** to mobilize airway secretions and facilitate expectoration: Often manual/mechanical percussion and postural drainage. Older children may use high-frequency chest wall compression device (vest therapy), mechanical chest percussors, or

oscillatory positive expiratory pressure (PEP) handheld devices (e.g., flutter valve and acapella).

2. **Aerosolized medications** to increase mucociliary clearance: recombinant human DNAase (dornase alfa), which cleaves nucleic material, and hypertonic saline nebs to hydrate airway mucus and stimulate cough

3. **Chronic antibiotics:** If *Pseudomonas aeruginosa* is persistently present in culture of airways, consider aerosolized aminoglycosides and/or chronic oral macrolide therapy.

4. **Intermittent use of IV antibiotics** when hospitalized for exacerbations. Common bacteria that cause exacerbations include *P. aeruginosa* and *Staphylococcus aureus*.

D. **Management of Common CF Complications**

1. **Pancreatic disease**
a. Pancreatic enzyme replacement therapy (PERT) prior to meals to improve digestion and intestinal absorption of dietary protein and fat
b. Nutritional supplementation to maintain body mass index (BMI) ≥50th percentile
c. Monitoring for CF-induced diabetes or liver disease

2. **Infertility:**
a. Absence of the vas deferens; however, assisted fertilization is possible using aspiration of viable sperm from testes
b. Women may have trouble becoming pregnant because of mucus-associated obstruction of the cervix.

3. **Decreased life expectancy;** survival continues to improve, and median predicted survival age is over 37 years.

X. OBSTRUCTIVE SLEEP APNEA SYNDROME (OSAS)[23-26]

Part of the spectrum of sleep-disordered breathing; characterized by prolonged partial and/or intermittent partial or complete upper airway obstruction with accompanying hypoxemia, hypercapnia, and/or sleep disruption. Alternate names include *obstructive hypoventilation*, *upper airway resistance syndrome*.

A. **Clinical Manifestations**

1. **Snoring** sometimes accompanied by snorts, gasps, or intermittent pauses in breathing.

2. **Increased respiratory effort** during sleep, disturbed or restless sleep with increased arousals and awakenings.

3. **Daytime cognitive and/or behavioral problems.** (Young children rarely present with daytime sleepiness.)

4. **Long-term complications** include neurocognitive impairment, behavioral problems, poor growth, and systemic and pulmonary hypertension.

5. **Risk factors include** adenotonsillar hypertrophy, obesity, family history of OSAS, craniofacial or laryngeal anomalies, prematurity, nasal/pharyngeal inflammation, cerebral palsy, and neuromuscular disease.

B. Diagnosis

1. **Screen for snoring** during routine well-child care.
2. **If a child snores on a regular basis** and has any of the complaints or findings shown in Box 24-2, clinicians should either (1) obtain a polysomnogram OR (2) refer the patient to a sleep specialist or otolaryngologist for more extensive evaluation.[23]

a. Polysomnography includes measurement of EEG, electrooculography (EOG), and electromyography (EMG) to monitor sleep stage and movement; ECG; chest wall and abdominal movement to assess respiratory effort; nasal/oral airflow; and transcutaneous or $ETco_2$ (ventilation) and pulse oximetry (oxygenation).

b. Diagnosis of OSAS by polysomnography is based on obstructive apnea-hypopnea index (AHI) and gas exchange abnormalities resulting from upper airway obstruction. Polysomnography is used to differentiate OSAS from benign snoring and other disorders that may disrupt sleep, including central hypoventilation syndrome, sleep-related respiratory failure related to neuromuscular or lung disease, and nocturnal seizures.

C. Treatment

1. **Tonsillectomy and adenoidectomy** are mainstays of treatment.
2. **Continuous positive airway pressure (CPAP) or bilevel positive airway pressure (BiPAP)** for patients who fail surgical therapy or are not candidates for surgery.

BOX 24-2

SYMPTOMS AND SIGNS OF OSAS

I. HISTORY

Frequent snoring (≥3 nights/week)
Labored breathing during sleep
Gasping/snorting noises or observed episodes of apnea
Sleep enuresis (especially secondary enuresis)
Sleeping in a seated position or with the neck hyperextended
Cyanosis
Headache on awakening
Daytime sleepiness
Attention-deficit/hyperactivity disorder
Learning problems

II. PHYSICAL EXAM

Underweight or overweight
Tonsillar hypertrophy
Adenoidal facies
Micrognathia/retrognathia
High-arched palate
Failure to thrive
Hypertension

Adapted from Marcus CL, Brooks LJ, Draper KA, et al. Diagnosis and management of childhood obstructive sleep apnea syndrome. *Pediatrics*. 2012;130:575-584.

3. **Weight loss in obese children.**
4. **Treatment of upper respiratory allergies.**

XI. SUDDEN INFANT DEATH SYNDROME[27]

Sudden death of an infant younger than 1 year that remains unexplained after a thorough case investigation, including performance of complete autopsy, examination of death scene, and review of clinical history. Thought to be caused when a genetically vulnerable infant is exposed to an exogenous stressor during a critical developmental period when there is immaturity of the cardiorespiratory system, autonomic nervous system, immune system, and arousal pathways, together with a failure of arousal responsiveness from sleep.

A. Epidemiology

1. **Incidence is** 0.56 per 1000 in the United States, 2–3 times higher in African American and Native American populations.
2. **Peak incidence is** at 2–4 months of age, with male predominance.

B. Risk Factors and Protective Factors (Box 24-3)

BOX 24-3

FACTORS ASSOCIATED WITH SUDDEN INFANT DEATH SYNDROME (SIDS)

Risk Factors	Protective Factors
Premature birth	Sleeping in supine position
In utero and postnatal smoke exposure	Sleeping on firm mattress
Side and prone sleeping	Pacifier use during sleep
Sleeping on soft mattress and bedding	Live and sleep in smoke-free zone
Overbundling	Sleep in same room as caregivers
Bed sharing	Breastfeeding
Recent infection	
Siblings with SIDS	
Low socioeconomic factors	

REFERENCES

1. Murray CB, Loughlin GM. Making the most of pulse oximetry. *Contemp Pediatr.*. 1995;12:45-52:55-57, 61-62.
2. Comber JT, Lopez BL. Examination of pulse oximetry in sickle cell anemia patients presenting to the emergency department in acute vasoocclusive crisis. *Am J Emerg Med.* 1996;14:16-18.
3. Salyer JW. Neonatal and pediatric pulse oximetry. *Respir Care.* 2003;48:386-396; discussion 397-398.
4. AAP Practice Guideline. Apnea, sudden infant death syndrome and home monitoring. *Pediatrics.* 2003;111(4 Pt 1):914-917.
5. Taussig L. *Pediatric Respiratory Medicine.* 2nd ed. Philadelphia: Mosby, 2008.
6. Blaisdell CJ, Goodman S, Clark K, et al. Pulse oximetry is a poor predictor of hypoxemia in stable children with sickle cell disease. *Arch Pediatr Adolesc Med.* 2000;154:900-903.
7. Schrier RW. *Renal and Electrolyte Disorders.* 7th ed. Philadelphia: Wolters Kluwer/Lippincott Williams & Wilkins, 2010.

8. Brenner BM, ed. *Brenner & Rector's The Kidney*. 8th ed. Philadelphia: Saunders, 2007.

9. Lanbertsten CJ. Transport of oxygen, CO_2, and inert gases by the blood. In: Mountcastle VB, ed. *Medical Physiology*. 14th ed. Mosby: St Louis, 1980.

10. Panitch HB. The pathophysiology of respiratory impairment in pediatric neuro-muscular diseases. *Pediatrics*. 2009;123:S215-S218.

11. Domènech-Clar R, López-Andreu JA, Compte-Torrero L, et al. Maximal static respiratory pressures in children and adolescents. *Pediatr Pulmonol*. 2003;35:126-132.

12. DeWolfe C. Apparent life-threatening event: a review. *Pediatr Clin North Am*. 2005;52:1127-1146.

13. McMillan JA, Feigin RD, DeAngelis CD, et al. *Oski's Pediatrics: Principles and Practice*. 4th ed. Philadelphia: Lippincott Williams and Wilkins, 2006.

14. Fu L, Moon R. Apparent life-threatening events: an update. *Pediatr Rev*. 2012:361-369.

15. NAEPP–Expert Panel Report 3. Guidelines for the Diagnosis and Management of Asthma http://www.nhlbi.nih.gov/guidelines/asthma/asthgdln.htm. August 2007. Accessed 27 July 2009.

16. AAP Clinical Practice Guideline. Diagnosis and management of bronchiolitis. *Pediatrics*. 2006;118:1774-1793.

17. Kair L, Leonard D, Anderson J. Bronchopulmonary dysplasia. *Pediatr in Rev*. 2012; 33(6):255-264.

18. Jobe A, Bancalari E. Bronchopulmonary dysplasia. *Am J Respir Crit Care Med*. 2001;163:1723-1729.

19. Allen J, Zwerdling R, Ehrenkranz R, et al. American Thoracic Society. Statement on the care of the child with chronic lung disease of infancy and childhood. *Am J Respir Crit Care Med*. 2003;168:356-396.

20. Montgomery G, Howenstine M. Cystic fibrosis. *Pediatr Rev*. 2009;30:302-310.

21. Farrell P. Guidelines for diagnosis of cystic fibrosis in newborns through older adults: Cystic Fibrosis Foundation Consensus Report. *J Pediatr*. 2008;153:S4-S14.

22. Flume PA, O'Sullivan BP, Robinson KA, et al. Cystic fibrosis pulmonary guidelines: chronic medicines for maintenance of lung health. *Am J Respir Crit Care Med*. 2007;176:957-969.

23. Marcus CL, Brooks LJ, Draper KA. Diagnosis and management of childhood obstructive sleep apnea syndrome. *Pediatrics*. 2012;130:575-584.

24. AAP Clinical Practice Guideline. Diagnosis and management of childhood obstructive sleep apnea. *Pediatrics*. 2002;109:704-712.

25. Carroll JL. Obstructive sleep-disordered breathing in children: new controversies, new directions. *Clin Chest Med*. 2003;24:261-282.

26. Wagner M, Torrez D. Interpretation of the polysomnogram in children. *Otolaryngol Clin North Am*. 2007;40:745-759.

27. Moon R, Horne R, Hauck F. Sudden infant death syndrome. *Lancet*. 2007;370:1578-1587.

24

Chapter 25

Radiology

Jessica Knight-Perry, MD

I. GENERAL PEDIATRIC PRINCIPLES

The amount of radiation children receive from medical sources is increasing. Considerations unique to the pediatric population are greater radiosensitivity of the thyroid gland, breast tissue, and gonads. Compared to adults, children have a longer lifespan in which to manifest radiation-related cancer. One computed tomography (CT) scan of the chest, for example, is equivalent to about 68 chest x-rays.[1]

A. Employ Judicious Use of CT

Consider ultrasound (US) or magnetic resonance imaging (MRI) whenever possible. If CT is indicated, remember the following to help minimize radiation exposure

1. **To limit exposure,** decrease tube voltage (kVp) and tube current (mA) through the development of child-size protocols.
2. **One scan (single phase) is often enough.**
3. **Scan only the indicated areas** (e.g., do not include pelvis if only abdomen is needed).
4. **Body CT scans without intravenous (IV) contrast are helpful** in delineating fine bony detail, calcifications, and lung parenchyma, but almost nothing else. If your clinical question concerns something other than these areas, and you cannot use IV contrast, then consider ultrasound as a substitute for CT.
5. For further information regarding appropriate use of radiation for the pediatric patient, please refer to www.imagegently.org.

II. HEAD [2]

Most intracranial processes, malformations, and tumors are best imaged with MRI. MRI is useful for neurodegenerative and demyelination disorders, diffuse axonal injury, neurocutaneous syndromes, structural lesions in focal seizure disorders, and vascular lesions. Compared to CT, MRI is more useful in detecting lesions in the posterior fossa.

A. Germinal Matrix Hemorrhage

Premature infants should undergo head US to detect intraventricular hemorrhage and periventricular leukomalacia and to screen for hydrocephalus and congenital abnormalities.

B. Congenital Malformations

Once detected on US, malformations are best further defined with MRI.

C. Congenital Infections

1. **Congenital infections such as herpes simplex virus (HSV) are best imaged with MRI.**

2. **Calcifications consistent with toxoplasmosis and cytomegalovirus (CMV) infection may be best detected with CT.** Calcifications in toxoplasmosis have a predilection for the basal ganglia and tend to be more diffuse than those of CMV, which primarily affects the periventricular region.

D. **Head Trauma**

1. **Best imaged by noncontrast CT to reveal skull fractures and subdural and epidural hematomas.** A head CT should be part of a physical abuse workup.
2. **Skull radiography is of limited value.**
3. **Multiple hemorrhages of various ages are best detected with MRI.**

E. **Ventriculoperitoneal (VP) Shunt Malfunction**

Initial imaging includes head CT to determine ventricle size. If signs of shunt malfunction are noted, radiographs of the length of the shunt (a shunt series) should follow to look for kinks or disconnections.

F. **Craniosynostosis**

Suture examination is best done initially with radiographs of the skull. If there are changes consistent with craniosynostosis, three-dimensional CT reconstructions should be obtained.

III. EYES [4]

A. **Orbital Cellulitis (Fig. 25-1)**

1. **Best imaged with contrast CT with orbital cuts.**
2. **To determine whether an infection is preseptal or postseptal,** a line is drawn from the medial to the lateral bony walls of the orbit on transverse cuts.

IV. SPINE

A. **Cervical Spine Trauma[3,4]**

1. **After immobilization in a collar,** lateral and anteroposterior (AP) radiographs of the cervical spine (C-spine) should be performed in all children who have sustained significant head trauma, deceleration injury, or undergone unwitnessed trauma. The C7 vertebral body and the C7–T1 junction must be visualized. C-spine injuries are most common from the occiput to C3 in children (especially subluxation at the atlanto-occipital joint or atlantoaxial joint in infants and toddlers) and in the lower C-spine in older children and adults.
2. **Flexion-extension films may be helpful,** especially in patients with Down syndrome, who are at risk for atlantoaxial subluxation.
3. **Odontoid views may be helpful in older children with suspected occipito-cervical injury** (e.g., whiplash).

B. **Reading C-spine Films[3,4]**

The following ABCDDS (or ABCDs) mnemonic is useful:

1. **Alignment:** Anterior vertebral body line, posterior vertebral body line, facet line, and spinous process line should each form a continuous line with smooth contour and no step-offs (Fig. 25-2).

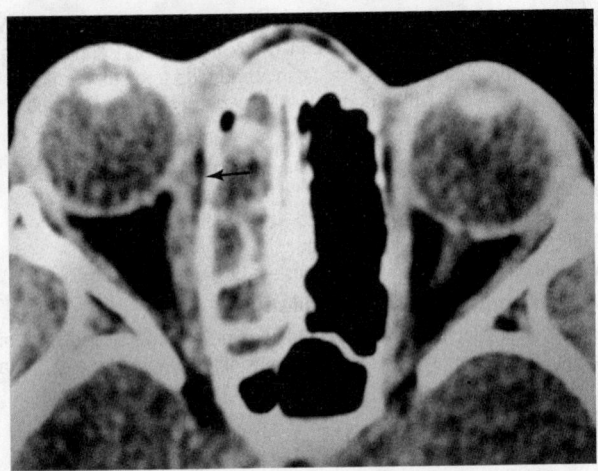

FIGURE 25-1
Orbital cellulitis with subperiosteal abscess. Preseptal and extracoronal portions of the medial right orbit are involved. Medial rectus muscle is slightly thickened and displaced, and a small focal fluid collection *(arrow)* representing a subperiosteal abscess is present. *(From Slovis TL. Caffey's Pediatric Diagnostic Imaging. 11th ed. Philadelphia: Mosby, 2008. Courtesy Kenneth D. Hopper, MD, Hershey, Pa.)*

2. **Bones:** Assess each bone looking for chips or fractures.
3. **Count:** Must see C7 body in its entirety.
4. **Dens:** Examine for chips or fractures.
5. **Disk spaces:** Should see consistent distance between each vertebral body.
6. **Soft tissue:** Assess for swelling, particularly in prevertebral area.

C. **Spinal Cord Injury without Radiographic Abnormality (SCIWORA)**[4,5]

1. **Definition:** A functional C-spine injury that cannot be excluded by abnormality on a radiograph; thought to be attributable to the increased mobility of a child's spine.
2. **Should be suspected in the setting of normal C-spine images when** clinical signs or symptoms (e.g., point tenderness, focal neurologic symptoms) suggest C-spine injury.
3. **If neurologic symptoms persist despite normal C-spine and flexion-extension views,** MRI is indicated to rule out swelling, contusion, or intramedullary hemorrhage of the cord.

D. **Spinal Dysraphism (e.g., myelocele, myelomeningocele)**

Initial imaging: Radiographs. Most often screened for with US. Abnormalities are followed by MRI.

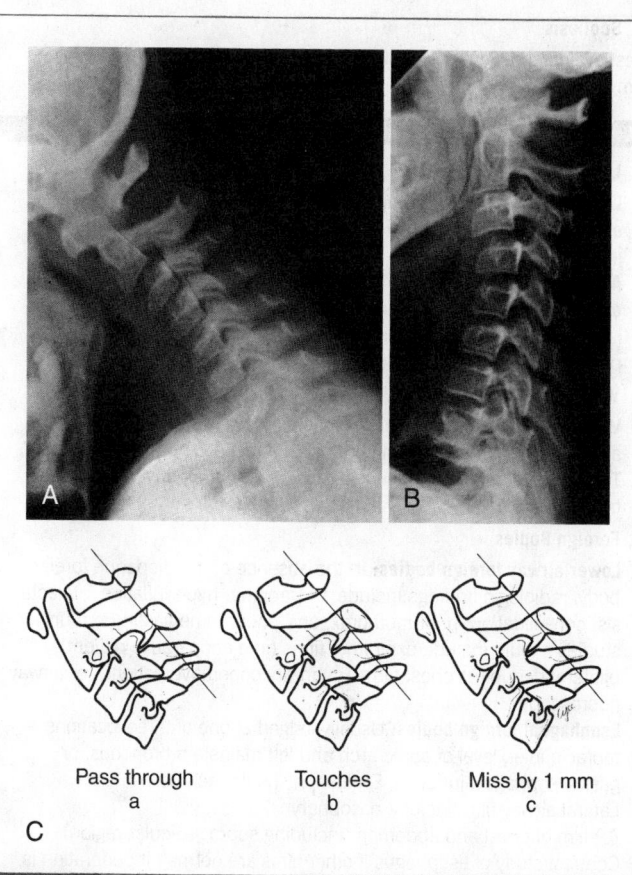

FIGURE 25-2

Normal cervical spine mobility in children. **A,** Normal forward shift of C2 on C3 in an asymptomatic 3-year-old girl. **B,** Normal forward shift of C3 on C4 (pseudosubluxation) in an asymptomatic 5-year-old girl. **C,** Normal limits of the posterior cervical line. Normal posterior cervical line can pass through or just behind the anterior cortex of C2 (*a*), touch the anterior cortex of C2 (*b*), or come within 1 mm of the anterior aspect of C2 (*c*). (*A and B from Sullivan CR, Bruwer AJ, Harris LE. Hypermobility of the cervical spine in children: a pitfall in the diagnosis of cervical dislocation. Am J Surg. 1958;95:636-640; C from Kuhns LR. Imaging of Spinal Trauma in Children: An Atlas and Text. Hamilton Ontario: BC Decker, 1998:31.*)

E. Scoliosis

Best evaluated by erect AP spine radiograph. Posteroanterior (PA) views can be used in postpubertal girls to decrease breast radiation dose.

V. AIRWAY [3]

A. Lateral Radiograph

1. **Lateral radiograph of the upper airway is the most useful film for evaluating a child with stridor.** If possible, should be obtained on inspiration.
2. **A radiologic workup should always include AP and lateral radiographs of the chest,** with inclusion of upper airway on the AP view. Diagnosis is based on airway radiologic examination in conjunction with clinical presentation (Table 25-1, Figs. 25-3 and 25-4).

B. Vascular Rings

1. **Vascular rings and other masses** that extrinsically obstruct the lower airways can be imaged with contrast-enhanced CT or MRI.
2. **Tracheomalacia and intrinsic masses** can be studied with bronchoscopy.

C. Foreign Bodies

1. **Lower airway foreign bodies:** In the absence of a radiopaque foreign body, radiologic findings include air trapping, hyperinflation, atelectasis, consolidation, pneumothorax, and pneumomediastinum. Further studies should include expiratory films (in a cooperative patient), bilateral decubitus chest films (in an uncooperative patient), or airway fluoroscopy.
2. **Esophageal foreign bodies:** Usually lodged at one of three locations—thoracic inlet, level of aortic arch and left mainstem bronchus, or gastroesophageal junction. Evaluation should include:
a. Lateral airway film (include nasopharynx)
b. AP film of chest and abdomen (including supraclavicular region)
c. Contrast study of esophagus if other films are normal. If perforation is suspected, use nonionic water-soluble contrast.

TABLE 25-1

DIAGNOSIS OF DISEASES BASED ON AIRWAY RADIOLOGIC EXAMINATION

Diagnosis	Findings on Airway Films
Croup	AP and lateral films with subglottic narrowing (*steeple sign*)
Epiglottitis	Enlarged, indistinct epiglottis on lateral film (*thumbprint sign*)
Vascular ring	AP and lateral films with narrowing; double or right aortic arch
Retropharyngeal abscess or pharyngeal mass	Soft tissue air or persistent enlargement of prevertebral soft tissues; more than half of a vertebral body above C3 and one vertebral body below C3
Immunodeficiency	Absence of adenoidal and tonsillar tissue after age 6 mo

AP, Anteroposterior.

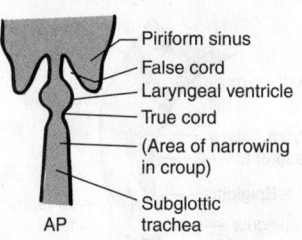

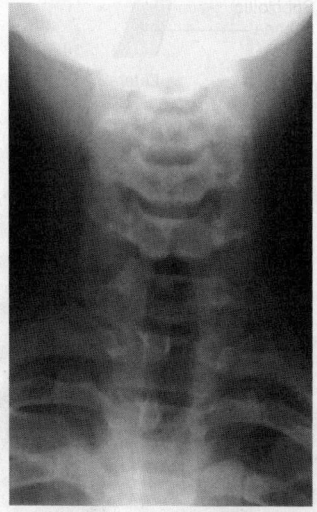

FIGURE 25-3

Anteroposterior (AP) neck film with normal anatomy on AP airway view.

VI. CHEST[3,4]

A. Posteroanterior and Lateral Radiographs

First images obtained when studying the chest (Figs. 25-5 and 25-6).

B. Pneumonia

1. **Lobar or segmental consolidation:** More typical of bacterial infections
2. **Hyperinflation, bilateral patchy or streaky densities, and peribronchial thickening:** More typical of nonbacterial disease

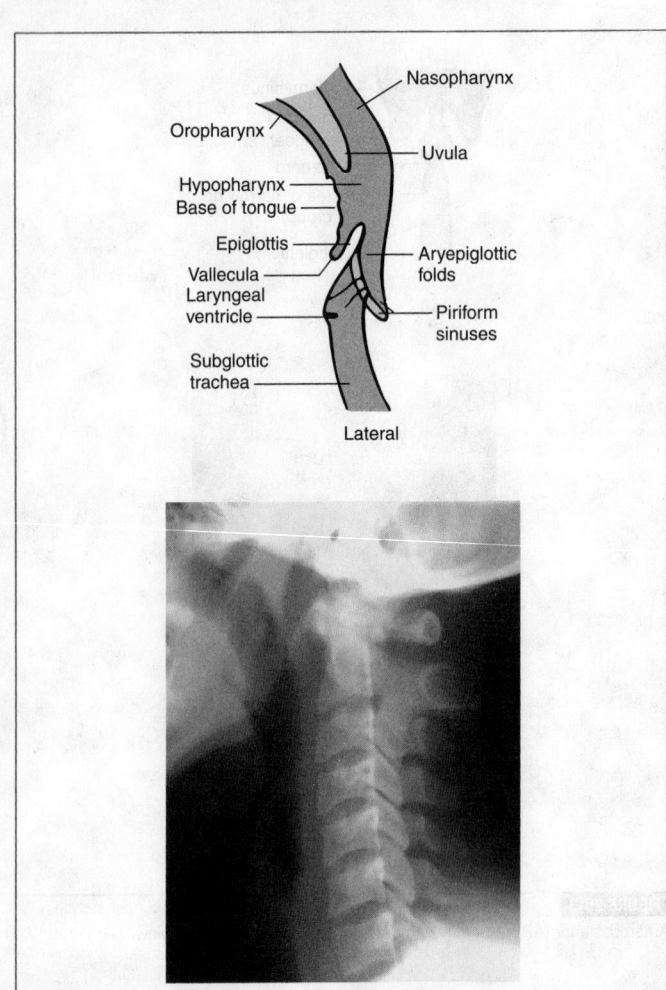

FIGURE 25-4
Lateral neck film with normal anatomy on lateral airway view.

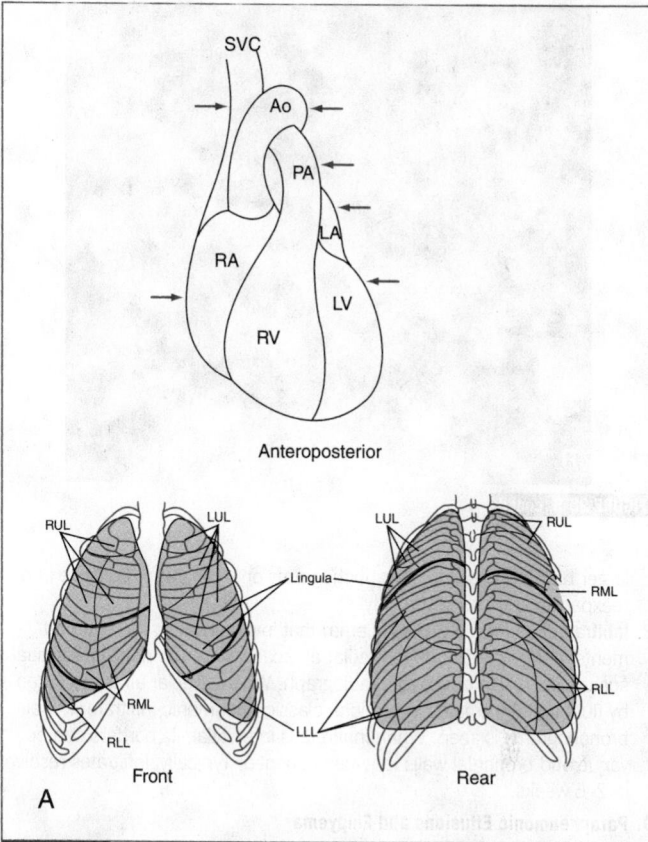

25

FIGURE 25-5

A, Normal lung and cardiac anatomy as seen on an anteroposterior chest radiograph. Arrows indicate contours seen on anteroposterior chest x-ray films **(B).** Ao, Aorta; LA, left atrium; LLL, left lower lobe; LUL, left upper lobe; LV, left ventricle; PA, pulmonary artery; RA, right atrium; RLL, right lower lobe; RML, right middle lobe; RUL, right upper lobe; RV, right ventricle; SVC, superior vena cava. *(Heart diagram modified from Kirks DR, Griscom NT.* Practical Pediatric Imaging: Diagnostic Radiology of Infants and Children. *3rd ed. Philadelphia: LIppincott-Raven, 1998.)*

Continued

C. Atelectasis vs. Infiltrate

1. **Atelectasis:** When air is removed from the lung, tissue collapses, resulting in volume loss on chest radiographs. If severe enough, mediastinum and/or diaphragm are pulled toward the lesion. Air may still remain in

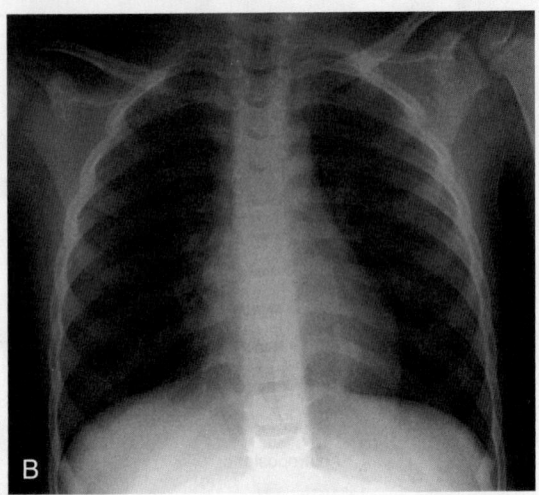

FIGURE 25-5, cont'd

larger bronchi, creating air bronchograms on radiograph. Collapse and reexpansion can occur quickly.
2. **Infiltrate:** Fluid (blood, pus, edema) that invades one of the compartments of the lung (bronchoalveolar air space or peribronchial interstitial space), seen as a density on radiograph. When alveolar air is displaced by fluid but air remains in bronchi, classic pneumonic infiltrate with air bronchograms is seen. When infiltrate is interstitial, its borders can be vague and bronchial walls may be thickened. Typically, infiltrates resolve in 2–6 weeks.

D. **Parapneumonic Effusions and Empyema**

Initially, PA and lateral radiographs are obtained. Lateral decubitus radiographs may also be helpful. Ultrasound is often the best modality for early identification of loculation, but a contrast-enhanced CT may be necessary to further delineate loculation or differentiate between pleural fluid and collapsed or consolidated tissue.

E. **Parenchymal Findings**
1. **Lung abscess, cavitary necrosis, lung contusions:** Best imaged with contrast-enhanced CT.
2. **Pneumatocele, fungal infections, interstitial lung disease:** Use non-contrast CT.

F. **Mediastinal Masses**

Mediastinal masses (thymus, lymphoma, bronchogenic cyst, neuroblastoma, neurofibroma) are initially imaged with plain films, followed by contrast-enhanced CT or MRI.

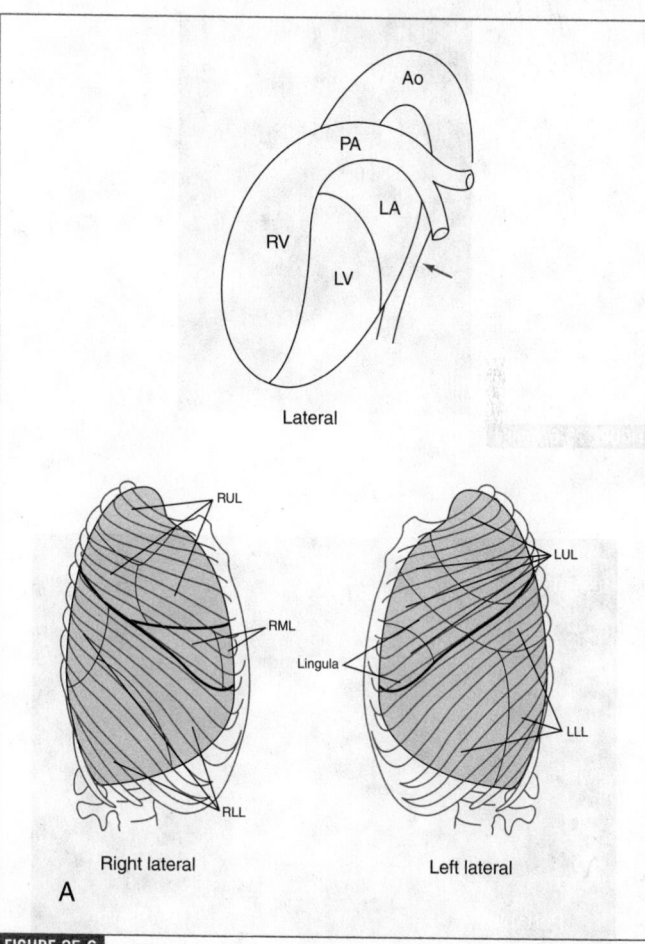

FIGURE 25-6

A, Normal lung and cardiac anatomy as seen on lateral chest radiograph. Arrow indicates contours seen on lateral chest x-ray films **(B)**. Ao, Aorta; LA, left atrium; LLL, left lower lobe; LUL, left upper lobe; LV, left ventricle; PA, pulmonary artery; RLL, right lower lobe; RML, right middle lobe; RUL, right upper lobe; RV, right ventricle. *(Heart diagram modified from Kirks DR, Griscom NT. Practical Pediatric Imaging: Diagnostic Radiology of Infants and Children. 3rd ed. Philadelphia: LIppincott-Raven, 1998.)*

Continued

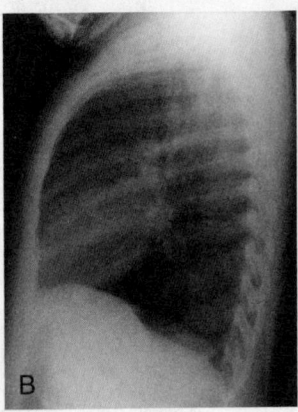

FIGURE 25-6, cont'd

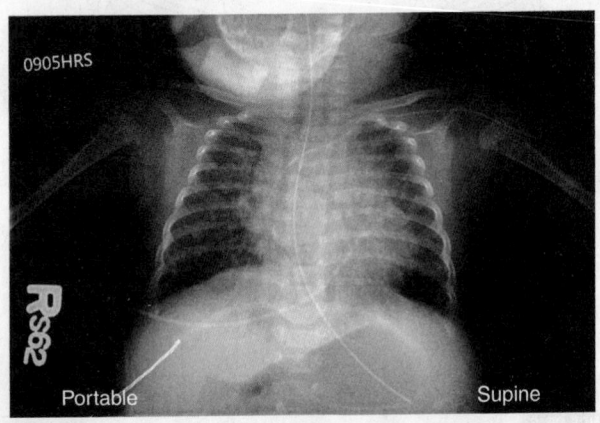

FIGURE 25-7

Central line placement on anteroposterior chest radiograph for line inserted in arm or neck.

G. Central Line Placement

On chest radiograph, central venous catheters entering from the neck or arm are ideally placed with catheter tip at junction of superior vena cava and right atrium. Some extension into right atrium is acceptable, but if catheter is noted to curve to patient's left on PA film, catheter may be positioned in right ventricle (Fig. 25-7). Catheters inserted below diaphragm should be placed with tip at level of diaphragm (Fig. 25-8).

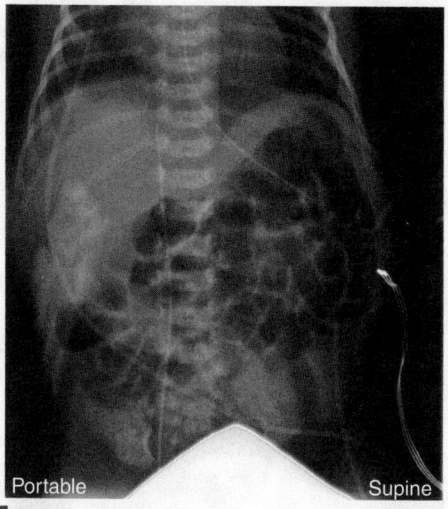

Portable   Supine

FIGURE 25-8

Central line placement on anteroposterior radiograph for line inserted below the diaphragm.

H. Endotracheal Tube (ETT) Placement

On chest radiograph, end of the ETT should rest about midway between thoracic inlet and carina. Lung fields should show symmetric aeration.

VII. HEART AND VESSELS [3]

A. Congenital Heart Disease

Most clearly defined by echocardiography, but initial PA and lateral chest radiograph may yield important clues:

1. **Position of aortic arch:** Left or right (Fig. 25-9)
2. **Situs:** Noting position of apex, stomach bubble, and liver
3. **Heart size:** With particular attention paid to lateral chest radiograph
4. **Pulmonary vascularity:** Increased or decreased flow in arteries and veins

B. Vessels

1. **Moving blood is detected by ultrasonographic frequency shifts.**
2. **Color Doppler flow imaging:** Can be used to evaluate deep vein thrombosis (DVT), vascular patency, intracranial blood flow (including transcranial Doppler [TCD] to screen for ischemic brain injury risk in sickle cell disease), cardiac shunt flow, transplant vascularity, veno-occlusive disease of the liver, and testicular perfusion in testicular torsion.
3. **Power Doppler** is particularly sensitive in detecting slow flow in small vessels (e.g., infant testes).

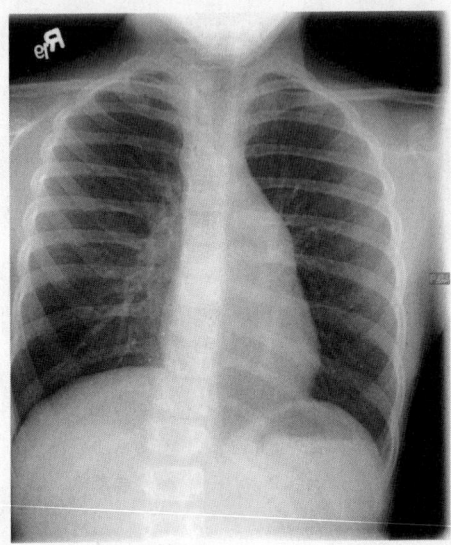

FIGURE 25-9
Right aortic arch as seen on anteroposterior chest radiograph.

C. Vessel Abnormalities

Can be studied with echocardiography/US, CT, and MRI. Use these modalities to detect coarctation of the aorta, aortic stenosis, pulmonary artery and vein abnormalities, vascular rings, arteriovenous malformations (AVMs), hemangiomas, aneurysms, and postoperative complications like thrombosis and stenosis.

VIII. ABDOMEN[3-5]

A. Neonatal Enterocolitis

Clinically diagnosed and followed by abdominal radiographs, which may show focal dilation, featureless loops, pneumatosis, and portal venous gas.

B. Esophageal Atresia and Tracheoesophageal Fistula (Fig. 25-10)

Studied initially with chest radiographs, which may reveal the air-distended esophageal atretic pouch, nasogastric tube curled up in this pouch, or excessive dilation of stomach as a result of fistula communication.

C. High Intestinal Obstruction

1. **Diagnosed with upper gastrointestinal (UGI) series:** Contrast is ingested, and esophagus, stomach, and duodenum are visualized.
   Causes: Esophageal webs and rings, masses, duodenal atresia or webs (Fig. 25-11), annular pancreas, midgut volvulus, and Ladd bands.

25

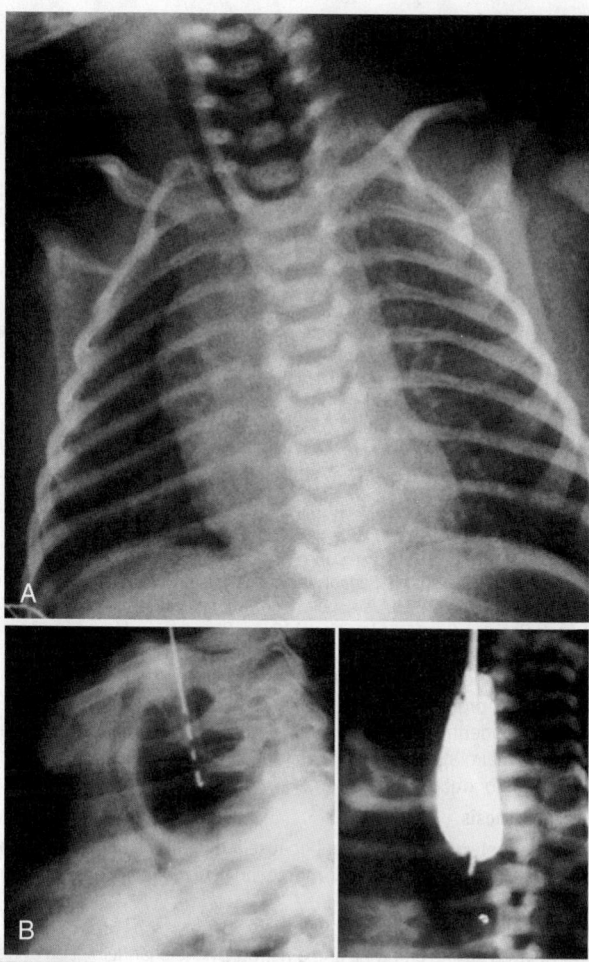

FIGURE 25-10

Esophageal atresia and tracheoesophageal fistula. **A,** Frontal chest examination reveals lucency over cervical and upper thoracic spine (blind-ending esophageal pouch filled with air) and air within stomach, typical for esophageal atresia with tracheoesophageal fistula. **B,** Tube has been placed in blind-ending pouch, and contrast material injected on subsequent film. Airway is bowed forward and in varying degrees of collapse on these two images. *(From Slovis TL.* Caffey's Pediatric Diagnostic Imaging. *11th ed. Philadelphia: Mosby, 2008.)*

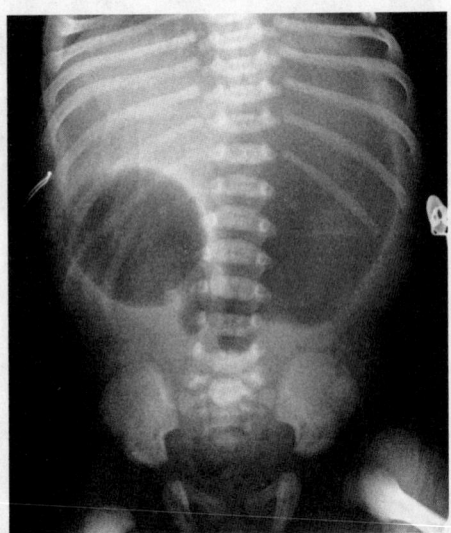

FIGURE 25-11
Newborn with duodenal atresia. Portable abdominal radiograph shows dilated stomach and proximal duodenum ("double-bubble" sign), with absent distal gas. *(From Slovis TL. Caffey's Pediatric Diagnostic Imaging. 11th ed. Philadelphia: Mosby, 2008.)*

2. **UGI** can also help evaluate hiatal hernias, varices, gastric outlet obstruction, motility problems, ulcerations, and reflux.
3. **During UGI,** identifying duodenojejunal junction (ligament of Treitz) helps diagnose malrotation. Normally the junction is to the left of spine, at or above level of duodenal bulb.

D. Pyloric Stenosis

1. **US is the preferred examination** because it directly visualizes the pyloric muscle. Normal pylorus is <17 mm in length, and its muscular wall is <4 mm in width (Fig. 25-12).
2. **Radiographs:** Show gastric distention.
3. **UGI:** Delayed gastric emptying and a narrow pyloric channel will be evident.

E. Bowel Obstruction

1. **Determination of large or small bowel obstruction:** Often aided by supine radiograph, prone radiograph, and either upright, supine cross-table lateral, or left lateral decubitus film to look for free air and air-fluid levels. Causes of obstruction: Adhesions, appendicitis, incarcerated inguinal hernias, Meckel diverticulum, intussusception.
2. **US can be helpful** in thin patients and female patients who have ovarian pathology in their differential for abdominal pain.
3. **CT with intravenous, oral, or rectal contrast is more useful** with an obese patient or when looking for perforated appendicitis or abscess.

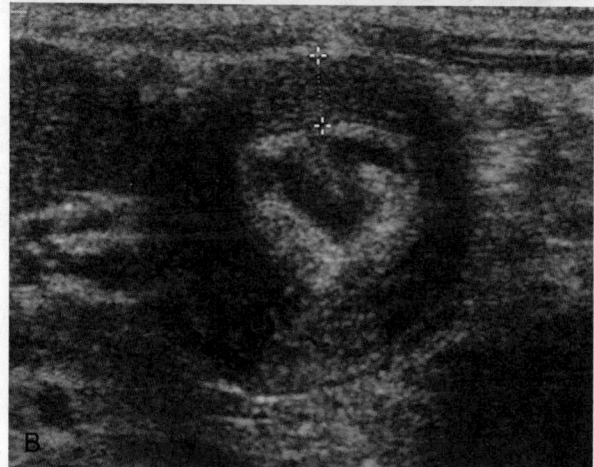

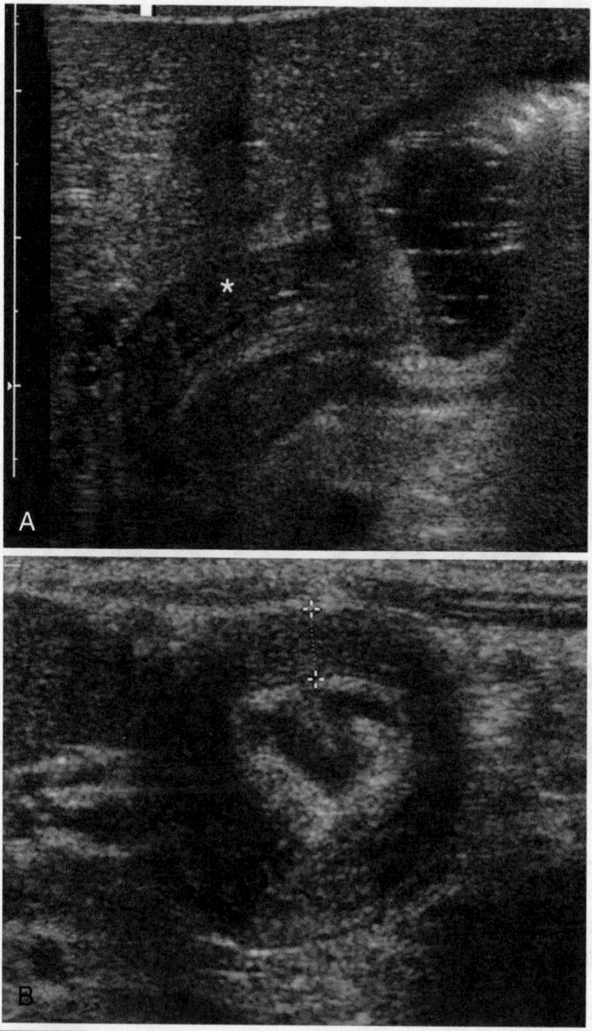

25

FIGURE 25-12

Abdominal ultrasound for diagnosis of hypertrophic pyloric stenosis. **A,** Ten minutes after dextrose solution was given, pyloric muscle *(asterisk)* was better seen, and canal length was easier to evaluate. **B,** "Doughnut" sign of hypertrophic pyloric stenosis in infant imaged in **A**. Fixed circumferential thickening of pylorus may resemble a dough-nut in image taken perpendicular to long axis of stomach. Calipers mark the anterior muscle, which measures more than 3 mm. Thickened mucosa is seen centrally. Note that echogenicity of the muscle perpendicular to ultrasound beam in near field and far field is greater than that seen in lateral aspects of thickened pyloric muscle. *(From Slovis TL. Caffey's Pediatric Diagnostic Imaging. 11th ed. Philadelphia: Mosby, 2008.)*

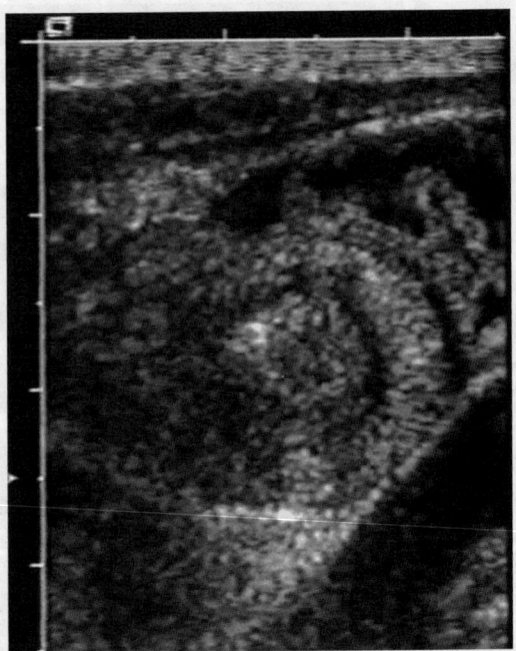

FIGURE 25-13

Abdominal ultrasound shows short segment intussusception. Longitudinal ultrasound image along right flank of an infant with proven viral gastroenteritis shows short-segment intussusception that occurred during the examination. Visible peristaltic activity of the intussusceptum within the intussuscipiens was visible in real time. Intussusception resolved spontaneously. *(From Slovis TL.* Caffey's Pediatric Diagnostic Imaging. *11th ed. Philadelphia: Mosby, 2008.)*

4. **Contrast enemas with dilute water-soluble agents** can also be useful in lower intestinal obstruction in the newborn.

F. **Intussusception**

1. **On abdominal radiographs,** particularly prone view, findings include minimal gas in right abdomen and ascending colon.
2. **US will show alternating rings.** Doppler will show flow in the intussuscepted mesentery, which will allow confirmation of the diagnosis as well as assessment of viability of the intussusceptum (Fig. 25-13).
3. **For fluoroscopy-guided therapeutic enema,** air insufflation is preferred, but other contrast agents may also be used. Reducing an intussusception with air or contrast is contraindicated if perforation is suspected.

G. **Meckel Diverticulum**

Suggested by painless lower GI bleeding; diagnosed by nuclear scintigraphy using technetium-99m (^{99m}Tc)-pertechnetate.

H. Abdominal Trauma

CT of abdomen and pelvis to detect solid organ injury, vascular extravasation, free fluid, bowel wall thickening, and organ laceration.

I. Biliary Atresia

1. **In neonates with jaundice,** US initially to distinguish biliary atresia from hepatitis. Gallbladder will be small or absent with biliary atresia.
2. **Hepatobiliary scintigraphy with** ^{99m}**Tc-iminodiacetate (HIDA) reveals** absence of radionuclide in GI tract, with biliary atresia.

J. Nasoduodenal (ND) Tube Placement

Visualize tube on a plain abdominal AP film passing through stomach, crossing midline, and passing into duodenal bulb (where tip of tube will just begin to point inferiorly). If it remains unclear whether tube is in duodenum or coiled in stomach, a lateral film is indicated (a properly placed ND tube tip will lie posterior, near the spine).

IX. GENITOURINARY TRACT [3]

A. Urinary Tract Infection (UTI)

1. **Initial febrile UTIs in children <5 years** require imaging to look for congenital anomalies (e.g., posterior urethral valves, ureterocele), vesicoureteral reflux, baseline renal measurements, and damage to kidney cortices.
2. **Workup first includes US to diagnose** hydronephrosis, ureteropelvic junction obstruction, posterior urethral valves, multicystic dysplastic kidneys, chronic pyelonephritis, renal fusion (horseshoe kidney), and renal cysts.
3. **If clinically indicated,** voiding cystourethrogram (VCUG) can be performed to diagnose vesicoureteral reflux, abnormalities of bladder or urethral function and anatomy (including ureterocele), and posterior urethral valves.
4. **Occasionally, dimercaptosuccinic acid (DMSA) scan** is useful in following renal cortical scarring and pyelonephritis.

B. Uterine and Ovarian Pathology

Transvaginal or transabdominal US should be performed if the clinical picture is suspicious for ovarian torsion, tubo-ovarian abscess (TOA), or ectopic pregnancy.

X. EXTREMITIES [3,5]

A. Trauma

1. **Adequate evaluation requires AP and lateral radiographs.** Restricting the film to include only the area of interest improves resolution (e.g., for a thumb injury, ask for an image of the thumb, not the hand).
2. **Comparison films of the uninvolved extremity are not necessary but may be helpful,** such as in evaluation of joint effusions (particularly hip), suspected osteomyelitis, or pyarthrosis and/or evaluation of subtle fractures, especially in areas of multiple ossification centers such as the elbow.

3. **Salter-Harris classification of growth-plate injury** (Table 25-2).

4. **Avulsion injuries tend to occur at the knee and pelvis.**

B. Stress Fractures

1. **Occur most often at the tibia, fibula, metatarsals, and calcaneus.**

2. **Radiography will show a band of sclerosis and new bone formation.**

3. **Skeletal scintigraphy is a sensitive method for making the diagnosis.**

C. Osteomyelitis

1. **Tends to occur at metaphysis of long bones and within flat bones.**

2. **Radiography will show deep soft-tissue swelling and bony changes** (may take 10 days to appear).

3. **Skeletal scintigraphy and MRI** will often be positive before radiographic changes are noticeable.

D. Hip Disorders

1. **Developmental hip dysplasia** (congenital hip dislocation) is imaged initially with US. Once femoral heads ossify, radiographs are more helpful (Fig. 25-14).

2. **Legg-Calvé-Perthes disease** (avascular necrosis of femoral head) can be imaged with AP and frog-leg lateral hip films as well as MRI and bone scintigraphy (Fig. 25-15).

3. **Slipped capital femoral epiphysis** (SCFE) will show femoral head displacementon frog-leg lateral and AP radiographs (Fig. 25-16).

E. Bone Lesions

1. **Osteochondroma:** Benign lesion that arises from the metaphysis of a long bone, most frequently the distal femur, proximal humerus, and proximal tibia. Composed of cortical and medullary bone with a cap of hyaline cartilage and is continous with the cortex and intramedullary cavity of the involved bone (Fig. 25-17).

2. **Unicameral bone cyst:** Benign lesion that appears on radiographs as a solitary, centrally located, lucent lesion located within the medullary portion of the bone and often extends to the physis. Tend to occur in the proximal femur or humerus (Fig. 25-18).

3. **Fibroma:** Benign lesion that appears on radiographs as a lucency in the metaphyseal cortex, highlighted by a sclerotic, often scalloped border (Fig. 25-19).

4. **Osteoma:** Benign lesion that appears on radiographs as a small, oval lucency in the metaphysis or diaphysis. Most frequently occurs in the proximal femur and tibia, although any bone can be involved, including vertebrae. Often present with gradually increasing pain that is worse at night (Fig. 25-20).

5. **Osteosarcoma:** Most common primary malignant bone tumor in children and adolescents >10 years of age. Lesion typically occurs at the metaphyses of long bones, and radiographs demonstrate sclerotic deconstruction, although sometimes lytic, with a classic sunburst pattern (Fig. 25-21).

TABLE 25-2

SALTER-HARRIS CLASSIFICATION OF GROWTH PLATE INJURY

Class I	Class II	Class III	Class IV	Class V
Fracture along growth plate	Fracture along growth plate with metaphyseal extension	Fracture along growth plate with epiphyseal extension	Fracture across growth plate, including metaphysis and epiphysis	Crush injury to growth plate without obvious fracture
I	II	III	IV	V

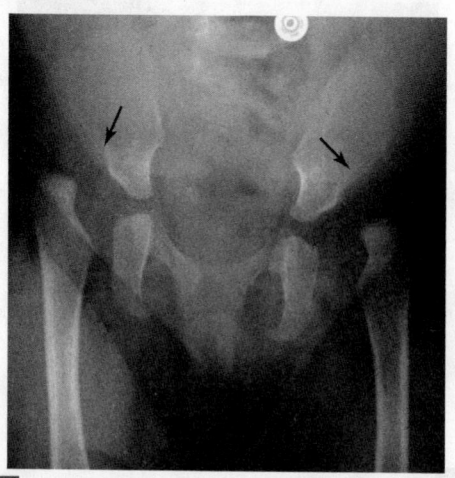

FIGURE 25-14

Neutral anteroposterior (AP) view of a 3-month-old girl shows bilateral shallow acetabula, dislocated hips, and early pseudoacetabulum formation *(arrows)*. (From Slovis TL. Caffey's Pediatric Diagnostic Imaging. *11th ed. Philadelphia: Mosby, 2008.*)

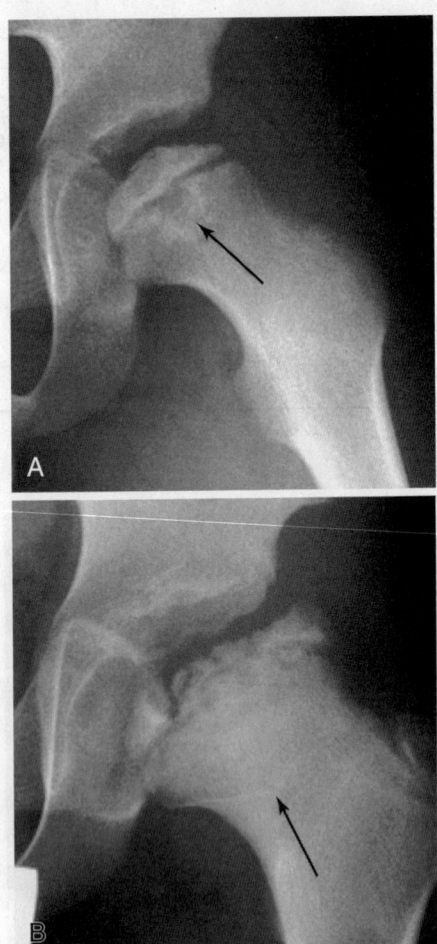

FIGURE 25-15

A 7-year-old boy with a limp and osteonecrosis of left proximal femoral epiphysis. **A,** Radiograph of left hip reveals a small, sclerotic proximal femoral epiphysis with an irregular joint surface. Metaphysis of proximal femur also shows cystic changes *(arrow)* that indicate a poor prognosis. **B,** At 18 months after presentation, radiograph of left hip reveals further fragmentation and continued lateral extrusion of epiphysis. Acetabulum is beginning to impinge on uncovered portion of lateral column, and incongruence of hip joint is apparent. The "sagging rope" sign *(arrow)*, produced by the outline of an abnormally oriented physis, indicates growth arrest. Widening of femoral neck is seen ("coxa magna"). *(From Slovis TL. Caffey's Pediatric Diagnostic Imaging. 11th ed. Philadelphia: Mosby, 2008.)*

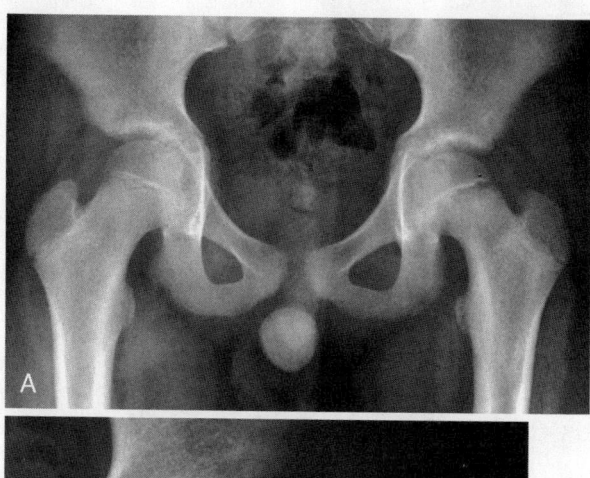

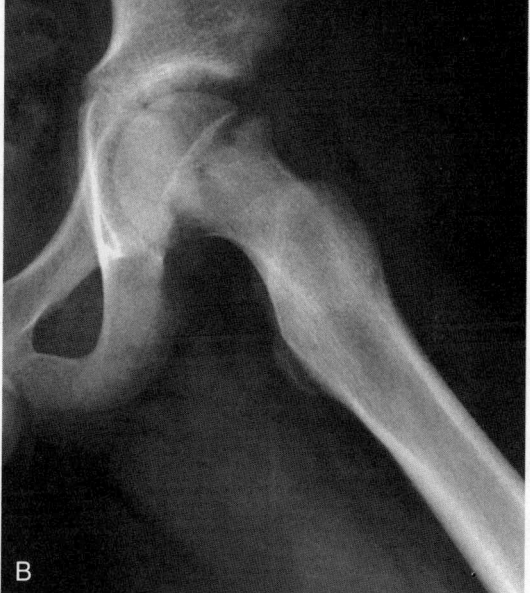

FIGURE 25-16

Slipped capital femoral epiphysis in 11-year-old boy with left hip pain. **A,** On anteroposterior view, growth plate of left proximal femur is wide and indistinct. No portion of left femoral head projects lateral to Klein line. Right proximal femur is normal. **B,** On lateral view, malalignment of femoral head and neck at growth plate is better seen. Femoral head is displaced posteromedially relative to femoral neck but is still in continuity. *(From Slovis TL. Caffey's Pediatric Diagnostic Imaging. 11th ed. Philadelphia: Mosby, 2008.)*

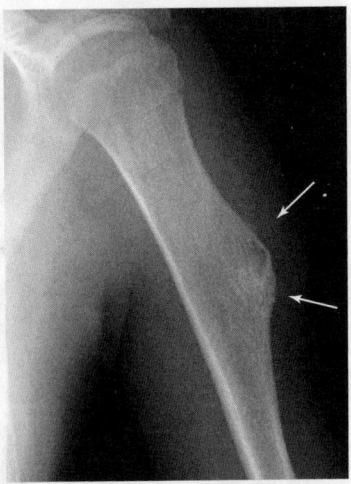

FIGURE 25-17

Sessile osteochondroma *(arrows)* of proximal humeral diaphysis in a 16-year-old girl. *(From Slovis TL. Caffey's Pediatric Diagnostic Imaging. 11th ed. Philadelphia: Mosby, 2008.)*

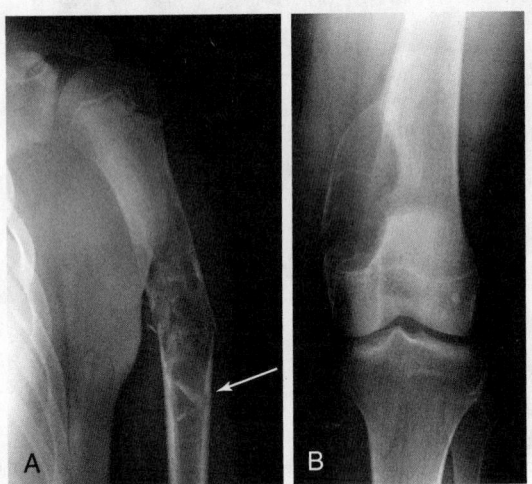

FIGURE 25-18

A, Simple bone cyst with pathologic fracture in a 12-year-old boy. Cyst has thinned and scalloped overlying cortex. A fallen fragment is noted *(arrow).* **B,** Aneurysmal bone cyst in a 13-year-old. Radiograph of knee shows an eccentric, expansile lucent lesion with a thin, bony shell involving medial aspect of distal femur. *(From Slovis TL. Caffey's Pediatric Diagnostic Imaging. 11th ed. Philadelphia: Mosby, 2008.)*

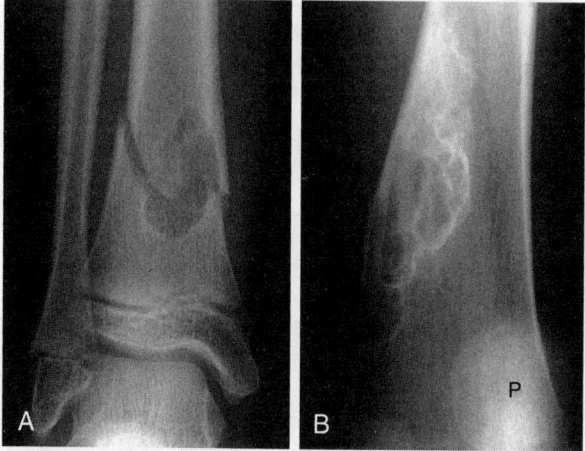

FIGURE 25-19

A, Pathologic fracture through a nonossifying fibroma in a 10-year-old boy. Lesion has well-defined, minimally sclerotic margins. **B,** Large, lobulated nonossifying fibroma in a 16-year-old boy; anteroposterior view of distal femur. Proximal portion of lesion is sclerotic, consistent with early involution. P, Patella. *(From Slovis TL. Caffey's Pediatric Diagnostic Imaging. 11th ed. Philadelphia: Mosby, 2008.)*

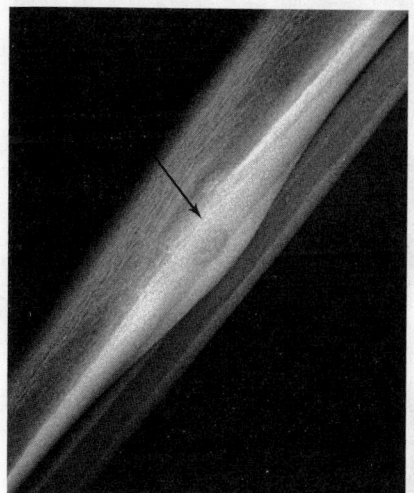

FIGURE 25-20

Osteoid osteoma of tibia in a 15-year-old girl. Radiograph shows cortical thickening posteriorly. Lucent nidus is faintly seen *(arrow)*. *(From Slovis TL. Caffey's Pediatric Diagnostic Imaging. 11th ed. Philadelphia: Mosby, 2008.)*

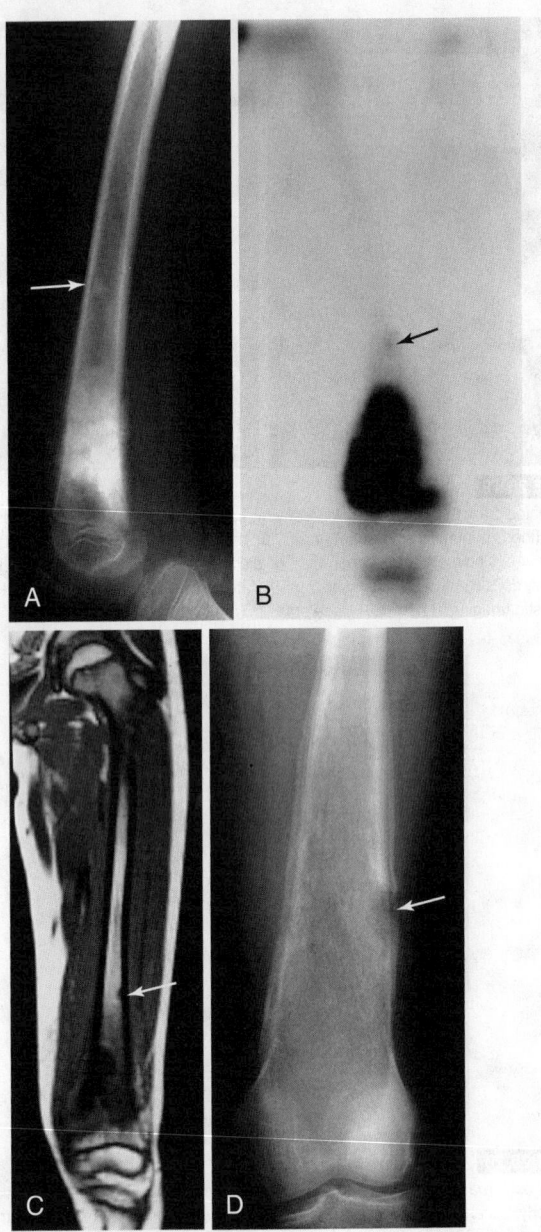

FIGURE 25-21

A, Lateral radiograph of femur of a 9-year-old boy with osteosarcoma shows a sclerotic intramedullary distal femoral tumor with slight periosteal new bone formation. A small, dense skip metastasis *(arrow)* is seen proximal to primary tumor of main tumor mass. Skip metastasis *(arrow)* is also seen on a technetium-99m methylene diphosphonate bone scan **(B)** and is shown as a cortical-based intramedullary lesion *(arrow)* on a coronal T1-weighted magnetic resonance image **(C). D,** Radiograph of femur of a 16-year-old boy with telangiectatic osteosarcoma shows large lesion in distal meta-diaphysis extending into epiphysis. Tumor is lytic rather than bone forming. There is mild periosteal reaction. There has been a recent incisional biopsy *(arrow)*. *(From Slovis TL.* Caffey's Pediatric Diagnostic Imaging. *11th ed. Philadelphia: Mosby, 2008.)*

6. **Ewing sarcoma:** Second most common primary malignant bone tumor in children and adolecents >10 years of age; most common primary malignant bone tumor in children <age 10. Lesion is typically in the diaphyses of long and flat bones, and radiographs demonstrate a lytic lesion with periosteal reaction, creating a classic lamellar "onion-skinning" appearance. CT or MRI of lesion may demonstrate a soft-tissue mass (Fig. 25-22).

F. **Bone Age**

Obtain a PA view of the left hand and wrist.

G. **Skeletal Survey**

1. **In cases of suspected child abuse,** should include lateral skull film with C-spine film, AP chest film (bone technique), oblique views of ribs, AP view of pelvis, abdominal film (bone technique) with lateral thoracic and lumbar spine, and AP long-bone films.

2. **Classic findings:** Multiple metaphyseal injuries (especially corner and bucket-handle fractures) and other fractures of various ages (Fig. 25-23). Suspicion should also be raised by fracture at unusual sites, such as posterior rib fractures or solitary spiral and transverse long-bone fractures with an inconsistent history of trauma (Fig. 25-24).

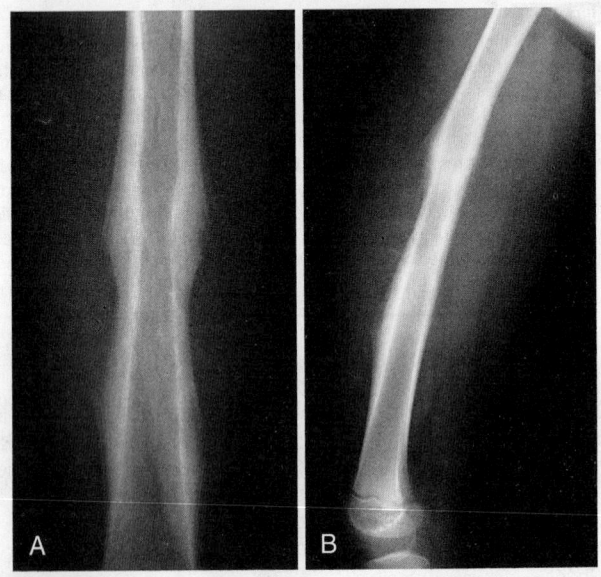

FIGURE 25-22

Anteroposterior **(A)** and lateral **(B)** radiographs of femur of a 6-year-old girl show a Ewing sarcoma arising from mid-diaphysis. Lamellar periosteal reaction and new bone formation are present, with Codman triangles at proximal and distal ends of tumor. Faint periosteal new bone extends perpendicularly into soft-tissue component of tumor. Medulla is not expanded. *(From Slovis TL.* Caffey's Pediatric Diagnostic Imaging. *11th ed. Philadelphia: Mosby, 2008.)*

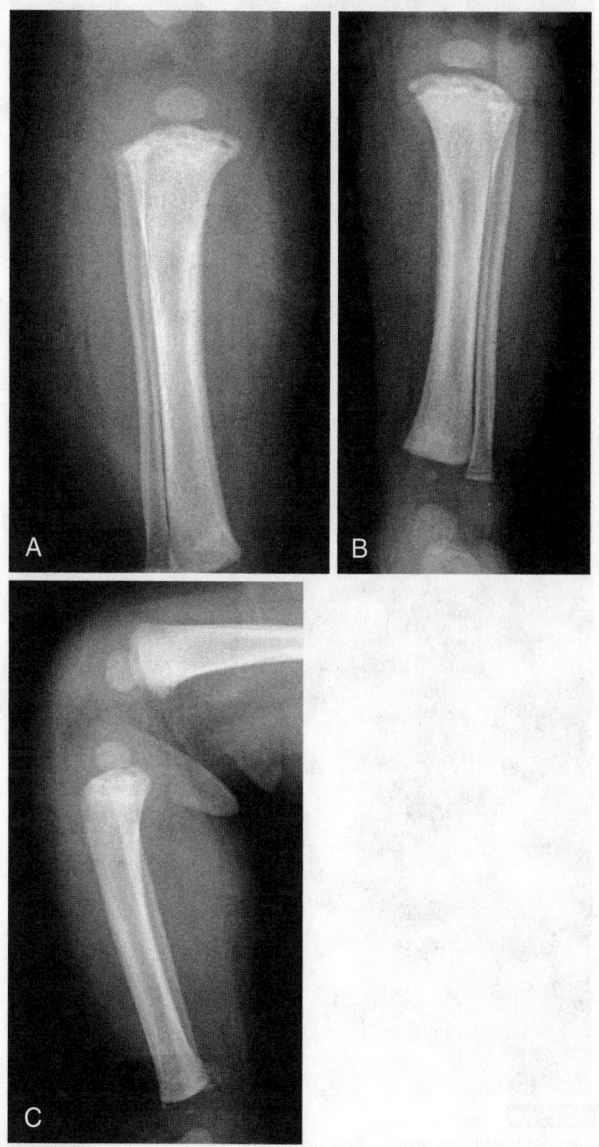

FIGURE 25-23

Anteroposterior right **(A)** and left **(B)** lower leg and lateral right **(C)** lower leg of 3-month-old male infant transferred with acute occipital skull fracture, classic metaphyseal lesions of distal femora and proximal and distal tibias, and 23 rib fractures. *(From Slovis TL. Caffey's Pediatric Diagnostic Imaging. 11th ed. Philadelphia: Mosby, 2008.)*

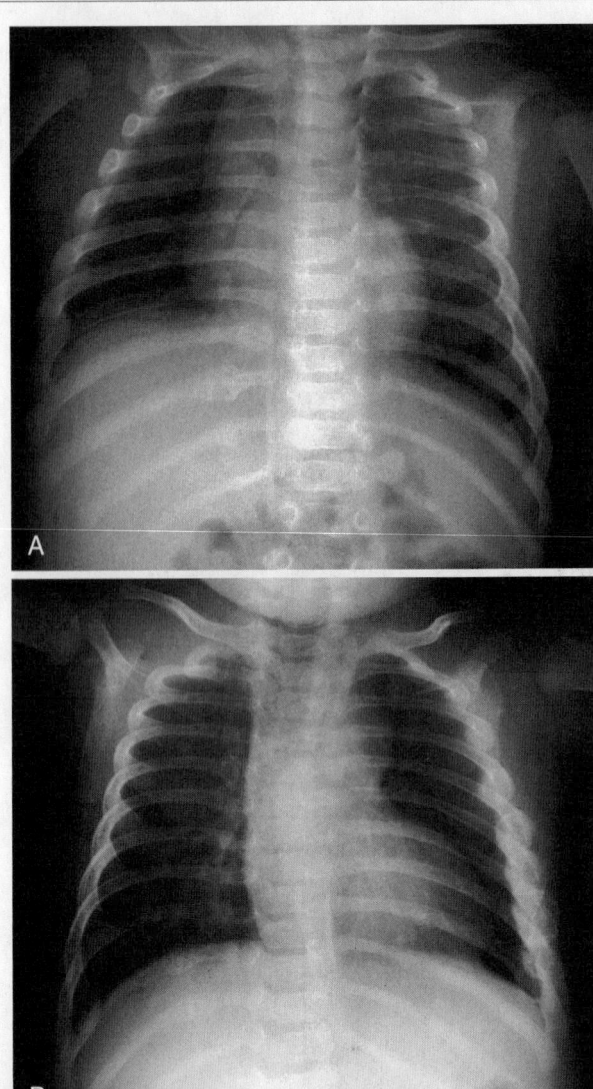

A 6-week-old male infant sent for an upper gastrointestinal series for evaluation of colicky pain was found to have healing rib fractures. **A,** Initial chest x-ray identifies healing fractures at the right 9th, 10th, and 11th ribs. **B,** Follow-up chest film 2 weeks later shows additional fractures, now healing, at lateral aspect of left 3rd through 9th ribs. Father admitted to shaking the infant. *(From Slovis TL. Caffey's Pediatric Diagnostic Imaging. 11th ed. Philadelphia: Mosby, 2008.)*

REFERENCES

1. Frush DP, Donnelly LF, Rosen NS. Computed tomography and radiation risks: what pediatric health care providers should know. *Pediatrics*. 2003;112:951-957.
2. Kirks DR, Griscom NT. *Practical Pediatric Imaging: Diagnostic Radiology of Infants and Children*. 3rd ed. Philadelphia: Lippincott-Raven, 1998.
3. Kuhn JP, Slovis T, Haller J. *Caffey's Pediatric Diagnostic Imaging*. 10th ed. St Louis: Mosby, 2003.
4. Donnelly LF. *Fundamentals of Pediatric Radiology*. Philadelphia: WB Saunders, 2001.
5. Slovis TL. *Caffey's Pediatric Diagnostic Imaging*. 11th ed. Philadelphia: Mosby, 2008.

Chapter 26

Rheumatology

Steven C. Marek, MD

⊘ See additional content on Expert Consult

I. WEBSITE

American College of Rheumatology: http://www.rheumatology.org/

II. LABORATORY STUDIES

Most laboratory studies used to diagnose rheumatic diseases are nonspecific, and results must be interpreted within the context of the full clinical picture. Once a diagnosis is established, however, they can be used to follow the condition's clinical course, indicating flares or remission of the rheumatic disease. Sensitivities and specificities of rheumatologic tests must be considered with any clinical decision (see Chapter 28).

A. Acute-Phase Reactants

1. **Overview:**
a. Indicate presence of inflammation when elevated.
b. Elevation is nonspecific and can result from trauma, infection, rheumatic diseases, or malignancy.[1]
c. Markers include erythrocyte sedimentation rate (ESR), C-reactive protein (CRP), platelet count, ferritin, haptoglobin, fibrinogen, serum amyloid A, and complement.[1,2]

2. **ESR:**
a. Measure of the rate of fall of red blood cells in anticoagulated blood within a vertical tube; reflects level of rouleaux formation caused by acute phase reactants.[1]
b. Can be falsely lowered in afibrinogenemia, anemia, and sickle cell disease; these states interfere with rouleaux formation.[2]
c. Levels vary depending on age, ethnicity, gender, and freshness of blood sample.[1]
d. Serial measurements may help in monitoring disease severity/activity in conditions such as systemic lupus erythematosus (SLE) and juvenile idiopathic arthritis (JIA).

3. **CRP**[1,3,4]:
a. Synthesized by the liver; assists in clearance of pathologic bacteria and damaged cells via activation of complement-mediated phagocytosis; mediates acute inflammation by altering cytokine release and is thought to prevent autoimmunity by binding to and masking autoantigens.
b. Increases and decreases rapidly owing to short half-life (≈18 hours).
c. Elevation is nonspecific, indicating only inflammation:
   (1) Most active phases of rheumatic disease result in elevation to 1–10 mg/dL.

(2) Level >10 mg/dL raises concern for bacterial infection or systemic vasculitis.

B. Autoantibodies (Table 26-1)

The positive predictive value of any autoantibody assay depends on clinical context. These studies can prove valuable in confirming clinical suspicion. However, in the absence of suspicion, they have low yield and may be misleading.

1. Antinuclear antibody (ANA):

a. Nonspecific test for rheumatic disease.[1]

b. Positive in ≈60%–70% of children with an autoimmune disease, but can be seen in ≈15%–35% of normal persons.

c. If positive, consider ordering individual autoantibodies (see Table 26-1).

d. Can be positive in nonrheumatic diseases:

    (1) Neoplasm

    (2) Infections (transiently positive): Mononucleosis, endocarditis, hepatitis, malaria

e. If positive in pauciarticular JIA, there is increased risk of uveitis.

2. Rheumatoid factor (RF)[1]:

a. Immunoglobulin (Ig)M antibodies to the Fc portion of IgG

b. Positive in rheumatic and nonrheumatic disease:

    (1) Rheumatic diseases: SLE, mixed cryoglobulinemia, JIA (rarely), mixed connective tissue disease, and Henoch-Schönlein purpura

    (2) Infections: Hepatitis B, bacterial endocarditis, tuberculosis, and toxoplasmosis, other, rubella, cytomegalovirus, and herpes (TORCH) infections

26

TABLE 26-1

AUTOANTIBODIES ASSOCIATED WITH COMMON RHEUMATOLOGIC DISEASES

Systemic Lupus Erythematosus (SLE)	Juvenile Idiopathic Arthritis*	Vasculitis	Polymyositis/ Dermatomyositis
• Antinuclear antibody (ANA) • Anti–double stranded DNA • Anti-Smith • Antiribonucleoprotein (anti-RNP) • Antimicrosomal • Antiphospholipids†	• Rheumatoid factor (RF) • Anti–cyclic citrullinated peptide (anti-CCP) • ANA	• Antineutrophil cytoplasmic antibody (ANCA)—cytoplasmic/ proteinase-3 (PR3) • ANCA—perinuclear/ MPO (myeloperoxidase)	• ANA • Anti–Jo-1

Mixed Connective Tissue Disease	Drug-Induced SLE	Sjögren Syndrome	Scleroderma
• ANA • Anti-RNP	• Antihistone	• ANA • Anti-Ro • Anti-La	• ANA • Anticentromere • Anti-RNP • Antitopoisomerase (anti–Scl-70)

*JIA is typically RF and CCP negative; when positive may indicate erosive disease.

†Antiphospholipids: anticardiolipin, lupus anticoagulant, and antiglycoprotein I.

Modified from Kliegman RM, Behrman RE, Jenson HB, et al. *Nelson Textbook of Pediatrics.* 18th ed. Philadelphia: Saunders Elsevier, 2007.

c. Negative RF: Does not rule out rheumatic disease
d. Prognostic importance in polyarticular JIA: Positive RF suggests more progressive disease (see Section III)

3. **Anti–cyclic citrullinated peptide (anti-CCP) antibodies:**
a. Currently being explored as an RF adjunct,[5-7] but routine use in the pediatric setting is not indicated until the full clinical significance in this population has been established.
b. Although pediatric studies are few, anti-CCP has been shown to have a high sensitivity and specificity for adult rheumatoid arthritis (RA).
c. Anti-CCP–positive juvenile rheumatoid arthritis (JRA) patients are usually also RF positive, as are females with late-onset polyarthritis.[7]
d. Anti-CCP positivity correlates with erosive joint disease in JIA.[8]

C. Complement[1,9]

The complement system is composed of a series of plasma proteins and cellular receptors that function together to mediate host defense and inflammation. Inflammatory processes may increase complement protein synthesis or increase their consumption.

1. **Total hemolytic complement level (CH_{50}):**
a. General measure of complement; also an acute-phase reactant
b. Increased in the acute phase response of numerous inflammatory states
c. Useful screening test for homozygous complement deficiency states
d. Typically decreased in SLE

2. **C3 and C4:**
a. Most common complement proteins assayed
b. May be increased or decreased in rheumatic diseases, depending on stage of disease or severity
c. Trends more instructive than isolated results

3. **Decreased levels of complement proteins:**
a. Indicator of immune complex formation:
   (1) Can occur in active SLE, some vasculitides, and multiple infections, including gram-negative sepsis, hepatitis, and pneumococcal infections.
   (2) Decreased levels typically signify more severe SLE, particularly with regard to renal disease.
b. Severe hepatic failure: Synthesis of complement proteins occurs primarily in the liver.
c. Congenital complement deficiency, which may predispose to development of autoimmune disease.

4. **Increased levels of complement proteins:**
a. Indicates the active phase of most rheumatic diseases (e.g., SLE, JIA, dermatomyositis)
b. May be seen in multiple infections (e.g., hepatitis, pneumococcal pneumonia) as part of the acute-phase response

D. Other Laboratory Studies

1. **Urinalysis:**
a. Renal involvement occurs in many rheumatic diseases.
b. Findings may include proteinuria, hematuria, or casts (see Chapter 19).

2. **Serum muscle enzymes**[2]:
a. Including aspartate aminotransferase (AST), lactate dehydrogenase (LDH), aldolase, and creatine kinase (CK)
b. Can be elevated in certain rheumatic diseases that cause muscle inflammation or destruction (e.g., dermatomyositis)
   NOTE: Patients with chronic ongoing myositis may have an elevated CK-MB fraction (noncardiac in origin) when serum CK levels are measured.
3. **Joint fluid analysis** (Fig. 26-1)[10]:
a. Important in the presence of an effusion, especially monoarticular disease.
b. Effusion can be seen in rheumatic and other disease processes (e.g., septic arthritis).

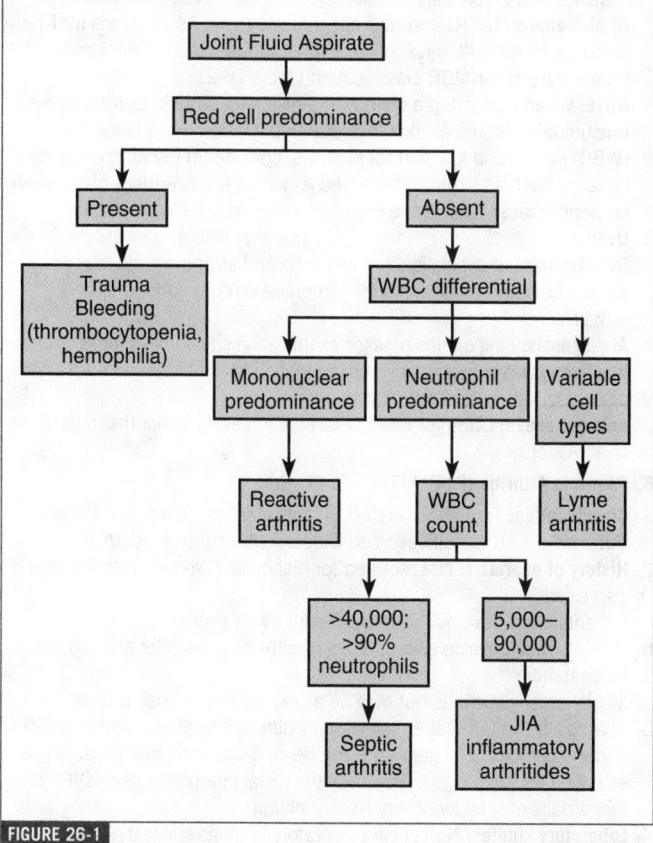

FIGURE 26-1

Joint fluid analysis algorithm. JRA, Juvenile rheumatoid arthritis; WBC, white blood cell. *(Data from Hay W, Levin M, Sondheimer J, et al. Current Pediatric Diagnosis and Treatment. 17th ed. New York: Lange Medical/McGraw-Hill, 2005.)*

III. ARTHRITIDES

A. Juvenile Rheumatoid Arthritis[1,2,9] and Juvenile Idiopathic Arthritis[12]

1. **Definition of arthritis:** Joint swelling or limitation/tenderness upon range of motion (ROM), lasting ≥6 weeks and not due to other identifiable cause[11]

2. **Diagnosis:**

a. Challenge of diagnosis: Children may not present with joint pain/swelling but other symptoms: morning stiffness, limp, refusal to walk, irritability, poor growth, or limb discrepancy.

b. Classical divisions: Based on clinical course over the first 6 months of illness in children <age 16 years, with arthritis present for at least 6 weeks.[1,2] Multiple classification systems exist; American College of Rheumatology (ACR) and International League of Associations for Rheumatology (ILAR) classifications are most widely used.[11] Divisions used here are based on ACR classification (Table 26-2).

NOTE: When evaluating a child with a history of chronic extremity pain (including nighttime awakenings due to pain), low white blood cell (WBC) count, and low-normal platelets, consider in the differential malignancy such as acute lymphocytic leukemia (even without blasts seen on peripheral smear). Bone marrow studies may be indicated.[13]

3. **Uveitis**
Development of uveitis is often insidious and asymptomatic, so routine pediatric ophthalmology screening is required for children with JIA:

a. **At diagnosis:** First ophthalmologic examination should be within 1 month.

b. **Inactive disease:** Frequency of examination varies based on ANA status, disease duration, and age at diagnosis.[18]

c. **Active disease:** Ophthalmologic examination every 3 months, regardless of ANA status.

B. Psoriatic Arthritis (PsA)[14,15]

1. **Classification:** Traditionally referred to as a *seronegative spondyloar-thropathy*; ILAR classification considers PsA a subtype of JIA.[11]

2. **History of psoriasis:** Not required for diagnosis *(psoriatic arthritis sine psoriasis)*:

a. Patients often have a first-degree relative with psoriasis.

b. Patients may develop skin findings months or years after arthritis onset.

3. **Presentation:**

a. Mostly an oligoarthritis but may be a polyarthritis or axial arthritis.

b. ±Sacroiliitis, inflammatory spinal pain/stiffness, synovitis, enthesitis, or dactylitis of toes or fingers (swelling beyond joint margins, producing a so-called sausage digit), especially the distal interphalangeal (DIP) joint.

c. Fingernails may show onycholysis or pitting.

4. **Laboratory studies:** No specific laboratory findings suggest a diagnosis of psoriatic arthritis, although markers of inflammation (CRP, ESR) may be helpful in tracking activity of disease. RF is usually negative.

TABLE 26-2

CLASSICAL DIVISIONS OF JUVENILE IDIOPATHIC ARTHRITIS[35]

	Pauciarticular	Polyarticular	Systemic-Onset
Frequency of cases	60%	30%	10%
Number of joints involved (in first 6 mo)	≤4	≥5	Variable
Age predominance	Type I: preschool age Type II: 9–11 yr	2–5 yr and 10–18 yr	None
Gender ratio (female/male)	Type I: 4:1 Type II: 1:20	3:1	1:1
Involved joints	Knees and ankles	Larger joints, symmetric involvement	Any, including hips
Chronic uveitis	20% (higher with [+] ANA)	5%	Rare
Extraarticular manifestations	Uveitis	Mild fever, hepatosplenomegaly, lymphadenopathy, subcutaneous nodules	Once- to twice-daily high-spiking fevers, hepatosplenomegaly, lymphadenopathy, polyserositis, pericarditis, and characteristic macular rash
Seropositivity			
ANA	75%–85%	40%–50%	10%
RF	10% (increases with age)	75%–85%	10%
Destructive arthritis	Rare	>50%	>50%
Major morbidities	Uveitis, leg length discrepancy		Pericarditis, pleuropericarditis, secondary amyloidosis, macrophage activation syndrome*
Prognosis	Excellent apart from eyesight	Poorer prognosis with RF seropositivity and later onset	Moderate to poor

*Macrophage activation syndrome (MAS) or reactive hematophagocytic lymphohistiocytosis: uncontrolled activation of T cells and macrophages, leading to rapid hepatic failure, encephalopathy, pancytopenia, purpura, mucosal bleeding, and renal failure. Paradoxically low erythrocyte sedimentation rate (ESR) with hypofibrinogenemia, elevated ferritin, and triglycerides, with disseminated intravascular coagulation (DIC).

ANA, Antinuclear antibody; RF, rheumatoid factor.

Modified from McMillan JA, Feigin RD, DeAngelis CD, et al. *Oski's Pediatrics.* 4th ed. Philadelphia, Lippincott Williams & Wilkins, 2006.

5. **Radiographic findings:** Blend of destruction and proliferation on plain films.
6. **Prognosis:** If left untreated, will result in a deforming combination of erosions and ankylosis within joints of digits.
7. **Major morbidities:** Chronic uveitis may develop; regular screening by an ophthalmologist recommended.

C. Reactive Arthritis[2]

1. **Definition:** Diverse group of inflammatory arthritides that follow a bacterial or viral infection, particularly involving respiratory, gastrointestinal (GI), and genitourinary tracts.

2. **Onset:** Infection typically precedes development of arthritis by 1–4 weeks; ≈80% of cases are preceded by gastroenteritis.

3. **Common precipitating organisms:** *Mycoplasma, Chlamydia, Yersinia, Salmonella, Shigella, Campylobacter, Neisseria gonorrhoeae,* Epstein-Barr virus (EBV), parvovirus B19, and enteroviruses.

4. **Presentation:** Sometimes accompanied by constitutional signs and symptoms (fever, weight loss, fatigue), as well as dermatologic and ophthalmologic findings.

5. **HLA-B27:**

a. Strong association between HLA-B27 and susceptibility to developing reactive arthritis after an infection with a bacterial arthritogenic organism

b. ≈50%–65% frequency seen in reactive arthritis

6. **Laboratory studies:**

a. ±Evidence of systemic inflammation (leukocytosis, thrombocytosis, elevated ESR and CRP).

b. Autoantibodies are typically absent.

c. Stool cultures, serum *Chlamydia pneumoniae* and *Mycoplasma* titers, and urinary *Chlamydia* DNA probe can be helpful. Negative stool culture does not exclude diagnosis of reactive arthritis secondary to an enteric organism.

d. Complement-deficient patients are at risk to develop gonorrheal arthritis, so complement levels should be measured in patients likely to be infected.

e. Consider enterovirus, EBV, and parvovirus B19 antibody titers.

f. Joint fluid analysis may be helpful to distinguish septic arthritis from reactive arthritis, especially in the case of *Salmonella* infection, where either a septic or reactive arthritis may develop (see Fig. 26-1).

7. **Prognosis:** Arthritis can last weeks to months, with eventual remission or development of recurrent episodes.

D. Management of Arthritis

1. **Pharmacologic agents**[1,2,7,13]: See Formulary for dosing guidelines and Table EC 26-A for related side effects and laboratory surveillance

a. Nonsteroidal antiinflammatory drugs (NSAIDs): First-line (e.g., naproxen, ibuprofen)

b. Disease-modifying antirheumatic drugs (DMARDs): Slow disease progression (e.g., methotrexate, sulfasalazine, hydroxychloroquine)

c. Biologic immunomodulators: Tumor necrosis factor (TNF) inhibitors (e.g., etanercept, infliximab, adalimumab); rituximab (anti-CD20); abatacept (modulates T-cell activation); and interleukin (IL)-1 receptor antagonist (anakinra, canakinumab)

d. Cytotoxic and immunosuppressive drugs: Cyclosporine and mycophenolate mofetil

e. Corticosteroids: Can be systemic or intraarticular

2. **Health maintenance**[1,7,13,16,17]:

a. Vaccines: Generally follow regular immunization schedule. Special considerations should be made for immunocompromised hosts (i.e., patients on biologic or immunosuppressive therapy; see Chapter 16). May have to postpone live viral vaccines.

TABLE 26-3

DIFFERENTIAL DIAGNOSIS FOR JOINT OR EXTREMITY PAIN

Rheumatologic	JIA; SLE; juvenile dermatomyositis; polyarteritis; scleroderma; Sjögren syndrome; Behçet's disease; Wegner granulomatosis; sarcoidosis; HSP; chronic recurrent multifocal osteomyelitis; juvenile ankylosing spondylitis; psoriatic arthritis
Infectious	Bacterial: *Staphylococcus aureus, Streptococcus pneumoniae, Neisseria gonorrhoeae, Haemophilus influenzae* Viral: parvovirus, rubella, mumps, EBV, hepatitis B Fungal Other: spirochetes, mycobacterial, endocarditis, Lyme
Immunodeficiencies	Hypogammaglobulinemia; IgA deficiency; HIV
Congenital and Metabolic	Gout and pseudogout; mucopolysaccharidoses; hypothyroidism or hyperthyroidism; vitamin C or D deficiency; connective tissue disease; lysosomal storage diseases: Fabry and Farber; familial mediterranean fever
Bone and Cartilage	Trauma; patellofemoral syndrome; osteochondritis dissecans and avascular necrosis; SCFE; hypertrophic osteoarthropathy
Inflammatory and Reactive	Kawasaki syndrome; IBD; acute rheumatic fever; reactive arthritis; toxic synovitis; serum sickness
Neurologic and Pain Syndromes	Peripheral neuropathy; carpal tunnel syndrome; Charcot joints; fibromyalgia; depression with somatization; reflex sympathetic dystrophy
Neoplastic	Leukemia and lymphoma; neuroblastoma; hysticytosis; synovial tumors Bone tumors: osteosarcoma, Ewing sarcoma, osteoid osteoma

IBD, Inflammatory bowel disease; EBV, Epstein-Barr virus; HIV, human immunodeficiency virus; HSP, Henoch-Schönlein purpura; JIA, juvenile idiopathic arthritis; SCFE, slipped capital femoral epiphysis; SLE, systemic lupus erythematosus.
Modified from Kliegman RM, Stanton BF, St. Geme JW, et al. *Nelson Textbook of Pediatrics.* 19th ed. Philadelphia: Saunders Elsevier, 2011.

b. Prevention or minimization of osteopenia: Adequate calcium and vitamin D intake and weight-bearing activities.
c. Physical and occupational therapy: Important in maintaining joint ROM and strength of associated muscle groups, as well as decreasing pain and preventing joint deformity and contractures.
d. Orthopedic surgery: Necessary in some cases for pain control, improvement in function, or contracture.

E. Differential Diagnosis
See Table 26-3 for differential diagnosis of joint/extremity pain.

IV. SYSTEMIC LUPUS ERYTHEMATOSUS

An episodic multisystem autoimmune disease characterized by inflammation of blood vessels and connective tissue. Apart from drug-induced SLE, the etiology remains unknown.

A. American College of Rheumatology Classification Criteria (Table 26-4)

These are not strict *diagnostic* criteria, but *classification* criteria for research purposes. Use caution when applying them to pediatric and international/multiethnic patients; few studies validate ACR criteria for these populations.[19,20]

Note: In 2012 the SLICC criteria were published, but they are still being investigated.

TABLE 26-4

1997 UPDATE OF THE 1982 AMERICAN COLLEGE OF RHEUMATOLOGY REVISED CRITERIA FOR CLASSIFICATION OF SYSTEMIC LUPUS ERYTHEMATOSUS

Criterion	
Malar rash	Fixed erythema (flat or raised) over malar eminences, tending to spare nasolabial folds; telangiectasias
Discoid rash	Erythematous raised patches with adherent keratotic scaling and follicular plugging; atrophic scarring may occur in older lesions
Photosensitivity	Rash due to unusual reaction to sunlight (by patient history or physician observation)
Oral ulcers	Oral or nasopharyngeal ulceration, usually painless, observed by physician
Nonerosive arthritis	Involving two or more peripheral joints, characterized by tenderness, swelling, or effusion
Pleuritis or pericarditis	1. Pleuritis: history of pleuritic pain or rubbing heard by physician, or evidence of pleural effusion AND/OR 2. Pericarditis: documented by electrocardiogram or rub or evidence of pericardial effusion
Renal disorder	1. Persistent proteinuria > 0.5 g/day or > 3+ if quantitation not performed AND/OR 2. Cellular casts: may be red cell, hemoglobin, granular, tubular, or mixed
Neurologic disorder	Seizures or psychosis: in the absence of offending drugs, hypertension, or known metabolic derangements
Hematologic disorder	1. Hemolytic anemia with reticulocytosis AND/OR 2. Leukopenia: <4000/μL on ≥two occasions AND/OR Lymphopenia: <1500/μL on ≥two occasions AND/OR 3. Thrombocytopenia: <100,000/μL in the absence of offending drugs
Autoimmune markers	1. Anti-DNA: antibody to native DNA in abnormal titer AND/OR 2. Anti-Smith (Sm): presence of antibody to Sm nuclear antigen
Positive antinuclear antibody	An abnormal titer of antinuclear antibody by immunofluorescence or an equivalent assay at any point in time in the absence of drugs

Data from http://www.rheumatology.org/, which was modified from Tan E, Cohen AS, Fries JF, et al. The 1982 revised criteria for the classification of systemic lupus erythematosus. *Arthritis Rheum.* 1982;25:1271-1277.

B. Clinical Features and Management of SLE

1. Diagnosis:

a. Most often based on meeting 4 or more of the 11 classification criteria.

b. Do not exclude the possibility of an SLE diagnosis for a pediatric patient who does not fully meet these criteria.

c. Majority of pediatric patients with *incomplete SLE* (<4 criteria) will likely completely fulfill these criteria in subsequent years.

2. Epidemiology:

a. Females more commonly affected; onset usually at age 9–15 years (median age, 12 years).[19]

b. African Americans and Asian Americans more commonly affected than whites.[1]

3. **Laboratory studies and surveillance**[1,15]:
a. CBC with differential and direct Coombs.
b. Urinalysis and serum creatinine: Of note, renal disease is the leading cause of death in lupus patients. See Table EC 26-B for World Health Organization (WHO) classification of SLE nephritis.[21]
c. ESR or CRP: May be increased with active disease; CRP levels may not correlate with disease activity.[22]
d. Complement levels (C3, C4): Serial levels most useful. Congenital complement deficiencies may also be seen in SLE, especially in males. Decreasing complement levels may indicate renal disease.
e. Autoantibodies (see Table 26-1)[1]:
   (1) ANA: Most patients with positive ANA do not have SLE, but almost all patients with SLE have positive ANA.[5]
   (2) Anti-ds (double-stranded) DNA: Highly specific for SLE, seen in about 60% of patients. Titers rise/fall depending on disease activity and usually increase during development of lupus nephritis. Not associated with discoid or subacute cutaneous lupus.[5]
   (3) Anti-Sm: Highly specific for SLE; seen in ≈10%–30% of patients.

4. **Treatment**[1]:
a. NSAIDs: Targeted to treat arthralgia and arthritis (use with caution; lupus patients more susceptible to renal toxicity with these agents).
b. Hydroxychloroquine: treats milder manifestations (e.g., skin lesions, arthritis) and may lower lipid levels, decreasing risk for thromboembolic disease.
c. Corticosteroids: Used to treat symptoms and decrease autoantibody production.
d. Cytotoxic therapy: Reserved for more severe cases. Cyclophosphamide is used in patients with lupus nephritis, vasculitis, pulmonary hemorrhage, or central nervous system involvement.
e. DMARDs: Methotrexate, cyclosporine, mycophenolate mofetil.
f. Biologics: Agents that target cytokine production; includes anti-CD20/22 monoclonal antibodies (i.e., rituximab).

C. Drug-Induced SLE[1,2]

1. **Pathogenesis:**
a. Inciting drugs (including but not limited to): hydralazine, minocycline, ethosuximide, doxycycline, procainamide, isoniazid, chlorpromazine, phenytoin, carbamazepine
b. Usually resolves with discontinuation of drug

2. **Clinical and laboratory features:**
a. Most frequent clinical manifestations are cutaneous and pleuropericardial involvement.
b. Often associated with antihistone antibodies.

D. Neonatal SLE[1,21]

1. **Pathogenesis:** Neonates born to mothers with active SLE can develop a transient lupus-like syndrome in the perinatal period. Transplacental

passage of anti-Ro (anti–SS-A) and anti-La (anti–SS-B) (also seen in Sjögren syndrome) mediate disease process. Mothers are often asymptomatic but carry antibodies, so mothers are routinely screened for SS-A and SS-B.

2. **Clinical and laboratory features:**
a. Thrombocytopenia, hemolytic anemia.
b. Inflammatory features of neonatal lupus will resolve within 6 months as maternal autoantibodies are cleared.
c. Congenital heart block (associated with anti-Ro): *Permanent* condition; usually requires placement of a pacemaker.
d. Common cause of hydrops likely secondary to heart block or Coombs antibody-mediated immune anemia.

V. VASCULITIS

A. General (Table 26-5)[28]

1. **Definition:** Inflammation of a blood vessel wall. Systemic vasculitis syndromes, although rare, are a concern in childhood.
2. **Clinical presentation:** Variable, ranging from rash or fever of unknown origin to progressive multisystem failure.[23]
3. **Initial laboratory tests:** CBC, basic metabolic panel, liver function tests, acute phase reactants, stool guaiac, and complete urinalysis.
4. **Diagnosis:**
a. Small vessel vasculitis: Confirmed by biopsy. Magnetic resonance angiography (MRA) may also be helpful, but a negative test does not rule out disease.
b. Medium-large vessel vasculitis: MRA.

B. Henoch-Schönlein Purpura (HSP)[1,2,24,25]

1. **Epidemiology:**
a. Most common small-vessel vasculitis in children
b. More frequent in males than females
c. Typical age of onset 2–7 years
d. History of viral upper respiratory infection several weeks preceding onset of illness in half to two thirds of cases
2. **Presentation[2,19–21]:**
a. Nonthrobocytopenic palpable purpura:
   (1) Most common and frequently presenting feature.
   (2) Evolution of rash: Urticarial lesions progress to a maculopapular rash, followed by purpuric lesions involving ankles, buttocks, and elbows, beginning on lower extremities but can involve entire body.
   (3) New lesions can appear over 2–4 weeks, leaving a mixed-stage appearance.
b. Migratory polyarthritis and/or polyarthralgias:
   (1) Presenting feature in 25% of cases: Very tender and painful periarticular joint swelling of ankles and knees (most often), without effusion.

TABLE 26-5

CHILDHOOD VASCULITIS SYNDROMES

Vessel Size	Vasculitis Syndrome	Clinical and Distinguishing Features
Large arteries	Takayasu arteritis	Aortic arch involvement leading to aneurysms, thrombosis, and stenosis Predominantly seen in young women Hypertension is most common sign
Aorta and large branches directed toward major body regions	Giant cell (temporal arteritis)	Granulomatous inflammation of aorta and major branches, with predilection for extracranial branches of carotid artery
Medium-sized arteries	Kawasaki disease	Arteritis including large, medium, and small arteries; associated with mucocutaneous lymph node syndrome (see Chapter 7)
Renal, hepatic, coronary, and mesenteric arteries	Polyarteritis nodosa	Cutaneous lesions include livedo reticularis, tender nodules, purpura Hypertension, renal failure, abdominal pain, intestinal infarction, and cerebrovascular accidents are common complications
Small arterioles and venules	Microscopic polyangiitis	Rare in pediatrics p-ANCA or myeloperoxidase (MPO) positive Glomerulonephritis and pulmonary capillaritis Associated with streptococcal infection or URIs
Venules, capillaries, arterioles, and intraparenchymal distal arteries	Henoch-Schönlein purpura	Most common pediatric vasculitis IgA-dominant immune deposits, palpable purpura involving buttocks and lower extremities, colicky abdominal pain, arthralgias/arthritis
	Wegener granulomatosis	Necrotizing granulomatous vasculitis of small and medium-sized vessels Presents with respiratory tract and kidney involvement c-ANCA or proteinase-3 (PR3) positive May also involve medium-sized vessels
	Churg-Strauss syndrome	Eosinophil-rich and granulomatous inflammation involving respiratory tract; associated with asthma

cANCA, Cytoplasmic antineutrophil cytoplasmic antibody; IgA, immunoglobulin A; pANCA, perinuclear antineutrophil cytoplasmic antibody; URI, upper respiratory infection.

Modified from Kliegman RM, Behrman, RE, Jenson HB, et al. *Nelson Textbook of Pediatrics.* 18th ed. Philadelphia: Saunders Elsevier, 2007; Cassidy J, Petty R. *Textbook of Pediatric Rheumatology.* 5th ed. Philadelphia: WB Saunders, 2005; Kim S, Dedeoglu F. Update on pediatric vasculitis. *Curr Opin Pediatr.* 2005;17:695-702; and Dillon M, Ozen S. A new international classification of childhood vasculitis. *Pediatr Nephrol.* 2006;21:1219-1222.

26

(2) Joint involvement is transient with no permanent deformities.

c. Abdominal pain:
(1) Colicky in nature, secondary to hemorrhage and edema of small intestine.
(2) Intussusception results in about 2% of cases (usually ileoileal).
(3) Stool can be guaiac positive without obvious signs of intestinal bleeding.

d. Glomerulonephritis:
(1) Occurs in 20%–60% of patients; may develop months after onset or before development of rash
(2) Renal biopsy: Typically consistent with IgA nephropathy, but crescentic glomerulonephritis may also be seen.
(3) More common in males, patients with GI bleeding, factor VIII activity <80%, and in patients <age 4 years[27]

e. Other features: Acute scrotal inflammation (2%–38% of male patients), dorsal edema of feet, occult pulmonary involvement

3. **Diagnosis:** Based on clinical characteristics[2,23,24]

4. **Laboratory findings:** Can help exclude other diagnoses and illuminate specific organ involvement:

a. Hematologic: Normal to elevated platelet count, normal platelet function tests and bleeding time, normal coagulation studies.

b. Urinalysis: ±proteinuria and hematuria, but casts uncommon.

c. Antibodies: IgA levels may be elevated, especially in acute phase of disease.

d. Stool guaiac: May be positive.

e. Anti–streptolysin O titer: May be elevated.

f. Throat culture may be positive for group A β-hemolytic streptococcus, warranting antibiotic treatment.

5. **Treatment[23,24]:**

a. Supportive care: Adequate hydration, analgesia for joint pain.

b. Monitor vital signs because of GI bleeding and renal involvement.

c. Serial urinalyses at routine office visits.

d. Consider steroids, especially if GI and renal systems involved.

e. Prolonged immunosuppression may be necessary for renal disease (cyclophosphamide or azathioprine).

6. **Prognosis:** Typically self-limited course, but may recur in a minority (10%–20%) of cases.

C. Juvenile Dermatomyositis[1,2,9,35-38]

1. **Pathogenesis:**

a. Nonsuppurative vasculitis with inflammation of skin, GI tract, and striated muscle.

b. Unlike adult-onset form, juvenile dermatomyositis is not related to malignancy.

2. **Epidemiology:**

a. One study found the incidence to be 3.2 cases per million children per year; female/male ratio of 2.3:1.

b. Peak age of onset for juvenile form is 5–14 years.

3. **Presentation:**
a. Constitutional: Fever, fatigue, weight loss.
b. Musculoskeletal: Symmetric proximal muscle pain or weakness involving shoulder and pelvic girdles.
c. Dermatologic: Heliotropic rash involving upper eyelids (or malar rash); Gottron papules (thickened, erythematous, scaly rash on extensor surfaces of elbows, knees, metacarpophalangeal and proximal interphalangeal joints). Dystrophic cutaneous calcifications or photosensitivity may be present.
   (1) Dermatologic symptoms are required to diagnose dermatomyositis.
d. Respiratory: Dyspnea/tachypnea may be present (restrictive lung disease due to respiratory muscle weakness), indicating more severe disease and poorer prognosis.
e. Other: Dysphagia, periorbital edema, nailfold or eyelid rim capillary abnormalities (dilation, aneurysms, dropout).

4. **Laboratory studies:**
a. Elevated muscle enzymes: AST, ALT, CK, LDH, and aldolase; may be normal at diagnosis.[37]
b. ANA may be positive; acute-phase reactants (ESR, CRP) are often normal.[36]

5. **Diagnosis:**
a. Muscle biopsy: Gold standard for definitive diagnosis.
b. MRI: Often used to demonstrate affected areas: T1-weighted images may show fibrosis, atrophy, and fatty infiltration; T2-weighted images may demonstrate active myositis.

VI. GRANULOMATOUS DISEASE

A. Differential Diagnosis[30,31]

1. **Infectious causes:** Tuberculosis, atypical mycobacteria, including leprosy, histoplasmosis, coccidioidomycosis, brucellosis, chlamydia, tularemia, treponemal organisms, leishmaniasis, toxoplasmosis
2. **Environmental exposures:** Hypersensitivity pneumonitis, berylliosis, silicosis, other metals (aluminum and titanium), talc
3. **Immune dysregulation:** Wegener granulomatosis, primary biliary cirrhosis, Churg-Strauss syndrome, sarcoidosis, Takayasu arteritis, Crohn's disease, chronic granulomatous disease
4. **Other:** Malignancy, foreign bodies, medications

B. Sarcoidosis[2,31-34]

1. **Pathophysiology:** Multisystem infiltrative noncaseating granulomatous disease of unknown etiology
2. **Epidemiology:**
a. Before puberty (very rare): Primarily affects caucasians.
b. During and after puberty: Predominantly affects African Americans.
c. Incidence increases with age, peaking between 20 and 40 years of age.
d. Males and females affected equally.

3. **Two forms of pediatric sarcoidosis:**
a. Before puberty (usually <age 4): May be familial; dominated by skin, musculoskeletal, and eye involvement
b. During or after puberty: Very similar to adult disease; dominated by lung, lymphatic, eye, and systemic involvement
4. **Presentation:** Lymphadenopathy is most common initial manifestation
a. General: Weight loss, fever, anorexia, fatigue
b. Musculoskeletal: Usually only seen in young children. Tenosynovitis and polyarthritis, mostly of wrists, knees, and ankles[32]
c. Pulmonary: Dyspnea on exertion, chest pain, chronic dry cough, wheezing or stridor, bilateral hilar lymphadenopathy with or without parenchymal disease on chest x-ray or computed tomography (CT), and restrictive pattern with impaired gas exchange on pulmonary function tests
d. Ophthalmologic: Bilateral uveitis (anterior, posterior, or panuveitis), band keratopathy, synechiae, iris nodules, cataracts, glaucoma, chorioretinitis, conjunctivitis, papilledema
e. Dermatologic: Erythema nodosum, plaques, maculopapules, subcutaneous nodules
f. Lymphatic: Hilar, mediastinal, and mobile, nontender peripheral lymphadenopathy
g. Neurologic: Headache, seizures, cranial nerve (CN VI, VII, VIII) palsies, pseudotumor cerebri, obstructive hydrocephalus, hemiparesis:
   (1) CN VII palsy: Most common neurologic manifestation in adolescent/adult form.[33]
   (2) Magnetic resonance imaging (MRI) may show mass lesion(s), periventricular white matter lesions, nodular or diffuse leptomeningeal enhancement.[34]
h. Cardiovascular: Arrhythmia, valvular disease, vasculitis of any size vessel
i. Renal: Renal failure (due to hypercalcemia or parenchymal infiltration) and nephrolithiasis
j. GI: Hepatosplenomegaly, elevated transaminases, hyperbilirubinemia due to parenchymal and biliary tree infiltration, parotitis, and rarely intestinal obstruction with rectal prolapse
k. Endocrine: Pituitary dysfunction (e.g., diabetes insipidus, hypercalcemia)
5. **Laboratory studies:** Nonspecific:
a. Hypercalcemia (due to pulmonary alveolar macrophage hydroxylation of vitamin D to active 1,25 dihydroxy form).
b. Elevated serum angiotensin-converting enzyme (ACE; produced by epithelial cells in granulomata).
c. Leukopenia, increased immunoglobulins, and eosinophilia are common.
6. **Initial evaluation:** Thorough history and physical examination, chest x-ray or CT, complete metabolic panel, pulmonary function testing, electrocardiogram, and ophthalmologic (slit-lamp) examination
7. **Diagnosis:** Biopsy demonstrating noncaseating granulomas in absence of other known cause
8. **Treatment:** Glucocorticoids standard; methotrexate, azathioprine secondary alternatives

REFERENCES

1. Kliegman RM, Stanton BF, St. Geme JW, et al. *Nelson Textbook of Pediatrics.* 19th ed. Philadelphia: Saunders Elsevier, 2011.
2. Cassidy J, Petty R. *Textbook of Pediatric Rheumatology.* 5th ed. Philadelphia: Saunders, 2005.
3. Marnell L, Mold C, Du Clos TW, et al. C-reactive protein: ligands, receptors and role in inflammation. *Clin Immunol.* 2005;117:104-111.
4. Rhodes B, Fürnrohr B, Vyse T. C-reactive protein in rheumatology: biology and genetics. *Nat Rev Rheumatol.* 2011;7:282-289.
5. Bosch X, Guilabert A, Font J. Antineutrophil cytoplasmic antibodies. *Lancet.* 2006;368:404-418.
6. van Venrooij W, Zendman AJ. Anti-CCP2 antibodies: an overview and perspective of the diagnostic abilities of this serological marker for early rheumatoid arthritis. *Clin Rev Allergy Immunol.* 2008;34:36-39.
7. Habib HM, Mosaad YM, Youssef HM, et al. Anti-cyclic citrullinated peptide antibodies in patients with juvenile idiopathic arthritis. *Immunol Invest.* 2008;37:849-857.
8. Gupta R, Thabah MM, Vaidya B. Anti-cyclic citrullinated peptide antibodies in juvenile idiopathic arthritis. *Indian J Pediatr.* 2010;77:41-44.
9. Harris ED, Budd RC, Genovese MC, et al. *Kelley's Textbook of Rheumatology.* 7th ed. Philadelphia: Elsevier Saunders, 2005.
10. Hay W, Levin M, Sondheimer J, et al. *Current Pediatric Diagnosis and Treatment.* 17th ed. New York: Lange Medical/McGraw-Hill, 2007.
11. Petty RE, Southwood TR, Manners P, et al. International League of Associations for Rheumatology classification of juvenile idiopathic arthritis: second revision, Edmonton, 2001. *J Rheumatol.* 2004;31:390-392.
12. Prakken B, Albani S, Martini A. Juvenile idiopathic arthritis. *Lancet.* 2011;377:2138-2149.
13. Jones OY, Spender CH, Bowyer SL, et al. A multicenter case-control study on predictive factors distinguishing childhood leukemia from juvenile rheumatoid arthritis. *Pediatrics.* 2006;117:840-844.
14. Helliwell P, Taylor WJ. Classification and diagnostic criteria for psoriatic arthritis. *Ann Rheum Dis.* 2005;64:3-8.
15. Stoll ML, Zurakowski D, Nigrovic LE, et al. Patients with juvenile psoriatic arthritis comprise two distinct populations. *Arthritis Rheum.* 2006;54:3564-3572.
16. Dell'Era L, Esposito S, Corona F. Vaccination of children and adolescents with rheumatic diseases. *Rheumatology.* 2011;50:1358-1365.
17. Milojevic D, Ilowite N. Treatment of rheumatic diseases in children: special considerations. *Rheum Dis Clin North Am.* 2002;28:461-482.
18. Cassidy J, Kivlin J, Lindsley C, et al. Ophthalmologic examinations in children with juvenile rheumatoid arthritis. *Pediatrics.* 2006;117:1843-1845.
19. Tan EM, Cohen AS, Fries JF, et al. The 1982 revised criteria for the classification of systemic lupus erythematosus. *Arthritis Rheum.* 1982;25:1271-1277.
20. Bader-Meunier B, Armengaud JB, Haddad E. Initial presentation of childhood-onset systemic lupus erythematosus: a French multicenter study. *J Pediatr.* 2005;146:648-653.
21. Petri M, Magder L. Classification criteria for systemic lupus erythematosus: a review. *Lupus.* 2004;13:829-837.
22. Williams RC, Harmon ME, Burlingame R. Studies of serum C-reactive protein in systemic lupus erythematosus. *J Rheumatol.* 2005;32:454-461.
23. Gross WL, Trabandt A, Reinhold-Keller T, et al. Diagnosis and evaluation of vasculitis. *Rheumatology.* 2000;39:245-252.

24. Sundel R, Szer I. Vasculitis in childhood. *Rheum Dis Clin North Am.* 2002;28: 625-654.

25. Saulsbury FT. Clinical update: Henoch-Schönlein purpura. *Lancet.* 2007;369: 976-978.

26. McMillan JA, Feigin RD, DeAngelis CD, et al. *Oski's Pediatrics.* 4th ed. Philadelphia: Lippincott Williams & Wilkins, 2006.

27. Sano H, Izumida M, Ogawa Y, et al. Risk factors of renal involvement and significant proteinuria in Henoch-Schönlein purpura. *Eur J Pediatr.* 2002;161:196-201.

28. Kim S, Dedeoglu F. Update on pediatric vasculitis. *Curr Opin Pediatr.* 2005;17:695-702.

29. Dillon M, Ozen S. A new international classification of childhood vasculitis. *Pediatr Nephrol.* 2006;21:1219-1222.

30. Frosch M, Foell D. Wegener granulomatosis in childhood and adolescence. *Eur J Pediatr.* 2004;163:425-434.

31. Iannuzzi MC, Rybicki BA, Teirstein AS. Sarcoidosis. *N Engl J Med.* 2007;357:2153-2165.

32. Lindsley C, Petty R. Overview and report on international registry of sarcoid arthritis in children. *Curr Rheumatol Rep.* 2000;2:343-348.

33. Baumann R, Robertson W. Neurosarcoid presents differently in children than in adults. *Pediatrics.* 2003;112:e480-e486.

34. Nowak D, Widenka D. Neurosarcoidosis: a review of its intracranial manifestation. *J Neurol.* 2001;248:363-372.

35. Mendez EP, Lipton R, Ramsey-Goldman R. US incidence of juvenile dermatomyositis, 1995-1998: results from the National Institute of Arthritis and Musculoskeletal and Skin Diseases Registry. *Arthritis Rheum.* 2003;49:300-305.

36. McCann LJ, Juggins AD, Maillard SM, et al. The Juvenile Dermatomyositis National Registry and Repository (UK and Ireland)—clinical characteristics of children recruited within the first 5 years. *Rheumatology.* 2006;45:1255-1260.

37. Ravelli A, Ruperto N, Trail L. Clinical assessment in juvenile dermatomyositis. *Autoimmunity.* 2006;39:197-203.

38. Feldman BM, Rider LG, Reed AM, et al. Juvenile dermatomyositis and other idiopathic inflammatory myopathies of childhood. *Lancet.* 2008;371:2201-2212.

39. International Study Group for Behçet's Disease. Criteria for diagnosis of Behçet's Disease. *Lancet.* 1990;335:1078-1080.

40. Gaffney K, Scott DGI. Azathioprine and Cyclophosphamide in the Treatment of Rheumatoid Arthritis. *Br J Rheumatol.* 1998;37:824-836.

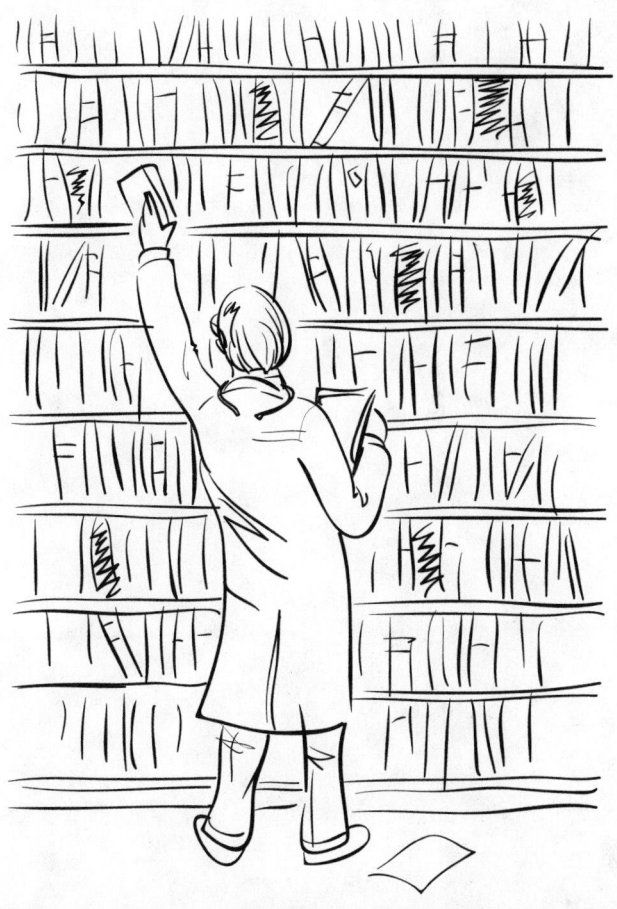

PART III

Chapter 27

Blood Chemistries and Body Fluids

Branden Engorn, MD, and Jamie Flerlage, MD

Determining normal reference ranges of laboratory studies in pediatric patients poses some major challenges. Available literature is often limited because of the small sample sizes of patients in many studies that have been used to derive these suggested normal ranges. **Please use great caution and be aware of this limitation when interpreting pediatric laboratory studies.**

The values that follow are compiled from both published literature and the Johns Hopkins Hospital Department of Pathology. Normal values vary with the analytic method used. Consult your laboratory for its analytic method and range of normal values and for less commonly used parameters, which are beyond the scope of this text. Additional normal laboratory values may be found in Chapters 10, 14, and 15.

A special thanks to Lori Sokoll, PhD, and Athena Kantartzis, PhD, for their guidance in preparing this chapter.

I. REFERENCE VALUES (TABLE 27-1)

TABLE 27-1

REFERENCE VALUES

	Conventional Units	SI Units
ALANINE AMINOTRANSFERASE (ALT)[1,2]		
(Major sources: Liver, skeletal muscle, and myocardium)		
Infant <12 mo	13–45 U/L	13–45 U/L
1–3 yr	5–45 U/L	5–45 U/L
4–6 yr	10–25 U/L	10–25 U/L
7–9 yr	10–35 U/L	10–35 U/L
10–11 yr		
Female	10–30 U/L	10–30 U/L
Male	10–35 U/L	10–35 U/L
12–13 yr		
Female	10–30 U/L	10–30 U/L
Male	10–55 U/L	10–55 U/L
14–15 yr		
Female	5–30 U/L	5–30 U/L
Male	10–45 U/L	10–45 U/L
>16 yr		
Female	5–35 U/L	5–35 U/L
Male	10–40 U/L	10–40 U/L

TABLE 27-1

REFERENCE VALUES (Continued)

	Conventional Units	SI Units
ALBUMIN		
(See Proteins)		
ALDOLASE[3]		
(Major sources: Skeletal muscle and myocardium)		
10–24 mo	3.4–11.8 U/L	3.4–11.8 U/L
2–16 yr	1.2–8.8 U/L	1.2–8.8 U/L
Adult	1.7–4.9 U/L	1.7–4.9 U/L
ALKALINE PHOSPHATASE[4]		
(Major sources: Liver, bone, intestinal mucosa, placenta, and kidney)		
Infant	150–420 U/L	150–420 U/L
2–10 yr	100–320 U/L	100–320 U/L
Adolescent male	100–390 U/L	100–390 U/L
Adolescent female	100–320 U/L	100–320 U/L
Adult	30–120 U/L	30–120 U/L
AMMONIA[2]		
(Heparinized venous specimen on ice analyzed within 30 min)		
Newborn	90–150 mcg/dL	64–107 µmol/L
0–2 wk	79–129 mcg/dL	56–92 µmol/L
Infant/child	29–70 mcg/dL	21–50 µmol/L
Adult	15–45 mcg/dL	11–32 µmol/L
AMYLASE[15]		
(Major sources: Pancreas, salivary glands, and ovaries)		
0–14 days	3–10 U/L	3–10 U/L
15 days–13 wk	2–22 U/L	2–22 U/L
13 wk–1 yr	3–50 U/L	3–50 U/L
>1 yr	25–101 U/L	25–101 U/L
ANTINUCLEAR ANTIBODY (ANA)[2] IMMUNOFLUORESCENCE ASSAY (IFA)		
Negative	<1:40	
Patterns with clinical correlation:		
Centromere: CREST*		
Nucleolar: Scleroderma		
Homogeneous: Systemic lupus erythematosus (SLE)		
ANTISTREPTOLYSIN O TITER[5]		
(Fourfold rise in paired serial specimens is significant.)		
Newborn	Similar to mother's value	
6–24 mo	≤50 Todd units/mL	
2–4 yr	≤160 Todd units/mL	
≥5 yr	≤330 Todd units/mL	

TABLE 27-1

REFERENCE VALUES (Continued)

	Conventional Units	SI Units

ASPARTATE AMINOTRANSFERASE (AST)[2]

(Major sources: Liver, skeletal muscle, kidney, myocardium, and erythrocytes)

0–10 days	47–150 U/L	47–150 U/L
10 days–24 mo	9–80 U/L	9–80 U/L
>24 mo		
Female	13–35 U/L	13–35 U/L
Male	15–40 U/L	15–40 U/L

BICARBONATE[2,4]

Newborn	17–24 mEq/L	17–24 mmol/L
Infant	19–24 mEq/L	19–24 mmol/L
2 mo–2 yr	16–24 mEq/L	16–24 mmol/L
>2 yr	22–26 mEq/L	22–26 mmol/L

BILIRUBIN (TOTAL)[4,6]

(Please see Chapter 18 for more complete information about neonatal hyperbilirubinemia and acceptable bilirubin values.)

Cord:		
Term and preterm	<2 mg/dL	<34 µmol/L
0–1 days:		
Term and preterm	<8 mg/dL	<137 µmol/L
1–2 days:		
Preterm	<12 mg/dL	<205 µmol/L
Term	<11.5 mg/dL	<197 µmol/L
3–5 days:		
Preterm	<16 mg/dL	<274 µmol/L
Term	<12 mg/dL	<205 µmol/L
Older infant:		
Preterm	<2 mg/dL	<34 µmol/L
Term	<1.2 mg/dL	<21 µmol/L
Adult	<1.5 mg/dL	<20.5 µmol/L

BILIRUBIN (CONJUGATED)[2–4]

Neonate	<0.6 mg/dL	<10 µmol/L
Infants/children	<0.2 mg/dL	<3.4 µmol/L

BLOOD GAS, ARTERIAL (BREATHING ROOM AIR)[2]

	pH	Pao_2 (mmHg)	$Paco_2$ (mmHg)	HCO_3^- (mEq/L)
Cord blood	7.28 ± 0.05	18.0 ± 6.2	49.2 ± 8.4	14–22
Newborn (birth)	7.11–7.36	8–24	27–40	13–22
5–10 min	7.09–7.30	33–75	27–40	13–22
30 min	7.21–7.38	31–85	27–40	13–22
60 min	7.26–7.49	55–80	27–40	13–22
1 day	7.29–7.45	54–95	27–40	13–22
Child/adult	7.35–7.45	83–108	32–48	20–28

Continued

27

TABLE 27-1

REFERENCE VALUES (Continued)

BLOOD GAS, ARTERIAL (BREATHING ROOM AIR)²

	pH	Pao_2 (mmHg)	$Paco_2$ (mmHg)	HCO_3^- (mEq/L)

NOTE: Venous blood gases can be used to assess acid-base status, not oxygenation. Pco_2 averages 6–8 mmHg higher than $Paco_2$, and pH is slightly lower. Peripheral venous samples are strongly affected by the local circulatory and metabolic environment. Capillary blood gases correlate best with arterial pH and moderately well with $Paco_2$.

	Conventional Units	SI Units
C-REACTIVE PROTEIN⁴	0–0.5 mg/dL	
CALCIUM (TOTAL)²		
Premature neonate	6.2–11 mg/dL	1.55–2.75 mmol/L
0–10 days	7.6–10.4 mg/dL	1.9–2.6 mmol/L
10 days–24 mo	9–11 mg/dL	2.25–2.75 mmol/L
24 mo–12 yr	8.8–10.8 mg/dL	2.2–2.7 mmol/L
12–18 yr	8.4–10.2 mg/dL	2.1–2.55 mmol/L
CALCIUM (IONIZED)³		
0–1 mo	3.9–6.0 mg/dL	1.0–1.5 mmol/L
1–6 mo	3.7–5.9 mg/dL	0.95–1.5 mmol/L
1–18 yr	4.9–5.5 mg/dL	1.22–1.37 mmol/L
Adult	4.75–5.3 mg/dL	1.18–1.32 mmol/L

CARBON DIOXIDE (CO_2 CONTENT)²

(See Blood Gas, Arterial)

CARBON MONOXIDE (CARBOXYHEMOGLOBIN)

Nonsmoker	0.5%–1.5% of total hemoglobin
Smoker	4%–9% of total hemoglobin
Toxic	20%–50% of total hemoglobin
Lethal	>50% of total hemoglobin

	Conventional Units	SI Units
CHLORIDE (SERUM)³		
0–6 mo	97–108 mEq/L	97–108 mmol/L
6–12 mo	97–106 mEq/L	97–106 mmol/L
Child/adult	97–107 mEq/L	97–107 mmol/L

CHOLESTEROL

(See Lipids)

CREATINE KINASE (CREATINE PHOSPHOKINASE)²

(Major sources: Myocardium, skeletal muscle, smooth muscle, and brain)

Newborn	145–1,578 U/L	145–1578 U/L
>6 wk–adult male	20–200 U/L	20–200 U/L
>6 wk–adult female	20–180 U/L	20–180 U/L

TABLE 27-1

REFERENCE VALUES (Continued)

	Conventional Units	SI Units
CREATININE (SERUM)[2] (Enzymatic)		
Cord	0.6–1.2 mg/dL	53–106 µmol/L
Newborn	0.3–1.0 mg/dL	27–88 µmol/L
Infant	0.2–0.4 mg/dL	18–35 µmol/L
Child	0.3–0.7 mg/dL	27–62 µmol/L
Adolescent	0.5–1.0 mg/dL	44–88 µmol/L
Adult male	0.9–1.3 mg/dL	80–115 µmol/L
Adult female	0.6–1.1 mg/dL	53–97 µmol/L
ERYTHROCYTE SEDIMENTATION RATE (ESR)[2]		
Child	0–10 mm/hr	
Adult male	0–15 mm/hr	
Adult female	0–20 mm/hr	
FERRITIN[2]		
Newborn	25–200 ng/mL	56–450 pmol/L
1 mo	200–600 ng/mL	450–1350 pmol/L
2–5 mo	50–200 ng/mL	112–450 pmol/L
6 mo–15 yr	7–140 ng/mL	16–315 pmol/L
Adult male	20–250 ng/mL	45–562 pmol/L
Adult female	10–120 ng/mL	22–270 pmol/L
FIBRINOGEN		
(See Chapter 14)		
FOLATE (SERUM)[3]		
Newborn	16–72 ng/mL	16–72 nmol/L
Child	4–20 ng/mL	4–20 nmol/L
Adult	10–63 ng/mL	10–63 nmol/L
FOLATE (RBC)[2]		
Newborn	150–200 ng/mL	340–453 nmol/L
Infant	74–995 ng/mL	168–2254 nmol/L
2–16 yr	>160 ng/mL	>362 nmol/L
>16 yr	140–628 ng/mL	317–1422 nmol/L
GALACTOSE[2]		
Newborn	0–20 mg/dL	0–1.11 mmol/L
Older child	<5 mg/dL	<0.28 mmol/L
GAMMA-GLUTAMYL TRANSFERASE (GGT)[2,5]		
(Major sources: Liver [biliary tree] and kidney)		
Cord	37–193 U/L	37–193 U/L
0–1 mo	13–147 U/L	13–147 U/L
1–2 mo	12–123 U/L	12–123 U/L
2–4 mo	8–90 U/L	8–90 U/L
4 mo–10 yr	5–32 U/L	5–32 U/L

Continued

TABLE 27-1

REFERENCE VALUES (Continued)

	Conventional Units	SI Units
GAMMA-GLUTAMYL TRANSFERASE (GGT) (Continued)		
10–15 yr	5–24 U/L	5–24 U/L
Adult male	11–49 U/L	11–49 U/L
Adult female	7–32 U/L	7–32 U/L
GLUCOSE (SERUM)[2,5]		
Preterm	20–60 mg/dL	1.1–3.3 mmol/L
Newborn, <1 day	40–60 mg/dL	2.2–3.3 mmol/L
Newborn, >1 day	50–90 mg/dL	2.8–5.0 mmol/L
Child	60–100 mg/dL	3.3–5.5 mmol/L
>16 yr	70–105 mg/dL	3.9–5.8 mmol/L
HAPTOGLOBIN[2]		
Newborn	5–48 mg/dL	50–480 mg/L
>30 days	26–185 mg/dL	260–1850 mg/L
HEMOGLOBIN A$_{1c}$[7]		
Normal	4.5%–5.6%	
At risk for diabetes	5.7%–6.4%	
Diabetes mellitus	≥6.5%	
HEMOGLOBIN F, % TOTAL HEMOGLOBIN (MEAN [SD])[2]		
1 day	77.0 (7.3)	
5 days	76.8 (5.8)	
3 wk	70.0 (7.3)	
6–9 wk	52.9 (11)	
3–4 mo	23.2 (16)	
6 mo	4.7 (2.2)	
8–11 mo	1.6 (1.0)	
Adult	<2.0	
IRON[2]		
Newborn	100–250 mcg/dL	17.9–44.8 µmol/L
Infant	40–100 mcg/dL	7.2–17.9 µmol/L
Child	50–120 mcg/dL	9.0–21.5 µmol/L
Adult male	65–175 mcg/dL	11.6–31.3 µmol/L
Adult female	50–170 mcg/dL	9.0–30.4 µmol/L
LACTATE[2,3]		
Capillary blood:		
0–90 days	9–32 mg/dL	1.1–3.5 mmol/L
3–24 mo	9–30 mg/dL	1.0–3.3 mmol/L
2–18 yr	9–22 mg/dL	1.0–2.4 mmol/L
Venous	4.5–19.8 mg/dL	0.5–2.2 mmol/L
Arterial	4.5–14.4 mg/dL	0.5–1.6 mmol/L
LACTATE DEHYDROGENASE (AT 37°C)[2]		
(Major sources: Myocardium, liver, skeletal muscle, erythrocytes, platelets, and lymph nodes)		
0–4 days	290–775 U/L	290–775 U/L
4–10 days	545–2000 U/L	545–2000 U/L

TABLE 27-1

REFERENCE VALUES (Continued)

	Conventional Units	SI Units
LACTATE DEHYDROGENASE (Continued)		
10 days–24 mo	180–430 U/L	180–430 U/L
24 mo–12 yr	110–295 U/L	110–295 U/L
>12 yr	100–190 U/L	100–190 U/L
LEAD[2]		
Child	<10 mcg/dL	<0.48 µmol/L
LIPASE[3]		
0–30 days	6–55 U/L	6–55 U/L
1–6 mo	4–29 U/L	4–29 U/L
6–12 mo	4–23 U/L	4–23 U/L
>1 yr	3–32 U/L	3–32 U/L

	Cholesterol (mg/dL)			LDL (mg/dL)			HDL (mg/dL)	
	Desirable	Borderline	High	Optimal	Near/Above optimal	Border-line	High	Desirable
LIPIDS[8,9]								
Child/adolescent	<170	170–199	>200	<110		110–129	>130	>35
Adult	<200	200–239	<240	<100	100–129	130–159	>160	40–60

	Conventional Units	SI Units
MAGNESIUM[2]	1.6–2.4 mg/dL	0.63–1.05 mmol/L
METHEMOGLOBIN[2]	0.78% (±0.37%) of total hemoglobin	
OSMOLALITY[2]	275–295 mOsm/kg (neonates as low as 266)	275–295 mmol/kg
PHENYLALANINE[2]		
Preterm	2.0–7.5 mg/dL	121–454 µmol/L
Newborn	1.2–3.4 mg/dL	73–206 µmol/L
Adult	0.8–1.8 mg/dL	48–109 µmol/L
PHOSPHORUS[2]		
0–9 days	4.5–9.0 mg/dL	1.45–2.91 mmol/L
10 days–24 mo	4–6.5 mg/dL	1.29–2.10 mmol/L
3–9 yr	3.2–5.8 mg/dL	1.03–1.87 mmol/L
10–15 yr	3.3–5.4 mg/dL	1.07–1.74 mmol/L
>15 yr	2.4–4.4 mg/dL	0.78–1.42 mmol/L
PORCELAIN[10]	9.0–24.11 mg/dL	9.0–28.13 mmol/L
POTASSIUM[2]		
Preterm	3.0–6.0 mEq/L	3.0–6.0 mmol/L
Newborn	3.7–5.9 mEq/L	3.7–5.9 mmol/L
Infant	4.1–5.3 mEq/L	4.1–5.3 mmol/L
Child	3.4–4.7 mEq/L	3.4–4.7 mmol/L
Adult	3.5–5.1 mEq/L	3.5–5.1 mmol/L

Continued

TABLE 27-1					

REFERENCE VALUES (Continued)

	Conventional Units			SI Units	

PREALBUMIN³

Newborn	7–39 mg/dL	
1–6 mo	8–34 mg/dL	
6 mo–4 yr	12–36 mg/dL	
4–6 yr	12–30 mg/dL	
6–19 yr	12–42 mg/dL	

PROTEIN ELECTROPHORESIS (g/dL)²

Age	Total Protein	Albumin	α-1	α-2	β	γ
Cord	4.8–8.0					
Premature	3.6–6.0					
Newborn	4.6–7.0					
0–15 day	4.4–7.6	3.0–3.9	0.1–0.3	0.3–0.6	0.4–0.6	0.7–1.4
15 day–1 yr	5.1–7.3	2.2–4.8	0.1–0.3	0.5–0.9	0.5–0.9	0.5–1.3
1–2 yr	5.6–7.5	3.6–5.2	0.1–0.4	0.5–1.2	0.5–1.1	0.5–1.7
3–16 yr	6.0–8.0	3.6–5.2	0.1–0.4	0.5–1.2	0.5–1.1	0.5–1.7
≥16 yr	6.0–8.3	3.9–5.1	0.2–0.4	0.4–0.8	0.5–1.0	0.6–1.2

	Conventional Units	SI Units
PYRUVATE³	0.7–1.32 mg/dL	0.08–0.15 mmol/L

RHEUMATOID FACTOR² <30 U/mL

SODIUM¹

<1 yr	130–145 mEq/L	130–145 mmol/L
>1 yr	135–147 mEq/L	135–147 mmol/L

TOTAL IRON-BINDING CAPACITY (TIBC)²

Infant	100–400 mcg/dL	17.9–71.6 μmol/L
Adult	250–425 mcg/dL	44.8–76.1 μmol/L

TOTAL PROTEIN

(See Proteins)

TRANSAMINASE (SGOT)

(See Aspartate aminotransferase [AST])

TRANSAMINASE (SGPT)

(See Alanine aminotransferase [ALT])

TRANSFERRIN²

Newborn	130–275 mg/dL	1.30–2.75 g/L
3 mo–16 yr	203–360 mg/dL	2.03–3.6 g/L
Adult	215–380 mg/dL	2.15–3.8 g/L

TABLE 27-1

REFERENCE VALUES (Continued)

TOTAL TRIGLYCERIDE[3]

	Conventional Units (mg/dL)		SI Units (mmol/L)	
	Male	Female	Male	Female
0–7 days	21–182	28–166	0.24–2.06	0.32–1.88
8–30 days	30–184	30–165	0.34–2.08	0.34–1.86
31–90 days	40–175	35–282	0.45–1.98	0.4–3.19
91–180 days	45–291	50–355	0.51–3.29	0.57–4.01
181–365 days	45–501	36–431	0.51–5.66	0.41–4.87
1–3 yr	27–125	27–125	0.31–1.41	0.31–1.41
4–6 yr	32–116	32–116	0.36–1.31	0.36–1.31
7–9 yr	28–129	28–129	0.32–1.46	0.32–1.46
10–19 yr	24–145	37–140	0.27–1.64	0.42–1.58

	Conventional Units	SI Units
TROPONIN-I[3]		
0–30 days	<4.8 mcg/L	
31–90 days	<0.4 mcg/L	
3–6 mo	<0.3 mcg/L	
7–12 mo	<0.2 mcg/L	
1–18 yr	<0.1 mcg/L	
UREA NITROGEN[1,2]		
Premature (<1 wk)	3–25 mg/dL	1.1–8.9 mmol/L
Newborn	2–19 mg/dL	0.7–6.7 mmol/L
Infant/child	5–18 mg/dL	1.8–6.4 mmol/L
Adult	6–20 mg/dL	2.1–7.1 mmol/L
URIC ACID[3,5]		
0–30 days	1.0–4.6 mg/dL	0.059–0.271 mmol/L
1–12 mo	1.1–5.6 mg/dL	0.065–0.33 mmol/L
1–5 yr	1.7–5.8 mg/dL	0.1–0.35 mmol/L
6–11 yr	2.2–6.6 mg/dL	0.13–0.39 mmol/L
Male 12–19 yr	3.0–7.7 mg/dL	0.18–0.46 mmol/L
Female 12–19 yr	2.7–5.7 mg/dL	0.16–0.34 mmol/L
VITAMIN A (RETINOL)[2,3]		
Preterm	13–46 mcg/dL	0.46–1.61 μmol/L
Full term	18–50 mcg/dL	0.63–1.75 μmol/L
1–6 yr	20–43 mcg/dL	0.7–1.5 μmol/L
7–12 yr	20–49 mcg/dL	0.9–1.7 μmol/L
13–19 yr	26–72 mcg/dL	0.9–2.5 μmol/L
VITAMIN B$_1$ (THIAMINE)[2]	4.5–10.3 mcg/dL	106–242 μmol/L
VITAMIN B$_2$ (RIBOFLAVIN)	4–24 mcg/dL	106–638 nmol/L
VITAMIN B$_{12}$ (COBALAMIN)[2]		
Newborn	160–1300 pg/mL	118–959 pmol/L
Child/adult	200–835 pg/mL	148–616 pmol/L

Continued

27

TABLE 27-1

REFERENCE VALUES (Continued)

	Conventional Units	SI Units
VITAMIN C (ASCORBIC ACID)[2]	0.4–2.0 mg/dL	23–114 μmol/L
VITAMIN D₃ (1,25-DIHY-DROXY-VITAMIN D)[2]	16–65 pg/mL	42–169 pmol/L
VITAMIN E[1,2,3]		
Preterm	0.5–3.5 mg/L	1–8 μmol/L
Full term	1.0–3.5 mg/L	2–8 μmol/L
1–12 yr	3.0–9.0 mg/L	7–21 μmol/L
13–19 yr	6.0–10.0 mg/L	14–23 μmol/L
ZINC[2]	70–120 mcg/dL	10.7–18.4 mmol/L

*CREST: **C**alcinosis, **R**aynaud syndrome, **E**sophageal dysmotility, **S**clerodactyly, **T**elangiectasia.

II. EVALUATION OF BODY FLUIDS

A. Evaluation of Transudate versus Exudate (Table 27-2)

B. Evaluation of Cerebrospinal Fluid (Table 27-3)

C. Evaluation of Synovial Fluid (Table 27-4)

TABLE 27-2

EVALUATION OF TRANSUDATE VS. EXUDATE (PLEURAL, PERICARDIAL, OR PERITONEAL FLUID)

Measurement*	Transudate	Exudate†
Protein (g/dL)	<3.0	>3.0
Fluid/serum ratio	<0.5	≥0.5
LDH (IU)	<200	≥200
Fluid/serum ratio (isoenzymes not useful)	<0.6	≥0.6
WBCs‡	<10,000/μL	>10,000/μL
RBCs	<5000	>5000
Glucose	>40	<40
pH§	>7.2	<7.2

*Always obtain serum for glucose, LDH, protein, amylase, etc.

†All of the following criteria do not have to be met for consideration as an exudate.

‡In peritoneal fluid, WBC count >800/μL suggests peritonitis.

§Collect anaerobically in a heparinized syringe.

NOTE: Amylase >5000 U/mL or pleural fluid/serum ratio >1 suggests pancreatitis.

LDH, Lactate dehydrogenase; RBCs, red blood cells; WBCs, white blood cells.

Data from Nichols DG, Ackerman AD, Carcillo JA, et al. *Rogers Textbook of Pediatric Intensive Care.* 4th ed. Baltimore: Williams & Wilkins, 2008.

SAMPLE ENTRY

regnancy: Refer to explanation of pregnancy categories (see p. 648).
east: Refer to explanation of breast-feeding categories (see p. 648).
idney: Indicates need for caution or need for dose adjustment in renal impairment (see also Chapter 31).
iver: Indicates need for caution or need for dose adjustment in hepatic impairment.
ow supplied

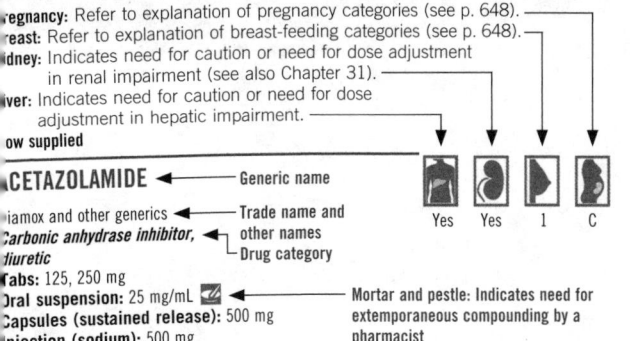

Yes   Yes   1   C

CETAZOLAMIDE ← Generic name

iamox and other generics ← Trade name and other names
Carbonic anhydrase inhibitor, ← Drug category
diuretic
Tabs: 125, 250 mg
Oral suspension: 25 mg/mL ← Mortar and pestle: Indicates need for extemporaneous compounding by a pharmacist
Capsules (sustained release): 500 mg
Injection (sodium): 500 mg
Contains 2.05 mEq Na/500 mg drug

Diuretic (PO, IV)
   Child: 5 mg/kg/dose once daily or every other day
   Adult: 250–375 mg/dose once daily or every other day

Glaucoma
   Child:
      PO: 8–30 mg/kg/24 hr ÷ Q6–8 hr
      IM/IV: 20–40 mg/kg/24 hr ÷ Q6 hr; **max. dose:** 1000 mg/24 hr
   Adult:
      PO (simple chronic; open-angle): 1000 mg/24 hr ÷ Q6 hr
      IV (acute secondary; closed-angle): For rapid decrease in intraocular pressure, administer 500 mg/dose IV

Seizures (extended-release product not recommended):
Child and adult: 8–30 mg/kg/24 hr ÷ Q6–12 hr PO; **max. dose:** 1 g/24 hr

Urine alkalinization:
   Adult: 5 mg/kg/dose PO repeated BID–TID over 24 hr.
Management of hydrocephalus (see remarks): Start with 20 mg/kg/24 hr ÷ Q8 hr PO/IV; may increase to 100 mg/kg/24 hr up to a **max. dose** of 2 g/24 hr.

Pseudotumor cerebri (PO; see remarks):
Child: Start with 25 mg/kg/24 hr ÷ once daily–QID, increase by 25 mg/kg/24 hr until clinical response or as tolerated up to a maximum of 100 mg/kg/24 hr.
Adolescent: Start with 1 g/24 hr ÷ once daily–QID, increase by 250 mg/24 hr until clinical response or as tolerated up to a maximum of 4 g/24 hr.

Drug dosing

Contraindicated in hepatic failure, severe renal failure (GFR <10 mL/min), and hypersensitivity to sulfonamides.
   $T_{1/2}$: 2–6 hr; **do not use** sustained release capsules in seizures; IM injection may be painful; bicarbonate replacement therapy may be required during long-term use (see *Citrate or Sodium Bicarbonate*). For use in pseudotumor cerebri, doses of 60 mg/kg/24 hr may be required.
   Possible side effects (more likely with long-term therapy) include GI irritation, paresthesias, sedation, hypokalemia, acidosis, reduced urate secretion, aplastic anemia, polyuria, and development of renal calculi.
   May increase toxicity of cyclosporine. Aspirin may increase toxicity of acetazolamide. May decrease the effects of salicylates, lithium, and phenobarbital. False-positive urinary protein may occur with several assays. **Adjust dose in renal failure (see Chapter 31).**

Brief remarks about side effects, drug interactions, precautions, therapeutic monitoring, and other relevant information

TABLE 27-3

EVALUATION OF CEREBROSPINAL FLUID

Age[4,11]	WBC Count/µL (median)	95th Percentile
0–28 days	0–12*(3)	19
29–56 days	0–6* (2)	9
Child	0–7	

	Conventional Units	SI Units
GLUCOSE[4,12]		
Preterm	24–63 mg/dL	1.3–3.5 mmol/L
Term	34–119 mg/dL	1.9–6.6 mmol/L
Child	40–80 mg/dL	2.2–4.4 mmol/L
PROTEIN[4,12,13]		
Preterm	65–150 mg/dL	0.65–1.5 g/L
0–14 days	79 (±23) mg/dL†	0.79 (±0.23) g/L†
15–28 days	69 (±20) mg/dL†	0.69 (±0.20) g/L†
29–42 days	58 (±17) mg/dL†	0.58 (±0.17) g/L†
43–56 days	53 (±17) mg/dL†	0.53 (±0.17) g/L†
Child	5–40 mg/dL	5–40 mg/dL

OPENING PRESSURE (LATERAL RECUMBENT POSITION[4,14])

Newborn	8–11 cm H_2O
1–18 yr	11.5–28 cm H_2O*
Respiratory variations	0.5–1 cm H_2O

*Up to 90th percentile.
†Mean (±SD).
WBC, White blood cell.

TABLE 27-4

CHARACTERISTICS OF SYNOVIAL FLUID IN THE RHEUMATIC DISEASES

Group	Condition	Synovial Complement	Color/Clarity	Viscosity	Mucin Clot	WBC Count	PMN (%)	Miscellaneous Findings
Noninflammatory	Normal	N	Yellow Clear	↑↑	G	<200	<25	
	Traumatic arthritis	N	Xanthochromic Turbid	↑	F–G	<2000	<25	Debris
	Osteoarthritis	N	Yellow Clear	↑	F–G	1000	<25	
Inflammatory	Systemic lupus erythematosus	↓	Yellow Clear	N	N	5000	10	Lupus cells
	Rheumatic fever	N–↑	Yellow Cloudy	↑	F	5000	10–50	
	Juvenile rheumatoid arthritis	N–↓	Yellow Cloudy	↑	Poor	15,000–20,000	75	
	Reiter syndrome	↑	Yellow Opaque	↑	Poor	20,000	80	Reiter cells
Pyogenic	Tuberculous arthritis	N–↑	Yellow-white Cloudy	↑	Poor	25,000	50–60	Acid-fast bacteria
	Septic arthritis	↑	Serosanguineous Turbid	↓	Poor	50,000–300,000	>75	Low glucose, bacteria

F, Fair; G, good; H, high; N, normal; PMN, polymorphonuclear leukocyte; WBC, white blood cell; ↓, decreased; ↑, increased.
From Cassidy JT, Petty RE. *Textbook of Pediatric Rheumatology.* 5th ed. Philadelphia: WB Saunders, 2005.

III. CONVERSION FORMULAS

A. Temperature

1. **To convert degrees Celsius to degrees Fahrenheit:**

$$([9/5] \times \text{Temperature}) + 32$$

2. **To convert degrees Fahrenheit to degrees Celsius:**

$$(\text{Temperature} - 32) \times (5/9)$$

B. Length and Weight

1. **Length:** To convert inches to centimeters, multiply by 2.54.
2. **Weight:** To convert pounds to kilograms, divide by 2.2.

REFERENCES

1. Meites S, ed. *Pediatric Clinical Chemistry.* 3rd ed. Washington, DC: American Association for Clinical Chemistry, 1989.
2. Wu Alan HB. *Tietz Guide to Laboratory Tests.* 4th ed. Philadelphia: WB Saunders, 2006.
3. Soldin SJ, Brugnara C, Wong EC. *Pediatric Reference Intervals.* 6th ed. Washington, DC: Americal Association for Clinical Chemistry Press, 2007.
4. McMillan JA. *Oski's Pediatrics: Principles and Practice.* 4th ed. Philadelphia: JB Lippincott, 2006.
5. Kleigman RM, Behrman RE, Jenson HB, et al. *Nelson Textbook of Pediatrics.* 18th ed. Philadelphia: WB Saunders, 2007.
6. Chernecky CC, Berger BJ. *Laboratory Tests and Diagnostic Procedures.* 5th ed. St Louis: Elsevier, 2008.
7. American Diabetes Association. Diagnosis and classification of diabetes mellitus—2010. *Diabetes Care.* 2010;33:S62-S69.
8. National Cholesterol Education Program (NCEP). Highlights of the report of the Expert Panel on Blood Cholesterol Levels in Children and Adolescents. NCEP Expert Panel on Blood Cholesterol Levels in Children and Adolescents. *Pediatrics.* 1992;89:495-501.
9. Executive Summary of the Third Report of the National Cholesterol Education Program (NCEP) Expert Panel on Detection, Evaluation, and Treatment of High Blood Cholesterol in Adults (Adult Treatment Panel III). *JAMA.* 2001;285:2486-2497.
10. Engorn, BM, Flerlage, JE. *Best Times of Our Lives: KME and TTF.* Baltimore: Johns Hopkins University Press, 2013-2014.
11. Kestenbaum LA, Ebberson J, Zorc JJ, et al. Defining cerebrospinal fluid white blood cell count reference values in neonates and young infants. *Pediatrics.* 2010;125:257-264.
12. Sarff LD, Platt LH, McCracken GH. Cerebrospinal fluid evaluation in neonates: comparison of high-risk infants with and without meningitis. *J Pediatr.* 1976;883:473-477.
13. Shah SS, Ebberson J, Kestenbaum LA, et al. Age-specific reference values for cerebrospinal fluid protein concentration in neonates and young infants. *J Hosp Med.* 2011;6:22-27.
14. Avery RA, Shah SS., Licht DJ.Reference range for cerebrospinal fluid opening pressure in children. *N Engl J Med.* 2010;363:891-893.
15. Colantonio DA, Kyriakopoulou L, Chan MK, et al. Closing the gaps in pediatric laboratory reference intervals: a CALIPER database of 40 biochemical markers in a healthy and multiethnic population of children. *Clin Chem.* 2012;58:854-868.

Chapter 28

Biostatistics and Evidence-Based Medicine

Kari Bjornard, MD, MPH

I. WEBSITES

A. Evidence-Based Resources

Centre for Evidence Based Medicine: http://www.cebm.net
Cochrane Reviews: http://www.thecochranelibrary.com/view/0/index.html
JAMA evidence: www.jamaevidence.com
Johns Hopkins University Welch Medical Library: Evidence Based
    Medicine Resources: http://www.welch.jhu.edu/internet/ebr.html
National Guideline Clearing House: http://guideline.gov/
University of Washington Healthlinks: Evidence-Based Practice:
    http://libguides.hsl.washington.edu/ebp

B. Statistics Resources and Software

BMJ Statistics at Square One:
http://www.bmj.com/collections/statsbk/index.dtl
EpiInfo: http://www.cdc.gov/epiinfo/
Open Epi: http://www.OpenEpi.com/OE2.3/Menu/OpenEpiMenu.htm

II. EVIDENCE-BASED MEDICINE

Evidence-based medicine refers to the method of integrating individual clinical expertise with the best available evidence from systematic research. It typically involves the following framework[1]:

A. Formulate the clinical question:

1. **Describe the patient or problem,** deciding whether the evidence you seek is on therapy, diagnosis or screening, prognosis, etiology or causation, cost-effectiveness, or a qualitative study.
2. **Describe the intervention** under consideration.
3. **Compare the intervention** with an alternative or standard of care if applicable.
4. **Formulate a specific outcome** of interest.

B. Search for the evidence to answer that question:

1. **Define search terms** that fit the clinical question.
2. **Develop your search strategy** using PubMed or other primary search sources. National Guideline Clearing House is a public resource for evidence-based practice guidelines: http://guideline.gov/.
3. **Review your results** and apply methodological filters to target the right type of study.

C. Critically appraise the evidence—decide whether the study findings are valid and whether they are important to your question:

1. **Therapy:**
a. Were patient groups randomized for treatment?
b. Were groups comparable and treated equally aside from the allocated treatment?
c. Were study subjects and investigators blinded?
d. Were all patients entering the trial accounted for in the groups they were randomized to (intention to treat)?
e. How large was the treatment effect (see Section III C. 5–7), and how precise was the estimate of the treatment effect?

2. **Diagnosis:**
a. Was the test compared with an independent blind reference (gold) standard of diagnosis?
b. Was the test evaluated in an appropriate spectrum of patients?

3. **Prognosis:**
a. Were study patients defined early in their course and followed up over a sufficient time?
b. How likely are these outcomes over a defined time period, and how precise are estimates of prognosis?

4. **Guidelines for judging causality of an association between a variable and outcome[3]:**
a. Is there a temporal relationship?
b. What is the strength of association?
c. Is there a dose/response relationship?
d. Were the findings replicated?
e. Is there biological plausibility?
f. Are there alternative explanations?
g. What happens with cessation of exposure?
h. Is this explanation consistent with other knowledge?
i. How specific is the association?

5. **For more comprehensive criteria or other types of studies,** use appropriate appraisal frameworks.[1]

D. Apply the evidence to the clinical question:

If the evidence is valid and important, integrate it with your clinical expertise. Decide whether patients in the study were similar to your individual patient and whether:

1. **Patient will benefit from the therapy** and accept its regimen and consequences
2. **Test is available, affordable, accurate, and precise**
3. **Study findings will impact what to tell or offer the patient**

III. BIOSTATISTICS FOR MEDICAL LITERATURE

A. Statistical Tests: Table 28-1

1. **Different statistics apply to test a hypothesis of whether observed differences are statistically significant:**

TABLE 28-1

SOME COMMONLY USED STATISTICAL TESTS[2]

Parametric Test	Nonparametric Test	Purpose of Test	Example
Two-sample (unpaired) t test	Mann-Whitney U test	Compares two independent samples	To compare girls' heights with boys' heights
One-sample (paired) t test	Wilcoxon matched pairs test	Compares two sets of observations on a single sample	To compare weight of infants before and after a feeding
One-way analysis of variance (F test) using total sum of squares (ANOVA)	Kruskall-Wallis analysis of variance by ranks	Effectively, a generalization of the paired t or Wilcoxon matched pairs test where three or more sets of observations are made on a single sample	To determine whether plasma glucose level is higher 1 hour, 2 hours, or 3 hours after a meal
Two-way analysis of variance (ANOVA)	Two-way analysis of variance by ranks	As above, but tests the influence (and interaction) of two different covariates	In the above example, to determine whether the results differ in male and female subjects
χ^2 test	Fisher's exact test	Tests the null hypothesis that the distribution of a discontinuous variable is the same in two (or more) independent samples	To assess whether male or female adolescents are more likely to smoke
Product moment correlation coefficient (Pearson's r)	Spearman's rank correlation coefficient (r_σ)	Assesses the strength of the straight-line association between two continuous variables	To assess whether and to what extent plasma HbA_{1c} concentration is related to plasma triglyceride concentration in diabetic patients
Regression by least squares method	Nonparametric regression (various tests)	Describes the numerical relation between two quantitative variables, allowing one value to be predicted from the other	To see how peak expiratory flow rate varies with height
Multiple regression by least squares method	Nonparametric regression (various tests)	Describes the numerical relationship between a dependent variable and several predictor variables (covariates)	To determine whether and to what extent a person's age, body fat, and sodium intake determine his or her blood pressure

Modified from Greenhalgh T. How to read a paper. Statistics for the non-statistician. I: different types of data need different statistical tests. *BMJ*. 1997;315:364-366.

a. *Parametric statistical tests* are more powerful and used when data follow a normal distribution. *Nonparametric tests* are used when a normal distribution cannot be assumed; they rank data rather than taking absolute differences into account.

b. *Paired tests* are performed on paired data—for example, when the same parameter or observation is measured twice on each study subject, often before and after an intervention. *Unpaired tests* compare values from independent samples.

c. A *two-tailed test* has to be performed whenever an intervention could potentially lead to either an increase or decrease of the parameter. When the difference can go in only one direction, a *one-tailed test* can be used, which has greater statistical power.

2. ***Correlation* and *regression* describe the degree of linear association between two quantitative variables,** but they do not imply causation

a. *Correlation* measures the strength of association between two values, expressed by the *correlation coefficient r*, also termed *Pearson's correlation coefficient*.

b. As a next step of describing association, the *regression equation* constructs the optimal straight line illustrating the correlation and allows prediction of a (dependent) variable from a known (independent) variable. The method of *multiple regression* is used when there are multiple independent variables. Multiple regression accounts for influences of various factors on the outcome.

3. **α (Alpha—significance level of statistical test):**

a. Definition: Probability of finding a statistical association by chance alone when in reality there is no association (type I error).

b. The level of α is typically set at ≤0.05 but can be set where a study determines, which allows interpretation with 95% certainty that a detected association is true.

c. The *P* value (probability of a difference occurring by chance) is complementary to α. If *P* is less than the significance level (typically set at ≤0.05), the detected association is unlikely to be due to chance alone.

4. **Power (of a statistical test):**

a. β (Beta) = probability of finding no statistical association when there truly is one (type II error)

b. Power = $1 - β$ = probability of finding a statistical association when there truly is one

c. Power typically set at a minimum of 0.80, which allows interpretation with 80% certainty that a detected lack of association is true

5. **Sample size:** Number of subjects required in a study to detect a certain (expected) effect magnitude with a sufficiently high power and sufficiently low α.

6. **Confidence interval (95%):** Describes the 95% certainty that the reported interval contains the true population value. When confidence intervals (CIs) for groups overlap, they do not differ in a statistically significant manner.

7. **Confounding:** Variable associated with both the disease and the exposure variable, which can cause a misperceived relationship between the disease and exposure. Can be controlled for by matching, blinding, and randomization.
8. **Effect modification (interaction):** Variable that affects or modifies the observed effect of a risk factor or exposure on disease status
a. Stratification can elucidate effect modification if there is a difference in the risk ratio across strata.

B. Study Design Comparison (Table 28-2)

TABLE 28-2

STUDY DESIGN COMPARISON

Design Type	Definition	Advantages	Disadvantages
Case-control (often called retrospective)	Define diseased subjects (cases) and non-diseased subjects (controls); compare proportion of cases with exposure (risk factor) with proportion of controls with exposure (risk factor)	Good for rare diseases Small sample size Shorter study times (not followed over time) Less expensive	Highest potential for biases (recall, selection, and others) Weak evidence for causality No prevalence, PPV, NPV
Cohort (usually prospective; occasionally retrospective)	In study population, define exposed group (with risk factor) and non-exposed group (without risk factor) Over time, compare proportion of exposed group with outcome (disease) with proportion of non-exposed group with outcome (disease)	Defines incidence Stronger evidence for causality Decreases biases (sampling, measurement, reporting)	Expensive Long study times May not be feasible for rare diseases/outcomes Factors related to exposure and outcome may falsely alter effect of exposure on outcome (confounding)
Cross-sectional	In study population, concurrently measure outcome (disease) and risk factor Compare proportion of diseased group with risk factor with proportion of non-diseased group with risk factor	Defines prevalence Short time to complete	Selection bias Weak evidence for causality

TABLE 28-2

STUDY DESIGN COMPARISON (Continued)

Design Type	Definition	Advantages	Disadvantages
Clinical trial (experiment)	In study population, assign (randomly) subjects to receive treatment or receive no treatment Compare rate of outcome (e.g., disease cure) between treatment and nontreatment groups	Randomized blinded trial is gold standard Randomization reduces confounding Best evidence for causality	Expensive Risks of experimental treatments in humans Longer study time Not suitable for rare outcomes/diseases
Meta-analysis (type of systematic review)	Collates data from multiple independent studies to maximize precision and power in testing for statistical significance	Higher statistical power Can control for inter-study variation	Possible bias in exclusion of published studies or publication bias

NPV, Negative predictive value; PPV, positive predictive value.

C. Measurements of Disease Occurrence and Treatment Effects (Table 28-3)

1. Prevalence:
a. Proportion of study population who have a disease (at one point in time)
b. Number of total cases in a population (old and new) at a specific time, divided by total population at that time
c. Prevalence = incidence x duration of disease
d. In cross-sectional studies (see Table 28-3):

$$(A + B)/(A + B + C + D)$$

2. Incidence:
a. Number of new cases in study population who newly develop an outcome (disease) per total study population at risk per given time period
b. Number of new cases divided by the total population over a given time period
c. For cohort studies and clinical trials (see Table 28-3):

$$(A + B)/(A + B + C + D)$$

3. Relative risk (RR):
a. Ratio of incidence of disease among people with risk factor to incidence of disease among people without risk factor
b. For cohort studies or clinical trials (see Table 28-3):

$$[A/(A + C)]/[B/(B + D)]$$

c. Values:
   (1) RR = 1: No effect of exposure (or treatment) on outcome (or disease)
   (2) RR < 1: Exposure or treatment protective against outcome
   (3) RR > 1: Exposure or treatment increases probability of outcome

TABLE 28-3

GRID FOR CALCULATIONS IN CLINICAL STUDIES

	Exposure or Risk Factor or Treatment	
Disease or Outcome	**Positive**	**Negative**
Positive	A	B
Negative	C	D

4. **Odds ratio (OR):**
a. For case-control studies, ratio of [odds of having risk factor in people with disease (A/B)] to [odds of having risk factor in people without disease (C/D)] (see Table 28-3):

$$(A/B)/(C/D) = (A \times D)/(B \times C)$$

b. OR approximates RR when disease is rare (incidence < 0.10):
    (1) OR = 1: No association between risk factor and disease
    (2) OR < 1: Suggests that risk factor is protective against disease
    (3) OR > 1: Suggests association between risk factor and disease

5. **Absolute risk reduction (ARR), absolute risk difference:**
a. Definition: Absolute difference the treatment makes, expressed as difference between (risk of the outcome in control group) minus (risk of the outcome in treatment group)

6. **Relative risk reduction (RRR):**
a. Definition: Clinical significance of treatment effect, expressed as (absolute risk reduction) divided by (risk of the outcome in control group), or 1 − RR

7. **Number needed to treat (NNT):**
a. Definition: Number of patients to be treated with treatment under question to prevent one undesirable outcome expressed as the inverse of the ARR, or 1 ÷ ARR

D. **Measurements of Test Validity and Reliability (Table 28-4)**

1. **Sensitivity (Sens):**
a. Proportion of all diseased who have positive test (see Table 28-4):

$$A/(A + C)$$

b. Measures the ability of the test to correctly identify those who have the disease. Use highly sensitive test to help exclude a disease. (Low false-negative rate. Desirable for screening tests.) Not affected by disease prevalence.

2. **Specificity (Spec):**
a. Proportion of all non-diseased who have a negative test (see Table 28-4):

$$D/(B + D)$$

b. Measures the ability of the test to correctly identify those who do not have the disease. Use highly specific test to help confirm a disease. (Low false-positive rate.) Not affected by disease prevalence.

TABLE 28-4

TABLE 28-4

GRID FOR EVALUATING A CLINICAL TEST

	Disease Status	
Test Result	**Positive**	**Negative**
Positive	A (true positive)	B (false positive)
Negative	C (false negative)	D (true negative)

3. **Positive predictive value (PPV):**
a. Proportion of all those with positive tests who truly have disease (see Table 28-4):

$$A/(A + B)$$

b. Increased PPV with higher disease prevalence and higher specificity (and to a lesser degree, higher sensitivity)

4. **Negative predictive value (NPV):**
a. Proportion of all those with negative tests who truly do not have disease (see Table 28-4):

$$D/(C + D)$$

b. Increased NPV with lower prevalence (rarer disease) and higher sensitivity

5. **Likelihood ratio (LR):**
a. LR positive: Ability of positive test result to confirm diseased status:
$$\text{LR positive} = (\text{Sens})/(1 - \text{Spec})$$

b. LR negative: Ability of negative test result to confirm nondiseased status:
$$\text{LR negative} = (\text{Spec})/(1 - \text{Sens})$$
$$[\text{Alternative LR negative} = (1 - \text{Sens})/\text{Spec}]$$

c. Good tests have LR ≥10. (Good tests have LR ≤0.1 if using alternative LR-negative formula.) Physical examination findings often have LR of about 2.

d. LR should not be affected by disease prevalence. Can be used to calculate increase in probability of disease from baseline prevalence with positive test (LR positive) and decrease in probability of disease from baseline prevalence with negative test (using alternative LR negative) for any level of disease prevalence.

28

REFERENCES

1. Straus SE, Richardson WS, Glasziou P, et al. *Evidence-Based Medicine*. 3rd ed. Edinburgh: Churchill Livingstone, 2005.
2. Greenhalgh T. How to read a paper. Statistics for the non-statistician. I: different types of data need different statistical tests. *BMJ*. 1997;315:364-366.
3. Gordis L. From association to causation: deriving inferences from epidemiologic studies. In: *Epidemiology*. 4th ed. Philadelphia: Elsevier Saunders, 2009.
4. Rosner B. In: Rosner B. *Fundamentals of Biostatistics*. 6th ed. Belmont, Calif: Duxbury Press, 2006.

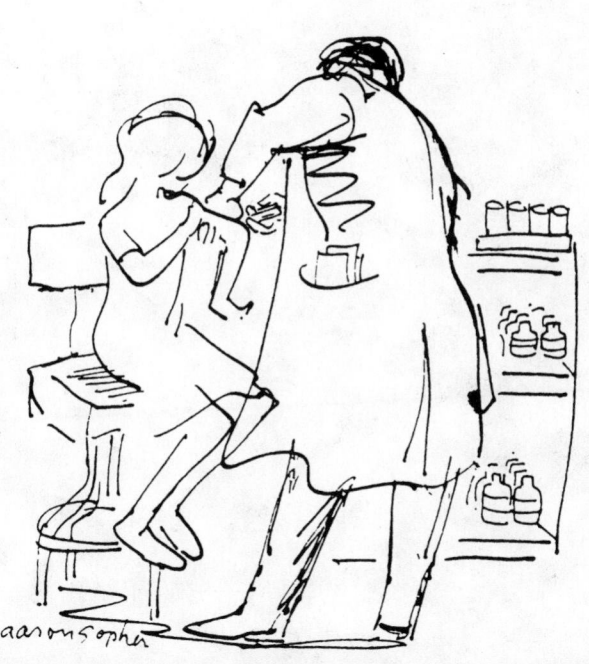

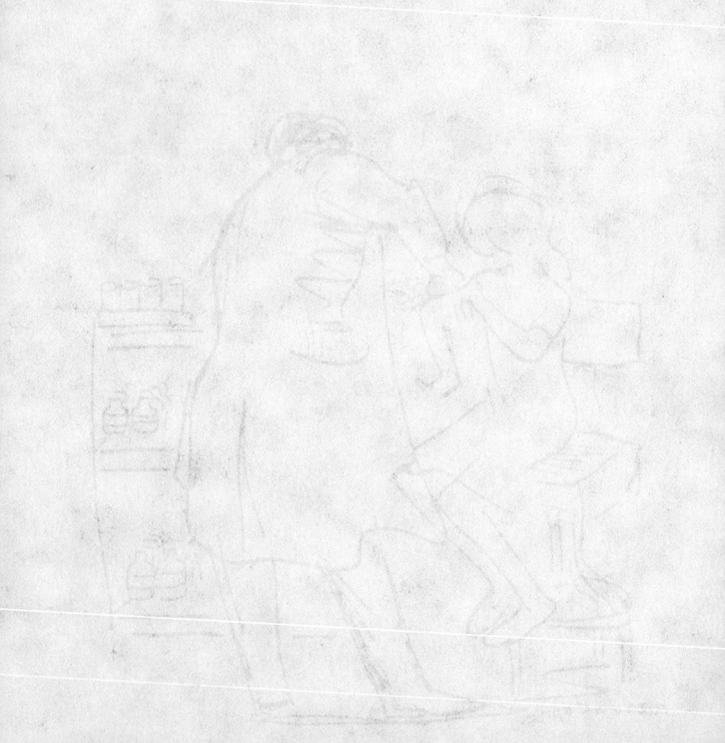

Chapter 29

Drug Dosages

Carlton K.K. Lee, PharmD, MPH;
Branden Engorn, MD; and Jamie Flerlage, MD

I. NOTE TO READER

The authors have made every attempt to check dosages and medical content for accuracy. Because of the incomplete data on pediatric dosing, many drug dosages will be modified after the publication of this text. We recommend that the reader check product information and published literature for changes in dosing, especially for newer medicines. The U.S. Food and Drug Administration (FDA) provides the following pediatric drug information data sources:

New Pediatric Labeling Information: www.fda.gov/NewPedLabeling

Drug Safety Reporting Updates: www.fda.gov/PedDrugSafety

Pediatric Study Characteristics Database: www.fda.gov/PedStudies

To prevent prescribing errors, the use of abbreviations has been greatly discouraged. The following is a list of abbreviations The Joint Commission considers prohibited for use.

29

THE JOINT COMMISSION

Official "Do Not Use" List*

Do Not Use	Potential Problem	Use Instead
U (unit)	Mistaken for "0" (zero), the number "4" (four) or "cc"	Write "unit"
IU (International Unit)	Mistaken for IV (intravenous) or the number 10 (ten)	Write "International Unit"
Q.D., QD, q.d., qd (daily)	Mistaken for each other	Write "daily"
Q.O.D., QOD, q.o.d., qod (every other day)	Period after the Q mistaken for "I" and the "O" mistaken for "I"	Write "every other day"
Trailing zero (X.0 mg)† Lack of leading zero (.X mg)	Decimal point is missed	Write X mg Write 0.X mg
MS	Can mean morphine sulfate or magnesium sulfate	Write "morphine sulfate" Write "magnesium sulfate"
MSO₄ and MgSO₄	Confused for one another	

*Applies to all orders and all medication-related documentation that is handwritten (including free-text computer entry) or on preprinted forms.

†Exception: A "trailing zero" may be used only where required to demonstrate the level of precision of the value being reported, such as for laboratory results, imaging studies that report size of lesions, or catheter/tube sizes. It may not be used in medication orders or other medication-related documentation.

Additional Abbreviations, Acronyms, and Symbols (For possible future inclusion in the Official "Do Not Use" List)

Do Not Use	Potential Problem	Use Instead
> (greater than) < (less than)	Misinterpreted as the number "7" (seven) or the letter "L" Confused for one another	Write "greater than" Write "less than"
Abbreviations for drug names	Misinterpreted due to similar abbreviations for multiple drugs	Write drug names in full
Apothecary units	Unfamiliar to many practitioners Confused with metric units	Use metric units
@	Mistaken for the number "2" (two)	Write "at"
cc	Mistaken for U (units) when poorly written	Write "mL" or "ml" or "milliliters" ("mL" is preferred)
µg	Mistaken for mg (milligrams), resulting in one thousand–fold overdose	Write "mcg" or "micrograms"

II. SAMPLE ENTRY

ACETAZOLAMIDE
Diamox and generics
Carbonic anhydrase inhibitor, diuretic

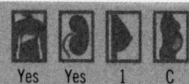

Yes   Yes   1   C

Tabs: 125, 250 mg
Oral suspension: 25 mg/mL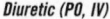
Capsules (extended release): 500 mg
Injection (sodium): 500 mg
Contains 2.05 mEq Na/500 mg drug

Diuretic (PO, IV)
   Child: 5 mg/kg/dose once daily or every other day
   Adult: 250–375 mg/dose once daily or every other day
Glaucoma
   Child:
      PO: 8–30 mg/kg/24 hr ÷ Q6–8 hr
      IM/IV: 20–40 mg/kg/24 hr ÷ Q6 hr; **max. dose:** 1000 mg/24 hr
   Adult:
      PO (simple chronic; open-angle): 1000 mg/24 hr ÷ Q6 hr
      IV (acute secondary; closed-angle): For rapid decrease in intraocular pressure, administer
      500 mg/dose IV
Seizures (extended-release product not recommended):
   Child and adult: 8–30 mg/kg/24 hr ÷ Q6–12 hr PO; **max. dose:** 1 g/24 hr
Urine alkalinization:
   Adult: 5 mg/kg/dose PO repeated BID–TID over 24 hr
Management of hydrocephalus (see remarks): Start with 20 mg/kg/24 hr ÷ Q8 hr PO/IV; may
increase to 100 mg/kg/24 hr up to a **max. dose** of 2 g/24 hr.
Pseudotumor cerebri (PO; see remarks):
   Child: Start with 25 mg/kg/24 hr ÷ once daily–QID; increase by 25 mg/kg/24 hr until clinical
   response or as tolerated up to a **maximum** of 100 mg/kg/24 hr.
   Adolescent: Start with 1 g/24 hr ÷ once daily–QID; increase by 250 mg/24 hr until clinical response
   or as tolerated up to a **maximum** of 4 g/24 hr.

Contraindicated in hepatic failure, severe renal failure (GFR < 10 mL/min), and
hypersensitivity to sulfonamides.

$T_{1/2}$: 2–6 hr; **do not use** sustained-release capsules in seizures; IM injection may be painful;
bicarbonate replacement therapy may be required during long-term use (see *Citrate* or *Sodium
Bicarbonate*). For use in pseudotumor cerebri, doses of 60 mg/kg/24 hr may be required.

Possible side effects (more likely with long-term therapy) include GI irritation, paresthesias, sedation,
hypokalemia, acidosis, reduced urate secretion, aplastic anemia, polyuria, and development of renal
calculi.

May increase toxicity of cyclosporine. Aspirin may increase toxicity of acetazolamide. May decrease the
effects of salicylates, lithium, and phenobarbital. False-positive urinary protein may occur with
several assays. **Adjust dose in renal failure (see Chapter 31).**

III. EXPLANATION OF BREAST-FEEDING CATEGORIES

See sample entry on p. 647.
1 Compatible
2 Use with caution
3 Unknown with concerns
X Contraindicated
? Safety not established

IV. EXPLANATION OF PREGNANCY CATEGORIES

A Adequate studies in pregnant women have not demonstrated a risk to the fetus in the first trimester of pregnancy, and there is no evidence of risk in later trimesters.

B Animal studies have not demonstrated a risk to the fetus, but there are no adequate studies in pregnant women; or animal studies have shown an adverse effect, but adequate studies in pregnant women have not demonstrated a risk to the fetus during the first trimester of pregnancy, and there is no evidence of risk in later trimesters.

C Animal studies have shown an adverse effect on the fetus, but there are no adequate studies in humans; or there are no animal reproduction studies and no adequate studies in humans.

D There is evidence of human fetal risk, but the potential benefits from the use of the drug in pregnant women may be acceptable despite its potential risks.

X Studies in animals or humans demonstrate fetal abnormalities or adverse reaction; reports indicate evidence of fetal risk. The risk of use in pregnant women clearly outweighs any possible benefit.

V. DRUG INDEX

Trade Names	Generic Name
1,25-dihydroxycholecalciferol	Calcitriol
2-PAM*	Pralidoxime Chloride
3TC*	Lamivudine
5-aminosalicylic acid	Mesalamine
5-ASA	Mesalamine
5-FC*	Flucytosine
5-Fluorocytosine*	Flucytosine
8-Arginine Vasopressin*	Vasopressin
9-Fluorohydrocortisone*	Fludrocortisone Acetate
27% Elemental Ca	Calcium Chloride
A-200	Pyrethrins
Abelcet	Amphotericin B Lipid Complex
Absorica	Isotretinoin
Abstra	Fentanyl
Accolate	Zafirlukast
AccuNeb (prediluted nebulized solution)	Albuterol
Accutane	Isotretinoin
Acetadote	Acetylcysteine

*Common abbreviation or other name (not recommended for use when writing a prescription).

Trade Names	Generic Name
Acticin	Permethrin
Actigall	Ursodiol
Actiq	Fentanyl
Activase	Alteplase
Acular, Acular LS	Ketorolac
Acuvail	Ketorolac
Aczone	Dapsone
Adalat CC	Nifedipine
Adderall, Adderall XR	Dextroamphetamine + Amphetamine
Adenocard	Adenosine
Adoxa	Doxycycline
Adrenaline	Epinephrine HCl
Advair Diskus, Advair HFA	Fluticasone Propionate and Salmeterol
Advil, Children's Advil	Ibuprofen
Aerospan	Flunisolide
Afrin	Oxymetazoline
AK-Poly-Bac Ophthalmic	Bacitracin + Polymyxin B
AK-Spore H.C. Otic	Polymyxin B Sulfate, Neomycin Sulfate, Hydrocortisone
AK-Sulf	Sulfacetamide Sodium Ophthalmic
AKTob	Tobramycin
AK-Tracin Ophthalmic	Bacitracin
Albuminar	Albumin, Human
Albutein	Albumin, Human
Aldactone	Spironolactone
Aleve [OTC]	Naproxen/Naproxen Sodium
Allegra, Allegra ODT	Fexofenadine
Allegra-D 12 Hour, Allegra-D 24 Hour	Fexofenadine + Pseudoephedrine
Allergen Ear Drops	Antipyrine and Benzocaine
Alloprim	Allopurinol
Almacone, Almacone II Double Strength	Aluminum Hydroxide with Magnesium Hydroxide
Alsuma	Sumatriptan Succinate
AlternaGEL	Aluminum Hydroxide
Alu-Cap	Aluminum Hydroxide
Alvesco	Ciclesonide
AmBisome	Amphotericin B, Liposomal
Amicar	Aminocaproic Acid
Amikin	Amikacin Sulfate
Amnesteem	Isotretinoin
Amoclan	Amoxicillin-Clavulanic Acid
Amoxil	Amoxicillin
Amphadase	Hyaluronidase
Amphocin	Amphotericin B
Amphojel	Aluminum Hydroxide
Anacin	Aspirin
Anaprox	Naproxen/Naproxen Sodium
Ancef	Cefazolin
Ancobon	Flucytosine
Anectine	Succinylcholine
Antilirium	Physostigmine Salicylate

*Common abbreviation or other name (not recommended for use when writing a prescription).

29

Trade Names	Generic Name
Antipyrine and Benzocaine Otic	Antipyrine and Benzocaine
Antizol	Fomepizole
Anzemet	Dolasetron
Apresoline	Hydralazine Hydrochloride
Apriso	Mesalamine
Aquachloral Supprettes	Chloral Hydrate
Aquasol A	Vitamin A
Aquasol E	Vitamin E
Aquavit-E	Vitamin E
Aralen	Chloroquine HCl/Phosphate
Aranesp	Darbepoetin Alfa
Arbinoxa	Carbinoxamine
Arestin	Minocycline
Aridol	Mannitol
Aristospan	Triamcinolone
ASA*	Aspirin
Asacol, Asacol HD	Mesalamine
Asmanex Twisthaler	Mometasone Furoate
Asprin Free Anacin	Acetaminophen
Astelin	Azelastine
Astepro	Azelastine
Astragraf XL	Tacrolimus
Ativan	Lorazepam
AtroPen	Atropine Sulfate
Atrovent	Ipratropium Bromide
Augmentin, Augmentin ES-600, Augmentin XR	Amoxicillin-Clavulanic Acid
Auralgan (available in Canada)	Antipyrine and Benzocaine
Auro Ear Drops	Carbamide Peroxide
Avinza	Morphine Sulfate
Avita	Tretinoin
Ayr Saline	Sodium Chloride—Inhaled Preparations
Azactam	Aztreonam
Azasan	Azathioprine
Azasite	Azithromycin
Azo-Standard [OTC]	Phenazopyridine HCl
Azulfidine, Azulfidine EN-Tabs	Sulfasalazine
Baciguent Topical	Bacitracin
Bactrim	Sulfamethoxazole and Trimethoprim
Bactroban, Bactroban Nasal	Mupirocin
BAL*	Dimercaprol
Beconase AQ	Beclomethasone Dipropionate
Benadryl	Diphenhydramine
Benzac AC Wash 2 ½, 5, 10; Benzac 5, 10	Benzoyl Peroxide
Beta-Val	Betamethasone
Bethkis	Tobramycin
Biaxin, Biaxin XL	Clarithromycin
Bicillin C-R, Bicillin C-R 900/300	Penicillin G Preparations—Penicillin G Benzathine and Penicillin G Procaine
Bicillin L-A	Penicillin G Preparations—Benzathine

*Common abbreviation or other name (not recommended for use when writing a prescription).

Trade Names	Generic Name
Bio-Statin	Nystatin
Bioxiverz	Neostigmine
Bleph 10	Sulfacetamide Sodium Ophthalmic
Brevibloc	Esmolol HCl
Brevoxyl Creamy Wash	Benzoyl Peroxide
Brisdelle	Paroxetine
British anti-Lewisite	Dimercaprol
Bufferin	Aspirin
Bumex	Bumetanide
Buminate	Albumin, Human
Cafcit	Caffeine Citrate
Cafergot	Ergotamine Tartrate + Caffeine
Calcidol	Ergocalciferol
Caldolor	Ibuprofen
Calan, Calan SR	Verapamil
Calciferol	Ergocalciferol
Calcijex	Calcitriol
Calcionate	Calcium Glubionate
Calciquid	Calcium Glubionate
Cal-Citrate	Calcium Citrate
Calcium disodium versenate	Edetate (EDTA) Calcium Disodium
Cal-Glu	Calcium Gluconate
Cal-Lac	Calcium Lactate
Calphron	Calcium Acetate
Camphorated opium tincture	Paregoric
Canasa	Mesalamine
Cancidas	Caspofungin
Cankaid	Carbamide Peroxide
Capoten	Captopril
Carafate	Sucralfate
Carbatrol	Carbamazepine
Cardene, Cardene SR	Nicardipine
Cardizem, Cardizem SR, Cardizem CD, Cardizem LA	Diltiazem
Carnitor	Carnitine
Catapres, Catapres TTS	Clonidine
Cathflo Activase	Alteplase
Caysten	Aztreonam
Ceclor, Ceclor CD	Cefaclor
Cecon	Ascorbic Acid
Cedax	Ceftibuten
Cefotan	Cefotetan
Ceftin	Cefuroxime Axetil
Cefzil	Cefprozil
Celestone	Betamethasone
CellCept	Mycophenolate Mofetil
Cephulac	Lactulose
Ceptaz	Ceftazidime
Cerebyx	Fosphenytoin
Chemet	Succimer

*Common abbreviation or other name (not recommended for use when writing a prescription).

29

Trade Names	Generic Name
Chloromycetin	Chloramphenicol
Chlor-Trimeton	Chlorpheniramine Maleate
Cholestyramine Light	Cholestyramine
Chronulac	Lactulose
Ciloxan ophthalmic	Ciprofloxacin
Cipro, Cipro XR, Ciprodex, Cipro HC Otic	Ciprofloxacin
Citracel	Calcium Citrate
Claforan	Cefotaxime
Claravis	Isotretinoin
Claritin, Claritin Children's Allergy, Claritin RediTabs	Loratadine
Claritin-D 12 Hour, Claritin-D 24 Hour	Loratadine + Pseudoephedrine
Cleocin-T, Cleocin	Clindamycin
Cogentin	Benztropine Mesylate
Colace	Docusate
Colocort	Hydrocortisone
CoLyte	Polyethylene Glycol—Electrolyte Solution
Compazine	Prochlorperazine
Concerta	Methylphenidate HCl
Copegus	Ribavirin
Cordarone	Amiodarone HCl
Cordron-D NR, Cordron-D	Carbinoxamine + Pseudoephedrine
Coreg, Coreg CR	Carvedilol
Cortef	Hydrocortisone
Cortenema	Hydrocortisone
Cortifoam	Hydrocortisone
Cortisporin Otic	Polymyxin B Sulfate, Neomycin Sulfate, Hydrocortisone
Co-Trimoxazole	Sulfamethoxazole and Trimethoprim
Coumadin	Warfarin
Covera-HS	Verapamil
Cozaar	Losartan
Crolom	Cromolyn
Cruex	Clotrimazole
Cuprimine	Penicillamine
Curosurf	Surfactant, Pulmonary/Poractant Alfa
Cutivate	Fluticasone Propionate
Cuvposa	Glycopyrrolate
Cyanoject	Cyanocobalamin/Vitamin B_{12}
Cyclogyl	Cyclopentolate
Cyclomydril	Cyclopentolate with Phenylephrine
Cyomin	Cyanocobalamin/Vitamin B_{12}
Cytovene	Ganciclovir
D-3, D3-5, D3-50	Cholecalciferol
Dantrium	Dantrolene
Daraprim	Pyrimethamine
Daytrana	Methylphenidate HCl
DDAVP*	Desmopressin Acetate
DDS*	Dapsone
D Drops	Cholecalciferol
Debrox	Carbamide Peroxide

*Common abbreviation or other name (not recommended for use when writing a prescription).

Trade Names	Generic Name
Decadron	Dexamethasone
Deltasone	Prednisone
Delzicol	Mesalamine
Deodorized tincture of opium	Opium Tincture
Depacon	Valproic Acid
Depakene	Valproic Acid
Depakote, Depakote ER	Divalproex Sodium
Depen	Penicillamine
Depo-Medrol	Methylprednisolone
Depo-Provera	Medroxyprogesterone
Depo-Sub Q Provera 104	Medroxyprogesterone
Desquam-E 5, Desquam-E 10	Benzoyl Peroxide
Desyrel (previously available as)	Trazodone
Dexedrine Spansules	Dextroamphetamine
DexFerrum	Iron—Injectable Preparations (iron dextran)
Dexpak Taperpak	Dexamethasone
DextroStat	Dextroamphetamine ± Amphetamine
Di-5-ASA*	Olsalazine
Dialume	Aluminum Hydroxide
Diaminodiphenylsulfone	Dapsone
Diamox	Acetazolamide
Diastat, Diastat AcuDial	Diazepam
Diflucan and others	Fluconazole
Digibind, DigiFab	Digoxin Immune Fab (Ovine)
Digitek	Digoxin
Dilacor XR	Diltiazem
Dilantin, Dilantin Infatab	Phenytoin
Dilaudid, Dilaudid-HP	Hydromorphone HCl
Di-mesalazine	Olsalazine
Dimetapp Children's Cold and Allergy	Brompheniramine with Phenylephrine
Diovan	Valsartan
Dipentum	Olsalazine
Diprolene, Diprolene AF	Betamethasone
Diprosone	Betamethasone
DisperMox	Amoxicillin
Ditropan, Ditropan XL	Oxybutynin Chloride
Diuril	Chlorothiazide
DMSA [dimercaptosuccinic acid]*	Succimer
Dobutrex (previously available as)	Dobutamine
Dolophine	Methadone HCl
Dopram	Doxapram HCl
Doryx	Doxycycline
Doxidan	Bisacodyl
Dramamine, Children's Dramamine	Dimenhydrinate
Drisdol	Ergocalciferol
Dulcolax	Bisacodyl
Dulera	Mometasone Furoate + Formoterol Fumarate
Duraclon	Clonidine
Duragesic	Fentanyl

29

*Common abbreviation or other name (not recommended for use when writing a prescription).

Trade Names	Generic Name
Duramist 12-Hr Nasal	Oxymetazoline
Duricef	Cefadroxil
Dycill	Dicloxacillin Sodium
Dynacin	Minocycline
Dyrenium	Triamterene
EC-Naprosyn	Naproxen
Efidac/24-Pseudoephedrine	Pseudoephedrine
Elavil	Amitriptyline
Elidel	Pimecrolimus
Elimite	Permethrin
Eliphos	Calcium Acetate
Elitek	Rasburicase
Elixophyllin	Theophylline
Elocon	Mometasone Furoate
Emfamil D-Vi-Sol	Cholecalciferol
EMLA, Eutectic mixture of lidocaine and prilocaine	Lidocaine and Prilocaine
E-Mycin	Erythromycin Preparations
Enbrel	Etanercept
Endocet	Oxycodone and Acetaminophen
Endodan	Oxycodone and Aspirin
Enemeez	Docusate
Enlon	Edrophonium Chloride
Entocort EC	Budesonide
Enuloase	Lactulose
Epaned	Enalapril Maleate
EpiPen	Epinephrine HCl
Epitol	Carbamazepine
Epivir, Epivir-HBV	Lamivudine
Epogen	Epoetin Alfa
Epsom salts	Magnesium Sulfate
Ergomar	Ergotamine Tartrate
Ery-Ped	Erythromycin
Erythrocin, Pediamycin, E-Mycin, Ery-Ped	Erythromycin
Erythropoietin	Epoetin Alfa
Eryzole	Erythromycin Ethylsuccinate and Acetylsulfisoxazole
Exalgo	Hydromorphone HCl
Extina	Ketoconazole
Famvir	Famciclovir
Fansidar	Pyrimethamine + Sulfadoxine
Felbatol	Felbamate
Fentora	Fentanyl
Feosol	Iron—Oral Preparations (Ferrous sulfate)
Fergon	Iron—Oral Preparations (Ferrous sulfate)
Fer-In-Sol	Iron—Oral Preparations (Ferrous gluconate)
Ferrlecit	Iron—Injectable Preparations (Ferric gluconate)
Feverall	Acetaminophen
Fiberall	Psyllium
First-Lansoprazole	Lansoprazole
First-Omeprazole	Omeprazole

*Common abbreviation or other name (not recommended for use when writing a prescription).

Trade Names	Generic Name
FK506	Tacrolimus
Flagyl, Flagyl ER	Metronidazole
Flebogamma DIF	Immune Globulin
Fleet Babylax	Glycerin
Fleet Laxative, Fleet Bisacodyl	Bisacodyl
Fleet Mineral Oil	Mineral Oil
Fleet, Fleet Phospho-Soda	Sodium Phosphate
Fletcher's Castoria	Senna/Sennosides
Flonase HFA	Fluticasone Propionate
Florinef Acetate	Fludrocortisone Acetate
Flovent Diskus	Fluticasone Propionate
Floxin, Floxin Otic	Ofloxacin
Flumadine	Rimantadine
Fluohydrisone	Fludrocortisone Acetate
Fluoritab	Fluoride
Focalin, Focalin XR	Dexmethylphenidate
Folvite	Folic Acid
Foradil Aerolizer	Formoterol
Fortamet	Metformin
Fortaz	Ceftazidime
Fortical Nasal Spray	Calcitonin—Salmon
Foscavir	Foscarnet
Fulvicin U/F, Fulvicin P/G	Griseofulvin
Fungizone	Amphotericin B
Furadantin	Nitrofurantoin
Gabitril	Tiagabine
Gablofen	Baclofen
Galzin	Zinc Salts, Systemic
Gamaplex	Immune Globulin
Gamma benzene hexachloride*	Lindane
Gammaked	Immune Globulin
Garamycin	Gentamicin
Gastrocrom	Cromolyn
Gas-X	Simethicone
Gengraf	Cyclosporine Modified
GlucaGen, Glucagon Emergency Kit	Glucagon HCl
Glucophage, Glucophage XR	Metformin
Gly-Oxide	Carbamide Peroxide
Glycate	Glycopyrrolate
GoLYTELY	Polyethylene Glycol—Electrolyte Solution
Gralise	Gabapentin
Granisol	Granisetron
Grifulvin V	Griseofulvin
Grisactin	Griseofulvin
Gris-PEG	Griseofulvin
Gyne-Lotrimin 3, Gyne-Lotrimin	Clotrimazole
H.P. Acthar Gel	Corticotropin
Haldol, Haldol Decanoate 50, Haldol Decanoate 100	Haloperidol
Hecoria	Tacrolimus

*Common abbreviation or other name (not recommended for use when writing a prescription).

Trade Names	Generic Name
Hexadrol	Dexamethasone
Horizant	Gabapentin
Humatin	Paromomycin Sulfate
Hydro-Tussin CBX	Carbinoxamine + Pseudoephedrine
Hylenex	Hyaluronidase
Hypersal	Sodium Chloride—Inhaled Preparations
Imitrex	Sumatriptan Succinate
Imodium, Imodium AD	Loperamide
Imuran	Azathioprine
Inapsine	Droperidol
Inderal, Inderal LA	Propranolol
Indocin, Indocin SR, Indocin IV	Indomethacin
Infasurf	Surfactant, Pulmonary/Calfactant
INFeD	Iron—Injectable Preparations (iron dextran)
INH*	Isoniazid
Intal (previously available as)	Cromolyn
Intropin (previously available as)	Dopamine
Intuniv	Guanfacine
Invanz	Ertapenem
Iosat	Potassium Iodide
Iquix	Levofloxacin
IsonaRif	Isoniazid
Isoptin SR	Verapamil
Isopto Carpine	Pilocarpine HCl
Isopto Hyoscine	Scopolamine Hydrobromide
Isuprel	Isoproterenol
Jantoven	Warfarin
Kadian	Morphine Sulfate
Kantrex	Kanamycin
Kaopectate	Bismuth Subsalicylate
Kao-Tin	Bismuth Subsalicylate
Kapvay	Clonidine
Kayexalate	Sodium Polystyrene Sulfonate
Keflex	Cephalexin
Kemstro	Baclofen
Kenalog	Triamcinolone
Keppra, Keppra XR	Levetiracetam
Ketalar	Ketamine
Kionex	Sodium Polystyrene Sulfonate
Klonopin	Clonazepam
Klout	Pyrethrins with Piperonyl Butoxide
Kondremul	Mineral Oil
Konsyl	Psyllium
K-PHOS Neutral	Phosphorus Supplements
Kristalose	Lactulose
Kytril	Granisetron
Lamictal, Lamictal ODT, Lamictal XR	Lamotrigine
Laniazid	Isoniazid
Lanoxin	Digoxin

*Common abbreviation or other name (not recommended for use when writing a prescription).

Trade Names	Generic Name
Lariam	Mefloquine HCl
Lasix	Furosemide
Lax-Pills	Senna/Sennosides
Lazanda	Fentanyl
L-Carnitine	Carnitine
Levaquin, Quixin, Iquix	Levofloxacin
Levocarnitine	Carnitine
Levophed and others	Norepinephrine Bitartrate
Lialda	Mesalamine
Licide	Pyrethrins with Piperonyl Butoxide
Lidoderm	Lidocaine
Lioresal	Baclofen
Liquid Pred	Prednisone
Lithobid	Lithium
L-M-X	Lidocaine
Loniten (previously available as)	Minoxidil
Lopressor, Toprol-XL	Metoprolol
Lotrimin AF	Clotrimazole
Lotrimin AF	Miconazole
Lovenox	Enoxaparin
Luminal	Phenobarbital
Luride	Fluoride
Luvox CR	Fluvoxamine
Maalox, Maalox Maximum Strength Liquid	Aluminum Hydroxide with Magnesium Hydroxide
Macrobid	Nitrofurantoin
Macrodantin	Nitrofurantoin
Mag-200, Mag-Ox 400, Uro-Mag	Magnesium Oxide
Marinol	Dronabinol
Maxidex	Dexamethasone
Maxipime	Cefepime
Maxivate	Betamethasone
Maxolon	Metoclopramide
Medrol, Medrol Dosepack	Methylprednisolone
Mefoxin	Cefoxitin
Mephyton	Phytonadione/Vitamin K_1
Mepron	Atovaquone
Merrem	Meropenem
Mestinon	Pyridostigmine Bromide
Metadate ER	Methylphenidate HCl
Metamucil	Psyllium
Methadose	Methadone HCl
Methylin, Methylin ER	Methylphenidate HCl
Metozolv	Metoclopramide
MetroCream	Metronidazole
MetroGel, MetroGel-Vaginal	Metronidazole
MetroLotion	Metronidazole
Miacalcin, Miacalcin Nasal Spray	Calcitonin—Salmon
Micatin	Miconazole
Microzide	Hydrochlorothiazide

*Common abbreviation or other name (not recommended for use when writing a prescription).

29

Trade Names	Generic Name
Milk of Magnesia	Magnesium Hydroxide
Millipred	Prednisolone
Minocin	Minocycline
Mintezol	Thiabendazole
Mintox	Aluminum Hydroxide with Magnesium Hydroxide
MiraLax	Polyethylene Glycol—Electrolyte Solution
Monistat	Miconazole
Motrin, Children's Motrin	Ibuprofen
MS Contin	Morphine Sulfate
Mucomyst	Acetylcysteine
Mucosol	Acetylcysteine
Murine Ear	Carbamide Peroxide
Myambutol	Ethambutol HCl
Mycamine	Micafungin Sodium
Mycelex, Mycelex-7	Clotrimazole
Mycobutin	Rifabutin
Mycostatin	Nystatin
Myfortic	Mycophenolate Sodium
Mylanta Gas	Simethicone
Mylanta, Mylanta Extra Strength	Aluminum Hydroxide with Magnesium Hydroxide
Mylicon	Simethicone
Myorisan	Isotretinoin
Mysoline	Primidone
Nallpen	Nafcillin
Naprelan	Naproxen/Naproxen Sodium
Naprosyn, Naprosen DR	Naproxen/Naproxen Sodium
Narcan	Naloxone
Nasacort AQ	Triamcinolone
Nasalcrom	Cromolyn
Nasarel	Flunisolide
Nascobal	Cyanocobalamin/Vitamin B_{12}
Nasonex	Mometasone Furoate
Nebcin	Tobramycin
NebuPent	Pentamidine Isethionate
Nembutal	Pentobarbital
NeoBenz Micro	Benzoyl Peroxide
Neo-fradin	Neomycin Sulfate
Neo-Polycin	Neomycin/Polymyxin B/Bacitracin
NeoProfen (IV)	Ibuprofen
Neoral	Cyclosporine
Neosporin, Neosporin Ophthalmic, Neo To Go	Neomycin/Polymyxin B/Bacitracin
Neosporin GU Irrigant	Neomycin/Polymyxin B
Neo-Synephrine	Phenylephrine HCl
Neo-Synephrine 12-Hr Nasal	Oxymetazoline
Nephron	Epinephrine, Racemic
Neupogen, G-CSF	Filgrastim
Neurontin	Gabapentin
Neut	Sodium Bicarbonate
Nexiclon XR	Clonidine

*Common abbreviation or other name (not recommended for use when writing a prescription).

Trade Names	Generic Name
Nexium	Esomeprazole
Nexterone	Amiodarone HCl
Niacor	Niacin (Vitamin B_3)
Niaspan	Niacin (Vitamin B_3)
Nicotinic acid	Niacin (Vitamin B_3)
Nifediac CC	Nifedipine
Niferex	Iron—Oral Preparations
Nilstat	Nystatin
Nipride (previously available as)	Nitroprusside
Nitro-Bid	Nitroglycerin
Nitro-Dur	Nitroglycerin
Nitro-Mist	Nitroglycerin
Nitropress	Nitroprusside
Nitrostat	Nitroglycerin
Nitro-Time	Nitroglycerin
Nix	Permethrin
Nizoral, Nizoral A-D	Ketoconazole
Noriate	Metronidazole
Normal Serum Albumin (Human)	Albumin, Human
Normodyne	Labetalol
Noroxin	Norfloxacin
Norvasc	Amlodipine
Nostrilla	Oxymetazoline
NuCort	Hydrocortisone
NuLYTELY	Polyethylene Glycol—Electrolyte Solution
Nutr-E-Sol	Vitamin E/α-Tocopherol
NVP*	Nevirapine
Nydrazid	Isoniazid
OCL*	Polyethylene Glycol—Electrolyte Solution
Ocean	Sodium Chloride—Inhaled Preparations
Ocuflox	Ofloxacin
Ocusulf-10	Sulfacetamide Sodium Ophthalmic
Omnaris	Ciclesonide
Ofirmev	Acetaminophen
Omeprazole and Syrspend SF Alka	Omeprazole
Omnicef	Cefdinir
Omnipaque 140, Omnipaque 180, Omnipaque 240, Omnipaque 300, and Omnipaque 350	Iohexol
Omnipen	Ampicillin
Onfi	Clobazam
Onmel	Itraconazole
Opticrom	Cromolyn
Optivar	Azelastine
Oralone	Corticosteroid
Oramorph SR	Morphine Sulfate
Orapred, Orapred ODT	Prednisolone
Oraqix	Lidocaine and Prilocaine
Orasone	Prednisone
OraVerse	Phentolamine Mesylate

29

*Common abbreviation or other name (not recommended for use when writing a prescription).

Trade Names	Generic Name
Orazinc	Zinc Salts, Systemic
Os-Cal	Calcium Carbonate
Osmitrol	Mannitol
OsmoPrep	Sodium Phosphate
Oxtellar	Oxcarbazepine
Oxy-5, Oxy-10	Benzoyl Peroxide
OxyContin	Oxycodone
Oxytrol	Oxybutynin Chloride
Pacerone	Amiodarone HCl
Palasbumin	Albumin, Human
Palgic	Carbinoxamine
Pamelor	Nortriptyline Hydrochloride
Pamix	Pyrantel Pamoate
Panadol	Acetaminophen
Paracetamol	Acetaminophen
Pataday	Olopatadine
Patanase	Olopatadine
Patanol	Olopatadine
Pathocil	Dicloxacillin Sodium
Paxil, Paxil CR	Paroxetine
Pediaflor	Fluoride
Pedia-Lax	Glycerin
Pediamycin	Erythromycin Preparations
Pediapred	Prednisolone
Pediazole	Erythromycin Ethylsuccinate and Acetylsulfisoxazole
PediOtic	Polymyxin B Sulfate, Neomycin Sulfate, Hydrocortisone
Pentam 300	Pentamidine Isethionate
Pentasa	Mesalamine
Pepcid, Pepcid AC [OTC], Maximum Strength Pepcid AC [OTC], Pepcid Complete [OTC], Pepcid RPD	Famotidine
Pepto-Bismol	Bismuth Subsalicylate
Percocet	Oxycodone and Acetaminophen
Percodan	Oxycodone and Aspirin
Perforomist	Formoterol
Periactin (previously available as)	Cyproheptadine
Periostat	Doxycycline
Pexeva	Paroxetine
Pfizerpen	Penicillin G Preparations—Aqueous Potassium and Sodium
PGE$_1$*	Alprostadil
Phazyme	Simethicone
Phenergan	Promethazine
Phenytek	Phenytoin
PhosLo	Calcium Acetate
Phoslyra	Calcium Acetate
Pilopine HS	Pilocarpine HCl
Pima	Potassium Iodide
Pin-Rid	Pyrantel Pamoate

*Common abbreviation or other name (not recommended for use when writing a prescription).

Trade Names	Generic Name
Pin-X	Pyrantel Pamoate
Pipracil	Piperacillin
Pitressin	Vasopressin
Plaquenil	Hydroxychloroquine
Polymox	Amoxicillin
Polysporin Ophthalmic	Bacitracin + Polymyxin B
Polysporin Topical	Bacitracin + Polymyxin B
Polytrim Ophthalmic Solution	Polymyxin B Sulfate and Trimethoprim Sulfate
Posture-D	Calcium Phosphate, Tribasic
Potassium Phosphate	Phosphorus Supplements
Precidex	Dexmedetomidine
Prelone	Prednisolone
Prevacid, Prevacid SoluTab	Lansoprazole
Prevalite	Cholestyramine
Prilosec, Prilosec OTC	Omeprazole
Primacor	Milrinone
Primaxin IV	Imipenem and Cilastatin
Principen	Ampicillin
Prinivil	Lisinopril
Privagen	Immune Globulin
ProAir HFA	Albuterol
Procanbid	Procainamide
Procardia, Procardia XL	Nifedipine
ProCentra	Dextroamphetamine Sulfate
Procrit	Epoetin Alfa
Proglycem	Diazoxide
Prograf	Tacrolimus
Pronestyl	Procainamide
Pronto	Pyrethrins
Prostaglandin E_1	Alprostadil
Prostigmin	Neostigmine
Prostin VR Pediatric	Alprostadil
Protonix	Pantoprazole
Protopam	Pralidoxime Chloride
Protopic	Tacrolimus
Protostat	Metronidazole
Proventil, Proventil HFA (aerosol inhaler)	Albuterol
Provera	Medroxyprogesterone
Prozac, Prozac Weekly	Fluoxetine Hydrochloride
Pseudo Carb Pediatric	Carbinoxamine + Pseudoephedrine
PTU*	Propylthiouracil
Pulmicort Respules, Pulmicort Flexhaler	Budesonide
Pulmozyme	Dornase Alfa/DNase
Pyrazinoic acid amide	Pyrazinamide
Pyridium	Phenazopyridine HCl
Pyrinyl	Pyrethrins
Qnasl	Beclomethasone Dipropionate
Quelicin, Quelicin-1000	Succinylcholine
Questran, Questran Light	Cholestyramine

*Common abbreviation or other name (not recommended for use when writing a prescription).

Trade Names	Generic Name
Quinidex	Quinidine
Quixin	Levofloxacin
QVAR*	Beclomethasone Dipropionate
Raniclor	Cefaclor
Rapamune	Sirolimus
Rayos	Prednisone
Rebetol	Ribavirin
Reese's Pinworm	Pyrantel Pamoate
Regitine	Phentolamine Mesylate
Reglan	Metoclopramide
Regonal	Pyridostigmine Bromide
Renova	Tretinoin
Resectisol	Mannitol
Restasis	Cyclosporine, Cyclosporine Microemulsion, Cyclosporine Modified
Retin-A, Retin-A Micro	Tretinoin
Retrovir, AZT	Zidovudine
Revatio	Sildenafil
Reversol	Edrophonium Chloride
Revonto	Dantrolene
R-Gene 10	Arginine Chloride
Rhinaris	Sodium Chloride—Inhaled Preparations
Rhinocort Aqua Nasal Spray	Budesonide
Ribaspheres	Ribavirin
RID	Pyrethrins
Rifadin	Rifampin
Rifamate	Isoniazid + Rifampin
Rifater	Pyrazinamide + Isoniazid + Rifampin
Rimactane	Rifampin
Riomet	Metformin
Risperdal, Risperdal M-Tab, Risperdal Consta	Risperidone
Ritalin, Ritalin SR, Ritalin LA	Methylphenidate HCl
Robinul	Glycopyrrolate
Rocaltrol	Calcitriol
Rocephin	Ceftriaxone
Rogaine, Men's Rogaine Extra Strength	Minoxidil
Romazicon	Flumazenil
Rowasa, SfRowasa	Mesalamine
Roxanol	Morphine Sulfate
Roxicet	Oxycodone and Acetaminophen
Roxicodone	Oxycodone
Roxilox	Oxycodone and Acetaminophen
RuLox Plus	Aluminum Hydroxide with Magnesium Hydroxide
S-2 Inhalant	Epinephrine, Racemic
Sabril	Vigabatrin
Salagen	Pilocarpine HCl
Salicylazosulfapyridine	Sulfasalazine
Sal-Tropine	Atropine Sulfate
Sancuso	Granisetron

*Common abbreviation or other name (not recommended for use when writing a prescription).

Trade Names	Generic Name
Sandimmune	Cyclosporine
Sandostatin, Sandostatin LAR Depot	Octreotide Acetate
Sani-Supp	Glycerin
Sarafem	Fluoxetine Hydrochloride
SAS*	Sulfasalazine
Scopace	Scopolamine Hydrobromide
Selsun and others	Selenium Sulfide
Senna-Gen	Senna/Sennosides
Senokot	Senna/Sennosides
Septra	Sulfamethoxazole and Trimethoprim
Serevent Diskus	Salmeterol
Sildec	Carbinoxamine + Pseudoephedrine
Silvadene	Silver Sulfadiazine
Simply Saline	Sodium Chloride—Inhaled Preparations
Singulair	Montelukast
Slo-Niacin	Niacin (Vitamin B_3)
Slow FE	Iron—Oral Preparations
Sodium Phosphate	Phosphorus Supplements
Solodyn	Minocycline
Solu-cortef	Hydrocortisone
Solu-Medrol	Methylprednisolone
Soluspan	Betamethasone
Sporanox	Itraconazole
SPS*	Sodium Polystyrene Sulfonate
SSD Cream, SSD AF Cream	Silver Sulfadiazine
SSKI*	Potassium Iodide
Stadol	Butorphanol
Stavzor	Valproic Acid
Stimate	Desmopressin Acetate
Stomach Relief, Stomach Relief Max St, Stomach Relief Plus	Bismuth Subsalicylate
Strattera	Atomoxetine
Streptase	Streptokinase
Sublimaze	Fentanyl
Sudafed	Pseudoephedrine
Sulfatrim	Sulfamethoxazole and Trimethoprim
Sulfazine, Sulfazine EC	Sulfasalazine
Sunkist Vitamin C	Ascorbic Acid
Suprax	Cefixime
Surfak	Docusate
Surfaxin	Surfactant, Pulmonary/Lucinactant
Survanta	Surfactant, Pulmonary/Beractant
Symbicort	Budesonide and Formoterol
Symmetrel	Amantadine Hydrochloride
Synagis	Palivizumab
Synercid	Quinupristin and Dalfopristin
Synthroid	Levothyroxine T_4
Tagamet, Tagamet HB [OTC]	Cimetidine
Tambocor	Flecainide Acetate

*Common abbreviation or other name (not recommended for use when writing a prescription).

Trade Names	Generic Name
Tamiflu	Oseltamivir Phosphate
Tapazole	Methimazole
Tazicef	Ceftazidime
Tazidime	Ceftazidime
Tegretol, Tegretol-XR	Carbamazepine
Tempra	Acetaminophen
Tenex	Guanfacine
Tenormin	Atenolol
Tensilon	Edrophonium Chloride
Tetrahydrocannabinol	Dronabinol
THC*	Dronabinol
Theo-24	Theophylline
Theochron	Theophylline
Thera-Ear	Carbamide Peroxide
Therazene	Silver Sulfadiazine
Thorazine	Chlorpromazine
ThyroSave	Potassium Iodide
ThyroShield	Potassium Iodide
Tiazac	Diltiazem
Tigan	Trimethobenzamide HCl
Timentin	Ticarcillin and Clavulanate
Tinactin	Tolnaftate
Tirosint	Levothyroxine
Tisit	Pyrethrins
TMP-SMX*	Sulfamethoxazole and Trimethoprim
TOBI, TOBI Podhaler	Tobramycin
Tobrex	Tobramycin
Tofranil, Tofranil-PM	Imipramine
Topamax	Topiramate
Topiragen	Topiramate
Toprol-XL	Metoprolol
Totacillin	Ampicillin
tPA*	Alteplase
Trandate	Labetalol
Transderm Scop	Scopolamine Hydrobromide
Trianex	Corticosteroid
Triaz	Benzoyl Peroxide
Triderm	Corticosteroid
Trileptal	Oxcarbazepine
Trilisate and others	Choline Magnesium Trisalicylate
TriLyte	Polyethylene Glycol—Electrolyte Solution
Trimethoprim-Sulfamethoxazole	Sulfamethoxazole and Trimethoprim
Trimox	Amoxicillin
Trokenndi XR	Topiramate
Tums	Calcium Carbonate
Tylenol	Acetaminophen
Tylenol #1, #2, #3, #4	Codeine and Acetaminophen
Tylox	Oxycodone and Acetaminophen
Uceris	Budesonide

*Common abbreviation or other name (not recommended for use when writing a prescription).

Trade Names	Generic Name
Unasyn	Ampicillin/Sulbactam
Unithroid, Unithroid Direct	Levothyroxine
Urecholine	Bethanechol Chloride
Uro-KP-Neutral	Phosphorus Supplements
Urolene Blue	Methylene Blue
Urso 250, Urso Forte	Ursodiol
Vagistat-3	Miconazole
Valcyte	Valganciclovir
Valium	Diazepam
Valtrex	Valacyclovir
Vancocin	Vancomycin
Vantin	Cefpodoxime Proxetil
VariZig	Varicella-Zoster Immune Globulin (Human)
Vasotec	Enalapril Maleate
Vasotec IV	Enalaprilat
Veetids	Penicillin V Potassium
Venofer	Iron—Injectable Preparations (iron sucrose)
Ventolin HFA	Albuterol
Veramyst	Fluticasone Propionate
Verelan, Verelan PM	Verapamil
Veripred	Prednisolone
Vermox	Mebendazole
Versed (previously available as)	Midazolam
VFEND	Voriconazole
Viagra	Sildenafil
Vibramycin	Doxycycline
Vimpat	Lacosamide
Viramune, Viramune XR	Nevirapine
Virazole	Ribavirin
Visicol	Sodium Phosphate
Visine LR	Oxymetazoline
Vistaril	Hydroxyzine
Vistide	Cidofovir
Vitamin B_1	Thiamine
Vitamin B_2	Riboflavin
Vitamin B_{12}	Cyanocobalamin/Vitamin B_{12}
Vitamin B_3	Niacin/Vitamin B_3
Vitamin B_6	Pyridoxine
Vitamin C	Ascorbic Acid
Vitrase	Hyaluronidase
Vitrasert	Ganciclovir
VoSpire ER	Albuterol
Vyvanse	Lisdexamfetamine
VZIG	Varicella-Zoster Immune Globulin (Human)
WinRho-SDF	Rho (D) Immune Globulin Intravenous (Human)
Wycillin	Penicillin G Preparations—Procaine
Wymox	Amoxicillin
Xolegel	Ketoconazole
Xopenex, Xopenex HFA	Levalbuterol

*Common abbreviation or other name (not recommended for use when writing a prescription).

Trade Names	Generic Name
Xylocaine	Lidocaine
Zantac, Zantac 75 [OTC], Zantac 150 Maximum Strength [OTC]	Ranitidine HCl
Zarontin	Ethosuximide
Zaroxolyn	Metolazone
Zegerid	Omeprazole
Zemuron	Rocuronium
Zenatane	Isotretinoin
Zenzedi	Dextroamphetamine Sulfate
Zestril	Lisinopril
Zetonna	Ciclesonide
Zinacef	Cefuroxime
Zirgan	Ganciclovir
Zithromax, Zithromax TRI-PAK, Zithromax Z-PAK, Zmax	Azithromycin
Zoderm	Benzoyl Peroxide
Zofran	Ondansetron
Zolicef	Cefazolin
Zoloft	Sertraline HCl
Zonegran	Zonisamide
ZORprin	Aspirin
Zosyn	Piperacillin with Tazobactam
Zovirax	Acyclovir
Zyloprim	Allopurinol
Zyrtec, Children's Zyrtec	Cetirizine
Zyrtec-D 12 Hour	Cetirizine + Pseudoephedrine
Zyvox	Linezolid

*Common abbreviation or other name (not recommended for use when writing a prescription).

ACETAMINOPHEN
Tylenol, Tempra, Panadol, Feverall, Aspirin-Free Anacin,
Paracetamol, Ofirmev, and many others
Analgesic, antipyretic

| Yes | Yes | 1 | B/C |

Tabs [OTC]: 325, 500, 650 mg
Chewable tabs [OTC]: 80, 160 mg; some may contain phenylalanine
Infant drops, solution/suspension [OTC]: 80 mg/0.8 mL
Child suspension/syrup [OTC]: 160 mg/5 mL
Oral liquid [OTC]: 160, 166.7 mg/5 mL; may contain 7% alcohol
   Extra-strength: 166.7 mg/5 mL
Elixir [OTC]: 160 mg/5 mL
Caplet [OTC]: 160, 500, 650 mg
Extended-release caplet/geltab [OTC]: 650 mg
Gelcap [OTC]: 500 mg
Capsules [OTC]: 500 mg
Dispersible tabs (Tylenol Children's Meltaways) [OTC]: 80 mg
Suppositories [OTC]: 80, 120, 325, 650 mg
Injection:
   Ofirmev: 10 mg/mL (100 mL)

PO/PR:
   Neonate: 10–15 mg/kg/dose PO/PR Q6–8 hr. Some advocate loading doses of 20–25 mg/kg/dose for PO dosing or 30 mg/kg/dose for PR dosing.
   Pediatric: 10–15 mg/kg/dose PO/PR Q4–6 hr; **max. dose:** 90 mg/kg/24 hr. For rectal dosing, some may advocate a 40–45 mg/kg/dose loading dose.

Dosing by weight (preferred) or age (PO/PR Q4–6 hr):

Weight (lb)	Weight (kg)	Age	Dosage (mg)
6–11	2.7–5	0–3 mo	40
12–17	5.1–7.7	4–11 mo	80
18–23	7.8–10.5	1–2 yr	120
24–35	10.6–15.9	2–3 yr	160
36–47	16–21.4	4–5 yr	240
48–59	21.5–26.8	6–8 yr	320
60–71	26.9–32.3	9–10 yr	400
72–95	32.4–43.2	11 yr	480

   Adult: 325–650 mg/dose
   Max. dose: 4 g/24 hr, 5 doses/24 hr

IV:
   Term neonate and infant < 1 yr: Labeled dosing from the UK and pharmacokinetic studies recommend 7.5–15 mg/kg/dose Q6 hr IV up to a **maximum** of 60 mg/kg/24 hr (see *Pediatr Anesth.* 2009;19:329-337). A phase 3 study is currently in progress in children <2 yr of age. See www.clinicaltrials.gov for updated information.
   Child (≥2–12 yr) and adolescent/adult < 50 kg: 15 mg/kg/dose Q6 hr, **OR** 12.5 mg/kg/dose Q4 hr IV up to a **maximum** of 75 mg/kg/24 hr.
   Adolescent and adult (≥50 kg): 1000 mg Q6 hr, **OR** 650 mg Q4 hr up to a **maximum** of 4000 mg/24 hr.

Does not possess anti-inflammatory activity. **Use with caution** in patients with known G6PD deficiency.

$T_{1/2}$: 1–3 hr, 2–5 hr in neonates; metabolized in the liver; see Chapter 2 and acetylcysteine for management of overdosage.

Some preparations contain alcohol (7%–10%) and/or phenylalanine; all suspensions should be shaken before use.

Continued

For explanation of icons, see p. 648

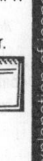

ACETAMINOPHEN *continued*

May decrease the activity of lamotrigine and increase the activity/toxicity of busulfan, warfarin, and zidovudine. Barbiturates, phenytoin, rifampin, and anticholinergic agents (e.g., scopolamine) may decrease the effect of acetaminophen. Increased risk for hepatotoxicity may occur with barbiturates, carbamazepine, phenytoin, carmustine (with high acetaminophen doses), and chronic alcohol use. **Adjust dose in renal failure (see Chapter 31).**

FOR IV USE: Administer dose undiluted over 15 min. Most common side effects with IV use include nausea, vomiting, constipation, pruritus, agitation, and atelectasis in children; and nausea, vomiting, headache, and insomnia in adults.

Pregnancy category "B" for PO and PR routes and "C" for IV route.

ACETAZOLAMIDE
Diamox and generics
Carbonic anhydrase inhibitor, diuretic

Yes Yes 1 C

Tabs: 125, 250 mg
Oral suspension: 25 mg/mL
Capsules (extended release): 500 mg
Injection (sodium): 500 mg
Contains 2.05 mEq Na/500 mg drug

Diuretic (PO, IV)
  Child: 5 mg/kg/dose once daily or every other day
  Adult: 250–375 mg/dose once daily or every other day
Glaucoma
  Child:
    PO: 8–30 mg/kg/24 hr ÷ Q6–8 hr
    IM/IV: 20–40 mg/kg/24 hr ÷ Q6 hr; **max. dose:** 1000 mg/24 hr
  Adult:
    PO (simple chronic; open-angle): 1000 mg/24 hr ÷ Q6 hr
    IV (acute secondary; closed-angle): For rapid decrease in intraocular pressure, administer 500 mg/dose IV
Seizures (extended-release product not recommended):
  Child and adult: 8–30 mg/kg/24 hr ÷ Q6–12 hr PO; **max. dose:** 1 g/24 hr
Urine alkalinization:
  Adult: 5 mg/kg/dose PO repeated BID–TID over 24 hr
Management of hydrocephalus (see remarks): Start with 20 mg/kg/24 hr ÷ Q8 hr PO/IV; may increase to 100 mg/kg/24 hr up to a **max. dose** of 2 g/24 hr.
Pseudotumor cerebri (PO; see remarks):
  Child: Start with 25 mg/kg/24 hr ÷ once daily–QID; increase by 25 mg/kg/24 hr until clinical response or as tolerated up to a **maximum** of 100 mg/kg/24 hr.
  Adolescent: Start with 1 g/24 hr ÷ once daily–QID; increase by 250 mg/24 hr until clinical response or as tolerated up to a **maximum** of 4 g/24 hr.

Contraindicated in hepatic failure, severe renal failure (GFR < 10 mL/min), and hypersensitivity to sulfonamides.

$T_{1/2}$: 2–6 hr; **do not use** sustained-release capsules in seizures; IM injection may be painful; bicarbonate replacement therapy may be required during long-term use (see *Citrate* or *Sodium Bicarbonate*). For use in pseudotumor cerebri, doses of 60 mg/kg/24 hr may be required.

Possible side effects (more likely with long-term therapy) include GI irritation, paresthesias, sedation, hypokalemia, acidosis, reduced urate secretion, aplastic anemia, polyuria, and development of renal calculi.

A

ACETAZOLAMIDE *continued*

May increase toxicity of cyclosporine. Aspirin may increase toxicity of acetazolamide. May decrease the effects of salicylates, lithium, and phenobarbital. False-positive urinary protein may occur with several assays. **Adjust dose in renal failure (see Chapter 31).**

ACETYLCYSTEINE
Mucomyst, Mucosol, Acetadote
Mucolytic, antidote for acetaminophen toxicity

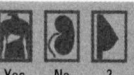

Yes   No   ?   B

Solution inhalation or oral use: 100 mg/mL (10%) (10, 30 mL) or 200 mg/mL (20%) (4, 10, 30 mL); contains EDTA

Injectable (Acetadote): 200 mg/mL (20%) (30 mL); contains EDTA 0.5 mg/mL

Acetaminophen poisoning (see Chapter 2 for additional information):

PO: 140 mg/kg × 1, followed by 70 mg/kg/dose Q4 hr for a total of 17 doses. Repeat dose if vomiting occurs within 1 hr of administration.

IV: 150 mg/kg ×1 diluted in D₅W or D₅W/½NS administered over 60 min, followed by 50 mg/kg diluted in D₅W administered over 4 hr, then 100 mg/kg diluted in D₅W administered over 16 hr. Recommended weight-based drug dilution volumes:

Weight (kg)	Volume of D₅W or D₅W/½NS for 150 mg/kg Loading Dose Administered Over 60 min	Volume of D₅W for 50 mg/kg Second Dose Administered Over 4 hr	Volume of D₅W for 100 mg/kg Third Dose Administered Over 16 hr
≤20	3 mL/kg	7 mL/kg	14 mL/kg
>20–<40	100 mL	250 mL	500 mL
≥40	200 mL	500 mL	1000 mL

Nebulizer:

Infant: 1–2 mL of 20% solution (diluted with equal volume of H₂O, or sterile saline to equal 10%), or 2–4 mL of 10% solution; administer TID–QID

Child: 3–5 mL of 20% solution (diluted with equal volume of H₂O, or sterile saline to equal 10%), or 6–10 mL of 10% solution; administer TID–QID

Adolescent: 5–10 mL of 10% or 20% solution; administer TID–QID

Distal intestinal obstruction syndrome in cystic fibrosis:

Adolescent and adult: 10 mL of 20% solution (diluted in a sweet drink) PO QID with 100 mL of 10% solution PR as an enema once daily–QID

Use with caution in asthma. For nebulized use, give inhaled bronchodilator 10–15 min before use and follow with postural drainage and/or suctioning after acetylcysteine administration. Prior hydration is essential for distal intestinal obstruction syndrome treatment.

May induce bronchospasm, stomatitis, drowsiness, rhinorrhea, nausea, vomiting, and hemoptysis. Anaphylactoid reactions have been reported with IV use.

For IV use, elimination T₁/₂ is longer in newborns (11 hr) than in adults (5.6 hr). T₁/₂ is increased by 80% in patients with severe liver damage (Child-Pugh score of 7–13) and biliary cirrhosis (Child-Pugh score of 5–7).

For oral administration, chilling the solution and mixing with carbonated beverages, orange juice, or sweet drinks may enhance palatability.

ACTH

See Corticotropin

ACYCLOVIR
Zovirax and generics
Antiviral

No   Yes   1   B

Capsules: 200 mg
Tabs: 400, 800 mg
Oral suspension: 200 mg/5 mL; may contain parabens
Ointment: 5% (15, 30 g)
Cream: 5% (2, 5 g)
Injection in powder (with sodium): 500, 1000 mg
Injection in solution (with sodium): 50 mg/mL
Contains 4.2 mEq Na/1 g drug

IMMUNOCOMPETENT:

Neonatal (HSV and HSV encephalitis; birth–3 mo):
   <35 wk postconceptional age: 40 mg/kg/24 hr ÷ Q12 hr IV × 14–21 days
   ≥35 wk postconceptional age: 60 mg/kg/24 hr ÷ Q8 hr IV × 14–21 days
   Oral therapy for HSV suppression and neurodevelopment after treatment with IV acyclovir for 14–21 days: 300 mg/m²/dose Q8 hr PO × 6 mo

HSV encephalitis (duration of therapy: 14–21 days):
   Birth–3 mo: Use above IV dosage.
   3 mo–12 yr: 60 mg/kg/24 hr ÷ Q8 hr IV; some experts recommend 45 mg/kg/24 hr ÷ Q8 hr IV
   ≥12 yr: 30 mg/kg/24 hr ÷ Q8 hr IV

Mucocutaneous HSV (including genital, ≥12 yr):
   Initial infection:
      IV: 15 mg/kg/24 hr or 750 mg/m²/24 hr ÷ Q8 hr × 5–7 days
      PO: 1000–1200 mg/24 hr ÷ 3–5 doses per 24 hr × 7–10 days. For pediatric dosing, use 40–80 mg/kg/24 hr ÷ Q6–8 hr × 5–10 days (**max. pediatric dose:** 1000 mg/24 hr).
   Recurrence (≥12 yr):
      PO: 1000 mg/24 hr ÷ 5 doses per 24 hr × 5 days, or 1600 mg/24 hr ÷ Q12 hr × 5 days, or 2400 mg/24 hr ÷ Q8 hr × 2 days
   Chronic suppressive therapy (≥12 yr):
      PO: 800 mg/24 hr ÷ Q12 hr for up to 1 year

Zoster:
   IV (all ages): 30 mg/kg/24 hr or 1500 mg/m²/24 hr ÷ Q8 hr × 7–10 days
   PO (≥12 yr): 4000 mg/24 hr ÷ 5×/24 hr × 5–7 days

Varicella:
   IV (≥2 yr): 30 mg/kg/24 hr or 1500 mg/m²/24 hr ÷ Q8 hr × 7–10 days
   PO (≥2 yr): 80 mg/kg/24 hr ÷ QID × 5 days (begin treatment at earliest signs/symptoms); **max. dose:** 3200 mg/24 hr

Max. dose of oral acyclovir in children = 80 mg/kg/24 hr.

IMMUNOCOMPROMISED:

HSV:
   IV (all ages): 750–1500 mg/m²/24 hr ÷ Q8 hr × 7–14 days
   PO (≥2 yr): 1000 mg/24 hr ÷ 3–5 times/24 hr × 7–14 days; **max. dose** for child: 80 mg/kg/24 hr

HSV prophylaxis:
   IV (all ages): 750 mg/m²/24 hr ÷ Q8 hr during risk period
   PO (≥2 yr): 600–1000 mg/24 hr ÷ 3–5 times/24 hr during risk period; **max. dose** for child: 80 mg/kg/24 hr

Varicella or zoster:
   IV (all ages): 1500 mg/m²/24 hr ÷ Q8 hr × 7–10 days

ACYCLOVIR *continued*

PO (consider using valacyclovir or famciclovir for better absorption):
   Infant and child: 20 mg/kg/dose (**max.** 800 mg) Q6 hr × 7–10 days
   Adolescent and adult: 20 mg/kg/dose (**max.** 800 mg) 5 times daily × 7–10 days
Max. dose of oral acyclovir in children = 80 mg/kg/24 hr.
TOPICAL:
   Apply 0.5-inch ribbon of 5% ointment for 4-inch-square surface area 6 times a day × 7 days.

See most recent edition of the AAP *Red Book* for further details. **Use with caution** in patients with preexisting neurologic or **renal impairment (adjust dose; see Chapter 31)** or dehydration. Adequate hydration and slow (1 hr) IV administration are essential to prevent crystallization in renal tubules. **Do not use** topical product on the eye or for prevention of recurrent HSV infections. Oral absorption is unpredictable (15%–30%); consider using valacyclovir or famciclovir for better absorption. Use ideal body weight for obese patients when calculating dosages. Resistant strains of HSV and VZV have been reported in immunocompromised patients (e.g., advanced HIV infection).

Can cause renal impairment; has been infrequently associated with headache, vertigo, insomnia, encephalopathy, GI tract irritation, elevated liver function tests, rash, urticaria, arthralgia, fever, and adverse hematologic effects. Probenecid decreases acyclovir renal clearance. Acyclovir may increase the concentration of tenofovir and meperidine (and its metabolite [normeperidine]).

ADDERALL

See Dextroamphetamine ± Amphetamine

ADENOSINE
Adenocard and generics
Antiarrhythmic

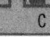

No   No   ?   C

Injection: 3 mg/mL (2, 4 mL); preservative free

Supraventricular tachycardia:
   Neonate: 0.05 mg/kg by rapid IV push over 1–2 seconds; may increase dose by 0.05 mg/kg increments Q2 min to **max.** of 0.25 mg/kg.
   Child: 0.1–0.2 mg/kg (**initial max. dose:** 6 mg) by rapid IV push over 1–2 seconds; may increase dose by 0.05 mg/kg increments Q2 min to **max.** of 0.25 mg/kg (up to 12 mg), or until termination of SVT. **Max. subsequent single dose:** 12 mg.
   Adolescent and adults ≥50 kg: 6 mg rapid IV push over 1–2 seconds; if no response after 1–2 min, give 12 mg rapid IV push. May repeat a second 12-mg dose after 1–2 min if required. **Max. single dose:** 12 mg.

Contraindicated in 2nd- and 3rd-degree AV block or sick sinus syndrome unless pacemaker placed. **Use with caution** in combination with digoxin (enhanced depressant effects on SA and AV nodes). If necessary, doses may be administered IO.

Follow each dose with NS flush. $T_{1/2}$: <10 seconds.

May precipitate bronchoconstriction, especially in asthmatics. Side effects include transient asystole, facial flushing, headache, shortness of breath, dyspnea, nausea, chest pain, and lightheadedness. Carbamazepine and dipyridamole may increase effects/toxicity of adenosine. Methylxanthines (e.g., caffeine, theophylline) may decrease effects of adenosine.

For explanation of icons, see p. 648

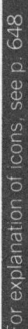

ALBUMIN, HUMAN
Albuminar, Albutein, Buminate, Plasbumin, Normal Serum
Albumin (Human), and many others
Blood product derivative, plasma volume expander

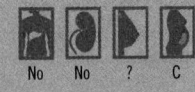

No   No   ?   C

Injection: 5% (50 mg/mL) (50, 100, 250, 500, mL); 25% (250 mg/mL) (20, 50, 100 mL); both concentrations contain 130–160 mEq Na/L

Hypoalbuminemia:
   Child: 0.5–1 g/kg/dose IV over 30–120 min; repeat Q1–2 days PRN
   Adult: 25 g/dose IV over 30–120 min; repeat Q1–2 days PRN
   Max. dose: 2 g/kg/24 hr
Hypovolemia:
   Child: 0.5–1 g/kg/dose IV rapid infusion; may repeat PRN; **max. dose:** 6 g/kg/24 hr
   Adult: 25 g/dose IV rapid infusion; may repeat PRN; **max. dose:** 250 g/48 hr

Contraindicated in cases of CHF or severe anemia; rapid infusion may cause fluid overload; hypersensitivity reactions may occur; may cause rapid increase in serum sodium levels.
Caution: 25% concentration contraindicated in preterm infants owing to risk of IVH. For infusion, use 5-micron filter or larger. Both 5% and 25% products are isotonic but differ in oncotic effects. Dilutions of the 25% product should be made with D₅W or NS; **avoid sterile water as a diluent.**

ALBUTEROL
Proventil, VoSpire ER (sustained-release tabs);
ProAir HFA, Proventil HFA, Ventolin HFA (aerosol inhaler);
AccuNeb (prediluted nebulized solution); and many others
β₂-Adrenergic agonist

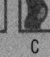

No   No   1   C

Tabs: 2, 4 mg
Sustained-release tabs: 4, 8 mg
Oral solution: 2 mg/5 mL (473 mL)
Aerosol inhaler (HFA): 90 mcg/actuation (60 actuations/inhaler) (8.5 g)
Nebulization solution (dilution required): 0.5% (5 mg/mL) (0.5, 20 mL)
Prediluted nebulized solution: 0.63 mg in 3 mL NS, 1.25 mg in 3 mL NS, and 2.5 mg in 3 mL NS (0.083%); some preparations may be preservative free.

Inhalations (nonacute use; see remarks):
   Aerosol (HFA): 2 puffs (90 mcg) Q4–6 hr PRN
   Nebulization:
     <1 yr: 0.05–0.15 mg/kg/dose Q4–6 hr
     1–5 yr: 1.25–2.5 mg/dose Q4–6 hr
     5–12 yr: 2.5 mg/dose Q4–6 hr
     >12 yr: 2.5–5 mg/dose Q4–8 hr
For use in acute exacerbations, more aggressive dosing may be used.
Oral (discouraged [see remarks]):
   2–6 yr: 0.3 mg/kg/24 hr PO ÷ TID; **max. dose:** 12 mg/24 hr
   6–12 yr: 6 mg/24 hr PO ÷ TID; **max. dose:** 24 mg/24 hr
   >12 yr and adult: 2–4 mg/dose PO TID–QID; **max. dose:** 32 mg/24 hr

Inhaled doses may be given more frequently than indicated. In such cases, consider cardiac monitoring and monitoring of serum potassium (hypokalemia). Systemic effects are dose related. Please verify concentration of nebulization solution used.

ALBUTEROL *continued*

Safety and efficacy for the treatment of symptoms or bronchospasms associated with obstructive airway disease have not been demonstrated for children <4 yr of age (either dose studied was not optimal in this age or drug is not effective in this age group).

Use of oral dosage form is discouraged owing to increased side effects and decreased efficacy compared to inhaled formulations.

Possible side effects include tachycardia, palpitations, tremor, insomnia, nervousness, nausea, and headache.

Use of tube spacers or chambers may enhance efficacy of metered dose inhalers and have been proven to be just as effective and sometimes safer than nebulizers.

ALLOPURINOL
Zyloprim, Alloprim, and generics
Uric acid–lowering agent, xanthine oxidase inhibitor

Yes   Yes   1   C

Tabs: 100, 300 mg
Oral suspension: 20 mg/mL
Injection (Alloprim): 500 mg
Contains ≈ 1.45 mEq Na/500 mg drug

For use in tumor lysis syndrome, see Chapter 22.
Child:
  Oral: 10 mg/kg/24 hr PO ÷ BID–QID; **max. dose:** 800 mg/24 hr
  Injectable: 200 mg/m²/24 hr IV ÷ Q6–12 hr; **max. dose:** 600 mg/24 hr
Adult:
  Oral: 200–800 mg/24 hr PO ÷ BID–TID
  Injectable: 200–400 mg/m²/24 hr IV ÷ Q6–12 hr; **max. dose:** 600 mg/24 hr

Adjust dose in renal insufficiency (see Chapter 31). Must maintain adequate urine output and alkaline urine.

Drug interactions: Increases serum theophylline level; may increase the incidence of rash with ampicillin and amoxicillin; increased risk of toxicity with azathioprine, didanosine, and mercaptopurine; increased risk of hypersensitivity reactions with ACE inhibitors and thiazide diuretics. Use with didanosine is **contraindicated** owing to increased risk for didanosine toxicity. Rhabdomyolysis has been reported with clarithromycin use.

Side effects include rash, neuritis, hepatotoxicity, GI disturbance, bone marrow suppression, and drowsiness.

IV dosage form is very alkaline and must be **diluted to a minimum concentration** of 6 mg/mL and infused over 30 min.

For explanation of icons, see p. 648

ALPROSTADIL
Prostin VR Pediatric, Prostaglandin E₁, PGE₁
Prostaglandin E₁, vasodilator

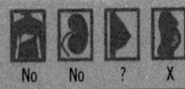

No   No   ?   X

Injection: 500 mcg/mL (1 mL); contains dehydrated alcohol

Neonate:
  Initial: 0.05–0.1 mcg/kg/min. Advance to 0.2 mcg/kg/min if necessary.
  Maintenance: When increase in PaO_2 is noted, decrease immediately to lowest effective dose.
  Usual dosage range: 0.01–0.4 mcg/kg/min; doses above 0.4 mcg/kg/min not likely to produce
  additional benefit.
To prepare infusion: See inside front cover.

For palliation only. Continuous vital sign monitoring essential. May cause apnea
  (10%–12%, especially in those weighing <2 kg at birth), fever, seizures, flushing,
  bradycardia, hypotension, diarrhea, gastric outlet obstruction, and reversible cortical
  proliferation of long bones (with prolonged use). May decrease platelet aggregation.

ALTEPLASE
Activase, Cathflo Activase, tPA
Thrombolytic agent, tissue plasminogen activator

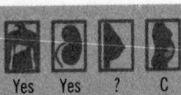

Yes   Yes   ?   C

Injection:
  Cathflo Activase: 2 mg
  Activase: 50 mg (29 million units), 100 mg (58 million units)
  Contains L-arginine and polysorbate 80.

Occluded IV catheter:
Aspiration method: Use 1 mg/1 mL concentration as follows:
  Central venous line (dosage per lumen, treating one lumen at a time):
    <30 kg: Instill a volume equal to 110% of internal lumen volume of the catheter
    NOT exceeding 2 mg.
    ≥30 kg: 2 mg each lumen.
  Subcutaneous port: Instill a volume equal to 110% of internal lumen and line volume of
    the port **NOT exceeding** 2 mg.
Instill into catheter over 1–2 min and leave in place for 2 hr before attempting blood withdrawal. After
2 hr, attempts to withdraw blood may be made Q2 hr for 3 attempts. Dose may be repeated once in 24
hours using a longer catheter dwell time of 3–4 hr. After 3–4 hr (repeat dose), attempts to withdrawal
blood may be made Q2 hr for 3 attempts. **DO NOT** infuse into patient.
Systemic thrombolytic therapy (use in consultation with a hematologist [see remarks]): Dosage
regimens ranging from lower dosages (0.01 mg/kg/hr) to higher dosages (0.1–0.6 mg/kg/hr) have been
reported (*Chest.* 2008;133:887S-968S). The length of continuous infusion is variable; patients may
respond to longer or shorter courses of therapy.

Current use in the pediatric population is limited. May cause bleeding, rash, and
  increase prothrombin time.
THROMBOLYTIC USE: History of stroke, transient ischemic attacks, other neurologic
  disease, and hypertension are **contraindications for adults** but considered **relative
  contraindications for children.** Monitor fibrinogen, thrombin clotting time, PT, and APTT when used
  as a thrombolytic. For systemic thrombosis therapy, efficacy has been reported at 40%–97%, with

ALTEPLASE *continued*

the risk for bleeding at 3%–27%. Poor efficacy in VTE in children has been recently reported. **Use with caution** in severe hepatic or renal dysfunction (systemic use only).

Newborns have reduced plasminogen levels (≈50% of adult values) that decrease the thrombolytic effects of alteplase. Plasminogen supplementation may be necessary.

ALUMINUM HYDROXIDE
Amphojel, Alu-Cap, Dialume, AlternaGEL and various generics
Antacid, phosphate binder

No   Yes   ?   ?

Oral suspension [OTC]: 320 mg/5 mL (473 mL)
Oral tablet: 300, 600 mg
Oral capsule (Alu-Cap): 400 mg
Each 5 mL suspension contains < 0.13 mEq Na.

Antacid:
  Child: 300–900 mg PO 1–3 hr PC and HS
  Adult: 600–1200 mg PO 1–3 hr PC and HS; **max. dose:** 3600 mg/24 hr
Prophylaxis against GI bleeding (mL volume dosages are based on the 320 mg/5 mL oral suspension concentration):
  Neonate: 1 mL/kg/dose PO Q4 hr PRN
  Infant: 2–5 mL PO Q1–2 hr
  Child: 5–15 mL PO Q1–2 hr
  Adult: 30–60 mL PO Q1–2 hr
Hyperphosphatemia (administer all doses between meals and titrate to normal serum phosphorus):
  Child: 50–150 mg/kg/24 hr ÷ Q4–6 hr PO
  Adult: 300–600 mg TID–QID PO between meals and QHS
Max. dose (all ages): 3000 mg/24 hr

Use with caution in patients with renal failure and upper GI hemorrhage.
Interferes with absorption of several orally administered medications, including digoxin, ethambutol, indomethacin, isoniazid, naproxen, mycophenolate, tetracyclines, fluoroquinolones (e.g., ciprofloxacin), and iron. Generally, **do not** take oral mediations within 1–2 hours of taking aluminum hydroxide dose unless specified.
May cause constipation, decreased bowel motility, encephalopathy, and phosphorus depletion.

ALUMINUM HYDROXIDE WITH MAGNESIUM HYDROXIDE
Maalox, Maalox Maximum Strength Liquid, Mylanta, Mylanta Extra Strength, Almacone, Almacone Double Strength, RuLox, and many others generics (see remarks)
Antacid

No   Yes   ?   ?

Chewable tabs [OTC]: (Al[OH]$_3$ and Mg[OH]$_2$)
  Almacone: 200 mg AlOH, 200 mg MgOH, and 20 mg simethicone
Oral suspension [OTC] (see remarks):
  Maalox, Mylanta, and Almacone: Each 5 mL contains 200 mg AlOH, 200 mg MgOH, and 20 mg simethicone (150, 360, 720 mL).
  RuLox: Each 5 mL contains 200 mg AlOH, 200 mg MgOH, and 25 mg simethicone (355 mL).
  Mylanta Extra Strength, Maalox Maximum Strength liquid, and Almacone Double Strength: Each 5 mL contains 400 mg AlOH, 400 mg MgOH, and 40 mg simethicone (360, 480 mL).

Continued

ALUMINUM HYDROXIDE WITH MAGNESIUM HYDROXIDE *continued*

Mylanta Ultimate Strength: Each 5 mL contains 500 mg AlOH, 500 mg MgOH (360 mL)
Many other combinations exist.
Contains 0.03–0.06 mEq Na/5 mL

Same as for aluminum hydroxide preparations. **Do not use** combination
product for hyperphosphatemia.

May have laxative effect. May cause hypokalemia. **Use with caution** in patients
with renal insufficiency (magnesium), gastric outlet obstruction.
Interferes with absorption of benzodiazepines, chloroquine, digoxin, naproxen, mycophenolate,
phenytoin, quinolones (e.g., ciprofloxacin), tetracyclines, and iron. Generally, **do not take** oral
mediations within 1–2 hr of taking antacid dose unless specified.
DO NOT use Maalox Total Relief (bismuth subsalicylate), Mylanta Supreme Liquid (calcium carbonate +
magnesium hydroxide), Maalox Regular Strength Chewable Tablets and Children's Mylanta Chewable
Tablets (calcium carbonate), Maalox Maximum Strength Chewable (calcium carbonate and simethicone),
Mylanta Gas (simethicone); these products do not contain aluminum hydroxide and magnesium hydroxide.

AMANTADINE HYDROCHLORIDE
Symmetrel and others
Antiviral agent

 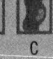 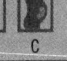

Yes   Yes   3   C

Capsule: 100 mg
Tabs: 100 mg
Oral solution or syrup: 50 mg/5 mL (480 mL); may contain parabens

*Influenza A prophylaxis and treatment (for treatment, it is best to initiate
therapy immediately after symptom onset, within 2 days [see remarks]):*
   1–9 yr: 5 mg/kg/24 hr PO ÷ BID; **max. dose:** 150 mg/24 hr
   >9 yr:
      <40 kg: 5 mg/kg/24 hr PO ÷ BID; **max. dose** 200 mg/24 hr
      ≥40 kg: 200 mg/24 hr ÷ BID
Alternative dosing for influenza A prophylaxis:
   Child >20 kg and adult: 100 mg/24 hr PO ÷ BID
Prophylaxis (duration of therapy):
   Single exposure: At least 10 days
   Repeated/uncontrolled exposure: Up to 90 days
   Use with influenza A vaccine when possible.
Symptomatic treatment (duration of therapy):
   Continue for 24–48 hr after disappearance of symptoms.

Do not use in first trimester of pregnancy. **Use with caution** in patients with liver
disease, seizures, renal disease, CHF, peripheral edema, orthostatic hypotension, history
of recurrent eczematoid rash, and in those receiving CNS stimulants. **Adjust dose in patients
with renal insufficiency (see Chapter 31).**
CDC has reported resistance to influenza A and recommendations against use for treatment and
prophylaxis. Check with local microbiology laboratories and CDC for seasonal susceptibility/
resistance. Individuals immunized with live attenuated influenza vaccine should not receive
amantadine prophylaxis for 14 days after the vaccine.
May cause dizziness, anxiety, depression, mental status change, rash (livedo reticularis), nausea,
orthostatic hypotension, edema, CHF, and urinary retention. Impulse control disorder has been
reported. Neuroleptic malignant syndrome has been reported with abrupt dose reduction or
discontinuation (especially if patient is receiving neuroleptics).

A

FORMULARY

AMIKACIN SULFATE
Amikin and many generics
Antibiotic, aminoglycoside

No   Yes   1   D

Injection: 250 mg/mL; may contain sodium bisulfite

Initial empirical dosage; patient specific dosage defined by therapeutic drug
monitoring (see remarks).
Neonates: See the following table.

Postconceptional Age (wk)	Postnatal Age (days)	Dose (mg/kg/dose)	Interval (hr)
≤29*	0–7	18	48
	8–28	15	36
	>28	15	24
30–33	0–7	18	36
	>7	15	24
34–37	0–7	15	24
	>7	15	18–24†
≥38	0–7	15	24
	>7	15	12–18

*Or significant asphyxia, PDA, indomethacin use, poor cardiac output, reduced renal function.
†Use Q36 hr interval for HIE patients receiving whole-body therapeutic cooling.

Infant and child: 15–22.5 mg/kg/24 hr ÷ Q8 hr IV/IM; infants and patients requiring higher doses
(e.g., cystic fibrosis) may receive initial doses of 30 mg/kg/24 hr ÷ Q8 hr IV/IM
Cystic fibrosis (if available, use patient's previous therapeutic mg/kg dosage):
 Conventional Q8 hr dosing: 30 mg/kg/24 hr ÷ Q8 hr IV
 High-dose extended interval (once daily) dosing (limited data): 30–35 mg/kg/24 hr Q24 hr IV
 Adult: 15 mg/kg/24 hr ÷ Q8–12 hr IV/IM
 Initial max. dose: 1.5 g/24 hr, then monitor levels

Use with **caution** in preexisting renal, vestibular, or auditory impairment;
concomitant anesthesia or neuromuscular blockers; neurotoxic, concomitant neurotoxic,
ototoxic, or nephrotoxic drugs; sulfite sensitivity; and dehydration. **Adjust dose in renal
failure (see Chapter 31).** Longer dosing intervals may be necessary for neonates receiving
indomethacin for PDAs and for all patients with poor cardiac output. Rapidly eliminated
in patients with cystic fibrosis, burns, and in febrile neutropenic patients. CNS penetration
is poor beyond early infancy.

Therapeutic levels (using conventional dosing): Peak, 20–30 mg/L; trough 5–10 mg/L. Recommended
serum sampling time at steady state: trough within 30 min before third consecutive dose and peak
30–60 minutes after administration of third consecutive dose. Peak levels of 25–30 mg/L have been
recommended for CNS, pulmonary, bone, life-threatening, *Pseudomonas* infections, and in febrile
neutropenic patients.

Therapeutic levels for cystic fibrosis using high-dose extended interval (once daily) dosing: Peak, 80 to
120 mg/L; trough, <10 mg/L. Recommended serum sampling time: trough within 30 minutes before
dose and peak 30 to 60 minutes after administration of dose.

For initial dosing in obese patients, use an adjusted body weight (ABW). ABW = Ideal body weight +
0.4 (Total body weight − Ideal body weight).

May cause ototoxicity, nephrotoxicity, neuromuscular blockade, and rash. Loop diuretics may potentiate
ototoxicity of all aminoglycoside antibiotics.

For explanation of icons, see p. 648

AMINOCAPROIC ACID
Amicar and generics
Hemostatic agent

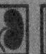
Yes   Yes   ?   C

Tabs: 500, 1000 mg
Oral liquid/syrup: 250 mg/mL (240, 480 mL); may contain 0.2% methylparaben and 0.05% propylparaben
Injection: 250 mg/mL (20 mL); contains 0.9% benzyl alcohol

Child (IV/PO):
Loading dose: 100–200 mg/kg
Maintenance: 100 mg/kg/dose Q4–6 hr; **max. dose:** 30 g/24 hr
Adult (IV/PO): 4–5 g during the first hour, followed by 1 g/hr × 8 hr or until bleeding is controlled.
Max. dose: 30 g/24 hr

Contraindications: DIC, hematuria. **Use with caution** in patients with cardiac, renal, or hepatic disease. Should not be given with factor IX complex concentrates or antiinhibitor coagulant concentrates because of risk for thrombosis. Dose should be reduced by 75% in oliguria or end-stage renal disease. Hypercoagulation may be produced when given in conjunction with oral contraceptives.

May cause nausea, diarrhea, malaise, weakness, headache, decreased platelet function, hypotension, and false increase in urine amino acids. Elevation of serum potassium may occur, especially in patients with renal impairment.

AMINOPHYLLINE
Various generic products
Bronchodilator, methylxanthine

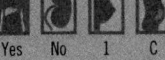
Yes   No   1   C

Injection: 25 mg/mL (79% theophylline) (10, 20 mL)
Note: Pharmacy may dilute IV dosage forms to enhance accuracy of neonatal dosing.

Neonatal apnea:
Loading dose: 5–6 mg/kg IV
Maintenance dose: 1–2 mg/kg/dose Q6–8 hr, IV
Asthma exacerbation and reactive airway disease:
IV loading: 6 mg/kg IV over 20 min (each 1.2 mg/kg dose raises the serum theophylline concentration 2 mg/L)
IV maintenance: Continuous IV drip:
Neonate: 0.2 mg/kg/hr
6 wk–6 mo: 0.5 mg/kg/hr
6 mo–1 yr: 0.6–0.7 mg/kg/hr
1–9 yr: 1–1.2 mg/kg/hr
9–12 yr and young adult smoker: 0.9 mg/kg/hr
>12 yr healthy nonsmoker: 0.7 mg/kg/hr
The above total daily doses may also be administered IV ÷ Q4–6 hr.

Consider mg of theophylline available when dosing aminophylline. For oral route of administration, use theophylline.

Monitoring serum levels is essential, especially in infants and young children. Intermittent dosing for infants and children 1–5 yr may require Q4 hr dosing regimen owing to enhanced metabolism/clearance. Side effects: restlessness, GI upset, headache, tachycardia, seizures (may occur in absence of other side effects with toxic levels).

AMINOPHYLLINE *continued*

Therapeutic level (theophylline): For asthma, 10–20 mg/L; for neonatal apnea, 6–13 mg/L.
Recommended Guidelines for obtaining levels:

IV bolus: 30 min after infusion

IV continuous: 12–24 hr after initiation of infusion

PO liquid, immediate-release tab:

Peak: 1 hr post dose

Trough: Just before dose

PO sustained-release:

Peak: 4 hr post dose

Trough: Just before dose

Ideally, obtain levels after steady state has been achieved (after at least 1 day of therapy). Liver impairment, cardiac failure, and sustained high fever may increase theophylline levels. See *Theophylline* for drug interactions.

Use in breast-feeding may cause irritability in infant. It is recommended to avoid breast-feeding for 2 hr after IV or 4 hr after immediate-release oral intermittent dose.

AMIODARONE HCL
Cordarone, Pacerone, Nexterone, and various generics
Antiarrhythmic, Class III

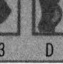

| Yes | No | 3 | D |

Tabs: 100, 200, 400 mg
Oral suspension: 5 mg/mL
Injection: 50 mg/mL (3, 9, 18 mL) (contains 20.2 mg/mL benzyl alcohol and 100 mg/mL polysorbate 80 or Tween 80)
Premixed injection (Nexterone): 1.5 mg/mL (100 mL) (iso-osmotic solution, each 1 mL contains 15 mg sulfobutyl ether β-cyclodextrin, 0.362 mg citric acid, 0.183 mg sodium citrate, and 42.1 mg dextrose), 1.8 mg/mL (200 mL) (iso-osmotic solution, each 1 mL contains 18 mg sulfobutyl ether β-cyclodextrin, 0.362 mg citric acid, 0.183 mg sodium citrate, and 41.4 mg dextrose)
Contains 37% iodine by weight.

See algorithms in front cover of book for arrest dosing.
Child PO for tachyarrhythmia:

<1 yr: 600–800 mg/1.73 m²/24 hr ÷ Q12–24 hr × 4–14 days and/or until adequate control achieved, then reduce to 200–400 mg/1.73 m²/24 hr.

≥1 yr: 10–15 mg/kg/24 hr ÷ Q12–24 hr × 4–14 days and/or until adequate control achieved, then reduce to 5 mg/kg/24 hr ÷ Q12–24 hr if effective.

Child IV for tachyarrhythmia (limited data):

5 mg/kg (**max. dose:** 300 mg) over 30 min, followed by a continuous infusion starting at 5 mcg/kg/min; infusion may be increased up to a **max. dose** of 15 mcg/kg/min or 20 mg/kg/24 hr.

Adult PO for ventricular arrhythmias:

Loading dose: 800–1600 mg/24 hr ÷ Q12–24 hr for 1–3 wk

Maintenance: 600–800 mg/24 hr ÷ Q12–24 hr × 1 mo, then 200 mg Q12–24 hr

Use lowest effective dose to minimize adverse reactions.

Adult IV for ventricular arrhythmias:

Loading dose: 150 mg over 10 min (15 mg/min), followed by 360 mg over 6 hr (1 mg/min), followed by a maintenance dose of 0.5 mg/min. Supplemental boluses of 150 mg over 10 min may be given for breakthrough VF or hemodynamically unstable VT, and the maintenance infusion may be increased to suppress the arrhythmia. **Max. dose:** 2.1 g/24 hr.

For explanation of icons, see p. 648

Continued

AMIODARONE HCL *continued*

Used in the resuscitation algorithm for ventricular fibrillation/pulseless ventricular tachycardia **(see front cover for arrest dosing and back cover for PALS algorithm).** Overall use of this drug may be limited to its potentially life-threatening side effects and the difficulties associated with managing its use.

Contraindicated in severe sinus node dysfunction, marked sinus bradycardia, second- and third-degree AV block. **Use with caution** in hepatic impairment.

Long elimination half-life (40–55 days). Major metabolite is active.

Increases cyclosporine, digoxin, phenytoin, tacrolimus, warfarin, calcium channel blocker, theophylline, and quinidine levels. Amiodarone is a cytochrome P450 3A3/4 substrate and inhibits CYP 3A3/4, 2C9, and 2D6. Risk of rhabdomyolysis is increased when used with simvastatin at doses >20 mg/24 hr and lovastatin at doses >40 mg/24 hr.

Proposed therapeutic level with chronic oral use: 1–2.5 mg/L.

Asymptomatic corneal microdeposits should appear in all patients. Alters liver enzymes, thyroid function. Pulmonary fibrosis reported in adults. May cause worsening of preexisting arrhythmias with bradycardia and AV block. May also cause hypotension, anorexia, nausea, vomiting, dizziness, paresthesias, ataxia, tremor, SIADH, and hypothyroidism or hyperthyroidism. Drug rash with eosinophilia and systemic symptoms (DRESS) have been reported.

Intravenous continuous infusion concentration for peripheral administration should not exceed 2 mg/mL and **must be diluted** with D_5W. The intravenous dosage form can leach out plasticizers such as DEHP. To reduce potential exposure to plasticizers in pregnant women and children at the toddler stages of development and younger, alternative methods of IV drug administration should be used.

Oral administration should be consistent with regard to meals, because food increases the rate and extent of oral absorption.

AMITRIPTYLINE
Elavil and generics
Antidepressant, tricyclic

   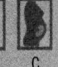

Yes   No   2   C

Tabs: 10, 25, 50, 75, 100, 150 mg
Oral suspension: 1 mg/mL

Antidepressant:
Child: Start with 1 mg/kg/24 hr ÷ TID PO for 3 days; then increase to 1.5 mg/kg/24 hr.
Dose may be gradually increased to a **max. dose** of 5 mg/kg/24 hr if needed.
Monitor ECG, BP, and heart rate for doses >3 mg/kg/24 hr.
Adolescent: 10 mg TID PO and 20 mg QHS; dose may be gradually increased up to a **max. dose** of 200 mg/24 hr if needed.
Adult: 40–100 mg/24 hr ÷ QHS–BID PO; dose may be gradually increased up to 300 mg/24 hr if needed; gradually decrease dose to lowest effective dose when symptoms are controlled.

Augment analgesia for chronic pain:
Child: Initial 0.1 mg/kg/dose QHS PO; increase as needed and tolerated over 2–3 wk to 0.5–2 mg/kg/dose QHS.

Migraine prophylaxis (limited data):
Child: Initial 0.1–0.25 mg/kg/dose QHS PO; increase as needed and tolerated Q2 wk by 0.1–0.25 mg/kg/dose up to a **max. dose** of 2 mg/kg/24 hr or 75 mg/24 hr. For doses >1 mg/kg/24 hr, divide daily dose BID and monitor ECG.
Adult: Initial 10–25 mg/dose QHS PO; reported range of 10–400 mg/24 hr.

AMITRIPTYLINE *continued*

Contraindicated in narrow-angle glaucoma, seizures, severe cardiac disorders, and patients who received MAO inhibitors within 14 days.

$T_{1/2}$ = 9–25 hr in adults. Maximum antidepressant effects may not occur for 2 wk or more after initiation of therapy. **Do not abruptly discontinue therapy in patients receiving high doses for prolonged periods.**

Therapeutic levels (sum of amitriptyline and nortriptyline): 100–250 ng/mL. Recommended serum sampling time: obtain a single level 8 hr or more after an oral dose (after 4–5 days of continuous dosing). Amitriptyline is a substrate for CYP 450 1A2, 2C9, 2C19, 2D6, and 3A3/4 and inhibitor for CYP 450 1A2, 2C19, 2C9, 2D6, and 2E1. Rifampin can decrease amitriptyline levels. Amitriptyline may increase side effects of tramadol.

Side effects include sedation, urinary retention, constipation, dry mouth, dizziness, drowsiness, liver enzyme elevation, and arrhythmia. May discolor urine (blue/green). QHS dosing during first weeks of therapy will reduce sedation. Monitor ECG, BP, CBC at start of therapy and with dose changes. Decrease dose if PR interval reaches 0.22 sec, QRS reaches 130% of baseline, HR rises above 140/min, or if BP is >140/90. Tricyclics may cause mania. For antidepressant use, monitor for clinical worsening of depression and suicidal ideation/behavior after initiation of therapy or after dose changes.

AMLODIPINE
Norvasc
Calcium channel blocker, antihypertensive

Yes   No   ?   C

Tabs: 2.5, 5, 10 mg
Oral suspension: 1 mg/mL

Child:
Hypertension: Start with 0.1 mg/kg/dose (**max. dose:** 5 mg) PO once daily–BID; dosage may be gradually increased to a **max. dose** of 0.6 mg/kg/24 hr up to 20 mg/24 hr.
An effective antihypertensive dose for 6–17 year olds of 2.5–5 mg once daily has been reported; doses >5 mg have not been evaluated.

Adult:
Hypertension: 5–10 mg/dose once daily PO; use 2.5 mg/dose once daily PO in patients with hepatic insufficiency.
Max. dose: 10 mg/24 hr

Use with caution in combination with other antihypertensive agents. Younger children may require higher mg/kg doses than older children and adults. A BID dosing regimen may provide better efficacy in children.

Reduce dose in hepatic insufficiency. Allow 5–7 days of continuous initial dose therapy before making dosage adjustments because of the drug's gradual onset of action and lengthy elimination half-life. Amlodipine is a substrate for CYP 450 3A4 and **should be used with caution** with 3A4 inhibitors such as protease inhibitors and azole antifungals (e.g., fluconazole, ketoconazole). May increase levels and toxicity of cyclosporine and simvastatin.

Dose-related side effects include edema, dizziness, flushing, fatigue, and palpitations. Other side effects include headache, nausea, abdominal pain, and somnolence.

For explanation of icons, see p. 648

AMMONIUM CHLORIDE
Various generics
Diuretic, urinary acidifying agent

Yes   Yes   ?   C

Injection: 5 mEq/mL (26.75%) (20 mL); contains EDTA
1 mEq = 53 mg

Urinary acidification:
   Child: 75 mg/kg/24 hr ÷ Q6 hr IV; **max. dose:** 6 g/24 hr
   Adult: 1.5 g/dose Q6 hr IV
Drug administration: Dilute to concentration ≤0.4 mEq/mL. Infusion **not to exceed** 50 mg/kg/hr
or 1 mEq/kg/hr.

Contraindicated in hepatic or renal insufficiency and primary respiratory acidosis.
   Use with caution in infants.
May produce acidosis, hyperammonemia, and GI irritation. Monitor serum chloride level,
acid/base status, and serum ammonia.

AMOXICILLIN
Amoxil, Trimox, Wymox, Polymox, Moxatag and generics
Antibiotic, aminopenicillin

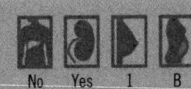

No   Yes   1   B

Oral suspension: 125, 250 mg/5 mL (80, 100, 150 mL); and 200, 400 mg/5 mL (50, 75, 100 mL)
Caps: 250, 500 mg
Tablets: 500, 875 mg
Chewable tabs: 125, 200, 250, 400 mg; may contain phenylalanine
Extended-release tabs (Moxatag [see remarks]): 775 mg

Neonate to ≤3 mo: 20–30 mg/kg/24 hr ÷ Q12 hr PO
Child:
   Standard dose: 25–50 mg/kg/24 hr ÷ Q8–12 hr PO
   High dose (resistant Streptococcus pneumoniae): 80–90 mg/kg/24 hr ÷ BID PO
   Max. dose: 2–3 g/24 hr
Adult:
   Mild/moderate infections: 250 mg/dose Q8 hr PO OR 500 mg/dose Q12 hr PO
   Severe infections: 500 mg/dose Q8 hr PO OR 875 mg/dose Q12 hr PO
   Max. dose: 2–3 g/24 hr
Tonsillitis/pharyngitis (Streptococcus pyogenes): 50 mg/kg/24 hr ÷ Q12 hr PO ×10 days; **max. dose:**
1 g/24 hr.
Extended-release tablets (Moxatag): 775 mg once daily PO × 10 days is indicated for children ≥12 yr
and adults.
Recurrent otitis media prophylaxis: 20 mg/kg/dose QHS PO
SBE prophylaxis: See Chapter 7.
Early Lyme disease:
   Child: 50 mg/kg/24 hr ÷ Q8 hr PO × 14–21 days; **max. dose:** 1.5 g/24 hr
   Adult: 500 mg/dose Q8 hr PO × 14–21 days

Renal elimination. **Adjust dose in renal failure (see Chapter 31).** Serum levels about twice
those achieved with equal dose of ampicillin. Fewer GI effects but otherwise similar to
ampicillin. Side effects: rash and diarrhea. Rash may develop with concurrent EBV infection.
May increase warfarin's effect by increasing INR.
High-dose regimen, increasingly useful, is recommended in respiratory infections, acute otitis media,
and sinusitis, owing to increasing incidence of penicillin-resistant pneumococci. Chewable tablets
may contain phenylalanine and should not be used by phenylketonurics.

AMOXICILLIN–CLAVULANIC ACID
Augmentin, Amoclan, Augmentin ES-600, Augmentin XR,
and various generic products
Antibiotic, aminopenicillin with β-lactamase inhibitor

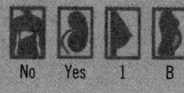

No   Yes   1   B

Tabs:
 For TID dosing: 250, 500 mg (with 125 mg clavulanate)
 For BID dosing: 875 mg amoxicillin (with 125 mg clavulanate); Augmentin XR: 1 g amoxicillin
 (with 62.5 mg clavulanate)
Chewable tabs:
 For BID dosing: 200, 400 mg amoxicillin (28.5 and 57 mg clavulanate, respectively); contains
 saccharin and aspartame
Oral suspension:
 For TID dosing: 125, 250 mg amoxicillin/5 mL (31.25 and 62.5 mg clavulanate/5 mL, respectively)
 (75, 100, 150 mL); contains saccharin
 For BID dosing: 200, 400 mg amoxicillin/5 mL (28.5 and 57 mg clavulanate/5 mL, respectively)
 (50, 75, 100 mL); 600 mg amoxicillin/5 mL (Augmentin ES-600 contains 42.9 mg clavulanate/5
 mL) (50, 75, 125, 200 mL); contains saccharin and/or aspartame
Contains 0.63 mEq K$^+$ per 125 mg clavulanate (Augmentin ES-600 contains 0.23 mEq K$^+$ per
42.9 mg clavulanate)

Dosage based on amoxicillin component (see remarks for resistant S. pneumoniae).
Infant 1–<3 mo: 30 mg/kg/24 hr ÷ Q12 hr PO (recommended dosage form is 125 mg/5 mL
suspension)

Child ≥3 mo:
 TID dosing (see remarks): 20–40 mg/kg/24 hr ÷ Q8 hr PO
 BID dosing (see remarks): 25–45 mg/kg/24 hr ÷ Q12 hr PO
 Augmentin ES-600:
 ≥3 mo and <40 kg: 90 mg/kg/24 hr ÷ Q12 hr PO × 10 days
Adult: 250–500 mg/dose Q8 hr PO or 875 mg/dose Q12 hr PO for more severe and respiratory infections
 Augmentin XR:
 ≥16 yr and adult: 2 g Q12 hr PO × 10 days for acute bacterial sinusitis or × 7–10 days for
 community-acquired pneumonia

Clavulanic acid extends the activity of amoxicillin to include β-lactamase–producing strains of
Haemophilus influenzae, Moraxella catarrhalis, Neisseria gonorrhoeae, and some
Staphylococcus aureus and may increase the risk for diarrhea. See *Amoxicillin* for additional
comments. **Adjust dose in renal failure (see Chapter 31). Contraindicated** in patients with
a history of cholestatic jaundice/hepatic dysfunction associated with amoxicillin–clavulanic
acid. Augmentin XR is **contraindicated** in patients with CrCl <30 mL/min.
The BID dosing schedule is associated with less diarrhea. For BID dosing, the 875-mg, 1-g tablets; the
200-mg, 400-mg chewable tablets; or the 200-mg/5 mL, 400-mg/5 mL, 600-mg/5 mL suspensions
should be used. These BID dosage forms contain phenylalanine and **should not be used** by
phenylketonurics. For TID dosing, the 250-mg, 500-mg tablets; or the 125-mg/5 mL, 250-mg/5 mL
suspensions should be used.
Higher doses of 80–90 mg/kg/24 hr (amoxicillin component) have been recommended for resistant
strains of *S. pneumoniae* in acute otitis media (use BID formulations containing 7:1 ratio of
amoxicillin to clavulanic acid or Augmentin ES-600).
The 250 or 500 mg tablets **cannot** be substituted for Augmentin XR.

For explanation of icons, see p. 648

AMPHOTERICIN B (CONVENTIONAL)
Fungizone, Amphocin, and various generics
Antifungal, polyene

Yes   Yes   ?   B

Injection: 50-mg vials

IV: Mix with D_5W to concentration 0.1 mg/mL (peripheral administration) or 0.25 mg/mL (central line only). pH > 4.2. Infuse over 2–6 hr.

Optional test dose: 0.1 mg/kg/dose IV up to **max. dose** of 1 mg (followed by remaining initial dose).

Initial dose: 0.5–1 mg/kg/24 hr; if test dose NOT used, infuse first dose over 6 hr and monitor frequently during the first several hours.

Increment: Increase as tolerated by 0.25–0.5 mg/kg/24 hr once daily or every other day. Use larger dosage increment (0.5 mg once daily) for critically ill patients.

Usual maintenance:
  Once-daily dosing: 0.5–1 mg/kg/24 hr once daily
  Every-other-day dosing: 1.5 mg/kg/dose every other day

Max. dose: 1.5 mg/kg/24 hr

Intrathecal: 25–100 mcg Q48–72 hr. Increase to 500 mcg as tolerated.

Bladder irrigation for urinary tract mycosis: 5–15 mg in 100 mL sterile water for irrigation at 100–300 mL/24 hr. Instill solution into bladder, clamp catheter for 1–2 hr, then drain; repeat TID–QID for 2–5 days.

Monitor renal, hepatic, electrolyte, and hematologic status closely. Hypercalciuria, hypokalemia, hypomagnesemia, RTA, renal failure, acute hepatic failure, hypotension, and phlebitis may occur. **For dosing information in renal failure, see Chapter 31.**

Common infusion-related reactions include fever, chills, headache, hypotension, nausea, vomiting; may premedicate with acetaminophen and diphenhydramine 30 min before and 4 hr after infusion. Meperidine useful for chills. Hydrocortisone, 1 mg/mg ampho (**max. dose:** 25 mg) added to bottle may help prevent immediate adverse reactions. Use total body weight for obese patients when calculating dosages.

Salt loading with 10–15 mL/kg of NS infused before each dose may minimize the risk of nephrotoxicity. Maintaining sodium intake of >4/kg/24 hr in premature neonates may also reduce risk for nephrotoxicity. Nephrotoxic drugs (e.g., aminoglycosides, chemotherapeutic agents, cyclosporine) may result in synergistic toxicity. Hypokalemia may increase toxicity of neuromuscular blocking agents and cardiac glycosides.

AMPHOTERICIN B LIPID COMPLEX
Abelcet, ABLC
Antifungal, polyene

Yes   Yes   ?   B

Injection: 5 mg/mL (20 mL)
(formulated as a 1:1 molar ratio of amphotericin B to lipid complex composed of dimyristoylphosphatidylcholine and dimyristoylphosphatidylglycerol)

IV: 2.5–5 mg/kg/24 hr once daily
  For visceral leishmaniasis that failed to respond to or relapsed after treatment with antimony compound, a dosage of 1–3 mg/kg/24 hr once daily × 5 days has been used.

Mix with D_5W to concentration 1 or 2 mg/mL for fluid-restricted patients.

Infusion rate: 2.5 mg/kg/hr; shake infusion bag Q2 hr if total infusion time exceeds 2 hr. **Do not** use an in-line filter.

Monitor renal, hepatic, electrolyte, and hematologic status closely. Thrombocytopenia, anemia, leukopenia, hypokalemia, hypomagnesemia, diarrhea, respiratory failure, rash, nephrotoxicity, and increases in liver enzymes and bilirubin may occur. See conventional amphotericin for drug interactions.

A

AMPHOTERICIN B LIPID COMPLEX *continued*

Highest concentrations achieved in spleen, lung, and liver from human autopsy data from one heart
transplant patient. CNS/CSF levels are lower than amphotericin B, liposomal (AmBisome). In animal
models, concentrations are higher in the liver, spleen, and lungs but the same in the kidneys when
compared with conventional amphotericin B. Pharmacokinetics in renal and hepatic impairment
have not been studied.

Common infusion-related reactions include fever, chills, rigors, nausea, vomiting, hypotension, and
headache; may premedicate with acetaminophen, diphenhydramine, and meperidine (see
Amphotericin B remarks).

AMPHOTERICIN B, LIPOSOMAL
AmBisome
Antifungal, polyene

Yes   Yes   ?   B

Injection: 50 mg (vials); contains soy, 900 mg sucrose
(formulated in liposomes composed of hydrogenated soy phosphatidylcholine, cholesterol,
distearoylphosphatidylglycerol, and α-tocopherol)

Systemic fungal infections: 3–5 mg/kg/24 hr IV once daily; an upper dosage limit of
10 mg/kg/24 hr has been suggested based on pharmacokinetic endpoints and risk for
hypokalemia. However, dosages as high as 15 mg/kg/24 hr have been used. Dosages as
high as 10 mg/kg/24 hr have been used in patients with *Aspergillus*.
Empirical therapy for febrile neutropenia: 3 mg/kg/24 hr IV once daily
Cryptococcal meningitis in HIV: 6 mg/kg/24 hr IV once daily
Leishmaniasis (a repeat course may be necessary if infection does not clear):
  Immunocompetent: 3 mg/kg/24 hr IV on days 1 to 5, 14, and 21
  Immunocompromised: 4 mg/kg/24 hr IV on days 1 to 5, 10, 17, 24, 31, and 38
Mix with D₅W to concentration of 1–2 mg/mL (0.2–0.5 mg/mL may be used for infants and small
children).
Infusion rate: Administer dose over 2 hr; infusion may be reduced to 1 hr if well tolerated. A ≥1-micron
in-line filter may be used.

Closely monitor renal, hepatic, electrolyte, and hematologic status. Thrombocytopenia, anemia,
leukopenia, tachycardia, hypokalemia, hypomagnesemia, hypocalcemia, hyperglycemia,
diarrhea, dyspnea, rash, low back pain, nephrotoxicity, and increases in liver enzymes and
bilirubin may occur. Rhabdomyolysis has been reported. Safety and effectiveness in neonates
have not been established. See conventional *Amphotericin* for drug interactions.
Compared with conventional amphotericin B, higher concentrations found in liver and spleen; similar
concentrations found in lungs and kidneys. CNS/CSF concentrations are higher than other
amphotericin B products. Pharmacokinetics in renal and hepatic impairment have not been studied.
Common infusion-related reactions include fever, chills, rigors, nausea, vomiting, hypotension, and
headache; may premedicate with acetaminophen, diphenhydramine, and meperidine (see
Amphotericin B remarks).
False elevations of serum phosphate have been reported with the PHOSm assay (used in Beckman
Coulter analyzers).

For explanation of icons, see p. 648

AMPICILLIN
Omnipen, Principen, Totacillin, and generics
Antibiotic, aminopenicillin

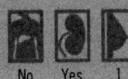

No   Yes   1   B

Oral suspension: 125 mg/5 mL, 250 mg/5 mL (100, 200 mL)
Caps: 250, 500 mg
Injection: 125, 250, 500 mg; 1, 2, 10 g
Contains 3 mEq Na/1 g IV drug

Neonate (IM/IV):

  <7 days:
    <2 kg: 50–100 mg/kg/24 hr ÷ Q12 hr
    ≥2 kg: 75–150 mg/kg/24 hr ÷ Q8 hr
    Group B streptococcal meningitis: 200–300 mg/kg/24 hr ÷ Q8 hr
  ≥7 days:
    <1.2 kg: 50–100 mg/kg/24 hr ÷ Q12 hr
    1.2–2 kg: 75–150 mg/kg/24 hr ÷ Q8 hr
    >2 kg: 100–200 mg/kg/24 hr ÷ Q6 hr
    Group B streptococcal meningitis: 300 mg/kg/24 hr ÷ Q4–6 hr
Infant/child:
  Mild/moderate infections:
    IM/IV: 100–200 mg/kg/24 hr ÷ Q6 hr
    PO: 50–100 mg/kg/24 hr ÷ Q6 hr; **max. PO dose:** 2–3 g/24 hr
  Severe infections: 200–400 mg/kg/24 hr ÷ Q4–6 hr IM/IV
  Community-acquired pneumonia in a fully immunized patient (IV/IM):
    Streptococcus pneumoniae *penicillin MIC ≤ 2.0:* 150–200 mg/kg/24 hr ÷ Q6 hr
    Streptococcus pneumoniae *penicillin MIC ≥ 4.0:* 300–400 mg/kg/24 hr ÷ Q6 hr
Max. IV/IM dose: 12 g/24 hr
Adult:
  IM/IV: 500–3000 mg Q4–6 hr
  PO: 250–500 mg Q6 hr
Max. IV/IM dose: 14 g/24 hr
SBE prophylaxis:
  Moderate-risk patients:
    Child: 50 mg/kg/dose × 1 IV/IM 30 min before procedure; **max. dose:** 2 g/dose
    Adult: 2 g/dose × 1 IV/IM 30 min before procedure
  High-risk patients with GU and GI procedures: Above doses PLUS gentamicin 1.5 mg/kg × 1
  (**max. dose:** 120 mg) IV within 30 min of starting procedure.

Use higher doses with shorter dosing intervals to treat CNS disease and severe infection.
  CSF penetration occurs only with inflamed meninges. **Adjust dose in renal failure**
  (see Chapter 31).
Produces the same side effects as penicillin, with cross-reactivity. Rash commonly seen at 5–10 days,
  and rash may occur with concurrent EBV infection or allopurinol use. May cause interstitial nephritis,
  diarrhea, and pseudomembranous enterocolitis. Chloroquine reduces ampicillin's oral absorption.

AMPICILLIN/SULBACTAM
Unasyn and generics
Antibiotic, aminopenicillin with β-lactamase inhibitor

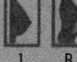

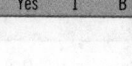
No   Yes   1   B

Injection:
   1.5 g = ampicillin 1 g + sulbactam 0.5 g
   3 g = ampicillin 2 g + sulbactam 1 g
   15 g = ampicillin 10 g + sulbactam 5 g
Contains 5 mEq Na per 1.5 g drug combination

Dosage based on ampicillin component:
Neonate:
   Premature (based on pharmacokinetic data): 100 mg/kg/24 hr ÷ Q12 hr IM/IV
   Full-term: 100 mg/kg/24 hr ÷ Q8 hr IM/IV
Infant ≥ 1 mo:
   Mild/moderate infections: 100–150 mg/kg/24 hr ÷ Q6 hr IM/IV
   Meningitis/severe infections: 200–300 mg/kg/24 hr ÷ Q6 hr IM/IV
Child:
   Mild/moderate infections: 100–200 mg/kg/24 hr ÷ Q6 hr IM/IV
   Meningitis/severe infections: 200–400 mg/kg/24 hr ÷ Q4–6 hr IM/IV
Adult: 1–2 g Q6–8 hr IM/IV
Max. dose: 8 g ampicillin/24 hr

Similar spectrum of antibacterial activity to ampicillin, with the added coverage of
   β-lactamase–producing organisms. Total sulbactam dose should not exceed 4 g/24 hr.
Use higher doses with shorter dosing intervals to treat CNS disease and severe infection.
   Adjust dose in renal failure (see Chapter 31). CSF distribution and side effects similar to
   ampicillin.

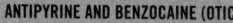

ANTIPYRINE AND BENZOCAINE (OTIC)
Allergen Ear Drops, Antipyrine and Benzocaine Otic, Aurodex,
Autoguard Otic, Auralgan (available in Canada), and generics
Otic analgesic, cerumenolytic

No   No   2   C

Otic solution: Antipyrine 5.4%, benzocaine 1.4% (10, 15 mL); may contain oxyquinoline sulfate

Otic analgesia: Fill external ear canal (2–4 drops) Q1–2 hr PRN. After instillation of solution,
   a cotton pledget should be moistened with solution and inserted into the meatus.
Cerumenolytic: Fill external ear canal (2–4 drops) TID–QID for 2–3 days.

Benzocaine sensitivity may develop; not intended for prolonged use. **Contraindicated** if
   tympanic membrane perforated or PE tubes in place. Local reactions (e.g., burning, stinging)
   and hypersensitivity reactions may occur. Risk of benzocaine-induced methemoglobinemia
   may be increased in infants ≤3 mo of age.

For explanation of icons, see p. 648.

ARGININE CHLORIDE—INJECTABLE PREPARATION
R-Gene 10
Metabolic alkalosis agent, urea cycle disorder treatment agent, growth hormone diagnostic agent

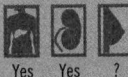

Yes Yes ? B

Injection: 10% (100 mg/mL) arginine hydrochloride contains 47.5 mEq chloride per 100 mL (300 mL)
Osmolality: 950 mOsmol/L

Used as a secondary alternative agent for patients who are unresponsive or unable to receive sodium chloride and potassium chloride.
  Correction of hypochloremia: Arginine chloride dose in mEq = 0.2 × Patient's weight (kg) × [103 − Patient's serum chloride in mEq/L]. Administer ½ to ⅔ of the calculated dose and reassess.
Drug administration: **Do not exceed** an IV infusion rate of 1 g/kg/hr (4.75 mEq/kg/hr). Drug may be administered without further dilution but should be diluted to reduce risk of tissue irritation.

Contraindicated in renal or hepatic failure. **Use with extreme caution;** overdosages may result in hyperchloremic metabolic acidosis, cerebral edema, and death. Hypersensitivity reactions, including anaphylaxis, and hematuria have been reported.

Arginine hydrochloride is metabolized to nitrogen-containing products for renal excretion. Excess arginine increases production of nitric oxide (NO) to cause vasodilation/hypotension. Closely monitor acid-base status. Hyperglycemia, hyperkalemia, GI disturbances, IV extravasation, headache, and flushing may occur.

In addition to its use for chloride supplementation, arginine is used in urea cycle disorder therapy (to increase arginine levels and prevent breakdown of endogenous proteins) and as a diagnostic agent for growth hormone (stimulates pituitary release of growth hormone).

ASCORBIC ACID
Vitamin C, Sunkist Vitamin C, and many others
Water-soluble vitamin

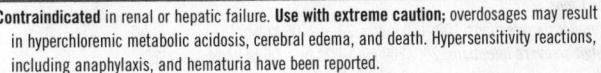

No No 1 A/C

Tabs [OTC]: 100, 250, 500 mg, 1 g
Chewable tabs (Sunkist Vitamin C and others) [OTC]: 100, 250, 500 mg; some may contain aspartame
Tabs (timed-release) [OTC]: 0.5, 1, 1.5 g
Caps [OTC]: 500, 1000 mg
Extended-release caps [OTC]: 500 mg
Injection: 500 mg/mL; may contain sodium hydrosulfite
Oral liquid [OTC]: 500 mg/5 mL (120, 480 mL)
Crystals [OTC]: 1 g per ¼ teaspoonful (170 g, 1000 g)
Some products may contain ≈ 5 mEq Na/1 g drug and/or calcium.

Scurvy (PO/IM/IV/SC):
  Child: 100–300 mg/24 hr ÷ once daily–BID for at least 2 wk
  Adult: 100–250 mg once daily–BID for at least 2 wk
U.S. Recommended Daily Allowance (RDA):
  See Chapter 21.

Adverse reactions: Nausea, vomiting, heartburn, flushing, headache, faintness, dizziness, hyperoxaluria. Use high doses with **caution** in G6PD patients. May cause false-negative and false-positive urine glucose determinations with glucose oxidase and cupric sulfate tests, respectively.

May increase absorption of aluminum hydroxide and increase adverse/toxic effects of deferoxamine. May reduce effects of amphetamines.

Oral dosing is preferred with or without food. IM route is the preferred parenteral route. Protect the injectable dosage form from light.

Pregnancy Category changes to "C" if used in doses above the RDA.

ASPIRIN
ASA, Anacin, Bufferin, and various trade names and generics
Nonsteroidal anti-inflammatory agent, antiplatelet
agent, analgesic

Yes   Yes   2   D

Tabs [OTC]: 325, 500 mg
Tabs, enteric-coated [OTC]: 81, 325, 500, 650 mg
Tabs, time-release [OTC]: 81, 650 mg
Tabs, buffered [OTC]: 325, 500 mg; may contain magnesium, aluminum, and/or calcium
Tabs, chewable [OTC]: 81 mg
Gum [OTC]: 227.5 mg (12s)
Suppository [OTC]: 300, 600 mg

Analgesic/antipyretic: 10–15 mg/kg/dose PO/PR Q4–6 hr up to total of 60–80 mg/kg/24 hr
Max. dose: 4 g/24 hr
Anti-inflammatory: 60–100 mg/kg/24 hr PO ÷ Q6–8 hr
Kawasaki disease: 80–100 mg/kg/24 hr PO ÷ QID during febrile phase until patient defervesces, then decrease to 3–5 mg/kg/24 hr PO QAM. Continue for at least 8 wk or until both platelet count and ESR are normal.

Do not use in children <16 yr for treatment of varicella or flulike symptoms (risk for Reye syndrome), in combination with other NSAIDs, or in severe renal failure. **Use with caution** in bleeding disorders, renal dysfunction, gastritis, and gout. May cause GI upset, allergic reactions, liver toxicity, and decreased platelet aggregation.

Drug interactions: May increase effects of methotrexate, valproic acid, and warfarin, which may lead to toxicity (protein displacement). Buffered dosage forms may decrease absorption of ketoconazole and tetracycline. GI bleeds have been reported with concurrent use of SSRIs (e.g., fluoxetine, paroxetine, sertraline).

Therapeutic levels: Antipyretic/analgesic, 30–50 mg/L; anti-inflammatory, 150–300 mg/L. Tinnitus may occur at levels of 200–400 mg/L. Recommended serum sampling time at steady state; obtain trough level just before dose after 1–2 days of continuous dosing. Peak levels obtained 2 hr (for non–sustained-release dosage forms) after a dose may be useful for monitoring toxicity. **Adjust dose in renal failure (see Chapter 31).**

Breast-feeding considerations:
  High-dose aspirin regimens: Use of an alternative drug is recommended.
  Low-dose (75–162 mg/24 hr) aspirin regimens: Avoid breast-feeding for 1–2 hr after a dose.

ATENOLOL
Tenormin and various generics
β₁-Adrenergic blocker, selective

No   Yes   2   D

Tab: 25, 50, 100 mg
Oral suspension: 2 mg/mL

Child and adolescent: 0.5–1 mg/kg/dose PO once daily–BID; **max. dose:** 2 mg/kg/24 hr up to 100 mg/24 hr
Adult:
  PO: 25–100 mg/dose PO once daily; **max. dose:** 100 mg/24 hr

Contraindicated in pulmonary edema, cardiogenic shock. May cause bradycardia, hypotension, second- or third-degree AV block, dizziness, fatigue, lethargy, and headache. **Use with caution** in diabetes and asthma. Wheezing and dyspnea have occurred when daily dosage exceeds

Continued

ATENOLOL *continued*

100 mg/24 hr. Postmarketing evaluation reports a temporal relationship for causing elevated LFTs and/or bilirubin, hallucinations, psoriatic rash, thrombocytopenia, visual disturbances, and dry mouth. **Avoid** abrupt withdrawal of the drug. Does not cross the blood-brain barrier; lower incidence of CNS side effects compared with propranolol. Neonates born to mothers receiving atenolol during labor or while breast-feeding may be at risk for hypoglycemia.

Use with disopyramide, amiodarone, or digoxin may enhance bradycardic effects. **Adjust dose in renal impairment (see Chapter 31).**

ATOMOXETINE
Strattera
Norepinephrine reuptake inhibitor, attention deficit hyperactivity disorder agent

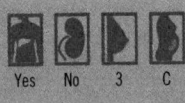

Yes | No | 3 | C

Capsules: 10, 18, 25, 40, 60, 80, 100 mg

Child ≥ 6 yr and adolescent ≤ 70 kg (see remarks):
Start with 0.5 mg/kg/24 hr PO QAM and increase after a minimum of 3 days to ≈ 1.2 mg/kg/24 hr PO ÷ QAM or BID (morning and late afternoon/early evening).
Max. daily dose: 1.4 mg/kg/24 hr or 100 mg, whichever is less
If used with a strong CYP 450 2D6 inhibitor (e.g., fluoxetine, paroxetine, quinidine) or in patients with reduced CYP 450 2D6 activity: Maintain above initial dose for 4 wk, and increase to a max. of 1.2 mg/kg/24 hr only if symptoms do not improve and initial dose is tolerated.

Child ≥ 6 yr and adolescent > 70 kg (see remarks):
Start with 40 mg PO QAM and increase after a minimum of 3 days to ≈ 80 mg/24 hr PO ÷ QAM or BID (morning and late afternoon/early evening). After 2–4 wk, dose may be increased to a **max.** of 100 mg/24 hr if needed.
If used with a strong CYP 450 2D6 inhibitor (e.g., fluoxetine, paroxetine, quinidine) or in patients with reduced CYP 450 2D6 activity: Maintain above initial dose for 4 wk, and increase to 80 mg/24 hr only if symptoms do not improve and initial dose is tolerated.

Contraindicated in patients with narrow-angle glaucoma, pheochromocytoma, and severe cardiac disorders. **Do not** administer with or within 2 wk after discontinuing an MAO inhibitor; fatal reactions have been reported. **Use with caution** in hypertension, tachycardia, cardiovascular or cerebrovascular diseases, or with concurrent albuterol therapy. Increased risk of suicidal thinking has been reported; closely monitor for clinical worsening, agitation, aggressive behavior, irritability, suicidal thinking or behaviors, and unusual changes in behavior when initiating (first few months) or at times of dose changes (increases or decreases). Atomoxetine is a CYP 450 2D6 substrate.

Doses >1.2 mg/kg/24 hr in patients ≤70 kg have not been shown to be of additional benefit. Reduce dose (initial and target doses) by 50% and 75% for patients with moderate (Child-Pugh Class B) and severe (Child-Pugh Class C) hepatic insufficiency, respectively. Effectiveness beyond 9 weeks and safety beyond 1 year have not been evaluated by controlled trials in children.

Major side effects include GI discomfort, vomiting, fatigue, anorexia, dizziness, and mood swings. Hypersensitivity reactions, aggression, irritability, allergic reactions, and severe liver injury have also been reported. Consider interrupting therapy in patients who are not growing or gaining weight satisfactorily.

Doses may be administered with or without food. Atomoxetine can be discontinued without tapering.

A

ATOVAQUONE
Mepron
Antiprotozoal

Yes   Yes   3   C

Oral suspension: 750 mg/5 mL (210 mL); contains benzyl alcohol

Pneumocystis jirovecii (carinii) *pneumonia* (PCP):
Treatment (21-day course):
  Child: 30–40 mg/kg/24 hr PO ÷ BID with fatty foods; **max. dose:** 1500 mg/24 hr. Infants 3–24 mo may require higher doses of 45 mg/kg/24 hr.
  Adult: 750 mg/dose PO BID
Prophylaxis (first episode and recurrence):
  Child 1–3 mo or >24 mo: 30 mg/kg/24 hr PO once daily; **max. dose:** 1500 mg/24 hr
  Child 4–24 mo: 45 mg/kg/24 hr PO once daily: **max. dose:** 1500 mg/24 hr
  Adult: 1500 mg/dose PO once daily
Toxoplasma gondii:
  Child:
    First episode prophylaxis and recurrence prophylaxis: Use PCP prophylaxis dosages ± pyrimethamine 1 mg/kg/dose (**max.** 25 mg/dose) PO once daily PLUS leucovorin 5 mg PO Q3 days.
  Adult:
    Treatment: 1500 mg/dose PO BID ± (sulfadiazine 1000–1500 mg PO Q6 hr or pyrimethamine PLUS leucovorin).
    First episode prophylaxis: 1500 mg/dose PO once daily ± pyrimethamine 25 mg PO once daily PLUS leucovorin 10 mg PO once daily.
    Recurrence prophylaxis: 750 mg/dose PO Q6–12 hr ± pyrimethamine 25 mg PO once daily PLUS leucovorin 10 mg PO once daily.

Not recommended in the treatment of severe PCP (lack of clinical data). Patients with GI disorders or severe vomiting and who cannot tolerate oral therapy should consider alternative IV therapies. Rash, pruritus, sweating, GI symptoms, LFT elevation, dizziness, headache, insomnia, anxiety, cough, and fever are common. Anemia, Stevens-Johnson syndrome, hepatitis, renal/urinary disorders, and pancreatitis have been reported.

Metoclopramide, rifampin, rifabutin, and tetracycline may decrease atovaquone levels. Shake oral suspension well before dispensing all doses. Take all doses with high-fat foods to maximize absorption.

ATROPINE SULFATE
Sal-Tropine, AtroPen, and many other generic products
Anticholinergic agent

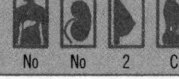

No   No   2   C

Tabs (Sal-Tropine): 0.4 mg
Injection: 0.05, 0.1, 0.4, 0.8, 1 mg/mL
Injection (auto-injector):
  AtroPen 0.25 mg: Delivers a single 0.25-mg (0.3 mL) dose (yellow-colored pen)
  AtroPen 0.5 mg: Delivers a single 0.5-mg (0.7 mL) dose (blue-colored pen)
  AtroPen 1 mg: Delivers a single 1-mg (0.7 mL) dose (dark red–colored pen)
  AtroPen 2 mg: Delivers a single 2-mg (0.7 mL) dose (green-colored pen)
Ointment (ophthalmic): 1% (1, 3.5 g)
Solution (ophthalmic): 1% (2, 5, 15 mL)

For explanation of icons, see p. 648

Continued

ATROPINE SULFATE *continued*

Preintubation dose:
Neonate: 0.01-0.02 mg/kg/dose IV (over 1 min)/IM prior to other premedications.
Child: 0.01 mg/kg/dose IV/IM, **min. dose:** 0.1 mg/dose; **max. dose:** 0.4 mg/dose;
may repeat Q4–6 hr PRN
Adult: 0.5 mg/dose IV/IM

Cardiopulmonary resuscitation/bradycardia (see remarks):
Neonate: 0.01-0.03 mg/kg/dose IV/IM Q10-15 min PRN up to a total **maximum** of 0.04 mg/kg.
Administer IV over 1 min.
Child: 0.02 mg/kg/dose IV Q5 min × 2–3 doses PRN; **min. dose:** 0.1 mg/dose; **max. single dose:**
0.5 mg in children, 1 mg in adolescents; **max total dose:** 1 mg children, 2 mg adolescents
Adult: 0.5–1 mg/dose IV Q5 min; **max. total dose:** 2 mg

Bronchospasm: 0.025–0.05 mg/kg/dose (**max. dose:** 2.5 mg/dose) in 2.5 mL NS Q6–8 hr via nebulizer

Nerve agent and insecticide poisoning for muscarinic symptoms (organophosphate or carbamate poisoning) (IV/IM/ET; dilute in 1–2 mL NS for ET administration):
Child: 0.05–0.1 mg/kg Q5–10 min until bronchial or oral secretions terminate
Adult: 2–5 mg/dose Q5–10 min until bronchial or oral secretions terminate

AtroPen device (IM route): Inject as soon as exposure is known or suspected. Give 1 dose for mild symptoms and 2 additional doses (total 3 doses) in rapid succession 10 min after the first dose for severe symptoms as follows:
Child < 6 mo (<7 kg): 0.25 mg
Child 6 mo–4 yr (7–18 kg): 0.5 mg
Child 4–10 yr (18–41 kg): 1 mg
Child > 10 yr and adult (≥41 kg): 2 mg

Ophthalmic (uveitis):
Child: (0.5% solution; prepared by diluting equal volume of the 1% atropine ophthalmic solution
with artificial tears) 1–2 drops in each eye once daily–TID
Adult: (1% solution) 1–2 drops in each eye once daily–QID

Contraindicated in glaucoma, obstructive uropathy, tachycardia, and thyrotoxicosis. **Use with caution** in patients sensitive to sulfites.

Recommended minimum dosage of 0.1 mg for neonates for bradycardia is currently
recommended by PALS for concerns of paradoxical bradycardia. However, use of this minimum dose
could result in an overdose. Additionally, data suggest the minimum 0.1 mg dose may not be
warranted for the pre-intubation indication as well.

Side effects include dry mouth, blurred vision, fever, tachycardia, constipation, urinary retention, CNS
signs (dizziness, hallucinations, restlessness, fatigue, headache).

In case of bradycardia, may give via endotracheal tube (dilute with NS to volume of 1–2 mL and follow
each dose with 1 mL NS) or intraosseous (IO) route. Use injectable solution for nebulized use; can be
mixed with albuterol for simultaneous administration.

AURALGAN

See Antipyrine and Benzocaine

A

AZATHIOPRINE
Imuran, Azasan, and generics
Immunosuppressant

Yes   Yes   3   D

Oral suspension: 50 mg/mL
Tabs:
  Imuran and generics: 50 mg (scored)
  Azasan: 75, 100 mg (scored)
Injection: 100 mg (20 mL)

Immunosuppression:
Child and adult:
  Initial: 3–5 mg/kg/24 hr IV/PO once daily
  Maintenance: 1–3 mg/kg/24 hr IV/PO once daily

Increased risk for hepatosplenic T-cell lymphoma has been reported in adolescents and young adults. Toxicity: bone marrow suppression, rash, stomatitis, hepatotoxicity, alopecia, arthralgias, and GI disturbances.

Use ¼–⅓ dose when given with allopurinol. Dose reduction or discontinuance is recommended in patients with low or absent thiopurine methyl transferase (TPMT) activity. Severe anemia has been reported when used in combination with captopril or enalapril. Monitor CBC, platelets, total bilirubin, alkaline phosphatase, BUN, and creatinine. Pancytopenia and bone marrow suppression have been reported with concomitant use of pegylated interferon and ribavirin in patients with hepatitis C. **Adjust dose in renal failure (see Chapter 31).**

Administer oral doses with food to minimize GI discomfort. To minimize infant exposure via breast milk, avoid breast-feeding for 4–6 hr after administering a maternal dose.

AZELASTINE
Astelin, Astepro, Opitvar, and generics
Antihistamine

Yes   Yes   ?   C

Nasal spray:
  0.1% (Astelin, Astepro): 137 mcg/spray (200 actuations per 30 mL); contains benzalkonium chloride and EDTA
  0.15% (Astepro): 205.5 mcg/spray (200 actuations per 30 mL); contains benzalkonium chloride and EDTA
Ophthalmic drops (Opitvar): 0.05% (0.5 mg/mL) (6 mL); contains benzalkonium chloride

Seasonal allergic rhinitis:
0.1% strength:
  Child 5–11 yr: 1 spray each nostril BID
  ≥12 yr and adult: 1–2 sprays each nostril BID
0.15% strength: Use similar dosing for 0.1% strength, or 2 sprays per nostril once daily for only children ≥12 yr and adults.
Ophthalmic:
  ≥3 yr and adult: Instill 1 drop into each affected eye BID.

Use with caution in asthmatics. Reduced dosages have been recommended in patients with renal and hepatic dysfunction. Optivar **should not be used** to treat contact lens–related irritation. Soft contact lens users should wait at least 10 min after dose instillation before they insert their lenses.

Continued

AZATHIOPRINE *continued*

Drowsiness may occur despite the nasal route of administration (**avoid** concurrent use of alcohol or CNS depressants). Bitter taste, nausea, nasal burning, pharyngitis, weight gain, fatigue, nasal sores, and epistaxis may also occur with nasal route. Eye burning and stinging have been reported in about 30% of patients receiving the ophthalmic dosage form.

AZITHROMYCIN
Zithromax, Zithromax TRI-PAK, Zithromax Z-PAK, Zmax
(extended-release oral suspension), Azasite, and generics
Antibiotic, macrolide

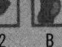 Yes Yes 2 B

Tablets: 250, 500, 600 mg
   TRI-PAK: 500 mg (3s as unit dose pack)
   Z-PAK: 250 mg (6s as unit dose pack)
Oral suspension: 100 mg/5 mL (15 mL), 200 mg/5 mL (15, 22.5, 30 mL)
Oral Powder (Sachet): 1 g (3s, 10s)
Extended-release oral suspension (microspheres):
   Zmax: 2 g reconstituted with 60 mL of water
Injection: 500 mg; contains 9.92 mEq Na/1 g drug
Ophthalmic solution (Azasite): 1% (2.5 mL)

Infant and child:
   Otitis media (≥6 mo):
      5-day regimen: 10 mg/kg PO on day 1 (**max. dose:** 500 mg), followed by 5 mg/kg/24 hr PO once daily (**max. dose:** 250 mg/24 hr) on days 2–5
      3-day regimen: 10 mg/kg/24 hr PO once daily × 3 days (**max. dose:** 500 mg/24 hr)
      1-day regimen: 30 mg/kg/24 hr PO × 1 (**max. dose:** 1500 mg/24 hr)
   Community-acquired pneumonia (≥6 mo):
      Tablet or oral suspension: Use otitis media 5-day regimen.
      Extended-release oral suspension (Zmax): 60 mg/kg (**max. dose:** 1500 mg) PO × 1.
   Pharyngitis/tonsillitis (2–15 yr): 12 mg/kg/24 hr PO once daily × 5 days (**max. dose:** 500 mg/24 hr)
   Acute sinusitis (≥6 mo): 10 mg/kg/dose (**max. dose:** 500 mg) PO once daily × 3 days
   Pertussis:
      Infant < 6 mo: 10 mg/kg/dose PO once daily × 5 days
      ≥6 mo: 10 mg/kg/dose (**max. dose:** 500 mg) PO × 1, followed by 5 mg/kg/ (**max. dose:** 250 mg) PO once daily on days 2–5
   Mycobacterium avium complex in HIV (see www.aidsinfo.nih.gov/guidelines for most current recommendations):
      Prophylaxis for first episode: 20 mg/kg/dose PO Q7 days (**max. dose:** 1200 mg/dose); alternatively, 5 mg/kg/24 hr PO once daily (**max. dose:** 250 mg/dose) with or without rifabutin
      Prophylaxis for recurrence: 5 mg/kg/24 hr PO once daily (**max. dose:** 250 mg/dose), plus ethambutol 15 mg/kg/24 hr (**max. dose:** 900 mg/24 hr) PO once daily with or without rifabutin 5 mg/kg/24 hr (**max. dose:** 300 mg/24 hr)
      Treatment: 10–12 mg/kg/24 hr PO once daily (**max. dose:** 500 mg/24 hr) × 1 month or longer, plus ethambutol 15–25 mg/kg/24 hr (**max. dose:** 1 g/24 hr) PO once daily with or without rifabutin 10–20 mg/kg/24 hr (**max. dose:** 300 mg/24 hr)
   Endocarditis prophylaxis: 15 mg/kg/dose (**max. dose:** 500 mg) PO × 1, 30–60 min before procedure
   Anti-inflammatory agent in cystic fibrosis:
      25–39 kg: 250 mg PO every Monday, Wednesday, and Friday
      ≥40 kg: 500 mg PO every Monday, Wednesday, and Friday

AZITHROMYCIN *continued*

Adolescent and adult:

Pharyngitis, tonsillitis, skin, and soft-tissue infection: 500 mg PO on day 1, then 250 mg/24 hr PO on days 2–5

Mild/moderate bacterial COPD exacerbation: Above 5-day dosing regimen *OR* 500 mg PO once daily × 3 days

Community-acquired pneumonia:

Tablets: 500 mg PO on day 1, then 250 mg/24 hr PO on days 2–5

Extended-release oral suspension (Zmax): Single dose of 2 g PO

IV and tablet regimen: 500 mg IV once daily × 2 days, followed by 500 mg PO once daily to complete a 7–10 day regimen (IV and PO)

Sinusitis:

Tablets: 500 mg PO once daily × 3 days

Extended-release oral suspension (Zmax): Single dose of 2 g PO

Uncomplicated chlamydial cervicitis or urethritis: Single dose of 1 g PO

Gonococcal cervicitis or urethritis: Single 2-g dose PO

Acute PID (chlamydia): 500 mg IV once daily × 1–2 days, followed by 250 mg PO once daily to complete a 7-day regimen (IV and PO).

Mycobacterium avium *complex in HIV (see* www.aidsinfo.nih.gov/guidelines *for most recent recommendations):*

Prophylaxis for first episode: 1200 mg PO Q7 days, with or without rifabutin 300 mg PO once daily

Prophylaxis for recurrence: 500 mg PO once daily, plus ethambutol 15 mg/kg/dose PO once daily, with or without rifabutin 300 mg PO once daily

Treatment: 500–600 mg PO once daily, with ethambutol 15 mg/kg/dose PO once daily, with or without rifabutin 300 mg PO once daily

Endocarditis prophylaxis: 500 mg PO × 1, 30–60 min before procedure

Anti-inflammatory agent in cystic fibrosis: Use same dosing as in children.

Ophthalmic:

≥1 yr and adult: Instill 1 drop into affected eye(s) BID (8–12 hr apart) × 2 days, followed by 1 drop once daily for the next 5 days.

Contraindicated in hypersensitivity to macrolides and history of cholestatic jaundice/hepatic dysfunction associated with prior use. **Use with caution** in impaired hepatic function, GFR < 10 mL/min (limited data), hypokalemia, hypomagnesemia, bradycardia, arrhythmias, prolonged QT intervals, and receiving medications that can cause the aforementioned conditions of caution. Can cause increase in hepatic enzymes, cholestatic jaundice, GI discomfort, and pain at injection site (IV use). Compared with other macrolides, less risk for drug interactions. Nelfinavir may increase azithromycin levels; monitor for liver enzyme abnormalities and hearing impairment. Vomiting, diarrhea, and nausea have been reported at higher frequency in otitis media with 1-day dosing regimen. Exacerbations of myasthenia gravis/syndrome have been reported. CNS penetration is poor.

Aluminum- and magnesium-containing antacids decrease absorption. Tablet and oral suspension dosage forms may be administered with or without food. Extended-release oral suspension should be taken on an empty stomach (at least 1 hr before or 2 hr after a meal). Intravenous administration is over 1–3 hr; **do not** give as a bolus or IM injection.

Ophthalmic use: Do not wear contact lenses. Eye irritation is the most common side effect.

For explanation of icons, see p. 648

AZTREONAM
Azactam, Cayston
Antibiotic, monobactam

No Yes 1 B

Injection: 1, 2 g
Frozen injection: 1 g/50 mL 3.4% dextrose, 2 g/50 mL 1.4% dextrose (iso-osmotic solutions)
Each 1 g drug contains ≈ 780 mg L-arginine
Nebulizer solution (Cayston): 75 mg powder to be reconstituted with the supplied diluent of 1 mL
0.17% sodium chloride (28-day course kit contains 84 sterile vials of Cayston and 88 ampules of
diluent)

Neonate:
30 mg/kg/dose:
<1.2 kg and 0–4 wk age: Q12 hr IV/IM
1.2–2 kg and 0–7 days: Q12 hr IV/IM
1.2–2 kg and >7 days: Q8 hr IV/IM
>2 kg and 0–7 days: Q8 hr IV/IM
>2 kg and >7 days: Q6 hr IV/IM
Child: 90–120 mg/kg/24 hr ÷ Q6–8 hr IV/IM
Cystic fibrosis: 150–200 mg/kg/24 hr ÷ Q6–8 hr IV/IM
Adult:
Moderate infections: 1–2 g/dose Q8–12 hr IV/IM
Severe infections: 2 g/dose Q6–8 hr IV/IM
Max. dose: 8 g/24 hr
Inhalation:
Cystic fibrosis prophylaxis therapy:
≥7 yr and adult: 75 mg TID (minimum 4 hr between doses) administered in repeated cycles
of 28 days on drug, followed by 28 days off drug. Administer each dose with the Altera Nebulizer
System.

Typically indicated in multidrug-resistant aerobic gram-negative infections when β-lactam
therapy is contraindicated. Well-absorbed IM. **Use with caution** in arginase deficiency. Low
cross-allergenicity between aztreonam and other β-lactams. Adverse reactions:
thrombophlebitis, eosinophilia, leukopenia, neutropenia, thrombocytopenia, elevation of liver
enzymes, hypotension, seizures, and confusion. Good CNS penetration. Probenecid and
furosemide increase aztreonam levels. **Adjust dose in renal failure (see Chapter 31).**
INHALATIONAL USE: Cough, nasal congestion, wheezing, pharyngolaryngeal pain, pyrexia, chest
discomfort, abdominal pain and vomiting may occur. Bronchospasm has been reported. Use the
following order of administration: bronchodilator first, chest physiotherapy, other inhaled
medications (if indicated), and aztreonam last.

BACITRACIN ± POLYMYXIN B
Bacitracin: AK-Tracin Ophthalmic, Baciguent Topical, and others
Bacitracin plus polymyxin B: AK-Poly-Bac Ophthalmic, Polysporin
Ophthalmic, Polysporin Topical, and others
Antibiotic, topical

No No ? C

BACITRACIN:
Ophthalmic ointment: 500 units/g (3.5 g)
Topical ointment (OTC): 500 units/g (15, 30 g)

BACITRACIN ± POLYMYXIN B *continued*

BACITRACIN IN COMBINATION WITH POLYMYXIN B:
Ophthalmic ointment: 500 units bacitracin + 10,000 units polymyxin B/g (3.5 g)
Topical ointment: 500 units bacitracin + 10,000 units polymyxin B/g (15, 30 g)

BACITRACIN
Child and adult:

   Topical: Apply to affected area 1–5 times/24 hr.
   Ophthalmic: Apply 0.25- to 0.5-inch ribbon into conjunctival sac of infected eye(s) Q3–12 hr; frequency depends on severity of infection. Administer Q3–4 hr × 7–10 days for mild/moderate infections.
BACITRACIN + POLYMYXIN B
Child and adult:
   Topical: Apply ointment or powder to affected area once daily to TID.
   Ophthalmic: Apply 0.25–0.5 inch ribbon into conjunctival sac of infected eye(s) Q3–12 hr; frequency depends on severity of infection. Administer Q3–4 hr × 7–10 days for mild/moderate infections.

Hypersensitivity reactions to bacitracin and/or polymyxin B can occur. **Do not use** topical ointment for eyes. Side effects may include rash, itching, burning, and edema. Ophthalmic dosage form may cause temporary blurred vision and retard corneal healing. For neomycin-containing products, see Neomycin/Polymyxin B ± Bacitracin.

BACLOFEN
Lioresal, Gablofen, Kemstro, and others
Centrally acting skeletal muscle relaxant

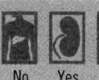 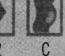
No   Yes   2   C

Tabs: 10, 20 mg
Disintegrating oral tabs (Kemstro): 10, 20 mg; contains phenylalanine
Oral suspension: 5, 10 mg/mL
Intrathecal injection (Lioresal, Gablofen): 50 mcg/mL (1 mL), 0.5 mg/mL (20 mL), 2 mg/mL (5 mL); preservative free

Oral: Dosage increments, if tolerated, are made at 3-day intervals until desired effect or max. dose is achieved. Initiate first dosage level at QHS, followed by Q12 hr and then Q8 hr.
Dosage increments are made by first increasing the QHS dosage, followed by the morning dosage and then the remaining midday dosage.
Child (PO, see remarks):
   <20 kg: Start at 2.5 mg QHS, increase in 2.5 mg increments if needed up to recommended **max. dose** below.
   ≥20–50 kg: Start at 5 mg QHS, increase in 5 mg increments if needed up to recommended **max. dose** below.
   >50 kg: Start at 10 mg QHS, increase in 10 mg increments if needed up to recommended max. dose below.
   Recommended max. PO dose:
     <8 yr: 60 mg/24 hr
     8–16 yr: 80 mg/24 hr
     >16 yr: 120 mg//24 hr
Adult (PO):
   Start at 5 mg TID, increase in 5-mg increments if needed up to a maximum of 80 mg/24 hr.
Intrathecal continuous infusion maintenance therapy (not well established):
   <12 yr: Average dose of 274 mcg/24 hr (range: 24–1199 mcg/24 hr) has been reported.
   ≥12 yr and adult: Most required 300–800 mcg/24 hr (range: 12–2003 mcg/24 hr with limited experience at doses >1000 mcg/24 hr).

For explanation of icons, see p. 648

Continued

BACLOFEN *continued*

Avoid abrupt withdrawal of drug. **Use with caution** in patients with seizure disorders, impaired renal function. About 70%–80% of drug is excreted unchanged in urine. Administer oral doses with food or milk.

Adverse effects: Drowsiness, fatigue, nausea, vertigo, psychiatric disturbances, rash, urinary frequency, hypotonia. **Avoid** abrupt withdrawal of intrahecal therapy to prevent potential life-threatening events (rhabdomyolysis, multiple organ-system failure, death). Cases of intrathecal mass at the tip of implanted catheter leading to withdrawal symptoms have been reported. Inadvertent subcutaneous injection may occur with improper access of the reservior refill septum and may result in overdose.

Usual oral dosage range observed from a single institution retrospective review in 87 patients include:

2 yr: 10–20 mg/24 hr to a **maximum** of 40 mg/24 hr
2–7 yr: 20–30 mg/24 hr to a **maximum** of 60 mg/24 hr
≥8 yr: 30–40 mg/24 hr to a **maximum** of 120 mg/24 hr

BECLOMETHASONE DIPROPIONATE
QVAR, Beconase AQ, Qnasl
Corticosteroid

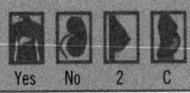

Yes	No	2	C

Inhalation, oral:
    QVAR: 40 mcg/inhalation (7.3 g provides 100 inhalations, 8.7 g provides 120 inhalations), 80 mcg/inhalation (4.2 g provides 50 inhalations, 7.3 g provides 100 inhalations, 8.7 g provides 120 inhalations); CFC-free product (HFA)
Inhalation, nasal:
    Beconase AQ: 42 mcg/inhalation (25 g provides 200 metered doses)
    Qnasl: 80 mcg/inhalation (8.7 g provides 120 metered doses)

Oral inhalation (QVAR):
    5–11 yr: Start at 40 mcg BID; **max. dose:** 80 mcg BID.
    ≥12 yr and adult:
        Corticosteroid naïve: Start at 40–80 mcg BID; **max. dose:** 320 mcg BID.
        Previous corticosteroid use: Start at 40–160 mcg BID; **max. dose:** 320 mcg BID.
Nasal inhalation:
    Beconase AQ:
        6–12 yr: Start with 1 spray (42 mcg) each nostril BID; may increase to 2 sprays each nostril BID if needed. Once symptoms are controlled, decrease dose to 1 spray each nostril BID.
        >12 yr and adult: 1–2 spray(s) (42–84 mcg) each nostril BID.
    Qnasl:
        >12 yr and adult: 2 sprays (160 mcg) each nostril once daily; **max. dose:** 4 sprays (320 mcg)/24 hr.

Oral inhalation route **not recommended** for children <5 yr, and nasal route **not recommended** for children <6 yr because safety and efficacy are unknown. Dose should be titrated to lowest effective dose. **Avoid** using higher than recommended doses.

Cytochrome P450 (CYP 450) 3A4 inhibitors (e.g., ketoconazole, erythromycin, protease inhibitors) or significant hepatic impairment may increase systemic exposure of beclomethasone.

Monitor for hypothalamic, pituitary, adrenal, or growth suppression and hypercorticism. Instruct patient to rinse mouth and gargle with water after oral inhalation; may cause thrush. Consider using with tube spacers for oral inhalation.

BENZOYL PEROXIDE
Benzac AC, Benzac AC Wash 5; Brevoxyl Creamy Wash,
Desquam-E 5, Desquam-E 10, NeoBenz Micro, Oxy-5, Oxy-10,
and many other products
Topical acne product

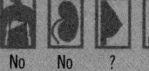
No   No   ?   C

Liquid wash: 5% (120, 150, 200 mL), 10% (120, 150, 240 mL)
Liquid cream wash: 4% (180 g), 8% (180 g)
Bar: 5% [OTC] (113 g), 10% [OTC] (106, 113 g)
Lotion: 4% (297 g), 5% [OTC] (30 mL), 6% (170, 340 g), 8% (297 g), 10% [OTC] (30 mL, 85, 170, 340 g)
Cleanser: 6% (170, 340 g), 8% (300 g)
Cleanser/Mask: [OTC] 3.5% (125 mL)
Cream: 5% [OTC] (18 g), 10% [OTC] (30 g)
Gel: 2.5% (50 g), 4% (42.5 g), 5% [OTC] (42.5, 60, 90 g), 7% (45 g), 10% (42.5, 60, 90 g)
NOTE: Some preparations may contain alcohol and come in combination packs of cleansers and creams at various strengths.
Combination product with erythromycin (Benzamycin and others):
　Gel: 30 mg erythromycin and 50 mg benzoyl peroxide/g (0.8, 23.3, 46 g); some preparations may
　contain 20% alcohol
Combination product with clindamycin:
　Gel:
　　BenzaClin and generics: 10 mg clindamycin and 50 mg benzoyl peroxide/g (25, 35, 50 g); some
　　preparations may contain methylparaben.
　　Duac: 12 mg clindamycin and 50 mg benzoyl peroxide/g (45 g); Duac CS is packaged with a
　　bottle of soap-free cleanser lotion containing PEG 75, sodium cocoyl isethionate steraryl
　　alcohol, and parabens.
　　Acanya: 12 mg clindamycin and 25 mg benzoyl peroxide/g (50 g).

Child ≥ 12 yr and adult:
　Cleansers (liquid wash or bar): Wet affected area before application. Apply and wash once
　daily–BID; rinse thoroughly and pat dry. Modify dose frequency or concentration to control
　amount of drying or peeling.
　Lotion, cream, or gel: Cleanse skin and apply small amounts over affected areas once daily initially;
　increase frequency to BID–TID if needed. Modify dose frequency or concentration to control drying or
　peeling.
Combination products:
　Benzamycin, BenzaClin, and generics: Apply BID (morning and evening) to affected areas after
　washing and drying skin.
　Duac: Apply QHS to affected areas after washing and drying skin.
　Acanya: Apply pea-sized amount once daily.

Contraindicated in patients with known history of hypersensitivity to product's components
(benzoyl peroxide, clindamycin, or erythromycin). **Avoid** contact with mucous membranes and
eyes. May cause skin irritation, stinging, dryness, peeling, erythema, edema, and contact
dermatitis. Anaphylaxis has been reported with products containing clindamycin and benzoyl
peroxide.
Concurrent use with tretinoin (Retin-A) will increase risk of skin irritation. Products containing
clindamycin and erythromycin should not be used in combination.
Any single application resulting in excessive stinging or burning may be removed with mild soap and
water. Lotion, cream, and gel dosage forms should be applied to dry skin.

For explanation of icons, see p. 648

BENZTROPINE MESYLATE
Cogentin and various generics
*Anticholinergic agent, drug-induced dystonic reaction
antidote, antiparkinsonian agent*

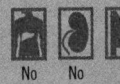 No  No  ? ?

Injection: 1 mg/mL (2 mL)
Tabs: 0.5, 1, 2 mg

Drug-induced extrapyramidal symptoms (PO/IM/IV):
>3 yr: 0.02–0.05 mg/kg/dose once daily–BID
Adult: 1–4 mg/dose once daily–BID
Acute dystonic reaction (phenothiazines) (IM/IV):
Child: 0.02 mg/kg/dose (**max. dose:** 1 mg) × 1
Adult: 1–2 mg/dose × 1

Contraindicated in myastenia gravis, GI/GU obstruction, untreated narrow-angle glaucoma, and peptic ulcer. Use IV route **only** when PO and IM routes are not feasible. May cause anticholinergic side effects, especially constipation and dry mouth. Drug interactions: potentiation of CNS depressant effects when used with CNS depressants, enhance CNS side effects of amantadine, inhibit response of neuroleptics. This medication has not been formally assigned a pregnancy category by the FDA.
Onset of action: 15 min for IV/IM and 1 hr for PO
Oral doses should be administered with food to decrease GI upset.

BERACTANT

See Surfactant, pulmonary

BETAMETHASONE
Beta-Val, Celestone, Celestone Soluspan, Diprolene,
Diprolene AF, Diprosone, Maxivate, and many others
Corticosteroid

  No No 3 C

Betamethasone base (Celestone):
Oral solution: 0.6 mg/5 mL (120 mL); contains alcohol
Na Phosphate and Acetate (Celestone Soluspan):
Injection suspension: 6 mg/mL (3 mg/mL Na phosphate + 3 mg/mL betamethasone acetate) (5 mL); may contain benzalkonium chloride and EDTA
Dipropionate (Diprosone, Maxivate, and others):
Topical cream: 0.05% (15, 45, 50 g)
Topical gel: 0.05% (15, 50 g)
Topical lotion: 0.05% (30, 60 mL); may contain 46.8% alcohol and propylene glycol
Topical ointment: 0.05% (15, 45, 50 g)
Valerate (Beta-Val and others):
Topical cream: 0.1% (15, 45 g)
Topical foam: 1.2 mg/g (50, 100 g); may contain 60.4% ethanol, cetyl alcohol, stearyl alcohol, and propylene glycol
Topical lotion: 0.1% (60 mL); may contain 47.5% isopropyl alcohol
Topical ointment: 0.1% (15, 45 g)
Dipropionate augmented (Diprolene, Diprolene AF, and others):
Topical cream: 0.05% (15, 45, 50 g); contains propylene glycol
Topical gel: 0.05% (15, 50 g); contains propylene glycol

BETAMETHASONE *continued*

Topical lotion: 0.05% (30, 60 mL); contains 30% isopropyl alcohol
Topical ointment: 0.05% (15, 45, 50 g); contains propylene glycol

All dosages should be adjusted based on patient response and severity of condition (see remarks).
Anti-inflammatory:
  Child:
    Oral: 0.0175–0.25 mg/kg/24 hr or 0.5–7.5 mg/m²/24 hr ÷ Q6–8 hr
    IM: 0.0175–0.125 mg/kg/24 hr or 0.5–7.5 mg/m²/24 hr ÷ Q6–12 hr
  Adolescent and adult:
    Oral: 2.4–4.8 mg/24 hr ÷ Q6–12 hr; may range from 0.6–7.2 mg/24 hr depending on disease being treated
    IM: 0.6–9 mg/24 hr ÷ Q12–24 hr
Topical (use smallest amount for shortest period of time to avoid adrenal suppression and reassess diagnosis if no improvement is achieved after 2 weeks; see remarks):
  Valerate and dipropionate forms:
    Child and adult: Apply to affected areas once daily–BID
  Dipropionate augmented forms:
    ≥13 yr–adult: Apply to affected areas once daily–BID
    Max. dose: 14 days and
      Cream and ointment: 45 g/week
      Gel: 50 g/week
      Lotion: 50 mL/week

Use with caution in hypothyroidism, cirrhosis, and ulcerative colitis. See Chapter 10 for relative steroid potencies and doses based on body surface area. Betamethasone is inadequate when used alone for adrenocortical insuficiency because of its minimal mineralocorticoid properties. Like all steroids, may cause hypertension, pseudotumor cerebri, acne, Cushing syndrome, adrenal axis suppression, GI bleeding, hyperglycemia, and osteoporosis.

Na phosphate and acetate injectable suspension recommended for IM, intraarticular, intrasynovial, intralessional, soft-tissue use only; but **not** for IV use. **Topical betamethasone dipropionate augmented (Diprolene and Diprolene AF) is not recommended in children ≤12 yr owing to higher risk for adrenal suppression.**

Injectable dosage form is used in premature labor to stimulate fetal lung maturation.

BETHANECHOL CHLORIDE
Urecholine and other brand names
Cholinergic agent

No   No   ?   C

Tabs: 5, 10, 25, 50 mg
Oral suspension: 1, 5 mg/mL

Child:
  Abdominal distention/urinary retention: 0.6 mg/kg/24 hr ÷ Q6–8 hr PO
  Gastroesophageal reflux: 0.1–0.2 mg/kg/dose 30 min–1 hr before meals and QHS PO; max. dose: 4 doses/24 hr
Adult:
  Urinary retention: 10–50 mg Q6–12 hr PO

Contraindicated in asthma, mechanical GI or GU obstruction, peptic ulcer disease, hyperthyroidism, cardiac disease, and seizure disorder. May cause hypotension, nausea (administer doses on an empty stomach to minimize nausea), bronchospasm, salivation,

Continued

BETHANECHOL CHLORIDE *continued*

flushing, and abdominal cramps. **Warning: Severe hypotension may occur when given with ganglionic blockers (e.g., trimethaphan). Atropine is the antidote.**

BICITRA

See Citrate Mixtures

BISACODYL
Dulcolax, Fleet Laxative, Fleet Bisacodyl, Doxidan, and various other names
Laxative, stimulant

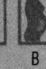
No   No   1   B

Tabs (enteric-coated): 5 mg
Suppository: 10 mg
Enema (Fleet Bisacodyl): 10 mg/30 mL (37.5 mL)
Delayed released tabs (Doxidan): 5 mg

Oral:
   Child (3–12 yr): 0.3 mg/kg/dose or 5–10 mg × 1 administered 6 hr before desired effect;
   max. dose: 30 mg/24 hr
   Adolescent and adult (>12 yr): 5–15 mg × 1 administered 6 hr before desired effect;
   max. dose: 30 mg/24 hr
Rectal suppository (as a single dose):
   <2 yr: 5 mg
   2–11 yr: 5–10 mg
   >11 yr and adult: 10 mg
Rectal enema (as a single dose):
   ≥12 yr and adult: 30 mL

Do not use in newborn period. Instruct patient/parent that tablets should be swallowed whole, **not** chewed or crushed; **not** to be taken within 1 hr of antacids or milk. May cause abdominal cramps, nausea, vomiting, and rectal irritation. Oral usually effective within 6–10 hr; rectal usually effective within 15–60 min.

Antacids may decrease the effect of bisacodyl and may cause premature release of the delayed-release formulation before reaching large intestine.

BISMUTH SUBSALICYLATE
Pepto-Bismol, Kaopectate, Kaopectate Extra Strength, Kao-Tin, Stomach Relief, Stomach Relief Max St, Stomach Relief Plus, and many others (see remarks)
Antidiarrheal, gastrointestinal ulcer agent

No   Yes   2   C/D

Liquid [OTC]:
   Kaopectate, Pepto-Bismol, Stomach Relief, and others: 262 mg/15 mL (240, 360, 480 mL)
   Kaopectate Extra Strength, Stomach Relief Max St, and Stomach Relief Plus: 525 mg/15mL
   (240, 480 mL)
Chewable tabs [OTC]: 262 mg; may contain aspartame
Contains 102 mg salicylate per 262-mg tablet, or 129 mg salicylate per 15 mL of 262-mg/15 mL liquid.

BISMUTH SUBSALICYLATE *continued*

Diarrhea:
  Child: 100 mg/kg/24 hr ÷ 5 equal doses for 5 days; **max. dose:** 4.19 g/24 hr
  Dosage by age: Give following dose Q30 min–1 hr PRN up to a **max. dose** of 8 doses/24 hr:
    3–5 yr: 87.3 mg (⅓ tablet or 5 mL of 262 mg/15 mL)
    6–8 yr: 174.7 mg (⅔ tablet or 10 mL of 262 mg/15 mL)
    9–11 yr: 262 mg (1 tablet or 15 mL of 262 mg/15 mL)
    ≥12 yr–adult: 524 mg (2 tablets or 30 mL of 262 mg/15 mL)
Helicobacter pylori gastric infection (in combination with ampicillin and metronidazole or with
tetracycline and metronidazole for adults; doses not well established for children):
  <10 yr: 262 mg PO QID × 6 wk
  ≥10 yr –adult: 524 mg PO QID × 6 wk

Generally not recommended in children <16 yr with chicken pox or flulike symptoms (risk for
  Reye syndrome); in combination with other nonsteroidal anti-inflammatory drugs,
  anticoagulants, or oral antidiabetic agents; or in severe renal failure. **Use with caution** in
  bleeding disorders, renal dysfunction, gastritis, and gout. May cause darkening of tongue
  and/or black stools, GI upset, impaction, and decreased platelet aggregation.
Drug combination appears to have antisecretory and antimicrobial effects, with some anti-inflammatory
  effects. Absorption of bismuth is negligible, whereas roughly 80% of salicylate is absorbed. Decreases
  absorption of tetracycline. Pregnancy category changes to "D" if used during third trimester.
DO NOT use Children's Pepto (calcium carbonate) since it does not contain bismuth subsalicylate.
  Avoid use in renal failure (see Chapter 31).

BROMPHENIRAMINE WITH PHENYLEPHRINE
Dimetapp Children's Cold and Allergy, and many other products
Antihistamine + decongestant
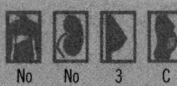
No   No   3   C

Oral syrup (Dimetapp Children's Cold and Allergy) [OTC]: Brompheniramine 1 mg + phenylephrine
2.5 mg/5 mL (237 mL)
Chewable tab (Dimetapp Children's Cold and Allergy) [OTC]: Brompheniramine 1 mg +
phenylephrine 2.5 mg

All doses based on brompheniramine component.
  2–<6 yr: 1 mg Q4 hr PO up to a **max. dose** of 6 mg/24 hr
  6–12 yr: 2 mg Q4 hr PO up to a **max. dose** of 12 mg/24 hr
  ≥12 yr: 4 mg Q4 hr PO up to a **max. dose** of 24 mg/24 hr
*Alternatively, dosing based on specific dosage forms/products. CAUTION: These products are
available in different concentrations.*
  Oral, elixir (Dimetapp Children's Cold and Allergy):
    6–<12 yr: 10 mL Q4 hr PO up to a **max. dose** of 60 mL/24 hr
    ≥12 yr: 20 mL Q4 hr PO up to a **max. dose** of 120 mL/24 hr
  Oral, chewable tab (Dimetapp Children's Cold and Allergy):
    6–<12 yr: Chew 2 tablets Q4 hr PO; **max. dose:** 6 doses/24 hr
    ≥12 yr: Chew 4 tablets Q4 hr PO; **max. dose:** 6 doses/24 hr

Generally not recommended for treating URIs for infants. No proven benefit for infants and young
  children with URIs. Over-the-counter (OTC or nonprescription) use of this product is **not
  recommended** for children <6 years owing to reports of serious adverse effects (cardiac and
  respiratory distress, convulsions, and hallucinations) and fatalities (from unintentional overdosages,
  including combined use of other OTC products containing the same active ingredients).

Continued

For explanation of icons, see p. 648

BROMPHENIRAMINE WITH PHENYLEPHRINE *continued*

Contraindicated with use of MAO inhibitors (concurrent use and within 14 days after discontinuing MAO inhibitor). **Use with caution** in narow-angle glaucoma, bladder neck obstruction, asthma, pyloroduodenal obstruction, symptomatic prostatic hypertrophy, hypertension, coronary artery disease, diabetes mellitus, and thyroid disease. Discontinue use 48 hours before allergy skin testing. May cause drowsiness, fatigue, CNS excitation, xerostomia, blurred vision, and wheezing.

BUDESONIDE
Pulmicort Respules, Pulmicort Flexhaler, Rhinocort Aqua
Nasal Spray, Entocort EC, Uceris, and generics
Corticosteroid

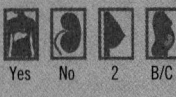

Yes   No   2   B/C

Nasal spray (Rinocort Aqua): 32 mcg/actuation (8.6 g, delivers approx. 120 sprays)
Nebulized inhalation suspension (Pulmicort Respules and generics): 0.25 mg/2 mL, 0.5 mg/2 mL (30s)
Oral inhalation powder:
    Pulmicort Flexhaler: 90 mcg/metered dose (165 mg, delivers 60 doses), 180 mcg/metered dose (225 mg, delivers 120 doses); contains lactose
Enteric-coated caps (Entocort EC and generics): 3 mg
Extended-release tabs (Uceris): 9 mg

Nebulized inhalation suspension:
    Child 1–8 yr:
        No prior steroid use: 0.5 mg/24 hr ÷ once daily–BID; **max. dose:** 0.5 mg/24 hr
        Prior inhaled steroid use: 0.5 mg/24 hr ÷ once daily–BID; **max. dose:** 1 mg/24 hr
        Prior oral steroid use: 1 mg/24 hr ÷ once daily–BID; **max. dose:** 1 mg/24 hr
    NIH Asthma Guideline 2007 recommendations (divide doses once daily–TID):
        Child 0–4 yr:
            Low dose: 0.25–0.5 mg/24 hr
            Medium dose: >0.5–1 mg/24 hr
            High dose: >1 mg/24 hr
        Child 5–11 yr:
            Low dose: 0.5 mg/24 hr
            Medium dose: 1 mg/24 hr
            High dose: 2 mg/24 hr
Oral inhalation:
    Pulmicort Flexhaler:
        Child ≥ 6 yr: Start at 180 mcg BID; **max. dose:** 720 mcg/24 hr.
        Adult: Start at 180–360 mcg BID; **max. dose:** 1440 mcg/24 hr.
Nasal inhalation (≥6 yr and adult):
    Rhinocort Aqua (initial): 1 spray in each nostril once daily. Increase dose as needed up to
    max. dose.
    Max. nasal dose: 6–11 yr: 128 mcg/24 hr (4 sprays/24 hr); ≥12 yr and adult: 256 mcg/24 hr
    (8 sprays/24 hr)
Crohn's disease (Encort EC):
    Child ≥ 6 yr: Data are limited; following dosages have been reported, but additional studies are
    warranted.
        Active disease: 9 mg PO once daily × 7–8 wk
        Maintenance of remission: 6 mg PO once daily × 3–4 wk
    A report in 10- to 19-year-old patients demonstrated higher remission rates with an induction dose of 12
    mg PO once daily × 4 wk, followed by 9 mg PO once daily × 3 wk, followed by 6 mg PO once daily × 3 wk.

BUDESONIDE *continued*

Adult:

Active disease: 9 mg PO QAM × 8 wk; if remission is not achieved, a second 8-week course may be given.

Maintenance of remission: 6 mg PO once daily for up to 3 mo. If symptom control is maintained at 3 mo, taper dosage to compete cessation. Remission therapy beyond 3 mo has not been shown to provide substantial clinical benefit.

Ulcerative colitis, induction of remission (Uceris):

Adult: 9 mg PO QAM for up to 8 weeks

Reduce maintenance dose to as low as possible to control symptoms. May cause pharyngitis, cough, epistaxis, nasal irritation, and HPA-axis suppression. Instruct patient to rinse mouth after each use via the oral inhalation route. Nebulized budesonide has been shown effective in mild to moderate croup at doses of 2 mg × 1. Ref: *N Engl J Med*. 331:285.

Hypersensitivity reactions (including anaphylaxis) have been reported with the inhaled route. Anaphylactic reactions and benign intracranial hypertension have been reported with oral administration.

CYP 450 3A4 inhibitors (e.g., ketoconazole, erythromycin, protease inhibitors) or significant hepatic impairment may increase systemic exposure of budesonide (inhalation and PO routes)

Onset of action for oral inhalation and nebulized suspension is within 1 day and 2–8 days, respectively, with peak effects at 1–2 wk and 4–6 wk, respectively.

For nasal use, onset of action is seen after 1 day, with peak effects after 3–7 days of therapy. Discontinue therapy if no improvement in nasal symptoms after 3 wk of continuous therapy.

Pregnancy category is "B" for inhalation routes of administration and "C" for oral route. Instruct patient/parent that oral capsule dosage form should be swallowed whole, **not** chewed or crushed.

BUDESONIDE AND FORMOTEROL
Symbicort
Corticosteroid and long-acting β₂-adrenergic agonist

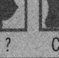
Yes   No   ?   C

Aerosol inhaler:

80 mcg budesonide + 4.5 mcg formoterol fumarate dihydrate (6.9 g delivers 60 inhalations, 10.2 g delivers about 120 inhalations)

160 mcg budesonide + 4.5 mcg formoterol fumarate dihydrate (6 g delivers 60 inhalations, 10.2 g delivers about 120 inhalations)

5–11 yr (NIH Asthma Guideline 2007 recommendations): 2 inhalations BID of 80 mcg budesonide + 4.5 mcg fomoterol; **max. dose:** 4 inhalations/24 hr

≥12 yr and adult:

No prior inhaled steroid use: Start with 2 inhalations BID of 80 mcg budesonide + 4.5 mcg fomoterol **OR** 160 mcg budesonide + 4.5 mcg fomoterol, depending on severity.

Prior low to medium doses of inhaled steroid use: Start with 2 inhalations BID of 80 mcg budesonide + 4.5 mcg fomoterol.

Prior medium to high doses of inhaled steroid use: Start with 2 inhalations BID of 160 mcg budesonide + 4.5 mcg fomoterol.

Max. dose: 2 inhalations of 160 mcg budesonide + 4.5 mcg formoterol BID

See *Budesonide* and *Fomoterol* for remarks. Should only be used for patients not adequately controlled on other asthma-controller medications (e.g., low- to medium-dose inhaled corticosteroids) or whose disease severity requires use of two maintenance therapies. Titrate to lowest effective strength after asthma is adequately controlled. Proper patient education, including dosage administration technique is essential; see patient package insert for detailed instructions. Instruct patient to rinse mouth after each use.

For explanation of icons, see p. 648

BUMETANIDE
Bumex and other generics
Loop diuretic

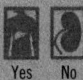

Yes   No   ?   C/D

Tabs: 0.5, 1, 2 mg
Injection: 0.25 mg/mL (2, 4, 10 mL); some preparations may contain 1% benzyl alcohol

Neonate and infant (see remarks): PO/IM/IV
≤6 mo: 0.01–0.05 mg/kg/dose once daily or every other day
Infant and child: PO/IM/IV
>6 mo: 0.015–0.1 mg/kg/dose once daily–BID; **max. dose:** 10 mg/24 hr
Adult:
PO: 0.5–2 mg/dose once daily–BID
IM/IV: 0.5–1 mg over 1–2 min. May give additional doses Q2–3 hr PRN
Usual max. dose (PO/IM/IV): 10 mg/24 hr

Cross-allergenicity may occur in patients allergic to sulfonamides. Dosage reduction may be necessary in patients with hepatic dysfunction. Administer oral doses with food.

Side effects include cramps, dizziness, hypotension, headache, electrolyte losses (hypokalemia, hypocalcemia, hyponatremia, hypochloremia), and encephalopathy. May also lead to metabolic alkalosis. Serious skin reactions (e.g., Stevens-Johnson, TEN) have been reported.

Drug elimination has been reported to be slower in neonates with respiratory disorders compared with neonates without. May displace bilirubin in critically ill neonates. **Maximal** diuretic effect for infants ≤6 mo has been reported at 0.04 mg/kg/dose, with greater efficacy seen at lower dosages.

Pregnancy category changes to "D" if used in pregnancy-induced hypertension.

BUTORPHANOL
Stadol and other generics
Narcotic, analgesic

   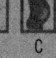

Yes   Yes   3   C

Injection: 1 mg/mL (1 mL), 2 mg/mL (1, 2, 10 mL)
Nasal solution: 10 mg/mL (2.5 mL); 1 mg per spray

Child: 0.03–0.05 mg/kg/dose (**max. dose:** 2 mg/dose) IV Q3–4 hr PRN
Adult:
IV: 1 mg/dose Q3–4 hr PRN; usual dosage range: 0.5–2 mg Q3–4 hr PRN
IM: 2 mg/dose Q3–4 hr PRN; usual dosage range: 1–4 mg Q3–4 hr PRN
Intranasal: 1 spray (1 mg) in one nostril × 1; an additional 1-mg dose may be given at 1–1.5 hr if needed. This 2-dose sequence may be repeated in 3–4 hr if needed. Alternatively, patient may receive 2 mg initially (1 mg in each nostril) only if they remain recumbent if drowsiness or dizziness occurs; an additional dose may be given 3–4 hr later.

A synthetic mixed agonist/antagonist opioid analalgesic. **Contraindicated** in patients hypersensitive to benzethonium chloride. **Use with caution** in hypotension, thyroid dysfunction, renal or hepatic impairment, and concomitant CNS depressants. **Suggested dosage reduction** in renal impairment (IV/IM): 75% of usual dose for GFR 10–50 mL/min and 50% of usual dose for GFR <10 mL/min, with an increase in dosage interval based on duration of clinical effects. A 50% IV/IM dosage reduction with increased dosage interval has been recommended in hepatic dsyfunction. Reduced dosage for intranasal administration for both renal and hepatic impairment: initial dose should not exceed 1 mg.

Common side effects include drowsiness, dizziness, insomnia (nasal spray), nausea, vomiting, nasal congestion (nasal spray).

Onset of action: 5–10 min (IV); 0.5–1 hr (IM); and within 15 min (intranasal)
Duration: 3–4 hr (IV/IM) and 4–5 hr (intranasal)

CAFFEINE CITRATE
Cafcit and others
Methylxanthine, respiratory stimulant

Yes   Yes   2   C

Injection: 20 mg/mL (3 mL)
Oral liquid: 20 mg/mL (3 mL), also available as powder for compounding 10, 20 mg/mL
20 mg/mL caffeine citrate salt = 10 mg/mL caffeine base

Doses expressed in mg of caffeine citrate.
Neonatal apnea:
   Loading dose: 20–25 mg/kg IV/PO × 1
   Maintenance dose: 5–10 mg/kg/dose PO/IV Q24 hr, to begin 24 hr after loading dose

Avoid use in symptomatic cardiac arrhythmias. **Do not use** caffeine benzoate formulation; it has been associated with kernicterus in neonates. **Use with caution** in impaired renal or hepatic function.
Therapeutic levels: 5–25 mg/L. Cardiovascular, neurologic, or GI toxicity reported at serum levels >50 mg/L. Recommended serum sampling time: obtain trough level within 30 minutes before a dose. Steady state is typically achieved 3 wk after initiation of therapy. Levels obtained before steady state are useful for preventing toxicity.
For IV administration, give loading dose over 30 min and maintenance dose over 10 min.

CALCITONIN—SALMON
Miacalcin, Miacalcin Nasal Spray, Fortical Nasal Spray
Hypercalcemia antidote, antiosteoporotic

No   No   ?   C

Injection: 200 U/mL (2 mL); contains phenol
Nasal spray: 200 U/metered dose (3.7 mL, provides at least 30 doses); may contain benzyl alcohol

Hypercalcemia (see remarks):
   Adult: Start with 4 U/kg/dose IM/SC Q12 hr; if response is unsatisfactory after 1 or 2 days, increase dose to 8 U/kg/dose Q12 hr. If response remains unsatisfactory after 2 more days, increase to a **max. dose** of 8 U/kg/dose Q6 hr.
Paget disease (see remarks):
   Adult: Start with 100 U IM/SC once daily initially, followed by a usual maintenance dose of 50 U once daily **OR** 50–100 U Q1–3 days.

Contraindicated in patients sensitive to salmon protein or gelatin. Because of hypersensitivity risk (e.g., bronchospasm, airway swelling, anaphylaxis), skin test is recommended before starting IM/SC therapy. For skin test, prepare a 10 U/mL dilution with normal saline, administer 0.1 mL intradermally, and observe for 15 min for wheal or significant erythema. Tachyphylaxis has been reported after 2–3 days of use for treatment of hypercalcemia of malignancy.
Nausea, abdominal pain, diarrhea, flushing, and inflammation at injection site has been reported with IM/SC route of administration.
Intranasal use currently indicated for postmenopausal osteoporosis in adults. Nasal irritation (alternate nostrils to reduce risk), rhinitis, epistaxis may occur with intranasal product.
Tremors has been reported with both intranasal and injectable routes of administration.
If injection volume exceeds 2 mL, use IM route and multiple sites of injection.

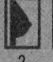 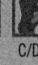

CALCITRIOL
1,25-dihydroxycholecalciferol, Rocaltrol, Calcijex, and generics
Active form vitamin D, fat soluble

No   No   2   C/D

Caps: 0.25, 0.5 mcg; may contain parabens
Oral solution: 1 mcg/mL (15 mL)
Injection: (Calcijex and others) 1 mcg/mL (1 mL); contains EDTA

Hypoparathyroidism (evaluate dosage at 2–4 wk intervals):
   Child > 1 yr and adult: initial dose of 0.25 mcg/dose PO once daily. May increase daily
   dosage by 0.25 mcg at 2- to 4-wk intervals. Usual maintenance dosage as follows:
     <1 yr: 0.04–0.08 mcg/kg/dose PO once daily
     1–5 yr: 0.25–0.75 mcg/dose PO once daily
     >6 yr and adult: 0.5–2 mcg/dose PO once daily
Renal failure: See National Kidney Foundation guidelines at http://www.kidney.org/professionals/kdoqi/
guidelinespedbone/guide9.htm.

Most potent vitamin D metabolite available. Should not be used to treat 25-OH vitamin D
   deficiency; use cholecalciferol or ergocalciferol. Monitor serum calcium, phosphorus, and PTH
   in dialysis patients. **Avoid** concomitant use of Mg^{2+}-containing antacids. IV dosing applies if
   patient undergoing hemodialysis.
Contraindicated in patients with hypercalcemia, vitamin D toxicity. Side effects include weakness,
   headache, vomiting, constipation, hypotonia, polydipsia, polyuria, myalgia, metastatic calcification,
   etc. Allergic reactions, including anaphylaxis, have been reported.
Pregnancy category changes to D if used in doses above the recommended daily allowance.

  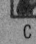

CALCIUM ACETATE
PhosLo, Calphron, Eliphos, Phoslyra, and generics;
25% elemental Ca
Calcium supplement, phosphorous-lowering agent

No   Yes   2   C

Tabs: 667 mg (169 mg elemental Ca)
Capsules: 667 mg (169 mg elemental Ca)
Oral solution (Phoslyra): 667 mg/5 mL (473 mL) (169 mg elemental Ca per 5 mL); contains
methylparabens and propylene glycol
Each 1 g of salt contains 12.7 mEq (250 mg) elemental Ca.

Doses expressed in mg of calcium acetate.
Hyperphosphatemia:
   Adult: Start with 1334 mg PO with each meal. Dosage may be increased gradually to bring serum
   phosphorous levels below 6 mg/dL, so long as hypercalcemia does not occur. Most patients require
   2001–2668 mg PO with each meal.

Contraindicated in ventricular fibrillation. **Use with caution** in renal impairment;
   hypercalcemia may develop in end-stage renal failure. Nausea and hypercalcemia may occur.
   About 40% of dose is systemically absorbed under fasting conditions and up to 30% in
   nonfasting conditions. May reduce absorption of tetracyclines, iron, and effectiveness of
   polystyrene sulfonate. May potentiate effects of digoxin.
Administer with meals and plenty of fluids for use as a phosphorus-lowering agent. Calcium is
   excreted in breast milk and is not expected to harm the infant, provided maternal serum calcium is
   appropriately monitored.

CALCIUM CARBONATE
Tums, Os-Cal, Children's Pepto, and many others;
40% elemental Ca
Calcium supplement, antacid

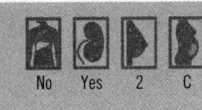

No   Yes   2   C

Tab, chewable [OTC]: 400, 500, 600, 750, 1000, 1250 mg
Children's Pepto [OTC]: 400 mg
Tab [OTC]: 500, 600, 650, 1250, 1500 mg
Oral suspension [OTC]: 1250 mg/5 mL
Caps [OTC]: 200, 364, 1250 mg
Powder [OTC]: 800 mg/2 g (480 g)
Each 1 g of salt contains 20 mEq elemental Ca (400 mg elemental Ca).

Hypocalcemia (Doses expressed in mg of elemental calcium. To convert to mg of salt, divide elemental dose by 0.4):
Neonate: 50–150 mg/kg/24 hr ÷ Q4–6 hr PO; **max. dose** 1 g/24 hr
Child: 45–65 mg/kg/24 hr PO ÷ QID
Adult: 1–2 g/24 hr PO ÷ TID–QID
Antacid (Doses expressed in mg of calcium carbonate):
2–5 yr: 400 mg PO as symptoms occur; **max. dose** 1200 mg/24 hr
>6–11 yr: 800 mg PO as symptoms occur; **max. dose** 2400 mg/24 hr
>11 yr and adult: 1000–3000 mg PO as symptoms occur; **max. dose** 7500 mg/24 hr

See *Calcium Acetate* for **contraindications, precautions** and drug interactions. Side effects: constipation, hypercalcemia, hypophosphatemia, hypomagnesemia, nausea, vomiting, headache, and confusion. Some products may contain trace amounts of sodium. Administer with plenty of fluids. For use as a phosphorus-lowering agent, administer with meals. Calcium is excreted in breast milk and is not expected to harm the infant, provided maternal serum calcium is appropriately monitored.

CALCIUM CHLORIDE
Various generics; 27% elemental Ca
Calcium supplement

No   Yes   2   C

Injection: 100 mg/mL (10%) (1.36 mEq Ca/mL); 1 g of salt contains 13.6 mEq (273 mg) elemental Ca
Each 1 g of salt contains 13.5 mEq (270 mg) elemental Ca.

Doses expressed in mg of CaCl.
Cardiac arrest or calcium channel blocker toxicity:
Infant/child: 20 mg/kg/dose IV Q10 min PRN; if effective, an infusion of 20–50 mg/kg/hr may be used
Adult: 500–1000 mg/dose IV Q10 min PRN *OR* 2–4 mg/kg/dose Q10 min PRN
MAXIMUM IV ADMINISTRATION RATES:
IV push: Do not exceed 100 mg/min (over 10–20 sec in cardiac arrest).
IV infusion: Do not exceed 45–90 mg/kg/hr with a **max. concentration** of 20 mg/mL.

Contraindicated in ventricular fibrillation. **Not recommended** for asystole and electromechanical dissociation. **Use with caution** in renal impairment; hypercalcemia may develop in end-stage renal failure. May potentiate effects of digoxin.
Use IV with extreme caution. Extravasation may lead to necrosis. Hyaluronidase may be helpful for extravasation. Central-line administration is preferred IV route of administration. **Do not use** scalp veins. **Do not administer via IM or SC routes.**
Rapid IV infusion associated with bradycardia, hypotension, and peripheral vasodilation. May cause hyperchloremic acidosis.
Calcium is excreted in breast milk and is not expected to harm the infant, provided maternal serum calcium is appropriately monitored.

see p. 648

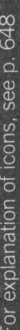

CALCIUM CITRATE
Cal-Citrate, Citracal, and generics; 21% elemental Ca
Calcium supplement

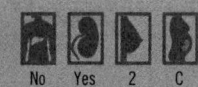
No   Yes   2   C

Tabs [OTC]: 950 mg (200 mg elemental), 1150 mg calcium citrate (250 mg elemental Ca)
Caps [OTC]:
   As elemental calcium: 180, 225 mg
Granules [OTC]:
   As elemental calcium: 760 mg/teaspoonful or 3.5 g of granules (480 g)
   Each 1 g of salt contains 10.6 mEq (211 mg) elemental Ca.
   Some products may be combined with vitamin D.

*Doses expressed as mg of elemental calcium. To convert to mg of salt, divide elemental
dose by 0.21.*
Hypocalcemia:
   Neonate: 50–150 mg/kg/24 hr ÷ Q4–6 hr PO; **max. dose** 1 g/24 hr
   Child: 45–65 mg/kg/24 hr PO ÷ QID
   Adult: 1–2 g/24 hr PO ÷ TID–QID

See *Calcium Acetate* for **contraindications, precautions**, and drug interactions. Side effects:
   constipation, hypercalcemia, hypophosphatemia, hypomagnesemia, nausea, vomiting,
   headache, and confusion.
Administer with meals for use as a phosphorus-lowering agent or with use of the granule dosage form.
   For hypocalcemia, do not administer with or before meals/food, and take plenty of fluids.
Calcium is excreted in breast milk and is not expected to harm the infant, provided maternal serum
   calcium is appropriately monitored.

CALCIUM GLUBIONATE
Calcionate, Calciquid, and generics; 6.4% elemental Ca
Calcium supplement

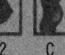
No   Yes   2   C

Syrup [OTC]: 1.8 g/5 mL (480 mL) (1.2 mEq Ca/mL)
Each 1 g of salt contains 3.2 mEq (64 mg) elemental Ca.

Doses expressed in mg calcium glubionate.
Hypocalcemia:
   Neonate: 1200 mg/kg/24 hr PO ÷ Q4–6 hr
   Infant/child: 600–2000 mg/kg/24 hr PO ÷ QID; **max. dose** 9 g/24 hr
   Adult: 6–18 g/24 hr PO ÷ QID

See *Calcium Acetate* for **contraindications, precautions**, and drug interactions. Side effects
   include GI irritation, dizziness, and headache. High osmotic load of syrup (20% sucrose) may
   cause diarrhea.
Best absorbed when given before meals. Absorption inhibited by high phosphate load.
Calcium is excreted in breast milk and is not expected to harm the infant, provided maternal serum
   calcium is appropriately monitored.

C

CALCIUM GLUCONATE
Cal-Glu and various generics; 9% elemental Ca
Calcium supplement

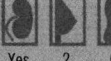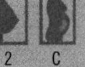

No   Yes   2   C

Tabs [OTC]: 50, 500, 648 mg
Caps (Cal-Glu) [OTC]: 500 mg
Injection: 100 mg/mL (10%) (0.45 mEq Ca2+/mL)
Each 1 g of salt contains 4.5 mEq (90 mg) elemental Ca

Doses expressed in mg calcium gluconate.
Maintenance/hypocalcemia:
  Neonate: IV: 200–800 mg/kg/24 hr ÷ Q6 hr
  Infant:
    IV: 200–500 mg/kg/24 hr ÷ Q6 hr
    PO: 400–800 mg/kg/24 hr ÷ Q6 hr
  Child: 200–500 mg/kg/24 hr IV or PO ÷ Q6 hr
  Adult: 0.5–8 g/24 hr IV or PO ÷ Q6 hr
For cardiac arrest:
  Infant and child: 100 mg/kg/dose IV Q10 min
  Adult: 1.5–3 g/dose IV Q10 min
  Max. dose: 3 g/dose
For tetany:
  Neonate, infant, child: 100–200 mg/kg dose IV over 5–10 min, repeat dose 6 hr later if needed;
    max. dose 500 mg/kg/24 hr
  Adult: 0.5–2 g IV over 10–30 min; repeat dose 6 hr later if needed
MAXIMUM IV ADMINISTRATION RATES:
  IV push: Do not exceed 100 mg/min (over 10–20 sec in cardiac arrest)
  IV infusion: Do not exceed 200 mg/min with a **maximum** concentration of 50 mg/mL

Contraindicated in ventricular fibrillation. **Use with caution** in renal impairment; hypercalcemia may develop in end-stage renal failure. **Avoid** peripheral infusion; extravasation may cause tissue necrosis. IV infusion associated with hypotension and bradycardia; also associated with arrhythmias in digitalized patients. May reduce absorption of tetracycline, iron, and effectiveness of polystyrene sulfonate with oral route of administration.
May precipitate when used with bicarbonate. **Do not use scalp veins. Do not administer IM or SC.**
Calcium is excreted in breast milk and is not expected to harm the infant, provided maternal serum calcium is appropriately monitored.

CALCIUM LACTATE
Cal-Lac and various generics; 13% elemental Ca
Calcium supplement

No   Yes   2   C

Tabs [OTC]: 100, 325, 650 mg
Caps (Cal-Lac) [OTC]: 500 mg
Each 1 g salt contains 6.5 mEq (130 mg) elemental Ca

Doses expressed in mg of calcium lactate.
Hypocalcemia:
  Neonate/Infant: 400–500 mg/kg/24 hr PO ÷ Q4–6 hr
  Child: 500 mg/kg/24 hr PO ÷ Q6–8 hr
  Adult: 1.5–3 g PO Q8 hr
  Max. dose: 9 g/24 hr

Continued

CALCIUM LACTATE *continued*

See *Calcium Acetate* for **contraindications**, **precautions**, and drug interactions. May cause
 constipation, headache, and hypercalcemia.
Give with or following meals and with plenty of fluids. **Do not** dissolve tablets in milk.
Calcium is excreted in breast milk and is not expected to harm the infant, provided maternal serum
 calcium is appropriately monitored.

CALCIUM PHOSPHATE, TRIBASIC
Posture-D; 39% elemental Ca
Calcium supplement

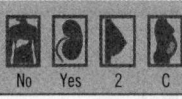

No   Yes   2   C

Tabs [OTC]: 600 mg elemental calcium and 280 mg phosphorus; with 500 IU vitamin D and 50 mg
 magnesium
Oral suspension: 10 mg elemental calcium/1 mL
NOTE: Pharmacy may crush tablets into a powder to enhance drug delivery for children unable to
 swallow tablets and to accommodate smaller doses.

Doses expressed as mg of elemental calcium.
Hypocalcemia:
 Neonate: 20–80 mg/kg/24 hr ÷ Q4–6 hr PO; **max. dose** 1 g/24 hr
 Child: 45–65 mg/kg/24 hr PO ÷ Q6 hr
 Adult: 1–2 g/24 hr PO ÷ Q6–8 hr

Contraindicated in ventricular fibrillation. **Use with caution** in renal impairment;
 hypercalcemia may develop in end-stage renal failure (avoid use in dialysis with
 hypercalcemia), history of kidney stones, and parathyroid disorders. May cause constipation,
 GI disturbances, and hypercalcemia. See *Calcium Acetate* for drug interactions.
Give with or following meals and with plenty of fluids. Keep in mind the amounts of vitamin D and
 magnesium your respective dosage may provide.
Calcium is excreted in breast milk and is not expected to harm the infant, provided maternal serum
 calcium is appropriately monitored.

CALFACTANT

See Surfactant, pulmonary

CAPTOPRIL
Capoten and various generics
Angiotensin-converting enzyme inhibitor, antihypertensive

No   Yes   2   D

Tabs: 12.5, 25, 50, 100 mg
Oral suspension: 0.75, 1 mg/mL

Neonate: 0.01–0.05 mg/kg/dose PO Q8–12 hr.
Infant < 6 mo: Initially 0.01–0.5 mg/kg/dose PO BID–TID; titrate upward if needed;
max. dose: 6 mg/kg/24 hr.
Child: Initially 0.3–0.5 mg/kg/dose PO BID–TID; titrate upward if needed; **max. dose** 6 mg/kg/24 hr
 up to 450 mg/24 hr.
Adolescent and adult: Initially 12.5–25 mg/dose PO BID–TID; increase weekly if necessary by 25 mg/
dose to **max. dose** of 450 mg/24 hr. Usual dosage range: 25–100 mg/24 hr ÷ BID.

CAPTOPRIL *continued*

Onset within 15–30 min of administration. Peak effect within 1–2 hr. **Adjust dose with renal failure (see Chapter 31).** Should be administered on an empty stomach 1 hr before or 2 hr after meals. Titrate to minimal effective dose. Lower doses should be used in patients with sodium and water depletion due to diuretic therapy.

Use with caution in collagen vascular disease and concomitant potassium-sparing diuretics. **Avoid use** with dialysis with high-flux membranes; anaphylactoid reactions have been reported. May cause rash, proteinuria, neutropenia, cough, angioedema (head, neck, and intestinal), hyperkalemia, hypotension, or diminution of taste perception (with long-term use). Known to decrease aldosterone and increase renin production. Do not coadminister with angiotensin receptor blockers or aliskiren, because use has been associated with increased risks for hypotension, hyperkalemia, and acute renal failure. Captopril is a CYP P450 2D6 substrate.

Captopril should be discontinued as soon as possible when pregnancy is detected.

CARBAMAZEPINE
Epitol, Tegretol, Tegretol-XR, Carbatrol, and various generics
Anticonvulsant

Yes Yes 2 D

Tabs: 200 mg
Chewable tabs: 100 mg
Extended-release tabs (Tegretol-XR and generics): 100, 200, 400 mg
Extended-release caps (Carbatrol and generics): 100, 200, 300 mg
Oral suspension: 100 mg/5 mL (10, 450 mL); may contain propylene glycol

See remarks regarding dosing intervals for specific dosage forms:
<6 yr:
  Initial: 10–20 mg/kg/24 hr PO ÷ BID–TID (QID for suspension)
  Increment: Q5–7 days up to **max. dose** of 35 mg/kg/24 hr PO
6–12 yr:
  Initial: 10 mg/kg/24 hr PO ÷ BID up to **max. dose** 100 mg/dose BID
  Increment: 100 mg/24 hr at 1-wk intervals (÷TID–QID) until desired response is obtained
  Maintenance: 20–30 mg/kg/24 hr PO ÷ BID–QID; usual maintenance dose is 400–800 mg/24 hr; **max. dose** 1000 mg/24 hr
>12 yr and adult:
  Initial: 200 mg PO BID
  Increment: 200 mg/24 hr at 1-wk intervals (÷BID–QID) until desired response is obtained
  Maintenance: 800–1200 mg/24 hr PO ÷ BID–QID
Max. dose:
  Child 12–15 yr: 1000 mg/24 hr
  Child > 15 yr: 1200 mg/24 hr
  Adult: 1.6–2.4 g/24 hr

Contraindicated for patients taking MAO inhibitors or who are sensitive to tricyclic antidepressants. Should **not** be used in combination with clozapine, owing to increased risk for bone marrow suppression and agranulocytosis. Increased risk for severe dermatologic reactions (e.g., SJS and TEN) has been associated with the HLA-B*1502 (prevalent among persons of Asian descent) and HLA-A*3101 (prevalent among Japanese, Native American, Southern Indian, and some Arabic ancestry) alleles.

Erythromycin, diltiazem, verapamil, cefixime, cimetidine, itraconazole, aprepitant, and INH may increase serum levels. Carbamazepine may decrease activity of warfarin, doxycycline, oral

Continued

CARBAMAZEPINE *continued*

contraceptives, cyclosporine, theophylline, phenytoin, benzodiazepines, ethosuximide, and valproic acid. Carbamazepine is a CYP 450 3A3/4 substrate and inducer of CYP 450 1A2, 2C, and 3A3/4. The enzyme-inducing effects may increase effects/toxicity of cyclophosphamide.

Suggested dosing intervals for specific dosage forms:

Extended-release tabs or caps, BID; chewable and immediate-release tabs, BID–TID; suspension, QID.

Doses may be administered with food. **Do not** crush or chew extended-release dosage forms. Shake bottle thoroughly before dispensing oral suspension dosage form, and **do not** administer simultaneously with other liquid medicines or diluents.

Drug metabolism typically increases after the first month of therapy initiation, owing to hepatic autoinduction.

Therapeutic blood levels: 4–12 mg/L. Recommended serum sampling time: Obtain trough level within 30 min before an oral dose. Steady state is typically achieved 1 month after initiation of therapy (after enzymatic autoinduction). Levels obtained before steady state are useful for preventing toxicity. Blood levels of 7–10 mg/L have been recommended for bipolar disorders.

Side effects include sedation, dizziness, diplopia, aplastic anemia, neutropenia, urinary retention, nausea, SIADH, and Stevens-Johnson syndrome. Suicidal behavior or ideation and onychomadesis have been reported. Pretreatment CBCs and LFTs are suggested. Patient should be monitored for hematologic and hepatic toxicity. **Adjust dose in renal impairment (see Chapter 31).**

See Chapter 2 for management of ingestions.

CARBAMIDE PEROXIDE
Debrox, Murine Ear, Auro Ear Drops, Thera-Ear Gly-Oxide, and generics
Cerumenolytic, topical oral analgesic

No   No   ?   ?

Otic solution [OTC]: 6.5% (15, 30 mL); may contain propylene glycol or alcohol
Oral liquid [OTC]: 10% (Gly-Oxide) (15, 60 mL)

Cerumenolytic:
  <12 yr: Tilt head sideways and instill 1–5 drops (according to patient size) into affected ear; retain drops in ear for several minutes. Remove wax by gently flushing ear with warm water, using a soft rubber bulb ear syringe. Dose may be repeated BID PRN for up to 4 days.
  ≥12 yr: Following the same instructions from above, instill 5–10 drops into affected ear BID PRN for up to 4 days.

Oral analgesic (see remarks):
  ≥3 yr (able to follow instructions): Instill several drops of the oral liquid to affected area and expectorate after 2–3 min, **OR** place 10 drops on tongue and mix with saliva, swish for several minutes, and expectorate. Administer up to QID, after meals and QHS, for **up to 7 days.**

Otic solution: Contraindicated if tympanic membrane perforated; after otic surgery; ear discharge, drainage, pain, irritation or rash; or PE tubes in place. Tip of applicator should not enter ear canal when used as a cerumenolytic.

Oral liquid: Prolonged use may result in fungal overgrowth. **Do not** rinse the mouth or drink for at least 5 min when using oral preparation.

Pregnancy category has not been formally assigned by the FDA.

C

CARBINOXAMINE
Arbinoxa, Palgic, and generics
Antihistamine

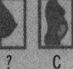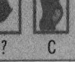

No   No   ?   C

Liquid: 4 mg/5 mL (473 mL); may contain propylene glycol
Tabs: 4 mg

Child (PO [see remarks]): 0.2–0.4 mg/kg/24 hr PO ÷ TID–QID; alternative dosing by age (**do not exceed** 0.4 mg/kg/24 hr):

  2–3 yr: 2 mg TID–QID
  3–6 yr: 2–4 mg TID–QID
  ≥6 yr: 4–6 mg TID–QID
Adult: 4–8 mg PO TID–QID

Generally not recommended for treating URIs for infants. No proven benefit for infants and young children with URIs. **The FDA does not recommend use for URIs in children <2 yr because of reports of increased fatalities.**

Contraindicated in acute asthma, hypersensitivity with other ethanolamine antihistamines, MAO inhibitors, severe hypertension, narrow-angle glaucoma, severe coronary artery disease, and urinary retention. Be aware that combination decongestant products may exist.

May cause drowsiness, vertigo, dry mucus membranes, and headache. Contact dermatitis and CNS excitation have been reported.

CARNITINE
Levocarnitine, Carnitor, Carnitor SF, ʟ-Carnitine, and generics
Nutritional supplement, amino acid

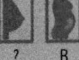

No   Yes   ?   B

Tabs: 250, 330 mg
Caps: 250 mg
Oral solution: 100 mg/mL (118 mL); contains methyl- and prophylparabens; Carnitor SF is a sugar-free product.
Injection: 200 mg/mL (5, 12.5 mL) (preservative free)

Primary carnitine deficiency:
  Oral:
    Child: 50–100 mg/kg/24 hr PO ÷ Q8–12 hr; increase slowly as needed and tolerated to **max. dose** of 3 g/24 hr.
    Adult: 330 mg to 1 g/dose BID–TID PO; **max. dose** 3 g/24 hr.
  IV:
    Child and adult: 50 mg/kg as loading dose; may follow with 50 mg/kg/24 hr IV infusion (for severe cases); maintenance: 50 mg/kg/24 hr ÷ Q4–6 hr; increase to **max. dose** of 300 mg/kg/24 hr if needed.

May cause nausea, vomiting, abdominal cramps, diarrhea, and body odor. Seizures have been reported in patients with or without a history of seizures. Safety in end-stage renal disease (ESRD) has not been established. High doses to severely compromised renal function or ESRD on dialysis may result in accumulation of potentially toxic metabolites (trimethylamine and trimethylamine-*N*-oxide).

Give bolus IV infusion over 2–3 min.

For explanation of icons, see p. 648

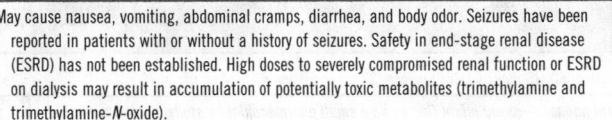

CARVEDILOL
Coreg, Coreg CR, and generics
Adrenergic antagonist (α and β), antihypertensive

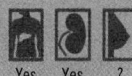
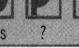

Yes   Yes   ?   C

Tabs: 3.125, 6.25, 12.5, 25 mg
Extended-release caps (Coreg CR): 10, 20, 40, 80 mg
Oral suspension: 0.1, 1.25, 1.67 mg/mL

Heart failure:
Immediate-release dosage forms (tablets and oral suspension [see remarks]):
Infant, child, adolescent: Start at 0.05–0.2 mg/kg/24 hr PO ÷ BID. Dose may be titrated at 1- or 2-wk intervals as needed up to a **maximum** of 2 mg/kg/24 hr or 50 mg/24 hr. Reported usual effective dose: 0.2–1 mg/kg/24 hr.
Adult: Start at 3.125 mg PO BID × 2 wk; if needed and tolerated, may increase to 6.25 mg BID. Dose may be doubled Q2 wk if needed to the following **maximum doses:**
Mild/moderate heart failure: <85 kg, 25 mg BID; ≥ 85 kg, 50 mg BID
Severe heart failure: 25 mg BID
Extended-release capsules:
Adult: Start at 10 mg PO once daily × 2 wk; if needed and tolerated, double the dose Q2 wk up to a **maximum** of 80 mg once daily.
Hypertension:
Adult:
Immediate-release dosage forms: Start at 6.25 mg PO BID; dose may be doubled every 1–2 wk up to a **maximum** of 25 mg PO BID.
Extended-release capsules: Start at 20 mg PO once daily × 1–2 wk; if needed and tolerated, increase to 40 mg PO once daily. If needed, dose may be further increased in 2-wk intervals up to a **maximum** of 80 mg/24 hr.

Contraindicated in asthma or related bronchospastic disease, sick sinus syndrome, second- or third-degree heart block, severe bradycardia, cardiogenic shock, decompensated cardiac failure requiring IV inotropic therapy, and severe hepatic impairment (Child-Pugh class C).

Use with caution in mild/moderate hepatic impairment (Child-Pugh class A or B), renal insufficiency, thyrotoxicosis, ischemic heart disease, diabetes, and cataract surgery. **Avoid abrupt withdrawal** of medication.

Children <3.5 years old may have faster carvedilol clearance and may require higher dosages or TID dosing. Carvedilol is a CYP 450 2D6 substrate. Digoxin, disopyramide, and dipyridamole may increase bradycardic effects.

Bradycardia, postural hypotension, peripheral edema, weight gain, hyperglycemia, diarrhea, dizziness, and fatigue are common. Hypersensitivity reactions have been reported. Chest pain, headache, vomiting, edema, and dyspnea have also been reported in children. Administering doses with food can reduce risk for orthostatic hypotension.

CASPOFUNGIN
Cancidas
Antifungal, echinocandin

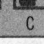

Yes   No   ?   C

Injection: 50, 70 mg; contains sucrose (39 mg in 50 mg vial and 54 mg in 70 mg vial)

Preterm neonate—<3 mo infant (based on a small pharmacokinetic study, achieving similar plasma exposure as seen in adults receiving 50 mg/24 hr): 25 mg/m²/dose IV once daily. Alternatively, 1 mg/kg/dose IV once daily × 2 days, followed by 2 mg/kg/dose IV once daily has been reported in a case series with excellent microbiological results.

CASPOFUNGIN *continued*

3 mo infant–17 yr (see remarks): 70 mg/m²/dose IV loading dose on day 1, followed by 50 mg/m²/dose IV once-daily maintenance dose. Increase maintenance dose to 70 mg/m²/dose if response is inadequate or if patient is receiving an enzyme-inducing medication (see remarks).
Maximum loading and maintenance dose: 70 mg/dose
Adolescent and adult (see remarks):
Loading dose: 70 mg IV × 1
Maintenance dose:
Usual: 50 mg IV once daily. If tolerated and response is inadequate or if patient is receiving an enzyme-inducing medication (see remarks), increase to 70 mg IV once daily.
Hepatic insufficiency (Child-Pugh score 7–9): 35 mg IV once daily

Use with caution in hepatic impairment and concomitant enzyme-inducing drugs. Higher maintenance doses (70 mg/m²/dose in children and 70 mg in adults) are recommended for concomitant use of enzyme inducers, such as carbamazepine, dexamethasone, phenytoin, nevirapine, efavirenz, or rifampin. Use Mosteller formula for calculating BSA.

Most common adverse effects (>10%) in children include fever, diarrhea, rash, elevated ALT/AST, hypokalemia, hypotension, and chills. May also cause facial swelling, nausea/vomiting, headache, infusion site phlebitis, and LFT elevation. Anaphylaxis and possible histamine-related reactions (angioedema, bronchospasm, and warmth sensation) have been reported. Hepatobiliary adverse effects have been reported in pediatric patients with serious underlying medical conditions.

Reduce daily dose by 30% in moderate hepatic impairment (Child-Pugh score 7–9).

Use with cyclosporine may cause transient increase in LFTs and caspofungin level elevations. May decrease tacrolimus levels.

Administer doses by slow IV infusion over 1 hr. **Do not** mix or co-infuse with other medications, and **avoid** using dextrose-containing diluents (e.g., D₅W).

CEFACLOR
Ceclor, Ceclor CD, Raniclor, and generics
Antibiotic, cephalosporin (second generation)

No   Yes   1   B

Caps: 250, 500 mg
Extended-release tabs (Ceclor CD): 500 mg
Chewable tabs (Raniclor): 125, 187, 250, 375 mg; contains phenylalanine
Oral suspension: 125 mg/5 mL (75, 150 mL), 187 mg/5 mL (100 mL), 250 mg/5 mL (75, 150 mL), 375 mg/5 mL (100 mL)

Child > 1 mo old (use regular-release dosage forms): 20–40 mg/kg/24 hr PO ÷ Q8 hr; **max. dose** 2 g/24 hr
Q12 hr dosage interval option for otitis media: 40 mg/kg/24 hr
Q12 hr dosage interval option for pharyngitis: 20 mg/kg/24 hr
Adult: 250–500 mg/dose PO Q8 hr; **max. dose** 4 g/24 hr
Extended-release tablets: 500 mg/dose PO Q12 hr

Use with caution in patients with penicillin allergy or renal impairment. Side effects include elevated LFTs, bone marrow suppression, and moniliasis. Probenecid may increase cefaclor concentrations. May cause positive Coombs test or false-positive test for urinary glucose. Serum sickness reactions have been reported in patients receiving multiple courses of cefaclor.

Do not crush, cut, or chew extended-release tablets. Doses should be given on an empty stomach. **Extended-release tablets not recommended for children. Adjust dose in renal failure (see Chapter 31).**

For explanation of icons, see p. 648

CEFADROXIL
Duricef and generics
Antibiotic, cephalosporin (first generation)

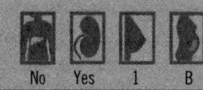

No   Yes   1   B

Oral suspension: 250, 500 mg/5 mL (75, 100 mL)
Tabs: 1 g
Caps: 500 mg

Infant and child: 30 mg/kg/24 hr PO ÷ Q12 hr (daily dose may be administered once daily for
group A β-hemolytic streptococci pharyngitis/tonsillitis); **max. dose** 2 g/24 hr
*Bacterial endocarditis prophylaxis for dental and upper airway procedures: 50 mg/kg/dose
(max. dose 2 g) × 1 PO 1 hr before procedure*
Adolescent and adult: 1–2 g/24 hr PO ÷ Q12–24 hr (administer Q12 hr for complicated UTIs);
max. dose 2 g/24 hr
Bacterial endocarditis prophylaxis for dental and upper airway procedures: 2 g × 1 PO 1 hr
before procedure

See *Cephalexin* for **precautions** and interactions. Rash, nausea, vomiting, and diarrhea are
common. Transient neutropenia, and vaginitis have been reported. **Adjust dose in renal
failure (see Chapter 31).**

CEFAZOLIN
Ancef, Zolicef, and generics
Antibiotic, cephalosporin (first generation)

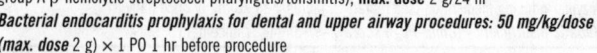

Yes   Yes   1   B

Injection: 0.5, 1, 5, 10, 20 g
Frozen injection: 1 g/50 mL 5% dextrose (iso-osmotic solution)
Contains 2.1 mEq Na/g drug

Neonate IM, IV:
Postnatal age ≤ 7 days: 40 mg/kg/24 hr ÷ Q12 hr
Postnatal age > 7 days:
≤2000 g: 40 mg/kg/24 hr ÷ Q12 hr
>2000 g: 60 mg/kg/24 hr ÷ Q8 hr
Infant > 1 mo and child: 50–100 mg/kg/24 hr ÷ Q6–8 hr IV/IM; **max. dose** 6 g/24 hr
Adult: 2–6 g/24 hr ÷ Q6–8 hr IV/IM; **max. dose** 12 g/24 hr
Bacterial endocarditis prophylaxis for dental and upper respiratory procedures:
Infant and child: 50 mg/kg IV/IM (**max. dose** 1 g) 30 min before procedure
Adult: 1 g IV/IM 30 min before procedure

Use with caution in renal impairment or in penicillin-allergic patients. Does not penetrate well
into CSF. May cause phlebitis, leukopenia, thrombocytopenia, transient liver enzyme
elevation, and false-positive urine reducing substance (Clinitest) and Coombs tests.
For dosing in obese patients, use higher end of the dosing recommendation. **Adjust dose in renal
failure (see Chapter 31).**

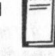

CEFDINIR
Omnicef
Antibiotic, cephalosporin (third generation)

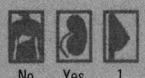

No   Yes   1   B

Caps: 300 mg
Oral suspension: 125 mg/5 mL (60, 100 mL), 250 mg/5 mL (60, 100 mL)

6 mo–12 yr:
   Otitis media, sinusitis, pharyngitis/tonsillitis: 14 mg/kg/24 hr PO ÷ Q12–24 hr;
   max. dose 600 mg/24 hr
   Uncomplicated skin infections (see remarks): 14 mg/kg/24 hr PO ÷ Q12 hr; **max. dose** 600 mg/24 hr
≥13 yr and adult:
   Bronchitis, sinusitis, pharyngitis/tonsillitis: 600 mg/24 hr PO ÷ Q12–24 hr
   Community-acquired pneumonia, uncomplicated skin infections (see remarks): 600 mg/24 hr
   PO ÷ Q12 hr

Use with caution in penicillin-allergic patients or in presence of renal impairment. Good gram-positive cocci activity. May cause diarrhea (especially in children <2 yr), headache, vaginitis, and false-positive urine reducing substance (Clinitest) and Coombs tests. Eosinophilia and abnormal liver function tests have been reported with higher than usual doses.

Once-daily dosing has not been evaluated in pneumonia and skin infections. Probenecid increases serum cefdinir levels. Avoid concomitant administration with iron and iron-containing vitamins and antacids containing aluminum or magnesium (space by 2 hr apart) to reduce risk for decreasing antibiotic's absorption. Doses may be taken without regard to food. **Adjust dose in renal failure (see Chapter 31).**

CEFEPIME
Maxipime and generics
Antibiotic, cephalosporin (fourth generation)

No   Yes   1   B

Injection: 0.5, 1, 2 g
Premixed injection: 1 g/50 mL, 2 g/100 mL (iso-osmotic dextrose solution)
Each 1 g drug contains 725 mg L-arginine.

Neonate:
   <14 days: 60 mg/kg/24 hr ÷ Q12 hr IV/IM
   ≥14 days: 100 mg/kg/24 hr ÷ Q12 hr IV/IM. For meningitis or *Pseudomonas* infections,
   use 150 mg/kg/24 hr ÷ Q8 hr IV/IM
Child ≥ 2 mo: 100 mg/kg/24 hr ÷ Q12 hr IV/IM
   Meningitis, fever, and neutropenia, or serious infections: 150 mg/kg/24 hr ÷ Q8 hr IV/IM.
   Max. dose 6 g/24 hr
Cystic fibrosis: 150 mg/kg/24 hr ÷ Q8 hr IV/IM, up to a **max. dose** of 6 g/24 hr
Adult: 1–4 g/24 hr ÷ Q12 hr IV/IM
   Severe infections: 6 g/24 hr ÷ Q8 hr IV/IM
   Max. dose: 6 g/24 hr

Use with caution in patients with penicillin allergy or renal impairment. Good activity against *Pseudomonas aeruginosa* and other gram-negative bacteria, plus most gram-positives (methicillin-sensitive *Staphylococcus aureus* [MRSA]). May cause thrombophlebitis, gastrointestinal discomfort, transient increases in liver enzymes, and false-positive urine reducing substance (Clinitest) and Coombs tests. Probenecid increases serum cefepime levels. Encephalopathy, myoclonus, seizures (including nonconvulsive status epilepticus), transient leukopenia, neutropenia, agranulocytosis, and thrombocytopenia have been reported. **Adjust dose in renal failure (see Chapter 31).**

For explanation of icons, see p. 648

CEFIXIME
Suprax
Antibiotic, cephalosporin (third generation)

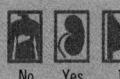 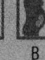

No   Yes   1   B

Oral suspension: 100 mg/5 mL (50, 75 mL)
Tabs: 400 mg

Infant (>6 mo) and child: 8 mg/kg/24 hr ÷ Q12–24 hr PO; **max. dose** 400 mg/24 hr
  Acute UTI: 16 mg/kg/24 hr ÷ Q12 hr on day 1, followed by 8 mg/kg/24 hr Q24 hr PO ×
  13 days. **Max. dose** 400 mg/24 hr
  Sexual victimization prophylaxis: 8 mg/kg PO × 1 (**max. dose** 400 mg) PLUS azithromycin 20 mg/kg
  PO × 1 (**max. dose** 1 g)
Adolescent and adult: 400 mg/24 hr ÷ Q12–24 hr PO
  Uncomplicated cervical, urethral, or rectal infections due to Neisseria gonorrhoeae: 400 mg × 1
  PO PLUS azithromycin 1 g PO × 1 **OR** doxycycline 100 mg PO BID × 7 days
  Sexual victimization prophylaxis: 400 mg PO × 1 PLUS azithromycin 1 g PO × 1 **OR** doxycycline 100
  mg BID PO × 7 days, PLUS metronidazole 2 g PO × 1, PLUS hepatitis B vaccine (if not immunized)

Use with caution in patients with penicillin allergy or renal failure. Adverse reactions include
diarrhea, abdominal pain, nausea, and headaches. Because of reduced bioavailability, **do not** use
tablets for treatment of otitis media. Probenecid increases serum cefixime levels. Unlike most
cephalosporins, drug is excreted unchanged in bile (5%–10%) and urine (50%). May increase
carbamazepine serum concentrations. May cause false-positive urine reducing substance test (Clinitest),
Coombs test, and nitroprusside test for ketones. **Adjust dose in renal failure (see Chapter 31).**

CEFOTAXIME
Claforan and generics
Antibiotic, cephalosporin (third generation)

   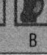 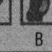

No   Yes   1   B

Injection: 0.5, 1, 2, 10 g
Frozen injection: 1 g/50 mL 3.4% dextrose, 2 g/50 mL 1.4% dextrose (iso-osmotic solutions)
Contains 2.2 mEq Na/g drug

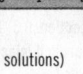

Neonate: IV/IM:
  Postnatal age ≤ 7 days:
    <2000 g: 100 mg/kg/24 hr ÷ Q12 hr
    ≥2000 g: 100–150 mg/kg/24 hr ÷ Q8–12 hr
  Postnatal age > 7 days:
    <1200 g: 100 mg/kg/24 hr ÷ Q12 hr
    1200–2000 g: 150 mg/kg/24 hr ÷ Q8 hr
    >2000 g: 150–200 mg/kg/24 hr ÷ Q6–8 hr
Infant and child (1 mo–12 yr and <50 kg): 100–200 mg/kg/24 hr ÷ Q6–8 hr IV/IM. Higher doses of
150–225 mg/kg/24 hr ÷ Q6–8 hr have been recommended for infections outside CSF due to
penicillin-resistant pneumococci.
  Meningitis: 200 mg/kg/24 hr ÷ Q6 hr IV/IM. Higher doses of 225–300 mg/kg/24 hr ÷ Q6–8 hr, in
  combination with vancomycin (dosed at CNS target levels), have been recommended for meningitis
  due to penicillin-resistant pneumococci.
  Max. dose: 12 g/24 hr
Child (>12 yr or ≥50 kg) and adult: 1–2 g/dose Q6–8 hr IV/IM
  Severe infection: 2 g/dose Q4–6 hr IV/IM
  Max. dose: 12 g/24 hr
  Uncomplicated gonorrhea: 0.5–1 g × 1 IM

CEFOTAXIME *continued*

Use with caution in penicillin allergy and renal impairment (reduce dosage). Toxicities similar to other cephalosporins: allergy, neutropenia, thrombocytopenia, eosinophilia, false-positive urine reducing substance (Clinitest) and Coombs tests, and elevated BUN, creatinine, and liver enzymes. Probenecid increases serum cefotaxime levels.
Good CNS penetration. **Adjust dose in renal failure (see Chapter 31).**

CEFOTETAN
Cefotan and generics
Antibiotic, cephalosporin (second generation)

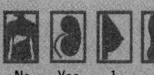

No   Yes   1   B

Injection: 1, 2, 10 g
Frozen injection: 1 g/50 mL 3.8% dextrose, 2 g/50 mL 2.2% dextrose (iso-osmotic solutions)
Contains 3.5 mEq Na/g drug

Infant and child (limited data): 40–80 mg/kg/24 hr ÷ Q12 hr IV/IM
Adolescent and adult: 2–4 g/24 hr ÷ Q12 hr IV/IM
  PID: 2 g Q12 hr IV × 24–48 hr after clinical improvement with doxycycline 100 mg Q12 hr PO/IV × 14 days
Max. dose (all ages): 6 g/24 hr
Preoperative prophylaxis (30–60 min before procedure):
  Child: 40 mg/kg/dose (**max. dose** 2 g/dose) IV
  Adult: 1–2 g IV

Use with caution in penicillin-allergic patients or in presence of renal impairment. Has good anaerobic activity. May cause disulfiram-like reaction with ethanol, increase effects/toxicities of anticoagulants, false-positive urine reducing substance test (Clinitest), and false elevations of serum and urine creatinine (Jaffe method). Hemolytic anemia has been reported. Good anaerobic activity but poor CSF penetration. **Adjust dose in renal failure (see Chapter 31).**

CEFOXITIN
Mefoxin and generics
Antibiotic, cephalosporin (second generation)

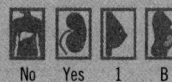

No   Yes   1   B

Injection: 1, 2, 10 g
Frozen injection: 1 g/50 mL 4% dextrose, 2 g/50 mL 2.2% dextrose (iso-osmotic solutions)
Contains 2.3 mEq Na/g drug

Neonate: 90–100 mg/kg/24 hr ÷ Q8 hr IM/IV
Infant and child:
  Mild/moderate infections: 80–100 mg/kg/24 hr ÷ Q6–8 hr IM/IV
  Severe infections: 100–160 mg/kg/24 hr ÷ Q4–6 hr IM/IV
Adult: 1–2 g/dose Q6–8 hr IM/IV
  PID: 2 g IV Q6h × 24–48 hr after clinical improvement. Doxycycline 100 mg Q12 hr PO/IV × 14 days is also initiated at the same time.
Max. dose (all ages): 12 g/24 hr

Use with caution in penicillin-allergic patients or in presence of renal impairment. Has good anaerobic activity but poor CSF penetration. Probenecid increases serum cefoxitin levels. May cause false-positive urine reducing substance tests (Clinitest and other copper reduction methods) and false elevations of serum and urine creatinine (Jaffe and KDA methods).
Adjust dose in renal failure (see Chapter 31).

For explanation of icons, see p. 648

CEFPODOXIME PROXETIL
Vantin and generics
Antibiotic, cephalosporin (third generation)

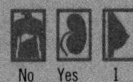

No   Yes   I   B

Tabs: 100, 200 mg
Oral suspension: 50, 100 mg/5 mL (50, 75, 100 mL)

2 mo–12 yr:
   Otitis media: 10 mg/kg/24 hr PO ÷ Q12–24 hr × 5 days; **max. dose** 400 mg/24 hr
   Pharyngitis/tonsillitis: 10 mg/kg/24 hr PO ÷ Q12 hr × 5–10 days; **max. dose** 200 mg/24 hr
   Acute maxillary sinusitis: 10 mg/kg/24 hr PO ÷ Q12 hr × 10 days; **max. dose** 400 mg/24 hr
≥13 yr–adult:
   Exacerbation of chronic bronchitis, community-acquired pneumonia, and sinusitis: 400 mg/24 hr
   PO ÷ Q12 hr × 10 days (14 days for pneumonia)
   Pharyngitis/tonsillitis: 200 mg/24 hr PO ÷ Q12 hr × 5–10 days
   Skin/skin structure infection: 800 mg/24 hr PO ÷ Q12 hr × 7–14 days
   Uncomplicated gonorrhea: 200 mg PO × 1

Use with caution in penicillin-allergic patients or in presence of renal impairment. May cause
diarrhea, nausea, vomiting, vaginal candidiasis, and false-positive Coombs test.
Tablets should be administered with food to enhance absorption. Suspension may be administered
without regard to food. High doses of antacids or H2 blockers may reduce absorption. Probenecid
increases serum cefpodoxime levels.
Adjust dose in renal failure (see Chapter 31).

CEFPROZIL
Cefzil and generics
Antibiotic, cephalosporin (second generation)

No   Yes   I   B

Tabs: 250, 500 mg
Oral suspension: 125 mg/5 mL, 250 mg/5 mL (50, 75, 100 mL); contains aspartame and
phenylalanine

Otitis media:
   6 mo–12 yr: 30 mg/kg/24 hr PO ÷ Q12 hr
Pharyngitis/tonsillitis:
   2–12 yr: 15 mg/kg/24 hr PO ÷ Q12 hr
Acute sinusitis:
   6 mo–12 yr: 15–30 mg/kg/24 hr PO ÷ Q12–24 hr
Uncomplicated skin infections:
   2–12 yr: 20 mg/kg/24 hr PO Q24 hr
Other:
   ≥13 yr and adult: 500–1000 mg/24 hr PO ÷ Q12–24 hr
Max. dose (all ages): 1 g/24 hr

Use with caution in penicillin-allergic patients or in presence of renal impairment. Oral
suspension contains aspartame and phenylalanine and should not be used by
phenyketonurics. May cause nausea, vomiting, diarrhea, liver enzyme elevations, and false-
positive urine reducing substance tests (Clinitest and other copper reduction methods) and
Coombs test. Probenecid increases serum cefprozil levels. Absorption not affected by food.
Adjust dose in renal failure (see Chapter 31).

CEFTAZIDIME
Fortaz, Tazidime, Tazicef, Ceptaz (arginine salt),
and generics
Antibiotic, cephalosporin (third generation)

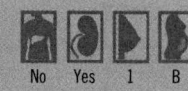

No   Yes   1   B

Injection: 0.5, 1, 2, 6, 10 g
Frozen injection: 1 g/50 mL 4.4% dextrose, 2 g/50 mL 3.2% dextrose (iso-osmotic solutions)
(Fortaz, Tazicef, Tazidime contains 2.3 mEq Na/g drug)
(Ceptaz contains 349 mg ʟ-arginine/g drug)

Neonate (IV/IM):
Postnatal age ≤ 7 days:
    <2000 g: 100 mg/kg/24 hr ÷ Q12 hr
    ≥2000 g: 100–150 mg/kg/24 hr ÷ Q8–12 hr
Postnatal age > 7 days:
    <1200 g: 100 mg/kg/24 hr ÷ Q12 hr
    ≥1200 g: 150 mg/kg/24 hr ÷ Q8 hr
Infant (>1 mo) and child: 100–150 mg/kg/24 hr ÷ Q8 hr IV/IM; **max. dose** 6 g/24 hr
Cystic fibrosis and meningitis: 150 mg/kg/24 hr ÷ Q8 hr IV/IM; **max. dose** 6 g/24 hr
Adult: 1–2 g/dose Q8–12 hr IV/IM; **max. dose** 6 g/24 hr

Use with caution in penicillin-allergic patients or in presence of renal impairment. Good
Pseudomonas coverage and CSF penetration. May cause rash, liver enzyme elevations, and
false-positive urine reducing substance tests (Clinitest and other copper reduction methods)
and Coombs test. Probenecid increases serum ceftazidime levels. **Adjust dose in renal
failure (see Chapter 31).**

CEFTIBUTEN
Cedax
Antibiotic, cephalosporin (third generation)

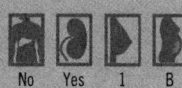

No   Yes   1   B

Oral suspension: 90 mg/5 mL (60, 90, 120 mL), 180 mg/5 mL (60 mL); contains sodium benzoate
Caps: 400 mg

Child (>6 mo):
Otitis media and pharyngitis/tonsillitis: 9 mg/kg/24 hr (**max. dose** 400 mg/24 hr) PO
once daily × 10 days
≥12 yr and adult: 400 mg PO once daily × 10 days; **max. dose** 400 mg/24 hr

Use with caution in penicillin-allergic patients or in presence of renal impairment. May cause
GI symptoms and elevations in eosinophils and BUN. Stevens-Johnson syndrome has been
reported. Gastric acid–lowering medications (e.g., ranitidine, omeprazole) may enhance
bioavailability of ceftibutin.
Oral suspension should be administered 2 hr before or 1 hr after a meal. **Adjust dose in renal failure
(see Chapter 31).**

CEFTRIAXONE
Rocephin and generics
Antibiotic, cephalosporin (third generation)

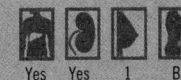

Yes   Yes   1   B

Injection: 0.25, 0.5, 1, 2, 10 g
Frozen injection: 1 g/50 mL 3.8% dextrose, 2 g/50 mL 2.4% dextrose (iso-osmotic solutions)
Contains 3.6 mEq Na/g drug

Neonate:
  Gonococcal ophthalmia or prophylaxis: 25–50 mg/kg/dose IM/IV × 1; **max. dose**
  125 mg/dose

Infant (>1 mo) and child:
  Mild/moderate infections: 50–75 mg/kg/24 hr ÷ Q12–24 hr IM/IV; **max. dose** 2 g/24 hr
  Meningitis (including penicillin-resistant pneumococci): 100 mg/kg/24 hr IM/IV ÷ Q12 hr;
  max. dose 2 g/dose and 4 g/24 hr
  Penicillin-resistant pneumococci outside of CSF: 80–100 mg/kg/24 hr ÷ Q12–24 hr; **max. dose**
  2 g/dose and 4 g/24 hr
  Acute otitis media: 50 mg/kg IM × 1; **max. dose** 1 g
Adult: 1–2 g/dose Q12–24 hr IV/IM; **max. dose** 2 g/dose and 4 g/24 hr
  Uncomplicated gonorrhea or chancroid: 250 mg IM × 1
Bacterial endocarditis prophylaxis for dental and upper respiratory procedures:
  Infant and child: 50 mg/kg IV/IM (**max. dose** 1 g) 30 min before procedure
  Adult: 1 g IV/IM 30 min before procedure

Contraindicated in neonates with hyperbilirubinemia. **Do not** administer with IV calcium-containing solutions or products (mixed or administered simultaneously via different lines) in neonates (<28 days old) because of risk of precipitation of ceftriaxone-calcium salt. Cases of fatal reactions with calcium-ceftriaxone precipitates in lung and kidneys in term and preterm neonates have been reported. **Do not** administer simultaneously with IV calcium-containing solutions via a Y-site for any age group. IV calcium-containing products may be administered sequentially only when the infusion lines are thoroughly flushed between infusions with a compatible fluid.

Use with caution in penicillin allergy; patients with gallbladder, biliary tract, liver, or pancreatic disease; presence of renal impairment; or in neonates with continuous dosing (risk for hyperbilirubinemia). In neonates, consider using an alternative third-generation cephalosporin with similar activity. Unlike other cephalosporins, ceftriaxone is significantly cleared by the biliary route (35%–45%).

Rash, injection site pain, diarrhea, and transient increase in liver enzymes are common. May cause reversible cholelithiasis, sludging in gallbladder, and jaundice. May interfere with serum and urine creatinine assays (Jaffe method) and cause false-positive urinary protein and urinary reducing substances (Clinitest).

For IM injections, dilute drug with either sterile water for injection or 1% lidocaine to a concentration of 250 or 350 mg/mL (250 mg/mL has lower incidence of injection site reactions). Assess potential risk/benefit for using lidocaine as a diluent; see *Lidocaine* for additional remarks.

CEFUROXIME (IV, IM)/CEFUROXIME AXETIL (PO)
CEFUROXIME AXETIL (PO)
IV: Zinacef and generics
PO: Ceftin and generics
Antibiotic, cephalosporin (second generation)

No   Yes   1   B

Injection: 0.75, 1.5, 7.5 g
Frozen injection: 1.5 g/50 mL water (iso-osmotic solutions)
Injectable dosage forms contain 2.4 mEq Na/g drug
Tabs: 250, 500 mg
Oral suspension: 125, 250 mg/5 mL (50, 100 mL); may contain aspartame

IM/IV:
  Neonate: 50–100 mg/kg/24 hr ÷ Q12 hr
  Infant (>3 mo)/child: 75–150 mg/kg/24 hr ÷ Q8 hr
  Adult: 750–1500 mg/dose Q8 hr
  Max. dose: 9 g/24 hr
PO (see remarks):
  Child (3 mo–12 yr):
    Pharyngitis and tonsillitis:
      Oral suspension: 20 mg/kg/24 hr ÷ Q12 hr; **max. dose** 500 mg/24 hr
      Tabs: 125 mg PO Q12 hr
    Otitis media, impetigo, and maxillary sinusitis:
      Oral suspension: 30 mg/kg/24 hr ÷ Q12 hr; **max. dose** 1 g/24 hr
      Tabs: 250 mg Q12 hr
    Lyme disease (alternative to doxycycline or amoxicillin):
      Oral suspension: 30 mg/kg/24 hr (**max. dose** 500 mg/24 hr) ÷ Q12 hr × 14–28 days
  Child (≥13 yr):
    Sinusitis, otitis media, pharyngitis, and tonsillitis:
      Tabs: 250 mg Q12 hr
  Adult: 250–500 mg BID; **max. dose** 1 g/24 hr

Use with caution in penicillin-allergic patients or in presence of renal impairment. May cause
GI discomfort; thrombophlebitis at infusion site; false-positive urine reducing substance
tests (Clinitest and other copper reduction methods) and Coombs test; and may interfere with
serum and urine creatinine determinations by the alkaline picrate method. **Not
recommended for meningitis.**

Tablets and oral suspension are **NOT** bioequivalent and are **NOT** substitutable on a mg/mg basis.
Administer suspension with food. Concurrent use of antacids, H2 blockers, and proton-pump
inhibitors may decrease oral absorption. **Adjust dose in renal failure (see Chapter 31).**

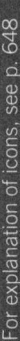

CEPHALEXIN
Keflex and generics
Antibiotic, cephalosporin (first generation)

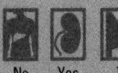

No   Yes   1   B

Caps: 250, 500, 750 mg
Tabs: 250, 500 mg
Oral suspension: 125 mg/5 mL, 250 mg/5 mL (100, 200 mL)

Infant and child: 25–100 mg/kg/24 hr PO ÷ Q6 hr. Less frequent dosing (Q8–12 hr) can be used for uncomplicated infections.
   Otitis media: 75–100 mg/kg/24 hr PO ÷ Q6 hr.
   Streptococcal pharyngitis and skin infections: 25–50 mg/kg/24 hr PO ÷ Q6–12 hr. Total daily dose may be divided Q12 hr for streptococcal pharyngitis (>1 yr).
Adult: 1–4 g/24 hr PO ÷ Q6 hr
Max. dose (all ages): 4 g/24 hr
Bacterial endocarditis prophylaxis for dental and upper respiratory procedures:
   Infant and child: 50 mg/kg PO (**max. dose** 2 g) 1 hr before procedure
   Adult: 2 g PO 1 hr before procedure

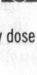

Some cross-reactivity with penicillins. **Use with caution** in renal insufficiency. May cause GI discomfort, false-positive urine reducing substance tests (Clinitest and other copper reduction methods) and Coombs test, false elevation of serum theophylline levels (HPLC method), and false urinary protein test. Probenecid increases serum cephalexin levels, and concomitant administration with cholestyramine may reduce cephalexin absorption. May increase effects of metformin.

Administer doses on an empty stomach, 2 hr before or 1 hr after meals. **Adjust dose in renal failure (see Chapter 31).**

CETIRIZINE ± PSEUDOEPHEDRINE
Zyrtec, Children's Zyrtec, and generics
In combination with pseudoephedrine: Zyrtec-D 12 Hour
Antihistamine, less sedating

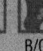

Yes   Yes   ?   B/C

Oral solution or syrup [OTC]: 5 mg/5 mL (120, 473 mL)
Tabs [OTC]: 5, 10 mg
Capsule (Liquid-filled [OTC]): 10 mg
Chewable tabs [OTC]: 5, 10 mg
In combination with pseudoephedrine (PE):
Extended-release tabs (Zyrtec-D 12 Hour [OTC]): 5 mg cetirizine + 120 mg PE

Cetirizine (see remarks for dosing in hepatic impairment):
   6 mo and <2 yr: 2.5 mg PO once daily; dose may be increased for children 12–23 mo to a **max. dose** of 2.5 mg PO Q12 hr.
   2–5 yr: Initial dose, 2.5 mg PO once daily; if needed, may increase dose to a **max. dose** of 5 mg/24 hr once daily or divided BID.
   ≥6 yr–adult: 5–10 mg PO once daily.
Cetirizine in combination with pseudoephedrine (PE) (see remarks for dosing in hepatic impairment):
   ≥12 yr and adult: Zyrtec-D 12 Hour: 1 tablet PO BID

CETIRIZINE ± PSEUDOEPHEDRINE *continued*

Generally **not recommended** for treating URIs for infants. No proven benefit for infants and young children with URIs. **The FDA does not recommend use for URIs in children <2 yr because of reports of increased fatalities.**

May cause headache, pharyngitis, GI symptoms, dry mouth, and sedation. Aggressive reactions and convulsions have been reported. Has **NOT** been implicated in causing cardiac arrhythmias when used with other drugs that are metabolized by hepatic microsomal enzymes (e.g., ketoconazole, erythromycin).

In hepatic impairment, the following doses have been recommended:
  Cetirizine:
    <6 yr: Use **not recommended**
    6–11 yr: <2.5 mg PO once daily
    ≥12 yr–adult: 5 mg PO once daily
  Cetirizine in combination with pseudoephedrine:
    ≥12 yr–adult: 1 tablet PO once daily

Doses may be administered without regard to food. For Zyrtec-D 12 Hour, see *Pseudoephedrine* for additional remarks. Pregnancy category is "B" for cetirizine and "C" when combined with pseudoephedrine. **Dosage adjustment is recommended in renal impairment (see Chapter 31).**

CHARCOAL, ACTIVATED

See Chapter 2

CHLORAL HYDRATE
Aquachloral Supprettes and generics
Sedative, hypnotic

Yes   Yes   2   C

Oral suspension: 100 mg/mL

Check with your pharmacy for availability of this medication in the United States.

Infant and child:
  Sedative: 25–50 mg/kg/24 hr PO/PR ÷ Q6–8 hr; **max. dose** 500 mg/dose
  Sedation for procedures: 50–75 mg/kg/dose PO/PR 30–60 min before procedure; may repeat in 30 min if needed to up to a total **max. dose** of 120 mg/kg or 1 g total for infants and 2 g total for children
Adult:
  Sedative: 250 mg/dose TID PO/PR
  Hypnotic: 500–1000 mg/dose PO/PR; **max. dose** 2 g/24 hr

Contraindicated in patients with hepatic or renal disease. **Avoid** use if GFR < 50 mL/min (see Chapter 31). **Use with caution** in combination with IV furosemide (vasodilation) or warfarin (potentiates warfarin). May cause GI irritation, paradoxical excitement, hypotension, and myocardial/respiratory depression. Chronic administration in neonates can lead to accumulation of active metabolites. Requires same monitoring as other sedatives.

Has no analgesic effects. Peak effects occur within 30–60 min. **Do not exceed** 2 wk of chronic use. **Avoid** use in moderate/severe renal failure. Sudden withdrawal may cause delirium tremens.

For explanation of icons, see p. 648

CHLORAMPHENICOL
Chloromycetin and generics
Antibiotic

Yes Yes 3 C

Injection: 1 g
Contains 2.25 mEq Na/g drug

Neonate IV:
  Loading dose: 20 mg/kg
  Maintenance dose (first dose should be given 12 hours after loading dose):
    ≤7 days: 25 mg/kg/24 hr Q24 hr
    >7 days:
      ≤2 kg: 25 mg/kg/24 hr Q24 hr
      >2 kg: 50 mg/kg/24 hr ÷ Q12 hr
Infant/child/adult: 50–75 mg/kg/24 hr IV ÷ Q6 hr
  Meningitis: 75–100 mg/kg/24 hr IV ÷ Q6 hr
Max. dose (all ages): 4 g/24 hr

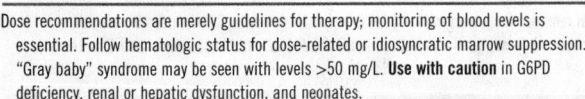

Dose recommendations are merely guidelines for therapy; monitoring of blood levels is essential. Follow hematologic status for dose-related or idiosyncratic marrow suppression. "Gray baby" syndrome may be seen with levels >50 mg/L. **Use with caution** in G6PD deficiency, renal or hepatic dysfunction, and neonates.

Concomitant use of phenobarbital and rifampin may lower chloramphenicol serum levels. Phenytoin may increase chloramphenicol serum levels. Chloramphenicol may increase effects/toxicity of phenytoin, chlorpropamide, cyclosporine, tacrolimus, and oral anticoagulants; may decrease absorption of vitamin B_{12}. Chloramphenicol is an inhibitor of CYP 450 2C9.

Therapeutic levels: Peak, 15–25 mg/L for meningitis; 10–20 mg/L for other infections. Trough, 5–15 mg/L for meningitis; 5–10 mg/L for other infections. Recommended serum sampling time: trough (IV/PO), within 30 min before next dose; peak (IV), 30 min after the end of infusion. Time to achieve steady state: 2–3 days for newborns, 12–24 hr for children and adults. **NOTE:** Higher serum levels may be achieved using oral rather than IV route.

CHLOROQUINE PHOSPHATE
Aralen and generics
Amebicide, antimalarial

Yes Yes 2 C

Tabs: 250, 500 mg as phosphate (150, 300 mg base, respectively)
Oral suspension: 16.67 mg/mL as phosphate (10 mg/mL base), 15 mg/mL as phosphate (9 mg/mL base)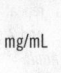

Doses expressed in mg of chloroquine base:
  Malaria prophylaxis (start 1 wk before exposure and continue for 4 wk after leaving endemic area):
    Infant and child: 5 mg/kg/dose PO every wk; **max. dose** 300 mg/dose
    Adult: 300 mg/dose PO every wk
  Malaria treatment (chloroquine-sensitive strains):
    For treatment for malaria, consult with ID specialist or see latest edition of AAP *Red Book.*
    Infant and child: 10 mg/kg/dose (**max. dose** 600 mg/dose) PO × 1, followed by 5 mg/kg/dose (**max. dose** 300 mg/dose) 6 hr later, and then once daily for 2 days.
    Adult: 600 mg/dose PO × 1, followed by 300 mg/dose 6 hr later, and then once daily for 2 days.

CHLOROQUINE PHOSPHATE *continued*

Use with caution in liver disease, preexisting auditory damage or seizures, G6PD deficiency,
psoriasis, porphyria, or concomitant hepatotoxic drugs. May cause nausea, vomiting, ECG
abnormalities, prolonged QT interval, blurred vision, retinal and corneal changes (reversible
corneal opacities), headaches, confusion, skeletal muscle weakness, increased liver enzymes,
and hair depigmentation. Steven-Johnson syndrome, TEN, and anaphylactic reactions have
been reported.

Antacids, ampicillin, and kaolin may decrease absorption of chloroquine (allow 4-hr interval between
these drugs and chloroquine). Cimetidine may increase effects/toxicity of chloroquine. May increase
serum cyclosporine levels. Coadministration with mefloquine may increase risk of convulsions. May
reduce antibody response to intradermal human diploid-cell rabies vaccine.

Adjust dose in renal failure (see Chapter 31).

CHLOROTHIAZIDE
Diuril and generics
Thiazide diuretic

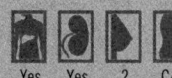

Yes   Yes   2   C/D

Tabs: 250, 500 mg
Oral suspension: 250 mg/5 mL (237 mL); contains 0.5% alcohol, 0.12% methylparaben, 0.02%
propylparaben, and 0.1% benzoic acid
Injection: 500 mg; contains 5 mEq Na/1 g drug

<6 mo:
  PO: 20–40 mg/kg/24 hr ÷ Q12 hr
  IV: Start at 2–8 mg/kg/24 hr ÷ Q12 hr, may increase to 20–40 mg/kg/24 hr ÷ Q12 hr
  if needed.
≥6 mo:
  PO: 10–20 mg/kg/24 hr ÷ Q12 hr; **maximum PO dose** by age:
    6 mo–2 yr: 375 mg/24 hr
    2–12 yr: 1 g/24 hr
    >12 yr: 2 g/24 hr
  IV: Start at 4 mg/kg/24 hr ÷ Q12–24 hr; may increase to 20 mg/kg/24 hr ÷ Q12 hr if needed.
Adult: 500–2000 mg/24 hr ÷ Q12–24 hr PO/IV; alternative IV dosing: some may respond to intermittent
dosing on alternate days or on 3–5 days each wk.

Use with caution in liver and severe renal disease. May increase serum calcium, bilirubin,
glucose, and uric acid. May cause alkalosis, pancreatitis, dizziness, hypokalemia, and
hypomagnesemia.

Avoid IM or SC administration.

Pregnancy category changes to D if used in pregnancy-induced hypertension.

For explanation of icons, see p. 648

C

FORMULARY

CHLORPHENIRAMINE MALEATE/DEXCHLORPHENIRAMINE MALEATE
Chlorpheniramine: Chlor-Trimeton, and generics
Dexchlorpheniramine: various generics
Antihistamine

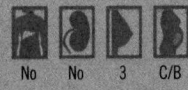

No   No   3   C/B

CHLORPHENIRAMINE MALEATE:
   Tabs [OTC]: 4 mg
   Caplets: 8 mg
   Chewable tab [OTC]: 2 mg
   Sustained-release tabs [OTC]: 12 mg
   Syrup [OTC]: 2 mg/5 mL (473 mL); may contain 5% alcohol and/or parabens
DEXCHLORPHENIRAMINE MALEATE:
   Syrup: 2 mg/5 mL (473 mL); may contain alcohol
   Sustained-release tabs: 6 mg

CHLORPHENIRAMINE MALEATE DOSING:
   Child < 12 yr: 0.35 mg/kg/24 hr PO ÷ Q4–6 hr or dose based on age as follows:
      2–5 yr: 1 mg/dose PO Q4–6 hr; **max. dose** 6 mg/24 hr
      6–11 yr: 2 mg/dose PO Q4–6 hr; **max. dose** 12 mg/24 hr
      ≥12 yr–adult: 4 mg/dose Q4–6 hr PO; **max. dose** 24 mg/24 hr
      Sustained-release: 12 mg PO Q12 hr
DEXCHLORPHENIRAMINE MALEATE DOSING:
   Immediate-release product:
      2–5 yr: 0.5 mg/dose PO Q4–6hr; **max. dose** 3 mg/24 hr
      6–11 yr: 1 mg/dose PO Q4–6 hr; **max. dose** 6 mg/24 hr
      ≥12 yr–adult: 2 mg/dose PO Q4–6 hr; **max. dose** 12 mg/24 hr
   Sustained-release product:
      ≥12 yr–adult: 6 mg PO QHS or Q8–10 hr; **max. dose** 12 mg/24 hr

Use with caution in asthma. May cause sedation, dry mouth, blurred vision, urinary retention, polyuria, and disturbed coordination. Young children may be paradoxically excited.
Combination over-the-counter (OTC or nonprescription) cough and cold products are **not recommended** for children <age 6; serious adverse effects (cardiac and respiratory distress, convulsions, and hallucinations) and fatalities (from unintentional overdosages, including combined use of other OTC products containing the same active ingredients) have been reported.
NOTE: Dexchlorpheniramine maleate doses are 50% of chlorpheniramine maleate and do not possess any significant advantages over other antihistamines.
Doses may be administered PRN. Administer doses with food. Sustained-release forms are **NOT recommended** in children <6 yr and should **NOT** be crushed, chewed, or dissolved.
Pregnancy category is "C" for chlorpheniramine and "B" for dexchlorpheniramine.

CHLORPROMAZINE
Thorazine and generics
Antiemetic, antipsychotic, phenothiazine derivative

No   No   3   C

Tabs: 10, 25, 50, 100, 200 mg
Injection: 25 mg/mL (1, 2 mL); contains 2% benzyl alcohol

Psychosis:
   Child > 6 mo:
      PO: 2.5–6 mg/kg/24 hr ÷ Q4–6 hr; **max. PO dose:** 500 mg/24 hr
      IM/IV: 2.5–4 mg/kg/24 hr ÷ Q6–8 hr

CHLORPROMAZINE *continued*

> **Max. IM/IV dose:**
> > ***<5 yr:*** 40 mg/24 hr
> > ***5–12 yr:*** 75 mg/24 hr

Adult:
> ***PO:*** 10–25 mg/dose Q4–6 hr; **max. dose** 2 g/24 hr
> ***IM/IV:*** Initial, 25 mg; if needed, repeat with 25–50 mg/dose Q1–4 hr up to a **max. dose** of 400 mg/dose Q4–6 hr

Antiemetic:
> **Child (≥6 mo):**
> > ***IV/IM/PO:*** 0.5–1 mg/kg/dose Q6–8 hr PRN
> > **Max. IM/IV/PO dose:**
> > > ***<5 yr:*** 40 mg/24 hr
> > > ***5–12 yr:*** 75 mg/24 hr

> **Adult:**
> > ***IV/IM:*** 25–50 mg/dose Q4–6 hr PRN
> > ***PO:*** 10–25 mg/dose Q4–6 hr PRN

Adverse effects include drowsiness, jaundice, lowered seizure threshold, extrapyramidal/anticholinergic symptoms, hypotension (more with IV), arrhythmias, agranulocytosis, and neuroleptic malignant syndrome. May potentiate effect of narcotics, sedatives, and other drugs. Monitor BP closely. ECG changes include prolonged PR interval, flattened T waves, and ST depression; do not use in combination with fluoxetine, haloperidol, citalopram, and other drugs that can prolong QT interval. **Do not administer oral liquid dosage form simultaneously with carbamazepine oral suspension;** an orange rubbery precipitate may form.

CHOLECALCIFEROL
D-3, D3-5, D3-50, D Drops, Enfamil D-Vi-Sol, and many others
Vitamin D₃

No　No　2　A/D

Tablet [OTC]: 400, 1000, 2000, 3000, 5000, 25,000 IU
Softgel caps [OTC]: 1000, 2000, 4000, 5000, 10,000, 25,000 IU
Caps: 1000, 2000, 5000 IU
> **D3–5:** 5000 IU
> **D3–50:** 50,000 IU

Oral drops (D Drops) [OTC]: 400, 1000, 2000 IU/drop (10 mL)
Oral liquid: (Enfamil D-Vi-Sol): 400 IU/mL (50 mL)

Dietary supplementation (see Chapter 21 for additional information):
> **Preterm:** 400–800 IU/24 hr PO
> **Infant (<1 yr):** 400 IU/24 hr PO
> **Breast-fed neonate and infant:** 400 IU/24 hr PO
> **Child (≥1 yr) and adolescent:** 600 IU/24 hr PO

Vitamin D deficiency and/or rickets (with calcium and phosphorus supplementation; decrease dose (all ages) to 400 IU once daily when radiologically proven healing is achieved):
> ***<1 mo:*** 1000 IU/24 hr PO × 2–3 mo
> ***1–12 mo:*** 1000–5000 IU/24 hr PO × 2–3 mo
> ***>12 mo:*** 5000–10,000 IU/24 hr PO × 2–3 mo

Continued

CHOLECALCIFEROL *continued*

Renal failure (CKD stages 2–5) and 25-OH vitamin D levels ≤ 30 ng/mL (monitor serum 25-OH vitamin D and corrected calcium/phosphorus one month after initiation and Q3 mo thereafter):
   Child (PO):
      25-OH vitamin D < 5 ng/mL: 8000 IU/24 hr × 4 wk, followed by 4000 IU/24 hr × 2 mo; **OR** 50,000 IU weekly × 4 wk, followed by 50,000 IU twice monthly for 3 mo
      25-OH vitamin D 5–15 ng/mL: 4000 IU/24 hr × 12 wk; **OR** 50,000 IU every other wk × 12 wk
      25-OH vitamin D 16–30 ng/mL: 2000 IU/24 hr × 3 mo; **OR** 50,000 IU monthly × 3 mo
      Maintenance dose (after repletion): 200–1000 IU once daily

Biological potency and oral absorption may be greater than ergocalciferol (vitamin D_2). Requires activation by the liver (25-hydroxylation) and kidney (1-hydroxylation) to the active form, calcitriol.

Monitor serum Ca^{2+}, PO_4, 25-OH vitamin D (goal level for infant and child: ≥20 ng/mL) and alkaline phosphate. Serum Ca^{2+}, PO_4 product should be <70 mg/dL to avoid ectopic calcification. Serum 25-OH vitamin D level of ≥35 ng/mL has been used in cystic fibrosis patients to decrease risk of hyperparathyroidism and bone loss.

Toxic effects in infants may result in nausea, vomiting, constipation, abdominal pain, loss of appetite, polydipsia, polyuria, muscle weakness, muscle/joint pain, confusion, and fatigue; renal damage may also occur.

Pregnancy category changes to "D" if used in doses above the U.S. RDA.

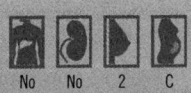

CHOLESTYRAMINE
Questran, Questran Light, Cholestyramine Light, Prevalite, and generics
Antilipemic, binding resin

No   No   2   C

Powder for oral suspension:
   Questran and generics: 4 g anhydrous resin per 9 g powder (9, 378 g)
   Questran Light: 4 g anhydrous resin per 6.4 g powder with aspartame (210, 239 g)
   Cholestyramine Light: 4 g anhydrous resin per 5.7 g powder with aspartame (210, 239 g)
   Prevalite: 4 g anhydrous resin per 5.5 g powder with aspartame (5.5, 231 g)

All doses based in terms of anhydrous resin. Titrate dose based on response and tolerance.
   Child: 240 mg/kg/24 hr ÷ TID; doses normally **do not exceed** 8 g/24 hr (higher doses do not provide additional benefit). Give PO as slurry in water, juice, or milk before meals.
   Adult: 3–4 g of cholestyramine BID–QID; **max. dose** 24 g/24 hr.

In addition to the use for managing hypercholesterolemia, drug may be used for itching associated with elevated bile acids and diarrheal disorders associated with excess fecal bile acids or *Clostridium difficile* (pseudomembranous colitis). May also be applied topically for diaper dermatitis by preparing a 5% or 10% topical product with hydrophilic topical ointment (Aquaphor); other compounded topical formulations exist (e.g., Butt paste: cholestyramine, sucralfate, zinc oxide, and Eucerin).

May cause constipation, abdominal distention, vomiting, vitamin deficiencies (A, D, E, K), and rash. Hyperchloremic acidosis may occur with prolonged use.

Give other oral medications 4–6 hr after cholestyramine or 1 hr before dose to avoid decreased absorption.

CHOLINE MAGNESIUM TRISALICYLATE
Trilisate and generics
Nonsteroidal anti-inflammatory agent

No Yes ? C/D

Combination of choline salicylate and magnesium salicylate (1:1.24 ratio, respectively); strengths expressed in terms of mg salicylate:
  Tabs: 500, 750, 1000 mg
  Oral liquid: 500 mg/5 mL (240 mL)

Dose based on total salicylate content.
Child: 30–60 mg/kg/24 hr PO ÷ TID–QID
Adult: 500 mg–1.5 g/dose PO once daily–TID

Avoid use in patients with suspected varicella or influenza, owing to concerns of Reye syndrome.
  Use with caution in severe renal failure because of risk for hypermagnesemia, or in peptic ulcer disease. Less GI irritation than aspirin and other NSAIDs. No antiplatelet effects.
Pregnancy category changes to "D" if used during the third trimester.
Therapeutic salicylate levels, see *Aspirin.* 500 mg choline magnesium trisalicylate is equivalent to 650 mg aspirin.

CICLESONIDE
Alvesco, Omnaris, Zetonna
Corticosteroid

Yes No 2 C

Aerosol inhaler (Alvesco): 80 mcg/actuation (6.1 g = 60 doses), 160 mcg/actuation (6.1 g = 60 doses)
Nasal spray:
  Omnaris (nasal suspension): 50 mcg/actuation (12.5 g = 120 doses)
  Zetonna (nasal aerosol solution): 37 mcg/actuation (6.1 g = 60 doses)

Intranasal (allergic rhinitis):
  Omnaris:
    2–11 yr (limited data): 1–2 sprays (50–100 mcg) per nostril once daily. **Max. dose:** 200 mcg/24 hr. 2 sprays (100 mcg) per nostril once daily is approved for use in children ≥6 yr for seasonal allergic rhinitis.
    ≥12 yr and adult: 2 sprays (100 mcg) per nostril once daily. **Max. dose:** 200 mcg/24 hr.
  Zetonna:
    ≥12 yr and adult: 1 spray (37 mcg) per nostril once daily. **Max. dose:** 74 mcg/24 hr.
Oral inhalation (asthma):
  ≥5 yr and adult (limited data; see below for current FDA-labeled dosage information): The following regimen has been suggested by the Global Strategy for Asthma Management and Prevention):
    Low dose: 80–160 mcg/24 hr
    Medium dose: >160–320 mcg/24 hr
    High dose: >320 mcg/24 hr up to a **maximum** of 640 mcg/24 hr
  ≥12 yr and adult:
    Prior use with bronchodilator only: 80 mcg/dose BID; **max. dose** 320 mcg/24 hr
    Prior use with inhaled corticosteroid: 80 mcg/dose BID; **max. dose** 640 mcg/24 hr
    Prior use with oral corticosteroid: 320 mcg/dose BID; **max. dose** 640 mcg/24 hr

Continued

CICLESONIDE *continued*

Ciclesonide is a prodrug hydrolyzed to an active metabolite, des-ciclesonide, via esterases in nasal mucosa and lungs; further metabolism is via hepatic CYP 3A4 and 2D6. Concurrent use with ketoconazole and other CYP 450 3A4 inhibitors may increase systemic des-ciclesonide levels. **Use with caution** and monitor in hepatic impairment.

Oral inhalation (asthma): Rinse mouth after each use. May cause headache, arthralgia, nasal congestion, nasopharyngitis, and URIs. Maximum benefit may not be achieved until 4 wk after initiation; consider dose increase if response is inadequate 4 wk after initial dosage.

Intranasal (allergic rhinitis): Clear nasal passages prior to use. May cause otalgia, epistaxis, nasopharyngitis, and headache. Monitor linear growth of pediatric patients routinely. Onset of action: 24–48 hours; further improvement observed over 1–2 wk in seasonal allergic rhinitis or 5 wk in perennial allergic rhinitis.

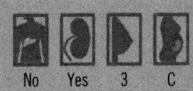

CIDOFOVIR
Vistide and generics
Antiviral

No   Yes   3   C

Injection: 75 mg/mL (5 mL); preservative free

Safety and efficacy has not been established in children.
CMV retinitis:
  Adult:
    Induction: 5 mg/kg IV once weekly × 2 with probenecid and hydration
    Maintenance: 5 mg/kg IV Q2 wk with probenecid and hydration
Adenovirus infection in immunocompromised oncology patients (limited data; see remarks):
  Child: 5 mg/kg/dose IV once weekly until PCR negative. Administer oral probenecid 1–1.25 g/m²/dose (rounded to the nearest 250-mg interval) 3 hr before and 1 hr and 8 hr after each dose of cidofovir. Also give IV normal saline at 3 times maintenance fluid 1 hr before and 1 hr after cidofovir, followed by 2 times maintenance fluid for an additional 2 hr. For patients with renal dysfunction (see remarks), give 1 mg/kg/dose IV 3 times weekly until PCR negative.
BK virus hemorrhagic cystitis (limited data): 1 mg/kg/dose IV once weekly without probenecid.

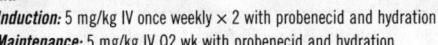

Contraindicated in hypersensitivity to probenecid or sulfa-containing drugs; sCr > 1.5 mg/dL, CrCl ≤ 55 mL/min, urine protein ≥ 100 mg/dL (2+ proteinuria), direct intraocular injection of cidofovir, and concomitant nephrotoxic drugs. **Renal impairment is the major dose-limiting toxicity.** IV NS prehydration and probenecid must be used (unless not indicated) to reduce risk of nephrotoxicity. May also cause nausea, vomiting, headache, rash, metabolic acidosis, uveitis, decreased intraocular pressure, and neutropenia.

Reported criteria for defining renal dysfunction in children include sCr > 1.5 mg/dL, GFR < 90 mL/min/1.73 m², and >2+ proteinuria. For adults, reduce dose to 3 mg/kg if sCr increases 0.3–0.4 mg/dL from baseline. Discontinue therapy if sCr increases ≥0.5 mg/dL from baseline or with development of ≥3+ proteinuria.

Administer doses via IV infusion over 1 hr at a concentration ≤8 mg/mL.

C

CIMETIDINE
Tagamet, Tagamet HB [OTC], and generics
Histamine-2 antagonist

   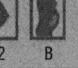
Yes   Yes   2   B

Tabs: 200 [OTC], 300, 400, 800 mg
Oral solution: 300 mg/5 mL (240 mL); may contain 2.8% alcohol

Neonate: 5–20 mg/kg/24 hr PO ÷ Q6–12 hr
Infant: 10–20 mg/kg/24 hr PO ÷ Q6–12 hr
Child: 20–40 mg/kg/24 hr PO ÷ Q6 hr
Adult: 300 mg/dose PO QID **OR** 400 mg/dose PO BID **OR** 800 mg/dose PO QHS
Ulcer prophylaxis: 400–800 mg PO QHS

Diarrhea, rash, myalgia, confusion, neutropenia, gynecomastia, elevated liver function tests, or dizziness may occur. **Use with caution** in hepatic and renal impairment (**adjust dose in renal failure; see Chapter 31**).

Inhibits CYP 450 1A2, 2C9, 2C19, 2D6, 2E1, and 3A4 isoenzymes; therefore increases levels and effects of many hepatically metabolized drugs (i.e., theophylline, phenytoin, lidocaine, diazepam, warfarin). Cimetidine may decrease absorption of iron, ketoconazole, and tetracyclines.

CIPROFLOXACIN
Cipro, Cipro XR, Ciloxan ophthalmic, Cetraxal, Ciprodex, Cipro HC Otic, and generics
Antibiotic, quinolone

No   Yes   2   C

Tabs: 100, 250, 500, 750 mg
Extended-release tabs (Cipro XR): 500, 1000 mg
Oral suspension: 250 mg/5 mL (100 mL), 500 mg/5 mL (100 mL)
Injection: 10 mg/mL (40 mL)
Premixed injection: 200 mg/100 mL 5% dextrose, 400 mg/100 mL 5% dextrose (iso-osmotic solutions)
Ophthalmic solution: 3.5 mg/mL (2.5, 5, 10 mL)
Ophthalmic ointment: 3.3 mg/g (3.5 g)
Otic suspension:
  Cetraxal: 0.5 mg/0.25 mL (14s)
  With dexamethasone (Ciprodex): 3 mg/mL ciprofloxacin + 1 mg/mL dexamethasone (7.5 mL); contains benzalkonium chloride
  With hydrocortisone (Cipro HC Otic): 2 mg/mL ciprofloxacin + 10 mg/mL hydrocortisone (10 mL); contains benzyl alcohol

Child:
PO: 20–30 mg/kg/24 hr ÷ Q12 hr; **max. dose** 1.5 g/24 hr
IV: 20–30 mg/kg/24 hr ÷ Q12 hr; **max. dose** 800 mg/24 hr
Complicated UTI or pyelonephritis (×10–21 days):
  PO: 20–40 mg/kg/24 hr ÷ Q12 hr; **max. dose** 1.5 g/24 hr
  IV: 18–30 mg/kg/24 hr ÷ Q8 hr; **max. dose** 1.2 g/24 hr
Cystic fibrosis:
  PO: 40 mg/kg/24 hr ÷ Q12 hr; **max. dose** 2 g/24 hr
  IV: 30 mg/kg/24 hr ÷ Q8 hr; **max. dose** 1.2 g/24 hr
Anthrax (see remarks):
  Inhalational/systemic/cutaneous: Start with 20–30 mg/kg/24 hr ÷ Q12 hr IV (**max. dose** 800 mg/24 hr) and convert to oral dosing with clinical improvement at 20–30 mg/kg/24 hr ÷ Q12 hr PO (**max. dose** 1 g/24 hr). Duration of therapy: 60 days (IV and PO combined)

Continued

CIPROFLOXACIN *continued*

Child:
   Postexposure prophylaxis: 20–30 mg/kg/24 hr ÷ Q12 hr PO × 60 days; **max. dose** 1 g/24 hr
Adult:
   PO:
      Immediate-release: 250–750 mg/dose Q12 hr
      Extended-release (Cipro XR):
         Uncomplicated UTI/cystitis: 500 mg/dose Q24 hr
         Complicated UTI/uncomplicated pyelonephritis: 1000 mg/dose Q24 hr
   IV: 200–400 mg/dose Q12 hr; 400 mg/dose Q8 hr for more severe/complicated infections
   Anthrax (see remarks):
      Inhalational/systemic/cutaneous: Start with 400 mg/dose Q12 hr IV, and convert to oral dosing
         with clinical improvement at 500 mg/dose Q12 hr PO. Duration of therapy: 60 days (IV and PO
         combined).
      Postexposure prophylaxis: 500 mg/dose Q12 hr PO × 60 days.
Ophthalmic solution:
   ≥1 yr and adult: 1–2 drops Q2 hr while awake × 2 days, then 1–2 drops Q4 hr while awake ×
   5 days
Ophthalmic ointment:
   ≥2 yr and adult: Apply 0.5-inch ribbon TID × 2, then BID × 5 days
Otic:
   Cetraxal:
      Acute otitis externa (≥1 yr and adult): 0.25 mL to affected ear(s) BID × 7 days
   Ciprodex:
      Acute otitis media with tympanostomy tubes or acute otitis externa (≥6 mo and adult): 4 drops
      to affected ear(s) BID × 7 days
   Cipro HC Otic:
      Otitis externa (>1 yr and adult): 3 drops to affected ear(s) BID × 7 days

Can cause GI upset, renal failure, and seizures. GI symptoms, headache, restlessness,
   and rash are common side effects. Peripheral neuropathy has been reported.
   Use with caution in children <18 yr (like other quinolones, tendon rupture can occur during
   or after therapy, especially with concomitant corticosteroid use), alkalinized urine (crystalluria),
   seizures, excessive sunlight (photosensitivity), and renal dysfunction **(adjust systemic dose in renal
   failure; see Chapter 31). Do not use otic suspension with perforated tympanic membranes and
   with viral infections of the external ear canal.**
For dosing in obese patients, use an adjusted body weight (ABW). ABW = Ideal body weight + 0.45
   (Total body weight − Ideal body weight).
Combinational antimicrobial therapy is recommended for anthrax. For penicillin-susceptible strains,
   consider changing to high-dose amoxicillin (25–35 mg/kg/dose TID PO). See www.bt.cdc.gov for the
   latest information.
Inhibits CYP 450 1A2. Ciprofloxacin can increase effects and/or toxicity of caffeine, methotrexate,
   theophylline, warfarin, tizanidine (excessive sedation and dangerous hypotension), and cyclosporine.
   Probenecid increases ciprofloxacin levels.
Do not administer antacids or other divalent salts with or within 2–4 hr of oral ciprofloxacin dose.

C

FORMULARY

CITRATE MIXTURES
Alkalinizing agent, electrolyte supplement

No Yes ? ?

Each mL of oral solution contains the following mEq of electrolyte:

	Na	K	Citrate or HCO₃
Tricitrates* (480 mL)	1	1	2
Cytra-K*† (480 mL)	0	2	2
Cytra-2* or Sodium Citrate/Citric Acid* (480 mL)	1	0	1
Oracit (15, 30, 500 mL)	1	0	1

*Sugar-free

†Also available as a powder for oral solution; each packet of powder must be diluted before use and contains 30 mEq each of potassium and citrate/HCO₃ (100 packets per box)

Dilute dose in water or juice.
All mEq doses based on citrate.
Infant and child (PO): 2–3 mEq/kg/24 hr ÷ Q6–8 hr or 5–15 mL/dose Q6–8 hr (after meals and before bedtime)
Adult (PO): 100–200 mEq/24 hr ÷ Q6–8 hr or 15–30 mL/dose Q6–8 hr (after meals and before bedtime)

Contraindicated in severe renal impairment and acute dehydration. **Use with caution** in patients already receiving potassium supplements or who are sodium restricted. May have laxative effect and cause hypocalcemia and metabolic alkalosis.

Adjust dose to maintain desired pH. 1 mEq of citrate is equivalent to 1 mEq HCO₃ in patients with normal hepatic function.

CLARITHROMYCIN
Biaxin, Biaxin XL, and generics
Antibiotic, macrolide

Yes Yes 2 C

Film tablets: 250, 500 mg
Extended-release tablets (Biaxin XL): 500 mg
Granules for oral suspension: 125, 250 mg/5 mL (50, 100 mL)

Infant and child:
Acute otitis media, pharyngitis/tonsillitis, pneumonia, acute maxillary sinusitis, or uncomplicated skin infections: 15 mg/kg/24 hr PO ÷ Q12 hr; **max. dose** 1 g/24 hr
Pertussis (≥1 mo): 15 mg/kg/24 hr PO ÷ Q12 hr × 7 days; **max. dose** 1 g/24 hr
Bacterial endocarditis prophylaxis: 15 mg/kg (**max. dose** 500 mg) PO 1 hr before procedure
Mycobacterium avium complex (MAC):
  Prophylaxis (1st episode and recurrence): 15 mg/kg/24 hr PO ÷ Q12 hr
  Treatment: 15 mg/kg/24 hr PO ÷ Q12 hr with other antimycobacterial drugs
  Max. dose: 1 g/24 hr
Adolescent and adult:
Pharyngitis/tonsillitis, acute maxillary sinusitis, bronchitis, pneumonia, or uncomplicated skin infections:
  Immediate-release: 250–500 mg/dose Q12 hr PO
  Extended-release (Biaxin XL): 1000 mg Q24 hr PO (currently not indicated for pharyngitis/tonsillitis or uncomplicated skin infections)

For explanation of icons, see p. 648

Continued

CLARITHROMYCIN *continued*

Adult:

Pertussis: 500 mg (immediate-release)/dose Q12 hr PO × 7 days

Bacterial endocarditis prophylaxis: 500 mg PO 1 hr before procedure

MAC:

Prophylaxis (1st episode and recurrence): 500 mg/dose Q12 hr PO

Treatment: 500 mg Q12 hr PO with other antimycobacterial drugs

Helicobacter pylori GI infection: 250 mg Q12 hr to 500 mg Q8 hr PO with omeprazole or ranitidine and bismuth; or amoxicillin and omeprazole or lansoprazole.

Contraindicated in patients allergic to erythromycin and history of cholestatic jaundice/hepatic dysfunction with prior use. As with other macrolides, clarithromycin has been associated with QT prolongation and ventricular arrhythmias, including ventricular tachycardia and torsades de pointes. May cause cardiac arrhythmias in patients also receiving cisapride. Side effects: diarrhea, nausea, abnormal taste, dyspepsia, abdominal discomfort (less than erythromycin but greater than azithromycin), and headache. Rare cases of anaphylaxis, hepatic dysfunction, rhabdomyolysis, Stevens-Johnson syndrome, and toxic epidermal necrolysis have been reported. May increase effects/toxicity of carbamazepine, theophylline, cyclosporine, digoxin, ergot alkaloids, fluconazole, tacrolimus, triazolam, and warfarin. Substrate and inhibitor of CYP 450 3A4, and inhibits CYP 1A2.

Adjust dose in renal failure (see Chapter 31). Doses, regardless of dosage form, may be administered with food.

CLINDAMYCIN
Cleocin-T, Cleocin, and generics
Antibiotic, lincomycin derivative

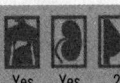 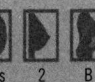

Yes   Yes   2   B

Caps: 75, 150, 300 mg

Oral solution: 75 mg/5 mL (100 mL)

Injection: 150 mg/mL (contains 9.45 mg/mL benzyl alcohol)

Premixed injection in 5% dextrose: 300 mg/50 mL, 600 mg/50 mL, 900 mg/50 mL

Solution, topical (Cleocin-T): 1% (30, 60 mL); may contain 50% isopropyl alcohol

Gel, topical (Cleocin-T): 1% (30, 60 g); may contain methylparaben

Lotion, topical (Cleocin-T): 1% (60 mL); may contain methylparaben

Foam, topical: 1% (50, 100 g); contains 58% ethanol

See *Benzoyl Peroxide* for combination topical product (clindamycin and benzoyl peroxide)

Vaginal cream: 2% (40 g); may contain benzyl alcohol

Vaginal suppository: 100 mg (3s)

Neonate:

IV/IM: 5 mg/kg/dose with the following dosage intervals:

≤7 days:

≤2 kg: Q12 hr

>2 kg: Q8 hr

>7 days:

<1.2 kg: Q12 hr

1.2–2 kg: Q8 hr

>2 kg: Q6 hr

Child:

PO: 10–30 mg/kg/24 hr ÷ Q6–8 hr; **max. dose** 1.8 g/24 hr

IM/IV: 25–40 mg/kg/24 hr ÷ Q6–8 hr; **max. dose** 4.8 g/24 hr

CLINDAMYCIN *continued*

Child:

> *Bacterial endocarditis prophylaxis:* 20 mg/kg (**max. dose** 600 mg) × 1 PO or IV; 1 hr before procedure with PO route and 30 min before procedure with IV route.

Adult:

> *PO:* 150–450 mg/dose Q6–8 hr; **max. dose** 1.8 g/24 hr
>
> *IM/IV:* 1200–1800 mg/24 hr IM/IV ÷ Q6–12 hr; **max. dose** 4.8 g/24 hr
>
> *Bacterial endocarditis prophylaxis:* 600 mg ×1 PO or IV; 1 hr before procedure with PO route and 30 min before procedure with IV route.

Topical (≥12 yr and adult): apply to affected area BID.

Bacterial vaginosis (adolescent and adult):

> *Suppositories:* 100 mg/dose QHS × 3 days
>
> *Vaginal cream (2%):* 1 applicator dose (5 g) QHS for 3 or 7 days in nonpregnant patients and for 7 days in pregnant patients in second and third trimesters.

Not indicated in meningitis; CSF penetration is poor.

Pseudomembranous colitis may occur up to several weeks after cessation of therapy. May cause diarrhea, rash, Stevens-Johnson syndrome, granulocytopenia, thrombocytopenia, or sterile abscess at injection site.

Clindamycin may increase the neuromuscular blocking effects of tubocurarine, pancuronium. **Do not exceed** IV infusion rate of 30 mg/min; hypotension, cardiac arrest has been reported with rapid infusions.

Dosage reduction may be required in severe renal or hepatic disease but not necessary in mild/moderate conditions. Oral liquid preparation may not be palatable; consider use of oral capsules as a sprinkle onto applesauce or pudding.

CLOBAZAM
Onfi
Benzodiazepine, anticonvulsant

  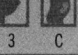

Yes | No | 3 | C

Tabs: 10, 20 mg
Oral suspension: 2.5 mg/mL (120 mL); contains parabens, polysorbate 80 and propylene glycol

Lennox-Gastaut (adjunctive therapy [see remarks]):

Child (≥2 yr) and adult (PO): Dosage increments (if needed) should not be more rapid than Q7 days.

Weight (kg)	Initial Dose	Dose at Day 8 (if needed)	Dose at Day 15 (if needed)
≤30 kg	5 mg once daily	5 mg BID	10 mg BID (**max. dose**)
>30 kg	5 mg BID	10 mg BID	20 mg BID (**max. dose**)

Dosage adjustment for mild/moderate hepatic impairment (Child-Pugh score 5–9) and individuals with poor CYP 450 2C19 activity (PO):

Weight (kg)	Initial Dose	First Dose Increment (if needed)	Second Dose Increment (if needed)	Third Dose Increment (if needed)
≤30 kg	5 mg once daily × ≥14 days	5 mg BID × ≥7 days	10 mg BID (**max. dose**)	N/A
>30 kg	5 mg once daily × ≥7 days	5 mg BID × ≥7 days	10 mg BID × ≥7 days	20 mg BID (**max. dose**)

N/A = Not applicable.

For explanation of icons, see p. 648

Continued

CLOBAZAM *continued*

Seizures (generalized or partial, as monotherapy or adjunctive therapy; limited data and prescribing information from Canada and the UK):

Infant and child (<2 yr): Start at 0.5–1 mg/kg/24 hr (**max. dose** 5 mg/24 hr) PO ÷ BID; if needed and tolerated, slowly increase dosage at 5–7 day intervals up to the **maximum** of 10 mg/kg/24 hr.

2–16 yr: Start at 5 mg PO once daily; if needed and tolerated, slowly increase dosage at 5–7 day intervals up to the **maximum** of 40 mg/kg/24 hr. Usual dosage range: 10–20 mg/24 hr or 0.3–1 mg/kg/24 hr ÷ BID.

Use with caution in hepatic impairment (dose adjustment may be needed). **Do not discontinue use abruptly** because seizures/withdrawal symptoms may occur. Common side effects include constipation, drooling, ataxia, drowsiness, insomnia, aggressive behavior, cough and fever. Stevens-Johnson syndrome, TEN, leukopenia, and thrombocytopenia have been reported.

Do not use in combination with azelastine, olanzapine, sodium oxybate, and thioridazine; increased risk of adverse events. Proton-pump inhibitors, azole antifungal agents (e.g., itraconazole, ketoconazole), St. John's wort, grapefruit juice, CNS depressants, cimetidine, and calcium channel blockers may increase the effects/toxicity of clobazam. Carbamazepine, rifamycin derivatives (e.g., rifampin), and theophylline may decrease the effects of clobazam. Clobazam is a major substrate for CYP 450 2C19 and P-glycoprotein, minor substrate for CYP 450 2B6 and 3A4, inhibitor of CYP 450 2D6, and inducer of CYP 3A4. Carefully review patient's medication profile for other drug interactions each time clobazam is initiated or when a new drug is added to a regimen containing clobazam.

Doses may be taken with or without food. Tablets may be crushed and mixed with applesauce.

CLONAZEPAM
Klonopin and others
Benzodiazepine, anticonvulsant

  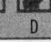 Yes Yes 3 D

Tabs: 0.5, 1, 2 mg
Disintegrating oral tabs: 0.125, 0.25, 0.5, 1, 2 mg; contains phenylalanine
Oral suspension: 100 mcg/mL

Infant and child: <10 yr or <30 kg:
Initial: 0.01–0.03 mg/kg/24 hr ÷ Q8 hr PO. **Maximum initial dose:** 0.05 mg/kg/24 hr.
Increment: 0.25–0.5 mg/24 hr Q3 days, up to **maximum maintenance dose** of 0.1–0.2 mg/kg/24 hr ÷ Q8 hr.
Child ≥ 10 yr or ≥ 30 kg and adult:
Initial: 1.5 mg/24 hr PO ÷ TID
Increment: 0.5–1 mg/24 hr Q3 days; **max. dose** 20 mg/24 hr

Contraindicated in severe liver disease and acute narrow-angle glaucoma. Drowsiness, behavior changes, increased bronchial secretions, GI, CV, GU, and hematopoietic toxicity (thrombocytopenia, leukopenia) may occur. Monitor for depression, suicidal behavior/ideation, and unusual changes in behavior/mood. **Use with caution** in patients with renal impairment. **Do not discontinue abruptly.** $T_{1/2}$: 24–36 hr.

Proposed therapeutic levels (not well established): 20–80 ng/mL. Recommended serum sampling time: Obtain trough level within 30 min before an oral dose. Steady state is typically achieved after 5–8 days of continuous therapy using the same dose.

Carbamazepine, phenytoin, and phenobarbital may decrease clonazepam levels and effect. Drugs that inhibit CYP 450 3A4 isoenzymes (e.g., erythromycin) may increase clonazepam levels and effects/toxicity.

C

FORMULARY

CLONIDINE
Catapres, Kapvay, Nexiclon XR, Catapres TTS, Duraclon,
and generics
Central α-adrenergic agonist, antihypertensive

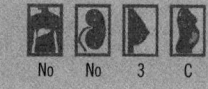

No   No   3   C

Tabs: 0.1, 0.2, 0.3 mg
Oral suspension: 20, 100 mcg/mL
Transdermal patch (Catapres TTS and generics): 0.1, 0.2, 0.3 mg/24 hr (7-day patch); contains
metallic components (see remarks)
Injection, epidural (Duraclon and generics): 100, 500 mcg/mL (10 mL); preservative free
Extended-release oral preparations:
  Extended-release oral tab:
    Kapvay and generics: 0.1, 0.2 mg; also available as dose pack blister cards, 60 tablets
    each of 0.1 and 0.2 mg tablets
    Nexiclon XR: 0.17 mg; for Q24 hr dosing
  Extended-release oral liquid (Nexiclon XR): 0.09 mg/mL (118 mL); for Q24 hr dosing

Hypertension (use immediate-release products unless noted):
  Child (PO): 5–10 mcg/kg/24 hr ÷ Q8–12 hr initially; if needed, increase at 5–7 day intervals
  to 5–25 mcg/kg/24 hr ÷ Q6 hr; **max. dose** 25 mcg/kg/24 hr up to 0.9 mg/24 hr.
  ≥12 yr and adult (PO): 0.1 mg BID initially; increase in 0.1 mg/24 hr increments at weekly intervals
  until desired response is achieved (usual range: adolescent, 0.2–0.6 mg/24 hr ÷ BID; adult,
  0.1–0.8 mg/24 hr ÷ BID). **Max. dose:** 2.4 mg/24 hr.
  Transdermal patch:
    Child: Conversion to patch only after establishing an optimal oral dose first. Use a transdermal
    dosage closest to the established total oral daily dose.
    Adult: Initial 0.1 mg/24 hr patch for first wk. May increase dose by 0.1 mg/24 hr at 1–2 wk
    intervals PRN. Usual range: 0.1–0.3 mg/24 hr. Each patch last for 7 days. Doses >0.6 mg/24 hr
    do not provide additional benefit.
ADHD (Child ≥ 6 yr and adolescent):
  Immediate-release product (PO): Start with 0.05 mg QHS; if needed, increase by 0.05 mg every
  3–7 days up to a **max. dose** of 0.4 mg/24 hr. Titrated doses may be divided TID–QID.
  Extended-release product (Kapvay, PO): Start with 0.1 mg QHS; if needed, increase by 0.1 mg every
  7 days by administering the dose BID up to a **maximum** of 0.4 mg/24 hr. Depending on dosage level,
  BID dosing should be either the same amount or with the higher dosage given at bedtime. If therapy
  is to be discontinued, slowly reduce dosage at ≤0.1 mg every 3 to 7 days to avoid withdrawal.
Neonatal abstinence syndrome, adjunctive therapy (use immediate-release product; limited data):
  0.5–1 mcg/kg/dose Q4–6 hr PO; use Q6 hr interval for preterm neonates.

Side effects: Dry mouth, dizziness, drowsiness, fatigue, constipation, anorexia, arrhythmias,
and local skin reactions with patch. May worsen sinus node dysfunction and AV block,
especially for patients taking other sympatholytic drugs. **Do not abruptly discontinue;**
signs of sympathetic overactivity may occur; taper gradually over >1 wk.
β-Blockers may exacerbate rebound hypertension during and after withdrawal of clonidine. If patient is
receiving both clonidine and a β-blocker and clonidine is to be discontinued, the β-blocker should
be withdrawn several days before tapering the clonidine. If converting from clonidine to a β-blocker,
introduce the β-blocker several days after discontinuing clonidine (after taper).
Monitor heart rate when used with digitalis, calcium channel blockers, and β-blockers. Use with
diltiazem or verapamil may result in sinus bradycardia. Use with neuroleptics may induce/exacerbate
orthostatic hypotension, dizziness, and fatigue.
$T_{1/2}$: 44–72 hr (neonate), 6–20 hr (adult). Onset of action (antihypertensive): 0.5–1 hr for oral route, 2–3
days for transdermal route. **Do not** use transdermal route while patient is undergoing an MRI procedure;
transdermal patches contain metals and may result in serious patient burns when undergoing MRI.

For explanation of icons, see p. 648

CLOTRIMAZOLE
Lotrimin AF, Gyne-Lotrimin 3, Gyne-Lotrimin 7, and generics
Antifungal, imidazole

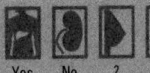

Yes No ? B/C

Oral troche: 10 mg
Cream, topical [OTC]: 1% (15, 30, 45 g); contains benzyl alcohol
Solution, topical [OTC]: 1% (10, 30 mL)
Lotion, topical [OTC]: 1% (20 mL); contains benzyl alcohol
Vaginal suppository [OTC]: 200 mg
Vaginal cream [OTC]: 1% (45 g), 2% (21 g)

Topical: Apply to affected skin areas BID × 4–8 wk
Vaginal candidiasis (>12 yr and adult):
  Vaginal suppositories (may be used in combination with a vaginal cream applied onto the vulva once daily or BID):
    100 mg/dose intravaginally QHS × 7 days *OR*
    200 mg/dose intravaginally QHS × 3 days
  Vaginal cream:
    1 applicator dose (5 g) of 1% cream intravaginally QHS × 7–14 days, or
    1 applicator dose of 2% cream intravaginally QHS × 3 days
Thrush:
  >3 yr–adult: Slowly dissolve (15–30 min) 1 troche in mouth 5 times/24 hr × 14 days.

May cause erythema, blistering, or urticaria with topical use. Liver enzyme elevation, nausea, and vomiting may occur with troches. **Avoid use** of condoms and diaphragms with vaginal cream or suppository; latex can be weakened. **Do not use** troches for systemic infections.
Pregnancy category is "B" for topical and vaginal dosage forms and "C" for troches.

CODEINE
Various generics
Narcotic, analgesic, antitussive

Yes Yes 2 C/D

Tabs: 15, 30, 60 mg; as sulfate
Oral suspension: 3 mg/mL

Analgesic (all doses PO PRN [see remarks]):
  Child: 0.5–1 mg/kg/dose Q4–6 hr; **max. dose** 60 mg/dose
  Adult: 15–60 mg/dose Q4–6 hr
Antitussive (all doses PO PRN [see remarks]): 1–1.5 mg/kg/24 hr ÷ Q4–6 hr; alternatively dose by age:
  2–5 yr: 2.5–5 mg/dose Q4–6 hr; **max. dose** 30 mg/24 hr
  6–12 yr: 5–10 mg/dose Q4–6 hr; **max. dose** 60 mg/24 hr
  ≥12 yr and adult: 10–20 mg/dose Q4–6 hr; **max. dose** 120 mg/24 hr

Use is considered **contraindicated** by the FDA for children in the postoperative period after a tonsillectomy and/or adenoidectomy. **Do not use** in children <2 yr old as antitussive. **Use with caution** in hypersensitivity reactions to other opioids, respiratory disorders, and severe liver or renal insufficiency. Side effects: CNS and respiratory depression, constipation, cramping, hypotension, and pruritus. May be habit forming.
Many **do not recommend** the use of codeine. Codeine's analgesic effect is due to its metabolism to morphine. Nursing infants whose mothers are taking codeine and are "ultra-rapid metabolizers" (CYP 450 2D6) of codeine may have a more rapid and complete conversion to morphine. This may increase the risk for morphine overdose in the nursing infant. Morphine overdose is also possible for individuals taking codeine and who are CYP 450 2D6 ultra-rapid metabolizers. See Chapter 6 for additional remarks.
Pregnancy risk factor changes to a "D" if used for prolonged periods or in high doses at term.

CORTICOTROPIN
Acthar HP
Adrenocorticotropic hormone

No   No   ?   C

Injection, repository gel: 80 U/mL (5 mL); contains phenol
1 unit = 1 mg

Infantile spasms (many regimens exist):
20–40 U/24 hr IM once daily × 6 wk or 150 U/m²/24 hr ÷ BID for 2 wk, followed by a
gradual taper
Anti-inflammatory:
≥2 yr and adolescent: 0.8 U/kg/24 hr ÷ Q12–24 hr IM

Contraindicated in acute psychoses, CHF, Cushing disease, TB, peptic ulcer, ocular herpes,
fungal infections, recent surgery, and sensitivity to porcine products. **Repository gel dosage
form is only for IM route.**
Hypersensitivity reactions may occur. Similar adverse effects as corticosteroids.

CORTISONE ACETATE
Various generics
Corticosteroid

No   No   ?   C/D

Tabs: 25 mg

Anti-inflammatory immunosuppressive:
Child: 2.5–10 mg/kg/24 hr ÷ Q6–8 hr PO
Adult: 25–300 mg/24 hr ÷ Q12–24 hr PO

May produce glucose intolerance, Cushing syndrome, edema, hypertension, adrenal suppression,
cataracts, hypokalemia, skin atrophy, peptic ulcer, osteoporosis, and growth suppression.
Pregnancy category changes to "D" if used in the first trimester.

CO-TRIMOXAZOLE

See SULFAMETHOXAZOLE AND TRIMETHOPRIM

CROMOLYN
Nasalcrom, Gastrocrom, Crolom, Opticrom, and various
generics; previously available as Intal
Antiallergic agent, mast cell stabilizer

Yes   Yes   1   B

Nebulized solution: 10 mg/mL (2 mL)
Oral concentrate (Gastrocrom and generics): 100 mg/5 mL
Ophthalmic solution (Crolom, Opticrom and generics): 4% (10 mL)
Nasal spray (Nasalcrom and generics) [OTC]: 4% (5.2 mg/spray) (100 sprays, 13 mL; 200 sprays,
26 mL); contains benzalkonium chloride and EDTA

Nebulization:
Child ≥ 2 yr and adult: 20 mg Q6–8 hr
Exercise-induced asthma: 20 mg × 1, 10–15 min before and no longer than 1 hr before exercise
Nasal:
Child ≥ 2 yr and adult: 1 spray each nostril TID–QID; **max. dose** 1 spray 6 times/24 hr
Ophthalmic:
Child > 4 yr and adult: 1–2 drops 4–6 times/24 hr

Continued

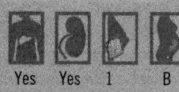

For explanation of icons, see p. 648

CROMOLYN *continued*

Food allergy/inflammatory bowel disease:
   2–12 yr: 100 mg PO QID; give 15–20 min AC and QHS; **max. dose** 40 mg/kg/24 hr
   >12 yr and adult: 200–400 mg PO QID; give 15–20 min AC and QHS
Systemic mastocytosis:
   Infant and child < 2 yr: 20 mg/kg/24 hr ÷ QID PO; **max. dose** 30 mg/kg/24 hr
   2–12 yr: 100 mg PO QID; give 30 min AC and QHS; **max. dose** 40 mg/kg/24 hr
   >12 yr and adult: 200 mg PO QID; give 30 min AC and QHS; **max. dose** 40 mg/kg/24 hr

May cause rash, cough, bronchospasm, and nasal congestion. May cause headache, diarrhea
with oral use. **Use with caution** in patients with renal or hepatic dysfunction.

Therapeutic response (PO route) often occurs within 2 wk, but a 4–6 wk trial may be needed to
determine maximum benefit. Oral concentrate can only be diluted in water. Nebulized solution can
be mixed with albuterol nebs.

CYANOCOBALAMIN/VITAMIN B₁₂
Cyanoject, Cyomin, Nascobal, Vitamin B₁₂, and generics
Vitamin (synthetic), water-soluble

No   No   1   A/C

Tabs [OTC]: 100, 250, 500, 1000 mcg
Extended-release tabs: 1000 mcg
Sublingual tabs: 2500 mcg
Lozenges [OTC]: 50, 100, 250, 500 mcg
Nasal spray (Nascobal): 500 mcg/spray (1.3 mL delivers 4 doses); contains benzalkonium chloride
Injection (Cyanoject, Cyomin): 1000 mcg/mL (1, 10, 30 mL); some preparations may contain benzyl
alcohol
Contains cobalt (4.35%)

U.S. RDA: See Chapter 21.
Vitamin B₍₁₂₎ deficiency, treatment:
   Child (IM or deep SC): 100 mcg/24 hr × 10–15 days
     Maintenance: At least 60 mcg/mo
   Adult (IM or deep SC): 30–100 mcg/24 hr × 5–10 days
     Maintenance: 100–200 mcg/mo
Pernicious anemia:
   Child (IM or deep SC): 30–50 mcg/24 hr for at least 14 days to a total dose of 1000–5000 mcg
     Maintenance: 100 mcg/month
   Adult (IM or deep SC): 100 mcg/24 hr × 7 days, followed by 100 mcg/dose every other day × 14
   days, then 100 mcg/dose Q3–4 days until remission is complete.
     Maintenance:
      IM/deep SC: 100–1000 mcg/mo
      Intranasal: 500 mcg in one nostril once weekly
      Sublingual: 1000–2000 mcg/24 hr

Contraindicated in optic nerve atrophy. May cause hypokalemia, hypersensitivity, pruritus, and
vascular thrombosis. Pregnancy category changes to "C" if used in doses above the RDA or if
administered by the intranasal route.

Prolonged use of acid-suppressing medications may reduce cyanocobalamin oral absorption.
Protect product from light. Oral route of administration is poorly absorbed and generally **not
recommended** for pernicious anemia and B₁₂ deficiency. IV route of administration is **not
recommended** because of more rapid elimination. See Chapter 21 for multivitamin preparations.

C

FORMULARY

CYCLOPENTOLATE
Cyclogyl and generics
Anticholinergic, mydriatic agent

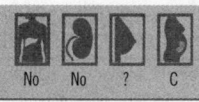

No   No   ?   C

Ophthalmic solution: 0.5%, 1%, 2% (2, 5, 15 mL); may contain benzalkonium chloride

Administer dose ≈ 40–50 min before examination/procedure.
  Infant: Use cyclopentolate/phenylphrine (Cyclomydril) because of lower cyclopentolate
concentration and reduced risk of systemic side effects.
  Child: 1 drop of 0.5%–1% OU, followed by repeat drop, if necessary, in 5 min.
  Adult: 1 drop of 1% OU followed by another drop OU in 5 min; use 2% solution for heavily pigmented iris.

Do not use in narrow-angle glaucoma. May cause a burning sensation, behavioral disturbance,
tachycardia, and loss of visual accommodation. Psychotic reactions and behavioral disturbances
have been reported in children. To minimize absorption, apply pressure over nasolacrimal sac for
at least 2 min. CNS and cardiovascular side effects are common with the 2% solution in
children. **Avoid** feeding infants within 4 hr of dosing to prevent potential feeding intolerance.
Onset of action: 15–60 min. Duration of action: 6–24 hr; complete recovery of accommodation may
take several days for some patients. Observe patient closely for at least 30 min after dose.

CYCLOPENTOLATE WITH PHENYLEPHRINE
Cyclomydril
Anticholinergic/sympathomimetic, mydriatic agent

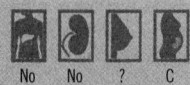

No   No   ?   C

Ophthalmic solution: 0.2% cyclopentolate and 1% phenylephrine (2, 5 mL); contains 0.1%
benzalkonium chloride, EDTA and boric acid

Administer dose ≈ 40–50 min before examination/procedure.
  Neonate–adult: 1 drop OU Q5–10 min; **max. dose** 3 drops per eye

Used to induce mydriasis. See *Cyclopentolate* for additional remarks.
Onset of action: 15–60 min. Duration of action: 4–12 hr.

**CYCLOSPORINE, CYCLOSPORINE MICROEMULSION,
CYCLOSPORINE MODIFIED**
Sandimmune, Gengraf, Neoral, Restasis, and generics
Immunosuppressant

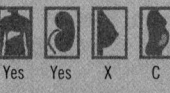

Yes   Yes   X   C

CYCLOSPORINE (Sandimmune and generics):
  Injection: 50 mg/mL; contains 32.9% alcohol and 650 mg/mL polyoxyethylated castor oil
  Oral solution: 100 mg/mL (50 mL); contains 12.5% alcohol
  Caps: 25, 50, 100 mg; contains 12.8% alcohol
CYCLOSPORINE MICROEMULSION (Neoral):
  Caps: 25, 100 mg
  Oral solution: 100 mg/mL (50 mL)
  Neoral products contain 11.9% alcohol
CYCLOSPORINE MODIFIED (Gengraf):
  Caps: 25, 100 mg; contains 12.8% alcohol
  Oral solution: 100 mg/mL (50 mL): Contains caster oil
OPHTHALMIC EMULSION (Restasis): 0.05% (0.4 mL as 30 single-use vials/box); preservative free

Continued

For explanation of icons, see p. 648

CYCLOSPORINE, CYCLOSPORINE MICROEMULSION,
CYCLOSPORINE MODIFIED *continued*

Neoral manufacturer recommends a 1:1 conversion ratio with Sandimmune. Because of its
better absorption, lower doses of Neoral and Gengraf may be required. Exact dosing will
vary depending on transplant type.

  Oral: 15 mg/kg/24 hr as a single dose given 4–12 hr pretransplantation; give same daily
  dose ÷ Q12–24 hr for 1–2 wk posttransplantation, then reduce by 5% per wk to 3–10 mg/kg/24 hr ÷
  Q12–24 hr.

  IV: 5–6 mg/kg/24 hr as a single dose given 4–12 hr pretransplantation; administer over 2–6 hr; give
  same daily dose posttransplantation until patient able to tolerate oral form.

  Ophthalmic:
    ≥16 yr and adult: Instill one drop onto affected eye(s) Q12 hr.

May cause nephrotoxicity, hepatotoxicity, hypomagnesemia, hyperkalemia, hyperuricemia,
hypertension, hirsutism, acne, GI symptoms, tremor, leukopenia, sinusitis, gingival
hyperplasia, and headache. Encephalopathy, convulsions, vision and movement disturbances,
and impaired consciousness have been reported, especially in liver transplant patients.
Psoriasis patients previously treated with PUVA and, to a lesser extent, methotrexate or other
immunosuppressive agents, UVB, coal tar, or radiation therapy are at increased risk for skin
malignancies when taking Neoral or Gengraf.

Opportunistic infections and activation of latent viral infections have been reported. BK virus–associated
nephropathy has been observed in renal transplant patients.

Use caution with concomitant use of other nephrotoxic drugs (e.g., amphotericin B, aminoglycosides,
NSAIDs, tacrolimus).

Plasma concentrations increased with the use of boceprevir, telaprevir, fluconazole, ketoconazole,
itraconazole, erythromycin, clarithromycin, voriconazole, nefazodone, diltiazem, verapamil,
nicardipine, carvedilol, and corticosteroids. Plasma concentrations decreased with the use of
carbamazepine, nafcillin, rifampin, oxcarbazepine, bosentin, phenobarbital, octreotide, and
phenytoin. May increase bosentan, methotrexate, repaglinide, and anthracycline antibiotics (e.g.,
doxorubicin, mitoxantrone, daunorubicin) levels. Use with nifedipine may result in gingival
hyperplasia. Cyclosporine is a substrate and inhibitor for CYP 450 3A4 and P-glycoprotein.

Children may require dosages 2–3 times higher than adults. Plasma half-life 6–24 hr.

Monitor trough levels (just before a dose at steady state). Steady state is generally achieved
after 3–5 days of continuous dosing. Interpretation will vary based on treatment protocol and assay
methodology (RIA monoclonal vs. RIA polyclonal vs. HPLC) as well as whole blood vs. serum sample.
Additional monitoring and dosage adjustments may be necessary in renal and hepatic impairment or
when changing dosage forms.

For ophthalmic use: Remove contact lens prior to use; lens may be inserted 15 min after dose
administration. May be used with artificial tears but must be separated by 15 min from one another.

CYPROHEPTADINE
Various generics; previously available as Periactin
Antihistamine

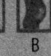

Yes   No   3   B

Tabs: 4 mg
Syrup: 2 mg/5 ml (473 mL); may contain alcohol

Antihistaminic uses:
  Child: 0.25 mg/kg/24 hr or 8 mg/m²/24 hr ÷ Q8–12 hr PO or by age:
    2–6 yr: 2 mg Q8–12 hr PO; **max. dose** 12 mg/24 hr
    7–14 yr: 4 mg Q8–12 hr PO; **max. dose** 16 mg/24 hr

CYPROHEPTADINE *continued*

Adult: Start with 12 mg/24 hr ÷ TID PO; dosage range, 12–32 mg/24 hr ÷ TID PO; **max. dose** 0.5 mg/kg/24 hr

Migraine prophylaxis: 0.25–0.4 mg/kg/24 hr ÷ BID–TID PO up to following **max. doses:**

2–6 yr: 12 mg/24 hr

7–14 yr: 16 mg/24 hr

Adult: 0.5 mg/kg/24 hr or 32 mg/24 hr

Appetite stimulation (see remarks):

≥2 yr and adolescent: 0.25 mg/kg/24 hr ÷ Q12 hr PO up to the following **max. dose by age:** 2–6 yr, 12 mg/24 hr; 7–14 yr, 16 mg/24 hr; ≥15 yr, 32 mg/24 hr

Alternative dosing by age:

4–8 yr (limited data): 2 mg Q8 hr PO

>13 yr and adult: Start with 2 mg Q6 hr PO; dose may be gradually increased to 8 mg Q6 hr over a 3-wk period.

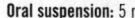

Contraindicated in neonates, patients currently on MAO inhibitors, and patients suffering from asthma, glaucoma, or GI/GU obstruction. May produce anticholinergic side effects, including sedation and appetite stimulation. Consider reducing dosage with hepatic insufficiency.

Allow 4–8 wk of continuous therapy for assessing efficacy in migraine prophylaxis. For use as an appetite stimulant, a dosing cycle of 3 wk on therapy, followed by 1 wk off therapy may enhance efficacy.

DANTROLENE
Dantrium, Revonto, and many generics
Skeletal muscle relaxant

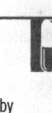

Yes No ? C

Cap: 25, 50, 100 mg
Oral suspension: 5 mg/mL
Injection (Dantrium, Revonto): 20 mg; contains 3 g mannitol/20 mg drug

Chronic spasticity:

Child: <5 yr

Initial: 0.5 mg/kg/dose PO BID

Increment: Increase frequency to TID–QID at 4- to 7-day intervals, then increase doses by 0.5 mg/kg/dose.

Max. dose: 3 mg/kg/dose PO BID–QID, up to 400 mg/24 hr

Malignant hyperthermia:

Prevention:

PO: 4–8 mg/kg/24 hr ÷ Q6 hr × 1–2 days before surgery, with last dose administered 3–4 hr before surgery

IV: 2.5 mg/kg over 1 hr beginning 1.25 hr before anesthesia; additional doses PRN

Treatment: 1 mg/kg IV, repeat PRN to **maximum cumulative dose** of 10 mg/kg, followed by a postcrisis regimen of 4–8 mg/kg/24 hr PO ÷ Q6 hr for 1–3 days

Contraindicated in active hepatic disease. Monitor transaminases for hepatotoxicity. **Use with caution** with cardiac or pulmonary impairment. May cause change in sensorium, drowsiness, weakness, diarrhea, constipation, incontinence, and enuresis. Rare cardiovascular collapse has been reported in patients receiving concomitant verapamil. May potentiate vecuronium-induced neuromuscular block.

Avoid unnecessary exposure of medication to sunlight. **Avoid** extravasation into tissues. A decrease in spasticity sufficient to allow daily function should be the therapeutic goal. Discontinue if benefits are not evident in 45 days.

For explanation of icons, see p. 648

DAPSONE
Aczone, Diaminodiphenylsulfone, DDS, and generics
Antibiotic, sulfone derivative

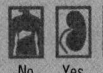 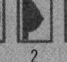 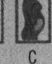

No   Yes   2   C

Tabs: 25, 100 mg
Oral suspension: 2 mg/mL
Topical gel (Aczone): 5% (30, 60, 90 g)

Pneumocystis jirovecii *(formerly carinii) treatment:*
   Child and adult: 2 mg/kg/24 hr PO once daily; **max. dose:** 100 mg/24 hr with trimethoprim
   15 mg/kg/24 hr PO ÷ TID

Pneumocystis jirovecii *(formerly* carinii) *prophylaxis (first episode and recurrence):*
   Child ≥ 1 mo: 2 mg/kg/24 hr PO once daily; **max. dose** 100 mg/24 hr. Alternative weekly dosing,
   4 mg/kg/dose PO Q7 days; **max. dose** 200 mg/dose.
   Adult: 100 mg/24 hr PO ÷ once daily–BID with or without pyrimethamine 50 mg PO Q7 days and
   leucovorin 25 mg PO Q7 days; other combination regimens with pyrimethamine and leucovorin may
   be used (see http://www.hivatis.org).

Toxoplasma gondii *prophylaxis (prevent first episode):*
   Child ≥ 1 mo: 2 mg/kg/24 hr (**max. dose:** 25 mg/24 hr) PO once daily with pyrimethamine
   1 mg/kg/24 hr (max. 25 mg/dose) PO once daily and leucovorin 5 mg PO Q3 days.
   Adult: 50 mg PO once daily with pyrimethamine 50 mg PO Q7 days and leucovorin 25 mg PO Q7
   days; other combination regimens with pyrimethamine and leucovorin may be used (see http://www.
   hivatis.org).

**Leprosy *(see* www.who.int/lep/disease/disease.htm *for latest recommendations, including
   combination regimens such as rifampin ± clofazimine):***
   Child: 1–2 mg/kg/24 hr PO once daily; **max. dose** 100 mg/24 hr
   Adult: 50–100 mg PO once daily

Acne vulgaris *(topical gel [Aczone]):*
   ≥12 yr: Apply small amount of topical gel onto clean, acne-affected areas BID.

Patients with HIV, glutathione deficiency, or G6PD deficiency may be at increased risk for
developing methemoglobinemia. Side effects include hemolytic anemia (dose related),
agranulocytosis, methemoglobinemia, aplastic anemia, nausea, vomiting, hyperbilirubinemia,
headache, nephrotic syndrome, and hypersensitivity reaction (sulfone syndrome). Cholestatic
jaundice, peripheral neuropathy, and suicidal intent have been reported with systemic use.

Didanosine, rifabutin, and rifampin decrease dapsone levels. Trimethoprim increases dapsone levels.
Pyrimethamine, nitrofurantoin, primaquine, and zidovudine increase risk for hematologic side
effects.

Oral suspension may not be absorbed as well as tablets.

TOPICAL USE: Dry skin, erythema, and peeling of skin may occur. Use of topical gel, followed by benzoyl
peroxide for acne, has resulted in temporary local discoloration (yellow/orange) of skin and facial
hair.

DARBEPOETIN ALFA
Aranesp
Erythropoiesis stimulating protein

  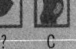

Yes   No   ?   C

Injection: 25, 40, 60, 100, 200, 300 mcg/1 mL (1 mL), 150 mcg/0.75 mL (0.75 mL)
Single-dose prefilled injection syringe (27-gauge ½-inch needle): 25 mcg/0.42 mL, 40 mcg/0.4 mL,
60 mcg/0.3 mL, 100 mcg/0.5 mL, 150 mcg/0.3 mL, 200 mcg/0.4 mL, 300 mcg/0.6 mL, 500 mcg/1 mL
Both dosage forms contain polysorbate (0.05 mg/mL)

D

DARBEPOETIN ALFA *continued*

Anemia in chronic renal failure (see remarks):
   Child (>1 yr) and adult:
      Receiving dialysis: Start with 0.45 mcg/kg/dose IV/SC once weekly, __OR__ 0.75 mcg/kg/dose IV/SC once Q2 wk; IV route is recommended for patients on hemodialysis. Adjust dose according to table that follows.
      Not receiving dialysis: Start with 0.45 mcg/kg/dose IV/SC once Q4 wk, and adjust dose according to table that follows:

Darbepoetin Alfa Dose Adjustment in Anemia Associated with Chronic Renal Failure

Response to Dose	Dose Adjustment
<1 g/dL increase in hemoglobin and below target range after 4 wk of therapy	Increase dose by 25% not more frequently than once monthly. Further increases, if needed, may be done at 4-wk intervals.
>1 g/dL increase in hemoglobin in any 2-wk period, or if hemoglobin exceeds and approaches 11 g/dL	Decrease dose by 25%.
Hemoglobin continues to increase despite dosage reduction.	Discontinue therapy; reinitiate therapy at a 25% lower dose of the previous dose after hemoglobin starts to decrease.

Anemia associated with chemotherapy (patients with nonmyeloid malignancies):
   Child (limited data) and adult (see remarks): Start with 2.25 mcg/kg/dose SC once weekly, and adjust dose according to table that follows:

Darbepoetin Alfa Dose Adjustment in Anemia Associated with Chemotherapy

Response to Dose	Dose Adjustment
<1 g/dL increase in hemoglobin and remains below 10 g/dL after 6 wk of therapy	Increase dose to 4.5 mcg/kg/dose once weekly SC/IV.
>1 g/dL increase in hemoglobin in any 2-wk period or when hemoglobin reaches a level needed to avoid transfusion	Decrease dose by 40%.
If hemoglobin exceeds a level needed to avoid transfusion	Hold therapy until hemoglobin approaches a level where transfusions may be required and restart at a reduced dose by 40%.
Lack or response after 8 wk or completion of chemotherapy	Discontinue therapy.

Conversion from Epoetin Alfa to Darbepoetin Alfa (see table below):

Previous Weekly Epoetin Alfa Dose (units/wk)[1]	PEDIATRIC Weekly Darbepoetin Alfa Dose (mcg/wk) Administered SC/IV Once Weekly[2]	ADULT Weekly Darbepoetin Alfa Dose (mcg/wk) Administered SC/IV Once Weekly[2]	ADULT Once Q2 wk Darbepoetin Alfa Dose (mcg Q2 wk) Administered SC/IV Once Q2 wk[3]
<1500	Insufficient data	6.25	12.5
1500–2499	6.25	6.25	12.5
2500–4999	10	12.5	25
5000–10,999	20	25	50
11,000–17,999	40	40	80
18,000–33,999	60	60	120
34,000–89,000	100	100	200
≥90,000	200	200	400

[1]. 200 units of epoetin alfa is equivalent to 1 mcg darbepoetin alfa.
[2]. If patient was receiving epoetin alfa 2–3 times weekly, darbepoetin alfa should be administered once weekly.
[3]. If patient was receiving epoetin alfa once weekly, darbepoetin alfa should be administered once Q2 wk.

For explanation of icons, see p. 648

DARBEPOETIN ALFA *continued*

Contraindicated in uncontrolled hypertension and patients hypersensitive to albumin/
polysorbate 80 or epoetin alfa. Darbepoetin alfa is not intended for patients requiring acute
correction of anemia. **Use with caution** in seizures and liver disease. Evaluate serum iron,
ferritin, and TIBC; concurrent iron supplementation may be necessary. Red cell aplasia and
severe anemia associated with neutralizing antibodies to erythropoietin have been reported.

USE IN CHRONIC RENAL FAILURE: In pediatric patients, higher doses may be needed for individuals
being switched from epoetin alfa compared with naïve patients. May cause edema, fatigue, GI
disturbances, headache, blood pressure changes, fever, cardiac arrhythmia/arrest, infections, and
myalgia. Higher risk for mortality and serious cardiovascular events have been reported with higher
targeted hemoglobin levels (>11 g/dL). If hemoglobin levels do not increase or reach targeted levels
despite appropriate dose titrations over a 12-wk period, (1) **do not** administer higher doses, and use
the lowest dose that will maintain hemoglobin levels to avoid the need for recurrent blood
transfusions; (2) evaluate and treat other causes of anemia; (3) always follow the dose adjustment
instructions; and (4) discontinue use if patient remains transfusion dependent.

USE IN CANCER: Use only for anemia due to myelosuppressive chemotherapy; not effective in reducing
the need for transfusions in patients with anemia not due to chemotherapy. Shortened survival and
time to tumor progression have been reported in patients with various cancers. May cause fatigue,
fever, edema, dizziness, headache, GI disturbances, arthralgia/myalgia, and rash. Use lowest dose
to avoid transfusions and **do not** exceed hemoglobin levels >12 g/dL; increased frequency of adverse
events, including mortality and thrombotic vascular events, have been reported. **Prescribers and
hospitals must enroll in and comply with the ESA APPRISE Oncology Program to prescribe and/or
dispense this drug to cancer patients.**

Monitor hemoglobin, BP, serum chemistries, and reticulocyte count. Increases in dose should not be
made more frequently than once a month. For IV administration, infuse over 1–3 min.

DEFEROXAMINE MESYLATE
Desferal and generics
Chelating agent

  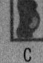

Yes Yes ? C

Injection: 500, 2000 mg

---

*Acute iron poisoning (if using IV route, convert to IM as soon as patient's clinical condition
permits [see remarks]):*
  Child:
    IV: 15 mg/kg/hr
    IM: 50 mg/kg/dose Q6 hr
    Max. dose: 6 g/24 hr
  Adult:
    IV: 15 mg/kg/hr
    IM: 1 g × 1, then 0.5 g Q4 hr × 2; may repeat 0.5 g Q4–12 hr
    Max. dose: 6 g/24 hr
Chronic iron overload (see remarks):
  Child and adolescent:
    IV: 20–40 mg/kg/dose over 8–12 hr once daily × 5–7 days per week; usual **max. doses** are
    40 mg/kg/24 hr (child) or 60 mg/kg/24 hr (adolescent)
    SC: 20–40 mg/kg/dose once daily as infusion over 8–12 hr; **max. dose** 2 g/24 hr

DEFEROXAMINE MESYLATE *continued*

Adult:
IV: 40–50 mg/kg/dose over 8–12 hr once daily × 5–7 days per week; **max. dose** 6 g/24 hr
IM: 0.5–1 g/dose once daily
SC: 1–2 g/dose once daily as infusion over 8–24 hr

Contraindicated in severe renal disease or anuria. **Not approved** for use in primary hemochromatosis. May cause flushing, erythema, urticaria, hypotension, tachycardia, diarrhea, leg cramps, fever, cataracts, hearing loss, nausea, and vomiting. Iron mobilization may be poor in children <3 yr. Serum creatinine elevation, acute renal failure, renal tubular disorders, and hepatic dysfunction have been reported.

Avoid use if GFR < 10 mL/min, and administer 25%–50% of usual dose if GFR is 10–50 mL/min or patient is receiving continuous renal replacement therapy (CRRT).

High doses and concomitant low ferritin levels have also been associated with growth retardation. Growth velocity may resume to pretreatment levels by reducing the dosage. Acute respiratory distress syndrome has been reported after treatment with excessively high IV doses in patients with acute iron intoxication or thalassemia. Toxicity risk has been reported with infusions >8 mg/kg/hr for >4 days for thalassemia, and with infusions of 15 mg/kg/hr for >1 day for acute iron toxicity. Pulmonary toxicity was not seen in 193 courses.

For IV infusion, **maximum rate:** 15 mg/kg/hr. Infuse IV infusion over 6–12 hr for mild/moderate iron intoxication and over 24 hr for severe cases, then reassess. SC route is via a portable controlled infusion device and is **not recommended** in acute iron poisoning.

DESMOPRESSIN ACETATE
DDAVP, Stimate, and generics
Vasopressin analog, synthetic; hemostatic agent

No No 2 B

Tabs: 0.1, 0.2 mg
Nasal solution (with rhinal tube): DDAVP, 100 mcg/mL (2.5 mL); contains 9 mg NaCl/mL
Injection: 4 mcg/mL (1, 10 mL); contains 9 mg NaCl/mL
Nasal spray:
  100 mcg/mL, 10 mcg/spray (50 sprays, 5 mL); contains 7.5 mg NaCl/mL
  Stimate: 1500 mcg/mL, 150 mcg/spray (25 sprays, 2.5 mL); contains 9 mg NaCl/mL
Conversion: 100 mcg = 400 IU arginine vasopressin

Diabetes insipidus (see remarks):
Oral:
  Child ≤ 12 yr: Start with 0.05 mg/dose BID; titrate to effect; usual dose range: 0.1–0.8 mg/24 hr.
  Child > 12 yr and adult: Start with 0.05 mg/dose BID; titrate dose to effect; usual dose range: 0.1–1.2 mg/24 hr ÷ BID–TID.
Intranasal (titrate dose to achieve control of excessive thirst and urination. Morning and evening doses should be adjusted separately for diurnal rhythm of water turnover):
  3 mo–12 yr: 5–30 mcg/24 hr ÷ once daily–BID
  >12 yr and adult: 10–40 mcg/24 hr ÷ once daily–TID
IV/SC:
  <12 yr (limited data): 0.1–1 mcg/24 hr ÷ once daily–BID; start with lower dose and increase as needed.
  ≥12 yr and adult: 2–4 mcg/24 hr ÷ BID

Continued

For explanation of icons, see p. 648

DESMOPRESSIN ACETATE *continued*

Hemophilia A and von Willebrand disease:
Intranasal: 2–4 mcg/kg/dose 2 hr before procedure
IV: 0.2–0.4 mcg/kg/dose over 15–30 min, administered 30 min before procedure
Nocturnal enuresis (≥6 yr [see remarks]):
Oral: 0.2 mg at bedtime, titrated to a **max. dose** of 0.6 mg to achieve desired effect

Use with caution in hypertension, patients at risk for water intoxication with hyponatremia, and coronary artery disease. May cause headache, nausea, seizures, blood pressure changes, hyponatremia, nasal congestion, abdominal cramps, and hypertension.

NOCTURNAL ENURESIS: Intranasal formulations are no longer indicated by the FDA for primary nocturnal enuresis (children are susceptible for severe hyponatremia and seizures) or in patients with a history of hyponatremia. Patients using tablets should reduce their fluid intake to prevent potential water intoxication and hyponatremia, and have their therapy interrupted during acute illnesses that may lead to fluid and/or electrolyte imbalance.

Injection may be used SC or IV at ≈ 10% of intranasal dose. Adjust fluid intake to decrease risk of water intoxication, and monitor serum sodium.

If switching stabilized patient from intranasal route to IV/SC route, use 10% of intranasal dose. Peak effects: 1–5 hr with intranasal route, 1.5–3 hr with IV route, and 2–7 hr with PO route.

DEXAMETHASONE
Decadron, Dexpak Taperpak, Hexadrol, Maxidex,
and many generics
Corticosteroid

 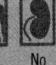 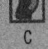

No   No   3   C

Tabs (Decadron and generics): 0.5, 0.75, 1, 1.5, 2, 4, 6 mg
Dexpak Taperpak: 1.5 mg (21 tabs [6 day], 35 tabs [10 day], 51 tabs [13 day])
Injection (sodium phosphate salt): 4, 10 mg/mL (some preparations contain benzyl alcohol or methyl/propyl parabens)
Elixir: 0.5 mg/5 mL (some preparations contain 5% alcohol)
Oral solution: 0.1, 1 mg/mL (some preparations contain 30% alcohol)
Ophthalmic solution: 0.1% (5 mL)
Ophthalmic suspension (Maxidex): 0.1% (5 mL)

Airway edema: 0.5–2 mg/24 hr IV/IM ÷ Q6 hr (begin 24 hr before extubation, and continue for 4–6 doses after extubation)

Croup: 0.6 mg/kg/dose PO/IV/IM × 1
Antiemetic (chemotherapy induced):
Initial: 10 mg/m²/dose IV; **max. dose** 20 mg
Subsequent: 5 mg/m²/dose Q6 hr IV
Anti-inflammatory:
Child: 0.08–0.3 mg/kg/24 hr PO, IV, IM ÷ Q6–12 hr
Adult: 0.75–9 mg/24 hr PO, IV, IM ÷ Q6–12 hr
Brain tumor–associated cerebral edema:
Loading dose: 1–2 mg/kg/dose IV/IM × 1
Maintenance: 1–1.5 mg/kg/24 hr ÷ Q4–6 hr; **max. dose** 16 mg/24 hr
Ophthalmic use (child and adult):
Ointment: Apply a thin coating of ointment to conjunctival sac of affected eye(s) TID–QID. When a favorable response is achieved, reduce daily dosage to BID and later to once daily as a maintenance dose sufficient to control symptoms.

DEXAMETHASONE *continued*

Solution: Instill 1 to 2 drops into conjunctival sac of affected eye(s) Q1 hr during the day and Q2 hr during the night as initial therapy. When a favorable response is achieved, reduce dosage to 1 drop Q4 hr. Further dose reduction to 1 drop TID–QID may be sufficient to control symptoms.

Suspension: Shake well before using. Instill 1–2 drops into conjunctival sacs of affected eye(s). For severe disease, drops may be used Q1 hr, then tapered to discontinuation as inflammation subsides. For mild disease, drops may be used ≤4–6 times/24 hr.

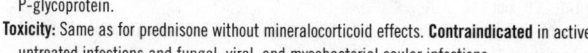

Not recommended for systemic therapy in prevention or treatment of chronic lung disease in infants with very low birth weight, owing to increased risk for adverse events (*Pediatrics*. 2002;109:330–338). Dexamethasone is a substrate of CYP P450 3A3/4 and P-glycoprotein.

Toxicity: Same as for prednisone without mineralocorticoid effects. **Contraindicated** in active untreated infections and fungal, viral, and mycobacterial ocular infections.

OPHTHALMIC USE: Use ophthalmic preparation only in consultation with an ophthalmologist. **Use with caution** in corneal/scleral thinning and glaucoma. Consider the possibility of persistent fungal infections of the cornea after prolonged use. Ophthalmic solution/suspension may be used in otitis externa.

Oral peak serum levels occur 1–2 hr and within 8 hr after IM administration. **For other uses, doses based on body surface area and dose equivalence to other steroids; see Chapters 10 and 30.**

DEXMEDETOMIDINE
Precedex
α-Adrenergic agonist, sedative

  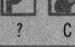

Yes   No   ?   C

Injection: 200 mcg/2 mL (2 mL); preservative free
Premixed injection: 200 mcg/50 mL (50 mL), 400 mcg/100 mL (100 mL); preservative free

NOTE: Maintenance infusion rate dosing metric is mcg/kg/hr.
ICU sedation:
  Child (limited data): 0.5–2 mcg/kg/dose IV × 1 over 10 min, followed by 0.2–1 mcg/kg/hr infusion titrated to effect. Children <1 yr of age may require higher dosages.
  Adult: 1 mcg/kg/dose IV × 1 over 10 min, followed by 0.2–0.7 mcg/kg/hr infusion and titrated to effect.
Procedural sedation:
  Child (limited data):
    IV: 2 mcg/kg/dose × 1 IV, followed by 1.5 mcg/kg/hr was administered to children with autism/pervasive developmental disorders for sedation for EEG.
    IM: 1–4.5 mcg/kg/dose × 1 IM was administered to children for sedation for EEG. Extremely anxious, inconsolable, aggressive, and noncompliant children received doses >2.5 mcg/kg; calm and relatively compliant children received doses ≤2.5 mcg/kg. A second lower repeat dose (≈2 mcg/kg/dose IM) was administered if adequate sedation was not achieved after 10 min after the first dose.
    Intranasal route (limited data): 1–2 mcg/kg/dose × 1 for premedication anesthesia induction.
  Adult: 1 mcg/kg/dose IV × 1 over 10 min, followed by 0.6 mcg/kg/hr titrated to effect; dosage has ranged from 0.2–1 mcg/kg/hr.

Continued

DEXMEDETOMIDINE *continued*

Use with caution with other vasodilating or negative chronotropic agents (additive pharmacodynamic effects), hepatic impairment (decrease drug clearance; consider dose reduction), advanced heart block, hypovolemia, diabetes mellitus, chronic hypertension, and severe ventricular dysfunction. Prolonged use >24 hr may be associated with tolerance and tachyphylaxis and dose-related side effects (ARDS, respiratory failure, agitation).

Hypotension, bradycardia, and dry mouth are common side effects. Transient hypertension has been observed during loading doses. **Do not** abruptly withdraw therapy; withdrawal symptoms (nausea, vomiting, agitation) are possible. Taper dose when discontinuing use.

Use with anesthetics, sedatives, hypnotics, and opioids may lead to enhanced effects; consider dosage reduction of dexmedetomidine. Dexmedetomidine is a CYP 450 2A6 substrate and a weak inhibitor of CYP 450 1A2, 2C9, and 3A4.

Onset of action for procedural sedation: IV or IM, 15 min; intranasal, 15–30 min. Duration of action for procedural sedation: IM, 1 hr; intranasal, 1–1.5 hr.

Use of this drug should be administered by individuals skilled in the management of patients in the ICU and OR. Concentrated IV solution must be diluted with NS to a concentration of 4 mcg/mL before administration. See Chapter 6 for additional information.

DEXMETHYLPHENIDATE
Focalin, Focalin XR, and generics
CNS stimulant

  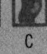

No   No   3   C

Tab (Focalin and generics): 2.5, 5, 10 mg
Extended-release caps (Focalin XR): 5, 10, 15, 20, 25, 30, 35, 40 mg

Attention deficit/hyperactivity disorder:

METHYLPHENIDATE NAIVE:

Age/Dosage Form	Initial Dose	Dosage Increase at Weekly Intervals (If Needed)	Daily Maximum Dose
≥6 yr and adolescent			
Immediate-release tabs*	2.5 mg PO BID	2.5–5 mg/24 hr	20 mg/24 hr (10 mg BID)
Extended-release caps†	5 mg PO once daily	5 mg/24 hr	30 mg/24 hr
Adult			
Immediate-release tabs*	2.5 mg PO BID	2.5–5 mg/24 hr	20 mg/24 hr (10 mg BID)
Extended-release caps†	10 mg PO once daily	10 mg/24 hr	40 mg/24 hr

*BID dosing.
†Once-daily dosing.

CONVERTING FROM METHYLPHENIDATE:
    ≥6 yr and adult: Start at 50% of the total daily dose of racemic methylphenidate with the following maximum doses:
        Immediate-release tabs (BID dosing): 20 mg/24 hr
        Extended-release caps (once-daily dosing): 30 mg/24 hr for ≥6 yr–adolescents; 40 mg/24 hr for adults

DEXMETHYLPHENIDATE *continued*

CONVERTING FROM IMMEDIATE-RELEASE TABS (BID) TO EXTENDED-RELEASE CAPS (once daily) DEXMETHYLPHENIDATE: Use the equivalent mg dosage amount.

Dexmethylphenidate is the ᴅ-enantiomer of methylphenidate and accounts for the majority of clinical effects for methylphenidate. **Contraindicated** in glaucoma, anxiety disorders, motor tics, and Tourette syndrome. **Do not** use with MAO inhibitors; hypertensive crisis may occur if used within 14 days of discontinuance of MAO inhibitor. See *Methylphenidate* for additional warnings and drug interactions.

Common side effects include abdominal pain, indigestion, appetite suppression, nausea, headache, insomnia, and anxiety.

Immediate-release tablets are dosed BID (minimum 4 hr between doses), and extended-release capsules are dosed once daily. Contents of the extended-release capsule may be sprinkled on a spoonful of applesauce and consumed immediately for those who are unable to swallow capsules.

DEXTROAMPHETAMINE ± AMPHETAMINE
Dexedrine, ProCentra, Zenzedi, and many generics
In combination with amphetamine: Adderall, Adderall XR, and generics
CNS stimulant, amphetamine

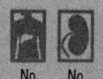

No No X C

Tabs (Zenzedi and generics): 2.5, 5, 7.5, 10 mg
Sustained-release caps (Dexedrine and generics): 5, 10, 15 mg
Oral solution (ProCentra and generics): 1 mg/mL (473 mL)
In combination with amphetamine (Adderall): Available as 1:1:1:1 mixture of dextroamphetamine sulfate, dextroamphetamine saccharate, amphetamine aspartate, and amphetamine sulfate salts (e.g., 5 mg tablet contains 1.25 mg dextroamphetamine sulfate, 1.25 mg dextroamphetamine saccharate, 1.25 mg amphetamine aspartate, and 1.25 mg amphetamine sulfate):
  Tabs: 5, 7.5, 10, 12.5, 15, 20, 30 mg
  Caps, extended-release (Adderal XR and generics): 5, 10, 15, 20, 25, 30 mg
  Oral suspension: 1 mg/mL

Dosages are in terms of mg of dextroamphetamine when using dextroamphetamine alone OR in terms of mg of the total dextroamphetamine and amphetamine salts when using Adderall. Non–extended-release dosage forms are usually given BID-TID (first dose on awakening and subsequent doses at intervals of 4–6 hr later). Extended/sustained-released dosage forms are usually given PO once daily, sometimes BID.
Attention deficit/hyperactivity disorder:
  3–5 yr: 2.5 mg/24 hr QAM; increase by 2.5 mg/24 hr at weekly intervals to a **max. dose** of 40 mg/24 hr ÷ once daily–TID.
  ≥6 yr: 5 mg/24 hr QAM; increase by 5 mg/24 hr at weekly intervals to a **max. dose** of 40 mg/24 hr ÷ once daily–TID.
Narcolepsy:
  6–12 yr: 5 mg/24 hr ÷ once daily–TID; increase by 5 mg/24 hr at weekly intervals to a **max. dose** of 60 mg/24 hr
  >12 yr and adult: 10 mg/24 hr ÷ once daily–TID; increase by 10 mg/24 hr at weekly intervals to a **max. dose** of 60 mg/24 hr

Use with caution in presence of hypertension or cardiovascular disease. **Avoid** use in known serious structural cardiac abnormalities, cardiomyopathy, serious heart rhythm abnormalities, coronary artery disease, or other serious cardiac problems that may increase

For explanation of icons, see p. 648

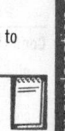

Continued

DEXTROAMPHETAMINE ± AMPHETAMINE *continued*

risk of sympathomimetic effects of amphetamines (sudden death, stroke, and MI have been reported). **Do not** give with MAO inhibitors or general anesthetics.

Not recommended for patients <age 3 yr. Medication should generally **not** be used in children <5 yr, because diagnosis of ADHD in this age group is extremely difficult (use in consultation with a specialist). Interrupt administration occasionally to determine need for continued therapy. Many side effects, including insomnia (**avoid** dose administration within 6 hr of bedtime), restlessness, anorexia, psychosis, visual disturbances, headache, vomiting, abdominal cramps, dry mouth, and growth failure. Paranoia, mania, peripheral vasculopathy (including Raynaud phenomenon), and auditory hallucination have been reported. Tolerance develops. Same guidelines as for methylphenidate apply.

DIAZEPAM
Valium, Diastat, Diastat AcuDial, and various generics
Benzodiazepine; anxiolytic, anticonvulsant

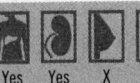

| Yes | Yes | X | D |

Tabs: 2, 5, 10 mg
Oral solution: 1 mg/mL, 5 mg/mL (contains 19% alcohol)
Injection: 5 mg/mL (contains 40% propylene glycol, 10% alcohol, 5% sodium benzoate, and 1.5% benzyl alcohol)
Rectal gel:
    Pediatric rectal gel (Diastat and generics): 2.5 mg (5 mg/mL concentration with 4.4-cm rectal tip delivery system; contains 10% alcohol, 1.5% benzyl alcohol, and propylene glycol); in twin packs
    Pediatric/Adult rectal gel (Diastat AcuDial and generics):
        4.4-cm rectal tip delivery system (Pediatric/Adult): 10 mg (5 mg/mL delivers set doses of either 5, 7.5, or 10 mg); contains 10% alcohol and 1.5% benzyl alcohol; in twin packs
        6-cm rectal tip delivery system (Adult): 20 mg (5 mg/mL delivers set doses of either 10, 12.5, 15, 17.5, 20 mg); contains 10% alcohol and 1.5% benzyl alcohol; in twin packs

Sedative/muscle relaxant:
  Child:
    IM or IV: 0.04–0.2 mg/kg/dose Q2–4 hr; **max. dose** 0.6 mg/kg within an 8-hr period
    PO: 0.12–0.8 mg/kg/24 hr ÷ Q6–8 hr
  Adult:
    IM or IV: 2–10 mg/dose Q3–4 hr PRN
    PO: 2–10 mg/dose Q6–12 hr PRN
Status epilepticus:
  Neonate: 0.3–0.75 mg/kg/dose IV Q15–30 min × 2–3 doses; max. total dose: 2 mg.
  Child > 1 mo: 0.2–0.5 mg/kg/dose IV Q15–30 min; **max. total dose** <5 yr, 5 mg; ≥5 yr, 10 mg. May repeat dosing in 2–4 hr as needed.
  Adult: 5–10 mg/dose IV Q10–15 min; **max. total dose** 30 mg in an 8-hr period. May repeat dosing in 2–4 hr as needed.
  Rectal dose (using IV dosage form): 0.5 mg/kg/dose, followed by 0.25 mg/kg/dose in 10 min PRN.
  Rectal gel: All doses rounded to nearest available dosage strength; repeat dose in 4–12 hr PRN.
    2–5 yr: 0.5 mg/kg/dose
    6–11 yr: 0.3 mg/kg/dose
    ≥12 yr and adult: 0.2 mg/kg/dose

Contraindicated in myasthenia gravis, severe respiratory insufficiency, severe hepatic failure, and sleep apnea syndrome. Hypotension and respiratory depression may occur. **Use with caution** in hepatic and renal dysfunction, glaucoma, shock, and depression. **Do not** use in combination with protease inhibitors. Concurrent use with CNS depressants, cimetidine, erythromycin, itraconazole, and valproic acid may enhance effects of diazepam. Diazepam is

D

DIAZEPAM *continued*

a substrate for CYP P450 2B6, 2C8, 2C9, and 3A5–7 and a minor substrate and inhibitor for CYP P450 2C19 and 3A3/4. The active desmethyldiazepam metabolite is a CYP P450 2C19 substrate.

Administer the conventional IV product undiluted no faster than 2 mg/min. **Do not** mix with IV fluids.

In status epilepticus, diazepam must be followed by long-acting anticonvulsants. Onset of anticonvulsant effect: 1–3 min with IV route, 2–10 min with rectal route. **For management of status epilepticus, see Chapter 1.**

DIAZOXIDE
Proglycem
Antihypoglycemic agent, antihypertensive agent

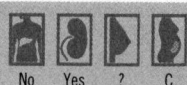

No   Yes   ?   C

Oral suspension: 50 mg/mL (30 mL); contains 7.25% alcohol

Hyperinsulinemic hypoglycemia (due to insulin-producing tumors; start at the lowest dose):
  Newborn and infant: 8–15 mg/kg/24 hr ÷ Q8–12 hr PO;
  usual range: 5–20 mg/kg/24 hr ÷ Q8 hr
  Child and adult: 3–8 mg/kg/24 hr ÷ Q8–12 hr PO

Hypoglycemia should be treated initially with IV glucose; diazoxide should be introduced only if refractory to glucose infusion. Should **not** be used in patients hypersensitive to thiazides unless benefit outweighs risk. **Use with caution** in renal impairment (clearance of drug is reduced); consider dosage reduction.

Sodium and fluid retention is common in young infants and adults and may precipitate CHF in patients with compromised cardiac reserve (usually responsive to diuretics). Hirsutism (reversible), GI disturbances, transient loss of taste, tachycardia, ketoacidosis, palpitations, rash, headache, weakness, and hyperuricemia may occur. Monitor BP closely for hypotension.

Hyperglycemic effect with PO administration occurs within 1 hr, with a duration of 8 hr.

DICLOXACILLIN SODIUM
Dycill, Pathocil, and generics
Antibiotic, penicillin (penicillinase-resistant)

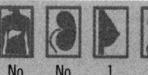

No   No   1   B

Caps: 250, 500 mg; contains 0.6 mEq Na/250 mg

Child (<40 kg) (see remarks):
  Mild/moderate infections: 12.5–50 mg/kg/24 hr PO ÷ Q6 hr
  Severe infections: 50–100 mg/kg/24 hr PO ÷ Q6 hr
  Max. dose: 2 g/24 hr
Child (≥40 kg) and adult: 125–500 mg/dose PO Q6 hr; **max. dose** 2 g/24 hr

Contraindicated in patients with a history of penicillin allergy. **Use with caution** in cephalosporin hypersensitivity. May cause nausea, vomiting, and diarrhea. Immune hypersensitivity has been reported.

Limited experience in neonates and very young infants. Higher doses (50–100 mg/kg/24 hr) are indicated after IV therapy for osteomyelitis.

May decrease effects of oral contraceptives and warfarin. Administer 1 hr before meals or 2 hr after meals.

For explanation of icons, see p. 648

DIGOXIN
Lanoxin, Lanoxin Pediatric, and generics
Antiarrhythmic agent, inotrope

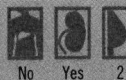

No   Yes   2   C

Tabs: 125, 250 mcg
Oral solution: 50 mcg/mL (60 mL); may contain 10% alcohol
Injection:
  Lanoxin Pediatric: 100 mcg/mL (1 mL); may contain propylene glycol and alcohol
  Lanoxin and generics: 250 mcg/mL (1, 2 mL); may contain propylene glycol and alcohol

Digitalizing: Total digitalizing dose (TDD) and maintenance doses in mcg/kg/24 hr (see table that follows):

DIGOXIN DIGITALIZING AND MAINTENANCE DOSES

	TDD		Daily Maintenance	
Age	PO	IV/IM	PO	IV/IM
Premature neonate	20	15	5	3–4
Full-term neonate	30	20	8–10	6–8
1 mo–<2 yr	40–50	30–40	10–12	7.5–9
2–10 yr	30–40	20–30	8–10	6–8
>10 yr and < 100 kg	10–15	8–12	2.5–5	2–3

Initial: ½ TDD, then ¼ TDD Q8–18 hr × 2 doses; obtain ECG 6 hr after dose to assess for toxicity.
Maintenance:
  <10 yr: Give maintenance dose ÷ BID.
  ≥10 yr: Give maintenance dose once daily.

Contraindicated in patients with ventricular dysrhythmias. Use should be **avoided** in patients with preserved left ventricular systolic function. **Use with caution** in renal failure, with calcium channel blockers (may result in heart block), and with adenosine (enhanced depressant effects on SA and AV nodes). May cause AV block or dysrhythmias. In patients treated with digoxin, cardioversion or calcium infusion may lead to ventricular fibrillation (pretreatment with lidocaine may prevent this). Patients with beri-beri heart disease may not respond to digoxin if underlying thiamine deficiency is not treated concomitantly. Decreased serum potassium and magnesium, or increased magnesium and calcium, may increase risk for digoxin toxicity. For signs and symptoms of toxicity, see Chapter 2.

Excreted via kidney; **adjust dose in renal failure (see Chapter 31)**. Therapeutic concentration: 0.8–2 ng/mL. Higher doses may be required for supraventricular tachycardia. Neonates, pregnant women, and patients with renal, hepatic, or heart failure may have falsely elevated digoxin levels due to the presence of digoxin-like substances.

Digoxin is a CYP 450 3A4 and P-glycoprotein substrate. Calcium channel blockers, carvedilol, amiodarone, quinidine, cyclosporine, itraconazole, and macrolide antibiotics may increase digoxin levels. Use with β-blockers may increase risk for bradycardia. Succinylcholine may cause arrhythmias in digitalized patients.

T$_{1/2}$: Premature infants, 61–170 hr; full-term neonates, 35–45 hr; infants, 18–25 hr; and children, 35 hr.

Recommended serum sampling at steady state: Obtain a single level from 6 hr post dose to just before next scheduled dose after 5–8 days of continuous dosing. Levels obtained before steady state may be useful in preventing toxicity.

FORMULARY

DIGOXIN IMMUNE FAB (OVINE)
DigiFab
Antidigoxin antibody

   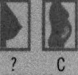

No Yes ? C

Injection: 40 mg

Dosing based on known amounts of digoxin acutely ingested:
First determine total body digoxin load (TBL):
  TBL (mg) = mg digoxin ingested × 0.8
Then, calculate digoxin immune Fab dose:
  Dose in number of digoxin immune Fab vials (DigiFab): # vials = TBL ÷ 0.5
  Dosing based on steady-state serum digoxin levels:

DIGIFAB DOSE (MG) FROM STEADY-STATE DIGOXIN LEVELS

Patient Weight (kg)	Serum Digoxin Concentration (ng/mL)						
	1	2	4	8	12	16	20
1	0.4 mg*	1 mg*	1.5 mg*	3 mg*	5 mg	6.5 mg	8 mg
3	1 mg*	2.5 mg*	5 mg	10 mg	14 mg	19 mg	24 mg
5	2 mg*	4 mg	8 mg	16 mg	24 mg	32 mg	40 mg
10	4 mg	8 mg	16 mg	32 mg	48 mg	64 mg	80 mg
20	8 mg	16 mg	32 mg	64 mg	96 mg	128 mg	160 mg
40	20 mg	40 mg	80 mg	120 mg	200 mg	280 mg	320 mg
60	20 mg	40 mg	120 mg	200 mg	280 mg	400 mg	480 mg
70	40 mg	80 mg	120 mg	240 mg	360 mg	440 mg	560 mg
80	40 mg	80 mg	120 mg	280 mg	400 mg	520 mg	640 mg
100	40 mg	80 mg	160 mg	320 mg	480 mg	640 mg	800 mg

*Use 1 mg/mL DigiFab concentration for dose accuracy.

Dosage administration:
Reconstitute each vial with 4 mL NS for a 10 mg/mL concentration and infuse IV dose over 30 min. If an infusion rate reaction occurs, stop infusion and restart at a a slower rate. In situations of cardiac arrest, DigiFab can be administered as a bolus injection, but expect an increased risk for infusion-related reactions. For smaller doses, vials may be reconstituted with 36 mL NS for a 1 mg/mL concentration.

Contraindicated if hypersensitive to sheep products. **Use with caution** in renal or cardiac failure. May cause rapidly developing severe hypokalemia, decreased cardiac output (due to withdrawal of digoxin's inotropic effects), rash, edema and phlebitis. Digoxin therapy may be reinstituted in 3–7 days when toxicity has been corrected. Digoxin immune FAB will interfere with digitalis immunoassay measurements, resulting in misleading concentrations.

DILTIAZEM
Cardizem, Cardizem SR, Cardizem CD, Cardizem LA, Matzim LA, Dilacor XR, Tiazac, and many others, including generics
Calcium channel blocker, antihypertensive

Yes Yes 1 C

Tabs: 30, 60, 90, 120 mg
Extended-release tabs:
  Cardizem LA: 120, 180, 240, 300, 360, 420 mg
  Matzim LA: 180, 240, 300, 360, 420 mg

Continued

For explanation of icons, see p. 648

DILTIAZEM *continued*

Extended-release caps:
Various generics: 60, 90, 120, 180, 240, 300, 360, 420 mg
Cardizem CD: 120, 180, 240, 300, 360 mg
Dilacor XR: 120, 180, 240 mg
Tiazac: 120, 180, 240, 300, 360, 420 mg
Oral liquid: 12 mg/mL
Injection: 5 mg/mL (5, 10, 25 mL)

Child: 1.5–2 mg/kg/24 hr PO ÷ TID–QID, **max. dose** 3.5 mg/kg/24 hr; **alternative max. doses** of 6 mg/kg/24 hr up to 360 mg/24 hr have been recommended.
Adolescent and adult:
   Immediate-release: 30–120 mg/dose PO TID–QID; usual range 180–360 mg/24 hr
   Extended-release: 120–360 mg/24 hr PO ÷ once daily–BID (BID dosing with Cardizem SR; once-daily dosing with Cardizem CD, Cardizem LA, Matzim LA, Dilacor XR, Tiazac); **max. dose** 540 mg/24 hr

Contraindicated in acute MI with pulmonary congestion, second- or third-degree heart block, and sick sinus syndrome. **Use with caution** in CHF or renal and hepatic impairment.
Dizziness, headache, edema, nausea, vomiting, heart block, and arrhythmias may occur.
Monitor heart rate with concurrent clonidine use (sinus bradycardia has been reported).
Diltiazem is a substrate and inhibitor of the CYP 450 3A4 enzyme system. May increase levels and/or effect of buspirone, cyclosporine, carbamazepine, fentanyl, digoxin, quinidine, tacrolimus, benzodiazepines, and β-blockers. Cimetidine and statins may increase diltiazem serum levels.
Rifampin may decrease diltiazem serum levels.
Maximal antihypertensive effect seen within 2 wk.

DIMENHYDRINATE
Dramamine, other brand names, and generics
Antiemetic, antihistamine

No   No   3   B

Tabs [OTC]: 50 mg
Chewable tabs [OTC]: 50 mg; contains 1.5 mg phenylalanine
Injection: 50 mg/mL; contains benzyl alcohol and propylene glycol

Child (<12 yr): 5 mg/kg/24 hr ÷ Q6 hr PO/IM/IV; alternative oral dosing by age:
   2–5 yr: 12.5–25 mg/dose Q6–8 hr PRN PO, with the **max. dosage** in the subsequent list
   6–12 yr: 25–50 mg/dose Q6–8 hr PRN PO, with the **max. dosage** in the subsequent list
≥12 yr and adult: 50–100 mg/dose Q4–6 hr PRN PO/IM/IV
MAXIMUM PO DOSE:
   2–5 yr: 75 mg/24 hr
   6–12 yr: 150 mg/24 hr
   ≥12 yr and adult: 400 mg/24 hr
MAXIMUM IM DOSE:
   Child: 300 mg/24 hr

Causes drowsiness and anticholinergic side effects. May mask vestibular symptoms and cause CNS excitation in young children. **Caution** when taken with ototoxic agents or history of seizures. **Use should be limited to management of prolonged vomiting of known etiology. Not recommended** in children <2 yr. Toxicity resembles anticholinergic poisoning.

DIMERCAPROL
BAL, British Anti-Lewisite, and generics
Heavy metal chelator (arsenic, gold, mercury, lead)

   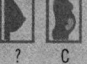
Yes   Yes   ?   C

Injection (in oil): 100 mg/mL; contains 20% benzyl benzoate and peanut oil (3 mL)

Give all injections deep IM.
Lead poisoning:
  Acute severe encephalopathy (lead level > 70 mcg/dL): 4 mg/kg/dose Q4 hr × 2–7 days,
  with the addition of Ca-EDTA (given at separate site) at the time of second dose.
  Less severe poisoning: 4 mg/kg × 1, then 3 mg/kg/dose Q4 hr × 2–7 days.
Arsenic or gold poisoning (see table below):

	Mild Cases	Severe Cases
Days 1 and 2	2.5 mg/kg/dose Q6 hr	3 mg/kg/dose Q4 hr
Day 3	2.5 mg/kg/dose Q12 hr	3 mg/kg/dose Q6 hr
Days 4–13	2.5 mg/kg/dose Q24 hr	3 mg/kg/dose Q12 hr

Mercury poisoning: 5 mg/kg × 1, then 2.5 mg/kg/dose once daily–BID × 10 days

Contraindicated in hepatic or renal insufficiency. May cause hypertension, tachycardia, GI
disturbance, headache, fever (30% of children), nephrotoxicity, transient neutropenia. Symptoms
are usually relieved by antihistamines. Urine should be kept alkaline to protect kidneys. **Use with
caution** with G6PD deficiency and peanut-sensitive patients. **Do not** use concomitantly with iron.

DIPHENHYDRAMINE
Benadryl and many other brand names and generics
Antihistamine

No   Yes   3   B

Elixir (OTC): 12.5 mg/5 mL; may contain 5.6% alcohol
Syrup (OTC): 12.5 mg/5 mL; some may contain 5% alcohol
Oral liquid/solution (OTC): 12.5 mg/5 mL
Caps/Tabs (OTC): 25, 50 mg
Tabs, orally disintegrating (OTC): 12.5 mg; contains aspartame, phenylalanine
Strips, orally disintegrating (OTC): 12.5, 25 mg; may contain <5% alcohol
Chewable tabs (OTC): 12.5 mg; contains aspartame, phenylalanine
Injection: 50 mg/mL
Cream (OTC): 1, 2% (30 g)
Topical gel (OTC): 1% (37.5 g), 2% (120 g)
Topical spray (OTC): 1,2 % (60 g)

*Severe allergic reaction (anaphylaxis) and dystonic reactions (including phenothiazine
toxicity) (PO/IM/IV):*
  Child: 1–2 mg/kg/dose Q6 hr; usual dose: 5 mg/kg/24 hr ÷ Q6 hr. **Max. dose:** 50 mg/dose
  and 300 mg/24 hr
  Adult: 25–50 mg/dose Q4–8 hr; **max. dose** 400 mg/24 hr
Sleep aid (PO/IM/IV): Administer dose 30 min before bedtime.
  2–11 yr: 1 mg/kg/dose; **max. dose** 50 mg/dose
  ≥12 yr: 50 mg

Contraindicated with concurrent MAO inhibitor use, acute attacks of asthma, and GI or urinary
obstruction. **Use with caution** in infants and young children, and **do not** use in neonates, owing to
potential CNS effects. Side effects include sedation, nausea, vomiting, xerostomia, blurred vision,
and other reactions common to antihistamines. CNS side effects more common than GI disturbances.
May cause paradoxical excitement in children. **Adjust dose in renal failure (see Chapter 31).**

DIVALPROEX SODIUM
Depakote, Depakote ER
Anticonvulsant

Yes   No   3   D/X

Delayed-release tabs: 125, 250, 500 mg
Extended-release tabs (Depakote ER): 250, 500 mg
Sprinkle caps: 125 mg

Dose: See Valproic Acid

See *Valproic Acid*. Preferred over valproic acid for patients on ketogenic diet. Depakote ER is
  prescribed for once-daily administration, whereas Depakote is typically prescribed BID.
  Depakote ER and Depakote are not bioequivalent; see package insert for dose conversion.
Efficacy was not established in separate randomized double-blinded placebo-controlled trials for the
  treatment of pediatric bipolar disorder (age 10–17 yr) and migraine prophylaxis (age 12–17 yr).
Pregnancy category is "X" when used for migraine prophylaxis and "D" for all other indications.

DOBUTAMINE
Various generics; previously available as Dobutrex
Sympathomimetic agent

No   No   ?   B

Injection: 12.5 mg/mL (20, 40 mL); contains sulfites
Prediluted injection in D_5W: 1 mg/mL (250 mL), 2 mg/mL (250 mL), 4 mg/mL (250 mL)

Continuous IV infusion (all ages): 2.5–15 mcg/kg/min
Max. dose: 40 mcg/kg/min
To prepare infusion: See IV infusions on page i.

Contraindicated in idiopathic hypertrophic subaortic stenosis (IHSS). Tachycardia, arrhythmias
  (PVCs), and hypertension may occasionally occur (especially at higher infusion rates). Correct
  hypovolemic states before use. Increases AV conduction, may precipitate ventricular ectopic activity.
Dobutamine has been shown to increase cardiac output and systemic pressure in pediatric patients of
  every age group. However, in premature neonates, dobutamine is less effective than dopamine in raising
  systemic blood pressure without causing undue tachycardia, and dobutamine has not been shown to
  provide any added benefit when given to such infants already receiving optimal infusions of dopamine.
Monitor BP and vital signs. $T_{1/2}$: 2 min. Peak effects in 10–20 min. Use with linezolid may potentially
  increase blood pressure.

DOCUSATE
Colace, Kao-Tin, Sur-Q-Lax, Enemeez, and many other brands
Stool softener, laxative

No   No   1   C/?

Available as docusate sodium:
  Caps [OTC]: 50, 100, 250 mg; sodium content (50 mg cap: 3 mg; 100 mg cap: ≈5 mg)
  Tabs [OTC]: 100 mg
  Syrup [OTC]: 20 mg/5 mL; may contain alcohol
  Oral liquid [OTC]: 10 mg/mL; contains 1 mg/mL sodium
  Rectal enema (Enemeez [OTC]): 283 mg/5 mL (5 mL); Enemeez Plus product contains benzocaine
Available as docusate calcium:
  Caps (Kao-Tin, Sur-Q-Lax [OTC]): 240 mg

DILTIAZEM *continued*

PO: (take with liquids)
  <3 yr: 10–40 mg/24 hr ÷ once daily–QID
  3–6 yr: 20–60 mg/24 hr ÷ once daily–QID
  6–12 yr: 40–150 mg/24 hr ÷ once daily–QID
  >12 yr and adult: 50–400 mg/24 hr ÷ once daily–QID
Rectal:
  Older child and adult: Add 50–100 mg of oral liquid (not syrup) to enema fluid (saline or oil retention enemas).

Oral dosage effective only after 1–3 days of therapy. Incidence of side effects is exceedingly low. Rash, nausea, and throat irritation have been reported. Oral liquid is bitter; give with milk, fruit juice, or formula to mask taste.

A few drops of the 10 mg/mL oral liquid may be used in the ear as a cerumenolytic. Effect is usually seen within 15 min.

Pregnancy category has not been formally assigned by the FDA but is considered a "C."

DOLASETRON
Anzemet
Antiemetic agent, 5-HT₃ antagonist

No   No   ?   B

Injection: 20 mg/mL (0.625, 5, 25 mL)
Tabs: 50, 100 mg
Oral suspension: 10 mg/mL

Chemotherapy-induced nausea and vomiting prevention:
  2 yr–adult: 1.8 mg/kg/dose PO up to a **max. dose** of 100 mg. Administer PO dose 60 min before chemotherapy. IV route of administration is considered contraindicated for this indication because of increased risk for QTc prolongation.
Postoperative nausea and vomiting prevention: Administer IV doses 15 min before cessation of anesthesia and PO doses 2 hr before surgery.
  2–16 yr:
    IV: 0.35 mg/kg/dose (**max. dose** 12.5 mg) × 1
    PO: 1.2 mg/kg/dose × 1 (**max. dose** 100 mg) × 1
  Adult:
    IV: 12.5 mg/dose × 1
    PO: 100 mg/dose × 1
Postoperative nausea and vomiting treatment: Administer IV at onset of nausea and vomiting.
  2–16 yr: 0.35 mg/kg/dose (**max. dose** 12.5 mg) IV
  Adult: 12.5 mg/dose IV

May cause hypotension and prolongation of cardiac conduction intervals, particularly QTc interval (dose-dependent effect). Common side effects include dizziness, headache, sedation, blurred vision, fever, chills, and sleep disorders. Rare cases of sustained supraventricular and ventricular arrhythmias, fatal cardiac arrest, and MI have been reported in children and adolescents.

Avoid use in patients with congenital long QTc syndrome, hypomagnesemia, hypokalemia, or with concurrent use of other drugs that increase QTc interval (e.g., erythromycin, cisapride). Drug's active metabolite (hydrodolasetron) is a substrate for CYP 450 2D6 and 3A3/4 isoenzymes; concomitant use of enzyme inhibitors (e.g., cimetidine) may increase risk for side effects, and use of enzyme inducers (e.g., rifampin) may decrease dolasetron's efficacy. Although no dosage adjustments are necessary, hydrodolasetron's clearance decreases 42% with severe hepatic impairment and 44% with severe renal impairment.

ECG monitoring is recommended in patients with electrolyte abnormalities, CHF, or bradyarrhythmias. IV doses may be administered undiluted over 30 sec.

DOPAMINE
Various generics; previously available as Intropin
Sympathomimetic agent

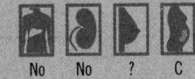

No   No   ?   C

Injection: 40, 80, 160 mg/mL (5, 10 mL)
Prediluted injection in D₅W: 0.8, 1.6, 3.2 mg/mL (250, 500 mL)

All ages:
Low dose: 2–5 mcg/kg/min IV; increases renal blood flow; minimal effect on heart rate
and cardiac output
Intermediate dose: 5–15 mcg/kg/min IV; increases heart rate, cardiac contractility, cardiac output,
and to a lesser extent, renal blood flow
High dose: >20 mcg/kg/min IV; α-adrenergic effects are prominent; decreases renal perfusion.
Max. dose recommended: 20–50 mcg/kg/min IV
To prepare infusion: See IV infusions on page i.

Do not use in pheochromocytoma, tachyarrhythmias, or hypovolemia. Monitor vital signs and
blood pressure continuously. Correct hypovolemic states. Tachyarrhythmias, ectopic beats,
hypertension, vasoconstriction, and vomiting may occur. **Use with caution** with phenytoin;
hypotension and bradycardia may be exacerbated. Use with linezolid may potentially increase
blood pressure.

Newborn infants may be more sensitive to vasoconstrictive effects of dopamine. Children <2 yr of age
clear dopamine faster and exhibit high variability in neonates.

Should be administered through a central line or large vein. Extravasation may cause tissue necrosis;
treat with phentolamine. **Do not** administer into an umbilical arterial catheter.

DORNASE ALFA/DNASE
Pulmozyme
Inhaled mucolytic

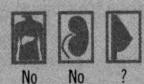

No   No   ?   B

Inhalation solution: 1 mg/mL (2.5 mL)

Cystic fibrosis:
Child > 5 yr and adult: 2.5 mg via nebulizer once daily. Some patients may benefit from
2.5 mg BID.

Contraindicated in patients with hypersensitivity to epoetin alfa. Voice alteration, pharyngitis,
laryngitis may result. These are generally reversible without dose adjustment. Safety and
efficacy has not been demonstrated in patients >1 year of continuous use.

Do not mix with other nebulized drugs. A β-agonist may be useful before administration to enhance
drug distribution. Chest physiotherapy should be incorporated into treatment regimen. The following
nebulizer compressor systems have been recommended for use: Pulmo-Aide, Pari-Proneb, Mobilaire,
Porta-Neb, or PariBaby. Use of the "Sidestream" nebulizer cup can significantly reduce medication
administration time.

DOXAPRAM HCL
Dopram and generics
CNS stimulant

No   No   ?   B

Injection: 20 mg/mL (20 mL); may contain 0.9% benzyl alcohol

Methylxanthine-refractory neonatal apnea: Load with 2.5–3 mg/kg over 15 min, followed by a continuous infusion of 1 mg/kg/hr titrated to lowest effective dose; **max. dose** 2.5 mg/kg/hr

Contraindicated in seizures, proven or suspected pulmonary embolism, head injuries, cerebral vascular accident, cerebral edema, cardiovascular or coronary artery disease, severe hypertension, pheochromocytoma, hyperthyroidism, and in patients with mechanical disorders of ventilation. **Do not** use with general anesthetic agents that can sensitize the heart to catecholamines (e.g., halothane, cyclopropane, enflurane) to reduce risk of cardiac arrhythmias, including ventricular tachycardia and ventricular fibrillation. **Do not** initiate doxapram until general anesthetic agent has been completely excreted.
Hypertension occurs with higher doses (>1.5 mg/kg/hr). May also cause tachycardia, arrhythmias, seizure, hyperreflexia, hyperpyrexia, abdominal distension, bloody stools, and sweating. **Avoid** extravasation into tissues.

DOXYCYCLINE
Adoxa, Vibramycin, Periostat, Doryx, many others, and generics
Antibiotic, tetracycline derivative

Yes   Yes   2   D

Caps: 20 (Periostat), 50, 75, 100, 150 mg
Tabs: 20 (Periostat), 50, 75, 100, 150 mg
Delayed-release caps: 40, 100 mg
Delayed-release tabs (Doryx): 80, 100, 150, 200 mg
Syrup: 50 mg/5 mL (60 mL); contains parabens
Oral suspension: 25 mg/5 mL (60 mL)
Injection: 100 mg

Initial:
≤45 kg: 2.2 mg/kg/dose BID PO/IV × 1 day to **max. dose** of 200 mg/24 hr
>45 kg: 100 mg/dose BID PO/IV × 1 day
Maintenance:
≤45 kg: 2.2–4.4 mg/kg/24 hr once daily–BID PO/IV
>45 kg: 100–200 mg/24 hr ÷ once daily–BID PO/IV
Max. dose: 200 mg/24 hr
PID:
Inpatient: 100 mg Q12 hr with cefotetan or cefoxitin, or ampicillin/sulbactam. Convert to oral therapy 24 hr after patient improves on IV to complete a 14-day total course (IV and PO).
Outpatient: 100 mg PO Q12 hr × 14 days with ceftriaxone, cefoxitin + probenecid, or other parenteral third-generation cephalosporin with or without metronidazole.
Anthrax (inhalation/systemic/cutaneous [see remarks]): Initiate therapy with IV route, and convert to PO route when clinically appropriate. Duration of therapy is 60 days (IV and PO combined):
≤8 yr or ≤45 kg: 2.2 mg/kg/dose BID IV/PO; **max. dose** 200 mg/24 hr
>8 yr and >45 kg: 100 mg/dose BID IV/PO

For explanation of icons, see p. 648

Continued

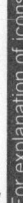

DOXYCYCLINE *continued*

Malaria prophylaxis (start 1–2 days before exposure, and continue for 4 wk after leaving endemic area):
>**8 yr:** 2 mg/kg/24 hr PO once daily; **max. dose** 100 mg/24 hr and **max. duration** of 4 mo
Adult: 100 mg PO once daily
Periodontitis:
Adult: 20 mg BID PO × ≤9 mo

Use with caution in hepatic and renal disease. Generally **not recommended** for use in children <8 yr owing to risk for tooth enamel hypoplasia and discoloration. However, the AAP *Redbook* recommends doxycycline as the drug of choice for rickettsial disease regardless of age. May cause GI symptoms, photosensitivity, hemolytic anemia, rash, and hypersensitivity reactions. Increased intracranial pressure (pseudotumor cerebri), TEN, erythema multiforme, and Stevens-Johnson syndrome have been reported.

Doxycycline is approved for treatment of anthrax *(Bacillus anthracis)* in combination with one or two other antimicrobials. If meningitis is suspected, consider using an alternative agent because of poor CNS penetration. Consider changing to high-dose amoxicillin (25–35 mg/kg/dose TID PO) for penicillin-susceptible strains. See www.bt.cdc.gov for the latest information.

Rifampin, barbiturates, phenytoin, and carbamazepine may increase clearance of doxycycline. Doxycycline may enhance the hypoprothrombinemic effect of warfarin. See *Tetracycline* for additional drug/food interactions and remarks.

Infuse IV over 1–4 hr. **Avoid** prolonged exposure to direct sunlight.

For periodontitis, take capsules ≥1 prior to meals, and take tablets ≥1 hr before or 2 hr after meals.

DRONABINOL
Marinol, Tetrahydrocannabinol, THC, and generics
Antiemetic

| Yes | No | X | C |

Caps: 2.5, 5, 10 mg; may contain sesame oil

Antiemetic:
Child and adult (PO): 5 mg/m^2/dose 1–3 hr before chemotherapy, then Q2–4 hr up to a **max. dose** of 6 doses/24 hr; doses may be gradually increased by 2.5 mg/m^2/dose increments up to a **max. dose** of 15 mg/m^2/dose if needed and tolerated.

Appetite stimulant:
Adult (PO): 2.5 mg BID 1 hr before lunch and dinner; if not tolerated, reduce dose to 2.5 mg QHS.
Max. dose: 20 mg/24 hr (**use caution** when increasing doses because of increased risk of dose-related adverse reactions at higher dosages).

Contraindicated in patients with history of substance abuse, mental illness, or allergy to sesame oil. **Use with caution** in heart disease, seizures, hepatic disease (reduce dose if severe). Side effects: euphoria, dizziness, difficulty concentrating, anxiety, mood change, sedation, hallucinations, ataxia, paresthesia, hypotension, excessively increased appetite, and habit-forming potential.

Onset of action: 0.5–1 hr; duration of psychoactive effects, 4–6 hr; appetite stimulation, 24 hr.

DROPERIDOL
Inapsine and generics
Sedative, antiemetic

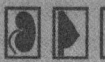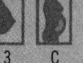

Yes Yes 3 C

Injection: 2.5 mg/mL (2 mL)

Antiemetic/sedation:
   Child: 0.03–0.07 mg/kg/dose IM or IV over 2–5 min; if needed, may give 0.1–0.15 mg/kg/dose; initial **max. dose** 0.1 mg/kg/dose, and subsequent **max. dose** 2.5 mg/dose.
      Dosage interval:
         Antiemetic: PRN Q4–6 hr.
         Sedation: Repeat dose in 15–30 min if necessary.
   Adult: 2.5–5 mg IM or IV over 2–5 min; initial **max. dose** is 2.5 mg.
      Dosage interval:
         Antiemetic: PRN Q3–4 hr.
         Sedation: Repeat dose in 15–30 min if necessary.

Use with caution in renal and hepatic impairment; 75% of metabolites are excreted renally, and drug is extensively metabolized in the liver. Side effects include hypotension, tachycardia, extrapyramidal side effects, such as dystonia, feeling of motor restlessness, laryngospasm, bronchospasm. May lower seizure threshold. **Fatal arrhythmias and QT interval prolongation has been associated with use.**
Onset in 3–10 min. Peak effects within 10–30 min. Duration: 2–4 hr. Often given as adjunct to other agents.

EDETATE (EDTA) CALCIUM DISODIUM
Calcium disodium versenate and generics
Chelating agent, antidote for lead toxicity

Yes Yes ? B

Injection: 200 mg/mL (5 mL)

Lead poisoning:
Lead level > 70 mcg/dL (use with dimercaprol): Initiate at the time of the second dimercaprol dose, and treat for 3–5 days. May repeat a course as needed after 2–4 days of no EDTA.
   IM: 1000–1500 mg/m²/24 hr ÷ Q4 hr
   IV: 1000–1500 mg/m²/24 hr as an 8–24 hour infusion or divided Q12 hr
   Use 1500 mg/m²/24 hr for 5 days in the presence of encephalopathy.
Lead level 20–70 mcg/dL: 1000 mg/m²/24 hr IV as an 8–24 hr infusion *OR* intermittent dosing divided Q12 hr × 5 days. May repeat course as needed after 2–4 days of no EDTA.
Max. daily dose: 75 mg/kg/24 hr

Edetate (EDTA) calcium disodium is NOT interchangeable with edetate disodium (Na₂EDTA); erroneous substitutions have led to fatalities. Prescribe this product by its full name and **avoid** the EDTA abbreviation to prevent dispensing errors.
May cause renal tubular necrosis. **Do not use** in the presence of anuria, hepatitis, and active renal disease. Dosage reduction is recommended with mild renal disease. Follow urinalysis and renal function. Monitor ECG continuously for arrhythmia when giving IV. Rapid IV infusion may cause sudden increase in intracranial pressure in patients with cerebral edema. May cause zinc and copper deficiency. Monitor Ca^{2+} and PO_4.
IM route preferred. Give IM with 0.5% procaine.

For explanation of icons, see p. 648

EDROPHONIUM CHLORIDE
Enlon, Tensilon
Anticholinesterase agent, antidote for neuromuscular blockade

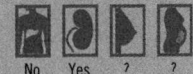

No   Yes   ?   ?

Injection: 10 mg/mL (15 mL) (contains 0.45% phenol and 0.2% sulfite)

Diagnosis for myasthenia gravis (IV [see remarks]):
  Neonate: 0.1 mg single dose
  Infant and child:
    Initial: 0.04 mg/kg/dose × 1
    Max. dose: 1 mg for <34 kg, 2 mg for ≥34 kg
    If no response after 1 min, may give 0.16 mg/kg/dose for a total of 0.2 mg/kg.
    Total max. dose: 5 mg for <34 kg, 10 mg for ≥34 kg
  Adult: 2-mg test dose IV; if no reaction, give 8 mg after 45 sec.

May precipitate cholinergic crisis, arrhythmias, and bronchospasm. Keep atropine available
in syringe, and have resuscitation equipment ready. Hypersensitivity to test dose
(fasciculations or intestinal cramping) is indication to stop giving drug. **Contraindicated** in
GI or GU obstruction, or arrhythmias. Dose may have to be reduced in chronic renal failure.
Reported doses for reversing neuromuscular blockade in children have ranged from 0.1–1.43 mg/kg/dose.
  Antagonism of nondepolarizing neuromuscular blocking drugs in children is more rapid than in adults.
Short duration of action with IV route (5–10 min). **Antidote:** atropine 0.01–0.04 mg/kg/dose.
Pregnancy category has not been established.

EMLA

See Lidocaine and Prilocaine

ENALAPRIL MALEATE (PO), ENALAPRILAT (IV)
Enalapril: Vasotec, Epaned, and other generics
Enalaprilat: Vasotec IV and other generics
Angiotensin-converting enzyme inhibitor, antihypertensive

No   Yes   2   D

Enalapril:
  Tabs: 2.5, 5, 10, 20 mg
  Oral suspension: 0.1, 1 mg/mL
  Epaned: 1 mg/mL (150 mL); contains parabens and saccharin
Enalaprilat:
  Injection: 1.25 mg/mL (1, 2 mL); contains benzyl alcohol

Hypertension:
  Infant and child:
    PO: 0.08 mg/kg/24 hr up to 5 mg/24 hr ÷ once daily; increase PRN over 2 wk
    Max. dose (higher doses have not been evaluated): 0.58 mg/kg/24 hr up to 40 mg/24 hr
    IV: 0.005–0.01 mg/kg/dose Q8–24 hr; **max. dose** 1.25 mg/dose
  Adolescent and adult:
    PO: 2.5–5 mg/24 hr once daily initially to **max. dose** of 40 mg/24 hr ÷ once daily–BID
    IV: 0.625–1.25 mg/dose IV Q6 hr; doses as high as 5 mg Q6 hr are reported to be tolerated for
    up to 36 hr.

Use with caution in bilateral renal artery stenosis. **Avoid use** with dialysis with high-flux
membranes; anaphylactoid reactions have been reported. Side effects: nausea, diarrhea,
headache, dizziness, hyperkalemia, hypoglycemia, hypotension, and hypersensitivity. Cough is
a reported side effect of ACE inhibitors.

FORMULARY

ENALAPRIL MALEATE (PO), ENALAPRILAT (IV) *continued*

Enalapril (PO) is converted to its active form (Enalaprilat) by the liver. Administer IV over 5 min. **Adjust dose in renal impairment (see Chapter 31).**

Nitritoid reactions have been in patients receiving concomitant IV gold therapy. Enalapril/enalaprilat should be discontinued as soon as possible when pregnancy is detected. If oliguria or hypotension occurs in a neonate with in utero exposure to enalapril/enalaprilat, exchange transfusions or dialysis may be necessary to reverse hypotension and/or support renal function.

ENOXAPARIN
Lovenox and generics
Anticoagulant, low-molecular-weight heparin

Yes   Yes   2   B

Injection: 100 mg/mL (3 mL); contains 15 mg/mL benzyl alcohol
Injection (prefilled syringes with 27-gauge, ½-inch needle): 30 mg/0.3 mL, 40 mg/0.4 mL, 60 mg/0.6 mL, 80 mg/0.8 mL, 100 mg/1 mL, 120 mg/0.8 mL, 150 mg/1 mL
Approximate anti–factor Xa activity: 100 IU per 1 mg

Initial empirical dosage; patient-specific dosage defined by therapeutic drug monitoring when indicated (see remarks).

DVT treatment:

Infant < 2 mo: 1.5 mg/kg/dose Q12 hr SC

Infant ≥ 2 mo–adult: 1 mg/kg/dose Q12 hr SC; alternatively, 1.5 mg/kg/dose Q24 hr SC can be used in adults.

Dosage adjustment for DVT treatment to achieve target anti–factor Xa low-molecular-weight heparin (LMWH) levels of 0.5–1 units/mL (see following table):

Anti–Factor Xa Level LMWH (units/mL)	Hold Next Dose?	Dose Change	Repeat Anti–Factor Xa Level LMWH?
<0.4	No	Increase by 25%	4 hr post next new dose
0.4	No	Increase by 10%	4 hr post next new dose
0.5	No	No	4 hr post next dose; if within therapeutic range, recheck 1 week later at 4 hr post dose
0.6–0.7	No	No	1 week later at 4 hr post dose
0.8–1	No	No	4 hr post next dose; if within therapeutic range, recheck 1 week later at 4 hr post dose
1.1–1.5	No	Decrease by 20%	4 hr post next new dose
1.6–2	3 hr	Decrease by 30%	Trough level (goal: <0.5) before next new dose and 4 hr post next new dose
>2	Until anti-factor Xa LMWH reaches 0.5 units/mL (levels can be measured Q12 hr until it reaches ≤0.5 units/mL).	When anti–factor Xa LMWH reaches 0.5 units/mL, dose may be restarted at a dose 40% less than originally prescribed.	4 hr post next new dose

ENOXAPARIN *continued*

DVT prophylaxis:
   Infant < 2 mo: 0.75 mg/kg/dose Q12 hr SC
   Infant ≥ 2 mo–child 18 yr: 0.5 mg/kg/dose Q12 hr SC; **max. dose** 30 mg/dose
   Patients with indwelling epidural catheters/neuraxial anesthesia (≥2 mo–child 18 yr): 1 mg/kg/dose Q24 hr SC; **max. dose** 40 mg/dose. Twice-daily dosing is **contraindicated** for these patients. See remarks.
   Adjust dosage for DVT prophylaxis to achieve target anti–factor Xa levels of 0.1–0.3 units/mL for all children.
   Adult:
      Knee or hip replacement surgery: 30 mg BID SC × 7–14 days; initiate therapy 12–24 hr after surgery, provided hemostasis is established. Alternatively for hip replacement surgery, 40 mg once daily SC × 7–14 days initially up to 3 wk thereafter; initiate therapy 9–15 hr before surgery.
      Abdominal surgery: 40 mg once daily SC × 7–12 days initiated 2 hr before surgery.
      Patients at risk due to severe restricted mobility during an acute illness: 40 mg once daily SC × 6–14 days.

Inhibits thrombosis by inactivating factor Xa without significantly affecting bleeding time, platelet function, PT, or APTT at recommended doses. Dosages of enoxaparin, heparin, or other LMWHs **cannot** be used interchangeably on a unit-for-unit (or mg-for-mg) basis because of differences in pharmacokinetics and activity. Peak anti–factor Xa LMWH activity is achieved 4 hr after a dose. **Anti–factor Xa LMWH is NOT THE SAME as unfractionated heparin anti–Xa level (used for monitoring heparin therapy).**

Contraindicated in major bleeding and drug-induced thrombocytopenia. **Use with caution** in uncontrolled arterial hypertension, bleeding diathesis, history of recurrent GI ulcers, diabetic retinopathy, and severe renal dysfunction (reduce dose by increasing dosage interval from Q12 hr to Q24 hr if GFR < 30 mL/min). Prophylactic use not recommended in patients with prosthetic heart valves (especially pregnant women) because of reports of fatalities in patients and fetuses. **Concurrent use with spinal or epidural anesthesia or spinal puncture has resulted in long-term or permanent paralysis; potential benefits must be weighed against risks.** May cause fever, confusion, edema, nausea, hemorrhage, thrombocytopenia, hypochromic anemia, and pain/erythema at injection site. Allergic reactions, headache, eosinophilia, alopecia, hepatocellular and cholestatic liver injury, and osteoporosis (long-term use) have been reported. **Protamine sulfate is the antidote;** 1 mg protamine sulfate neutralizes 1 mg enoxaparin.

DVT prophylaxis for patients with epidural catheters/neuraxial anesthesia: If placing needle, hold anticoagulation for 12 hr, and restart dosing no sooner than 4 hr after needle insertion. If removing catheter, hold anticoagulation for 12 hr, and restart dosing no sooner than 2 hr after catheter removal.

Recommended anti–factor Xa LMWH levels obtained 4 hr after subcutaneous dose after the third consecutive dose:
   DVT treatment: 0.5–1 units/mL
   DVT prophylaxis: 0.1–0.3 units/mL

Administer by deep SC injection by having patient lie down. Alternate administration between the left and right anterolateral and left and right posterolateral abdominal wall. See package insert for detailed SC administration recommendations. To minimize bruising, do not rub the injection site. IV or IM route of administration is not recommended.

For additional information, see *Chest.* 2008;133:887-968 and *Regional Anesth Pain Med.* 2003;28:172-197.

EPINEPHRINE HCL
Adrenalin, EpiPen, other brand names and generics
Sympathomimetic agent

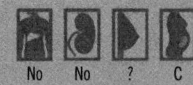

No   No   ?   C

Injection:
1:1000 (aqueous): 1 mg/mL (1, 30 mL)
1:10,000 (aqueous): 0.1 mg/mL (10 mL prefilled syringes with either 18G, 3.5-inch or 21G, 1.5-inch needles or 10-mL vials)

Autoinjector:
EpiPen and others: Delivers a single 0.3-mg (0.3-mL) dose (1 or 2 pack)
EpiPen Jr and others: Delivers a single 0.15-mg (0.3-mL) dose (1 or 2 pack)
Some preparations may contain sulfites.

Cardiac uses:
Neonate:
Asystole and bradycardia: 0.01–0.03 mg/kg of 1:10,000 solution (0.1–0.3 mL/kg) IV/ET Q3–5 min PRN

Infant and child:
Bradycardia/asystole and pulseless arrest: See page ii and PALS algorithms in back of book.
Bradycardia, asystole, and pulseless arrest (see remarks):
First dose: 0.01 mg/kg of 1:10,000 solution (0.1 mL/kg) IO/IV; **max. dose** 1 mg (10 mL). Subsequent doses Q3–5 min PRN should be the same. High-dose epinephrine after failure of standard dose has not been shown to be effective (see remarks). Must circulate drug with CPR. For ET route see below.
All ET doses: 0.1 mg/kg of 1:1000 solution (0.1 mL/kg) ET Q3–5 min

Adult:
Asystole: 1–5 mg IV/ET Q3–5 min
IV drip (all ages): 0.1–1 mcg/kg/min; titrate to effect; to prepare infusion, see inside front cover.

Respiratory uses:
Bronchodilator: 1:1000 (aqueous):
Infant and child: 0.01 mL/kg/dose SC (**max. single dose** 0.5 mL); repeat Q15 min × 3–4 doses or Q4 hr PRN
Adult: 0.3–0.5 mg (0.3–0.5 mL)/dose SC Q20 min × 3 doses
Nebulization (alternative to racemic epinephrine): 0.5 mL/kg of 1:1000 solution diluted in 3 mL NS. **Max. doses:** ≤4 yr, 2.5 mL/dose; >4 yr, 5 mL/dose

Hypersensitivity reactions (see remarks for IV dosing):
Child: 0.01 mg/kg/dose IM/SC up to a **max. dose** of 0.5 mg/dose Q20 min–4 hr PRN. If using EpiPen or EpiPen Jr, administer only via IM route using following dosage:
<30 kg: 0.15 mg
≥30 kg: 0.3 mg
Adult: Start with 0.1–0.5 mg IM/SC Q20 min–4 hr PRN; doses may be increased if necessary to a single **max. dose** of 1 mg.

High-dose rescue therapy for in-hospital cardiac arrest in children after failure of an initial standard dose has been reported to be of no benefit compared to standard dose (*N Engl J Med.* 2004;350:1722-1730).

Hypersensitivity reactions: For bronchial asthma and certain allergic manifestations (e.g., angioedema, urticaria, serum sickness, anaphylactic shock) use epinephrine SC. Patients with anaphylaxis may benefit from IM administration. Adult IV dose for hypersensitivity reactions or to relieve bronchospasm usually ranges from 0.1–0.25 mg injected slowly over 5–10 min Q5–15 min as needed. Neonates may be given a dose of 0.01 mg/kg body weight; for infants, 0.05 mg is an adequate initial dose, and this may be repeated at 20- to 30-min intervals in the management of asthma attacks.

Continued

EPINEPHRINE HCL *continued*

May produce arrhythmias, tachycardia, hypertension, headaches, nervousness, nausea, vomiting.
  Necrosis may occur at site of repeated local injection.
Concomitant use of noncardiac selective β-blockers or tricyclic antidepressants may enhance
  epinephrine's pressor response. Chlorpromazine may reverse pressor response.
ETT doses should be diluted with NS to a volume of 3–5 mL before administration. Follow with several
  positive-pressure ventilations.
EpiPen and EpiPen Jr should be administered IM into anterolateral aspect of thigh. See EpiPen product
  information for proper use of the device and to prevent injury and/or inadvertent dose administration
  to the individual administering the dose. Accidental injection into digits, hands, or feet may result in
  loss of blood flow to affected area.

EPINEPHRINE, RACEMIC
S-2 Inhalant and others
Sympathomimetic agent

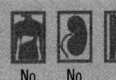 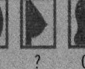

No   No   ?   C

Solution for inhalation (OTC): 2.25% (1.25% epinephrine base) (0.5, 15, 30 mL)
Contains edetate disodium and may contain sulfites

<4 yr:
  Croup (using 2.25% solution): 0.05 mL/kg/dose up to a **max. dose** of 0.5 mL/dose, diluted
  to 3 mL with NS. Given via nebulizer over 15 min PRN but **not** more frequently than Q1–2 hr.
≥4 yr: 0.5 mL/dose diluted to 3 mL with NS via nebulizer over 15 min Q3–4 hr PRN

Tachyarrhythmias, headache, nausea, palpitations reported. Rebound symptoms may occur.
  Cardiorespiratory monitoring should be considered if administered more frequently than
  Q1–2 hr.

EPOETIN ALFA
Erythropoietin, Epogen, Procrit
Recombinant human erythropoietin

   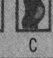

No   No   2   C

Injection (single-dose, preservative-free vials): 2000, 3000, 4000, 10,000, 40,000 U/mL (1 mL)
Injection (multidose vials): 10,000 U/mL (2 mL), 20,000 U/mL (1 mL); contains 1% benzyl alcohol
All dosage forms contain 2.5 mg albumin per 1 mL.

***Anemia in chronic renal failure (see remarks for dosage adjustment and withholding
  therapy):*** SC/IV (IV preferred for hemodialysis patients)
Initial dose:
  Child and adolescent: Start at 50 U/kg/dose 3 times per week. Reported dosage range for children
  (3 mo–20 yr) not requiring dialysis, 50–250 U/kg/dose 3 times per week. Reported dosage range
  for children receiving hemodialysis, 50–450 U/kg/dose 2–3 times per week.
  Adult: Start at 50–100 U/kg/dose 3 times per week.
Maintenance dose: Dose is individualized to achieve and maintain the lowest Hgb level sufficient to
  avoid transfusions and **not to exceed** 11 g/dL.
***Anemia in cancer (use until chemotherapy is completed; see remarks for dosage reduction and
  withholding therapy):***
  Initial dose:
    Child (5–18 yr): Start at 600 U/kg (**max. dose** 40,000 U) IV once weekly.
    Adult: Start at 150 U/kg/dose SC 3 times per week or 40,000 U SC once every week.

EPOETIN ALFA *continued*

Increasing doses (if needed):
Three-times-a-week dosing regimen (adult): If no increase in Hgb >1 g/dL, and Hgb remains <10 g/dL after initial 4 wk of therapy, increase dosage to 300 U/kg/dose 3 times per week.

Weekly dosing regimen: If no increase in Hgb >1 g/dL, and Hgb remains <10 g/dL after initial 4 wk of therapy:

Child: Increase dose to 900 U/kg/dose IV (**max. dose** 60,000 U) once weekly

Adult: 60,000 U SC once weekly

For all ages, discontinue use after 8 wk of therapy if transfusions are still required or no hemoglobin response is observed.

AZT-treated HIV patients (Hgb should not exceed 12 g/dL): SC/IV
Child: Reported dosage range in children (8 mo–17 yr), 50–400 U/kg/dose 2–3 times per wk.

Adult (with serum erythropoietin ≤500 milliunits/mL and receiving ≤4200 mg AZT per week): Start at 100 U/kg/dose 3 times per wk × 8 wk.

Dose increments (if needed): If response is not satisfactory in reducing transfusion requirements or increasing Hgb levels after 8 wk of therapy, dose may be increased by 50–100 U/kg/dose given 3 times per wk, and reevaluate every 4–8 wk thereafter. Patients are unlikely to respond to doses >300 U/kg/dose 3 times per wk.

For all ages, withhold therapy if Hgb > 12 g/dL, and resume therapy by decreasing dosage by 25% once Hgb falls below 11 g/dL. For adults, discontinue therapy if Hgb does not increase after 8 wk of the 300 U/kg/dose 3 times per wk.

Anemia of prematurity (many regimens exist):
250 U/kg/dose SC 3 times per wk × 10 doses; alternatively, 200–400 U/kg/dose IV/SC 3–5 times per wk for 2–6 wk (total dose per wk is 600–1400 U/kg). Administer with supplemental iron at 3–6 mg elemental iron/kg/24 hr.

Use the lowest dose to avoid transfusions. Increased risk for death, serious cardiovascular events, and thrombosis/stroke have been reported in patients treated with chronic kidney disease and hemoglobin levels > 11 g/dL. Increased risk for death, shortened survival and/or shortened time to tumor progression/regression, serious cardiovascular events, and thrombosis in various cancer patients, especially with Hgb levels >12 g/dL, have been reported with epoetin alfa and other erythropoiesis-stimulating agents.

Evaluate serum iron, ferritin, TIBC before therapy. Iron supplementation recommended during therapy unless iron stores are already in excess. Monitor Hct, BP, clotting times, platelets, BUN, serum creatinine. Peak effect in 2–3 wk.

DOSAGE ADJUSTMENT FOR ANEMIA IN CHRONIC RENAL FAILURE:

Reduce dose by ≥25%: when Hgb increases >1 g/dL in any 2-wk period. Dose reductions can be made more frequently than once every 4 weeks if needed.

Increase dose by 25%: when Hgb does not increase by 1 g/dL after 4 wk of therapy. Dosage increments should not be made more frequently than once every 4 wk.

Withholding therapy: When Hgb > 11 g/dL; restart therapy at a 25% lower dose after Hgb decreases to target levels or <11 g/dL.

Inadequate response after a 12-week dose escalation: Use minimum effective dosage that will maintain Hgb levels to avoid the need for recurrent blood transfusions, and evaluate other causes of anemia. Discontinue use if patient remains transfusion dependent.

DOSAGE REDUCTION ADJUSTMENT/WITHHOLDING THERAPY FOR ANEMIA IN CANCER:

If Hgb exceeds a level needed to avoid blood transfusion: Withhold dose and resume therapy at a reduced dosage by 25% when Hgb approaches a level where blood transfusions may be needed.

If Hgb increases >1 g/dL in any 2-wk period or Hgb reaches a level to avoid blood transfusion: Reduce dose by 25%.

May cause hypertension, seizure, hypersensitivity reactions, headache, edema, dizziness. SC route provides sustained serum levels compared to IV route. For IV administration, infuse over 1–3 min. Do not use multidose vial preparation for breast-feeding mothers because of concerns for benzyl alcohol.

For explanation of icons, see p. 648

ERGOCALCIFEROL
Drisdol, Calciferol, Calcidol, and other generics
Vitamin D₂

   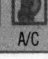

No   No   2   A/C

Caps: 50,000 IU (1.25 mg)
Tabs: 400, 2000 IU
Drops [OTC]: 8000 IU/mL (200 mcg/mL) (60 mL); contains propylene glycol
1 mg = 40,000 IU vitamin D activity

Dietary supplementation (see Chapter 21 for additional information):
  Preterm: 400–800 IU/24 hr PO
  Infant (<1 yr): 400 IU/24 hr PO
  Child (≥1 yr) and adolescent: 600 IU/24 hr PO
Renal failure (CKD stages 2–5) and 25-OH vitamin D levels < 30 ng/mL (monitor serum 25-OH
vitamin D and corrected calcium/phosphorus 1 mo after initiation and Q3 mo thereafter):
  25-OH vitamin D < 5 ng/mL:
    Child: 8000 IU/24 hr × 4 wk, followed by 4000 IU/24 hr × 2 mo; *OR* 50,000 IU weekly × 4 wk,
    followed by 50,000 IU twice monthly for 2 mo
  25-OH vitamin D 5–15 ng/mL:
    Child: 4000 IU/24 hr PO × 12 wk *OR* 50,000 IU every other wk × 12 wk
  25-OH vitamin D 16–30 ng/mL:
    Child: 2000 IU/24 hr PO × 3 mo *OR* 50,000 IU every mo × 3 mo
Vitamin D–dependent rickets:
  Child: 3000–5000 IU/24 hr PO; **max. dose** 60,000 IU/24 hr
Nutritional rickets:
  Child and adult with normal GI absorption: 2000–5000 IU/24 hr PO × 6–12 week
  Malabsorption:
    Child: 10,000–25,000 IU/24 hr PO
    Adult: 10,000–300,000 IU/24 hr PO
Vitamin D–resistant rickets (with phosphate supplementation):
  Child: initial dose 40,000–80,000 IU/24 hr PO; increase daily dose by 10,000–20,000 IU PO Q3–4 mo
  if needed.
  Adult: 10,000–60,000 IU/24 hr PO
Hypoparathyroidism (with calcium supplementation):
  Child: 50,000–200,000 IU/24 hr PO
  Adult: 25,000–200,000 IU/24 hr PO

Monitor serum Ca²⁺, PO₄, 25-OH vitamin D (goal level for infant and child: ≥20 ng/mL), and
alkaline phosphate. Serum Ca²⁺, PO₄ product should be <70 mg/dL to avoid ectopic
calcification. Titrate dosage to patient response. Watch for symptoms of hypercalcemia:
weakness, diarrhea, polyuria, metastatic calcification, nephrocalcinosis. Vitamin D₂ is
activated by 25-hydroxylation in liver and 1-hydroxylation in kidney.
Serum 25-OH vitamin D level of ≥35 ng/mL has been suggested in cystic fibrosis patients to decrease
risk of hyperparathyroidism and bone loss.
Pregnancy category changes to "C" if used in doses above U.S. RDA.

ERGOTAMINE TARTRATE ± CAFFEINE
Ergomar
In combination with caffeine: Cafergot, Migergot and other generics
Ergot alkaloid

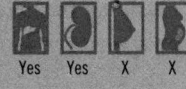

Yes   Yes   X   X

Sublingual tabs (Ergomar): 2 mg
In combination with caffeine:
    Tabs: 1 mg and 100 mg caffeine
    Suppository: 2 mg and 100 mg caffeine (12s)

Doses based on mg of ergotamine.
Older child and adolescent:
    PO/SL: 1 mg at onset of migraine attack, then 1 mg Q30 min PRN up to **max. dose** of
    3 mg per 24 hr; **do not exceed** 5 mg per wk.
Adult:
    PO/SL: 2 mg at onset of migraine attack, then 1–2 mg Q30 min up to 6 mg per 24 hr; **do not
    exceed** 10 mg per wk.
    Suppository: 2 mg at first sign of attack; follow with second 2-mg dose after 1 hr; **max. dose**
    4 mg per 24 hr, **not to exceed** 10 mg/wk.

Use with caution in renal or hepatic disease. May cause paresthesias, GI disturbance, angina-
like pain, rebound headache with abrupt withdrawal, or muscle cramps. **Contraindicated** in
pregnancy and has **not been recommended** in breast-feeding. Concurrent administration
with protease inhibitors, clarithromycin, erythromycin, or other CYP 450 3A4 inhibitors is
contraindicated owing to risk of ergotism (nausea, vomiting, vasospastic ischemia leading to
cerebral and peripheral ischemia).

ERTAPENEM
Invanz
Antibiotic, carbapenem

No   Yes   2   B

Injection: 1 g
Contains ≈ 6 mEq Na/g drug

3 mo–12 yr: 15 mg/kg/dose IV/IM Q12 hr; **max. dose** 1 g/24 hr
Adolescent and adult: 1 g IV/IM Q24 hr
    Recommended duration of therapy (all ages):
        Complicated intraabdominal infection: 5–14 days
        Complicated skin/subcutaneous tissue infections: 7–14 days
        Diabetic foot infection without osteomyelitis: up to 28 days
        Community-acquired pneumonia, complicated UTI/pyelonephritis: 10–14 days
        Acute pelvic infection: 3–10 days
        Surgical site prophylaxis for colorectal surgery: 1 g IV 1 hr before procedure

Ertapenem has poor activity against *Pseudomonas aeruginosa, Acinetobacter,* MRSA, and
Enterococcus. **Do not use** in meningitis; has poor CSF penetration. **Use with caution** with
CNS disorders, including seizures. Adjust dosage in renal impairment; see Chapter 31.
Diarrhea, infusion complications, nausea, headache, vaginitis, phlebitis/thrombophlebitis, and
vomiting are common. Seizures (primarily with renal insufficiency and/or CNS disorders such as
brain lesions and seizures), muscle weakness, gait disturbance, abnormal coordination, and DRESS
syndrome have been reported. Increased ALT, AST, and neutropenia have been reported in pediatric
clinical trials. Decreases valproic acid levels. Probenecid may increase ertapenem levels.
IM route requires reconstitution with 1% lidocaine and **should not** be administered IV. **Do not**
reconstitute or co-infuse with dextrose-containing solutions.

For explanation of icons, see p. 648

ERYTHROMYCIN ETHYLSUCCINATE AND ACETYLSULFISOXAZOLE
Pediazole, E.S.P., and other generics
Antibiotic, macrolide + sulfonamide derivative

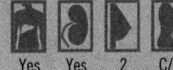

Yes   Yes   2   C/D

Oral suspension: 200 mg erythromycin and 600 mg sulfisoxazole/5 mL (100, 150, 200, 250 mL)

Otitis media:
≥2 mo: 50 mg/kg/24 hr (as erythromycin) and 150 mg/kg/24 hr (as sulfisoxazole) ÷
Q6–8 hr PO, *OR* give 1.25 mL/kg/24 hr ÷ Q6–8 hr PO
Max. dose: 2 g erythromycin, 6 g sulfisoxazole/24 hr
Adult: 400 mg erythromycin and 1200 mg sulfisoxazole Q6 hr PO

Contraindicated in liver dysfunction or porphyria. See adverse effects and drug interactions of
Erythromycin and *Sulfisoxazole*. **Not recommended** in infants <2 mo. **Do not use** in renal
impairment because dosage adjustments are inconsistent for sulfisoxazole and erythromycin.
Pregnancy category changes to "D" if administered near term.

ERYTHROMYCIN PREPARATIONS
Erythrocin, Pediamycin, E-Mycin, Ery-Ped, EES, and other generics
Ophthalmic ointment: Ilotycin, Romycin, and others
Antibiotic, macrolide

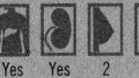

Yes   Yes   2   B

Erythromycin base:
  Tabs: 250, 500 mg
  Delayed-release tabs: 250, 333, 500 mg
  Delayed-release caps: 250 mg
  Topical ointment: 2% (25 g)
  Topical gel: 2% (30, 60 g); contains alcohol 92%
  Topical solution: 2% (60 mL); may contain 44%–66% alcohol
  Topical pad/swab: 2% (60s)
  Ophthalmic ointment: 0.5% (1, 3.5 g)
Erythromycin ethyl succinate (EES):
  Oral suspension: 200 mg/5 mL (100, 200 mL), 400 mg/5 mL (100 mL)
  Oral drops: 100 mg/2.5 mL (100 mL)
  Tabs: 400 mg
Erythromycin stearate:
  Tabs: 250 mg
Erythromycin lactobionate:
  Injection: 500, 1000 mg; may contain benzyl alcohol

Oral:
Neonate (use EES preparation):
  <1.2 kg: 20 mg/kg/24 hr ÷ Q12 hr PO
  ≥1.2 kg:
    0–7 days: 20 mg/kg/24 hr ÷ Q12 hr PO
    >7 days:
      1.2–2 kg: 30 mg/kg/24 hr ÷ Q8 hr PO
      ≥2 kg: 30–40 mg/kg/24 hr ÷ Q6–8 hr PO
  Chlamydial conjunctivitis and pneumonia: 50 mg/kg/24 hr ÷ Q6 hr PO × 14 days; max. dose 2 g/24 hr
Child (use base or EES preparation): 30–50 mg/kg/24 hr ÷ Q6–8 hr; **max. dose** 2 g/24 hr for base
preparations and 3.2 g/24 hr for EES preparations
  Pertussis: 40–50 mg/kg/24 hr ÷ Q6 hr PO × 14 days (**max. dose** 2 g/24 hr); use azithromycin for
infants <1 mo old.

ERYTHROMYCIN PREPARATIONS *continued*

Adult: 1–4 g/24 hr ÷ Q6 hr; **max. dose** 4 g/24 hr
Parenteral:
Child: 20–50 mg/kg/24 hr ÷ Q6 hr IV
Adult: 15–20 mg/kg/24 hr ÷ Q6 hr IV
Max. dose: 4 g/24 hr
Rheumatic fever prophylaxis: 500 mg/24 hr ÷ Q12 hr PO
Ophthalmic: Apply 0.5-inch ribbon to affected eye BID–QID. Apply as a one-time dose for prophylaxis of neonatal gonococcal ophthalmia.
Preoperative bowel preparation: 20 mg/kg/dose PO erythromycin base × 3 doses, with neomycin, 1 day before surgery
Prokinetic agent:
Infant and child: 10–20 mg/kg/24 hr PO ÷ TID–QID (QAC or QAC and QHS)

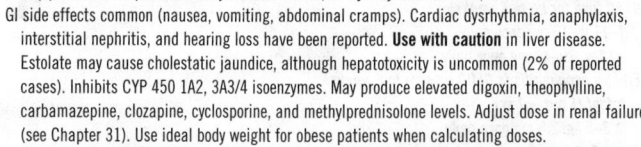

Avoid use in patients with known QT prolongation, proarrhythmic conditions (e.g., hypokalemia, hypomagnesemia, significant bradycardia), and receiving class IA or class III antiarrhythmic agents, astemizole, cisapride, pimozide, or terfenadine. Hypertrophic pyloric stenosis in neonates receiving prophylactic therapy for pertussis, life-threatening episodes of ventricular tachycardia associated with prolonged QTc interval, and exacerbation of myasthenia gravis have been reported. May produce false-positive urinary catecholamines, 17-hydroxycorticosteroids, and 17-ketosteroids.
GI side effects common (nausea, vomiting, abdominal cramps). Cardiac dysrhythmia, anaphylaxis, interstitial nephritis, and hearing loss have been reported. **Use with caution** in liver disease. Estolate may cause cholestatic jaundice, although hepatotoxicity is uncommon (2% of reported cases). Inhibits CYP 450 1A2, 3A3/4 isoenzymes. May produce elevated digoxin, theophylline, carbamazepine, clozapine, cyclosporine, and methylprednisolone levels. Adjust dose in renal failure (see Chapter 31). Use ideal body weight for obese patients when calculating doses.
Oral therapy should replace IV as soon as possible. Give oral doses after meals. Because of different absorption characteristics, higher oral doses of EES are needed to achieve therapeutic effects. **Avoid** IM route (pain, necrosis). For ophthalmic use, avoid ointment tip contact with eye or skin.

ERYTHROPOIETIN

See Epoetin Alfa

ESMOLOL HCL
Brevibloc and generics
β1-Adrenergic (selective) blocking agent, antihypertensive agent, class II antiarrhythmic

No   No   ?   C

Injection: 10 mg/mL (10 mL)
Injection, premixed infusion in iso-osmotic sodium chloride: 10 mg/mL (250 mL), 20 mg/mL (100 mL)

Postoperative hypertension: Titrate to response (limited information):
Loading dose: 500 mcg/kg IV over 1 min
Maintenance dose: 50–250 mcg/kg/min IV as infusion. Titrate doses upward 50–100 mcg/kg/min Q5–10 min as needed. Dosages as high as 1000 mcg/kg/min have been administered to children 1–12 yr.
SVT: Titrate to response (limited information).
Loading dose: 100–500 mcg/kg IV over 1 min
Maintenance dose: 25–100 mcg/kg/min IV as infusion. Titrate doses upward 50–100 mcg/kg/min Q5–10 min as needed. Dosages as high as 1000 mcg/kg/min have been administered.

Continued

For explanation of icons, see p. 648

ESMOLOL HCL *continued*

Contraindicated in sinus bradycardia, >first-degree heart block, and cardiogenic shock or heart failure. Short duration of action; $T_{1/2} = 2.9$–4.7 min for children and 9 min for adults. May cause bronchospasm, congestive heart failure, hypotension (at doses >200 mcg/kg/min), nausea, and vomiting. May increase digoxin (by 10%–20%) and theophylline levels. Morphine may increase esmolol level by 46%. Theophylline may decrease esmolol's effects.

Administer only in a monitored setting. Concentration for administration is typically ≤10 mg/mL, but 20 mg/mL has been administered in pediatric patients.

ESOMEPRAZOLE
Nexium and other
Gastric acid proton pump inhibitor

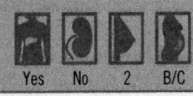

Yes   No   2   B/C

Caps, delayed-release: 20, 40 mg; contains magnesium (NOTE: Another delayed-release capsule product containing strontium may also be available.)
Powder for oral suspension: 2.5, 5, 10, 20, 40 mg packets (30s); contains magnesium
Injection: 20, 40 mg; contains EDTA

Child (PO):
   GERD (use for up to 8 weeks):
     1–11 yr: 10 mg once daily
     ≥12 yr: 20–40 mg once daily
   Erosive esophagitis in GERD (use up to 6 weeks):
     Infant (1 mo–<1 yr):
       3–5 kg: 2.5 mg once daily
       >5–7.5 kg: 5 mg once daily
       >7.5–12 kg: 10 mg once daily
     1–11 yr:
       <20 kg: 10 mg once daily
       ≥20 kg: 10 or 20 mg once daily
Child (IV):
   GERD with erosive esophagitis:
     Infant: 0.5-1 mg/kg/dose once daily
   Child 1–17 yr:
     <55 kg: 10 mg once daily
     ≥55 kg: 20-40 mg once daily
Adult (PO/IV):
   GERD: 20 or 40 mg once daily × 4–8 wk
   Prevention of NSAID-induced gastric ulcers: 20 or 40 mg once daily for up to 6 mo
   Pathologic hypersecretory conditions (e.g., Zollinger-Ellison syndrome): 40 mg BID; doses up to 240 mg/24 hr have been used.
   Hepatic impairment: Patients with severe hepatic function impairment (Child-Pugh class C) should not exceed 20 mg/24 hr.

Cross-allergic reactions with other proton-pump inhibitors (e.g., lansoprazole, pantoprazole, rabeprazole). **Use with caution** in liver impairment (see dosage adjustment recommendation in dosing section). GI disturbances and headache are common. Hypomagnesemia may occur with continuous use. Erythema multiforme, Stevens-Johnson syndrome, TEN, pancreatitis, and fractures of the hip, wrist, and spine (in adults >50 yr old receiving high doses or prolonged therapy >1 yr) have been reported. Drug is a substrate and inhibitor of CYP 450 2C19 and substrate of CYP 450 3A4. May decrease absorption or effects of atazanavir, clopidogrel, ketoconazole, itraconazole, and iron salts. May increase effect/toxicity of diazepam, midazolam, digoxin, carbamazepine, and warfarin. Voriconazole may increase

ESOMEPRAZOLE *continued*

effects of esomeprazole. May be used in combination with clarithromycin and amoxicillin for *Helicobacter pylori* infections.

Pregnancy category is a "B" for the magnesium-containing product and a "C" for the strontium-containing product.

Administer all oral doses before meals and 30 min before sucralfate (if receiving). **Do not** crush or chew capsules. IV doses may be given as fast as 3 min or infused over 10–30 min.

ETANERCEPT
Enbrel
Antirheumatic, immunomodulatory agent, tumor necrosis factor receptor p75 Fc fusion protein

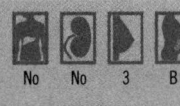

No   No   3   B

Prefilled injection: 25 mg (0.51 mL of 50 mg/mL solution), 50 mg (0.98 mL of 50 mg/mL solution); contains sucrose, L-arginine
Injection (powder): 25 mg with diluent (1 mL bacteriostatic water containing 0.9% benzyl alcohol); contains mannitol, sucrose, tromethamine

Juvenile idiopathic arthritis:
    Child 2–17 yr: 0.4 mg/kg/dose SC twice weekly administered 72–96 hr apart; **max. dose** 25 mg. Alternative once-weekly dose of 0.8 mg/kg/dose SC (**max. dose** 50 mg/wk and **max. single injection site dose** of 25 mg) may be used.
Rheumatoid arthritis, psoriatic arthritis, ankylosing spondylitis:
    Adult: 25 mg SC twice weekly administered 72–96 hr apart. Alternative once-weekly dose of 50 mg SC (**max. single injection site dose** of 25 mg) may be used.
Plaque psoriasis:
    Child and adolescent (4–17 yr; limited data): 0.8 mg/kg/dose (max. dose 50 mg) SC once weekly
    Adult: Start with 50 mg SC twice weekly administered 72–96 hr apart × 3 mo, followed by a reduced maintenance dose of 50 mg SC per wk. Starting doses of 25 mg or 50 mg per wk have also been shown to be effective.
    Max. single injection site dose: 25 mg

Contraindicated in serious infections, sepsis, or hypersensitivity to any of medication components. **Use with caution** in patients with history of recurrent infections or underlying conditions that may predispose them to infections (including concomitant immunosuppressive therapy), CNS demyelinating disorders, malignancies, immune-related diseases, and latex allergy. Common adverse effects in children include headache, abdominal pain, vomiting, and nausea. Injection site reactions (e.g., discomfort, itching, swelling), rhinitis, dizziness, rash, depression, infections (varicella, aseptic meningitis, rare cases of TB, and fatal/serious infections and sepsis), bone marrow suppression (e.g., aplastic anemia), vertigo, and CNS demyelinating disorder have also been reported. Malignancies (some fatal, and ≈ 50% were lymphomas) have been reported in children and adolescents.

Do not administer live vaccines concurrently with this drug. In JRA, it is recommended that before initiating therapy, the patient be brought up to date with all immunizations in agreement with current immunization guidelines.

Onset of action is 1–4 wk, with peak effects usually within 3 mo.

Patients must be properly instructed on preparing and administering the medication. Drug requires reconstitution by gently swirling its contents with the supplied diluent (**do not** shake or vigorously agitate) because some foaming will occur. Reconstituted solutions should be clear and colorless and used within 6 hr.

Drug is administered subcutaneously by rotating injection sites (thigh, abdomen, or upper arm) with a **max. single injection site dose** of 25 mg. Administer new injections ≥1 inch from an old site and never where the skin is tender, bruised, red, or hard.

For explanation of icons, see p. 648

ETHAMBUTOL HCL
Myambutol and generics
Antituberculosis drug

   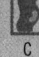

No   Yes   2   C

Tabs: 100, 400 mg

Tuberculosis:
> *Infant, child, adolescent, and adult:* 15–25 mg/kg/dose PO once daily or
> 50 mg/kg/dose PO twice weekly; **max. dose** 2.5 g/24 hr.

Nontuberculous mycobacterial infection and **Mycobacterium avium** *complex in AIDS (recurrence prophylaxis or treatment; use in combination with other medications):*
> *Infant, child, adolescent, and adult:* 15–25 mg/kg/24 hr PO once daily; **max. dose** 2.5 g/24 hr

May cause reversible optic neuritis, especially with larger doses. Obtain baseline ophthalmologic studies before beginning therapy and then monthly. Follow visual acuity, visual fields, and (red-green) color vision. **Do not use** in optic neuritis and in children whose visual acuity cannot be assessed. **Discontinue** if any visual deterioration occurs. Monitor uric acid, liver function, heme status, and renal function. Hyperuricemia, GI disturbances, and mania are common. Erythema multiforme has been reported. Coadministration with aluminum hydroxide can reduce ethambutol's absorption; space administration by 4 hr. Give with food. **Adjust dose with renal failure (see Chapter 31).**

ETHOSUXIMIDE
Zarontin and generics
Anticonvulsant

 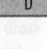

Yes   Yes   2   D

Caps: 250 mg
Syrup: 250 mg/5 mL (473 mL)

Oral:
> *≤6 yr:*
> > *Initial:* 15 mg/kg/24 hr ÷ BID; **max. dose** 500 mg/24 hr; increase as needed Q4–7 days.
> > *Usual maintenance dose:* 15–40 mg/kg/24 hr ÷ BID
> *>6 yr and adult:* 250 mg BID; increase by 250 mg/24 hr as needed Q4–7 days.
> > *Usual maintenance dose:* 20–40 mg/kg/24 hr ÷ BID
> **Max. dose (all ages):** 1500 mg/24 hr

Use with caution in hepatic and renal disease. Ataxia, anorexia, drowsiness, sleep disturbances, rashes, and blood dyscrasias are rare idiosyncratic reactions. May cause lupus-like syndrome; may increase frequency of grand mal seizures in patients with mixed-type seizures. Serious dermatologic reactions (e.g., Stevens-Johnson syndrome and DRESS) have been reported. May increase risk of suicidal thoughts/behavior. Cases of birth defects have been reported; ethosuximide crosses the placenta. Drug of choice for absence seizures.

Carbamazepine, phenytoin, primidone, phenobarbital, valproic acid, nevirapine, and ritonavir may decrease ethosuximide levels.

Therapeutic levels: 40–100 mg/L. $T_{1/2}$ = 24–42 hr. Recommended serum sampling time at steady state: obtain trough level within 30 min before next scheduled dose after 5–10 days of continuous dosing.

To minimize GI distress, may administer with food or milk. Abrupt withdrawal of drug may precipitate absence status.

FAMCICLOVIR
Famvir and generics
Antiviral

Yes   Yes   ?   B

Tabs: 125, 250, 500 mg

Adult:
Herpes zoster: 500 mg Q8 hr PO × 7 days; initiate therapy promptly as soon as diagnosis
is made (initiation within 48 hr after rash onset is ideal; currently no data for starting
treatment >72 hr after rash onset).
Genital herpes (first episode): 250 mg Q8 hr PO × 7–10 days
Recurrent genital herpes:
   Immunocompetent: 1000 mg Q12 hr PO × 1 day or 125 mg Q12 hr PO × 5 days; initiate therapy
   at first sign or symptom. Efficacy has not been established when treatment is initiated >6 hr
   after onset of symptoms or lesions.
   Immunocompromised: 500 mg Q8 hr PO × 7 days.
   Suppression of recurrent genital herpes (immunocompetent): 250 mg Q12 hr PO up to 1 yr,
   then reassess for HSV infection recurrence.
Recurrent herpes labialis:
   Immunocompetent: 1500 mg PO × 1
   Immunocompromised: 500 mg Q8 hr PO × 7 days
Recurrent mucocutaneous herpes in HIV: 500 mg Q12 hr PO × 7 days

Drug is converted to its active form (penciclovir). Hepatic impairment may impair/reduce
conversion of famciclovir to penciclovir. Better absorption than PO acyclovir.
May cause headache, diarrhea, nausea, and abdominal pain. Serious skin reactions (e.g., TEN
and Stevens-Johnson syndrome), angioedema, palpitations, cholestatic jaundice, and abnormal
LFTs have been reported. Concomitant use with probenecid and other drugs eliminated by active
tubular secretion may result in decreased penciclovir clearance. **Reduce dose in renal impairment
(see Chapter 31).**
Safety and efficacy in suppression of recurrent genital herpes have not been established beyond 1 yr.
No efficacy data available for children 1–<12 yr to support its use for genital herpes, recurrent
herpes labialis, and varicella. Efficacy has not been established for recurrent herpes labialis for
children 12–<18 yr. May be administered with or without food.

FAMOTIDINE
Pepcid, Pepcid AC [OTC], Maximum Strength Pepcid AC [OTC],
Pepcid Complete [OTC], Pepcid RPD, and generics
Histamine-2-receptor antagonist

No   Yes   1   B

Injection: 10 mg/mL (2, 4, 20, 50 mL); multidose vials contain 0.9% benzyl alcohol
Premixed injection: 20 mg/50 mL in iso-osmotic sodium chloride
Oral suspension: 40 mg/5 mL (contains parabens) (50 mL)
Tabs: 10 [OTC], 20 [OTC], 40 mg
Disintegrating oral tabs (Pepcid RPD): 20, 40 mg; contains aspartame
Chewable tabs (Pepcid Complete and others) [OTC]: 10 mg famotidine with 800 mg calcium
carbonate and 165 mg magnesium hydroxide; may contain aspartame

Neonate and <3 mo:
   IV: 0.25–0.5 mg/kg/dose Q24 hr
   PO: 0.5–1 mg/kg/dose Q24 hr
≥3 mo–1 yr (GERD): 0.5 mg/kg/dose PO Q12 hr

Continued

FAMOTIDINE *continued*

Child (1–12 yr):

IV: Initial: 0.6–0.8 mg/kg/24 hr ÷ Q8–12 hr up to a **max.** of 40 mg/24 hr

PO: Initial: 1–1.2 mg/kg/24 hr ÷ Q8–12 hr up to a **max.** of 40 mg/24 hr

Peptic ulcer: 0.5 mg/kg/24 hr PO QHS or ÷ Q12 hr up to a **max. dose** of 40 mg/24 hr

GERD: 1–2 mg/kg/24 hr PO ÷ Q12 hr up to a **max. dose** of 80 mg/24 hr

Adolescent and adult:

Duodenal ulcer:

PO: 20 mg BID or 40 mg QHS × 4–8 wk, then maintenance therapy at 20 mg QHS

IV: 20 mg BID

GERD: 20 mg BID PO × 6 wk

Esophagitis: 20–40 mg BID PO × 12 wk

A Q12-hr dosage interval is generally recommended, but infants and young children may require a Q8-hr interval because of enhanced drug clearance. Headaches, dizziness, constipation, diarrhea, and drowsiness have occurred. **Dosage adjustment is required in severe renal failure (see Chapter 31);** prolonged QT interval has been reported very rarely in patients with renal impairment whose dosage had not been adjusted appropriately.

Shake oral suspension well before each use. Disintegrating oral tablets should be placed on the tongue to be disintegrated and subsequently swallowed. Doses may be administered with or without food.

FELBAMATE
Felbatol and generics
Anticonvulsant

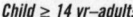

Yes   Yes   ?   C

Tabs: 400, 600 mg
Oral suspension: 600 mg/5 mL

Lennox-Gastaut for child 2–14 yr (adjunctive therapy):

Start at 15 mg/kg/24 hr PO ÷ TID–QID; increase dosage by 15 mg/kg/24-hr increments at weekly intervals up to a **max. dose** of 45 mg/kg/24 hr or 3600 mg/24 hr (whichever is less). See remarks for adjusting concurrent anticonvulsants.

Child ≥ 14 yr–adult:

Adjunctive therapy: Start at 1200 mg/24 hr PO ÷ TID–QID; increase dosage by 1200 mg/24 hr at weekly intervals up to a **max. dose** of 3600 mg/day. See remarks for adjusting concurrent anticonvulsants.

Monotherapy (as initial therapy): Start at 1200 mg/24 hr PO ÷ TID–QID. Increase dose under close clinical supervision at 600-mg increments Q2 wk to 2400 mg/24 hr. **Max. dose:** 3600 mg/24 hr.

Conversion to monotherapy: Start at 1200 mg/24 hr ÷ PO TID–QID for 2 wk. At wk 3, increase to 2400 mg/24 hr for 1 wk. At wk 3, increase to 3600 mg/24 hr. Reduce dose of other anticonvulsants by 33% at initiation of felbamate, and continue to reduce other anticonvulsants as clinically indicated at wk 2 when felbamate dose is increased.

Drug should be prescribed under strict supervision by a specialist. **Contraindicated** in blood dyscrasias or hepatic dysfunction (prior or current) and hypersensitivity to meprobamate. Aplastic anemia and hepatic failure leading to death have been associated with drug. May cause headache, fatigue, anxiety, GI disturbances, gingival hyperplasia, increased liver enzymes, and bone marrow suppression. Suicidal behavior or ideation have been reported. **Obtain serum levels of concurrent anticonvulsants.** Monitor liver enzymes, bilirubin, CBC with differential, platelets at baseline and Q1–2 wk. Doses should be decreased by 50% in renally impaired patients.

FELBAMATE *continued*

When initiating adjunctive therapy (all ages), doses of other antiepileptic drugs (AEDs) are reduced by 20% to control plasma levels of concurrent phenytoin, valproic acid, phenobarbital, and carbamazepine. Further reductions of concomitant AED dosage may be necessary to minimize side effects caused by drug interactions.

When converting to monotherapy, reduce other AEDs by one third at start of felbamate therapy. Then after 2 wk and at the start of increasing the felbamate dosage, reduce other AEDs by an additional one third. At wk 3, continue to reduce other AEDs as clinically indicated.

Carbamazepine levels may be decreased, whereas phenytoin and valproic acid levels may be increased. Phenytoin and carbamazepine may increase felbamate clearance; valproic acid may decrease its clearance.

Doses can be administered with or without food.

FENTANYL
Sublimaze, Duragesic, Fentora, Abstral, Actiq, Lazanda,
and many generics
Narcotic; analgesic, sedative

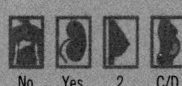

No   Yes   2   C/D

Injection: 50 mcg/mL
SR patch (Duragesic and others): 12.5, 25, 50, 75, 100 mcg/hr (5s)
Tabs for buccal administration:
Fentora: 100, 200, 400, 600, 800 mcg (28s)
Lozenge on a stick:
Actiq and others: 200, 400, 600, 800, 1200, 1600 mcg (30s)
Nasal solution:
Lazanda: 100 mcg/spray, 400 mcg/spray (5 mL; delivers 8 sprays)

Titrate dose to effect.
Neonate and younger infant:
 Sedation/analgesia: 1–4 mcg/kg/dose IV Q2–4 hr PRN
 Continuous IV infusion: 1–5 mcg/kg/hr; tolerance may develop
Older infant and child:
 Sedation/analgesia: 1–2 mcg/kg/dose IV/IM Q30–60 min PRN
 Continuous IV infusion: 1 mcg/kg/hr; titrate to effect; usual infusion range 1–3 mcg/kg/hr
To prepare infusion, use the following formula:

$$50 \times \frac{\text{Desired dose (mcg/kg/hr)}}{\text{Desired infusion rate (mL/hr)}} \times \text{Wt (kg)} = \frac{\text{mcg Fentanyl}}{50 \text{ mL fluid}}$$

Oral, breakthrough cancer pain for opioid-intolerant patients (see remarks):
 Buccal tabs (Fentora; ≥18 yr): Start with 100 mcg by placing tablet in the buccal cavity (above a rear molar, between upper cheek and gum) and letting tablet dissolve for 15–25 min. A second 100 mcg dose, if needed, may be administered 30 min after the start of first dose. If needed, increase dose initially in multiples of 100-mcg tablet when patients require >1 dose per breakthrough pain episode for several consecutive episodes. If titration requires >400 mcg/dose, use 200-mcg tabs.
 Lozenges (≥16 yr): Start with 200 mcg by placing lozenge in the mouth between cheek and lower gum. If needed, may repeat dose 15 min after the completion of first dose (30 min after start of prior dose). If therapy requires >1 lozenge per episode, consider increasing dose to the next higher strength. Do not give more than 2 doses for each episode of breakthrough pain, and reevaluate long-acting opioid therapy if patient requires >4 doses/24 hr.

Continued

For explanation of icons, see p. 648

FORMULARY

FENTANYL *continued*

Transdermal (see remarks): Safety has not been established in children <2 yr and should be administered in children ≥2 yr who are opioid tolerant. Use is **contraindicated** in acute or postoperative pain in opiate-naïve patients.

Opioid-tolerant child receiving at least 60 mg morphine equivalents/24 hr: Use 25 mcg/hr patch Q72 hr. Patch titration should not occur before 3 days of administration of initial dose or more frequently than Q6 days thereafter.

See Chapter 6 for equianalgesic dosing and PCA dosing.

Intranasal route for acute and preprocedure analgesia (see remarks):
    ≥1 yr–adolescent: 1–2 mcg/kg/dose intranasally (**max. dose** 50 mcg) Q1 hr PRN

Use with caution in bradycardia, respiratory depression, and increased intracranial pressure. **Adjust dose in renal failure (see Chapter 31).** Fatalities and life-threatening respiratory depression have been reported with inappropriate use (overdoses, use in opioid-naïve patients, changing patch too frequently and exposing patch to a heat source) of the transdermal route.

Highly lipophilic and may deposit into fat tissue. IV onset of action 1–2 min, with peak effects in 10 min. IV duration of action 30–60 min. Give IV dose over 3–5 min. Rapid infusion may cause respiratory depression and chest wall rigidity. Respiratory depression may persist beyond the period of analgesia. Transdermal onset of action 6–8 hr, with a 72-hr duration of action. See Chapter 6 for pharmacodynamic information with transmucosal and transdermal routes.

Buccal tabs and oral lozenges are indicated only for management of breakthrough cancer pain in patients already receiving and tolerant to opioid therapy. Buccal tabs (Fentora) and lozenge (Actiq) dosage forms are available through a restricted distribution program (REMS) and are **NOT** bioequivalent (see package insert for conversion).

Intranasal route of administration for analgesia has an onset of action at 10–30 min. Pediatric studies have demonstrated that intranasal fentanyl is equivalent to and better than morphine (PO/IV/IM) and equivalent to IV fentanyl for providing analgesia.

Fentanyl is a substrate for the CYP 450 3A4 enzyme. Be aware of medications that inhibit or induce this enzyme, for it may increase or decrease the effects of fentanyl, respectively.

Pregnancy category changes to "D" if drug is used for prolonged periods or in high doses at term.

FERRIC GLUCONATE

See Iron – Injectable Preparations

FERROUS SULFATE

See Iron - Oral Preparations

FEXOFENADINE ± PSEUDOEPHEDRINE
Allegra, Allegra ODT, Allegra-D 12 Hour, Allegra-D 24 Hour, and generics
Antihistamine, less-sedating ± decongestant

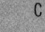

No   Yes   2   C

Tabs: 30, 60, 180 mg
Tabs, orally disintegrating (Allegra Allergy Childrens; ODT): 30 mg; contains phenylalanine
Oral suspension: 6 mg/mL (120 mL)
Extended-release tab in combination with pseudoephedrine (PE):
    Allegra-D 12 Hour: 60 mg fexofenadine + 120 mg pseudoephedrine
    Allegra-D 24 Hour: 180 mg fexofenadine + 240 mg pseudoephedrine

FEXOFENADINE ± PSEUDOEPHEDRINE *continued*

Fexofenadine:
6 mo–<2 yr: 15 mg PO BID
2–11 yr: 30 mg PO BID
≥12 yr–adult: 60 mg PO BID; 180 mg PO daily may be used in seasonal rhinitis.
Extended-release tabs of fexofenadine and pseudoephedrine:
≥12 yr–adult:
    Allegra-D 12 Hour: 1 tablet PO BID
    Allegra-D 24 Hour: 1 tablet PO once daily

May cause drowsiness, fatigue, headache, dyspepsia, nausea, and dysmenorrhea. Has **not** been implicated in causing cardiac arrhythmias when used with other drugs that are metabolized by hepatic microsomal enzymes (e.g., ketoconazole, erythromycin). **Reduce dose to 30 mg PO once daily for child 6–11 yr old and 60 mg PO once daily for ≥12 yr old if CrCl < 40 mL/min.** For use of Allegra-D 12 Hour and decreased renal function, an initial dose of 1 tablet PO once daily is recommended. Avoid use of Allegra-D 24 Hour in renal impairment. See *Pseudoephedrine* for additional remarks if using the combination product.
Medication as the single agent may be administered with or without food. **Do not** administer antacids with or within 2 hr of fexofenadine dose. The extended-release combination product should be swallowed whole without food.

FILGRASTIM
Neupogen, G-CSF
Colony-stimulating factor

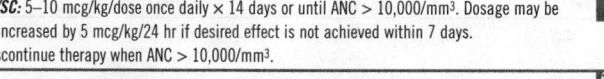

No   No   ?   C

Injection: 300 mcg/mL (1, 1.6 mL vials)
Injection, prefilled syringes with 27-gauge, ½-inch needles: 600 mcg/mL (300 mcg per 0.5 mL and 480 mcg per 0.8 mL) (10s)
All dosage forms are preservative free.

Individual protocols may direct dosing.
IV/SC: 5–10 mcg/kg/dose once daily × 14 days or until ANC > 10,000/mm³. Dosage may be increased by 5 mcg/kg/24 hr if desired effect is not achieved within 7 days.
Discontinue therapy when ANC > 10,000/mm³.

May cause bone pain, fever, and rash. Monitor CBC, uric acid, and LFTs. Thrombocytopenia and decreased bone density/osteoporosis in pediatric patients with severe chronic neutropenia have been reported. **Use with caution** in patients with malignancies with myeloid characteristics. **Contraindicated** for patients sensitive to *Escherichia coli*–derived proteins. **Do not** administer 24 hr before or after administration of chemotherapy.
SC routes of administration are preferred because of prolonged serum levels over IV route. If used via IV route and G-CSF final concentration < 15 mcg/mL, add 2 mg albumin/1 mL of IV fluid to prevent drug adsorption to the IV administration set.

FLECAINIDE ACETATE
Tambocor and generics
Antiarrhythmic, class Ic

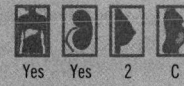

Yes   Yes   2   C

Tabs: 50, 100, 150 mg
Oral suspension: 5, 20 mg/mL

Child: Initial: 1–3 mg/kg/24 hr ÷ Q8 hr PO; usual range: 3–6 mg/kg/24 hr ÷ Q8 hr PO. Monitor serum levels to adjust dose if needed.

Continued

For explanation of icons, see p. 648

FLECAINIDE ACETATE *continued*

Adult:

Sustained V tach: 100 mg PO Q12 hr; may increase by 50 mg Q12 hr (100 mg/24 hr) Q4 days to **max. dose** of 600 mg/24 hr.

Paroxysmal SVT/paroxysmal AF: 50 mg PO Q12 hr; may increase dose by 50 mg Q12 hr Q4 days to **max. dose** of 300 mg/24 hr.

May aggravate LV failure, sinus bradycardia, preexisting ventricular arrhythmias. May cause AV block, dizziness, blurred vision, dyspnea, nausea, headache, and increased PR or QRS intervals. **Reserve for life-threatening cases. Use with caution** in renal and/or hepatic impairment.

Flecainide is a substrate for the CYP 450 2D6 enzyme. Be aware of medications that inhibit (e.g., certain SSRIs) or induce this enzyme, for it may increase or decrease effects of flecainide, respectively.

Therapeutic trough level: 0.2–1 mg/L. Recommended serum sampling time at steady state: Obtain trough level within 30 min before next scheduled dose after 2–3 days of continuous dosing for children; after 3–5 days for adults. **Adjust dose in renal failure (see Chapter 31).**

FLUCONAZOLE
Diflucan and generics
Antifungal agent

 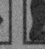

Yes   Yes   2   C/D

Tabs: 50, 100, 150, 200 mg
Injection: 2 mg/mL (50, 100, 200 mL); contains 9 mEq Na/2 mg drug
Oral suspension: 10 mg/mL (35 mL), 40 mg/mL (35 mL)

Neonate (IV/PO):

Loading dose: 12–25 mg/kg

Maintenance dose: 6–12 mg/kg, with the following dosing intervals (see table); use higher doses for severe infections of *Candida* strains with MICs >4–8 mcg/mL.

Postconceptional Age (wk)	Postnatal Age (days)	Dosing Interval (hr) & Time (hr) to Start First Maintenance Dose after Load
≤29	0–14	48
	>14	24
≥30	0–7	48
	>7	24

Child (IV/PO):

Indication	Loading Dose	Maintenance Dose (Q24 hr) to Begin 24 hr after Loading Dose
Oropharyngeal candidiasis	6 mg/kg	3 mg/kg
Esophageal candidiasis	12 mg/kg	6 mg/kg
Invasive systemic candidiasis and cryptococcal meningitis	12 mg/kg	6–12 mg/kg
Suppressive therapy for HIV infected with cryptococcal meningitis	6 mg/kg	6 mg/kg

Max. dose: 12 mg/kg/24 hr

Adult:

Oropharyngeal and esophageal candidiasis: Loading dose of 200 mg PO/IV, followed by 100 mg Q24 hr (24 hr after load); doses up to **max. dose** of 400 mg/24 hr should be used for esophageal candidiasis.

Systemic candidiasis and cryptococcal meningitis: Loading dose of 400 mg PO/IV, followed by 200–800 mg Q24 hr (24 hr after load).

Bone marrow transplant prophylaxis: 400 mg PO/IV Q24 hr

FLUCONAZOLE *continued*

Suppressive therapy, HIV infected, and cryptococcal meningitis: 200 mg PO/IV Q24 hr
Vaginal candidiasis: 150 mg PO × 1

Cardiac arrhythmias may occur when used with cisapride; concomitant use is **contraindicated**.
May cause nausea, headache, rash, vomiting, abdominal pain, hepatitis, cholestasis, and
diarrhea. Neutropenia, agranulocytosis, and thrombocytopenia have been reported. **Use with
caution** in hepatic or renal dysfunction and in patients with proarrhythmic conditions.
Inhibits CYP 450 2C9/10 and CYP 450 3A3/4 (weak inhibitor). May increase effects, toxicity, or levels of
cyclosporine, midazolam, phenytoin, rifabutin, tacrolimus, theophylline, warfarin, oral hypoglycemics,
and AZT. Rifampin increases fluconazole metabolism.
Pediatric to adult dose equivalency: Every 3 mg/kg-pediatric dosage is equal to 100-mg adult dosage.
Consider using higher doses in morbidly obese patients. **Adjust dose in renal failure (see Chapter 31).**
Pregnancy category is "C" for single 150-mg use for vaginal candidiasis; category "D" for all other
indications (high-dose use during first trimester of pregnancy may result in birth defects).

FLUCYTOSINE
Ancobon, 5-FC, 5-Fluorocytosine, and generics
Antifungal agent

No   Yes   3   C

Caps: 250, 500 mg
Oral liquid: 10 mg/mL

Neonate: 80–160 mg/kg/24 hr ÷ Q6 hr PO
Child and adult: 50–150 mg/kg/24 hr ÷ Q6 hr PO

Monitor CBC, BUN, serum creatinine, alkaline phosphatase, AST, and ALT. Common side
effects: nausea, vomiting, diarrhea, rash, CNS disturbance, anemia, leukopenia, and
thrombocytopenia. Use is **contraindicated** in the first trimester of pregnancy.
Therapeutic levels: 25–100 mg/L. Recommended serum sampling time at steady state: Obtain peak
level 2–4 hr after oral dose, after 4 days of continuous dosing. Peak levels of 40–60 mg/L have been
recommended for systemic candidiasis. Maintain trough levels above 25 mg/L. Prolonged levels
above 100 mg/L can increase risk for bone marrow suppression. Bone marrow suppression in
immunosuppressed patients can be irreversible and fatal.
Flucytosine interferes with creatinine assay tests using the dry-slide enzymatic method (Kodak
Ektachem analyzer). **Adjust dose in renal failure (see Chapter 31).**

FLUDROCORTISONE ACETATE
Florinef acetate, 9-Fluorohydrocortisone, Fluohydrisone,
and various generics
Corticosteroid

No   Yes   3   C

Tabs: 0.1 mg

Infant and child: 0.05–0.1 mg/24 hr once daily PO
Congenital adrenal hyperplasia: 0.05–0.3 mg/24 hr once daily PO
Adult: 0.05–0.2 mg/24 hr once daily PO

Contraindicated in CHF and systemic fungal infections. Has primarily mineralocorticoid
activity. **Use with caution** in hypertension, edema, or renal dysfunction. May cause
hypertension, hypokalemia, acne, rash, bruising, headaches, GI ulcers, and growth
suppression.
Monitor BP and serum electrolytes. See Chapter 10 for steroid potency comparison.

Continued

For explanation of icons, see p. 648

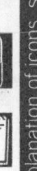

FLUDROCORTISONE ACETATE *continued*

Drug interactions: Drug's hypokalemic effects may induce digoxin toxicity; phenytoin and rifampin may increase fludrocortisone metabolism.

Doses 0.2–2 mg/24 hr have been used in the management of severe orthostatic hypotension in adults. Use a gradual dosage taper when discontinuing therapy.

FLUMAZENIL
Romazicon and generics
Benzodiazepine antidote

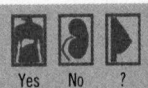

Yes   No   ?   C

Injection: 0.1 mg/mL (5, 10 mL); contains parabens

Benzodiazepine overdose (IV, see remarks):
  Child (limited data): 0.01 mg/kg (**max. dose** 0.2 mg) Q1 min PRN to a **max. total cumulative dose** of 1 mg. As an alternative for repeat bolus doses, a continuous infusion of 0.005–0.01 mg/kg/hr has been used.
  Adult: Initial dose of 0.2 mg over 30 sec; if needed, give 0.3 mg 30 sec later over 30 sec. Additional doses of 0.5 mg given over 30 sec Q1 min PRN up to a cumulative dose of 3 mg (**usual cumulative dose** 1–3 mg). Patients with only partial response to 3 mg may require additional slow titration to a total of 5 mg.

Reversal of benzodiazepine sedation (IV):
  Child: Initial dose of 0.01 mg/kg (**max. dose** 0.2 mg) given over 15 sec; if needed, after 45 sec, give 0.01 mg/kg (**max. dose** 0.2 mg) Q1 min to a **max. total cumulative dose** of 0.05 mg/kg or 1 mg, whichever is lower. Usual total dose: 0.08–1 mg (average 0.65 mg).
  Adult: Initial dose of 0.2 mg over 15 sec; if needed after 45 sec, give 0.2 mg Q1 min to a **max. total cumulative dose** of 1 mg. Doses may be repeated at 20-min intervals (**max. dose** of 1 mg per 20-min interval) up to a **max. dose** of 3 mg in 1 hr.

Does not reverse narcotics. Onset of benzodiazepine reversal occurs in 1–3 min. Reversal effects of flumazenil ($T_{1/2} \approx 1$ hr) may wear off sooner than benzodiazepine effects. If patient does not respond after cumulative 1–3 mg dose, suspect agent other than benzodiazepines.

May precipitate seizures, especially in patients taking benzodiazepines for seizure control or in patients with tricyclic antidepressant overdose. Fear and panic attacks in patients with history of panic disorders have been reported.

Use with caution in liver dysfunction; flumazenil's clearance is significantly reduced. Use normal dose for initial dose, and decrease dosage and frequency for subsequent doses.

See Chapter 2 for complete management of suspected ingestions.

FLUNISOLIDE
Nasal solution: Nasarel and generics
Oral inhaler: Aerospan
Corticosteroid

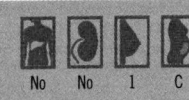

No   No   1   C

Nasal solution:
  Nasarel and generics: 25 mcg/spray (200 sprays/bottle) (25 mL)
Oral aerosol inhaler:
  Aerospan: 80 mcg/dose (60 doses/5.1 g, 120 doses/8.9 g); CFC-free (HFA)

FLUNISOLIDE *continued*

> *For all dosage forms, after symptoms are controlled, reduce to lowest effective*
> *maintenance dose (i.e., 1 spray each nostril once daily) to control symptoms.*

Nasal solution:
  Child (6–14 yr):
    Initial: 1 spray per nostril TID or 2 sprays per nostril BID; **max. dose** of 4 sprays per nostril/24 hr
  ≥15 yr and adult:
    Initial: 2 sprays per nostril BID; if needed, in 4–7 days, increase to 2 sprays per nostril TID; **max.**
    dose of 8 sprays per nostril/24 hr
Oral inhaler (see remarks):
  Aerospan:
    Child 6–11 yr: 1 puff BID; **max. dose** of 4 puffs/24 hr
    Adult: 2 puffs BID; **max. dose** of 8 puffs/24 hr

May cause a reduction in growth velocity. Shake inhaler or nasal solution well before use.
  Patients using nasal solution should clear nasal passages before use.
Do not use a spacer with Aerospan; product has a self-contained spacer. To prevent thrush,
  patient/parent should be instructed to rinse mouth after administering drug by inhaler.

FLUORIDE
Luride, Fluoritab, Pediaflor, and many others
Mineral

 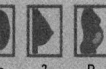

No   No   ?   B

Concentrations and strengths based on fluoride ion:
Oral drops: 0.125 mg/drop (30 mL), 0.25 mg/drop (24 mL), 0.5 mg/mL (50 mL)
Oral solution (rinse): 0.2, 2 mg/mL
Chewable tabs: 0.25, 0.5, 1 mg
Lozenges: 1 mg
See Chapter 21 for fluoride-containing multivitamins.

All doses/24 hr (see table below):
Recommendations from American Academy of Pediatrics and American Dental Association.

Age	Concentration of Fluoride in Drinking Water (ppm)		
	<0.3	**0.3–0.6**	**>0.6**
Birth–6 mo	0	0	0
6 mo–3 yr	0.25 mg	0	0
3–6 yr	0.5 mg	0.25 mg	0
6–16 yr	1 mg	0.5 mg	0

Contraindicated in areas where drinking water fluoridation is >0.7 ppm. **Acute overdose:** GI
  distress, salivation, CNS irritability, tetany, seizures, hypocalcemia, hypoglycemia,
  cardiorespiratory failure. Chronic excess use may result in mottled teeth or bone changes.
Take with food, but **not** milk, to minimize GI upset. The doses have been decreased owing to
  concerns over dental fluorosis.

FLUOXETINE HYDROCHLORIDE
Prozac, Sarafem, Prozac Weekly, and various generics
Antidepressant, selective serotonin reuptake inhibitor

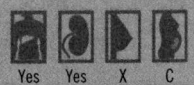

Yes   Yes   X   C

Oral solution: 20 mg/5 mL; may contain alcohol
Caps: 10, 20, 40 mg
Delayed-released caps (Prozac Weekly): 90 mg
Tabs: 10, 20, 60 mg

Depression:
  Child, 8–18 yr: Start at 10–20 mg once daily PO. If started on 10 mg/24 hr, may increase dose to 20 mg/24 hr after 1 wk. Use lower 10-mg/24 hr initial dose for lower-weight children; if needed, increase to 20 mg/24 hr after several weeks.
  Adult: Start at 20 mg once daily PO. May increase after several wk by 20-mg/24-hr increments to **max. dose** of 80 mg/24 hr. Doses >20 mg/24 hr should be divided BID.
Obsessive-compulsive disorder:
  Child, 7–18 yr:
    Lower-weight child: Start at 10 mg once daily PO. May increase after several wk. Usual dose range: 20–30 mg/24 hr. There is very minimal experience with doses >20 mg/24 hr and no experience with doses >60 mg/24 hr.
    Higher-weight child and adolescent: Start at 10 mg once daily PO and increase dose to 20 mg/24 hr after 2 wk. May further increase dose after several wk. Usual dose range: 20–60 mg/24 hr.
Bulimia:
  Adolescent (PO; limited data): 20 mg QAM × 3 days, then 40 mg QAM × 3 days, then 60 mg QAM.
  Adult: 60 mg QAM PO; it is recommended to titrate up to this dose over several days.
Premenstrual dysphoric disorder:
  Adult: Start at 20 mg once daily PO using the Sarafem product. **Max. dose:** 80 mg/24 hr. Systematic evaluation has shown that efficacy is maintained for periods of 6 mo at a dose of 20 mg/day. Reassess patients periodically to determine the need for continued treatment.

Contraindicated in patients taking MAO inhibitors (e.g., linezolid); possibility of seizures, hyperpyrexia, and coma. **Use with caution** in patients receiving diuretics, or with liver (reduce dose with cirrhosis) or renal impairment. May increase effects of tricyclic antidepressants. May cause headache, insomnia, nervousness, drowsiness, GI disturbance, and weight loss. Increased bleeding diathesis with unaltered prothrombin time may occur with warfarin. Hyponatremia has been reported. Monitor for clinical worsening of depression and suicidal ideation/behavior after initiation of therapy or after dose changes.

May displace other highly protein-bound drugs. Inhibits CYP 450 2C19, 2D6, and 3A3/4 drug metabolism isoenzymes, which may increase effects or toxicity of drugs metabolized by these enzymes. Use with serotonergic drugs (e.g., triptans, methylene blue) and drugs that impair serotonin metabolism (MAOIs) may increase risk for serotonin syndrome. Carefully review patients' medication profile for potential interactions.

Delayed-release capsule is currently indicated for depression and is dosed at 90 mg Q7 days. It is unknown whether weekly dosing provides same protection from relapse as daily dosing.

Breast-feeding is not recommended by the manufacturer; adverse events to nursing infants have been reported. Fluoxetine and metabolite are variable and are higher when compared with other SSRIs. Maternal use of SSRIs during pregnancy and postpartum may result in more difficult breast-feeding. Infants exposed to SSRIs during pregnancy may also have increased risk for persistent pulmonary hypertension of the newborn.

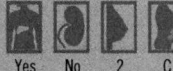

FORMULARY

FLUTICASONE PROPIONATE
Flonase HFA, Cutivate, Flovent Diskus, Veramyst, and selected generics
Corticosteroid

Yes   No   2   C

Nasal spray:
   Flonase and generics (as fluticasone propionate): 50 mcg/actuation (16 g = 120 doses)
   Veramyst (as fluticasone furoate): 27.5 mcg/actuation (10 g = 120 doses)
Topical cream (Cutivate and generics): 0.05% (15, 30, 60 g)
Topical ointment (Cutivate and generics): 0.005% (15, 30, 60 g)
Topical lotion (Cutivate and generics): 0.05% (60, 120 mL)
Aerosol inhaler (MDI) (Flovent HFA): 44 mcg/actuation (10.6 g), 110 mcg/actuation (12 g), 220 mcg/actuation (12 g); each inhaler provides 120 metered inhalations.
Dry-powder inhalation (DPI) (Flovent Diskus): 50 mcg/dose, 100 mcg/dose, 250 mcg/dose; all strengths come in a package of 15 Rotadisks; each Rotadisk provides 4 doses, for a total of 60 doses per package.

Intranasal (allergic rhinitis):
Fluticasone propionate (Flonase and others):
   ≥4 yr and adolescent: 1 spray (50 mcg) per nostril once daily. Dose may be increased to 2 sprays (100 mcg) per nostril once daily if inadequate response or severe symptoms. Reduce to 1 spray per nostril once daily when symptoms are controlled.
   Adult: Initial 200 mcg/24 hr (2 sprays [100 mcg]) per nostril once daily; *OR* 1 spray (50 mcg) per nostril BID. Reduce to 1 spray per nostril once daily when symptoms are controlled.
   Max. dose (4 yr–adult): 2 sprays (100 mcg) per nostril/24 hr
Fluticasone furoate (Veramyst):
   2–11 yr: 1 spray (27.5 mcg) per nostril once daily. If needed, dose may be increased to 2 sprays each nostril once daily. Reduce to 1 spray per nostril once daily when symptoms are controlled.
   ≥11 and adult: 2 sprays (55 mcg) each nostril once daily. Reduce to 1 spray per nostril once daily when symptoms are controlled.
   Max. dose(2 yr–adult): 2 sprays (55 mcg) per nostril/24 hr
Oral inhalation (asthma): **Divide all 24-hr doses BID.** If desired response is not seen after 2 wk of starting therapy, increase dosage. Then reduce to lowest effective dose when asthma symptoms are controlled. Administration of MDI with aerochamber enhances drug delivery.

RECOMMENDED DOSAGES FOR ASTHMA

Age	Previous Use of Bronchodilators Only (max. dose)	Previous Use of Inhaled Corticosteroid (max. dose)	Previous Use of Oral Corticosteroid (max. dose)
Child (4–11 yr)	MDI: 88 mcg/24 hr (176 mcg/24 hr) DPI: 100 mcg/24 hr (200 mcg/24 hr)	MDI: 88 mcg/24 hr (176 mcg/24 hr) DPI: 100 mcg/24 hr (200 mcg/24 hr)	Dose not available
≥12 yr and adult	MDI: 176 mcg/24 hr (880 mcg/24 hr) DPI: 200 mcg/24 hr (1000 mcg/24 hr)	MDI: 176–440 mcg/24 hr (880 mcg/24 hr) DPI: 200–500 mcg/24 hr (1000 mcg/24 hr)	MDI: 880 mcg/24 hr (1760 mcg/24 hr) DPI: 1000–2000 mcg/24 hr (2000 mcg/24 hr)

DPI, Dry-powder inhaler; MDI, metered dose inhaler.

Eosinophilic esophagitis (limited data; use oral HFA dosage form without spacer for PO administration):
   Child (1–10 yr): 220 mcg QID × 4 wk, then 220 mcg TID × 3 wk, then 220 mcg BID × 3 wk, and 220 mcg once daily × 2 wk

For explanation of icons, see p. 648

Continued

FLUTICASONE PROPIONATE *continued*

Child ≥ 11 and adolescent: 440 mcg QID × 4 wk, then 440 mcg TID × 3 wk, then 440 mcg BID × 3 wk, and 440 mcg once daily × 2 wk

Topical (reassess diagnosis if no improvement in 2 wk):

Cream (see Chapter 8 for topical steroid comparisons):

≥*3 mo and adult:* Apply thin film to affected areas once daily–BID; then reduce to a less potent topical agent when symptoms are controlled.

Lotion (see remarks):

≥*1 yr and adult:* Apply thin film to affected areas once daily. Safety of use has not been evaluated longer than 4 wk.

Ointment:

Adult: Apply thin film to affected areas BID.

Concurrent administration with ritonavir and other CYP 450 3A4 inhibitors may increase fluticasone levels, resulting in Cushing syndrome and adrenal suppression. **Use with caution** and monitor closely in hepatic impairment.

Intranasal: Clear nasal passages before use. May cause epistaxis and nasal irritation, which are usually transient. Taste and smell alterations, rare hypersensitivity reactions (angioedema, pruritus, urticaria, wheezing, dyspnea), and nasal septal perforation have been reported in postmarketing studies.

Oral inhalation: Rinse mouth after each use. May cause dysphonia, oral thrush, and dermatitis. Compared with beclomethasone, has been shown to have less of an effect on suppressing linear growth in asthmatic children. Eosinophilic conditions may occur with the withdrawal or decrease of oral corticosteroids after initiation of inhaled fluticasone.

Topical use: Avoid application/contact to face, eyes, and open skin. Occlusive dressings are not recommended; they may increase local side effects (irritation, folliculitis, acneiform eruptions, hypopigmentation, perioral dermatitis, contact dermatitis, secondary infection, skin atrophy, striae, hypertrichosis, miliaria). **Do not use** lotion dosage form with formaldehyde hypersensitivity.

FLUTICASONE PROPIONATE AND SALMETEROL
Advair Diskus, Advair HFA
Corticosteroid and long-acting β₂-adrenergic agonist

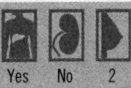

Yes   No   2   C

Dry-powder inhalation (DPI) (Advair Diskus; contains lactose):

100 mcg fluticasone propionate + 50 mcg salmeterol per inhalation (14, 60 inhalations)
250 mcg fluticasone propionate + 50 mcg salmeterol per inhalation (60 inhalations)
500 mcg fluticasone propionate + 50 mcg salmeterol per inhalation (60 inhalations)

Aerosol inhaler (MDI) (Advair HFA):

45 mcg fluticasone propionate + 21 mcg salmeterol per inhalation (8 g delivers 60 doses, 12 g delivers 120 doses)
115 mcg fluticasone propionate + 21 mcg salmeterol per inhalation (8 g delivers 60 doses, 12 g delivers 120 doses)
230 mcg fluticasone propionate + 21 mcg salmeterol per inhalation (8 g delivers 60 doses, 12 g delivers 120 doses)

Asthma:
Without prior inhaled steroid use:

Dry-powder inhalation (DPI):

4 yr–adult: Start with one inhalation BID of 100 mcg fluticasone propionate + 50 mcg salmeterol.

Aerosol inhaler (MDI):

≥*12 yr and adult:* 2 inhalations BID of 45 mcg fluticasone + 21 mcg salmeterol, *OR* 115 mcg fluticasone + 21 mcg salmeterol; **max. dose** is 2 inhalations BID of 230 mcg fluticasone + 21 mcg salmeterol.

FLUTICASONE PROPIONATE AND SALMETEROL *continued*

With prior inhaled steroid use (conversion from other inhaled steroids; see following table):

Inhaled Corticosteroid	Current Daily Dose	Recommended Strength of Fluticasone Propionate + Salmeterol Diskus (DPI) (Advair Diskus) Administered at 1 Inhalation BID	Recommended Strength of Fluticasone Propionate + Salmeterol Aerosol Inhaler (MDI) (Advair HFA) Administered at 2 Inhalations BID
Beclomethasone dipropionate (Qvar; CFC-free, HFA)	160 mcg	100 mcg + 50 mcg	45 mcg + 21 mcg
	320 mcg	250 mcg + 50 mcg	115 mcg + 21 mcg
	640 mcg	500 mcg + 50 mcg	230 mcg + 21 mcg
Budesonide	≤400 mcg	100 mcg + 50 mcg	45 mcg + 21 mcg
	800–1200 mcg	250 mcg + 50 mcg	115 mcg + 21 mcg
	1600 mcg	500 mcg + 50 mcg	230 mcg + 21 mcg
Flunisolide (Aerobid, Aerobid-M; containing CFCs)	≤1000 mcg	100 mcg + 50 mcg	45 mcg + 21 mcg
	1250–2000 mcg	250 mcg + 50 mcg	115 mcg + 21 mcg
Flunisolide (Aerospan; CFC-free, HFA)	≤320 mcg	100 mcg + 50 mcg	45 mcg + 21 mcg
	640 mcg	250 mcg + 50 mcg	115 mcg + 21 mcg
Fluticasone propionate aerosol (HFA)	≤176 mcg	100 mcg + 50 mcg	45 mcg + 21 mcg
	440 mcg	250 mcg + 50 mcg	115 mcg + 21 mcg
	660–880 mcg	500 mcg + 50 mcg	230 mcg + 21 mcg
Fluticasone propionate dry powder (DPI)	≤200 mcg	100 mcg + 50 mcg	45 mcg + 21 mcg
	500 mcg	250 mcg + 50 mcg	115 mcg + 21 mcg
	1000 mcg	500 mcg + 50 mcg	230 mcg + 21 mcg
Mometasone furoate	220 mcg	100 mcg + 50 mcg	45 mcg + 21 mcg
	440 mcg	250 mcg + 50 mcg	115 mcg + 21 mcg
	880 mcg	500 mcg + 50 mcg	230 mcg + 21 mcg
Triamcinolone	≤1000 mcg	100 mcg + 50 mcg	45 mcg + 21 mcg
	1100–1600 mcg	250 mcg + 50 mcg	115 mcg + 21 mcg

Max. doses:
> *Dry-powder inhalation (DPI):* 1 inhalation BID of 500 mcg fluticasone propionate + 50 mcg salmeterol
> *Aerosol inhaler (MDI):* 2 inhalations BID of 230 mcg fluticasone propionate + 21 mcg salmeterol

See *Fluticasone Propionate* and *Salmeterol* for remarks. Titrate to lowest effective strength after asthma is adequately controlled. Proper patient education, including dosage administration technique, is essential. See package insert for detailed instructions. Rinse mouth after each use.

FLUVOXAMINE
Luvox CR (previously available as Luvox), many generics
Antidepressant, selective serotonin reuptake inhibitor

Yes	No	2	C

Tabs: 25, 50, 100 mg
Extended-release capsules (Luvox CR and generics): 100, 150 mg

Obsessive compulsive disorder (use immediate-release tablets unless noted otherwise):
8–17 yr: Start at 25 mg PO QHS. Dose may be increased by 25 mg/24 hr Q7–14 days (slower titration for minimizing behavioral side effects). Total daily doses >50 mg/24 hr should be divided BID. Female patients may require lower dosages than males.

Continued

FLUVOXAMINE *continued*

> **Max. dose:** *Child: 8–11 yr:* 200 mg/24 hr; *child ≥ 12–17 yr:* 300 mg/24 hr
> *Adult:* Start at 50 mg PO QHS. Dose may be increased by 50 mg/24 hr Q4–7 days up to a **max. dose** of 300 mg/24 hr. Total daily doses >100 mg/24 hr should be divided BID.
> > *Extended-release capsule (adult):* Start at 100 mg PO QHS. Dose may be increased by 50 mg/24 hr Q7 days up to a **max. dose** of 300 mg/24 hr.

Contraindicated with coadministration of cisapride, pimozide, thioridazine, tizanidine, or MAO inhibitors. **Use with caution** in hepatic disease (dosage reduction may be necessary); drug is extensively metabolized by liver. Monitor for clinical worsening of depression and suicidal ideation/behavior after initiation of therapy or after dose changes.

Inhibits CYP 450 1A2, 2C19, 2D6, and 3A3/4, which may increase effects or toxicity of drugs metabolized by these enzymes. Dose-related use of thioridazine with fluvoxamine may cause prolongation of QT interval and serious arrhythmias. May increase warfarin plasma levels by 98% and prolong PT. May increase toxicity and/or levels of theophylline, caffeine, and tricyclic antidepressants. Side effects include headache, insomnia, somnolence, nausea, diarrhea, dyspepsia, and dry mouth.

Titrate to lowest effective dose. Consider benefits vs. potential risk for maternal use in breast-feeding. Maternal use during pregnancy and postpartum may result in breast-feeding difficulties.

FOLIC ACID
Folvite and many generics
Water-soluble vitamin

No	No	1	A/C

Tabs [OTC]: 0.4, 0.8, 1 mg
Caps: 0.4 mg [OTC], 0.8 mg [OTC], 5 mg, 20 mg
Oral solution: 50 mcg/mL
Injection: 5 mg/mL; contains 1.5% benzyl alcohol

For U.S. RDA, see Chapter 21.
Folic acid deficiency PO, IM, IV, SC (see following table):

Infant	Child 1–10 yr	Child ≥ 11 yr and Adult
INITIAL DOSE		
15 mcg/kg/dose; max. dose 50 mcg/24 hr	1 mg/dose	1 mg/dose
MAINTENANCE		
30–45 mcg/24 hr once daily	0.1–0.4 mg/24 hr once daily	0.4 mg/24 hr once daily Pregnant/lactating women: 0.8 mg/24 hr once daily

Normal levels: See Chapter 21. May mask hematologic effects of vitamin B_{12} deficiency but will not prevent progression of neurologic abnormalities. High-dose folic acid may decrease absorption of phenytoin.

Women of childbearing age considering pregnancy should take at least 0.4 mg once daily before and during pregnancy to reduce risk of neural tube defects in the fetus. Pregnancy category changes to "C" if used in doses above the RDA.

FOMEPIZOLE
Antizol and generics
Antidote for ethylene glycol or methanol toxicity

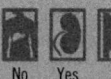 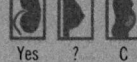

No   Yes   ?   C

Injection: 1 g/ mL (1.5 mL)

Child and adult not requiring hemodialysis (IV, all doses administered over 30 min):
  Loading dose: 15 mg/kg/dose × 1
  Maintenance: 10 mg/kg/dose Q12 hr × 4 doses, then 15 mg/kg/dose Q12 hr until ethylene glycol or methanol level decreases to <20 mg/dL and patient is asymptomatic, with normal pH.
Child and adult requiring hemodialysis (IV after recommended doses at intervals indicated here. Fomepizole is removed by dialysis. All doses administered IV over 30 min):
  Dosing at beginning of hemodialysis:
    If <6 hr since last fomepizole dose: **DO NOT** administer dose.
    If ≥6 hr since last fomepizole dose: Administer next scheduled dose.
  Dosing during hemodialysis: Administer Q4 hr or as continuous infusion of 1–1.5 mg/kg/hr.
  Dosing at the time hemodialysis is completed (based on time between last dose and end of hemodialysis):
    <1 hr: **DO NOT** administer dose at end of hemodialysis.
    1–3 hr: Administer half of next scheduled dose.
    >3 hr: Administer next scheduled dose.
  Maintenance dose off hemodialysis: Give next scheduled dose 12 hr from last dose administered.

Works by competitively inhibiting alcohol dehydrogenase. Safety and efficacy in pediatrics have not been established. **Contraindicated** in hypersensitivity to any components or other pyrazole compounds. Most frequent side effects include headache, nausea, and dizziness. Fomepizole is extensively eliminated by kidneys (**use with caution** in renal failure) and removed by hemodialysis.

Drug product may solidify at temperatures <25°C (77°F); vial can be liquefied by running it under warm water (efficacy, safety, and stability are not affected). All doses must be diluted with at least 100 mL of D_5W or NS to prevent vein irritation.

FORMOTEROL
Foradil Aerolizer, Perforomist
β₂-Adrenergic agonist (long-acting)

No   No   2   C

Inhalation powder in capsules (Foradil Aerolizer): 12 mcg (12s and 60s); contains lactose and milk proteins. Use with Aerolizer inhaler
Inhalation solution (Perforomist): 20 mcg/2 mL (60s)

≥5 yr and adult:
  Asthma/bronchodilation (should be used with an inhaled corticosteroid):
    Foradil Aerolizer: 12 mcg Q12 hr; **max. dose** of 24 mcg/24 hr (12 mcg spaced 12 hr apart)
  Prevention of exercise-induced asthma for patients NOT receiving maintenance long-acting β₂-agonists (e.g., formoterol or salmeterol):
    Foradil Aerolizer: 12 mcg 15 min before exercise. If needed, an additional dose may be given AFTER 12 hr. **Max. dose:** 24 mcg/24 hr (12 mcg spaced 12 hr apart). Consider alternative therapy if maximal dosage is not effective.

Continued

FORMOTEROL *continued*

Fast onset of action (1–3 min), with peak effects in 0.5–1 hr and long duration (up to 12 hr). Although long-acting β_2-adrenergic agonists may decrease the frequency of asthma episodes, they may make asthma episodes more severe when they occur. **Use with caution** in seizures, thyrotoxicosis, diabetes, ketoacidosis, aneurysm, and pheochromocytoma. Abdominal pain, dyspepsia, nausea, and tremor may occur.

Inhalation solution product (Perforomist) is indicated for COPD in adults (20 mcg Q12 hr; **max. dose** of 40 mcg/24 hr [20 mcg spaced 12 hr apart]).

WARNING: Long-acting β_2-agonists may increase risk of asthma-related death. Only use formoterol as additional therapy for patients not adequately controlled on other asthma-controller medications (e.g., low- to medium-dose inhaled corticosteroids) or whose disease severity clearly requires initiation of treatment with 2 maintenance therapies. Should **not** be used in conjunction with an inhaled long-acting β_2-agonist, and is **not** a substitute for inhaled or systemic corticosteroids. See Chapter 24 for recommendations for asthma controller therapy.

FOSCARNET
Foscavir and generics
Antiviral agent

No   Yes   3   C

Injection: 24 mg/mL (250, 500 mL)

HIV positive or exposed with the following infection (IV):
CMV disease:
  Infant and child:
    Induction: 180 mg/kg/24 hr ÷ Q8 hr in combination with ganciclovir; continue until symptom improvement and convert to maintenance therapy
    Maintenance: 90–120 mg/kg/dose Q24 hr
CMV retinitis (disseminated disease):
  Infant and child:
    Induction: 180 mg/kg/24 hr ÷ Q8 hr × 14–21 days with or without ganciclovir
    Maintenance: 90–120 mg/kg/24 hr once daily
  Adolescent and adult:
    Induction: 180 mg/kg/24 hr ÷ Q8–12 hr × 14–21 days
    Maintenance: 90–120 mg/kg/24 hr once daily
Acyclovir-resistant herpes simplex:
  Infant and child: 40 mg/kg/dose Q8 hr or 60 mg/kg/dose Q12 hr for up to 3 wk or until lesions heal
  Adolescent and adult: 40 mg/kg/dose Q8–12 hr × 14–21 days or until lesions heal
Varicella zoster unresponsive to acyclovir:
  Infant and child: 40–60 mg/kg/dose Q8 hr × 7–10 days
  Adolescent: 90 mg/kg/dose Q12 hr
Varicella zoster, progressive outer retinal necrosis:
  Infant and child: 90 mg/kg/dose Q12 hr in combination with ganciclovir IV and intravitreal foscarnet with or without ganciclovir
  Adolescent: 90 mg/kg/dose Q12 hr in combination with IV ganciclovir and intravitreal foscarnet and/or ganciclovir
Intravitreal route for progressive outer retinal necrosis (HIV positive or exposed):
  Child and adolescent: 1.2 mg/0.05 mL per dose twice weekly in combination with IV foscarnet and ganciclovir and/or intravitreal ganciclovir

FOSCARNET *continued*

Use with caution in patients with renal insufficiency. **Discontinue use** in adults if serum Cr ≥ 2.9 mg/dL. **Adjust dose in renal failure (see Chapter 31).**
May cause peripheral neuropathy, seizures, hallucinations, GI disturbance, increased LFTs, hypertension, chest pain, ECG abnormalities, coughing, dyspnea, bronchospasm, and renal failure (adequate hydration and avoiding nephrotoxic medications may reduce risk). Hypocalcemia (increased risk if given with pentamidine), hypokalemia, and hypomagnesemia may also occur. Use with ciprofloxacin may increase risk for seizures.

FOSPHENYTOIN
Cerebyx and generics
Anticonvulsant

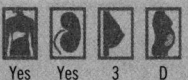

Yes   Yes   3   D

Injection: 50 mg phenytoin equivalent (75 mg fosphenytoin)/1 mL (2, 10 mL)
1 mg phenytoin equivalent provides 0.0037 mmol phosphate.

All doses are expressed as phenytoin sodium equivalents (PE) (see remarks for dose administration information):
Child: See Phenytoin and use the conversion of 1 mg phenytoin = 1 mg PE.
Adult:
   Loading dose:
      Status epilepticus: 15–20 mg PE/kg IV
      Nonemergent loading: 10–20 mg PE/kg IV/IM
      Nonemergent initial maintenance dose: 4–6 mg PE/kg/24 hr IV/IM ÷ once daily or BID

All doses should be prescribed and dispensed in terms of mg phenytoin sodium equivalents (PE) to avoid medication errors. Safety in pediatrics has not been fully established.
Use with caution in patients with renal or hepatic impairment and porphyria (consider amount of phosphate delivered by fosphenytoin in patients with phosphate restrictions). Drug is also metabolized to liberate small amounts of formaldehyde, which is considered clinically insignificant with short-term use (e.g., 1 wk). Side effects: hypokalemia (with rapid IV administration), slurred speech, dizziness, ataxia, rash, exfoliative dermatitis, nystagmus, diplopia, and tinnitus. Increased unbound phenytoin concentrations may occur in patients with renal disease or hypoalbuminemia; measure "free" or "unbound" phenytoin levels in these patients.
Abrupt withdrawal may cause status epilepticus. BP and ECG monitoring should be present during IV loading-dose administration. **Max. IV infusion rate:** 3 mg PE/kg/min up to a **max.** of 150 mg PE/min. Administer IM via 1 or 2 injection sites; IM route is **not recommended** in status epilepticus.
Therapeutic levels: 10–20 mg/L (free and bound phenytoin) *OR* 1–2 mg/L (free only). Recommended peak serum sampling times: 4 hr after an IM dose or 2 hr after an IV dose.
See *Phenytoin* remarks for drug interactions and additional side effects. Drug is more safely administered via peripheral IV than phenytoin.

For explanation of icons, see p. 648

FUROSEMIDE
Lasix and many generics
Loop diuretic

Yes   Yes   3   C/D

Tabs: 20, 40, 80 mg
Injection: 10 mg/mL (2, 4, 10 mL)
Oral solution: 10 mg/mL (60, 120 mL), 40 mg/5 mL (5, 500 mL)

IM, IV:
 Neonate (see remarks): 0.5–1 mg/kg/dose Q8–24 hr; **max. dose** 2 mg/kg/dose
 Infant and child: 1–2 mg/kg/dose Q6–12 hr
 Adult: 20–40 mg/24 hr ÷ Q6–12 hr; **max. dose** 600 mg/24 hr or 80 mg/dose
PO:
 Neonate: Bioavailability by this route is poor; doses of 1–4 mg/kg/dose once daily to BID have been used.
 Infant and child: Start at 2 mg/kg/dose; may increase by 1–2 mg/kg/dose no sooner than 6–8 hr after the previous dose. **Max. dose:** 6 mg/kg/dose. Dosages have ranged from 1–6 mg/kg/dose Q12–24 hr.
 Adult: 20–80 mg/dose Q6–12 hr; **max. dose** 600 mg/24 hr.
Continuous IV infusion:
 Infant and child: Start at 0.05 mg/kg/hr and titrate to effect.
 Adult: Start at 0.1 mg/kg/hr and titrate to effect; **max. dose** 0.4 mg/kg/hr.

Contraindicated in anuria and hepatic coma. **Use with caution** in hepatic disease (hepatic encephalopathy has been reported); cirrhotic patients may require higher doses than usual. Ototoxicity may occur in presence of renal disease (especially when used with aminoglycosides), with rapid IV injection (do not infuse >4 mg/min in adults), or with hypoproteinemia. May cause hypokalemia, alkalosis, dehydration, hyperuricemia, and increased calcium excretion. Prolonged use in premature infants and in children <4 yr may result in nephrocalcinosis. May increase risk for PDA in premature infants during the first week of life.

Furosemide-resistant edema in pediatric patients may benefit with the addition of metolazone. Some of these patients may have an exaggerated response, leading to hypovolemia, tachycardia, and orthostatic hypotension requiring fluid replacement. Severe hypokalemia has been reported with a tendency for diuresis persisting for up to 24 hr after discontinuing metolazone.

Max. rate of intermittent IV dose: 0.5 mg/kg/min. For patients receiving ECMO, **do not** administer IV doses directly into the ECMO circuit; medication is absorbed in the circuit, which may result in diminished effects and the need for higher doses.

Pregnancy category changes to "D" if used in pregnancy-induced hypertension.

GABAPENTIN
Neurontin, Gralise, Horizant, and generics
Anticonvulsant

No   Yes   2   C

Caps: 100, 300, 400 mg
Tabs: 300, 600, 800 mg
Slow-release/extended-release tabs (these dosage forms are **not** interchangeable with other gabapentin products; different pharmacokinetic profiles affect dosing interval [see specific product information for specific indications for use and dosage]):
 Gralise: 300, 600 mg
 Horizant (Gabapentin Enacarbil): 300, 600 mg
Oral solution: 250 mg/5 mL (470 mL)

GABAPENTIN *continued*

Seizures (maximum time between doses should not exceed 12 hr):
  3–12 yr (PO [see remarks]):
    Day 1: 10–15 mg/kg/24 hr ÷ TID, then gradually titrate dose upward to the following
      dosages over a 3-day period:
      3–4 yr: 40 mg/kg/24 hr ÷ TID
      ≥5–12 yr: 25–35 mg/kg/24 hr ÷ TID
      Dosages up to 50 mg/kg/24 hr have been well tolerated.
    >12 yr and adults (PO [see remarks]): Start with 300 mg TID; if needed, increase dose up to 1800
      mg/24 hr ÷ TID. Usual effective doses: 900–1800 mg/24 hr ÷ TID. Doses as high as 3.6 g/24 hr
      have been tolerated.
Neuropathic pain:
  Child (PO [limited data]):
    Day 1: 5 mg/kg/dose at bedtime
    Day 2: 5 mg/kg/dose BID
    Day 3: 5 mg/kg/dose TID, then titrate dose to effect. Usual dosage range: 8–35 mg/kg/24 hr.
    Maximum daily dose has not been evaluated.
  Adult (PO):
    Day 1: 300 mg at bedtime
    Day 2: 300 mg BID
    Day 3: 300 mg TID; then titrate dose to effect. Usual dosage range: 1800–2400 mg/24 hr; **max.
      dose** 3600 mg/24 hr.
    Postherpetic neuralgia: The above dosage regimen may be titrated up PRN for pain relief to a
      daily dose of 1800 mg/24 hr ÷ TID (efficacy has been shown from 1800–3600 mg/24 hr, but no
      additional benefit has been shown for doses >1800 mg/24 hr). The Gralise dosage form is
      designed for once-daily administration with the evening meal, whereas the Horizant dosage form
      is dosed once daily–BID. See specific product information for details.

Generally used as adjunctive therapy for partial and secondary generalized seizures and
  neuropathic pain.
Somnolence, dizziness, ataxia, fatigue, and nystagmus were common in use for seizures (≥12 yr).
  Viral infections, fever, nausea and/or vomiting, somnolence, and hostility have been reported in
  patients 3–12 yr receiving other antiepileptic drugs (AEDs). Dizziness, somnolence, and peripheral
  edema are common side effects in adults with postherpetic neuralgia. Suicidal behavior or ideation
  and multiorgan hypersensitivity (DRESS) have been reported.
Do not withdraw medication abruptly (withdraw gradually over a minimum of 1 wk). Drug is not
  metabolized by the liver and is primarily excreted unchanged in urine. Higher doses may be required
  for children <5 yr because of faster clearance in this age group.
May be taken with or without food. In TID dosing schedule, **interval between doses should not exceed
  12 hr. Adjust dose in renal impairment (see Chapter 31).**

GANCICLOVIR
Cytovene, Vitrasert, Zirgan, and others
Antiviral agent

   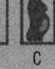

No   Yes   3   C

Injection: 500 mg; contains 4 mEq Na per 1 g drug
Intravitreal implant (sustained release over 5–8 mo):
Vitrasert: 4.5 mg
Ophthalmic gel (drops):
Zirgan: 0.15% (5 g); contains benzalkonium chloride

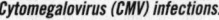

Cytomegalovirus (CMV) infections:
  Neonate (congenital CMV): 12 mg/kg/24 hr ÷ Q12 hr IV × 6 wk
  Child > 3 mo and adult:
    Induction therapy (duration 14–21 days): 10 mg/kg/24 hr ÷ Q12 hr IV
    IV maintenance therapy: 5 mg/kg/dose once daily IV for 7 days/wk *OR* 6 mg/kg/dose once daily IV for 5 days/wk
Prevention of CMV in transplant recipients:
  Child and adult:
    Induction therapy (duration 7–14 days): 10 mg/kg/24 hr ÷ Q12 hr IV
    IV maintenance therapy: 5 mg/kg/dose once daily IV for 7 days/wk *OR* 6 mg/kg/dose once daily IV for 5 days/wk for 100–120 days posttransplant
Prevention of CMV in HIV-infected individuals (see www.aidsinfo.nih.gov for latest recommendations and guidelines for CMV treatment as well):
  Recurrence prophylaxis:
    Infant, child, adolescent and adult: 5 mg/kg/dose IV once daily. Consider valganciclovir as an oral alternative.
CMV retinitis (intravitreal implant):
  ≥9 yr and adult: One implant lasts for 5–8 mo. As drug is depleted from implant, retinitis will progress; implant may be removed and replaced.
Herpetic keratitis (ophthalmic gel/drops):
  ≥2 yr and adult: Apply 1 drop onto affected eye(s) 5 times a day (≈Q3 hr while awake) until corneal ulcer is healed, then 1 drop TID × 7 days.

Limited experience with use in children <age 12. **Contraindicated** in severe neutropenia (ANC < 500/microliter) or severe thrombocytopenia (platelets < 25,000/microliter). **Use with extreme caution. Reduce dose in renal failure (see Chapter 31).** For oral route of administration, see *Valganciclovir.*

Common side effects: Neutropenia, thrombocytopenia, retinal detachment, confusion. Drug reactions alleviated with dose reduction or temporary interruption. Ganciclovir may increase didanosine and zidovudine levels, whereas didanosine and zidovudine may decrease ganciclovir levels. Immunosuppressive agents may increase hematologic toxicities. Amphotericin B and cyclosporine and tacrolimus increases risk for nephrotoxicity. Imipenem/cilastatin may increase risk for seizures.

Minimal dilution is 10 mg/mL and should be infused IV over ≥1 hr. IM and SC administration are **contraindicated** because of high pH (pH = 11).

GCSF

See Filgrastim

G

FORMULARY

GENTAMICIN
Garamycin and many generics
Antibiotic, aminoglycoside

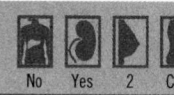

No   Yes   2   C/D

Injection: 10 mg/mL (2 mL), 40 mg/mL (2, 20 mL); some products may contain sodium metabisulfite
Premixed injection in NS: 40 mg (50 mL), 60 mg (50 mL), 70 mg (50 mL), 80 mg (50, 100 mL), 90 mg (100 mL), 100 mg (50, 100 mL), 120 mg (50, 100 mL)
Ophthalmic ointment: 0.3% (3.5 g)
Ophthalmic drops: 0.3% (5, 15 mL)
Topical ointment: 0.1% (15, 30 g)
Topical cream: 0.1% (15, 30 g)

Initial empirical dosage; patient-specific dosage defined by therapeutic drug monitoring (see remarks):
  Parenteral (IM or IV):
    Neonate/Infant (see table below):

Postconceptional Age (wk)	Postnatal Age (days)	Dose (mg/kg/dose)	Interval (hr)
≤29*	0–7	5	48
	8–28	4	36
	>28	4	24
30–33	0–7	4.5	36
	>7	4	24
34–37	0–7	4	24
	>7	4	18–24
≥38	0–7	4	24†
	>7	4	12–18

*Or significant asphyxia, PDA, indomethacin use, poor cardiac output, reduced renal function.
†Use Q36 hr interval for HIE patients receiving whole-body therapeutic cooling.

  Child: 7.5 mg/kg/24 hr ÷ Q8 hr
  Adult: 3–6 mg/kg/24 hr ÷ Q8 hr
  Cystic Fibrosis: 7.5–10.5 mg/kg/24 hr ÷ Q8 hr
Intrathecal/intraventricular (use preservative-free product only):
  Newborn: 1 mg once daily
  >3 mo: 1–2 mg once daily
  Adult: 4–8 mg once daily
Ophthalmic ointment: Apply Q8–12 hr
Ophthalmic drops: 1–2 drops Q2–4 hr

Use with caution in patients receiving anesthetics or neuromuscular blocking agents, and in patients with neuromuscular disorders. May cause nephrotoxicity and ototoxicity. Ototoxicity may be potentiated with the use of loop diuretics. Eliminated more quickly in patients with cystic fibrosis, neutropenia, and burns. **Adjust dose in renal failure (see Chapter 31).** Monitor peak and trough levels.

Therapeutic peak levels are 6–10 mg/L in general, and 8–10 mg/L in pulmonary infections, cystic fibrosis, neutropenia, osteomyelitis, and severe sepsis.

To maximize bactericidal effects, an individualized peak concentration to target a peak/MIC ratio of 8–10:1 may be applied.

Therapeutic trough levels: <2 mg/L. Recommended serum sampling time at steady state: trough within 30 min before third consecutive dose, and peak 30–60 min after administration of third consecutive dose.

For initial dosing in obese patients, use an adjusted body weight (ABW). ABW = Ideal body weight + 0.4 (Total body weight − Ideal body weight).

Pregnancy category is "C" for ophthalmic use and "D" with IV use.

For explanation of icons, see p. 648

GLUCAGON HCl
GlucaGen, Glucagon Emergency Kit
Antihypoglycemic agent
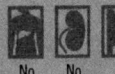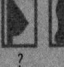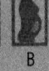
No   No   ?   B

Injection: 1 mg vial (requires reconstitution)
1 unit = 1 mg

Hypoglycemia (IM, IV, SC):
Neonate, infant, and child < 20 kg: 0.5 mg/dose (or 0.02–0.03 mg/kg/dose) Q20 min PRN
Child ≥ 20 kg and adult: 1 mg/dose Q20 min PRN
β-Blocker and calcium channel blocker overdose: Load with 0.05–0.15 mg/kg (usually ≈ 10 mg in adults) IV over 1 min, followed by an IV infusion of 0.05–0.1 mg/kg/hr.
Alternatively, 5-mg IV bolus Q5–10 min PRN up to 4 doses. If patient is responsive at a particular bolus dose, initiate an hourly IV infusion at that same responsive dose (e.g., if patient responded at 10 mg, start infusion of 10 mg/hr).

Use with caution in insulinoma and/or pheochromocytoma. Drug product is genetically engineered and identical to human glucagon. High doses have cardiac stimulatory effect and have had some success in β-blocker and calcium channel blocker overdose. May cause nausea, vomiting, urticaria, and respiratory distress. **Do not delay** glucose infusion; dose for hypoglycemia is 2–4 mL/kg of dextrose 25%.
Onset of action: IM, 8–10 min; IV, 1 min. Duration of action: IM, 12–27 min; IV, 9–17 min.

GLYCERIN
Pedia-Lax, Sani-Supp, Fleet Liquid Supp, and others
Osmotic Laxative
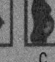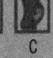
No   No   ?   C

Rectal solution [OTC]: 4 mL per application (6 doses), 7.5 mL per application (4 doses)
Suppository [OTC]:
Infant/pediatric: 1, 1.2 g (10s, 12s, 25s)
Adult: 2 g (10s, 12s, 24s, 25s, 50s)

Constipation:
Neonate: 0.5 mL/kg/dose rectal solution PR as an enema once daily PRN or half of infant suppository PR once daily PRN
Child < 6 yr: 2–5 mL rectal solution PR as an enema or 1 infant suppository PR once daily PRN
>6 yr–adult: 5–15 mL rectal solution PR as an enema or 1 adult suppository PR once daily PRN

Onset of action: 15–30 min. May cause rectal irritation, abdominal pain, bloating, and dizziness. Insert suppository high into rectum and retain for 15 min.

GLYCOPYRROLATE
Robinul, Cuvposa, Glycate, and generics
Anticholinergic agent
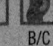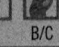
Yes   Yes   ?   B/C

Tabs: 1, 1.5, 2 mg
Oral solution (Cuvposa): 1 mg/5 mL; contains propylene glycol and parabens
Injection: 0.2 mg/mL (1, 2, 5, 20 mL); some multidose vials contain 0.9% benzyl alcohol

Respiratory antisecretory:
IM/IV:
Child: 0.004–0.01 mg/kg/dose Q4–8 hr

GLYCOPYRROLATE *continued*

Adult: 0.1–0.2 mg/dose Q4–8 hr
Max. dose: 0.2 mg/dose or 0.8 mg/24 hr
Oral:
Child: 0.04–0.1 mg/kg/dose Q4–8 hr
Adult: 1–2 mg/dose BID–TID
Reverse neuromuscular blockade:
Child and adult: 0.2 mg IV for every 1 mg neostigmine or 5 mg pyridostigmine

Use with caution in hepatic and renal disease, ulcerative colitis, asthma, glaucoma, ileus, or urinary retention. Atropine-like side effects: tachycardia, nausea, constipation, confusion, blurred vision, and dry mouth. These may be potentiated if given with other drugs with anticholinergic properties.

Onset of action: PO, within 1 hr; IM/SC, 15–30 min; IV, 1 min. Duration of antisialogogue effect: PO, 8–12 hr; IM/SC/IV, 7 hr.

Pregnancy category is "B" for the injection and tablet dosage forms and "C" for the oral solution.

GRANISETRON
Kytril, Granisol, Sancuso, and generics
Antiemetic agent, 5-HT₃ antagonist

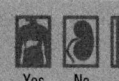

Yes No ? B

Injection: 1 mg/mL (1, 4 mL); 4-mL vials contain benzyl alcohol
Tabs: 1 mg
Oral liquid (Granisol): 0.2 mg/mL (30 mL); contains sodium benzoate
Transdermal patch (Sancuso): 3.1 mg/24 hr

Chemotherapy-induced nausea and vomiting:
IV:
Child ≥ 2 yr and adult: 10–20 mcg/kg/dose 15–60 min before chemotherapy; same dose may be repeated 2–3 times at ≥10-min intervals after chemotherapy (within 24 hr after chemotherapy) as a treatment regimen. **Max. dose:** 3 mg/dose or 9 mg/24 hr. Alternatively, a single 40-mcg/kg/dose 15–60 min before chemotherapy has been used.
PO:
Adult: 2 mg/24 hr ÷ once daily–BID; initiate first dose 1 hr before chemotherapy.
Postoperative nausea and vomiting prevention (dosed before anesthesia or immediately before anesthesia reversal) and treatment (IV; see remarks):
Adult: 1 mg × 1
Radiation-induced nausea and vomiting prevention:
Adult: 2 mg once daily PO administered 1 hr before radiation
Transdermal patch:
Prophylaxis for chemotherapy-induced nausea and vomiting (adult): Apply 1 patch 24–48 hr prior before chemotherapy. Patch may be worn up to 7 days, depending on chemotherapy regimen duration.

Use with caution in liver disease and preexisting cardiac conduction disorders and arrhythmias. May cause hypertension, hypotension, arrhythmias, agitation, and insomnia. Inducers or inhibitors of the CYP 450 3A3/4 drug metabolizing enzymes may increase or decrease, respectively, the drug's clearance. QT prolongation has been reported.

Safety and efficacy in pediatric patients for prevention of postoperative nausea and vomiting has not been established owing to lack of efficacy and QT prolongation in a prospective multicenter randomized double-blinded trial in 157 patients (2–16 years old).

Onset of action: IV, 4–10 min. Duration of action: IV, ≤24 hr.

GRISEOFULVIN
Grifulvin V, Griseofulvin Microsize, Grisactin, Gris-PEG, and generics
Antifungal agent

Yes   No   ?   C

Microsize:
   Tabs (Grifulvin V): 500 mg
   Oral suspension (Griseofulvin Microsize): 125 mg/5 mL (120 mL); contains 0.2% alcohol, parabens, and propylene glycol
Ultramicrosize (250 mg ultramicrosize is ≈ 500 mg microsize):
   Tabs (Gris-PEG): 125, 250 mg

Microsize:
  Child > 2 yr: 10–20 mg/kg/24 hr PO ÷ once daily–BID; give with milk, eggs, fatty foods. Some have recommended a higher dose of 20–25 mg/kg/24 hr PO for tinea capitis to improve efficacy, owing to to relative resistance of the organism.
  Adult: 500–1000 mg/24 hr PO ÷ once daily–BID
  Max. dose (all ages): 1 g/24 hr
Ultramicrosize:
  Child > 2 yr: 10–15 mg/kg/24 hr PO ÷ once daily–BID
  Adult: 330–750 mg/24 hr PO ÷ once daily–BID
  Max. dose (all ages): 750 mg/24 hr

Contraindicated in porphyria, pregnancy, and hepatic disease. Monitor hematologic, renal, and hepatic function. May cause leukopenia, rash, headache, paresthesias, and GI symptoms. Severe skin reactions (e.g., Stevens-Johnson syndrome, TEN), erythema multiforme, LFT elevations (AST, ALT, bilirubin), and jaundice have been reported. Possible cross-reactivity in penicillin-allergic patients. Usual treatment period is 8 wk for tinea capitis and 4–6 mo for tinea unguium. Photosensitivity reactions may occur. May reduce effectiveness or decrease level of oral contraceptives, warfarin, and cyclosporine. Induces CYP 450 1A2 isoenzyme. Phenobarbital may enhance clearance of griseofulvin. Coadministration with fatty meals will increase drug's absorption.

GUANFACINE
Intuniv, Tenex, and generics
α₂-Adrenergic agonist

Yes   Yes   3   B

Tabs: 1, 2 mg
Extended-release tabs: 1, 2, 3, 4 mg

Attention deficit hyperactivity disorder (see remarks):
  Immediate-release tab:
    ≥6 yr and adolescent:
      ≤45 kg: Start at 0.5 mg QHS; if needed and tolerated, increase dose every 3–4 days at 0.5 mg/24-hr increments by increasing dosing frequency to BID, TID, QID. **Max. dose:** 27--40.5 kg: 2 mg/24 hr and 40.5--45 kg: 3 mg/24 hr.
      >45 kg: Start at 1 mg QHS; if needed and tolerated, increase dose every 3–4 days at 1 mg/24-hr increments by increasing dosing frequency to BID, TID, QID. **Max. dose:** 4 mg/24 hr.
  Extended-release tab:
    6–17 yr: Start at 1 mg Q24 hr; if needed and tolerated, increase dose no more than 1 mg/wk up to **max. dose** of 4 mg/24 hr.

GUANFACINE *continued*

Use with strong CYP 450 3A4 inhibitors or inducers:

CYP 450 3A4 characteristic	Adding guanfacine with respective CYP 450 3A4 inducer/inhibitor already on board.	Adding respective CYP 450 3A4 inducer/inhibitor with guanfacine already on board.
Strong inducer (e.g., carbamazepine, phenytoin, rifampin, St. John's Wort)	Guanfacine may be titrated faster at 2 mg/wk; if needed and tolerated, up to a **max.** of 8 mg/24 hr.	Gradually double original guanfacine dose over 1–2 wk as tolerated. When the strong inducer is discontinued, decrease guanfacine dose by 50% over 1–2 weeks (**max. dose** 4 mg/24 hr).
Strong inhibitor (e.g., clarithromycin, azole antifungals)	Use lower **max.** daily guanfacine dose of 2 mg/24 hr.	Decrease guanfacine dose by 50%. When the strong inhibitor is discontinued, double the guanfacine dose (**max. dose** 4 mg/24 hr).

Use with caution in patients at risk for hypotension, bradycardia, heart block, and syncope. A dose-dependent hypotension and bradycardia may occur. Orthostatic hypotension and syncope have been reported. Somnolence, fatigue, insomnia, dizziness, and abdominal pain are common side effects.
Drug is a substrate for CYP 450 3A4. See dosing section for dosage adjustment with inhibitors and inducers.
Do not abruptly discontinue therapy. Dose reductions may be required with clinically significant renal or hepatic impairment. When converting from immediate-release tabs to extended-release tabs, **do not** convert on a mg-per-mg basis (there are differences in pharmacokinetic profiles), but discontinue the immediate-release, and titrate with the extended-release product using the recommended dosing schedule.

HALOPERIDOL
Haldol, Haldol Decanoate, and generics
Antipsychotic agent

Yes   Yes   3   C

Injection (IM use only):
Lactate: 5 mg/mL (1, 10 mL); may contain parabens
Decanoate (long-acting): 50, 100 mg/mL (1, 5 mL); in sesame oil with 1.2% benzyl alcohol
Tabs: 0.5, 1, 2, 5, 10, 20 mg
Oral solution: 2 mg/mL (15, 120 mL)

Child 3–12 yr:
PO: Initial dose at 0.025–0.05 mg/kg/24 hr ÷ BID–TID. If necessary, increase daily dosage by 0.25–0.5 mg/24 hr Q5–7 days PRN up to a **max. dose** of 0.15 mg/kg/24 hr. Usual maintenance doses for specific indications include:
    Agitation: 0.01–0.03 mg/kg/24 hr once daily PO
    Psychosis: 0.05–0.15 mg/kg/24 hr ÷ BID–TID PO
    Tourette syndrome: 0.05–0.075 mg/kg/24 hr ÷ BID–TID PO; may increase daily dose by 0.5 mg Q5–7 days
IM, as lactate, for 6–12 yr: 1–3 mg/dose Q4–8 hr; **max. dose** 0.15 mg/kg/24 hr
>12 yr:
    Acute agitation: 2–5 mg/dose IM as lactate *OR* 1–15 mg/dose PO; repeat in 1 hr PRN
    Psychosis: 2–5 mg/dose Q4–8 hr IM PRN *OR* 1–15 mg/24 hr ÷ BID–TID PO
    Tourette syndrome: 0.5–2 mg/dose BID–TID PO; 3–5 mg/dose BID–TID PO may be used for severe symptoms

For explanation of icons, see p. 648

Continued

HALOPERIDOL *continued*

Use with caution in patients with cardiac disease (risk of hypotension), renal or hepatic dysfunction, thyrotoxicosis, and in patients with epilepsy (drug lowers the seizure threshold). Extrapyramidal symptoms, drowsiness, headache, tachycardia, ECG changes, nausea, and vomiting can occur. Higher-than-recommended doses are associated with a higher risk of QT prolongation and torsades de pointes. Leukopenia/neutropenia, including agranulocytosis, has been reported.

Drug is metabolized by CYP 450 1A2, 2D6, and 3A3/4 isoenzymes. May also inhibit CYP 450 2D6 and 3A3/4 isoenzymes. Serotonin-specific reuptake inhibitors (e.g., fluoxetine) may increase levels and effects of haloperidol. Carbamazepine and phenobarbital may decrease levels and effects of haloperidol. Monitor for encephalopathic syndrome when used in combination with lithium.

Acutely aggravated patients may require doses as often as Q60 min. **Decanoate salt is given every 3–4 wk in doses that are 10–15 times the individual patient's stabilized oral dose.**

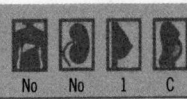

HEPARIN SODIUM
Various generics
Anticoagulant

No No 1 C

Injection:
Porcine intestinal mucosa: 1000, 2500, 5000, 10,000, 20,000 U/mL (Some products may be preservative-free; multidose vials contain benzyl alcohol.)
Lock flush solution (porcine based): 1, 10, 100 U/mL (Some products may be preservative-free or contain benzyl alcohol.)
Injection for IV infusion (porcine based):
D_5W: 40 U/mL (500 mL), 50 U/mL (500 mL), 100 U/mL (100, 250 mL); contains bisulfite
NS (0.9% NaCl): 2 U/mL (500, 1000 mL)
0.45% NaCl: 50 U/mL (250, 500 mL), 100 U/mL (250 mL); contains EDTA
120 U = approximately 1 mg

Anticoagulation empirical dosage (see Chapter 14 for dosage adjustments):
Continuous IV infusion (initial doses for goal *unfractionated* heparin (UFH) anti-Xa level of 0.3–0.7 units/mL):

Age	Loading Dose (IV)*	Initial IV Infusion Rate (units/kg/hr)
Neonate and infant < 1 yr	75 U/kg IV	28
Child ≤ 1–16 yr	75 U/kg IV (**max. dose 7700 U**)	20 (max. initial rate: 1650 U/hr)
>16 yr	70 U/kg IV (**max. dose 7700 U**)	15 (max. initial rate: 1650 U/hr)

*Do not give loading dose for stroke patients, and obtain aPTT 4 hr after loading dose.

DVT or PE prophylaxis:
Adult: 5000 U/dose SC Q8–12 hr until ambulatory
Heparin flush (doses should be less than heparinizing dose):
Younger child: Lower doses should be used to avoid systemic heparinization.
Older child and adult:
Peripheral IV: 1–2 mL of 10 U/mL solution Q4 hr
Central lines: 2–3 mL of 100 U/mL solution Q24 hr
TPN (central line) and arterial line: Add heparin to make final concentration of 0.5–1 U/mL.

Contraindicated in active major bleeding, known or suspected HIT, and concurrent epidural therapy. **Use with caution** if platelets <50,000/mm³. **Avoid** IM injections and other medications affecting platelet function (e.g., NSAIDs, ASA). Toxicities include bleeding, allergy, alopecia, and thrombocytopenia.

H

FORMULARY

HEPARIN SODIUM *continued*

Adjust dose with one of the following laboratory goals:

Unfractionated heparin (UFH) anti-Xa level: 0.3–0.7 units/mL

aPTT level (reagent specific to reflect anti-Xa level of 0.3–0.7 units/mL): 50–80 seconds.

These laboratory measurements are best measured 4–6 hr after initiation or changes in infusion rate.
Do not collect blood levels from the heparinized line or same extremity as site of heparin infusion. If *unfractionated* heparin anti-Xa or aPTT levels are not available, a ratio of aPTT 1.5–2.5 times control value has been used in the past. *Unfractionated* heparin anti-Xa level is NOT THE SAME as *low-molecular-weight* heparin (LMWH) anti-Xa (used for monitoring LMWH products such as enoxaparin).

Use preservative-free heparin in neonates. **Note**: heparin flush doses may alter APTT in small patients; consider using more dilute heparin in these cases.

Use actual body weight when dosing obese patients. Due to recent regulatory changes to the manufacturing process, heparin products may exhibit decreased potency.

Antidote: protamine sulfate (1 mg per 100 U heparin in previous 4 hr). For LMWH, see *Enoxaparin.*

HYALURONIDASE
Amphadase, Hylenex, Vitrase
Antidote, extravasation

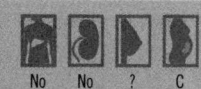

No   No   ?   C

Injection:
Amphadase: 150 U/mL (1 mL); bovine source and contains thimerosal
Hylenex: 150 U/mL (1 mL); recombinant human source; contains 1 mg albumin per 150 U
Vitrase: 200 U/mL (1.2 mL); ovine source, preservative-free
Pharmacy can make a 15 U/mL dilution.

Infant and child: Give 1 mL (150 U) by injecting 5 separate injections of 0.2 mL (30 U) at borders of extravasation site SC or intradermally, using a 25- or 26-gauge needle. Alternatively, a diluted 15 U/mL concentration has been used with the same dosing instructions.

Contraindicated in dopamine and α-agonist extravasation and hypersensitivity to the respective product sources (bovine or ovine). May cause urticaria. Patients receiving large amounts of salicylates, cortisone, ACTH, estrogens, or antihistamines may decrease the effects of hyaluronidase (larger doses may be necessary). Administer as early as possible (minutes to 1 hour) after IV extravasation.

HYDRALAZINE HYDROCHLORIDE
Apresoline and generics
Antihypertensive, vasodilator

No   Yes   1   C

Tabs: 10, 25, 50, 100 mg
Injection: 20 mg/mL (1 mL)
Oral liquid: 1.25, 4 mg/mL
Some dosage forms may contain tartrazines or sulfites.

Hypertensive crisis (may result in severe and prolonged hypotension, see Chapter 4 for alternatives).
Child: 0.1–0.2 mg/kg/dose IM or IV Q4–6 hr PRN; **max. dose** 20 mg/dose. Usual IV/IM dosage range is 1.7–3.5 mg/kg/24 hr
Adult: 10–40 mg IM or IV Q4–6 hr PRN

Continued

For explanation of icons, see p. 648

HYDRALAZINE HYDROCHLORIDE *continued*

Chronic hypertension:
Infant and child: Start at 0.75–1 mg/kg/24 hr PO ÷ Q6–12 hr (**max. dose** 25 mg/dose). If necessary, increase dose over 3–4 wk up to a **max. dose** of 5 mg/kg/24 hr for infants and 7.5 mg/kg/24 hr for children, or 200 mg/24 hr.
Adult: 10–50 mg/dose PO QID; **max. dose** of 300 mg/24 hr

Use with caution in severe renal and cardiac disease. Slow acetylators, patients receiving high-dose chronic therapy, and those with renal insufficiency are at highest risk of lupus-like syndrome (generally reversible). May cause reflex tachycardia, palpitations, dizziness, headaches, and GI discomfort. MAO inhibitors and β-blockers may increase hypotensive effects. Indomethacin may decrease hypotensive effects.

Drug undergoes first-pass metabolism. Onset of action: PO, 20–30 min; IV, 5–20 min. Duration of action: PO, 2–4 hr; IV, 2–6 hr. **Adjust dose in renal failure (see Chapter 31).**

HYDROCHLOROTHIAZIDE
Microzide, many generics, and previously available as Hydrodiuril
Diuretic, thiazide

No   Yes   2   B/D

Tabs: 12.5, 25, 50 mg
Caps (Microzide and generics): 12.5 mg

Edema:
Neonate and infant < 6 mo: 2–4 mg/kg/24 hr ÷ BID PO; **max. dose** 37.5 mg/24 hr
≥6 mo and child: 2 mg/kg/24 hr ÷ BID PO; **max. dose** 100 mg/24 hr
Adult: 25–100 mg/24 hr ÷ once daily–BID PO; **max. dose** 200 mg/24 hr
Hypertension:
Infant and child: Start at 0.5–1 mg/kg/24 hr once daily PO; dose may be increased to a **max. dose** of 3 mg/kg/24 hr up to 50 mg/24 hr.
Adult: 12.5–25 mg/dose once daily–BID PO; doses >50 mg/24 hr often result in hypokalemia.

See *Chlorothiazide*. May cause fluid and electrolyte imbalances and hyperuricemia. Drug may not be effective when creatinine clearance is <25–50 mL/min. Use with carbamazepine may result in symptomatic hyponatremia.

Hydrochlorothiazide is also available in combination with potassium-sparing diuretics (e.g., spironolactone), ACE inhibitors, angiotensin II receptor antagonists, hydralazine, methyldopa, reserpine, and β-blockers.

Pregnancy category is "D" if used in pregnancy-induced hypertension.

HYDROCORTISONE
Solu-Cortef, Cortef, Cortifoam, Colocort, Cortenema, NuCort, and many others, including generics
Corticosteroid

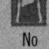

No   No   3   C/D

Hydrocortisone base:
Tabs (Cortef and generics): 5, 10, 20 mg
Oral suspension: 1, 2, 2.5 mg/mL
Rectal cream: 1% (30 g), 2.5% (30 g)
Rectal suspension (Colocort, Cortenema): 100 mg/60 mL (7s)
Topical ointment: 0.5% [OTC], 1% [OTC], 2.5%

HYDROCORTISONE *continued*

Topical cream: 0.5% [OTC], 1% [OTC], 2.5%
Topical lotion: 1% [OTC], 2.5%
Na Succinate (Solu-Cortef):
Injection: 100, 250, 500, 1000 mg/vial; contains benzyl alcohol
Acetate:
Topical ointment [OTC]: 0.5%, 1%
Topical cream [OTC]: 0.5%, 1%
Topical lotion (NuCort): 2% (60 g); contains benzyl alcohol
Rectal cream: 1%
Suppository: 25, 30 mg
Rectal foam aerosol (Cortifoam): 10% (90 mg/dose) (15 g)

Status asthmaticus:
Child:
Loading dose (optional): 4–8 mg/kg/dose IV; **max. dose** of 250 mg
Maintenance: 8 mg/kg/24 hr ÷ Q6 hr IV
Adult: 100–500 mg/dose Q6 hr IV
Physiologic replacement: see Chapter 10 for dosing.
Anti-inflammatory/immunosuppressive:
Child:
PO: 2.5–10 mg/kg/24 hr ÷ Q6–8 hr
IM/IV: 1–5 mg/kg/24 hr ÷ Q12–24 hr
Adolescent and adult:
PO/IM/IV: 15–240 mg/dose Q12 hr
Acute adrenal insufficiency: See Chapter 10 for dosing.
Topical use:
Child and adult: Apply to affected areas BID–QID, depending on severity.
Rectal use:
Adolescent and adult: Insert 1 application once daily–BID × 2–3 weeks.

Use with caution in immunocompromised patients; they should avoid exposure to
chickenpox or measles.
For doses based on body surface area and topical preparations (with comparisons),
see Chapters 10 and 30. Pregnancy category changes to "D" if used in first trimester.

HYDROMORPHONE HCL
Dilaudid, Dilaudid-HP, Exalgo, and generics
Narcotic, analgesic

Yes   Yes   3   C/D

Tabs: 2, 4, 8 mg
Extended-release tabs (Exalgo): 8, 12, 16, 32 mg
Injection: 1, 2, 4, 10 mg/mL (may contain methyl- and propylparabens)
Powder for injection (Dilaudid-HP): 250 mg
Suppository: 3 mg
Oral solution: 1 mg/mL

Analgesia, initial doses (titrate to effect):
Child (<50 kg):
IV: 0.015 mg/kg/dose Q4–6 hr PRN
PO: 0.03–0.08 mg/kg/dose Q4–6 hr PRN; **max. dose** 5 mg/dose

Continued

For explanation of icons, see p. 648

HYDROMORPHONE HCL *continued*

Analgesia, initial doses (titrate to effect):

Adolescent (>50 kg) and adult:
   IM, IV, SC: 1–2 mg/dose Q4–6 hr PRN
   PO:
      Adolescent: 1–2 mg/dose Q4–6 hr PRN
      Adult: 2–4 mg/dose Q4–6 hr PRN

Refer to Chapter 6 for equianalgesic doses and for patient-controlled analgesia dosing. Less
   pruritus than morphine. Similar profile of side effects to other narcotics. **Use with caution** in
   infants and young children, and **do not use** in neonates (potential CNS effects). Dose
   reduction recommended in renal insufficiency or severe hepatic impairment. Pregnancy
   category changes to "D" if used for prolonged periods or in high doses at term.
Extended-release tab use requires Risk Evaluation and Mitigation Strategies (REMS)-based provision
   of safety information and postmarketing safety studies.

HYDROXYCHLOROQUINE
Plaquenil and generics
Antimalarial, antirheumatic agent
                                                      Yes   Yes   2   ?

Tabs: 200 mg (155 mg base)
Oral suspension: 25 mg/mL (19.375 mg/mL base)

All doses expressed in mg of hydroxychloroquine base.
*Malaria prophylaxis (start 2 wk before exposure and continue for 4 wk after leaving
endemic area):*
   Child: 5 mg/kg/dose PO once weekly; **max. dose** 310 mg
   Adult: 310 mg PO once weekly
Malaria treatment (acute uncomplicated cases):
For treatment of malaria, consult with ID specialist or see the latest edition of the AAP *Red Book.*
   Child: 10 mg/kg/dose (**max. dose** 620 mg) PO × 1, followed by 5 mg/kg/dose (**max. dose** 310 mg)
   6 hr later. Then 5 mg/kg/dose (**max. dose** 310 mg) Q24 hr × 2 doses, starting 24 hr after first
   dose.
   Adult: 620 mg PO × 1, followed by 310 mg 6 hr later. Then 310 mg Q24 hr × 2 doses, starting 24 hr
   after first dose.
Juvenile rheumatoid arthritis or systemic lupus erythematosus:
   Child: 2.325–3.875 mg/kg/24 hr (base) PO ÷ once daily–BID; **max. dose** of 310 mg/24 hr, **not to
   exceed** 5.425 mg/kg/24 hr.

Contraindicated in psoriasis, porphyria, retinal or visual field changes, and 4-aminoquinoline
   hypersensitivity. **Use with caution** in liver disease, G6PD deficiency, concomitant hepatic
   toxic drugs, renal impairment, metabolic acidosis, or hematologic disorders.
Long-term use in children is **not recommended**. May cause headaches, myopathy, GI disturbances,
   skin and mucosal pigmentation, agranulocytosis, visual disturbances, and increased digoxin serum
   levels. Use with aurothioglucose may increase risk for blood dyscrasias.
When used in combination with other immunosuppressive agents for SLE and JRA, lower doses of
   hydroxychloroquine can be used.
Pregnancy category has not been formally assigned by the FDA. The only situation where use is
   recommended during pregnancy is during suppression or treatment of malaria, when benefits
   outweigh risks.

HYDROXYZINE
Vistaril and various generics
Antihistamine, anxiolytic, antiemetic

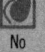

Yes   No   3   C

Tabs (HCl salt): 10, 25, 50 mg
Caps (pamoate salt): 25, 50, 100 mg
Oral syrup, solution (HCl salt): 10 mg/5 mL (120, 473 mL); may contain alcohol
Injection for IM use (HCl salt): 25, 50 mg/mL; may contain benzyl alcohol
NOTE: Pamoate and HCL salts are equivalent in regard to mg of hydroxyzine.

Pruritus and anxiety:
Oral:
  Child: 2 mg/kg/24 hr ÷ Q6–8 hr PRN
  Max. single dose:
    <6 yr: 12.5 mg,
    6–12 yr: 25 mg
    >12 yr: 100 mg
    Alternative dosing by age:
      <6 yr: 50 mg/24 hr ÷ Q6–8 hr PRN
      ≥6 yr: 50–100 mg/24 hr ÷ Q6–8 hr PRN
  Adult: 25 mg/dose TID–QID PRN; **max. dose** 600 mg/24 hr
IM:
  Child and adolescent: 0.5–1 mg/kg/dose Q4–6 hr PRN; **max. single dose** 100 mg
  Adult: 25–100 mg/dose Q4–6 hr PRN; **max. dose** 600 mg/24 hr

May potentiate barbiturates, meperidine, and other CNS depressants. May cause dry mouth, drowsiness, tremor, convulsions, blurred vision, and hypotension. May cause pain at injection site.

Increase dosage interval to Q24 hr or less in the presence of liver disease (e.g., primary biliary cirrhosis).

Onset of action within 15–30 min. Duration of action 4–6 hr. IV administration is **not recommended**.

IBUPROFEN
PO: Motrin, Advil, Children's Advil, Children's Motrin, and generics
IV: NeoProfen, Caldolor
Nonsteroidal anti-inflammatory agent

Yes   Yes   1   C/D

Oral suspension [OTC]: 100 mg/5 mL (60, 120, 480 mL)
Oral drops [OTC]: 40 mg/mL (15, 30 mL)
Chewable tabs [OTC]: 50, 100 mg
Caplets [OTC]: 100, 200 mg
Tabs: 100 [OTC], 200 [OTC], 400, 600, 800 mg
Capsules [OTC]: 200 mg
Injection:
  NeoProfen (lysine salt): 10 mg ibuprofen base/1 mL (2 mL)
  Caldolor: 100 mg/mL (4, 8 mL); contains 78 mg/mL arginine

PO:
Infant and child (≥6 mo):
  Analgesic/antipyretic: 5–10 mg/kg/dose Q6–8 hr PO; **max. dose** 40 mg/kg/24 hr
  JRA (6 mo–12 yr): 30–50 mg/kg/24 hr ÷ Q6 hr PO; **max. dose** 2400 mg/24 hr

Continued

IBUPROFEN *continued*

Adult:

> *Inflammatory disease:* 400–800 mg/dose Q6–8 hr PO; **max. dose** 800 mg/dose *OR* 3.2 g/24 hr
> *Pain/fever/dysmenorrhea:* 200–400 mg/dose Q4–6 hr PRN PO; **max. dose** 1.2 g/24 hr

IV:

> *Analgesic (≥17 yr and adult [see remarks]):* 400–800 mg/dose Q6 hr PRN; **max. dose** 3200 mg/24 hr
> *Antipyretic (≥17 yr and adult [see remarks]):* 400 mg/dose Q4–6 hr or 100–200 mg/dose Q4 hr PRN; **max. dose** 3200 mg/24 hr

Closure of ductus arteriosus:

> *<32 wk of gestation and 0.5–1.5 kg (use birth weight to calculate all doses and infuse all doses over 15 min [see remarks]):* 10 mg/kg/dose IV × 1, followed by 2 doses of 5 mg/kg/dose each after 24 and 48 hr. Hold second or third dose if urinary output is <0.6 mL/kg/hr; dosing should resume when laboratory studies indicate return of normal renal function. If ductus arteriosus fails to close or reopens, a second course of ibuprofen, use of IV indomethacin, or surgery may be necessary.

Contraindicated with active GI bleeding and ulcer disease. **Use caution** with aspirin hypersensitivity, hepatic/renal insufficiency, heart disease (risk for MI and stroke with prolonged use), dehydration, and in patients receiving anticoagulants. GI distress (lessened with milk), rashes, ocular problems, hypertension, granulocytopenia, and anemia may occur. Inhibits platelet aggregation. Consumption of more than three alcoholic beverages per day or use with corticosteroids or anticoagulants may increase risk for GI bleeding.

May increase serum levels and effects of digoxin, methotrexate, and lithium. May decrease effects of antihypertensives, aspirin (antiplatelet effects), furosemide, and thiazide diuretics. Pregnancy category changes to "D" if used in third trimester or near delivery.

IV USE for analgesia/antipyretic: Hydrate patient well before use. Doses must be diluted to a concentration ≤4 mg/mL with NS, D_5W, or LR and infused over ≥30 min. Most common reported side effects in clinical trials include nausea, flatulence, vomiting, and headache.

IV USE for PDA: Contraindicated in untreated infections, congenital heart diseases requiring a patent ductus arteriosus to facilitate satisfactory pulmonary and systemic blood flow, active intracranial or GI bleeds, thrombocytopenia, coagulation defects, suspected/active NEC, and significant renal impairment. **Use with caution** in hyperbilirubinemia. Not indicated for IVH prophylaxis. Renal side effects are generally less frequent and severe than with IV indomethacin.

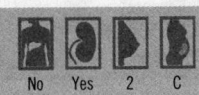

IMIPENEM AND CILASTATIN
Primaxin IV and generics
Antibiotic, carbapenem

| No | Yes | 2 | C |

Injection: 250, 500 mg; contains 3.2 mEq Na/g drug
Each 1 mg drug contains 1 mg imipenem and 1 mg cilastatin.

Neonate:

> *0–4 wk old and <1.2 kg:* 50 mg/kg/24 hr ÷ Q12 hr IV
> *<1 wk old and ≥1.2 kg:* 50 mg/kg/24 hr ÷ Q12 hr IV
> *≥1 wk old and ≥1.2 kg:* 75 mg/kg/24 hr ÷ Q8 hr IV

Child (4 wk–3 mo): 100 mg/kg/24 hr ÷ Q6 hr IV

Child (>3 mo): 60–100 mg/kg/24 hr ÷ Q6 hr IV; **max. dose** 4 g/24 hr

> *Cystic fibrosis:* 90 mg/kg/24 hr ÷ Q6 hr IV; **max. dose** 4 g/24 hr

Adult:

> *IV:* 1–4 g/24 hr ÷ Q6–8 hr; **max. dose** 4 g/24 hr or 50 mg/kg/24 hr, whichever is less
> *IM:* 500–750 mg/dose Q12 hr

IMIPENEM AND CILASTATIN *continued*

For IV use, give slowly over 30–60 min at a concentration ≤5 mg/mL to reduce risk for nausea (lowering rate may reduce severity). Adverse effects: thrombophlebitis, pruritus, urticaria, GI symptoms, seizures, dizziness, hypotension, elevated LFTs, blood dyscrasias, and penicillin allergy. Greater risk for seizures may occur with CNS infections, concomitant use with ganciclovir, higher doses, and renal impairment. CSF penetration is variable but best with inflamed meninges.
Do not administer with probenecid (increases imipenem/cilastatin levels) and ganciclovir (increased risk for seizures). May significantly reduce valproic acid levels. **Adjust dose in renal insufficiency (see Chapter 31).**

IMIPRAMINE
Tofranil, Tofranil-PM, and many generics
Antidepressant, tricyclic

Yes   Yes   3   ?

Tabs (HCI): 10, 25, 50 mg
Caps (Tofranil-PM, pamoate): 75, 100, 125, 150 mg; strengths are expressed as imipramine HCl equivalent.

Antidepressant:
Child:
Initial: 1.5 mg/kg/24 hr ÷ TID PO; increase 1–1.5 mg/kg/24 hr Q3–4 days to a **max. dose** of 5 mg/kg/24 hr.
Adolescent:
Initial: 25–50 mg/24 hr ÷ once daily–TID PO; **max. dose** 200 mg/24 hr. Dosages exceeding 100 mg/24 hr are generally not necessary.
Adult:
Initial: 75–100 mg/24 hr ÷ TID PO
Maintenance: 50–300 mg/24 hr QHS PO; **max. dose** 300 mg/24 hr
Enuresis (≥6 yr):
Initial: 10–25 mg QHS PO
Increment: 10–25 mg/dose at 1- to 2-wk intervals until max. dose for age or desired effect achieved. Continue × 2–3 mo, then taper slowly.
Max. doses:
  6–12 yr: 50 mg/24 hr
  ≥12 yr: 75 mg/24 hr
Augment analgesia for chronic pain:
Initial: 0.2–0.4 mg/kg/dose QHS PO; increase 50% Q2–3 days to a **max. dose** of 1–3 mg/kg/dose QHS PO.

Contraindicated in narrow-angle glaucoma and patients who used MAO inhibitors within 14 days. See Chapter 2 for management of toxic ingestion. Monitor for clinical worsening of depression and suicidal ideation/behavior after initiation of therapy or after dose changes.
Use with caution in renal or hepatic impairment. Side effects include sedation, urinary retention, constipation, dry mouth, dizziness, drowsiness, and arrhythmia. QHS dosing during first weeks of therapy will reduce sedation. Monitor ECG, BP, and CBC at start of therapy and with dose changes. Tricyclics may cause mania.
Therapeutic reference range (sum of imipramine and desipramine) = 150–250 ng/mL. Levels >1000 ng/mL are toxic, but toxicity may occur at levels >300 ng/mL.
Recommended serum sampling times at steady state: Obtain trough level within 30 min before next scheduled dose after 5–7 days of continuous therapy. Carbamazepine may reduce imipramine levels; cimetidine, fluoxetine, fluvoxamine, labetalol, and quinidine may increase imipramine levels.

Continued

IMIPRAMINE *continued*

Onset of antidepressant effects: 1–3 wk. **Do not discontinue abruptly** in patients receiving long-term high-dose therapy.

Pregnancy category has not been officially assigned by the FDA, but congenital anomalies have been reported in humans, with the causal relationship not established.

IMMUNE GLOBULIN
Immune globulins

No Yes ? C

IM preparations:
GamaSTAN S/D: 150–180 mg/mL (2, 10 mL); contains 0.21–0.32 M glycine; preservative free

IV preparations in solution:
Flebogamma DIF: 5% (50 mg/mL) (10, 50, 100, 200, 400 mL) 10% (100 mg/mL) (50, 100, 200 mL); contains 50 mg/mL sorbitol and ≤6 mg/mL polyethylene glycol; sucrose free
Gamunex-C: 10% (100 mg/mL) (10, 25, 50, 100, 200 mL); contains 0.16–0.24 M glycine; sucrose free
Gammagard liquid: 10% (100 mg/mL) (10, 25, 50, 100, 200 mL); contains 0.25 M glycine; sucrose free
Gammagard S/D ≤1 mcg/mL IgA: 5% (50 mg/mL) (100, 200 mL); contains 22.5 mg/mL glycine; sucrose and preservative free
Gammaked: 10% (100 mg/mL) (10, 25, 50, 100, 200 mL); contains 0.16–0.24 M glycine; sucrose free
Gamaplex: 5% (50 mg/mL) (50, 100, 200 mL); contains 50 mg/mL sorbitol, 6 mg/mL glycine, and 0.05 mg/mL polysorbate 80; sucrose free
Octagam: 5% (50 mg/mL) (20, 50, 100, 200, 500 mL); contains 100 mg/mL maltose; sucrose free
Privagen 10% (100 mg/mL) (50, 100, 200 mL); contains 210–290 mmol/L L-poline; sucrose free

IV preparations in powder for reconstitution:
Carimune NF: 3, 6, 12 g (contains 1.67 g sucrose and <20 mg NaCl per 1 g Ig); dilute to 3%, 6%, 9%, or 12%
Gammagard S/D: 2.5, 5, 10 g (contains 3 mg/mL albumin, 22.5 mg/mL glycine, 20 mg/mL glucose, 2 mg/mL polyethylene glycol, 1 mcg/mL tri-*n*-butyl phosphate, 1 mcg/mL octoxynol 9, and 100 mcg/mL polysorbate 80); dilute to 5% or 10%

Subcutaneous (SC) preparations:
Hizentra: 20% (200 mg/mL) (5, 10, 20 mL); contains 210–290 mmol/L L-proline, 10–30 mg/L polysorbate 80; sucrose and preservative free

See indications and doses in Chapter 15.
General guidelines for administration (see package insert of specific products):
IV: Begin infusion at 0.01 mL/kg/min, double rate every 15–30 min, up to **max.** of 0.08 mL/kg/min. If adverse reactions occur, stop infusion until side effects subside, and may restart at rate that was previously tolerated.
Subcutaneous (SC) preparation:
Converting to SC route from previous IV dosage for patients receiving IV immune globulin (IVIG) infusions at regular intervals for at least 3 mo (≥2 yr):
Initial weekly dose (start 1 wk after last IV dose):
Dose (g) = 1.53 × Previous IVIG dose in grams (g) ÷ number of weeks between IVIG doses
To convert the above dose in grams to milliliters of drug, multiply dose (g) by 5.
Adjust dose over time by clinical response and serum IgG trough levels. Obtain a previous trough level from IVIG therapy prior SC conversion, and repeat trough level 2–3 mo after initiating the SC route. A goal trough with the SC route of ≈ 290 mg/dL higher than a trough with the IV route has been recommended.

FORMULARY

IMMUNE GLOBULIN *continued*

SC administration: Injection sites include abdomen, thigh, upper arm, and/or lateral hip. Doses may be administered into multiple sites (spaced ≥2 inches apart) simultaneously. See following table.

Subcutaneous Product	Max. Simultaneous Injection sites	Max. Infusion Rate	Max. Infusion Volume
Hizentra	4	First infusion: 15 mL/hr per infusion site Subsequent infusions: 25 mL/hr per infusion site (max. 50 mL/hr for all simultaneous sites combined)	First 4 infusions: 15 mL per infusion site Subsequent infusions: 20–25 mL per infusion site

Use with caution in patients with increased risk of thrombosis (e.g., hypercoagulable states, prolonged immobilization, indwelling catheters, estrogen use, thrombosis history, cardiovascular risks, and hyperviscosity) or hemolysis (e.g., non-O blood type, associated inflammatory conditions, and receiving high cumulative doses of immune globulins over several days).

May cause flushing, chills, fever, headache, and hypotension. Hypersensitivity reaction may occur when IV form is administered rapidly. Maltose containing products may cause an osmotic diuresis. May cause **anaphylaxis** in IgA-deficient patients due to varied amounts of IgA. Some products are IgA depleted; consult a pharmacist.

To decrease risk of renal dysfunction, including acute renal failure, IV preparations containing sucrose should not be infused at a rate such that the amount of sucrose exceeds 3 mg/kg/min.

SC route provides higher serum trough levels, lower rate of adverse reactions, and shorter administration time than IV route. Use of adjusted body weight [ABW=Ideal body weight + 0.5 (Actual body weight − Ideal body weight)] for dosing in obese patients has been recommended.

Delay immunizations after immune globulin administration (see latest AAP *Red Book* for details).

INDOMETHACIN
Indocin, Indocin SR, Indocin I.V., and various generics
Nonsteroidal anti-inflammatory agent

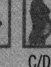

Yes   Yes   1   C/D

Caps: 25, 50 mg
Sustained-release caps (Indocin SR and other generics): 75 mg
Oral suspension: 25 mg/5 mL (237 mL); contains 1% alcohol
Suppositories: 50 mg (30s)
Injection (Indocin I.V. and other generics): 1 mg

Anti-inflammatory/rheumatoid arthritis:
Child (>= 2 yr): Start at 1–2 mg/kg/24 hr ÷ BID–QID PO; **max. dose** is the lesser of 4 mg/kg/24 hr or 200 mg/24 hr.
Adult: 50–150 mg/24 hr ÷ BID–QID PO; **max. dose** 200 mg/24 hr.
Closure of ductus arteriosus:
Infuse IV over 20–30 min:

Postnatal Age	Dose (mg/kg/dose Q12–24 hr)*		
	#1	#2	#3
<48 hr	0.2	0.1	0.1
2–7 days	0.2	0.2	0.2
>7 days	0.2	0.25	0.25

*Do not administer if urine output is <0.6 mL/kg/hr or anuric.

For infants <1500 g, 0.1–0.2 mg/kg/dose IV Q24 hr may be given for an additional 3–5 days.

Continued

For explanation of icons, see p. 648

INDOMETHACIN *continued*

Closure of ductuc arteriosus:

Intraventricular hemorrhage prophylaxis: 0.1 mg/kg/dose IV Q24 hr × 3 doses, initiated at 6–12 hr of age (give in consultation with a neonatologist).

Contraindicated in active bleeding, coagulation defects, necrotizing enterocolitis, and renal insufficiency (urine output < 0.6 mL/kg/hr). **Use with caution** in cardiac dysfunction, hypertension, heart disease (risk for MI and stroke with prolonged use), and renal or hepatic impairment. May cause (especially in neonates) decreased urine output, platelet dysfunction (thrombocytopenia), decreased GI blood flow, and reduce antihypertensive effects of β-blockers, hydralazine, and ACE inhibitors. **Fatal hepatitis reported in treatment of JRA.** Monitor renal and hepatic function before and during use.

Reduction in cerebral blood flow associated with rapid IV infusion; infuse all IV doses over 20–30 min. Sustained-release capsules are dosed once daily–BID. Pregnancy category changes to "D" if used for >48 hr or after 34-wk gestation or close to delivery.

INSULIN PREPARATIONS
Pancreatic hormone

   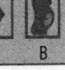

Yes   Yes   1   B

Many preparations, at concentrations of 100, 500 U/mL. See Chapter 10.
Diluted concentrations of 1 U/mL or 10 U/mL may be necessary for smaller doses in neonates and infants.

Hyperkalemia: See Chapter 11.
DKA: See Chapter 10.

When using insulin drip with new IV tubing, fill tubing with insulin infusion solution and wait 30 min before connecting tubing to patient. Then flush the line and connect IV line to patient to start infusion. This will ensure proper drug delivery. **Adjust dose in renal failure (see Chapter 31). Use with caution** and monitor closely in hepatic impairment.

IODIDE

See Potassium Iodide

IOHEXOL
Omnipaque 140, Omnipaque 180, Omnipaque 240,
Omnipaque 300, and Omnipaque 350
Radiopaque agent, contrast media

Yes   Yes   3   B

Injection:
Omnipaque 140: 302 mg iohexol equivalent to 140 mg iodine/mL (50 mL)
Omnipaque 180: 388 mg iohexol equivalent to 180 mg iodine/mL (10, 20 mL)
Omnipaque 240: 518 mg iohexol equivalent to 240 mg iodine/mL (10, 20, 50, 100, 150, 200 mL)
Omnipaque 300: 647 mg iohexol equivalent to 300 mg iodine/mL (10, 30, 50, 75, 100, 125, 150 mL)
Omnipaque 350: 755 mg iohexol equivalent to 350 mg iodine/mL (50, 75, 100, 125, 150, 200, 250 mL)

Contrast-enhanced CT scan of abdomen:
Oral (administered before IV dose):
Child: Mix 20 mL of Omnipaque 350 with 500 mL of noncarbonated beverage of patient's choice (apple juice works well for younger patients). Administer diluted contrast media PO 30–60 min before IV dose and image acquisition, using the following dosage:
<6 mo: 40–60 mL
6–18 mo: 120–160 mL

IOHEXOL *continued*

> ***18 mo–3 yr:*** 165–240 mL
> ***3 yr–12 yr:*** 250–360 mL
> ***>12 yr:*** 480–520 mL
> ***Adult:*** Mix 50 mL of Omnipaque 350 with half gallon of noncarbonated beverage of patient's choice. Give 2–4 cups containing 480 mL (16 oz) of diluted contrast media PO 20–40 min before IV dose and image acquisition.

IV (administered after PO dose):
> ***Child:*** 1–2 mL/kg IV of Omnipaque 240 or Omnipaque 300 given 30–60 min after oral dose
> **Max. dose:** 3 mL/kg
> ***Adult:*** 100–150 mL IV of Omnipaque 300 given 20–40 min after oral dose

Use with caution in dehydration, previous allergic reaction to a contrast medium, iodine sensitivity, asthma, hay fever, food allergy, CHF, severe liver or renal impairment, diabetic nephropathy, multiple myeloma, pheochromocytoma, hyperthyroidism, and sickle cell disease. Allergic reactions, arrhythmias, and nephrotoxicity have been rarely reported. Children at higher risk for adverse events with contrast medium administration may include those with asthma, sensitivity to medication and/or allergens, CHF, serum creatinine > 1.5 mg/dL, or <12 mo.

Use **NOT** recommended with drugs that lower seizure threshold (e.g., phenothiazines), amiodarone (increased risk of cardiotoxicity), and metformin (lactic acidosis and acute renal failure).

Many other uses exist; see package insert for additional information. Iohexol is particularly useful when barium sulfate is **contraindicated** in patients with suspected bowel perforation or those where aspiration of contrast medium is of concern. Oral dose is poorly absorbed from the normal GI tract (0.1%–0.5%); absorption increases with bowel perforation or bowel obstruction. Concentrations 302–755 mg iohexol/mL have osmolalities from 1.1–3 times that of plasma (285 mOsm/kg) and CSF (301 mOsm/kg) and may be hypertonic.

IPRATROPIUM BROMIDE
Atrovent and generics
Anticholinergic agent

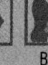

No   No   1   B

Aerosol (HFA): 17 mcg/dose (200 actuations per canister, 12.9 g)
Nebulized solution: 0.02% (500 mcg/2.5 mL) (25s, 30s, 60s)
Nasal spray: 0.03% (21 mcg per actuation, 30 mL); 0.06% (42 mcg per actuation, 15 mL)
In combination with albuterol:
> Nebulized solution (DuoNeb): 0.5 mg ipratropium bromide and 2.5 mg albuterol in 3 mL (30s, 60s)
> Aerosol (Combivent): 18 mcg ipratropium and 103 mcg albuterol per actuation (200 actuations per canister, 14.7 g)
> Inhalation spray (Combivent Respimat): 20 mcg ipratropium and 100 mcg albuterol per actuation (120 actuations per canister, 4 g)

Acute use in the ED or ICU:
Nebulizer treatments:
> ***<12 yr:*** 250 mcg/dose Q20 min × 3, then Q2–4 hr PRN
> ***≥12 yr:*** 500 mcg/dose Q30 min × 3, then Q2–4 hr PRN

Inhaler:
> ***Child and adult:*** 4–8 puffs PRN

Nonacute use:
Inhaler:
> ***<12 yr:*** 1–2 puffs Q6 hr; **max. dose** 12 puffs/24 hr
> ***≥12 yr:*** 2–3 puffs Q6 hr; **max. dose** 12 puffs/24 hr

Continued

For explanation of icons, see p. 648

IPRATROPIUM BROMIDE *continued*

Non-acute use:

 Nebulized treatments:

  Infant: 125–250 mcg/dose Q8 hr

  Child ≤ 12 yr: 250 mcg/dose Q6–8 hr

  >12 yr and adult: 250–500 mcg/dose Q6–8 hr

 Nasal spray:

  Allergic and nonallergic rhinitis:

   ≥6 yr and adult: 2 sprays of 0.03% strength (42 mcg) per nostril BID–TID

  Rhinitis associated with common cold (use up to a total of 4 days; safety and efficacy have not been evaluated >4 days):

   5–11 yr: 2 sprays of 0.06% strength (84 mcg) per nostril TID

   ≥12 yr and adult: 2 sprays of 0.06% strength (84 mcg) per nostril TID–QID

  Rhinitis associated with seasonal allergies (use up to a total of 3 weeks; safety and efficacy have not been evaluated >3 weeks):

   ≥5 yr and adult: 2 sprays of 0.06% strength (84 mcg) per nostril QID

> **Contraindicated** in soy or peanut allergy (for aerosol inhaler) and atropine hypersensitivity. **Use with caution** in narrow-angle glaucoma or bladder neck obstruction, though ipratropium has fewer anticholinergic systemic effects than atropine. May cause anxiety, dizziness, headache, GI discomfort, and cough with inhaler or nebulized use. Epistaxis, nasal congestion, and dry mouth/throat have been reported with nasal spray. Reversible anisocoria may occur with unintentional aerosolization of drug to eyes, particularly with mask nebulizers. Proven efficacy of nebulized solution in pediatrics is currently limited to reactive airway disease management in the ER and ICU areas. The combination product (Combivent) is currently approved for use only in adults and has not been studied in children.

Bronchodilation onset of action is 1–3 min, with peak effects within 1.5–2 hr and duration of action of 4–6 hr. Shake inhaler well before use with spacer. Nebulized solution may be mixed with albuterol (or use DuoNeb). Breast-feeding safety **extrapolated** from safety of atropine.

IRON DEXTRAN

See Iron – Injectable Preparations

IRON SUCROSE

See Iron – Injectable Preparations

IRON—INJECTABLE PREPARATIONS
Ferric gluconate: Ferrlecit and generics
Iron dextran: INFeD, DexFerrum
Iron sucrose: Venofer
Parenteral iron

No   No   2   B/C

Injection:

 Ferric gluconate (Ferrlecit and generics): 62.5 mg/mL (12.5 mg elemental Fe/mL) (5 mL); contains 9 mg/mL benzyl alcohol and 20% sucrose.

 Iron dextran (INFeD, DexFerrum): 50 mg/mL (50 mg elemental Fe/mL) (1, 2 mL); products containing phenol 0.5% are only for IM administration; products containing sodium chloride 0.9% can be administered via the IM or IV route.

 Iron sucrose (Venofer): 20 mg/mL (20 mg elemental Fe/mL) (2.5, 5, 10 mL); contains 300 mg/mL sucrose; preservative free.

IRON—INJECTABLE PREPARATIONS *continued*

Ferric gluconate (IV):

Iron-deficiency anemia in patents undergoing chronic hemodialysis who are receiving supplemental erythropoietin therapy (most require 8 doses at 8 sequential dialysis treatments to achieve a favorable response):

Child ≥ 6 yr: 1.5 mg/kg elemental Fe (0.12 mL/kg) IV; **max. dose** 125 mg elemental Fe/dose. Dilute dose in 25 mL NS and infuse over 1 hr.

Adult: 125 mg elemental Fe in 100 mL NS IV; infuse over 1 hr. Most require a minimal cumulative dose of 1 g elemental Fe administered over 8 sessions.

Iron dextran (IV or IM):

Iron-deficiency anemia:

Test dose: 25 mg (12.5 mg for infants) IV (over 5 min) or IM. May initiate treatment dose 1 hr after test dose.

Total replacement dose of iron dextran (mL) = 0.0476 × Lean body wt (kg) × (Desired Hb [g/dL] − Measured Hb [g/dL]) + 1 mL per 5 kg lean body weight (up to **max.** of 14 mL).

Acute blood loss: Total replacement dose of iron dextran (mL) = 0.02 × Blood loss (mL) × Hematocrit expressed as decimal fraction. Assumes 1 mL of RBC = 1 mg elemental iron. If no reaction to test dose, give remainder of replacement dose ÷ over 2–3 daily doses.

Max daily (IM) dose:

<5 kg: 0.5 mL (25 mg)

5–10 kg: 1 mL (50 mg)

>10 kg: 2 mL (100 mg)

IM administration: Use "Z-track" technique.

IV administration: Dilute in NS at a **max. concentration** of 50 mg/mL and infuse over 1–6 hr at a **max. rate** of 50 mg/min.

Iron sucrose (IV):

Iron-deficiency anemia in patients with chronic kidney disease:

Child (limited data from 14 children with ESRD on hemodialysis): 1 mg/kg/dialysis was adequate for correcting ferritin levels, and 0.3 mg/kg/dialysis was successful in maintaining ferritin levels between 193–250 mcg/L. Doses were administered during last hr of each dialysis; recommended frequency, 3 times a week. A 10-mg test dose was administered.

Adult:

Hemodialysis dependent: 100 mg elemental Fe 1–3 times a wk during dialysis up to a total cumulative dose of 1000 mg. May continue to administer at lowest dose to maintain target Hb, Hct, and iron levels.

Non–hemodialysis dependent: 200 mg elemental Fe on 5 different days over a 2-wk period (total cumulative dose: 1000 mg).

IV administration: May administer undiluted over 2–5 min. For an infusion, dilute each 100 mg with a **max.** of 100 mL NS and infuse over at least 15 min.

Oral therapy with iron salts is preferred; injectable routes are painful. Gluconate and sucrose salts may be better tolerated than iron dextran. Adverse effects include hypotension, GI disturbances, fever, rash, myalgia, arthralgias, cramps, and headaches. Hypersensitivity reactions (fatal anaphylaxis with iron dextran; use test dose before first therapeutic dose) have been reported.

IM administration is only possible with iron dextran salt. Follow infusion recommendations for specific product. Monitor vital signs during IV infusion. TIBC levels may not be meaningful within 3 wk after dosing.

Efficacy and safety of iron sucrose for maintenance therapy has been evaluated in children 2 yr and older with CKD and receiving erythropoietin therapy. Common side effects include headache, respiratory tract viral infection, peritonitis, vomiting, pyrexia, dizziness, and cough.

Pregnancy category is "B" for ferric gluconate and iron sucrose and "C" for iron dextran.

For explanation of icons, see p. 648

IRON—ORAL PREPARATIONS
Fergon, Fer-In-Sol, Feosol, Niferex, Slow FE, and many generics
Oral iron supplements

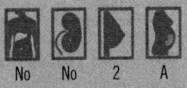

No   No   2   A

Ferrous sulfate (20% elemental Fe):
Drops and oral solution (Fer-In-Sol and generics) [OTC]: 75 mg (15 mg Fe)/1 mL (50 mL); contains 0.2% alcohol and sodium bisulfite
Oral elixir and liquid [OTC]: 220 mg (44 mg Fe)/5 mL; may contain 5% alcohol
Oral syrup [OTC]: 300 mg (60 mg Fe)/5 mL
Tabs [OTC]: 300 mg (60 mg Fe), 324 mg (65 mg Fe), 325 mg (65 mg Fe)
Extended-release tabs (Slow FE and generics) [OTC]: 140 mg (45 mg Fe), 160 mg (50 mg Fe), and 325 mg (65 mg Fe)
Ferrous gluconate (12% elemental Fe):
Tabs (Fergon and generics) [OTC]: 240 mg (27 mg Fe), 256 mg (28 mg Fe), 325 mg (36 mg Fe)
Ferrous fumarate (33% elemental Fe):
Tabs [OTC]: 90 mg (29.5 mg Fe), (324 mg (106 mg Fe), 325 mg (106 mg Fe), 456 mg (150 mg Fe)
Polysaccharide-iron complex and ferrous bis-glycinate chelate (Niferex and generics) (expressed in mg elemental Fe):
Caps [OTC]: 50, 150 mg; 150 mg strength may contain 50 mg vitamin C
Elixir [OTC]: 100 mg/5 mL (237 mL); contains 10% alcohol

Iron-deficiency anemia:
  Premature infant: 2–4 mg elemental Fe/kg/24 hr ÷ once daily–BID PO; **max. dose** 15 mg elemental Fe/24 hr
  Child: 3–6 mg elemental Fe/kg/24 hr ÷ once daily–TID PO
  Adult: 60–100 mg elemental Fe BID PO up to 60 mg elemental Fe QID
Prophylaxis:
  Child: Give dose below PO ÷ once daily–TID.
    Premature: 2 mg elemental Fe/kg/24 hr; **max. dose** 15 mg elemental Fe/24 hr
    Full term: 1–2 mg elemental Fe/kg/24 hr; **max. dose** 15 mg elemental Fe/24 hr
  Adult: Give 60–100 mg elemental Fe/24 hr PO ÷ once daily–BID.

Contraindicated in hemolytic anemia and hemochromatosis. **Avoid** use in GI tract inflammation.
Iron preparations are variably absorbed. Less GI irritation when given with or after meals.
  Vitamin C, 200 mg per 30 mg iron, may enhance absorption. Liquid iron preparations may stain teeth. Give with dropper or drink through straw. May produce constipation, dark stools (false-positive guaiac is controversial), nausea, and epigastric pain. Iron and tetracycline inhibit each other's absorption. Antacids may decrease iron absorption.

ISONIAZID
INH, Nydrazid, Laniazid, and generics
In combination with rifampin: Rifamate, IsonaRif
In combination with rifampin and pyrazinamide: Rifater
Antituberculous agent

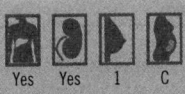

Yes   Yes   1   C

Tabs: 100, 300 mg
Syrup: 50 mg/5 mL (473 mL)
Injection: 100 mg/mL (10 mL); contains 0.25% chlorobutanol
In combination with rifampin:
Caps (Rifamate, IsonaRif): 150 mg isoniazid + 300 mg rifampin
In combination with rifampin and pyrazinamide:
Caps (Rifater): 50 mg isoniazid + 120 mg rifampin + 300 mg pyrazinamide

ISONIAZID *continued*

See most recent edition of the AAP *Red Book* for details and length of therapy.
Prophylaxis:
  Infant and child: 10 mg/kg (**max. dose** 300 mg) PO once daily. After 1 mo of daily therapy and in cases where daily compliance cannot be assured, may change to 20–40 mg/kg (**max. dose** 900 mg) per dose PO, given twice weekly.
  Adult: 300 mg PO once daily
Treatment:
  Infant and child:
    10–15 mg/kg (**max. dose** 300 mg) PO once daily or 20–30 mg/kg (**max. dose** 900 mg) per dose twice weekly with rifampin for uncomplicated pulmonary tuberculosis in compliant patients. Additional drugs are necessary in complicated disease.
  Adult:
    5 mg/kg (**max. dose** 300 mg) PO once daily or 15 mg/kg (**max. dose** 900 mg) per dose twice weekly with rifampin. Additional drugs are necessary in complicated disease.
For INH-resistant TB: Discuss with Health Department or consult ID specialist.

Should not be used alone for treatment. **Contraindicated** in acute liver disease and previous isoniazid-associated hepatitis. Peripheral neuropathy, optic neuritis, seizures, encephalopathy, psychosis, hepatic side effects may occur with higher doses, especially in combination with rifampin. Severe liver injury has been reported in children and adults treated for latent TB. Follow LFTs monthly. Supplemental pyridoxine (1–2 mg/kg/24 hr) is recommended. May cause false-positive urine glucose test.

Inhibits CYP 450 1A2, 2C9, 2C19, and 3A3/4 microsomal enzymes; decrease dose of carbamazepine, diazepam, phenytoin, and prednisone. Prednisone may decrease isoniazid's effects. Also a substrate and inducer of CYP 450 2E1 and may potentiate acetaminophen hepatotoxicity. Avoid daily alcohol use to reduce risk for isoniazid-induced hepatitis.

May be given IM (same as oral doses) when oral therapy is not possible. Administer oral doses 1 hr before and 2 hr after meals. Aluminum salts may decrease absorption.

ISOPROTERENOL
Isuprel
Adrenergic agonist

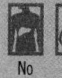

No   Yes   ?   C

Injection: 0.2 mg/mL (5, 10 mL); contains sulfites

NOTE: Dosage units for adults are in mcg/min, compared with mcg/kg/min for children.
IV infusion:
  Neonate–child: 0.05–2 mcg/kg/min; start at minimal dose and increase every 5–10 min by 0.1 mcg/kg/min until desired effect or onset of toxicity; **max. dose** 2 mcg/kg/min.
  Adult: 2–20 mcg/min; titrate to desired effect.

Use with caution in diabetes, hyperthyroidism, renal disease, CHF, ischemia, or aortic stenosis. May cause flushing, ventricular arrhythmias, profound hypotension, anxiety, and myocardial ischemia. Monitor heart rate, respiratory rate, and blood pressure. **Not** for treatment of asystole or for use in cardiac arrests unless bradycardia is due to heart block.

Continuous infusion for bronchodilation must be gradually tapered over a 24–48 hr period to prevent rebound bronchospasm. Tolerance may occur with prolonged use. Clinical deterioration, myocardial necrosis, CHF, and **death** have been reported with continuous infusion use in refractory asthmatic children.

For explanation of icons, see p. 648

ISOTRETINOIN
Accutane, Absorica, Amnesteem, Claravis, Myorisan, Zenatane
Retinoic acid, vitamin A derivative

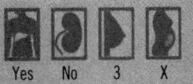

Yes   No   3   X

Caps: 10, 20, 30, 40 mg; may contain soybean oil, EDTA, and parabens

Cystic acne:
  Child (>12 yr) and adult: 0.5–2 mg/kg/24 hr ÷ BID PO × 15–20 wk or until total cyst count decreases by 70%, whichever comes first. Dosages as low as 0.05 mg/kg/24 hr have been reported to be beneficial.

Contraindicated during pregnancy; known teratogen. Use with caution in females during childbearing years. May cause conjunctivitis, xerosis, pruritus, photosensitivity reactions (avoid exposure to sunlight and use sunscreen), epistaxis, anemia, hyperlipidemia, pseudotumor cerebri (especially in combination with tetracyclines; avoid this combination), cheilitis, bone pain, muscle aches, skeletal changes, lethargy, nausea, vomiting, elevated ESR, mental depression, aggressive/violent behavior, and psychosis. Serious skin reactions (e.g., Stevens-Johnson syndrome, TEN) have been reported.

Elevation of liver enzymes may occur during treatment; a dosage reduction or continued treatment may result in normalization. Discontinue use if liver enzymes do not normalize or if hepatitis is suspected.

To avoid additive toxic effects, **do not** take vitamin A concomitantly. Increases clearance of carbamazepine. Hormonal birth control (oral , injectable, and implantable) failures have been reported with concurrent use. Monitor CBC, ESR, triglycerides, and LFTs.

Prescribers, site pharmacists, patients, and wholesalers must register with the iPLEDGE system (a risk minimization program) at www.ipledgeprogram.com or 1-866-495-0654 before doses are dispensed. Prescriptions may not be written for more than a 1-mo supply.

ITRACONAZOLE
Sporanox, Onmel, and generics
Antifungal agent

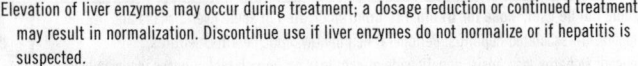

Yes   Yes   3   C

Caps (Sporanox and generics): 100 mg
Tabs (Onmel): 200 mg
Oral solution (Sporanox): 10 mg/mL (150 mL); contains saccharin and sorbitol

Neonate (limited data in full-term neonates treated for tinea capitis): 5 mg/kg/24 hr PO once daily × 6 wk
Child (limited data): 3–5 mg/kg/24 hr PO ÷ once daily–BID; dosages as high as 5–10 mg/kg/24 hr have been used for *Aspergillus* prophylaxis in chronic granulomatous disease. Population pharmacokinetic data in pediatric cystic fibrosis and bone marrow transplant patients suggest an oral liquid dosage of 10 mg/kg/24 hr PO ÷ BID **OR** oral capsule dosage of 20 mg/kg/24 hr PO ÷ BID to be more reliable for achieving trough plasma levels between 500 and 2000 ng/mL.
  Prophylaxis for recurrence of opportunistic disease in HIV:
    Coccidioides *spp.:* 2–5 mg/kg/dose PO Q12 hr; **max. dose** 400 mg/24 hr
    Cryptococcus neoformans: 5 mg/kg/dose PO Q24 hr; **max. dose** 200 mg/24 hr
    Histoplasma capsulatum: 5 mg/kg/dose PO Q12 hr; **max. dose** 400 mg/24 hr
  Treatment of opportunistic disease in HIV:
    Candidiasis: 5 mg/kg/24 hr PO ÷ Q12–24 hr; **max. dose** 400 mg/24 hr
    Coccidioides *spp.:* 5–10 mg/kg/dose PO BID × 3 days, followed by 2–5 mg/kg/dose PO BID; **max. dose** 400 mg/24 hr

FORMULARY

ITRACONAZOLE *continued*

Treatment of opportunistic disease in HIV (cont.):

Cryptococcus neoformans: 2.5–5 mg/kg/dose (**max. dose** 200 mg/dose) PO TID × 3 days, followed by 5–10 mg/kg/24 hr (**max. dose** 400 mg/24 hr) ÷ once to twice daily for a minimum of 8 wk

Histoplasma capsulatum: 2–5 mg/kg/dose (**max. dose** 200 mg/dose) PO TID × 3 days, followed by 2–5 mg/kg/dose (**max. dose** 200 mg/dose) PO BID × 12 mo

Adult:

Blastomycosis and nonmeningeal histoplasmosis: 200 mg PO once daily up to a **max. dose** of 400 mg/24 hr ÷ BID (**max. dose** 200 mg/dose)

Aspergillosis and severe infections: 600 mg/24 hr PO ÷ TID × 3–4 days, followed by 200–400 mg/24 hr ÷ BID; **max. dose** 600 mg/24 hr ÷ TID

Oral solution and capsule dosage form should **NOT** be used interchangeably; oral solution is more bioavailable. Only the oral solution has been demonstrated effective for oral and/or esophageal candidiasis. **Contraindicated** in CHF and certain interacting drugs (see below). **Use with caution** in hepatic and/or renal impairment, cardiac dysrhythmias, and azole hypersensitivity. May cause GI symptoms, headaches, rash, liver enzyme elevation, hepatitis, and hypokalemia.

Like ketoconazole, it inhibits activity of CYP 450 3A4 drug metabolizing isoenzyme. Thus, coadministration of cisapride, dofetilide, felodipine, methadone, nisoldipine, pimozide, quinidine, triazolam, lovastatin, simvastatin, ergot derivatives, and oral midazolam is **contraindicated**. See remarks at *Ketoconazole* for additional drug interaction information.

Steady-state trough serum concentrations of >250 ng/mL itraconazole and >1000 ng/mL hydroxyitraconazole (metabolite) have been recommended. Recommended serum sampling time at steady state: trough level after 2 wk of continuous dosing.

Administer oral solution on an empty stomach, but administer capsules with food. Achlorhydria reduces absorption of drug. **Do not** use oral liquid dosage form in patients with GFR <30 mL/min; the hydroxypropyl-β-cyclodextrin excipient has reduced clearance with renal failure.

KANAMYCIN
Kantrex and generics
Antibiotic, aminoglycoside

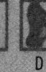

No   Yes   2   D

Injection: 333 mg/mL (3 mL); may contain sulfites

Neonate IV/IM administration (see following table):

Birth Weight (kg)	<7 days	≥7 days
<2	15 mg/kg/24 hr ÷ Q12 hr	22.5 mg/kg/24 hr ÷ Q8 hr
≥2	20 mg/kg/24 hr ÷ Q12 hr	30 mg/kg/24 hr ÷ Q8 hr

Infant and child: IM/IV: 15–30 mg/kg/24 hr ÷ Q8–12 hr

Adult: IV/IM: 15 mg/kg/24 hr ÷ Q8–12 hr

PO administration for GI bacterial overgrowth: 150–250 mg/kg/24 hr ÷ Q6 hr; **max. dose** 4 g/24 hr

Renal toxicity and ototoxicity may occur. Give over 30 min if IV route is used. Use with caution in neuromuscular disorders (e.g., infant botulism, myasthenia gravis), anesthesia and muscle-relaxant medications, and hypermagnesemia (may result in respiratory arrest). **Adjust dose in renal failure (see Chapter 31).** Poorly absorbed orally; PO used to treat GI bacterial overgrowth. Oral route is **contraindicated** in intestinal obstructions. **Avoid** use with loop diuretics.

Therapeutic levels: Peak, 15–30 mg/L; trough, <5–10 mg/L. Recommended serum sampling time at steady state: trough within 30 min before third consecutive dose, and peak 30–60 min after administration of third consecutive dose.

For explanation of icons, see p. 648

KETAMINE
Ketalar and various generics
General anesthetic

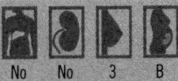

No   No   3   B

Injection: 10 mg/mL (20 mL), 50 mg/mL (10 mL), 100 mg/mL (5, 10 mL); contains benzelthonium chloride

Child (see remarks):
  Sedation:
    PO: 5 mg/kg × 1
    IV: 0.25–1 mg/kg
    IM: 2–5 mg/kg × 1
Adult:
  Analgesia with sedation:
    IV (see remarks): 0.2–1 mg/kg
    IM: 0.5–4 mg/kg

Contraindicated in elevated ICP, hypertension, aneurysms, thyrotoxicosis, CHF, angina, and psychotic disorders. May cause hypertension, hypotension, emergence reactions, tachycardia, laryngospasm, respiratory depression, and stimulation of salivary secretions. Cystitis has been reported with chronic use/abuse. IV use may induce general anesthesia. Coadministration of an anticholinergic agent may be added in situations of clinically significant hypersalivation in patients with impaired ability to mobilize secretions. Benzodiazepine may be used in the presence of a ketamine-associated recovery reaction (prophylaxis use in adults may be beneficial). Ondansetron prophylaxis can slightly reduce vomiting. See *Ann Emerg Med.* 2001;57:449-461 for additional use information in the emergency department.

Rate of IV infusion should **not** exceed 0.5 mg/kg/min and should **not** be administered in <60 sec. For additional information, including onset and duration of action, see Chapter 6.

Pregnancy category is considered by many as a "B" despite no formal designation by the FDA.

KETOCONAZOLE
Nizoral, Nizoral A-D, Xolegel, Extina, and generics
Antifungal agent, imidazole

Yes   No   2   C

Tabs: 200 mg
Oral suspension: 100 mg/5 mL
Cream: 2% (15, 30, 60 g); contains sulfites
Gel: 2% [Xolegel] (45 g); contains 34% alcohol
Shampoo: 1% [Nizoral A-D, OTC] (120, 210 mL), 2% (120 mL)
Foam: 2% [Extina] (50, 100 g)

Oral:
  Child ≥ 2 yr: 3.3–6.6 mg/kg/24 hr once daily
  Adult: 200–400 mg/24 hr once daily
  Max. dose: 800 mg/24 hr ÷ BID
Topical: 1–2 applications/24 hr
Shampoo (dandruff): Twice weekly, with at least 3 days between applications for up to 8 weeks PRN. Thereafter, intermittently as needed to maintain control.
Suppressive therapy against mucocutaneous candidiasis in HIV:
  Child: 5–10 mg/kg/24 hr ÷ once daily–BID PO; **max. dose** of 800 mg/24 hr ÷ BID
  Adolescent and adult: 200 mg/dose once daily PO

The systemic dosage form should not be first-line treatment for any fungal infection, owing to concerns of hepatotoxicity and adrenal gland effects (per FDA).

KETOCONAZOLE continued

Monitor LFTs in long-term use and adrenal function for patients at risk. Drugs that decrease gastric acidity will decrease absorption. May cause nausea, vomiting, rash, headache, pruritus, and fever. Hepatotoxicity (including fatal cases) has been reported; use with hepatic impairment is **contraindicated**. High doses may decrease adrenocortical function and serum testosterone levels. Hypersensitivity reactions (including anaphylaxis) have been reported with all dosage forms.

Safety and efficacy with topical use in seborrheic dermatitis for patients >age 12 yr has been established. Avoid topical use on breast or nipples in nursing mothers.

Inhibits CYP 450 3A4. **Contraindicated** when used with cisapride, mefloquine, quinidine, terfinadine, pimozide, any drug that can prolong QT interval (risk for cardiac arrhythmias), and HMG-CoA reductase inhibitors (e.g., simvastatin, lovastatin). Excessive sedation and prolonged hypnotic effects with triazolam (also **contraindicated**). May increase levels/effects of phenytoin, digoxin, cyclosporine, corticosteroids, nevirapine, protease inhibitors, and warfarin. Achlorhydria, phenobarbital, rifampin, isoniazid, H2 blockers, antacids, and omeprazole can decrease levels of oral ketoconazole.

Administering oral doses with food or acidic beverages and 2 hr before antacids will increase absorption.

To use shampoo, wet hair and scalp with water, apply sufficient amount to scalp, and gently massage for about 1 min. Rinse hair thoroughly, reapply shampoo, leave on scalp for an additional 3 min, then rinse.

KETOROLAC
Many generics (previously available as Toradol), Acular,
Acular LS, Acuvail
Nonsteroidal anti-inflammatory agent

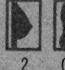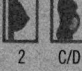

Yes | Yes | 2 | C/D

Injection: 15 mg/mL (1 mL), 30 mg/mL (1, 2, 10 mL); contains 10% alcohol and tromethamine
Tabs: 10 mg; contains tromethamine
Ophthalmic solution (all contain tromethamine):
Acular: 0.5% (5, 10 mL); contains benzalkonium chloride
Acular LS and generics: 0.4% (3, 5, 10 mL); contains benzalkonium chloride
Acuvail: 0.45% (0.4 mL; 30s); preservative free

Systemic use is not to exceed 3–5 days; regardless of administration route (IM, IV, PO).
IM/IV:
Child: 0.5 mg/kg/dose IM/IV Q6–8 hr. **Max. dose:** 30 mg Q6 hr or 120 mg/24 hr. Alternatively, manufacturer has recommended following doses for children aged 2–16 yr with moderate/severe acute pain:
IV: 0.5 mg/kg × 1; **max. dose** 15 mg
IM: 1 mg/kg × 1; **max. dose** 30 mg
Adult: 30 mg IM/IV Q6 hr; **max. dose** 120 mg/24 hr
PO:
Child > 16 yr (>50 kg) and adult: 10 mg PRN Q6 hr; **max. dose** 40 mg/24 hr
Ophthalmic (see remarks):
≥3 yr–adult: 1 drop in each affected eye QID

May cause GI bleeding, nausea, dyspepsia, drowsiness, decreased platelet function, and interstitial nephritis. **Not recommended** in patients at increased risk of bleeding. **Do not use** in hepatic or renal failure. **Use with caution** in heart disease (risk for MI and stroke with prolonged use).

Duration of therapy for ophthalmic use: 14 days after cataract surgery, and up to 4 days after corneal refractive surgery. Also indicated for ocular itching associated with seasonal allergic conjunctivitis. Bronchospasm or asthma exacerbations have been reported with ophthalmic use.

Pregnancy category changes to a "D" if used in the third trimester.

For explanation of icons, see p. 648

LABETALOL
Normodyne, Trandate, and various generics
Adrenergic antagonist (α and β), antihypertensive

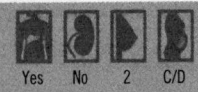

Yes No 2 C/D

Tabs: 100, 200, 300 mg
Injection: 5 mg/mL (4, 20, 40 mL); contains parabens
Oral suspension: 10, 40 mg/mL

Child (see remarks):
  PO: Initial: 1–3 mg/kg/24 hr ÷ BID. May increase up to a maximum of 12 mg/kg/24 hr up to 1200 mg/24 hr.
  IV: Hypertensive emergency (start at lowest dose and titrate to effect; see Chapter 4 for additional information):
    Intermittent dose: 0.2–1 mg/kg/dose Q10 min PRN; **max. dose** 40 mg/dose.
    Infusion (hypertensive emergencies): 0.4–1 mg/kg/hr to a **max. dose** of 3 mg/kg/hr. May initiate with a 0.2–1 mg/kg bolus; **max. bolus** 40 mg.
Adult (see remarks):
  PO: 100 mg BID; increase by 100 mg/dose Q2–3 days PRN to a **max. dose** of 2.4 g/24 hr. Usual range: 200–800 mg/24hr ÷ BID.
  IV: Hypertensive emergency (start at lowest dose and titrate to effect, with a **max. total dose** of 300 mg for both methods of administration):
    Intermittent dose: 20–80 mg/dose (begin with 20 mg) Q10 min PRN
    Infusion: 2 mg/min, increase to titrate to response

Contraindicated in asthma, pulmonary edema, cardiogenic shock, and heart block. May cause orthostatic hypotension, edema, CHF, bradycardia, AV conduction disturbances, bronchospasm, urinary retention, and skin tingling. **Use with caution** in hepatic disease (dose reduction may be necessary), diabetes, liver function test elevation, hepatic necrosis, and hepatitis. Cholestatic jaundice have been reported. Use with digitalis glycosides may increase risk for bradycardia.
Patient should remain supine for up to 3 hr after IV administration. Pregnancy category changes to "D" if used in second or third trimesters.
Onset of action: PO: 1–4 hr; IV: 5–15 min.

LACOSAMIDE
Vimpat
Anticonvulsant

Yes Yes ? C

Oral solution: 10 mg/mL (200, 465 mL); contains aspartame and propylene glycol
Tabs: 50, 100, 200 mg
Injection: 10 mg/mL (20 mL)

Child (3–18 yr; limited data in 18 patients with refractory partial seizures as adjunctive therapy with moderate response): Start at 1 mg/kg/24 hr PO ÷ BID. If needed, dose may be increased at weekly intervals by 1 mg/kg/24 hr, administered BID up to 10 mg/kg/24 hr. The final doses ranged from 2–10 mg/kg/24 hr. A retrospective trial in 16 patients 8–21 years old with focal seizures as adjunctive therapy received an average dose of 4.7 mg/kg/24 hr PO with moderate response.
A randomized placebo-controlled trial for lacosamide as an add-on therapy for patients 4–<17 yr with partial-onset seizures is evaluating the following dosages (see ww.clinicaltrials.gov for updates):
  <30 kg: 8–12 mg/kg/24 hr PO ÷ BID
  ≥30–<50 kg: 6–8 mg/kg/24 hr PO ÷ BID
  ≥50 kg: 150–200 mg PO BID

L

LACOSAMIDE *continued*

≥17 yr and adult:

Partial-onset seizures: Start at 50 mg BID IV/PO. If needed, dose may be increased at weekly intervals by 100 mg/24 hr, administered BID up to the usual maintenance dose of 200–400 mg/24 hr ÷ BID. Use same dose when converting from IV to PO and vice versa. IV use should be considered for temporary use.

Use with caution with known cardiac conduction problems (e.g., second-degree AV block), severe cardiac disease (e.g., MI or heart failure), concomitant use with drugs known to prolong PR interval, and renal (see Chapter 31) and hepatic impairment. In adults with GFR < 30 mL/min and ESRD, the maximum daily dosage is 300 mg/24 hr. Lacosamide is 95% excreted by the kidneys. Dose reduction may be necessary with hepatic or renal impairment and concurrent strong inhibitor of CYP 450 3A4 or 2C9 medication. Use is **not recommended** in severe hepatic impairment, and an adult **max. dose** of 300 mg/24 hr is recommended for mild/moderate hepatic impairment. Oral bioavailability is ≈ 100%.

Most common side effects in adults include diplopia, headache, dizziness, and nausea. Somnolence and irritability were frequently reported in pediatric studies. Patients should be advised of potential dizziness, ataxia, and syncope with use. Multiorgan hypersensitivity reactions (affecting skin, kidney, liver) and euphoria (high doses) have been reported. As with other AEDs, monitor for suicidal behavior and ideation.

Oral doses may be administered with or without food. IV doses should be administered over 30–60 min. **Do not** abruptly withdraw therapy; gradually taper to prevent potential seizures.

LACTULOSE
Cephulac, Chronulac, Enuloase, Kristalose, and generics
Ammonium detoxicant, hyperosmotic laxative

    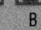

No   No   ?   B

Syrup: 10 g/15 mL (15, 30, 237, 473, 960, 1893 mL); contains galactose, lactose, and other sugars
Crystals for reconstitution (Kristalose): 10 g (30s), 20 g (30s)

Constipation:

Child: 1–3 mL/kg/24 hr PO ÷ BID; **max. dose** 60 mL/24 hr

Adult: 15–30 mL/24 hr PO once daily to a **max. dose** of 60 mL/24 hr

Portal systemic encephalopathy (adjust dose to produce 2–3 soft stools/day):

Infant: 2.5–10 mL/24 hr PO ÷ TID–QID

Child: 40–90 mL/24 hr PO ÷ TID–QID

Adult: 30–45 mL/dose PO TID–QID; acute episodes, 30–45 mL Q1–2 hr until 2–3 soft stools/day

Rectal (adult): 300 mL diluted in 700 mL water or NS in 30–60 min retention enema; may give Q4–6 hr

Contraindicated in galactosemia. **Use with caution** in diabetes mellitus. GI discomfort and diarrhea may occur. For portal systemic encephalopathy, monitor serum ammonia, serum potassium, and fluid status.

Adjust dose to achieve 2–3 soft stools per day. **Do not use** with antacids. Dissolve crystal dosage form with 4 ounces of water or juice. All doses may be administered with juice, milk, or water.

For explanation of icons, see p. 648

LAMIVUDINE
Epivir, Epivir-HBV, 3TC, and generics
Antiviral agent, nucleoside analog reverse transcriptase inhibitor

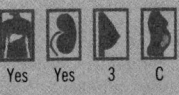

Yes Yes 3 C

Tabs: 100 mg (Epivir-HBV), 150, 300 mg
Oral solution: 5 mg/mL (Epivir-HBV) (240 mL), 10 mg/mL (Epivir) (240 mL); contains parabens

HIV: See www.aidsinfo.nih.gov/guidelines.
Prevention of maternal-fetal transmission to reduce nevirapine resistance (for infants born to mothers with no antiretroviral therapy before or during labor, infants born to mothers with only intrapartum antiretroviral therapy, infants born to mothers with suboptimal viral suppression at delivery, or infants born to mothers with known antiretroviral drug resistance):
Neonate: 2 mg/kg/dose PO BID × 7–14 days from birth
Chronic hepatitis B (see remarks):
2–17 yr: 3 mg/kg/dose PO once daily up to a **max. dose** of 100 mg/dose
≥18 and adult: 100 mg/dose PO once daily

See aidsinfo.nih.gov/guidelines for remarks for use in HIV.
May cause headache, fatigue, GI disturbances, rash, and myalgia/arthralgia. Lactic acidosis, severe hepatomegaly with steatosis, posttreatment exacerbations of hepatitis B and ALT elevations, pancreatitis, and emergence of resistant viral strains have been reported. Concomitant use with cotrimoxazole (TMP/SMX) may result in increased lamivudine levels.
Use Epivir-HBV product for chronic hepatitis B indication. Safety and effectiveness beyond 1 yr have not been determined. Patients with both HIV and hepatitis B should use the higher HIV doses along with an appropriate combination regimen.
May be administered with food. **Adjust dose in renal impairment (see Chapter 31).**

LAMOTRIGINE
Lamictal, Lamictal ODT, Lamictal XR, and generics
Anticonvulsant

  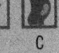

Yes Yes 2 C

Tabs: 25, 100, 150, 200 mg
Extended-release tabs (Lamictal XR and generics): 25, 50, 100, 200, 250, 300 mg
Chewable tabs: 2, 5, 25 mg
Orally disintegrated tabs (Lamictal ODT): 25, 50, 100, 200 mg
Oral suspension: 1 mg/mL

Child 2–12 yr, adjunctive therapy (see remarks):
WITH antiepileptic drugs (AEDs) other than carbamazepine, phenytoin, phenobarbital, primidone, or valproic acid (use immediate-release dosage forms):
Wk 1 and 2: 0.3 mg/kg/24 hr PO ÷ once daily–BID, rounded down to the nearest whole tablet
Wk 3 and 4: 0.6 mg/kg/24 hr PO ÷ BID, rounded down to the nearest whole tablet
Usual maintenance dose: 4.5–7.5 mg/kg/24 hr PO ÷ BID, titrated to effect. To achieve the usual maintenance dose, increase doses Q1–2 wk by 0.6 mg/kg/24 hr (rounded down to the nearest whole tablet) as needed.
Max. dose: 300 mg/24 hr ÷ BID
WITH enzyme-inducing AEDs WITHOUT valproic acid (use immediate-release dosage forms):
Wk 1 and 2: 0.6 mg/kg/24 hr PO ÷ BID, rounded down to the nearest whole tablet
Wk 3 and 4: 1.2 mg/kg/24 hr PO ÷ BID, rounded down to the nearest whole tablet

LAMOTRIGINE *continued*

Usual maintenance dose: 5–15 mg/kg/24 hr PO ÷ BID, titrated to effect. To achieve the usual maintenance dose, increase doses Q1–2 wk by 1.2 mg/kg/24 hr (rounded down to the nearest whole tablet) as needed.

Max. dose: 400 mg/24 hr ÷ BID

WITH AEDs WITH valproic acid (use immediate-release dosage forms):

Wk 1 and 2: 0.15 mg/kg/24 hr PO ÷ once daily–BID, rounded down to the nearest whole tablet (see following table)

Wk 3 and 4: 0.3 mg/kg/24 hr PO ÷ once daily–BID, rounded down to the nearest whole tablet (see following table)

Weight (kg)	Weeks 1 & 2	Weeks 3 & 4
6.7–14	2 mg every other day	2 mg once daily
14.1–27	2 mg once daily	4 mg/24 hr ÷ once daily–BID
27.1–34	4 mg/24 hr ÷ once daily–BID	8 mg/24 hr ÷ once daily–BID
34.1–40	5 mg once daily	10 mg/24 hr ÷ once daily–BID

Usual maintenance dose: 1–5 mg/kg/24 hr PO ÷ once daily–BID, titrated to effect. To achieve the usual maintenance dose, increase doses Q1–2 wk by 0.3 mg/kg/24 hr (rounded down to the nearest whole tablet) as needed. If adding lamotrigine with valproic acid alone, usual maintenance dose is 1–3 mg/kg/24 hr.

Max. dose: 200 mg/24 hr

>12 yr and adult adjunctive therapy:

WITH AEDs other than carbamazepine, phenytoin, phenobarbital, primidone, or valproic acid (use immediate-release dosage forms):

Wk 1 and 2: 25 mg once daily PO

Wk 3 and 4: 50 mg once daily PO

Usual maintenance dose: 225–375 mg/24 hr ÷ BID PO, titrated to effect. To achieve the usual maintenance dose, increase doses Q1–2 wk by 50 mg/24 hr as needed.

WITH enzyme-inducing AEDs WITHOUT valproic acid (use immediate-release dosage forms):

Wk 1 and 2: 50 mg once daily PO

Wk 3 and 4: 50 mg BID PO

Usual maintenance dose: 300–500 mg/24 hr ÷ BID PO, titrated to effect. To achieve the usual maintenance dose, increase doses Q1–2 wk by 100 mg/24 hr as needed. Doses as high as 700 mg/24 hr ÷ BID have been used.

WITH AEDs WITH valproic acid: (use immediate-release dosage forms):

Wk 1 and 2: 25 mg every other day PO

Wk 3 and 4: 25 mg once daily PO

Usual maintenance dose: 100–400 mg/24 hr ÷ once daily–BID PO, titrated to effect. To achieve the usual maintenance dose, increase doses Q1–2 wk by 25–50 mg/24 hr as needed. If adding lamotrigine to valproic acid alone, usual maintenance dose is 100–200 mg/24 hr.

Extended-release dosage form (Lamictal XR)

≥13 yr and adult adjunctive therapy (max. dose: increases after week 8: 100 mg/24 hr at weekly intervals; see remarks):

	Weeks 1 & 2	Weeks 3 & 4	Week 5	Week 6	Week 7	Maintenance Dose
Patient NOT receiving enzyme-inducing drugs (e.g., carbamazepine) *OR* valproic acid	25 mg once daily	50 mg once daily	100 mg once daily	150 mg once daily	200 mg once daily	300–400 mg once daily

For explanation of icons, see p. 648

Continued

LAMOTRIGINE *continued*

	Weeks 1 & 2	Weeks 3 & 4	Week 5	Week 6	Week 7	Maintenance Dose
Patients receiving enzyme-inducing drugs (e.g., carbamaze-pine) WITHOUT valproic acid	50 mg once daily	100 mg once daily	200 mg once daily	300 mg once daily	400 mg once daily	400–600 mg once daily
Patients receiving valproic acid	25 mg every other day	25 mg once daily	50 mg once daily	100 mg once daily	150 mg once daily	200–250 mg once daily

Converting from a single enzyme-inducing AED to lamotrigine monotherapy for child ≥16 yr and adult (titrate lamotrigine to maintenance dose; then gradually withdraw enzyme-inducing AED by 20% decrements over a 4-wk period; use immediate-release dosage forms):

   Wk 1 and 2: 50 mg once daily PO

   Wk 3 and 4: 50 mg BID PO

   Usual maintenance dose: 500 mg/24 hr ÷ BID PO, titrated to effect. To achieve the usual maintenance dose, increase doses Q1–2 wk by 100 mg/24 hr as needed.

Bipolar disease (use immediate-release dosage forms):
≥18 yr and adult (PO; see table below):

	Weeks 1 & 2	Weeks 3 & 4	Week 5	Week 6 and Thereafter
Patient NOT receiving enzyme-inducing drugs (e.g., carbamazepine) *OR* valproic acid	25 mg/24 hr	50 mg/24 hr	100 mg/24 hr	200 mg/24 hr (target dose)
Patents receiving enzyme-inducing drugs (e.g., carbamazepine) WITHOUT valproic acid	50 mg/24 hr	100 mg/24 hr ÷ once daily–BID	200 mg/24 hr PO ÷ once daily–BID	Week 6: 300 mg/24 hr ÷ once daily –BID Week 7 and thereafter: may increase to 400 mg/24 hr ÷ once daily–BID (target dose)*
Patients receiving valproic acid	25 mg every other day	25 mg/24 hr	50 mg/24 hr PO	100 mg/24 hr (target dose)†

*If carbamazepine or other enzyme-inducing drug is discontinued, maintain current lamotrigine dose for 1 week, then decrease daily lamotrigine dose in 100-mg increments at weekly intervals until 200 mg/24 hr.

†If valproic acid is discontinued, increase by 50-mg weekly intervals up to 200 mg/24 hr.

Enzyme-inducing AEDs include carbamazepine, phenytoin, and phenobarbital. Stevens-Johnson syndrome, toxic epidermal necrolysis, and other potentially life-threatening rashes have been reported in children (0.8%) and adults (0.3%) for adjunctive therapy in seizures. Reported rates for adults treated for bipolar/mood disorders as monotherapy and adjunctive therapy are 0.08% and 0.13%, respectively. May cause fatigue, drowsiness, ataxia, rash (especially with valproic acid), headache, nausea, vomiting, and abdominal pain. Diplopia, nystagmus, aseptic meningitis, and alopecia have also been reported. Use during the first 3 mo of pregnancy may result in a higher chance for cleft lip or cleft palate in the newborn. Suicidal behavior or ideation have been reported.

If converting from immediate-release to extended-release dosage form, initial dose of extended-release drug should match total daily dose of immediate-release drug and be administered once daily. Adjust dose as needed with recommended dosage guidelines.

LAMOTRIGINE *continued*

Reduce maintenance dose in renal failure. Reduce all doses (initial, escalation, and maintenance) in liver dysfunction defined by Child-Pugh grading system as follows:

Grade B: Moderate dysfunction, decrease dose by ≈ 50%

Grade C: Severe dysfunction, decrease dose by ≈ 75%

Withdrawal symptoms may occur if discontinued suddenly. A stepwise dose reduction over ≥2 wk (≈50% per week) is recommended unless safety concerns require a more rapid withdrawal.

Acetaminophen, carbamazepine, oral contraceptives (ethinylestradiol), phenobarbital, primidone, phenytoin, and rifampin may decrease levels of lamotrigine. Valproic acid may increase levels.

LANSOPRAZOLE
Prevacid, Prevacid SoluTab, First-Lansoprazole, and generics
Gastric acid pump inhibitor

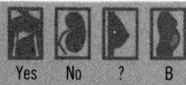

Yes   No   ?   B

Caps, delayed-release: 15, 30 mg
Tabs, disintegrating delayed-release (Prevacid SoluTab): 15, 30 mg; contains aspartame
Granules for delayed-release oral suspension: 15, 30 mg packets (30s)
Oral suspension (First-Lansoprazole): 3 mg/mL (90, 150, 300 mL); contains benzyl alcohol

1–11 yr (short-term treatment of GERD and erosive esophagitis, for up to 12 wk):
Initial dose:
    ≤30 kg: 15 mg PO once daily
    >30 kg: 30 mg PO once daily–BID
Subsequent dosage increase (if needed): May be increased up to 30 mg PO BID after ≥2 wk of therapy without response at initial dose level.
12 yr–adult:
    GERD: 15 mg PO once daily for up to 8 wk
    Erosive esophagitis: 30 mg PO once daily × 8–16 wk; *maintenance dose:* 15 mg PO once daily
    Duodenal ulcer: 15 mg PO once daily × 4 wk; *maintenance dose:* 15 mg PO once daily
    Gastric ulcer and NSAID-induced ulcer: 30 mg PO once daily for up to 8 wk
    Hypersecretory conditions: 60 mg PO once daily; dosage may be increased up to 90 mg PO BID, where doses >120 mg/24 hr are divided BID.

Common side effects include GI discomfort, headache, fatigue, rash, and taste perversion. Microscopic colitis resulting in watery diarrhea has been reported, and switching to an alternative proton pump inhibitor may be beneficial in resolving diarrhea.

Drug is a substrate for CYP 450 2C19 and 3A3/4. May decrease absorption of itraconazole, ketoconazole, iron salts, and ampicillin esters; may increase levels/effects of methotrexate, tacrolimus, and warfarin. Theophylline clearance may be enhanced. **Reduce dose in severe hepatic impairment.** May be used in combination with clarithromycin and amoxicillin for *Helicobacter pylori* infections.

In a multicenter double-blind parallel-group study in infants (1 mo–1 yr) with GERD, lansoprazole was no more effective than placebo.

Administer all oral doses before meals and 30 min before sucralfate. **Do not** crush or chew granules (all dosage forms). Capsule may be opened and intact granules administered in an acidic beverage or food (e.g., apple or cranberry juice, applesauce). **Do not** break or cut orally disintegrating tablets. Use of oral disintegrating tablets dissolved in water has been reported to clog and block oral syringes and feeding tubes (gastric and jejunostomy). For IV use, use a 1.2- micron inline filter.

For explanation of icons, see p. 648

LEVALBUTEROL
Xopenex, Xopenex HFA, and generics
β₂-Adrenergic agonist

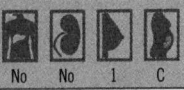

No   No   1   C

Prediluted nebulized solution: 0.31 mg in 3 mL, 0.63 mg in 3 mL, 1.25 mg in 3 mL (30s)
Concentrated nebulized solution: 1.25 mg/0.5 mL (0.5 mL) (30s)
Aerosol inhaler (MDI; Xopenex HFA): 45 mcg/actuation (15 g delivers 200 doses)

Nebulizer:
 ≤4 yr: Start at 0.31 mg inhaled Q4–6 hr PRN; dose may be increased up to 1.25 mg
 Q4–6 hr PRN.
 5–11 yr: Start at 0.31 mg inhaled Q8 hr PRN; dose may be increased to 0.63 mg Q8 hr PRN.
 ≥12 yr and adult: Start at 0.63 mg inhaled Q6–8 hr PRN; dose may be increased to 1.25 mg inhaled
 Q8 hr PRN.
Aerosol inhaler (MDI):
 ≥4 yr and adult: 2 puffs Q4–6 hr PRN
For use in acute exacerbations, more aggressive dosing may be used.

R-isomer of racemic albuterol. Side effects include tachycardia, palpitations, tremor, insomnia,
nervousness, nausea, and headache.
Current clinical data in children indicate levalbuterol is as effective as albuterol, with fewer
cardiac side effects at equipotent doses (0.31–0.63 mg levalbuterol ≈ 2.5 mg albuterol).
More frequent dosing may be necessary in asthma exacerbation.

LEVETIRACETAM
Keppra, Keppra XR, and generics
Anticonvulsant

No   Yes   2   C

Tabs: 250, 500, 750, 1000 mg
Extended-release tabs (Keppra XR): 500, 750 mg
Oral solution: 100 mg/mL (480 mL); dye free and contains parabens
Injection: 100 mg/mL (5 mL); contains 45 mg sodium chloride and 8.2 mg sodium acetate trihydrate
per 100 mg drug
Premixed injection: 500 mg/100 mL in 0.82% sodium chloride, 1000 mg/100 mL in 0.75% sodium
chloride, 1500 mg/100 mL in 0.54% sodium chloride

Partial seizures (adjunctive therapy using immediate-release dosage forms):

  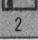

 Infant (1–5 mo): Start at 7 mg/kg/dose PO BID; increase by 7 mg/kg/dose BID every
 2 wk as tolerated to the recommended dose of 21 mg/kg/dose BID. An average daily dose
 of 35 mg/kg/24 hr was reported in clinical trials.
 Infant ≥ 6 mo–child 3 yr (>20 kg): Start at 10 mg/kg/dose PO BID; increase by 10 mg/kg/dose BID
 every 2 wk as tolerated to the recommended dose of 25 mg/kg/dose BID. An average daily dose of 47
 mg/kg/24 hr was reported in clinical trials.
 Child 4–15 yr: Start at 10 mg/kg/dose PO BID; increase by 10 mg/kg/dose BID every 2 wk as
 tolerated up to a **max. dose** of 30 mg/kg/dose BID or 3000 mg/24 hr. An average daily dose of 44
 mg/kg/24 hr was reported in clinical trials.
 Alternative dosing with oral tablets:
 20–40 kg: Start at 250 mg PO BID; increase by 250 mg BID every 2 wk as tolerated up to a
 maximum of 750 mg BID.
 >40 kg: Start at 500 mg PO BID; increase by 500 mg BID every 2 wk as tolerated up to a
 maximum of 1500 mg BID.
 16 yr–adult: Start at 500 mg PO BID; may increase by 500 mg/dose BID every 2 wk as tolerated up
 to a **max. dose** of 1500 mg BID.

L

FORMULARY

LEVETIRACETAM *continued*

Myoclonic seizure (adjunctive therapy using immediate-release dosage forms):
    ≥12 yr and adult: Start at 500 mg PO BID, then increase dosage by 500 mg/dose BID every 2 wk as tolerated to reach target dosage of 1500 mg BID.
Tonic-clonic seizure (primary generalized, adjunctive therapy; use immediate-release dosage forms):
    Child 6–15 yr: Start at 10 mg/kg/dose PO BID; increase by 10 mg/kg/dose BID every 2 wk as tolerated to reach the target dosage of 30 mg/kg/dose BID.
    16 yr–adult: Start at 500 mg PO BID; then increase dosage by 500 mg/dose BID every 2 wk as tolerated to reach the target dosage of 1500 mg BID.
Refractory seizures (add-on therapy [limited data]): See remarks.

Do not abruptly withdraw therapy to reduce risk for seizures. **Use with caution** in renal impairment **(reduce dose; see Chapter 31)**, hemodialysis, and neuropsychiatric conditions.
May cause loss of appetite, vomiting, dizziness, headaches, somnolence, agitation, depression, and mood swings. Drowsiness, fatigue, nervousness, and aggressive behavior have been reported in children. Nonpsychotic behavioral symptoms reported in children is ≈ 3 times greater than in adults (37.6% vs. 13.3%). Suicidal behavior or ideation, serious dermatologic reactions (e.g., Stevens-Johnson syndrome and TEN), and hematologic abnormalities have been reported. Levetiracetam may decrease carbamazepine's effects. Ginkgo may decrease levetiracetam's effects.
Use in children 6 mo–4 yr have been reported in refractory seizures of various types and as an add-on therapy. The following dosage had been used: Start at 5–10 mg/kg/24 hr PO ÷ BID–TID; if needed and tolerated, increase dose by 10 mg/kg/24 hr at weekly intervals up to a **max. dose** of 60 mg/kg/24 hr.
Drug has excellent PO absorption. For IV use, use similar immediate-release PO dosages only when oral route of administration is not feasible. Extended-release tablet is designed for once-daily administration at similar daily dosage of immediate-release forms (e.g., 1000 mg once daily of the extended-release tablet is equivalent to 500 mg BID of the immediate-release tablet).

LEVOCARNITINE

See Carnitine

LEVOFLOXACIN
Levaquin, Quixin, Iquix and generics
Antibiotic, quinolone

| No | Yes | 2 | C |

Tabs: 250, 500, 750 mg
Oral solution: 25 mg/mL (100, 200, 480 mL)
Injection: 25 mg/mL (20, 30 mL)
Premixed injection in D$_5$W: 250 mg/50 mL, 500 mg/100 mL, 750 mg/150 mL
Ophthalmic drops:
    Quixin: 0.5% (5 mL)
    Iquix: 1.5% (5 mL)

Child:
    <5 yr: 10 mg/kg/dose IV/PO Q12 hr; **max. dose** 500 mg/24 hr
    ≥5 yr: 10 mg/kg/dose IV/PO Q24 hr; **max. dose** 500 mg/24 hr
Recurrent or persistent acute otitis media (6 mo–<5 yr): 10 mg/kg/dose PO Q12 hr × 10 days; **max. dose** 500 mg/24 hr
Community-acquired pneumonia (IDSA/Pediatric Infectious Disease Society):
    6 mo–<5 yr: 8–10 mg/kg/dose PO/IV Q12 hr; **max. dose** 750 mg/24 hr
    5–12 yr: 8–10 mg/kg/dose PO/IV Q24 hr; **max. dose** 750 mg/24 hr

Continued

For explanation of icons, see p. 648

LEVOFLOXACIN *continued*

Inhalational anthrax (postexposure) and plague:
≥*6 mo and <50 kg:* 8 mg/kg/dose PO/IV Q12 hr; **max. dose** 500 mg/24 hr
>*50 kg:* 500 mg PO/IV once daily
Duration of therapy:
Inhalational anthrax (postexposure): 60 days
Plague: 10–14 days
Adult:
Community-acquired pneumonia: 500 mg PO/IV Q24 hr × 7–14 days; *OR* 750 mg PO/IV Q24 hr × 5 days
Complicated UTI/acute pyelonephritis: 250 PO/IV Q24 hr × 10 days; *OR* 750 mg PO/IV Q24 hr × 5 days
Uncomplicated UTI: 250 mg PO/IV Q24 hr × 3 days
Uncomplicated skin/skin structure infection: 500 mg PO/IV Q24 hr × 7–10 days
Acute bacterial sinusitis: 500 mg PO/IV Q24 hr × 10–14 days; *OR* 750 mg PO/IV Q24 hr × 5 days
Inhalational anthrax (post exposure) and plague: 500 mg PO/IV Q24 hr. **Duration of therapy:**
inhalational anthrax, 60 days; plague, 10–14 days.
Conjunctivitis:
≥*1 yr and adult:* Instill 1–2 drops of the 0.5% solution to affected eye(s) Q2 hr up to 8 times/24 hr
while awake for the first 2 days, then Q4 hr up to 4 times/24 hr while awake for the next 5 days.
Corneal ulcer:
≥*6 yr and adult:* Instill 1–2 drops of the 1.5% solution to affected eye(s) Q30 min–2 hr while awake
and 4 and 6 hr after retiring for the first 3 days, then Q1–4 hr while awake.

Contraindicated in hypersensitivity to other quinolones. **Avoid** in patients with history of QTc
prolongation or taking QTc-prolonging drugs, and excessive sunlight exposure. **Use with
caution** in diabetes, seizures, children <18 yr, and renal impairment **(adjust dose, see
Chapter 31).** Ophthalmic solution may cause GI disturbances, headache, and blurred vision.
Musculoskeletal disorders (e.g., arthralgia, arthritis, tendinopathy, and gait abnormality) may
occur. Peripheral neuropathy has been reported. Safety in pediatric patients treated >14 days
has not been evaluated. Like other quinolones, tendon rupture can occur during or after
therapy (risk increases with concurrent corticosteroids). Use with NSAIDs may increase risk of
CNS stimulation and seizures.
Infuse IV over 1–1.5 hr; **avoid** IV push or rapid infusion because of risk of hypotension. **Do not**
administer antacids or other divalent salts with or within 2 hr of oral levofloxacin dose; otherwise
may be administered with or without food.

LEVOTHYROXINE (T₄)
Synthroid, Tirosint, Unithroid, Unithroid Direct, and generics
Thyroid product

No No 1 A

Tabs: 25, 50, 75, 88, 100, 112, 125, 137, 150, 175, 200, 300 mcg
Caps (Tirosint): 13, 25, 50, 75, 88, 100, 112, 125, 137, 150 mcg
Injection: 100, 200, 500 mcg; preservative free
Oral suspension: 25 mcg/mL

Child PO dosing:
1–3 mo: 10–15 mcg/kg/dose once daily. If patient is at risk for developing cardiac failure,
start with lower dose of 25 mcg/24 hr. If patient has very low T₄ (<5 mcg/dL) use higher
12–17 mcg/kg/24 hr dose.
3–6 mo: 8–10 mcg/kg/dose once daily
6–12 mo: 6–8 mcg/kg/dose once daily
1–5 yr: 5–6 mcg/kg/dose once daily

LEVOTHYROXINE (T₄) *continued*

6–12 yr: 4–5 mcg/kg/dose once daily
>12 yr:
 Incomplete growth and prepuberty: 2–3 mcg/kg/dose once daily
 Complete growth and puberty: 1.7 mcg/kg/dose once daily
Child IM/IV dose: 50%–75% of oral dose once daily
Adult:
 PO: Start with 12.5–25 mcg/dose once daily. Increase by 25–50 mcg/24 hr at intervals of Q2–4 wk
 until euthyroid. Usual adult dose: 100–200 mcg/24 hr.
 IM/IV dose: 50% of oral dose once daily.
 Myxedema coma or stupor: 200–500 mcg IV × 1, then 75–300 mcg IV once daily; convert to oral
 therapy once patient is stabilized.

Contraindications include acute MI, thyrotoxicosis, and uncorrected adrenal insufficiency. May
cause hyperthyroidism, rash, growth disturbances, hypertension, arrhythmias, diarrhea, and
weight loss. Pseudotumor cerebri has been reported in children. Overtreatment may cause
craniosynostosis in infants and premature closure of epiphyses in children.

Total replacement dose may be used in children unless there is evidence of cardiac disease; in that
case, begin with one fourth of maintenance and increase weekly. Titrate dosage with clinical status
and serum T₄ and TSH. Increases effects of warfarin. Phenytoin, rifampin, carbamazepine, iron and
calcium supplements, antacids, and orlistat may decrease levothyroxine levels. Tricyclic
antidepressants and SSRIs may enhance toxic effects.

100 mcg levothyroxine = 65 mg thyroid USP. Administer oral doses on an empty stomach and tablets
with a full glass of water. Iron and calcium supplements and antacids may decrease absorption; do
not administer within 4 hr of these agents. Excreted in low levels in breast milk; preponderance of
evidence suggests no clinically significant effect in infants.

LIDOCAINE
Xylocaine, L-M-X, Lidoderm, and various generics
Antiarrhythmic class Ib, local anesthetic

   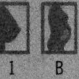

Yes   No   1   B

Injection: 0.5%, 1%, 1.5%, 2%, 4%, 5%, 10% (1% sol = 10 mg/mL)
IV infusion (in D₅W): 0.4% (4 mg/mL) (250, 500 mL); 0.8% (8 mg/mL) (250 mL)
Injection with epinephrine (some preparations may contain metasulfite or are preservative free):
 Injection with 1:50,000 epi: 2%
 Injection with 1:100,000 epi: 1%, 2%
 Injection with 1:200,000 epi: 0.5%, 1%, 1.5%, 2%
Ointment: 5% (30, 50 g)
Cream, topical: 3% (30, 85 g), 4% (L-M-X-4 and others) [OTC] (5, 15, 30, 45 g); may contain benzyl
alcohol
Cream, rectal: 5% (L-M-X-5 and others; 15, 30 g); contains benzyl alcohol
Gel (external): 2% (5, 10, 20, 30 mL), 3% (10, 30 mL), 4% (10, 30 , 113 g), 5% (10, 30, 113 g);
may contain benzyl alcohol, EDTA
Lotion: 3% (177 mL)
Solution (external): 4% (50 mL); may contain parabens
Oral solution (mouth/throat): 2% (4, 15, 100 mL)
Transdermal patch (Lidoderm): 5% (30s)
Topical 2.5% (with 2.5% prilocaine): See *Lidocaine and Prilocaine.*

Continued

For explanation of icons, see p. 648

LIDOCAINE *continued*

Anesthetic:
Injection:

Without epinephrine: **Max. dose** of 4.5 mg/kg/dose (up to 300 mg); do not repeat within 2 hr.

With epinephrine: **Max. dose** of 7 mg/kg/dose (up to 500 mg); do not repeat within 2 hr.

Topical:

Cream (child ≥ 2 yr and adult): Apply to affected intact skin areas BID–QID.

Gel or ointment (child ≥ 2 yr and adult): Apply to affected intact skin areas once daily–QID; **max. dose** 4.5 mg/kg up to 300 mg.

Patch (adult): Apply to most painful area with up to 3 patches at a time. Patch(es) may be applied for up to 12 hr in any 24-hr period.

Antiarrhythmic (infant, child, adolescent):

Bolus: 1 mg/kg/dose (**max. dose** 100 mg) slowly IV; may repeat in 10–15 min × 2; **max. total dose** 3–5 mg/kg within the first hr. ETT dose = 2–3 × IV dose.

Continuous infusion: 20–50 mcg/kg/min IV/IO (**do not** exceed 20 mcg/kg/min for patients with shock, CHF, hepatic disease, or cardiac arrest); see inside cover for infusion preparation. Administer a 1-mg/kg bolus when infusion is initiated if bolus has not been given within previous 15 min.

Oral use (viscous liquid):

Child (≥3 yr): Up to the lesser of 4.5 mg/kg/dose or 300 mg/dose, swish and spit Q3 hr PRN up to a **max. dose** of 4 doses per 12-hr period.

Adult: 15 mL, swish and spit Q3 hr PRN up to a **max. dose** of 8 doses/24 hr.

For cardiac arrest, amiodarone is the preferred agent over lidocaine; lidocaine may be used only when amiodarone is not available.

Contraindicated in Stokes-Adams attacks, SA, AV, or intraventricular heart block without a pacemaker. Side effects include hypotension, asystole, seizures, and respiratory arrest. Anaphylactic reactions have been reported.

CYP 450 2D6 and 3A3/4 substrate. Decrease dose in hepatic failure or decreased cardiac output. **Do not use** topically for teething. Prolonged infusion may result in toxic accumulation of lidocaine, especially in infants. **Do not use** epinephrine-containing solutions for treatment of arrhythmias.

Therapeutic levels 1.5–5 mg/L. Toxicity occurs at >7 mg/L. Toxicity in neonates may occur at >5 mg/L, owing to reduced protein binding of drug. Elimination $T_{1/2}$: premature infant, 3.2 hr; adult, 1.5–2 hr.

When using topical patch, avoid exposing application site to external heat sources; may increase risk for toxicity.

LIDOCAINE AND PRILOCAINE
EMLA, Oraqix, Eutectic mixture of lidocaine and prilocaine
Topical analgesic

Yes   Yes   ?   B

Cream: Lidocaine 2.5% + prilocaine 2.5% (5, 30 g)

Periodontal gel (Oraqix): Lidocaine 2.5% + prilocaine 2.5% (1.7 g in dental cartridges; 20s)

See Chapter 6 for general use information.

Neonate (≥37-wk gestation):

Painful procedures (e.g., IM injections): 1 g/site for at least 60 min

Circumcision: 1–2 g and cover with occlusive dressing for 60–90 min

Infant and child: The following are the recommended **max. doses** based on child's age and weight.

LIDOCAINE AND PRILOCAINE *continued*

Age and Weight	Maximum Total EMLA Dose (g)	Maximum Application Area (cm²)	Maximum Application Time
Birth–<3 mo or <5 kg	1	10	1 hr
3–12 mo and >5 kg*	2	20	4 hr
1–6 yr and >10 kg	10	100	4 hr
7–12 yr and >20 kg	20	200	4 hr

*If patient is >3 months and is not >5 kg, use max. total dose that corresponds to patient's weight.
EMLA, Eutectic mixture of local anesthetics.

Adult:
    Minor procedures: 2.5 g/site for at least 60 min
    Painful procedures: 2 g/10 cm² of skin for at least 2 hr

Should not be used in neonates <37 wk of gestation or infants <age 12 mo receiving treatment with methoglobin-inducing agents (e.g., sulfa drugs, acetaminophen, nitrofurantoin, nitroglycerin, nitroprusside, phenobarbital, phenytoin). **Use with caution** in patients with G6PD deficiency, patients treated with class I or III antiarrhythmic drugs (additive or toxic cardiac effects), and in patients with renal and hepatic impairment. Prilocaine has been associated with methemoglobinemia. Long duration of application, large treatment area, small patients, or impaired elimination may result in high blood levels.
Apply topically to intact skin and cover with occlusive dressing; **avoid** mucous membranes and eyes. Wipe off cream before procedure.

LINDANE
Gamma benzene hexachloride and various generics
Scabicidal agent, pediculocide

No   No   3   C

Shampoo: 1% (60 mL)
Lotion: 1% (60 mL)

Child and adult (see remarks):
    Scabies: Apply thin layer of lotion to skin. Bathe and rinse off medication in adults after 8–12 hr; children 6–8 hr. May repeat × 1 in 7 days PRN.
    Pediculosis capitis: Apply 15–30 mL of shampoo, lather for 4–5 min, rinse hair and comb with fine comb to remove nits. May repeat × 1 in 7 days PRN.
    Pediculosis pubis: May use lotion or shampoo (applied locally) as for scabies and pediculosis capitis (see above).

Contraindicated in premature infants and seizure disorders. **Use with caution** with drugs that lower seizure threshold. Systemically absorbed. Risk of toxic effects is greater in young children; use other agents (permethrin) in infants, young children (<2 yr), and during pregnancy. Lindane is considered second-line therapy owing to side-effect risk and reports of resistance.
May cause a rash; rarely may cause seizures or aplastic anemia. For scabies, change clothing and bed sheets after starting treatment, and treat family members. For pediculosis pubis, treat sexual contacts.
Avoid contact with face, urethral meatus, damaged skin, or mucous membranes. **Do not** use any covering that does not breathe (e.g., plastic lining or clothing) over the applied lindane.

For explanation of icons, see p. 648

LINEZOLID
Zyvox
Antibiotic, oxazolidinone

   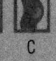

No   No   2   C

Tabs: 600 mg; contains ≈ 0.45 mEq Na per 200 mg drug
Oral suspension: 100 mg/5 mL (150 mL); contains phenylalanine and sodium benzoate and 0.8 mEq Na per 200 mg drug
Injection, premixed: 200 mg in 100 mL, 600 mg in 300 mL; contains 1.7 mEq Na per 200 mg drug

Neonate:
  <1 kg:
    <14 days old: 10 mg/kg/dose IV Q12 hr
    ≥14 days old: 10 mg/kg/dose IV Q8 hr
  ≥1 kg:
    <7 days old: 10 mg/kg/dose IV/PO Q12 hr
    ≥7 days old: 10 mg/kg/dose IV/PO Q8 hr
  ≥34 wk gestation and 0–28 days old: 10 mg/kg/dose IV/PO Q8 hr
Infant and child < 12 yr old:
  Pneumonia, bacteremia, bone/joint infections, septic thrombosis (MRSA), complicated skin/skin structure infections, vancomycin-resistant Enterococcus faecium (VRE) infections (including endocarditis): 10 mg/kg/dose IV/PO Q8 hr
  Uncomplicated skin/skin structure infections:
    <5 yr: 10 mg/kg/dose IV/PO Q8 hr
    5–11 yr: 10 mg/kg/dose IV/PO Q12 hr
  Max. dose for all indications <12 yr: 600 mg/dose
≥12 yr and adult: 600 mg Q12 hr IV/PO. 400 mg Q12 hr IV/PO may be used for adults with uncomplicated infection. **Duration of therapy:**
  MRSA infections: Variable based on response
  Pneumonia: 10–14 days for non-MRSA and 7–21 days (per clinical response) for MRSA
  Bacteremia: 10–28 days
  Bone/joint infections: 3–6 weeks
  Skin/skin structure infections: 10–14 days; longer for complicated cases
  Septic thrombosis (MRSA): 4–6 weeks
  VRE infections: 14–28 days, minimum of 8 weeks for endocarditis

Most common side effects include diarrhea, headache, and nausea. Anemia, leukopenia, pancytopenia, thrombocytopenia may occur in patients who are at risk for myelosuppression and receive regimens >2 wk. CBC monitoring recommended in these individuals. Pseudomembranous colitis and neuropathy (peripheral and optic) have also been reported. CSF penetration is variable in patients with VP shunts.

Do not use with SSRIs (e.g., fluoxetine, paroxetine), tricyclic antidepressants, venlafaxine, and trazodone; may cause serotonin syndrome. **Avoid** use with MAOIs (e.g., phenelzine) and in patients with uncontrolled hypertension, pheochromocytoma, thyrotoxicosis, and taking sympathomimetics or vasopressive agents (may elevate blood pressure). Patients must **use caution** when consuming large amounts of foods and beverages containing tyramine; may increase blood pressure. Dosing information in severe hepatic failure and renal impairment with multidoses have not been completed.

Protect all dosage forms from light and moisture. Oral suspension product must be gently mixed by inverting the bottle 3–5 times before each use (**do not shake**). All oral doses may be administered with or without food.

L

LISDEXAMFETAMINE
Vyvanse
CNS stimulant

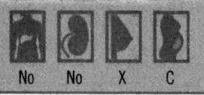

No   No   X   C

Capsules: 20, 30, 40, 50, 60, 70 mg

Attention deficit hyperactivity disorder:
Child ≥ 6 yr and adult: Start with 30 mg PO QAM. May increase dose by 10–20 mg/24 hr at weekly intervals if needed, up to a **max. dose** of 70 mg/24 hr.

Lisdexamfetamine is a prodrug of dextroamphetamine, which requires activation by intestinal/hepatic metabolism.

Contraindicated in amphetamine or sympathomimetic hypersensitivity, symptomatic cardiovascular disease, moderate/severe hypertension, hyperthyroidism, glaucoma, agitated states, drug/alcohol abuse history, and MAOIs (concurrent or use within 14 days). As with other CNS stimulant medications, serious cardiovascular events, including **death**, have been reported in patients with preexisting structural cardiac abnormalities or other serious heart problems. **Use with caution** in patients with hypertension, psychiatric conditions, and epilepsy. May cause insomnia, irritability, rash, appetite suppression/weight loss, dizziness, xerostomia, and GI disturbances. Dermatillomania, Stevens-Johnson syndrome, and TEN have been reported.

Urinary acidifying agents may reduce levels of amphetamines, and urinary alkalinizing agents may increase levels. May increase effects of TCAs; increase or decrease effects of guanfacine, phenytoin, and phenobarbital; and decrease effects of adrenergic blockers, antihistamines, and antihypertensives. Norepinephrine may increase effects of amphetamines.

See *Dextroamphetamine ± Amphetamine* for additional remarks.

LISINOPRIL
Prinivil, Zestril, and generics
Angiotensin converting enzyme inhibitor, antihypertensive

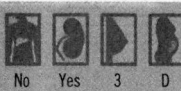

No   Yes   3   D

Tabs: 2.5, 5, 10, 20, 30, 40 mg
Oral suspension: 1, 2 mg/mL

Hypertension (see remarks):
Child (<6 yr; limited data): Use 6–16 yr dosing below.
6–16 yr: Start with 0.07–0.1 mg/kg/dose PO once daily; **max. initial dose** 5 mg/dose. If needed, titrate dose upward at 1–2 wk intervals to doses up to 0.61 mg/kg/24 hr or 40 mg/24 hr (higher doses have not been evaluated).
Adult: Start with 10 mg PO once daily. If needed, increase dose by 5–10 mg/24 hr at 1–2 wk intervals. Usual dosage range: 10–40 mg/24 hr. **Max. dose:** 80 mg/24 hr.

Use lower initial dose (50% of recommended dose) if using with a diuretic or in the presence of hyponatremia, hypovolemia, and severe CHF.

Contraindicated in hypersensitivity and history of angioedema with other ACE inhibitors. Do not use with aliskiren in patients with diabetes. **Avoid** use with dialysis with high-flux membranes; anaphylactoid reactions have been reported. **Use with caution** in aortic or bilateral renal artery stenosis. Side effects include cough, dizziness, headache, hyperkalemia, hypotension (especially with concurrent diuretic or antihypertensive agent use), rash, and GI disturbances. Mood alterations, including depressive symptoms, have been reported.

Continued

LISINOPRIL *continued*

Dual blockade of the renin-angiotensin system with lisinopril and angiotensin receptor antagonist (e.g., losartan) or aliskiren is associated with increased risk for hypotension, syncope, hyperkalemia, and renal impairment. Diabetic patients treated with oral antidiabetic agents should be monitored for hypoglycemia, especially during first month of use. NSAIDs (e.g., indomethacin) may decrease linsinopril's effects. **Adjust dose in renal impairment (see Chapter 31).**

Onset of action: 1 hr, with maximal effect in 6–8 hr. Lisinopril should be discontinued as soon as possible when pregnancy is detected.

LITHIUM
Lithobid and many generics (previously available as Eskalith)
Antimanic agent

No   Yes   X   D

Carbonate:
300 mg carbonate = 8.12 mEq lithium
Caps: 150, 300, 600 mg
Tabs: 300 mg
Extended-release tabs: 300 mg (Lithobid), 450 mg
Citrate:
Syrup: 8 mEq/5 mL (5, 500 mL); 5 mL is equivalent to 300 mg lithium carbonate

Child:
Initial (immediate-release dosage forms): 15–60 mg/kg/24 hr ÷ TID–QID PO.
Adjust as needed (weekly) to achieve therapeutic levels.
Adolescent: 600–1800 mg/24 hr ÷ TID–QID PO (divided BID using controlled/slow-release tablets).
Adult:
Initial: 300 mg TID PO. Adjust as needed to achieve therapeutic levels. Usual dose is about 300 mg TID–QID with immediate-release dosage form. For controlled/slow-release tablets, 900–1800 mg/24 hr PO ÷ BID.
Max. dose: 2400 mg/24 hr

Contraindicated in severe cardiovascular (including Brugada syndrome) or renal disease.
Decreased sodium intake or increased sodium wasting will increase lithium levels.
May cause goiter, nephrogenic diabetes insipidus, hypothyroidism, arrhythmias, or sedation at therapeutic doses.

Coadministration with thiazide diuretics, metronidazole, ACE inhibitors, or NSAIDs may increase risk for lithium toxicity. Iodine may increase risk for hypothyroidism. If used in combination with haloperidol, closely monitor neurologic toxicities, because an encephalopathic syndrome followed by irreversible brain damage has been reported.

Therapeutic levels: 0.6–1.5 mEq/L. In either acute or chronic toxicity, confusion and somnolence may be seen at levels of 2–2.5 mEq/L. **Seizures or death** may occur at levels >2.5 mEq/L. Recommended serum sampling: trough level within 30 min before next scheduled dose. Steady state is achieved within 4–6 days of continuous dosing. **Adjust dose in renal failure (see Chapter 31).**

L

FORMULARY

LOPERAMIDE
Imodium, Imodium A-D, and generics
Antidiarrheal

 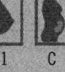

No   No   1   C

Caps [OTC]: 2 mg
Tabs [OTC]: 2 mg
Chewable tabs [OTC]: 2 mg
Caplets [OTC]: 2 mg
Oral liquid [OTC]: 1 mg/5 mL (120 mL); contains 0.5% alcohol
Oral suspension [OTC]: 1 mg/7.5 mL (120 mL); each 30 mL contains 16 mg of sodium

Acute diarrhea:
Child (initial doses within first 24 hr):
   2–5 yr (13–< 21 kg): 1 mg PO TID
   6–8 yr (21–27 kg): 2 mg PO BID
   9–11 yr (>27–43 kg): 2 mg PO TID
   Max. single dose: 2 mg
     Follow initial day's dose with 0.1 mg/kg/dose after each loose stool (not to exceed
     aforementioned initial doses).
≥12 yr and adult: 4 mg/dose × 1, followed by 2 mg/dose after each stool up to **max. dose** of 8
mg/24 hr for adolescents and 16 mg/24 hr for adults.
Chronic diarrhea:
Child: 0.08–0.24 mg/kg/24 hr ÷ BID–TID; **max. dose** 2 mg/dose

Contraindicated in acute dysentery, acute ulcerative colitis, bacterial enterocolitis due to
Salmonella, *Shigella*, *Campylobacter*, and *Clostridium difficile*, and abdominal pain in the
absence of diarrhea. **Avoid** use in children <2 yr owing to reports of paralytic ileus associated
with abdominal distention. Rare hypersensitivity reactions, including anaphylactic shock
have been reported. May cause nausea, rash, vomiting, constipation, cramps, dry mouth, and
CNS depression. **Discontinue use if no clinical improvement is observed within 48 hr.**
Naloxone may be administered for CNS depression.

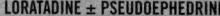

LORATADINE ± PSEUDOEPHEDRINE
Alavert, Claritin, Claritin Children's Allergy, Claritin RediTabs,
Claritin-D 12 Hour, Claritin-D 24 Hour, many others, and generics
Antihistamine, less sedating ± decongestant

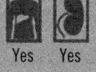

Yes   Yes   2   B

Tabs [OTC]: 10 mg
Chewable tabs (Claritin Children's Allergy) [OTC]: 5 mg; contains aspartame
Disintegrating tabs (RediTabs) [OTC]: 5, 10 mg; contains aspartame
Oral solution or syrup [OTC]: 1 mg/mL (120 mL); contains propylene glycol and sodium benzoate;
some preparations may contain metasulfite
Time-release tabs in combination with pseudoephedrine (PE):
  Claritin-D 12 Hour [OTC]: 5 mg loratadine + 120 mg PE
  Claritin-D 24 Hour [OTC]: 10 mg loratadine + 240 mg PE

Loratadine:
2–5 yr: 5 mg PO once daily
≥6 yr and adult: 10 mg PO once daily
Time-release tabs of loratadine and pseudoephedrine:
≥12 yr and adult (see remarks):
  Claritin-D 12 Hour: 1 tablet PO BID
  Claritin-D 24 Hour: 1 tablet PO once daily

For explanation of icons, see p. 648

LORATADINE ± PSEUDOEPHEDRINE *continued*

May cause drowsiness, fatigue, dry mouth, headache, bronchospasms, palpitations, dermatitis, and dizziness. Has **not** been implicated in causing cardiac arrhythmias when used with other drugs metabolized by hepatic microsomal enzymes (e.g., ketoconazole, erythromycin). May be administered safely in patients who have allergic rhinitis and asthma.

In hepatic and renal function impairment (GFR < 30 mL/min), prolong loratadine (single agent) dosage interval to every other day. **Adjust dose in renal failure (see Chapter 31).**

For time-release tablets of the combination product (loratadine and pseudoephedrine), prolong dosage interval in renal impairment (GFR < 30 mL/min) as follows: Claritin-D 12 Hour, 1 tablet PO once daily; Claritin-D 24 Hour, 1 tablet PO every other day. **Do not use** the combination product in hepatic impairment; component drugs cannot be individually titrated.

Administer doses on an empty stomach. For use of RediTabs, place tablet on tongue and allow it to disintegrate in the mouth with or without water. For Claritin-D products, also see remarks in *Pseudoephedrine*.

LORAZEPAM
Ativan and many generics
Benzodiazepine anticonvulsant

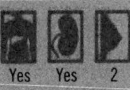

Yes   Yes   2   D

Tabs: 0.5, 1, 2 mg
Injection: 2, 4 mg/mL (each contains 2% benzyl alcohol and propylene glycol)
Oral solution: 2 mg/mL (30 mL); alcohol and dye free

Status epilepticus:
   Neonate, infant, child, and adolescent: 0.05–0.1 mg/kg/dose IV over 2–5 min.
   May repeat dose in 10–15 min. **Max. dose:** 4 mg/dose.
   Adult: 4 mg/dose given slowly over 2–5 min. May repeat in 10–15 min. Usual total **max. dose** in
   12-hr period is 8 mg.
Antiemetic adjunct therapy:
   Child: 0.02–0.05 mg/kg/dose IV Q6 hr PRN; **max. single dose** is 2 mg.
Anxiolytic/sedation:
   Infant and child: 0.05 mg/kg/dose Q4–8 hr PO/IV; **max. dose** is 2 mg/dose.
     May also give IM for preprocedure sedation.
   Adult: 1–10 mg/24 hr PO ÷ BID–TID

Contraindicated in narrow-angle glaucoma and severe hypotension. **Use with caution** in renal insufficiency (glucuronide metabolite clearance is reduced), hepatic insufficiency (may worsen hepatic encephalopathy; decrease dose with severe hepatic impairment), compromised pulmonary function, and use of CNS-depressant medications. May cause respiratory depression, especially in combination with other sedatives. May also cause sedation, dizziness, mild ataxia, mood changes, rash, and GI symptoms. Paradoxical excitation has been reported in children (10%–30% of patients <8 year old).

Significant respiratory depression and/or hypotension has been reported when used in combination with loxapine. Probenecid and valproic acid may increase the effects/toxicity of lorazepam, and oral contraceptive steroids may decrease lorazepam's effects.

Injectable product may be given rectally. Benzyl alcohol and propylene glycol may be toxic to newborns at high doses.

Onset of action for sedation: PO, 20–30 min; IM, 30–60 min; IV, 1–5 min. Duration of action: 6–8 hr.
Flumazenil is the antidote.

M

LOSARTAN
Cozaar and generics
Angiotensin II receptor antagonist

Yes   Yes   ?   C/D

Tabs: 25, 50, 100 mg
Oral suspension: 2.5 mg/mL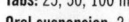
Contains 2.12 mg potassium per 25 mg drug

Hypertension (see remarks):
6–16 yr: Start with 0.7 mg/kg/dose (**max. dose** of 50 mg/dose) PO once daily.
Adjust dose to desired blood pressure response. **Max. dose:** 1.4 mg/kg/24 hr or 100 mg/24 hr.
≥17 yr and adult: Start with 50 mg PO once daily (use lower initial dose of 25 mg PO once daily if patient receiving diuretics, experiencing intravascular volume depletion, or has hepatic impairment). Usual maintenance dose is 25–100 mg/24 hr PO ÷ once daily–BID.

Use with caution in angioedema (current or past), excessive hypotension (volume depletion), hepatic (use lower starting dose) or renal (contains potassium) impairment, hyperkalemia, renal artery stenosis, and severe CHF. Not recommended in patients <age 6 yr or in children with GFR <30 mL/min/1.73 m². owing to lack of data.
Discontinue use as soon as possible when pregnancy is detected; injury and death to developing fetus may occur. Pregnancy category is "C" during first trimester but changes to "D" for second and third trimesters. Diarrhea, asthenia, dizziness, fatigue, and hypotension are common. Thrombocytopenia, rhabdomyolysis, and angioedema have been rarely reported. Losartan is a substrate for CYP 450 2C9 (major) and 3A4. Fluconazole and cimetidine may increase losartan effects/toxicity. Rifampin, phenobarbital, and indomethacin may decrease its effects. Losartan may increase risk of lithium toxicity. **Do not use** with aliskiren in patients with diabetes or with renal impairment (GFR < 60 mL/min). Dual blockade of the renin-angiotensin system with losartan and ACE inhibitors (e.g., captopril) or aliskiren is associated with increased risk for hypotension, syncope, hyperkalemia, and renal impairment.

LOW-MOLECULAR-WEIGHT HEPARIN

See Enoxaparin

LUCINACTANT

See Surfactant, pulmonary

MAGNESIUM CITRATE
Various generics
16.17% Elemental Magnesium
Laxative/cathartic

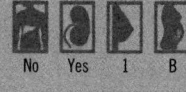
No   Yes   1   B

Oral solution [OTC]: 1.75 g/30 mL (300 mL); 5 mL = 3.9–4.7 mEq Mg
Tabs: 100 mg

Cathartic:
<6 yr: 2–4 mL/kg/24 hr PO ÷ once daily–BID
6–12 yr: 100–150 mL/24 hr PO ÷ once daily–BID
>12 yr and adult: 150–300 mL/24 hr PO ÷ once daily–BID

Use with caution in renal insufficiency (monitor magnesium level) and patients receiving digoxin. May cause hypermagnesemia, diarrhea, muscle weakness, hypotension, and respiratory depression. Up to about 30% of dose is absorbed. May decrease absorption of H2 antagonists, phenytoin, iron salts, tetracycline, steroids, benzodiazepines, and quinolone antibiotics.

For explanation of icons, see p. 648

MAGNESIUM HYDROXIDE
Milk of Magnesia and various generics
41.69% Elemental Magnesium
Antacid, laxative

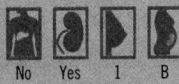

No   Yes   1   B

Oral liquid [OTC]: 400 mg/5 mL (Milk of Magnesia and others)
Concentrated oral liquid [OTC]: 2400 mg/10 mL (Milk of Magnesia concentrate)
Chewable tabs [OTC]: 400 mg
400 mg magnesium hydroxide is equivalent to 166.76 mg elemental magnesium.
Combination product with aluminum hydroxide: See *Aluminum Hydroxide.*

Laxative (all liquid mL doses based on 400 mg/5 mL magnesium hydroxide, unless noted otherwise):
Dose/24 hr ÷ once daily–QID PO
   <2 yr: 0.5 mL/kg
   2–5 yr: 5–15 mL *OR* 400–1200 mg (1–3 chewable tabs)
   6–11 yr: 15–30 mL *OR* 1200–2400 mg (3–6 chewable tabs)
   ≥12 yr and adult: 30–60 mL *OR* 2400–4800 mg (6–12 chewable tabs)
Antacid:
   Child:
      Liquid: 2.5–5 mL/dose once daily–QID PO
      Tabs: 400 mg once daily–QID PO
   Adult:
      Liquid: 5–15 mL/dose once daily–QID PO
      Concentrated liquid (800 mg/5 mL): 2.5–7.5 mL/dose once daily–QID PO
      Tabs: 400–1200 mg/dose once daily–QID PO

See *Magnesium Citrate.* **Use with caution** in renal insufficiency (monitor magnesium level) and patients receiving digoxin. Drink a full 8 oz of liquid with each dose of chewable tablets.

MAGNESIUM OXIDE
Mag-200, Mag-Ox 400, Uro-Mag, and generics
60.32% Elemental Magnesium
Oral magnesium salt

No   Yes   1   B

Tabs [OTC]: 200, 250, 400, 420, 500 mg
Caps (Uro-Mag [OTC]): 140 mg
400 mg magnesium oxide is equivalent to 241.3 mg elemental Mg or 20 mEq Mg.

Doses expressed in magnesium oxide salt.
Magnesium supplementation:
   Child: 5–10 mg/kg/24 hr ÷ TID–QID PO
   Adult: 400–800 mg/24 hr ÷ BID–QID PO
Hypomagnesemia:
   Child: 65–130 mg/kg/24 hr ÷ QID PO
   Adult: 2000 mg/24 hr ÷ QID PO

See *Magnesium Citrate.* **Use with caution** in renal insufficiency (monitor magnesium level) and patients receiving digoxin. For dietary recommended intake (U.S. RDA) for magnesium, see Chapter 21.

MAGNESIUM SULFATE
Epsom salts and others
9.9% Elemental Magnesium
Magnesium salt

No   Yes   1   D

Injection: 500 mg/mL (4 mEq/mL) (2, 10, 20, 50 mL)
Injection, prediluted in sterile water for injection; ready to use: 40 mg/mL (0.325 mEq/mL)
(50, 100, 500, 1000 mL); 80 mg/mL (0.65 mEq/mL) (50 mL)
Injection, prediluted in D₅W; ready to use: 10 mg/mL (0.081 mEq/mL) (100 mL); 20 mg/mL (0.163 mEq/mL) (500 mL)
Granules: Approx. 40 mEq Mg per 5 g (454, 1810 g)
500 mg magnesium sulfate is equivalent to 49.3 mg elemental Mg or 4.1 mEq Mg.

All doses expressed in magnesium sulfate salt.
Cathartic:
   Child: 0.25 g/kg/dose PO Q4–6 hr
   Adult: 10–30 g/dose PO Q4–6 hr
Hypomagnesemia or hypocalcemia:
IV/IM: 25–50 mg/kg/dose Q4–6 hr × 3–4 doses; repeat PRN; **max. single dose:** 2 g
PO: 100–200 mg/kg/dose QID PO
Daily maintenance:
   30–60 mg/kg/24 hr or 0.25–0.5 mEq/kg/24 hr IV
   Max. dose: 1 g/24 hr
Adjunctive therapy for moderate to severe reactive airway disease exacerbation (bronchodilation):
   Child: 25–75 mg/kg/dose (**max. dose:** 2 g) × 1 IV over 20 min
   Adult: 2 g/dose × 1 IV over 20 min

When given IV **beware** of hypotension, respiratory depression, complete heart block, and/or
hypermagnesemia. Calcium gluconate (IV) should be available as **antidote.** Use with caution
in patients with renal insufficiency (monitor magnesium levels) and patients on digoxin. **Serum
level–dependent toxicity** includes the following: >3 mg/dL: CNS depression; >5 mg/dL:
decreased deep tendon reflexes, flushing, somnolence; and >12 mg/dL: respiratory paralysis,
heart block.
Max. IV intermittent infusion rate: 1 mEq/kg/hr or 125 mg MgSO₄ salt/kg/hr
Pregnancy category is "D" because hypocalcemia, osteopenia, and fractures in the developing baby or
fetus have been reported in pregnant women receiving magnesium >5–7 days for preterm labor.

MANNITOL
Aridol, Osmitrol, Resectisol, and various generics
Osmotic diuretic

No   Yes   ?   C

Injection: 50, 100, 150, 200, 250 mg/mL (5%, 10%, 15%, 20%, 25%, respectively)
Irrigation solution (Resectisol): 50 mg/mL (5%)

Anuria/oliguria (child and adult):
   Test dose to assess renal function: 0.2 g/kg/dose (**max. dose:** 12.5 g) IV over 3–5 min. If
   there is no diuresis within 2 hr, discontinue mannitol.
   Initial: 0.5–1 g/kg/dose IV over 2–6 hr
   Maintenance: 0.25–0.5 g/kg/dose Q4–6 hr IV over 2–6 hr

Contraindicated in severe renal disease, active intracranial bleed, dehydration, and pulmonary
edema. May cause circulatory overload and electrolyte disturbances. For hyperosmolar
therapy, keep serum osmolality at 310–320 mOsm/kg.

For explanation of icons, see p. 648

Continued

MANNITOL *continued*

Caution: Drug may crystallize at low temperatures with concentrations ≥15%; redissolve crystals by warming solution up to 70°C with agitation. Use an in-line filter. May cause hypovolemia, headache, and polydipsia. Reduction in ICP occurs in 15 min and lasts 3–6 hr.

MEBENDAZOLE
Vermox and others
Anthelmintic

Yes No 1 C

Chewable tabs: 100 mg (may be swallowed whole or chewed) (boxes of 12s)

Child (>2 yr) and adult:
  Pinworms **(Enterobius):** 100 mg PO × 1, repeat in 2 wk if not cured.
  Hookworms, roundworms **(Ascaris),** *and whipworm* **(Trichuris):** 100 mg PO BID × 3 days.
  Repeat in 3–4 wk if not cured. Alternatively, may administer 500 mg PO × 1.
  Capillariasis: 200 mg PO BID × 20 days
  Visceral larva migrans (toxocariasis): 100–200 mg PO BID × 5 days
  Trichinellosis **(Trichinella spiralis):** 200–400 mg PO TID × 3 days, then 400–500 mg PO TID × 10
  days; use with steroids for severe symptoms.
  Ancylostoma caninum **(eosinophilic enterocolitis):** 100 mg PO BID × 3 days.
See latest edition of the AAP *Red Book* for additional information.

Experience in children <2 yr and in pregnancy is limited. May cause rash, headache, diarrhea, and abdominal cramping in cases of massive infection. Liver function test elevations and hepatitis have been reported with prolonged courses; monitor hepatic function with prolonged therapy. Family may need to be treated as a group. Therapeutic effect may be decreased if administered to patients receiving aminoquinolones, carbamazepine, or phenytoin. Cimetidine may increase effects/toxicity of mebendazole. Administer with food. Tablets may be crushed and mixed with food, swallowed whole, or chewed.

MEDROXYPROGESTERONE
Depo-Provera, Provera, and various generics; Depo-Sub Q
Provera 104
Contraceptive, progestin

Yes No 2 X

Tabs (Provera and generics): 2.5, 5, 10 mg
Injection, suspension as acetate:
  Depo-Provera and generics, for IM use only: 150 mg/mL (1 mL), 400 mg/mL (2.5 mL); may contain
  parabens
Injection, prefilled syringe as acetate:
  Depo-Sub Q Provera 104, for SC use only: 104 mg (0.65 mL of 160 mg/mL); contains parabens

Adolescent and adult:
  Contraception: Initiate therapy during first 5 days after onset of a normal menstrual period,
  within 5 days postpartum if not breast feeding, or if breast feeding, at 6-wk postpartum. When
  converting contraceptive method to Depo-Sub Q Provera, dose should be administered within 7 days
  after last day of using previous method (pill, ring, patch).
    IM (Depo-Provera): 150 mg Q3 mo
    SC (Depo-Sub Q Provera 104): 104 mg Q3 mo (Q12–14 wk)

MEDROXYPROGESTERONE *continued*

Adolescent and adult:

Amenorrhea: 5–10 mg PO once daily × 5–10 days

Abnormal uterine bleeding: 5–10 mg PO once daily × 5–10 days, initiated on 16th or 21st day of menstrual cycle

Endometriosis-associated pain (Depo-Sub Q Provera 104): 104 mg SC Q3 mo. **Do not use** >2 yr, owing to impact on bone mineral density.

Consider patient's risk for osteoporosis because of potential for decrease in bone mineral density with long-term use. **Contraindicated** in pregnancy, breast or genital cancer, liver disease, missed abortion, thrombophlebitis, thromboembolic disorders, cerebral vascular disease, and undiagnosed vaginal bleeding. **Use with caution** in patients with family history of breast cancer, depression, diabetes, and fluid retention. May cause dizziness, headache, insomnia, fatigue, nausea, weight increase, appetite changes, amenorrhea, and breakthrough bleeding. Cholestatic jaundice and increased ICP have been reported.

Aminoglutethimide may decrease medroxyprogesterone levels. May alter thyroid and liver function tests, prothrombin time, factors VII, VIII, IX and X, and metyrapone test.

Do not inject IM or SC product intravenously. Shake IM injection vial well before use, and administer in upper arm or buttock. Administer SC injection product into anterior thigh or abdomen. Administer oral doses with food.

MEFLOQUINE HCL
Lariam and generics
Antimalarial

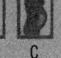

Yes   No   2   C

Tabs: 250 mg (228 mg base)

Doses expressed in mg mefloquine HCl salt

Malaria prophylaxis (start 1 wk before exposure and continue for 4 wk after leaving endemic area):

Child (PO, administered Q weekly):

<10 kg: 5 mg/kg

10–19 kg: 62.5 mg (¼ tablet)

20–30 kg: 125 mg (½ tablet)

31–45 kg: 187.5 mg (¾ tablet)

>45 kg: 250 mg (1 tablet)

Adult: 250 mg PO Q weekly

Malaria treatment (uncomplicated/mild infection, chloroquine-resistant *Plasmodium vivax***):**

Child ≥ 6 mo and > 5 kg: 15 mg/kg × 1 PO, followed by 10 mg/kg × 1 PO 12 hr later (**max. total dose:** 1250 mg)

Adult: 750 mg × 1 PO, followed by 500 mg × 1 PO 12 hr later

See latest edition of AAP *Red Book* for additional information.

Contraindicated in active or recent history of depression, anxiety disorders, psychosis or schizophrenia, seizures, or hypersensitivity to quinine or quinidine. **Use with caution** in cardiac dysrhythmias and neurologic disease. May cause dizziness, headache, syncope, psychiatric symptoms (e.g., anxiety, paranoia, depression, hallucinations, psychotic behavior), seizures, ocular abnormalities, GI symptoms, leukopenia, and thrombocytopenia. Most adverse events occur within 3 doses with prophylaxis use. Monitor liver enzymes and ocular examinations for therapies >1 yr.

Mefloquine is a substrate and inhibitor of P-glycoprotein and may reduce valproic acid levels. ECG abnormalities may occur when used in combination with quinine, quinidine, chloroquine,

Continued

For explanation of icons, see p. 648

MEFLOQUINE HCL *continued*

halofantrine, and β-blockers. If any of the aforementioned antimalarial drugs is used in the initial treatment of severe malaria, initiate mefloquine at least 12 hours after the last dose of any of these drugs. **Do not** initiate halofantrine or ketoconazole within 15 days of last dose of mefloquine. Use with chloroquine may increase risk for seizures. Rifampin may decrease mefloquine levels.

Do not take on an empty stomach. Administer with at least 240 mL (8 oz) water. Treatment failures in children may be related to vomiting of administered dose. If vomiting occurs <30 min after dose, administer a second full dose. If vomiting occurs 30–60 min after dose, administer an additional half-dose. If vomiting continues, monitor patient closely and consider alternative therapy.

MEROPENEM
Merrem and generics
Carbapenem antibiotic

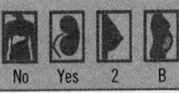

No   Yes   2   B

Injection: 0.5, 1 g
Contains 3.92 mEq Na/g drug

Neonate (IV):
  Non-CNS intraabdominal infections with meropenem MIC <4 mcg/mL based on population PK modeling:
    <32 wk' gestation:
      <14 days old: 20 mg/kg/dose IV Q12 hr
      ≥14 days old: 20 mg/kg/dose IV Q8 hr
    ≥32 wk' gestation:
      <14 days old: 20 mg/kg/dose IV Q8 hr
      ≥14 days old: 30 mg/kg/dose IV Q8 hr
  Non-CNS intraabdominal infections with meropenem MIC 4–8 mcg/mL (moderately resistant) from a single-dose PK simulation study:
    >30 wk' gestation and >7 days old: 40 mg/kg/dose IV Q8 hr
Infant ≥ 1–3 mo (IV):
  Non-CNS intraabdominal infections with meropenem MIC <4 mcg/mL based on population PK modeling: 20–30 mg/kg/dose IV Q8 hr
  Meningitis (recommended dose from 2004 IDSA meningitis practice guidelines): 40 mg/kg/dose Q8 hr
Infant ≥ 3 mo, child, and adolescent (IV):
  Skin and subcutaneous tissue infections: 30 mg/kg/24 hr ÷ Q8 hr; **max. dose:** 1.5 g/24 hr
  Intraabdominal and mild/moderate infections, and fever/neutropenia empirical therapy: 60 mg/kg/24 hr ÷ Q8 hr; **max. dose:** 3 g/24 hr
  Meningitis, severe infections, cystic fibrosis pulmonary exacerbations: 120 mg/kg/24 hr ÷ Q8 hr. **Max. dose:** 6 g/24 hr
Adult (IV):
  Skin and subcutaneous tissue infections: 1.5 g/24 hr ÷ Q8 hr
  Intraabdominal and mild/moderate infections, and fever/neutropenia empirical therapy: 1 g Q8 hr
  Meningitis and severe infections: 2 g ÷ Q8 hr

Contraindicated in patients sensitive to carbapenems or with a history of anaphylaxis to β-lactam antibiotics. **Use with caution** in meningitis and CNS disorders (may cause seizures) and renal impairment (**adjust dose [see Chapter 31]**). Drug penetrates well into CSF.

May cause diarrhea, rash, nausea, vomiting, oral moniliasis, glossitis, pain and irritation at IV injection site, and headache. Hepatic enzyme and bilirubin elevation, dermatologic reactions (including Stevens-Johnson syndrome and TEN), leukopenia, thrombocytopenia (in renal dysfunction) and neutropenia have been reported. Probenecid may increase serum meropenem levels. May reduce valproic acid levels.

M

MESALAMINE
Apriso, Asacol, Asacol HD, Canasa, Delzicol, Lialda, Pentasa, Rowasa, SfRowasa, and others; 5-aminosalicylic acid, 5-ASA
Salicylate, GI antiinflammatory agent

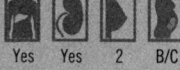

Yes Yes 2 B/C

Caps, controlled release:
  Pentasa: 250, 500 mg
  Delzicol: 400 mg
  Apriso: 375 mg; contains aspartame
Tabs, delayed-release: 400 mg (Asacol), 800 mg (Asacol HD), 1200 mg (Lialda)
Suppository (Canasa): 1000 mg (30s, 42s)
Rectal suspension (Rowasa, SfRowasa, and others): 4 g/60 mL; contains sulfites (SfRowasa is sulfite free) and sodium benzoate

Child:
  Caps, controlled release: 50 mg/kg/24 hr ÷ Q6–12 hr PO; **max. dose:** 1 g/dose
  Tabs, delayed-release: 50 mg/kg/24 hr ÷ Q8–12 hr PO; **max. dose:** 4.8 g/24 hr
Adult (ulcerative colitis):
  Caps, controlled release:
    Initial therapy: 1 g QID PO × 3–8 wk
    Maintenance therapy for remission:
      Apriso: 1.5 g QAM PO
      Pentasa: 1 g QID PO
  Tabs, delayed-release:
    Initial therapy:
      Asacol: 800 mg TID PO × 6 wk
      Asacol HD: 1.6 g TID PO × 6 wk
      Lialda: 2.4–4.8 g once daily PO up to 8 wk
    Maintenance therapy for remission:
      Asacol: 1.6 g/24 hr PO in divided doses
      Lialda: 2.4 g PO once daily
  Suppository: 1000 mg QHS PR × 3–6 wk, retaining each dose in rectum for 1–3 hr or longer if possible.
  Rectal suspension: 60 mL (4 g) QHS × 3–6 wk, retaining each dose for ≈ 8 hr; lying on left side during administration improves delivery to sigmoid colon.

Generally **not recommended** in children <16 yr with chicken pox or flulike symptoms (risk of Reye syndrome). **Contraindicated** in active peptic ulcer disease, severe renal failure, and salicylate hypersensitivity. Rectal suspension should not be used in patients with history of sulfite allergy. **Use with caution** in sulfasalazine hypersensitivity, impaired hepatic or renal function, pyloric stenosis, and concurrent thrombolytics. May cause headache, GI discomfort, pancreatitis, pericarditis, rash, and Stevens-Johnson syndrome.

Do not administer with lactulose or other medications that can lower intestinal pH. Oral capsules are designed to release medication throughout the GI tract, and oral tablets release medication at the terminal ileus and beyond. Mesalamine 400 mg PO is equivalent to 1 g sulfasalazine PO. Tablets should be swallowed whole.

May cause a false-positive urinary normetanephrine test. All products are pregnancy category "B" except for Asacol HD, which is pregnancy category "C."

For explanation of icons, see p. 648

METFORMIN
Glucophage, Glucophage XR, Glumetza, Fortamet, Riomet, and generics
Antidiabetic, biguanide

Yes   Yes   2   B

Tabs: 500, 850, 1000 mg
Tabs, extended release:
   Glucophage XR and others: 500, 750 mg
   Fortamet, Glumetza, and others: 500, 1000 mg
Oral suspension (Riomet): 100 mg/mL (120, 480 mL); contains saccharin

Administer all doses with meals (e.g., BID with morning and evening meals).

Child (10–16 yr) (see remarks): Start with 500 mg BID; may increase dose weekly by
   500 mg/24 hr in 2 divided doses up to a **max. dose** of 2000 mg/24 hr.

Child ≥ 17 yr and adult (see remarks):

   500 mg tabs: Start with 500 mg PO BID; may increase dose weekly by 500 mg/24 hr in 2 divided
      doses up to a **max. dose** of 2500 mg/24 hr. Administer 2500 mg/24 hr doses by dividing daily
      dose TID with meals.

   850 mg tabs: Start with 850 mg PO once daily with morning meal; may increase by 850 mg every 2
      wk up to a **max. dose** of 2550 mg/24 hr (first dosage increment: 850 mg PO BID; second dosage
      increment: 850 mg PO TID).

   Extended-release tabs: Start with 500 mg PO once daily with evening meal; may increase by 500
      mg every wk up to a **max. dose** of 2000 mg/24 hr (if glycemic control is not achieved at max.
      dose, divide dose to 1000 mg PO BID). If a dose > 2000 mg is needed, switch to non–extended-
      release tablets in divided doses, and increase dose to a **max. dose** of 2550 mg/24 hr.

Contraindicated in renal impairment, hepatic impairment (increased risk for lactic acidosis),
   CHF, metabolic acidosis, and during radiology studies using iodinated contrast media. **Use
   with caution** when transferring patients from chlorpropamide therapy (potential
   hypoglycemia risk) or for patients with excessive alcohol intake, hypoxemia, dehydration,
   surgical procedures, hepatic disease, anemia, and thyroid disease.

Fatal lactic acidosis (diarrhea, severe muscle pain, cramping, shallow and fast breathing, unusual
   weakness and sleepiness) and decrease in vitamin B_{12} levels have been reported. May cause GI
   discomfort (≈50% incidence), anorexia, and vomiting. Transient abdominal discomfort or diarrhea
   have been reported in 40% of pediatric patients. Cimetidine, furosemide, and nifedipine may
   increase effects/toxicity of metformin. In addition to monitoring serum glucose and glycosylated
   hemoglobin, monitor renal function and hematologic parameters (baseline and annual).

Adult patients initiated on 500 mg PO BID may also have their dose increased to 850 mg PO BID after
   2 wk.

COMBINATION THERAPY WITH SULFONYLUREAS: If patient has not responded to 4 wk of maximum
   doses of metformin monotherapy, consider gradual addition of an oral sulfonylurea, with continued
   maximum metformin dosing (even if failure with sulfonylurea has occurred). Attempt to identify
   minimum effective dosage for each drug (metformin and sulfonylurea), because the combination
   can increase risk for sulfonylurea-induced hypoglycemia. If patient does not respond to 1–3 mo of
   combination therapy with maximum metformin doses, consider discontinuing combination therapy
   and initiating insulin therapy.

Administer all doses with food.

METHADONE HCL
Dolophine, Methadose, and generics
Narcotic, analgesic

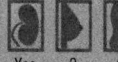

No   Yes   2   C

Tabs: 5, 10 mg
Tabs (dispersible): 40 mg
Oral solution: 5 mg/5 mL, 10 mg/5 mL; contains 8% alcohol
Concentrated. solution: 10 mg/mL
Injection: 10 mg/mL (20 mL), contains 0.5% chlorobutanol

Analgesia:
  Child: 0.7 mg/kg/24 hr PO, SQ, IM, or IV ÷ Q4–6 hr PRN for pain; **max. dose:** 10 mg/dose
  Adult: 2.5–10 mg/dose Q3–4 hr PO, SQ, IM, or IV PRN for pain
Detoxification or maintenance: See package insert.

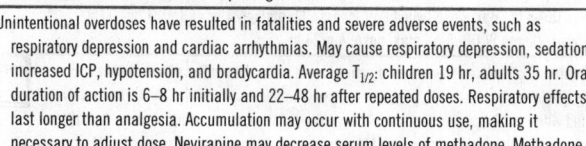

Unintentional overdoses have resulted in fatalities and severe adverse events, such as respiratory depression and cardiac arrhythmias. May cause respiratory depression, sedation, increased ICP, hypotension, and bradycardia. Average $T_{1/2}$: children 19 hr, adults 35 hr. Oral duration of action is 6–8 hr initially and 22–48 hr after repeated doses. Respiratory effects last longer than analgesia. Accumulation may occur with continuous use, making it necessary to adjust dose. Nevirapine may decrease serum levels of methadone. Methadone is a substrate for CYP 450 3A3/4, 2D6, and 1A2 and an inhibitor of 2D6.
See Chapter 6 for equianalgesic dosing and onset of action. **Adjust dose in renal failure (see Chapter 31).**

METHIMAZOLE
Tapazole and generics
Antithyroid agent

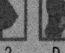

No   No   2   D

Tabs: 5, 10 mg

Hyperthyroidism:
  Child:
    Initial: 0.4–0.7 mg/kg/24 hr or 15–20 mg/m²/24 hr PO ÷ Q8 hr
    Maintenance: ⅓–⅔ of initial dose PO ÷ Q8 hr
    Max. dose: 30 mg/24 hr
  Adult:
    Initial: 15–60 mg/24 hr PO ÷ TID
    Maintenance: 5–15 mg/24 hr PO ÷ TID

Readily crosses placental membranes and distributes into breast milk (maternal doses ≤20 mg/24 hr considered safe, but data are insufficient to support safe use with maternal doses >20 mg/24 hr). Blood dyscrasias, dermatitis, hepatitis, arthralgia, CNS reactions, pruritus, nephritis, hypoprothrombinemia, agranulocytosis, headache, fever, and hypothyroidism may occur.
May increase effects of oral anticoagulants. When correcting hyperthyroidism, existing β-blocker, digoxin, and theophylline doses may have to be reduced to avoid potential toxicities.
Switch to maintenance dose when patient is euthyroid. Administer all doses with food.

For explanation of icons, see p. 648

METHYLDOPA
Various brand names
Central α-adrenergic blocker, antihypertensive

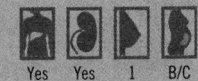

Yes   Yes   1   B/C

Tabs: 250, 500 mg
Injection: 50 mg/mL (5 mL); may contain sulfites
Oral suspension: 50 mg/mL

Hypertension:
 Child: 10 mg/kg/24 hr ÷ Q6–12 hr PO; increase PRN Q2 days. **Max. dose:**
 65 mg/kg/24 hr or 3 g/24 hr, whichever is less.
 Adult: 250 mg/dose BID–TID PO. Increase PRN Q2 days to **max. dose** of 3 g/24 hr.
Hypertensive crisis:
 Child: 2–4 mg/kg/dose IV. If no response within 4–6 hr, may increase dose to 5–10 mg/kg/dose IV;
 give doses Q6–8 hr. **Max. dose** (whichever is less): 65 mg/kg/24 hr or 3 g/24 hr.
 Adult: 250–1000 mg IV Q6–8 hr; **max. dose:** 4 g/24 hr

Contraindicated in pheochromocytoma and active liver disease. **Use with caution** if patient is
 receiving haloperidol, propranolol, lithium, or sympathomimetics. Positive Coombs test rarely
 associated with hemolytic anemia. Fever, leukopenia, sedation, memory impairment, hepatitis,
 GI disturbances, orthostatic hypotension, black tongue, and gynecomastia may occur. May
 interfere with laboratory tests for creatinine, urinary catecholamines, uric acid, and AST.
May increase AV blocking effects of β-blockers and antihypertensive effects of other antihypertensives.
 α$_2$-Antagonist antidepressants, serotonin/norepinephrine reuptake inhibitors, and methylphenidate
 may reduce antihypertensive effects of methyldopa. **Do not use** in combination with MAOIs (may
 enhance adverse effects of methyldopa). **Do not coadminister** oral doses with iron; decreases
 methyldopa absorption. **Adjust dose in renal failure (see Chapter 31).**
Pregnancy category is "C" for injectable dosage form and "B" for oral dosage forms.

METHYLENE BLUE
Many generics
Antidote, drug-induced methemoglobinemia and cyanide toxicity

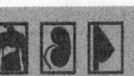

No   Yes   3   X

Injection: 10 mg/mL (1%) (1, 10 mL)

Methemoglobinemia:
 Child and adult: 1–2 mg/kg/dose or 25–50 mg/m^2/dose IV over 5 min. May repeat in 1 hr if
 needed.

At high doses, may cause methemoglobinemia. **Avoid** subcutaneous or intrathecal routes of
 administration. **Use with caution** in G6PD deficiency or renal insufficiency. May cause
 nausea, vomiting, dizziness, headache, diaphoresis, stained skin, and abdominal pain.
 Causes blue-green discoloration of urine and feces.
Serotonin syndrome has been reported with coadministration of SSRIs, SNRIs, or clomipramine. Use
 with bupropion, paroxetine, sertraline, duloxetine, vilazodone, venlafaxine, fluoxetine, or desipramine
 is considered contraindicated.

M

METHYLPHENIDATE HCL
Ritalin, Methylin, Metadate ER, Methylin ER, Concerta, Ritalin SR,
Metadate CD, Ritalin LA, Daytrana, Quillivant XR, and generics
CNS stimulant

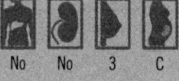

No   No   3   C

Tabs: 5, 10, 20 mg
Chewable tabs: 2.5, 5, 10 mg; contains phenylalanine
Oral solution (Methylin and generics): 1 mg/mL, 2 mg/mL; may contain propylene glycol
Oral suspension (Quillivant XR): 25 mg/5 mL (60, 120, 150, 180 mL); contains sodium benzoate
Extended-release tabs:
 8-hr duration (Metadate ER): 20 mg
 24-hr duration (Concerta): 18, 27, 36, 54 mg
Sustained-release tabs:
 8-hr duration (Ritalin SR): 20 mg
Extended-release caps:
 24-hr duration (Metadate CD, Ritalin LA): 10, 20, 30, 40, 50. 60 mg
Transdermal patch (Daytrana): 10 mg/9 hr (each 12.5 cm² patch contains 27.5 mg), 15 mg/9 hr
(each 18.75 cm² patch contains 41.3 mg), 20 mg/9 hr (each 25 cm² patch contains 55 mg),
30 mg/9 hr (each 37.5 cm² patch contains 82.5 mg) (30s)

Attention deficit hyperactivity disorder:
 Immediate-release oral dosage forms (Methylin, Ritalin [≥6 yr]):
  Initial: 0.3 mg/kg/dose (or 2.5–5 mg/dose) given before breakfast and lunch.
  May increase by 0.1 mg/kg/dose PO (or 5–10 mg/24 hr) weekly until maintenance
  dose achieved. May give extra afternoon dose if needed.
  Maintenance dose range: 0.3–1 mg/kg/24 hr
  Max. dose: 2 mg/kg/24 hr or 60 mg/24 hr
 Extended-release once-daily oral dosage form (Concerta [≥6 yr]):
  Methylphenidate-naïve patients: Start with 18 mg PO QAM for children and adolescents and
  18–36 mg PO QAM for adults. Dosage may be increased at weekly intervals in 18-mg increments
  up to the following **max. doses:**
   6–12 yr: 54 mg/24 hr
   13–17 yr: 72 mg/24 hr, **not to exceed** 2 mg/kg/24 hr
  Patients currently receiving methylphenidate: See following table.
Recommended Dose Conversion from Methylphenidate Regimens to Concerta

Previous Methylphenidate Daily Dose	Recommended Concerta Dose
5 mg PO BID–TID or 20 mg SR PO once daily	18 mg PO QAM
10 mg PO BID–TID or 40 mg SR PO once daily	36 mg PO QAM
15 mg PO BID–TID or 60 mg SR PO once daily	54 mg PO QAM
20 mg PO BID–TID	72 mg PO QAM

After a week of receiving above recommended Concerta dose, dose may be increased in 18-mg increments at weekly
intervals up to a **max.** of 54 mg/24 hr for 6–12 yr and 72 mg/24 hr (**not to exceed** 2 mg/kg/24 hr) for 13–17 yr.

 Other extended-release oral dosage forms:
  Metadate CD (≥6 yr): Start with 20 mg PO once daily; dosage may be increased at weekly
  intervals in 20-mg increments up to a **max. dose** of 60 mg/24 hr.
  Ritalin LA (≥6 yr): Start with 20 mg PO once daily; dosage may be increased at weekly intervals in
  10-mg increments up to a **max. dose** of 60 mg/24 hr.
 Transdermal patch (Daytrana): Apply to the hip 2 hr before effect is needed, and remove 9 hr later. Patch
 may be removed before 9 hr if shorter duration of effect is desired or if late-day adverse effects appear.

Continued

METHYLPHENIDATE HCL *continued*

Transdermal patch (Daytrana): .

    6–17 yr: Start with 10 mg/9-hr patch once daily. Increase dose PRN Q7 days by increasing to next dosage strength.

Contraindicated in glaucoma, anxiety disorders, motor tics, and Tourette syndrome. Medication should generally **not** be used in children <age 5 yr; diagnosis of ADHD in this age group is extremely difficult and should only be done in consultation with a specialist. Sudden death (children, adolescents, and adults), stroke (adults), and MI (adults) have been reported in patients with preexisting structural cardiac abnormalities or other serious heart problems. **Use with caution** in patients with hypertension, psychiatric conditions, and epilepsy. Insomnia, weight loss, anorexia, rash, nausea, emesis, abdominal pain, hypertension or hypotension, tachycardia, arrhythmias, palpitations, restlessness, headaches, fever, tremor, visual disturbances, and thrombocytopenia may occur. Abnormal liver function, cerebral arteritis and/or occlusion, peripheral vasculopathy (including Raynaud phenomenon), leukopenia and/or anemia, hypersensitivity reactions, transient depressed mood, paranoia, mania, auditory hallucination, priapism, and scalp hair loss have been reported. Skin irritation may occur, and contact dermatitis has been reported with transdermal route. High doses may slow growth by appetite suppression. GI obstruction has been reported with Concerta.

May increase serum concentrations/effects of tricyclic antidepressants, dopamine agonists (e.g., haloperidol), phenytoin, phenobarbital, and warfarin. May decrease effects of antihypertensive drugs. Effect of methylphenidate may be potentiated by MAOIs; hypertensive crisis may also occur if used within 14 days of discontinuance of MAOI.

Extended/sustained-release dosage forms have either an 8- or 24-hour interval (as stipulated previously). Concerta dosage form delivers 22.2% of its dose as an immediate-release product, with the remaining amounts as an extended-release product (e.g., 18-mg strength: 4 mg as immediate release and 14 mg as extended release). **Do not** consume alcohol with Ritalin LA or Metadate CD dosage forms; may result in more rapid release of drug. **Do not** expose transdermal application site to external heat sources (e.g., electric blankets, heating pads); may increase drug release.

METHYLPREDNISOLONE
Medrol, Medrol Dosepack, Solu-Medrol, Depo-Medrol, and generics
Corticosteroid

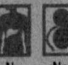   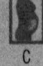

No   No   2   C

Tabs: 2, 4, 8, 16, 24, 32 mg
Tabs, dose pack (Medrol Dosepack and others): 4 mg (21s)
Injection, Na succinate (Solu-Medrol and others): 40, 125, 500, 1000, 2000 mg (IV or IM use); may contain benzyl alcohol
Injection, Acetate (Depo-Medrol and others): 20, 40, 80 mg/mL (IM repository); may contain polyethylene glycol (1, 5 mL)

Anti-inflammatory/immunosuppressive:
    PO/IM/IV: 0.5–1.7 mg/kg/24 hr ÷ Q6–12 hr
Asthma exacerbations (2007 National Heart, Lung, and Blood Institute Guideline Recommendations; dose until peak expiratory flow reaches 70% of predicted or personal best):
    Child ≤ 12 yr (IM/IV/PO): 1–2 mg/kg/24 hr ÷ Q12 hr (**max. dose:** 60 mg/24 hr). Higher alternative regimen of 1 mg/kg/dose Q6 hr × 48 hr, followed by 1–2 mg/kg/24 hr (**max. dose:** 60 mg/24 hr) ÷ Q12 hr has been suggested.
    >12 yr and adult (IV/IM/PO): 40–80 mg/24 hr ÷ Q12–24 hr

METHYLPREDNISOLONE *continued*

Outpatient asthma exacerbation burst therapy (longer durations may be necessary):
PO:
    Child ≤ 12 yr: 1–2 mg/kg/24 hr ÷ Q12–24 hr (**max. dose:** 60 mg/24 hr) × 3–10 days.
    Child > 12 yr and adult: 40–60 mg/24 hr ÷ Q12–24 hr × 3–10 days.
IM (use methylprednisolone acetate product) for patients vomiting or with adherence issues:
    Child ≤ 12 yr: 7.5 mg/kg (**max. dose:** 240 mg) IM × 1
    Child > 12 yr and adult: 240 mg IM × 1
Acute spinal cord injury:
    30 mg/kg IV over 15 min, followed in 45 min by a continuous infusion of 5.4 mg/kg/hr × 23 hr

See Chapter 30 for relative steroid potencies and doses based on BSA. Acetate form may also be used for intraarticular and intralesional injection and has longer times to max. effect and duration of action; it should **NOT** be given IV. Like all steroids, may cause hypertension, pseudotumor cerebri, acne, Cushing syndrome, adrenal axis suppression, GI bleeding, hyperglycemia, and osteoporosis.
Barbiturates, phenytoin, and rifampin may enhance methylprednisolone clearance. Erythromycin, itraconazole, and ketoconazole may increase methylprednisone levels. Methylprednisolone may increase cyclosporine and tacrolimus levels.

METOCLOPRAMIDE
Reglan, Maxolon, Metozolv, and many generics
Antiemetic, prokinetic agent

No   Yes   2   B

Tabs: 5, 10 mg
Tabs, orally disintegrating (ODT [Metozolv]): 5 mg
Injection: 5 mg/mL (2 mL)
Oral solution: 5 mg/5 mL

Gastroesophageal reflux (GER) or GI dysmotility:
    Infant and child: 0.1–0.2 mg/kg/dose up to QID IV/IM/PO; **max. dose:** 0.8 mg/kg/24 hr
    Adult: 10–15 mg/dose QAC and QHS IV/IM/PO
Antiemetic (all ages): Premedicate with diphenhydramine to reduce EPS.
    1–2 mg/kg/dose Q2–6 hr IV/IM/PO
Postoperative nausea and vomiting:
    Child: 0.1–0.2 mg/kg/dose Q6–8 hr PRN IV
    >14 yr and adult: 10 mg Q6–8 hr PRN IV

Contraindicated in GI obstruction, seizure disorder, pheochromocytoma, or in patients receiving drugs likely to cause extrapyramidal symptoms (EPS). May cause EPS, especially at higher doses. Sedation, headache, anxiety, depression, leukopenia, and diarrhea may occur. Neuroleptic malignant syndrome and tardive dyskinesia (increased risk with prolonged duration of therapy; avoid use >12 weeks) have been reported.
For GER, give 30 min before meals and at bedtime. **Reduce dose in renal impairment (see Chapter 31).**

For explanation of icons, see p. 648

METOLAZONE
Zaroxolyn and many generics
Diuretic, thiazide-like

   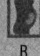

Yes   Yes   2   B

Tabs: 2.5, 5, 10 mg
Oral suspension: 0.25, 1 mg/mL

Dosage based on Zaroxolyn (for oral suspension, see remarks):
Child: 0.2–0.4 mg/kg/24 hr ÷ once daily–BID PO
Adult:
  Hypertension: 2.5–5 mg once daily PO
  Edema: 2.5–20 mg once daily PO

Contraindicated in patients with anuria, hepatic coma, or hypersensitivity to sulfonamides or thiazides. Use with caution in severe renal disease, impaired hepatic function, gout, lupus erythematosus, diabetes mellitus, and elevated cholesterol and triglycerides. Electrolyte imbalance, GI disturbance, hyperglycemia, marrow suppression, chills, hyperuricemia, chest pain, hepatitis, and rash may occur.

Oral suspensions have increased bioavailability; lower doses may be necessary when using these dosage forms. More effective than thiazide diuretics in impaired renal function; may be effective in GFRs as low as 20 mL/min. Furosemide-resistant edema in pediatric patients may benefit from addition of metolazone.

Pregnancy category changes to "D" if used for pregnancy-induced hypertension.

METOPROLOL
Lopressor, Toprol-XL, and generics
Adrenergic blocking agent (β₁-selective), class II antiarrhythmic

Yes   No   1   C

Tabs: 25, 50, 100 mg
Extended-release tabs (Toprol-XL and generics): 25, 50, 100, 200 mg
Oral liquid: 10 mg/mL
Injection: 1 mg/mL (5 mL)

Hypertension:
  Child ≥ 1 yr and adolescent:
    Non–extended-release oral dosage forms: Start at 1–2 mg/kg/24 hr PO ÷ BID; **max. dose:** 6 mg/kg/24 hr up to 200 mg/24 hr.
    Extended-release tabs (≥6 yr and adolescent): Start at 1 mg/kg/dose (**max. dose:** 50 mg) PO once daily; if needed, adjust dose up to a **max. dose** of 2 mg/kg/24 hr or 200 mg/24 hr once daily (higher doses have not been evaluated).
  Adult:
    Non–extended-release tabs: Start at 50–100 mg/24 hr PO ÷ once daily–BID; if needed, increase dosage at weekly intervals to desired blood pressure. Usual effective dosage range is 100–450 mg/24 hr. Doses >450 mg/24 hr have not been studied. Patients with bronchospastic diseases should receive the lowest possible daily dose ÷ TID.
    Extended-release tabs: Start at 25–100 mg/24 hr PO once daily; if needed, increase dosage at weekly intervals to desired blood pressure. Usual dosage range is 50–100 mg/24 hr. Doses >400 mg/24 hr have not been studied.

METOPROLOL continued

Contraindicated in sinus bradycardia, heart block >1st degree, sick sinus syndrome (except with functioning pacemaker), cardiogenic shock, and uncompensated CHF. **Use with caution** in hepatic dysfunction, peripheral vascular disease, history of severe anaphylactic hypersensitivity drug reactions, pheochromocytoma, and concurrent use with verapamil, diltiazem, or anesthetic agents that may decrease myocardial function. Should not be used with bronchospastic diseases. Reserpine and other drugs that deplete catecholamines (e.g., MAOIs) may increase effects of metoprolol. Metoprolol is a CYP 450 2D6 substrate.

Avoid abrupt cessation of therapy in ischemic heart disease; angina, ventricular arrhythmias, and MI have occurred. Common side effects include bradyarrhythmia, heart block, heart failure, pruritus, rash, GI disturbances, dizziness, fatigue, and depression. Bronchospasm, dyspnea, and elevations in transaminase, alkaline phosphatase, and LDH have all been reported.

METRONIDAZOLE
Flagyl, Flagyl ER, Protostat, MetroGel, MetroLotion, MetroCream, Noritate, MetroGel-Vaginal, and generics
Antibiotic, antiprotozoal

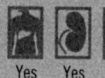
Yes Yes 3 B

Tabs: 250, 500 mg
Tabs, extended release (Flagyl ER): 750 mg
Caps: 375 mg
Oral suspension: 10 mg/mL or 50 mg/mL
Oral syrup: 5 mg/mL
Injection: 500 mg; contains 830 mg mannitol/g drug
Ready-to-use injection: 5 mg/mL (100 mL); contains 28 mEq Na/g drug
Gel, topical (MetroGel): 0.75% (28, 60 g)
Lotion (MetroLotion): 0.75% (60 mL); contains benzyl alcohol
Cream, topical:
  MetroCream: 0.75% (45 g); contains benzyl alcohol
  Noritate: 1% (30 g)
Gel, vaginal (MetroGel-Vaginal): 0.75% (70 g with 5 applicators)

Amebiasis:
Child: 35–50 mg/kg/24 hr PO ÷ TID × 10 days
Adult: 500–750 mg/dose PO TID × 10 days
Anaerobic infection:
Neonate, PO/IV:
  <7 days:
    <1.2 kg: 7.5 mg/kg/dose Q48 hr
    1.2–2 kg: 7.5 mg/kg/dose Q24 hr
    ≥2 kg: 15 mg/kg/24 hr ÷ Q12 hr
  ≥7 days:
    <1.2 kg: 7.5 mg/kg Q24 hr
    1.2–2 kg: 15 mg/kg/24 hr ÷ Q12 hr
    ≥2 kg: 30 mg/kg/24 hr ÷ Q12 hr
Infant/child/adult:
  IV/PO: 30 mg/kg/24 hr ÷ Q6 hr; **max. dose:** 4 g/24 hr

Continued

METRONIDAZOLE *continued*

Other parasitic infections:
  Infant/child: 15–30 mg/kg/24 hr PO ÷ Q8 hr
  Adult: 250 mg PO Q8 hr or 2 g PO × 1
Bacterial vaginosis:
  Adolescent and adult:
    PO:
      Immediate-release tabs: 500 mg BID × 7 days
      Extended-release tabs: 750 mg once daily × 7 days
    Vaginal: 5 g (1 applicator full) BID × 5 days
Giardiasis:
  Child: 15 mg/kg/24 hr PO ÷ TID × 5 days; **max. dose:** 750 mg/24 hr
  Adult: 250 mg PO TID × 5 days
Trichomoniasis: Treat sexual contacts.
  Child: 15 mg/kg/24 hr PO ÷ TID × 7 days; **max. dose:** 2000 mg/24 hr
  Adolescent/adult: 2 g PO × 1; **OR** 250 mg PO TID **OR** 375 mg PO BID × 7 days
Clostridium difficile *infection (IV may be less efficacious):*
  Child: 30 mg/kg/24 hr ÷ Q6 hr PO/IV x 10 days; **max. dose:** 2000 mg/24 hr
  Adult: 250–500 mg TID–QID PO × 10–14 days, or 500 mg Q8 hr IV × 10–14 days
Helicobacter pylori *infection (use in combination with amoxicillin and bismuth subsalicylate):*
  Child: 15–20 mg/kg/24 hr ÷ BID PO × 4 wk
  Adult: 250–500 mg TID PO × 14 days
Inflammatory bowel disease (as alternative to sulfasalazine):
  Adult: 400 mg BID PO
Topical use: Apply and rub a thin film into affected areas at the following frequencies specific to
  product concentration:
  0.75% cream: BID
  1% cream: Once daily

Avoid use in first-trimester pregnancy. **Use with caution** in patients with CNS disease, blood
dyscrasias, severe liver or **renal disease (GFR < 10 mL/min); see Chapter 31.** If using single
2-g dose in a breast-feeding mother, discontinue breast-feeding for 12 to 24 hours to allow
excretion of drug.

Nausea, diarrhea, urticaria, dry mouth, leukopenia, vertigo, metallic taste, and peripheral neuropathy
may occur. Candidiasis may worsen. May discolor urine. Patients **should not** ingest alcohol for
24–48 hr after dose (disulfiram-type reaction).

Single-dose oral regimen no longer recommended in bacterial vaginosis (poor efficacy). May increase
levels or toxicity of phenytoin, lithium, and warfarin. Phenobarbital and rifampin may increase
metronidazole metabolism.

IV infusion must be given slowly over 1 hr. For IV use in all ages, some references recommend a 15 mg/
kg loading dose.

MICAFUNGIN SODIUM
Mycamine
Antifungal, echinocandin

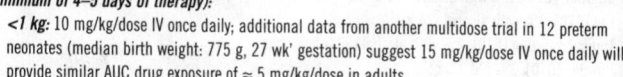

Yes   Yes   ?   C

Injection: 50, 100 mg; contains lactose

Invasive candidiasis (see remarks):
  Neonate and infant (based on a multidose pharmacokinetic and safety trial in 13 neonates/infants >48 hr and <120 days old with suspected or invasive candidiasis; minimum of 4–5 days of therapy):
    <1 kg: 10 mg/kg/dose IV once daily; additional data from another multidose trial in 12 preterm neonates (median birth weight: 775 g, 27 wk' gestation) suggest 15 mg/kg/dose IV once daily will provide similar AUC drug exposure of ≈ 5 mg/kg/dose in adults.
    ≥1 kg: 7 mg/kg/dose IV once daily
  Child and adolescent: 3–4 mg/kg/dose IV once daily; **max. dose:** 200 mg/dose
  Adult: 100–150 mg IV once daily
Esophageal candidiasis (see remarks):
  Child and adult:
    <50 kg: 3–4 mg/kg/dose IV once daily; **max. dose:** 200 mg/dose
    ≥50 kg: 150 mg IV once daily; mean duration for successful therapy was 15 days (range, 10–30 days).
Candida prophylaxis in hematopoietic stem cell transplant:
  Child and adult:
    <50 kg: 1.5 mg/kg/dose IV once daily; **max. dose:** 50 mg/dose
    ≥50 kg: 50 mg IV once daily
Invasive aspergillosis (see remarks; doses under investigation):
  Child and adult:
    <50 kg: 3–4 mg/kg/dose IV once daily; dosages as high as 7.5 mg/kg/24 hr have been tolerated.
    ≥50 kg: 150 mg IV once daily

Prior hypersensitivity to other echinocandins (anidulafungin, caspofungin) increases risk; anaphylaxis with shock has been reported. **Use with caution** in hepatic and renal impairment.

No dosing adjustments are required based on race or gender, or in patients with severe renal dysfunction or mild to moderate hepatic function impairment. Effect of severe hepatic function impairment on micafungin pharmacokinetics has not been evaluated. Higher dosage requirements in premature and young infants may be due to faster drug clearance secondary to lower protein binding. Higher treatment doses in infants and children have been reported at 8.6–12 mg/kg/dose IV once daily.

May cause GI disturbances, phlebitis, rash, hyperbilirubinemia, liver function test elevation, headache, fever, and rigor. Anemia, leukopenia, neutropenia, thrombocytopenia, and hemolysis have been reported. Micafungin is a CYP 450 3A isoenzyme substrate and weak inhibitor. May increase effects/toxicity of nifedipine and sirolimus.

For explanation of icons, see p. 648

MICONAZOLE
Topical products: Micatin, Lotrimin AF, and others
Vaginal products: Monistat, Vagistat-3, and others
Antifungal agent

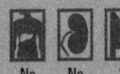

No   No   2   C

Cream [OTC]: 2% (15, 30, 90 g)
Lotion [OTC]: 2% (30, 60 mL)
Ointment [OTC]: 2% (28.4 g)
Solution [OTC]: 2% with alcohol (30.3 mL)
Gel [OTC]: 2% with alcohol (24 g)
Topical solution [OTC]: 2% with alcohol (30.3 mL)
Powder [OTC]: 2% (70, 90 g)
Spray, liquid [OTC]: 2% (105 mL); contains alcohol
Spray, powder [OTC]: 2% (85, 90, 100 g); contains alcohol
Vaginal cream [OTC]: 2% (15, 25, 45 g), 4% (15, 25 g)
Vaginal suppository [OTC]: 100 mg (7s), 200 mg (3s)
Vaginal combination packs:
  Monistat 1 Combination Pack [OTC]: 1200 mg suppository (1) and 2% cream (9 g)
  Monistat 3, Vagistat-3 [OTC]: 200 mg suppository (3s) and 2% cream (9 g)
  Monistat 7 [OTC]: 100 mg suppository (7s) and 2% cream (9 g)

Topical: Apply BID × 2–4 wk.
Vaginal:
  7-day regimen: 1 applicator full of 2% cream or 100 mg suppository QHS × 7 days
  3-day regimen: 1 applicator full of 4% cream or 200 mg suppository QHS × 3 days
  Monistat 1: 1200 mg suppository × 1 at bedtime or during the day

Use with caution in hypersensitivity to other imidazole antifungal agents (e.g., clotrimazole, ketoconazole). Side effects include pruritus, rash, burning, phlebitis, headaches, and pelvic cramps.

Drug is a substrate and inhibitor of the CYP 450 3A3/4 isoenzymes. Vaginal use with concomitant warfarin use has also been reported to increase warfarin's effect. Vegetable oil base in vaginal suppositories may interact with latex products (e.g., condoms and diaphragms); consider switching to vaginal cream.
Avoid contact with eyes.

MIDAZOLAM
Various generics; previously available as Versed
Benzodiazepine

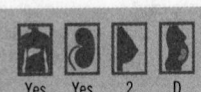

Yes   Yes   2   D

Injection: 1, 5 mg/mL; some preparations may contain 1% benzyl alcohol
Oral syrup: 2 mg/mL; contains sodium benzoate

Titrate to effect under controlled conditions. See Chapter 6 for additional routes of administration.
Sedation for procedures:
  Child:
    IV:
      6 mo–5 yr: 0.05–0.1 mg/kg/dose over 2–3 min. May repeat dose PRN in 2–3-min intervals up to a **max. total dose** of 6 mg. A total dose up to 0.6 mg/kg may be necessary for desired effect.
      6–12 yr: 0.025–0.05 mg/kg/dose over 2–3 min. May repeat dose PRN in 2–3 min intervals up to a **max. total dose** of 10 mg. A total dose up to 0.4 mg/kg may be necessary for desired effect.
      >12–16 yr: Use adult dose, up to **max. total dose** of 10 mg.

MIDAZOLAM *continued*

PO:

≥6 mo: 0.25–0.5 mg/kg/dose × 1. **Max. dose:** 20 mg. Younger patients (6 mo–5 yr) may require higher doses of 1 mg/kg/dose, whereas older patients (6–15 yr) may require only 0.25 mg/kg/dose. Use 0.25 mg/kg/dose for patients with cardiac or respiratory compromise, concurrent CNS-depressive drug, or high-risk surgery.

Adult:

IV: 0.5–2 mg/dose over 2 min. May repeat PRN in 2–3-min intervals until desired effect. Usual total dose: 2.5–5 mg; **max. total dose:** 10 mg.

Sedation with mechanical ventilation:

Intermittent:

Infant and child: 0.05–0.15 mg/kg/dose IV Q1–2 hr PRN

Continuous IV infusion (initial doses, titrate to effect):

Neonate:

<32 wk' gestation: 0.5 mcg/kg/min

≥32 wk' gestation: 1 mcg/kg/min

Infant and child: 1–2 mcg/kg/min

Refractory status epilepticus:

≥2 mo and child: Load with 0.15 mg/kg IV × 1, followed by a continuous infusion of 1 mcg/kg/min; titrate dose upward Q5 min to effect (mean dose of 2.3 mcg/kg/min [range, 1–18 mcg/kg/min] has been reported).

Contraindicated in patients with narrow angle glaucoma and shock. **Use with caution in CHF, renal impairment (adjust dose [see Chapter 31])**, pulmonary disease, hepatic dysfunction, and in neonates. Causes respiratory depression, hypotension, and bradycardia. Cardiovascular monitoring is recommended. Use lower doses or reduce dose when given in combination with narcotics or in patients with respiratory compromise.

Higher recommended dosage for younger patients (6 mo–5 yr) is attributed to water-soluble properties of midazolam and higher percentage of body water for younger patients.

Drug is a substrate for CYP 450 3A4. Serum concentrations may be increased by cimetidine, clarithromycin, diltiazem, erythromycin, itraconazole, ketoconazole, and protease inhibitors (use contraindicated). Sedative effects may be antagonized by theophylline. **Effects can be reversed by flumazenil.** For pharmacodynamic information, see Chapter 6.

MILRINONE
Primacor and generics
Inotrope

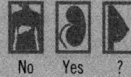

No Yes ? C

Injection: 1 mg/mL (10, 20, 50 mL)
Premixed injection in D₅W: 200 mcg/mL (100, 200 mL)

Child (limited data): 50 mcg/kg IV bolus over 15 min, followed by a continuous infusion of 0.25–0.75 mcg/kg/min and titrate to effect.
Adult: 50 mcg/kg IV bolus over 10 min, followed by a continuous infusion of 0.375–0.75 mcg/kg/min and titrate to effect. **Max. dose:** 1.13 mg/kg/24 hr.

Contraindicated in severe aortic stenosis, severe pulmonic stenosis, and acute MI. May cause headache, dysrhythmias, hypotension, hypokalemia, nausea, vomiting, anorexia, abdominal pain, hepatotoxicity, and thrombocytopenia. Pediatric patients may require higher mcg/kg/min doses because of a faster elimination $T_{1/2}$ and larger volume of distribution than adults. Hemodynamic effects can last up to 3–5 hr after discontinuation of infusion in children. **Reduce dose in renal impairment.**

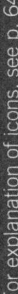

MINERAL OIL
Kondremul, Fleet Mineral Oil, and generics
Laxative, lubricant

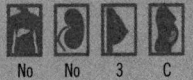

No　No　3　C

Liquid, oral [OTC]: 480 mL
Emulsion, oral (Kondremul [OTC]): 480 mL; each 5 mL Kondremul contains 2.5 mL mineral oil
Rectal liquid (Fleet Mineral Oil [OTC]): 133 mL

Constipation:
　Child 5–11 yr (see remarks):
　　Oral liquid: 5–15 mL/24 hr ÷ once daily–TID PO
　　Oral emulsion (Kondremul): 10–30 mL/24 hr ÷ once daily–TID PO
　　Rectal: 66.5 mL as single dose
　Child ≥ 12 yr and adult (see remarks):
　　Oral liquid: 15–45 mL/24 hr ÷ once daily–TID PO
　　Oral emulsion (Kondremul): 30–90 mL/24 hr ÷ once daily–TID PO
　　Rectal: 133 mL as single dose

May cause diarrhea, cramps, and lipid pneumonitis via aspiration. Use as a laxative **should not exceed** >1 wk. Onset of action is ≈ 6–8 hr. Higher doses may be necessary to achieve desired effect. **Use with caution** and **do not** give QHS dose in children <5 yr to minimize risk of aspiration. May impair absorption of fat-soluble vitamins, calcium, phosphorus, oral contraceptives, and warfarin. Emulsified preparations are more palatable and dosed differently than oral liquid preparation.
For disimpaction, doses up to 1 ounce (30 mL) per yr of age (**max. dose** of 240 mL) BID can be given.

MINOCYCLINE
Minocin, Dynacin, Arestin, Solodyn, and generics
Antibiotic, tetracycline derivative

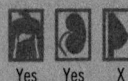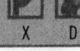

Yes　Yes　X　D

Tabs: 50, 75, 100 mg
Caps: 50, 75, 100 mg
Extended-release tabs (Solodyn): 45, 65, 90, 115, 135 mg
Caps (pellet filled): 50, 100 mg
Sustained-release microspheres (Arestin): 1 mg (12s)
Oral suspension: 50 mg/5 mL (60 mL); contains 5% alcohol

General infections:
　Child (8–12 yr): 4 mg/kg/dose × 1 PO, then 2 mg/kg/dose Q12 hr PO; **max. dose:** 200 mg/24 hr
　Adolescent and adult: 200 mg/dose × 1 PO, then 100 mg Q12 hr PO
Chlamydia trachomatis/Ureaplasma urealyticum:
　Adolescent and adult: 100 mg PO Q12 hr × 7 days
Acne (≥12 yr–adult):
　Immediate-release dosage forms: 50–100 mg PO once daily–BID
　Extended-release tabs:
　　45–54 kg: 45 mg PO once daily
　　55–77 kg: 65 mg PO once daily
　　78–102 kg: 90 mg PO once daily
　　103–125 kg: 115 mg PO once daily
　　126–136 kg: 135 mg PO once daily

MINOCYCLINE *continued*

Not recommended for children <8 yr and during last half of pregnancy (risk of permanent tooth discoloration). **Use with caution** in renal failure; lower dosage may be necessary. High incidence of vestibular dysfunction (30%–90%). Nausea, vomiting, allergy, increased ICP, photophobia and injury to developing teeth may occur. Hepatitis, including autoimmune hepatitis, liver failure, hypersensitivity reactions (e.g., anaphylaxis, Stevens-Johnson syndrome, erythema multiforme), and lupus-like syndrome have been reported.

May increase effects/toxicity of warfarin and decrease efficacy of live attenuated oral typhoid vaccine. May be administered with food but **NOT** with milk or dairy products. See *Tetracycline* for additional drug/food interactions and comments.

MINOXIDIL
Various generics (previously available as Loniten), Rogaine, Men's Rogaine Extra Strength
Antihypertensive agent, hair growth stimulant

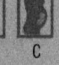
No   Yes   2   C

Tabs: 2.5, 10 mg
Topical solution:
  Rogaine and generics [OTC]: 2% (60 mL)
  Men's Rogaine Extra Strength and generics [OTC]: 5% (60, 120 mL); contains 30% alcohol
Topical aerosol foam:
  Men's Rogaine Extra Strength [OTC]: 5% (60 g); contains alcohol

Child < 12 yr:
Start with 0.1–0.2 mg/kg/24 hr PO once daily. **Max. dose:** 5 mg/24 hr. Dose may be increased in increments of 0.1–0.2 mg/kg/24 hr at 3-day intervals. Usual effective range: 0.25–1 mg/kg/24 hr PO ÷ once daily–BID. **Max. dose:** 50 mg/24 hr.

≥12 yr and adult:
Oral: Start with 5 mg once daily. Dose may be gradually increased at 3-day intervals. Usual effective range: 10–40 mg/24 hr ÷ once daily–BID. **Max. dose:** 100 mg/24 hr.

Topical (alopecia; see remarks):
Adult: Apply topically to the affected areas of the scalp BID (QAM and QHS).

Contraindicated in acute MI, dissecting aortic aneurysm, and pheochromocytoma. Concurrent use with a β-blocker and diuretic is recommended to prevent reflex tachycardia and reduce water retention, respectively. May cause drowsiness, dizziness, CHF, pulmonary edema, pericardial effusion, pericarditis, thrombocytopenia, leukopenia, Stevens-Johnson syndrome, and hypertrichosis (reversible) with systemic use.

Concurrent use of guanethidine may cause profound orthostatic hypotension; use with other antihypertensive agents may cause additive hypotension. Patients with renal failure or receiving dialysis may require a dosage reduction. Antihypertensive onset of action within 30 min and peak effects within 2–8 hr.

TOPICAL USE: Local irritation, contact dermatitis may occur. **Do not use** in conjunction with other topical agents (i.e., topical corticosteroids, retinoids, or petrolatum) or agents known to enhance cutaneous drug absorption. Onset of hair growth is 4 mo. Wash hands thoroughly after each application. The 5% solution is flammable.

For explanation of icons, see p. 648

MOMETASONE FUROATE ± FORMOTEROL FUMARATE
Asmanex Twisthaler, Nasonex, Elocon and other generic
topical products
In combination with formoterol: Dulera
Corticosteroid

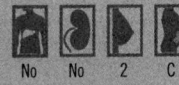

No   No   2   C

Nasal spray (Nasonex): 0.05%, 50 mcg per actuation (17 g = 120 doses)
Powder for inhalation, breath activated (Asmanex Twisthaler [see remarks]): 110 mcg per
actuation (7, 14, 30 units), 220 mcg per actuation (14, 60, 120 units); contains lactose
Topical cream and ointment (Elocon and generics): 0.1% (15, 45 g)
Topical lotion and solution (Elocon and others): 0.1% (30, 60 mL); contains isopropyl alcohol
In combination with formoterol:
Aerosol inhaler (Dulera):
   100 mcg mometasone furoate + 5 mcg formoterol fumarate dihydrate per inhalation (8.8 g
   delivers 60 inhalations, 13 g delivers 120 inhalations)
   200 mcg mometasone furoate + 5 mcg formoterol fumarate dihydrate per inhalation (8.8 g
   delivers 60 inhalations, 13 g delivers 120 inhalations)

MOMETASONE FUROATE:

Intranasal (allergic rhinitis): Patients with known seasonal allergic rhinitis should initiate
therapy 2–4 wk before anticipated pollen season.
   2–11 yr: 50 mcg (1 spray) each nostril once daily
   ≥12 yr and adult: 100 mcg (2 sprays) each nostril once daily
Oral inhalation:
   4–11 yr: Start with 110 mcg (1 inhalation) QHS of the 110 mcg inhaler regardless of prior therapy.
   Max. dose: 110 mcg/24 hr
   ≥12 yr and adult: max. effects may not be achieved until 1–2 wk or longer. Titrate doses to lowest
   effective dose once asthma stabilized.
      Previously treated with bronchodilators alone or with inhaled corticosteroids: Start with 220 mcg
      (1 inhalation) QHS. Dose may be increased up to a **max. dose** of 440 mcg/24 hr ÷ QHS or BID.
      Previously treated with oral corticosteroids: Start with 440 mcg BID; **max. dose:** 880 mcg/24 hr.
Topical (see Chapter 30 for topical steroid comparisons):
   Cream and ointment:
      ≥2 yr and adult: Apply a thin film to affected area once daily. Safety and efficacy for >3 wk has
      not been established for pediatric patients.
   Lotion:
      ≥12 yr and adult: Apply a few drops to affected area, massaging lightly into skin until it
      disappears, once daily.
MOMETASONE FUROATE + FORMOTEROL FUMARATE (Dulera):
   ≥12 yr and adult: Two inhalations BID of either 100 mcg mometasone + 5 mcg formoterol or 200
   mcg mometasone + 5 mcg formoterol based on prior asthma therapy (see table below). **Max. dose:**
   Two inhalations BID of 200 mcg mometasone + 5 mcg formoterol.

Previous Therapy	Recommended Starting Dose	Recommended Maximum Daily Dose
Medium-dose inhaled corticosteroids	100 mcg mometasone + 5 mcg formoterol: 2 inhalations BID	400 mcg mometasone + 20 mcg formoterol
High-dose inhaled corticosteroids	200 mcg mometasone + 5 mcg formoterol: 2 inhalations BID	800 mcg mometasone + 20 mcg formoterol

Concurrent administration with ketoconazole and other CYP 450 3A4 inhibitors (e.g., protease
inhibitors) may increase mometasone levels, resulting in Cushing syndrome and adrenal
suppression.

M

MOMETASONE FUROATE ± FORMOTEROL FUMARATE *continued*

INTRANASAL: Clear nasal passages and shake nasal spray well before each use. Onset of action for nasal symptoms of allergic rhinitis has been shown to occur within 11 hr after first dose. Nasal burning and irritation may occur. Nasal septal perforation and taste/smell disturbances have been rarely reported.

ORAL INHALATION (all forms): Rinse mouth after each use. Fever, allergic rhinitis, URI, UTI, GI discomfort, and sore throat have been reported in children. Musculoskeletal pain, oral candidiasis, arthralgia, and fatigue may occur. May potentially worsen fungal, bacterial, viral, or parasitic infection, tuberculosis, or ocular herpes simplex. Do not use Asmanex Twisthaler if allergic to milk proteins.

MOMETASONE + FORMOTEROL (Dulera): Breast-feeding information is currently unknown. Common side effects include nasopharyngitis, sinusitis, and headache. Angioedema and anaphylaxis have been reported. See *Formoterol* for additional remarks.

TOPICAL USE: HPA axis suppression and skin atrophy have been reported with cream and ointment use in infants 6–23 mo. Avoid application/contact to face, eyes, underarms, groin, and open skin. Occlusive dressings and use in diaper dermatitis are not recommended.

MONTELUKAST
Singulair and generics
Antiasthmatic, antiallergy leukotriene receptor antagonist

No   No   ?   B

Chewable tabs: 4, 5 mg; contains phenylalanine
Tabs: 10 mg
Oral granules: 4 mg per packet (30s)

Asthma and seasonal allergic rhinitis:
   Child (6 mo–5 yr): 4 mg (oral granules or chewable tablet) PO QHS; minimum age for use in asthma (per product label) is 12 mo.
   Child (6–14 yr): 5 mg (chewable tablet) PO QHS
   ≥15 yr and adult: 10 mg PO QHS
Prevention of exercise-induced bronchospasm (administer dose at least 2 hr before exercise; additional doses should not be administered within 24 hr):
   Child (6–14 yr): 5 mg (chewable tablet) PO
   ≥15 yr and adult: 10 mg PO

Chewable tablet dosage form is **contraindicated** in phenylketonuric patients. Side effects include headache, abdominal pain, dyspepsia, fatigue, dizziness, cough, and elevated liver enzymes. Diarrhea, epistaxis, eosinophilia, thrombocytopenia, hypersensitivity reactions (including Stevens-Johnson syndrome and TEN), pharyngitis, nausea, otitis, sinusitis, and viral infections have been reported in children. Neuropsychiatric events, including aggression, anxiety, dream abnormalities, hallucinations, depression, suicidal behavior, and insomnia have been reported.

Drug is a substrate for CYP 450 3A4 and 2C9. Phenobarbital and rifampin may induce hepatic metabolism to increase clearance of montelukast.

Doses may administered with or without food.

For explanation of icons, see p. 648

MORPHINE SULFATE
Roxanol, MS Contin, Oramorph SR, Avinza, Kadian, and many others
Narcotic, analgesic

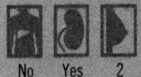

No   Yes   2   C/D

Oral solution: 10 mg/5 mL, 20 mg/5 mL
Concentrated oral solution: 100 mg/5 mL
Caps/tabs: 15, 30 mg
Controlled-release tabs (MS Contin, Oramorph SR): 15, 30, 60, 100, 200 mg
Extended-release tabs: 15, 30, 60, 100, 200 mg
Soluble tabs: 10, 15, 30 mg
Extended-release caps:
   Avinza (10% of dose as immediate release): 30, 45, 60, 75, 90, 120 mg
   Kadian: 10, 20, 30, 40, 50, 70, 80, 100, 130, 150, 200 mg
   Generics: 10, 20, 30, 50, 60, 80, 100 mg
Rectal suppository: 5, 10, 20, 30 mg
Injection: 0.5, 1, 2, 4, 5, 8, 10, 15, 25, 50 mg/mL

Titrate to effect.

Analgesia/tetralogy (cyanotic) spells:
   Neonate: 0.05–0.2 mg/kg/dose IM, slow IV, SC Q4 hr
   Neonatal opiate withdrawal: 0.08–0.2 mg/dose PO Q3–4 hr PRN
   Infant 1–6 mo:
      PO: 0.08–0.1 mg/kg/dose Q3–4 hr PRN
      IV: 0.025–0.03 mg/kg/dose Q2–4 hr PRN
   Infant > 6 mo and child:
      PO: 0.2–0.5 mg/kg/dose (**initial max. dose:** 15–20 mg/dose) Q4–6 hr PRN (immediate release) or 0.3–0.6 mg/kg/dose Q12 hr PRN (controlled release)
      IM/IV/SC: 0.1–0.2 mg/kg/dose Q2–4 hr PRN; **max. initial dose:** infant: 2 mg/dose; 1–6 yr: 4 mg/dose; 7–12 yr: 8 mg/dose; adolescent: 10 mg/dose
   Adult:
      PO: 10–30 mg Q4 hr PRN (immediate release) or 15–30 mg Q8–12 hr PRN (controlled release)
      IM/IV/SQ: 2–15 mg/dose Q2–6 hr PRN
Continuous IV infusion and SC infusion: Dosing ranges, titrate to effect.
   Neonate (IV route only): 0.01–0.02 mg/kg/hr
   Infant and child:
      Postoperative pain: 0.01–0.04 mg/kg/hr
      Sickle cell and cancer: 0.04–0.07 mg/kg/hr
   Adult: 0.8–10 mg/hr

To prepare infusion for neonates, infants, and children, use the following formula:

$$50 \times \frac{\text{Desired dose (mg/kg/hr)}}{\text{Desired infusion rate (mL/hr)}} \times \text{Wt (kg)} = \frac{\text{mg Morphine}}{50 \text{ mL Fluid}}$$

Dependence, CNS and respiratory depression, nausea, vomiting, urinary retention, constipation, hypotension, bradycardia, increased ICP, miosis, biliary spasm, and allergy may occur.
Naloxone may be used to reverse effects, especially respiratory depression. Causes histamine release, resulting in itching and possible bronchospasm. Low-dose naloxone infusion may be used for itching. Inflammatory masses (e.g., granulomas) have been reported with continuous infusions via indwelling intrathecal catheters.

See Chapter 6 for equianalgesic dosing. Pregnancy category changes to "D" if used for prolonged periods or in higher doses at term. Rectal dosing is same as oral dosing but is not recommended owing to poor absorption.

M

MORPHINE SULFATE *continued*

The FDA has recently announced safety labeling changes and postmarket study requirements for extended-release/long-acting opioid analgesics; see www.fda.gov/drugs/drugsafety for updated information. Controlled/sustained-release oral tablets must be administered whole. Controlled-release oral capsules may be opened and the entire contents sprinkled on applesauce immediately before ingestion. Be aware of the various oral solution concentrations; the concentrated oral solution (100 mg/5 mL) has been associated with accidental overdoses. **Adjust dose in renal failure (see Chapter 31).**

MUPIROCIN
Bactroban, Bactroban Nasal, and generics
Topical antibiotic

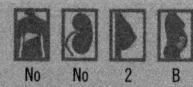

No   No   2   B

Ointment: 2% (22, 30 g); contains polyethylene glycol
Cream: 2% (15, 30 g); contains benzyl alcohol
Nasal ointment (Bactroban Nasal): 2% (1 g), as calcium salt

Topical (see remarks):
  ≥3 mo–adult: Apply small amount TID to affected area × 5–14 days. Topical ointment may be used in infants ≥2 mo for impetigo.
Intranasal (all ages; see remarks): Apply small amount intranasally BID × 5–10 days.

Avoid contact with eyes. Topical cream is **not** intended for use in lesions >10 cm in length or 100 cm² in surface area. **Do not use** topical ointment preparation on open wounds because of concerns about systemic absorption of polyethylene glycol. May cause minor local irritation and dry skin. Intranasal route may cause nasal stinging, taste disorder, headache, rhinitis, and pharyngitis.

If clinical response is not apparent in 3–5 days with topical use, reevaluate infection. Intranasal administration may be used to eliminate carriage of *Staphylococcus aureus*, including MRSA.

MYCOPHENOLATE
Mycophenolate mofetil: CellCept and generics
Mycophenolate sodium: Myfortic and generics
Immunosuppressant agent

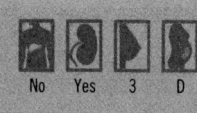

No   Yes   3   D

Mycophenolate mofetil:
  Caps: 250 mg
  Tabs: 500 mg
  Oral suspension: 200 mg/mL (160 mL); contains phenylalanine (0.56 mg/mL) and methylparabens
  Injection: 500 mg
Mycophenolate sodium:
  Tabs: 500 mg
  Delayed-release tabs (Myfortic): 180, 360 mg

Child (see remarks):
  Renal transplant:
    Caps, tabs, or suspension: 600 mg/m²/dose PO/IV BID up to a **max. dose** of 2000 mg/24 hr
    Alternatively, patients with BSAs ≥1.25 m² may be dosed as follows:
      1.25–1.5 m²: 750 mg PO BID
      >1.5 m²: 1000 mg PO BID

Continued

MYCOPHENOLATE *continued*

Child (see remarks):
  Renal transplant:
    Delayed-release tabs (Myfortic): 400–450 mg/m²/dose PO BID. **Max. dose:** 720 mg BID. This dosage form not recommended in patients with BSAs <1.19 m². Alternatively, patients with BSA ≥1.19 m² may be dosed as follows:
      1.19–1.58 m²: 540 mg PO BID
      >1.58 m²: 720 mg PO BID
  Nephrotic syndrome:
    Frequently relapsing: 12.5–18 mg/kg/dose PO BID up to a **max. dose** of 2000 mg/24 hr for 1–2 years, and taper prednisone regimen.
    Steroid dependent: 12–18 mg/kg/dose or 600 mg/m²/dose PO BID up to a **max. dose** of 2000 mg/24hr.
Adult (in combination with corticosteroids and cyclosporine; check specific transplantation protocol for specific dosage):
  IV: 2000–3000 mg/24 hr ÷ BID
  Oral:
    Caps, tabs, or suspension: 2000–3000 mg/24 hr PO ÷ BID
    Delayed-release tabs (Myfortic): 720–1080 mg PO BID

Check specific transplantation protocol for specific dosage. Mycophenolate mofetil is a prodrug for mycophenolic acid. Owing to differences in absorption, delayed-release tablets should **not** be interchanged with other oral dosage forms on an equivalent mg-to-mg basis. Increases risk of first-trimester pregnancy loss and increased risk of congenital malformations (especially external ear and facial abnormalities [e.g., cleft lip and palate] and anomalies of distal limbs, heart, and esophagus).

Common side effects may include headache, hypertension, diarrhea, vomiting, bone marrow suppression, anemia, fever, opportunistic infections, and sepsis. May increase risk for bacterial, fungal, protozoal, and viral infections, and lymphomas or other malignancies. GI bleeds and increased risk for rejection in heart transplant patients switched from calicineurin inhibitors (e.g., cyclosporine, tacrolimus) and CellCept to sirolimus and CellCept have been reported. Cases of progressive multifocal leukoencephalopathy (PML) and pure red cell aplasia (PRCA) have also been reported.

Use with caution in patients with active GI disease or renal impairment (GFR < 25 mL/min/1.73 m²) outside of the immediate posttransplant period. In adults with renal impairment, **avoid** doses >2 g/24 hr and observe carefully. Dose should be interrupted or reduced in the presence of neutropenia (ANC < 1.3 × 10³/μL). No dose adjustment is needed for patients experiencing delayed graft function postoperatively.

Drug interactions: (1) Displacement of phenytoin or theophylline from protein binding sites will decrease total serum levels and increase free serum levels of these drugs. Salicylates displace mycophenolate to increase free levels of mycophenolate. (2) Competition for renal tubular secretion results in increased serum levels of acyclovir, ganciclovir, probenecid, and mycophenolate (when any of these are used together). (3) **Avoid** live and live attenuated vaccines (including influenza); decreases vaccine effectiveness. (4) Proton-pump inhibitors may reduce mycophenolate levels.

Administer oral doses on an empty stomach. Cholestyramine and antacid use may decrease mycophenolic acid levels. Infuse IV doses over 2 hr. Oral suspension may be administered via NG tube with a minimum size of 8 French.

NAFCILLIN
Nallpen and generics
Antibiotic, penicillin (penicillinase resistant)

Yes Yes 2 B

Injection: 1, 2, 10 g; contains 2.9 mEq Na/g drug
Injection, premixed in iso-osmotic dextrose: 1 g in 50 mL, 2 g in 100 mL

Neonate (IM/IV):
  ≤7 days:
    <2 kg: 50 mg/kg/24 hr ÷ Q12 hr
    ≥2 kg: 75 mg/kg/24 hr ÷ Q8 hr
  >7 days:
    <1.2 kg: 50 mg/kg/24 hr ÷ Q12 hr
    1.2–2 kg: 75 mg/kg/24 hr ÷ Q8 hr
    ≥2 kg: 100 mg/kg/24 hr ÷ Q6 hr
Infant and child (IM/IV):
  Mild to moderate infections: 50–100 mg/kg/24 hr ÷ Q6 hr
  Severe infections: 100–200 mg/kg/24 hr ÷ Q4–6 hr; give 200 mg/kg/24 hr ÷ Q4–6 hr for
  staphylococcal endocarditis
  Max. dose: 12 g/24 hr
Adult:
  IV: 500–2000 mg Q4–6 hr
  IM: 500 mg Q4–6 hr
  Max. dose: 12 g/24 hr

Allergic cross-sensitivity with penicillin. **Oral route not recommended because of
unpredictable absorption.** Solutions containing dextrose may be **contraindicated** in patients
with known allergy to corn or corn products. High incidence of phlebitis with IV dosing. CSF
penetration is poor unless meninges are inflamed. **Use with caution** in patients with
combined renal and hepatic impairment (reduce dose by 33%–50%). Nafcillin may increase
elimination of cyclosporine and warfarin. Acute interstitial nephritis is rare. May cause rash,
bone marrow suppression, and false-positive urinary and serum proteins. Hypokalemia has
been reported.

NALOXONE
Narcan and many generics
Narcotic antagonist

  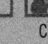

No No ? C

Injection: 0.4 mg/mL (1, 10 mL); some preparations may contain parabens
Injection, in syringe: 1 mg/mL (2 mL)

Opiate intoxication (IM/IV/SC, use 2–10 times IV dose for ETT route; see remarks):
  Neonate, infant, child ≤ 20 kg or ≤ 5 yr: 0.1 mg/kg/dose. May repeat PRN Q2–3 min.
  Child > 20 kg or > 5 yr: 2 mg/dose. May repeat PRN Q2–3 min.
  Continuous infusion (child and adult): 0.005 mg/kg loading dose, followed by infusion of 0.0025 mg/
  kg/hr has been recommended. A range of 0.0025–0.16 mg/kg/hr has been reported. Taper gradually
  to avoid relapse.
  Adult: 0.4–2 mg/dose. May repeat PRN Q2–3 min. Use 0.1- to 0.2-mg increments in opiate-
  dependent patients.

Continued For explanation of icons, see p. 648

NALOXONE *continued*

Opiate-induced pruritus (limited data): 0.25–2 mcg/kg/hr IV; a dose-finding study in 59 children suggests a minimum dose of 1 mcg/kg/hr when used as prophylactic therapy. Doses ≥3 mcg/kg/hr increase risk for reduced pain control.

Short duration of action may necessitate multiple doses. For severe intoxication, doses of 0.2 mg/kg may be required. If no response is achieved after a cumulative dose of 10 mg, reevaluate diagnosis. **In the nonarrest situation, use lowest dose effective (may start at 0.001 mg/kg/dose). See Chapter 6 for additional information.**

Will produce narcotic withdrawal syndrome in patients with chronic dependence. **Use with caution** in patients with chronic cardiac disease. Abrupt reversal of narcotic depression may result in nausea, vomiting, diaphoresis, tachycardia, hypertension, and tremulousness.

IV administration preferred. Onset of action may be delayed with other routes of administration.

NAPROXEN/NAPROXEN SODIUM
Naprosyn, Anaprox, EC-Naprosyn, Naprosyn DR, Naprelan,
Aleve [OTC], and many others
Nonsteroidal antiinflammatory agent

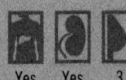 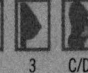

Yes   Yes   3   C/D

Naproxen:
    Tabs (Naprosyn and generics): 250, 375, 500 mg
    Delayed-release tabs (EC-Naprosyn, Naprosyn DR): 375, 500 mg
    Oral suspension: 125 mg/5 mL; contains 0.34 mEq Na/1 mL and parabens
Naproxen Sodium:
    Tabs:
        Aleve and others [OTC]: 220 mg (200 mg base); contains 0.87 mEq Na
        Anaprox and generics: 275 mg (250 mg base), 550 mg (500 mg base); contains 1 mEq, 2 mEq Na, respectively
    Controlled-release tabs (Naprelan): 412.5 mg (375 mg base), 550 mg (500 mg base), 825 mg (750 mg base)

All doses based on naproxen base.
Child > 2 yr:

    Analgesia: 5–7 mg/kg/dose Q8–12 hr PO
    JRA: 10–20 mg/kg/24 hr ÷ Q12 hr PO
    Usual max. dose: 1000 mg/24 hr
Adult:
    Analgesia (includes adolescents):
        Over-the-counter dosage forms: 200 mg Q8–12 hr PRN PO; if needed, 400 mg initial dose may be needed. **Max. dose:** 600 mg/24 hr.
        Prescription-strength dosage forms: 250 mg Q8–12 hr PRN (500 mg initial dose may be needed) ***OR*** 500 mg Q12 hr PRN PO. **Max. dose:** 1250 mg/24 hr for first day then 1000 mg/24 hr.
    Rheumatoid arthritis, ankylosing spondylitis:
        Immediate-release forms: 250–500 mg BID PO
        Delayed-release tabs (EC-Naprosyn, Naprosyn DR): 375–500 mg BID PO
        Controlled-release tabs (Naprelan): 750–1000 mg once daily PO. For patients converting from immediate and delayed-release forms, calculate daily dose and administer Naprelan as a single daily dose.
        Max. dose (all dosage forms): 1500 mg/24 hr

NAPROXEN/NAPROXEN SODIUM *continued*

Dysmenorrhea (adult):
500 mg × 1, then 250 mg Q6–8 hr PRN PO or 500 mg Q12 hr PRN PO; **max. dose:** 1250 mg/24 hr for first day, then 1000 mg/24 hr

Contraindicated in treating perioperative pain for coronary artery bypass graft surgery. May cause GI bleeding, thrombocytopenia, heartburn, headache, drowsiness, vertigo, and tinnitus. **Use with caution** in patients with GI disease, cardiac disease (risk for thrombotic events, MI, stroke), renal or hepatic impairment, and those receiving anticoagulants. See *Ibuprofen* for other side effects.

Pregnancy category changes to "D" if used in the third trimester or near delivery. Administer doses with food or milk to reduce GI discomfort.

NEOMYCIN SULFATE
Neo-fradin and generics
Antibiotic, aminoglycoside; ammonium detoxicant

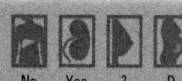

No   Yes   ?   D

Tabs: 500 mg
Oral solution (Neo-Fradin): 125 mg/5 mL (480 mL); contains parabens

Diarrhea:
Preterm and newborn: 50 mg/kg/24 hr ÷ Q6 hr PO
Hepatic encephalopathy:
Infant and child: 50–100 mg/kg/24 hr ÷ Q6–8 hr PO × 5–6 days; **max. dose:** 12 g/24 hr
Adult: 4–12 g/24 hr ÷ Q4–6 hr PO × 5–6 days
Bowel prep (in combination with erythromycin base):
Child: 90 mg/kg/24 hr PO ÷ Q4 hr × 2–3 days
Adult: 1 g Q1 hr PO × 4 doses, then 1 g Q4 hr PO × 5 doses; many other regimens exist.

Contraindicated in ulcerative bowel disease, intestinal obstruction, or aminoglycoside hypersensitivity. Monitor for nephrotoxicity and ototoxicity. Oral absorption is limited, but levels may accumulate. Consider dosage reduction in the presence of renal failure. May cause itching, redness, edema, colitis, candidiasis, or poor wound healing if applied topically. Prevalence of neomycin hypersensitivity has increased. May decrease absorption of penicillin V, vitamin B_{12}, digoxin, and methotrexate. May potentiate oral anticoagulants and adverse effects of other neurotoxic, ototoxic, or nephrotoxic drugs.

NEOMYCIN/POLYMYXIN B/± BACITRACIN
NEOMYCIN/POLYMYXIN B:
Neosporin GU Irrigant
NEOMYCIN/POLYMYXIN B + BACITRACIN:
Neosporin, Neo To Go, Neo-Polycin, Neosporin Ophthalmic, and generics
Topical antibiotic

No   No   ?   C/D

NEOMYCIN/POLYMYXIN B:
Solution, genitourinary irrigant: 40 mg neomycin sulfate, 200,000 U polymyxin B/mL (1, 20 mL); multidose vial contains methylparabens.

Continued

For explanation of icons, see p. 648

NEOMYCIN/POLYMYXIN B/± BACITRACIN *continued*

NEOMYCIN/POLYMYXIN B + BACITRACIN:
  Ointment, topical (Neosporin, Neo To Go) [OTC]: 3.5 mg neomycin sulfate, 400 U bacitracin, 5000 U polymyxin B/g (0.9, 15, 30, 454 g)
  Ointment, ophthalmic (Neosporin Ophthalmic): 3.5 mg neomycin sulfate, 400 U bacitracin, 10,000 U polymyxin B/g (3.5 g)

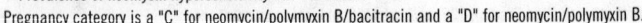

NEOMYCIN/POLYMYXIN B + BACITRACIN:
  Child and adult:
    Topical: Apply to minor wounds and burns once–twice daily
    Ophthalmic: Apply small amount to conjunctiva Q3–4 hr × 7–10 days, depending on severity of infection.
NEOMYCIN/POLYMYXIN B:
  Bladder irrigation:
    Child and adult: Mix 1 mL in 1000 mL NS and administer via a three-way catheter at a rate adjusted to patient's urine output. Do not exceed 10 days of continuous use.

Do not use for extended periods. May cause superinfection, delayed healing. See *Neomycin* for additional remarks. Ophthalmic preparation may cause stinging and sensitivity to bright light. **Avoid** use of bladder irrigant in patients with defects in the bladder mucosa or wall. Prevalence of neomycin hypersensitivity has increased.

Pregnancy category is a "C" for neomycin/polymyxin B/bacitracin and a "D" for neomycin/polymyxin B.

NEOSTIGMINE
Prostigmin, Bioxiverz, and generics
Anticholinesterase (cholinergic) agent

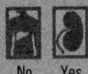 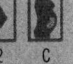

No   Yes   2   C

Tabs: 15 mg (bromide)
Injection: 0.5, 1 mg/mL (methylsulfate); may contain parabens or phenol

Myasthenia gravis diagnosis: Use with atropine (see remarks).
  Child: 0.025–0.04 mg/kg IM × 1
  Adult: 0.02 mg/kg IM × 1
Treatment:
  Child:
    IM/IV/SC: 0.01–0.04 mg/kg/dose Q2–4 hr PRN
    PO: 2 mg/kg/24 hr ÷ Q3–4 hr; **max. dose:** 375 mg/24 hr
  Adult:
    IM/IV/SC: 0.5–2.5 mg/dose Q1–3 hr PRN up to **max. dose** of 10 mg/24 hr
    PO: Start with 15 mg/dose TID. May increase every 1–2 days. Dosage requirements may vary from 15–375 mg/24 hr with an average of 150 mg/24 hr. Some patients may require as much as 30–40 mg Q2–4 hr.
Reversal of nondepolarizing neuromuscular blocking agents: Administer with atropine or glycopyrrolate.
  Infant: 0.025–0.1 mg/kg/dose IV
  Child: 0.025–0.08 mg/kg/dose IV
  Adult: 0.5–2.5 mg/dose IV
  Max. dose (all ages): 5 mg/dose

N

NEOSTIGMINE *continued*

Contraindicated in GI and urinary obstruction. **Caution** in asthmatics. May cause cholinergic crisis, bronchospasm, salivation, nausea, vomiting, diarrhea, miosis, diaphoresis, lacrimation, bradycardia, hypotension, fatigue, confusion, respiratory depression, and seizures. Titrate for each patient, but **avoid** excessive cholinergic effects.

For diagnosis of myasthenia gravis (MG), administer atropine 0.011 mg/kg/dose IV immediately before or IM (0.011 mg/kg/dose) 30 min before neostigmine. For treatment of MG, patients may need higher doses of neostigmine at times of greatest fatigue.

Antidote: Atropine 0.01–0.04 mg/kg/dose. Atropine and epinephrine should be available in the event of a hypersensitivity reaction.

Adjust dose in renal failure (see Chapter 31).

NEVIRAPINE
Viramune, Viramune XR, NVP, and generics
Antiviral, non-nucleoside reverse transcriptase inhibitor

Yes Yes 3 B

Tabs: 200 mg
Extended-release tabs (Viramune XR): 400 mg
Oral suspension: 10 mg/mL (240 mL); contains parabens

HIV: See www.aidsinfo.nih.gov/guidelines
Prevention of vertical transmission during high-risk situations (women who received no antepartum antiretroviral prophylaxis, women with suboptimal viral suppression at delivery, or women with known antiretroviral drug-resistant virus) and in combination with zidovudine (see Chapter 17 for additional information):
Newborn: 3 doses (based on birth weight) in the first week of life; dose 1: within 0–48 hr of birth; dose 2: 48 hr after dose 1; dose 3: 96 hr after dose 2
  Birth weight 1.5–2 kg: 8 mg/dose PO
  Birth weight > 2 kg: 12 mg/dose PO

See www.aidsinfo.nih.gov/guidelines for additional remarks.
Use with caution in patients with hepatic or renal dysfunction. **Contraindicated** in moderate/severe hepatic impairment (Child-Pugh Class B or C) and postexposure (occupational or non-occupational) prophylaxis regimens. Most frequent side effects include: rash (may be life-threatening, including Stevens-Johnson syndrome; permanently discontinue and never restart), fever, abnormal liver function tests, headache, and nausea. **Discontinue therapy** if any of the following occurs: severe rash; rash with fever, blistering, oral lesions, conjunctivitis, or muscle aches. Permanently discontinue and do not restart therapy if symptomatic hepatitis, severe transaminase elevations, or hypersensitivity reactions occur.

Life-threatening hepatotoxicity has been reported, primarily during first 12 wk of therapy. Patients with increased serum transaminase or history of hepatitis B or C infection before nevirapine are at greater risk for hepatotoxicity. Women, including pregnant women, with CD4 counts >250 cells/mm^3 or men with CD4 counts >400 cells/mm^3 are at risk for hepatotoxicity. Monitor liver function tests (obtain transaminases immediately after development of hepatitis signs/symptoms, hypersensitivity reactions, or rash) and CBCs. Hypophosphatemia has been reported.

Nevirapine induces the CYP 450 3A4 drug-metabolizing isoenzyme to cause an autoinduction of its own metabolism within the first 2–4 wk of therapy and has the potential to interact with many drugs. **Carefully review patients' drug profile for other drug interactions each time nevirapine is initiated or when a new drug is added to a regimen containing nevirapine.**

Doses can be administered with food and concurrently with didanosine.

For explanation of icons, see p. 648

NIACIN/VITAMIN B₃
Niacor, Niaspan, Slo-Niacin, Nicotinic acid, Vitamin B₃,
and many generics
Vitamin, water soluble

Yes Yes ? A/C

Tabs [OTC]: 50, 100, 250, 500 mg
Timed or extended-release tabs [all OTC except 1000 mg]: 250, 500, 750, 1000 mg
Timed or extended-release caps [OTC]: 250, 500 mg

US RDA: See Chapter 21.
Pellagra (PO):
  Child: 50–100 mg/dose TID
  Adult: 50–100 mg/dose TID–QID
Max. dose: 500 mg/24 hr

Contraindicated in hepatic dysfunction, active peptic ulcer, and severe hypotension. Use with
caution in unstable angina, acute MI (especially if receiving vasoactive drugs), renal
dysfunction, and in patients with history of jaundice, hepatobiliary disease, or peptic ulcer.
Adverse reactions of flushing, pruritus, or GI distress may occur with PO administration. May
cause hyperglycemia, hyperuricemia, blurred vision, abnormal liver function tests, dizziness,
and headaches. Burning sensation of the skin, skin discoloration, hepatitis, and elevated
creatine kinase have been reported. May cause false-positive urine catecholamines
(fluorometric methods) and urine glucose (Benedict's reagent).
Pregnancy category changes to "C" if used in doses above the RDA or for typical doses used for lipid
disorders. **See Chapter 21 for multivitamin preparations.**

NICARDIPINE
Cardene IV, Cardene SR, and generics
Calcium channel blocker, antihypertensive

Yes Yes 2 C

Caps (immediate-release): 20, 30 mg
Sustained-release caps (Cardene SR): 30, 60 mg
Injection (Cardene IV): 0.1 mg/mL (200 mL), 0.2 mg/mL (200 mL), 2.5 mg/mL (10 mL;
also available in generic)

Child (see remarks):
  Hypertension:
    Continuous IV infusion: Start at 0.5–1 mcg/kg/min; dose may be increased as needed
    every 15–30 min up to a **max.** of 4–5 mcg/kg/min.
Adult:
  Hypertension:
    Oral:
      Immediate release: 20 mg PO TID; dose may be increased after 3 days to 40 mg PO TID if
      needed.
      Sustained release: 30 mg PO BID; dose may be increased after 3 days to 60 mg PO BID if
      needed.
    Continuous IV infusion: Start at 5 mg/hr; increase dose as needed by 2.5 mg/hr Q5–15 min up to
    a **max. dose** of 15 mg/hr. After attainment of desired BP, decrease infusion to 3 mg/hr and adjust
    rate as needed to maintain desired response.

NICARDIPINE continued

Reported use in children has been limited to a small number preterm infants, infants, and children. **Contraindicated** in advanced aortic stenosis. **Avoid** systemic hypotension in patients after an acute cerebral infarct or hemorrhage. **Use with caution** in hepatic or renal dysfunction by carefully titrating dose. The drug undergoes significant first-pass metabolism through the liver and is excreted in the urine (60%).

May cause headache, dizziness, asthenia, peripheral edema, and GI symptoms. Cimetidine increases effects/toxicity of nicardipine. **See Nifedipine for additional drug and food interactions.**

Onset of action for PO administration is 20 min, with peak effects in 0.5–2 hr. IV onset of action is 1 min. Duration of action after a single IV or PO dose is 3 hr. To reduce risk for venous thrombosis, phlebitis, and vascular impairment with IV administration, do not use small veins (e.g., dorsum of hand or wrist). Avoid intraarterial administration or extravasation. For additional information, see Chapter 4.

NIFEDIPINE
Adalat CC, Nifediac CC, Procardia, Procardia XL, and
many generics
Calcium channel blocker, antihypertensive

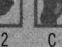

No No 2 C

Caps (Procardia and generics): 10 mg (0.34 mL), 20 mg (0.45 mL)
Sustained-release tabs (Adalat CC, Nifediac CC, Procardia XL, and others): 30, 60, 90 mg
Oral suspension: 1, 4 mg/mL

Child (see remarks for precautions):
  Hypertensive urgency: 0.1–0.25 mg/kg/dose Q4–6 hr PRN PO/SL; **max. dose:** 10 mg/dose
  or 1–2 mg/kg/24 hr
  Hypertension:
    Sustained-release tabs: Start with 0.25–0.5 mg/kg/24 hr (**max. dose:** 30–60 mg/24 hr) ÷
    Q12–24 hr. May increase to **max. dose** of 3 mg/kg/24 hr up to 120 mg/24 hr.
  Hypertrophic cardiomyopathy (infant): 0.6–0.9 mg/kg/24 hr ÷ Q6–8 hr PO/SL
Adult:
  Hypertension:
    Sustained-release tabs: Start with 30 mg PO once daily; usual range: 30–60 mg once daily. May
    increase to **max. dose** of 90 mg/24 hr for Adalat CC and 120 mg/24 hr for Procardia XL.
  Angina:
    Caps: Start with 10 mg/dose PO TID. May increase to 30 mg/dose PO TID–QID. **Max. dose:**
    180 mg/24 hr.

Use of immediate-release dosage form in children is controversial and has been abandoned by some. **Use with caution** in children with acute CNS injury, owing to increased risk for stroke, seizure, and altered level of consciousness. To prevent rapid decrease in blood pressure in children, an initial dose of ≤0.25 mg/kg is recommended.

Use with caution in patients with CHF, aortic stenosis, GI obstruction/narrowing (bezoar formation), and cirrhosis (reduced drug clearance). May cause severe hypotension, peripheral edema, flushing, tachycardia, headaches, dizziness, nausea, palpitations, and syncope. Acute generalized exanthematous pustulosis has been reported.

Although overall use in adults has been abandoned, the immediate-release dosage form is **contraindicated** in adults with severe obstructive coronary artery disease or recent MI, and in hypertensive emergencies.

Continued

NIFEDIPINE *continued*

Nifedipine is a substrate for CYP 450 3A3/4 and 3A5–7. **Do not administer** with grapefruit juice; may increase bioavailability and effects. Itraconazole and ketoconazole may increase nifedipine levels/effects. CYP 3A inducers (e.g., rifampin, rifabutin, phenobarbital, phenytoin, carbamazepine) may reduce nifedipine's effects. Nifedipine may increase phenytoin, cyclosporine, and digoxin levels. For hypertensive emergencies, **see Chapter 4**.

For sublingual administration, capsule must be punctured and liquid expressed into mouth. A small amount is absorbed via the SL route. Most effects are due to swallowing and oral absorption. **Do not** crush or chew sustained-release tablet dosage form.

NITROFURANTOIN
Furadantin, Macrodantin, Macrobid, and generics
Antibiotic

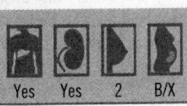

Yes   Yes   2   B/X

Caps (macrocrystals; Macrodantin and generics): 25, 50, 100 mg
Caps (dual-release; Macrobid): 100 mg (25 mg macrocrystal/75 mg monohydrate)
Oral suspension (Furadantin and generics): 25 mg/5 mL (230 mL); contains parabens and saccharin

Child (>1 mo; oral suspension or macrocrystals):
Treatment: 5–7 mg/kg/24 hr ÷ Q6 hr PO; **max. dose:** 400 mg/24 hr
UTI prophylaxis: 1–2 mg/kg/dose QHS PO; **max. dose:** 100 mg/24 hr
≥12 yr and adult:
Macrocrystals: 50–100 mg/dose Q6 hr PO
Dual-release (Macrobid): 100 mg/dose Q12 hr PO
UTI prophylaxis (macrocrystals): 50–100 mg/dose PO QHS

Contraindicated in severe renal disease, infants <1 mo of age, GFR <60 mL/min (reduced drug distribution the urine), active/previous cholestatic jaundice/hepatic dysfunction, and pregnant women at term. **Use with caution** in G6PD deficiency, anemia, lung disease, and peripheral neuropathy. May cause nausea, hypersensitivity reactions (including vasculitis), vomiting, cholestatic jaundice, headache, hepatotoxicity, polyneuropathy, and hemolytic anemia.

Anticholinergic drugs and high-dose probenecid may increase nitrofurantoin toxicity. Magnesium salts may decrease nitrofurantoin absorption. Causes false-positive urine glucose with Clinitest.

Pregnancy category changes to "X" at term (38–42 wk' gestation). Breast-feeding in mothers receiving nitrofurantoin is not recommended for infants <1 and those with G6PD deficiency; use in infants ≥1 mo and without G6PD deficiency is compatible.

NITROGLYCERIN
Nitro-Bid, Nitrostat, Nitro-Time, Nitro-Dur, NitroMist,
and many others
Vasodilator, antihypertensive

Yes   Yes   ?   C

Injection: 5 mg/mL (10 mL); may contain alcohol or propylene glycol
Prediluted injection in D₅W: 100 mcg/mL, 200 mcg/mL, 400 mcg/mL (250, 500 mL)
Sublingual tabs (Nitrostat and others): 0.3, 0.4, 0.6 mg
Sustained-release caps (Nitro-Time and others): 2.5, 6.5, 9 mg
Ointment, topical (Nitro-Bid): 2% (1, 30, 60 g)

NITROGLYCERIN *continued*

Patch (Nitro-Dur and others): 2.5 mg/24 hr (0.1 mg/hr), 5 mg/24 hr (0.2 mg/hr), 7.5 mg/24 hr
(0.3 mg/hr), 10 mg/24 hr (0.4 mg/hr), 15 mg/24 hr (0.6 mg/hr), 20 mg/24 hr (0.8 mg/hr)
Spray, translingual (NitroMist and others): 0.4 mg per metered spray (4.1, 8.5 g; delivers 90 and
230 doses, respectively); contains butane (flammable)

NOTE: The IV dosage units for children are in mcg/kg/min, compared with mcg/min for adults.
Child:
   Continuous IV infusion: Begin with 0.25–0.5 mcg/kg/min; may increase by 0.5–1 mcg/kg/min
   Q3–5 min PRN. Usual dose: 1–5 mcg/kg/min. **Max. dose:** 20 mcg/kg/min.
Adult:
   Continuous IV infusion: 5 mcg/min IV, then increase Q3–5 min PRN by 5 mcg/min up to 20 mcg/min.
   If no response, increase by 10 mcg/min Q3–5 min PRN up to a **max.** of 400 mcg/min.
   Sublingual: 0.2–0.6 mg Q5 min; **max.** of three doses in 15 min
   Oral: 2.5–9 mg BID–TID; up to 26 mg QID
   Ointment: Apply 1–2 inches Q8 hr, up to 4–5 inches Q4 hr.
   Patch: 0.2–0.4 mg/hr initially, then titrate to 0.4–0.8 mg/hr. Apply new patch daily (tolerance is
   minimized by removing patch for 10–12 hr/24 hr).

Contraindicated in glaucoma, severe anemia, and concurrent phosphodiesterase-5 inhibitor
(e.g., sildenafil). In small doses (1–2 mcg/kg/min) acts mainly on systemic veins and
decreases preload. At 3–5 mcg/kg/min acts on systemic arterioles to decrease resistance.
May cause headache, flushing, GI upset, blurred vision, and methemoglobinemia. **Use with
caution** in severe renal impairment, increased ICP, and hepatic failure. IV nitroglycerin may
antagonize anticoagulant effect of heparin.
Decrease dose gradually in patients receiving drug for prolonged periods to **avoid** withdrawal reaction.
Must use polypropylene infusion sets to **avoid** adsorption of drug to plastic tubing. Use in
heparinized patients may result in a decrease of PTT, with subsequent rebound effect upon
discontinuation of nitroglycerin.
Onset (duration) of action: IV: 1–2 min (3–5 min); sublingual: 1–3 min (30–60 min); PO sustained
release: 40 min (4–8 hr); topical ointment: 20–60 min (2–12 hr); and transdermal patch: 40–60
min (18–24 hr).

NITROPRUSSIDE
Nitropress (previously available as Nipride)
Vasodilator, antihypertensive

Yes   Yes   ?   C

Injection: 25 mg/mL (2 mL)

Child and adult: IV, continuous infusion
   Dose: Start at 0.3–0.5 mcg/kg/min, titrate to effect. Usual dose is 3–4 mcg/kg/min.
   Max. dose: 8–10 mcg/kg/min

Contraindicated in patients with decreased cerebral perfusion and in situations of
compensatory hypertension (increased ICP). Monitor for hypotension and acidosis.
Dilute with D₅W and protect from light.
Nitroprusside is nonenzymatically converted to cyanide, which is converted to thiocyanate. Cyanide
may produce metabolic acidosis and methemoglobinemia; thiocyanate may produce psychosis and
seizures. Monitor thiocyanate levels if used for >48 hr or if dose ≥ 4 mcg/kg/min. **Thiocyanate
levels should be <50 mg/L.** Monitor **cyanide levels (toxic levels > 2 mcg/mL)** in patients with
hepatic dysfunction and thiocyanate levels in patients with renal dysfunction.
Onset of action is 2 min, with a 1- to 10-min duration of effect.

For explanation of icons, see p. 648

NOREPINEPHRINE BITARTRATE
Levophed and generics
Adrenergic agonist

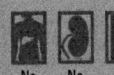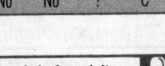

No   No   ?   C

Injection: 1 mg/mL as norepinephrine base (4 mL); contains sulfites

NOTE: *The dosage units for children are in mcg/kg/min, compared with mcg/min for adults.*
  Child: Continuous IV **infusion doses as norepinephrine base.** Start at 0.05–0.1 mcg/kg/min. Titrate to effect. **Max. dose:** 2 mcg/kg/min.
  Adult: Continuous IV infusion **doses as norepinephrine base.** Start at 4 mcg/min and titrate to effect. Usual dosage range: 8–12 mcg/min.

May cause cardiac arrhythmias, hypertension, hypersensitivity, headaches, vomiting, uterine contractions, and organ ischemia. May cause decreased renal blood flow and urine output. Avoid extravasation into tissues; may cause severe tissue necrosis. If this occurs, treat locally with phentolamine.

NORFLOXACIN
Noroxin
Antibiotic, quinolone

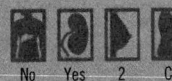

No   Yes   2   C

Tabs: 400 mg
Oral suspension: 20 mg/mL

Child:
  UTI (limited data in children 5 mo–19 yr [see remarks]): 9–14 mg/kg/24 hr PO ÷ Q12 hr. **Max. dose:** 800 mg/24 hr. For UTI prophylaxis, give 2–6 mg/kg/24 hr.
Adult:
  UTI: 400 mg PO Q12 hr (× 7–10 days for uncomplicated cases and × 10–21 days for complicated cases)
  Prostatitis: 400 mg PO Q12 hr × 28 days

Like other quinolones, there is concern regarding development of arthropathy. Norfloxacin does **not** adequately treat *Chlamydia* co-infections. UTI dosing can be used for BK virus nephropathy in immunocompromised patients. Fluoroquinolones are no longer recommended for gonorrhea by the CDC owing to resistance. **Use with caution** in children <18 yr, seizures, proarrhythmic conditions, diabetes, patients receiving Class Ia or Class III antiarrhythmics and impaired renal function **(adjust dose in renal failure; see Chapter 31).**
Inhibits CYP 450 1A2. May increase serum cyclosporine and theophylline levels and decrease mycophenolate levels. May prolong PT in patients on warfarin. Nitrofurantoin may decrease norfloxacin's antibacterial effects. Probenecid may increase norfloxacin's effects/toxicity. See *Ciprofloxacin* for common side effects and other drug interactions. QTc prolongation, peripheral neuropathy, and tendon rupture (with all ages, especially with corticosteroid use) have been reported.
Administer oral doses on an empty stomach.

NORTRIPTYLINE HYDROCHLORIDE
Pamelor and various generics
Antidepressant, tricyclic

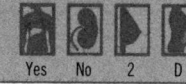

Yes No 2 D

Caps: 10, 25, 50, 75 mg; may contain benzyl alcohol, EDTA
Oral solution: 10 mg/5 mL; contains up to 4% alcohol

Depression:
  Child 6–12 yr: 1–3 mg/kg/24 hr ÷ TID–QID PO **OR** 10–20 mg/24 hr ÷ TID–QID PO
  Adolescent: 1–3 mg/kg/24 hr ÷ TID–QID PO **OR** 30–50 mg/24 hr ÷ TID–QID PO
  Adult: 75–100 mg/24 hr ÷ TID–QID PO
  Max. dose (all ages): 150 mg/24 hr
Nocturnal enuresis:
  6–7 yr (20–25 kg): 10 mg PO QHS
  8–11 yr (26–35 kg): 10–20 mg PO QHS
  >11 yr (36–54 kg): 25–35 mg PO QHS

See *Imipramine* for contraindications and common side effects. Also contraindicated with linezolid or IV methylene because of increased risk for serotonin syndrome. Fewer CNS and anticholinergic side effects than amitriptyline. Lower doses and slower dose titration is recommended in hepatic impairment. Therapeutic antidepressant effects occur in 7–21 days. Monitor for clinical worsening of depression and suicidal ideation/behavior after initiation of therapy or after dose changes. **Do not** discontinue abruptly. Nortriptyline is a substrate for the CYP 450 1A2 and 2D6 drug-metabolizing enzymes. Rifampin may increase metabolism of nortriptyline.

Therapeutic nortriptyline levels for depression: 50–150 ng/mL. Recommended serum sampling time: obtain a single level 8 or more hr after an oral dose (after 4 days of continuous dosing for children and after 9–10 days for adults).
Administer with food to decrease GI upset.

NYSTATIN
Bio-Statin, Mycostatin, Nilstat, and generics
Antifungal agent

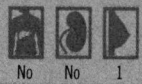

No No 1 A/C

Tabs: 500,000 U
Caps: 500,000, 1,000,000 U
Oral suspension: 100,000 U/mL (5, 60, 480 mL)
Cream/ointment: 100,000 U/g (15, 30 g)
Topical powder: 100,000 U/g (15, 30 g)
Vaginal tabs: 100,000 U (15s)

Oropharyngeal candidiasis:
  Preterm infant: 0.5 mL (50,000 U) to each side of mouth QID
  Term infant: 1 mL (100,000 U) to each side of mouth QID
  Child/adult:
    Oral suspension: 4–6 mL (400,000–600,000 U), swish and swallow QID
Vaginal:
  Adolescent and adult: 1 tab QHS × 14 days
Topical: Apply to affected areas BID–QID.

Continued

NYSTATIN *continued*

May produce diarrhea and GI side effects. Local irritation, contact dermatitis and Stevens-Johnson syndrome have been reported. Treat until 48–72 hr after resolution of symptoms. Drug is poorly absorbed through GI tract. **Do not** swallow troches whole (allow to dissolve slowly). Oral suspension should be swished about the mouth and retained in mouth as long as possible before swallowing.

Pregnancy category is "A" for vaginal product and "C" for oral and topical products.

OCTREOTIDE ACETATE
Sandostatin, Sandostatin LAR Depot, and generics
Somatostatin analog, antisecretory agent

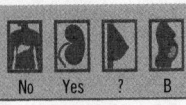

| No | Yes | ? | B |

Injection (amps): 0.05, 0.1, 0.5 mg/mL (1 mL)
Injection (multidose vials): 0.2, 1 mg/mL (5 mL); contains phenol
Injection, microspheres for suspension (Sandostatin **LAR Depot**): 10, 20, 30 mg (in kits with 2 mL diluent and 1.5-inch, 20-gauge needles)

Infant and child (limited data):
  Intractable diarrhea:
    IV/SC: 1–10 mcg/kg/24 hr ÷ Q12–24 hr. Dose may be increased within the recommended range by 0.3 mcg/kg/dose Q3 days as needed. **Max. dose:** 1500 mcg/24 hr.
    IV continuous infusion: 1 mcg/kg/dose bolus, followed by 1 mcg/kg/hr has been used in diarrhea associated with graft-versus-host disease.

Cholelithiasis, hyperglycemia, hypoglycemia, hypothyroidism, nausea, diarrhea, abdominal discomfort, headache, dizziness, and pain at injection site may occur. Growth hormone suppression may occur with long-term use. Bradycardia, thrombocytopenia, and increased risk for pregnancy in patients with acromegaly and pancreatitis have been reported. Cyclosporine levels may be reduced in patients receiving this drug. May increase effects/toxicity of bromocriptine.

Patients with severe renal failure requiring dialysis may require dosage adjustments owing to an increase in half-life. Effects of hepatic dysfunction on octreotide have not been evaluated.

Sandostatin LAR Depot is administered once every 4 wk **only** by the IM route and is currently indicated for use in adults who have been stabilized on IV/SC therapy. See package insert for details.

OFLOXACIN
Floxin, Floxin Otic, Ocuflox, and generics
Antibiotic, quinolone

   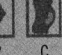

| Yes | Yes | 2 | C |

Otic solution (Floxin Otic and generics): 0.3% (5, 10 mL)
Ophthalmic solution (Ocuflox and generics): 0.3% (5, 10 mL); may contain benzalkonium chloride
Tabs: 200, 300, 400 mg

Otic use:
  Otitis externa:
    6 mo–12 yr: 5 drops to affected ear(s) once daily × 7 days
    ≥13 yr–adult: 10 drops to affected ear(s) once daily × 7 days
  Chronic suppurative otitis media:
    ≥12 yr–adult: 10 drops to affected ear(s) BID × 14 days
  Acute otitis media with tympanostomy tubes:
    1–12 yr: 5 drops to affected ear(s) BID × 10 days

OFLOXACIN *continued*

Ophthalmic use (>1 yr to adult):
  Conjunctivitis: 1–2 drops to affected eye(s) Q2–4 hr while awake × 2 days, then QID for an additional 5 days
  Corneal ulcer: 1–2 drops to affected eye(s) Q30 min while awake and Q4–6 hr while asleep at night × 2 days, followed by Q1 hr while awake × 5 days, and then QID until treatment completed

Pruritus, local irritation, taste perversion, dizziness, earache have been reported with otic use. Ocular burning/discomfort is frequent with ophthalmic use. Consult with ophthalmology in corneal ulcers.

When using otic solution, warm solution by holding bottle in hand for 1–2 min. Cold solutions may result in dizziness. For otitis externa, patient should lie with affected ear upward before instillation and remain in same position after dose administration for 5 min to enhance drug delivery. For acute otitis media with tympanostomy tubes, patient should lie in same position before instillation, and the tragus should be pumped 4 times after the dose to assist in drug delivery to middle ear.

For systemic use, adjust dose in severe renal or hepatic impairment (max. dose: 400 mg/24 hr). Systemic use of ofloxacin is typically replaced by its S-isomer, levofloxacin, which has a more favorable side-effect profile than ofloxacin. See *Levofloxacin.*

OLOPATADINE
Patanol, Pataday, Patanase
Antihistamine

No   No   ?   C

Ophthalmic solution:
  Patanol: 0.1% (5 mL); contains benzalkonium chloride
  Pataday: 0.2% (2.5 mL); contains benzalkonium chloride
Nasal spray (Patanase): 0.6% (30.5 g provides 240 metered spray doses); contains benzalkonium chloride

Allergic conjunctivitis:
  ≥3 yr and adult:
    0.1% solution (Patanol): 1 drop in affected eye(s) BID (spaced 6–8 hr apart)
    0.2% solution (Pataday): 1 drop in affected eye(s) once daily
Allergic rhinitis:
  6–11 yr: Inhale 1 spray into each nostril BID.
  ≥12 yr and adult: Inhale 2 sprays into each nostril BID.

Ocular use: DO NOT use while wearing contact lenses; wait at least 10 min after instilling drops before inserting lenses. Ocular side effects include burning or stinging, dry eye, foreign body sensation, hyperemia, keratitis, lid edema, and pruritus. May also cause headaches, asthenia, pharyngitis, rhinitis, and taste perversion.

Nasal use: common side effects include bitter taste and headaches. Nasal ulceration, epistaxis, nasal septal perforation, throat pain and postnasal drip have been reported.

For explanation of icons, see p. 648

OLSALAZINE
Dipentum, Di-mesalazine, Di-5-ASA
Salicylate, GI anti-inflammatory agent

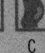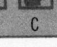

Yes   Yes   2   C

Caps: 250 mg

Ulcerative colitis:
   Child: Consider using sulfasalazine instead (see remarks).
   Adult: 500 mg PO BID

Drug is converted to 5-aminosalicylic acid (mesalamine) by colonic bacteria; 1 g olsalazine
generally delivers 0.9 g of mesalamine to the colon. Only 1%–3% of olsalazine is
systemically absorbed.

Contraindicated in salicylate hypersensitivity. **Use with caution** in severe liver disease, renal
   dysfunction, sulfasalazine hypersensitivity, and bronchial asthma. Diarrhea is the most common
   dose-related side effect. May also cause GI discomfort, headaches, rash, dizziness, and increased
   risk of bleeding with low-molecular-weight heparins or heparinoids and warfarin. Use with
   6-mercaptopurine or thioguanine may increase risk of myelosuppression. Pancreatitis in children
   and hepatotoxicity have been reported. Monitor urinalysis and renal function.

Administer all doses with food to enhance efficacy.

Use in children (2–18 yr) has been limited to a trial where olsalazine 30 mg/kg/24 hr (**max. dose:** 2
   g/24 hr) was found to be less efficacious than sulfasalazine 60 mg/kg/24 hr (**max. dose:** 4 g/24 hr)
   in treating mild/moderate ulcerative colitis. This may suggest inadequate dosing in this trial;
   additional studies are needed.

OMEPRAZOLE
Prilosec, Prilosec OTC, First-Omeprazole, Omeprazole and Syrspend
SF Alka, and generics
In combination with sodium bicarbonate: Zegerid
Gastric acid pump inhibitor

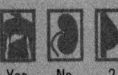

Yes   No   2   C

Caps, sustained-release: 10, 20, 40 mg
Tabs, delayed-release [OTC]: 20 mg
Oral suspension:
   First-Omeprazole: 2 mg/mL (90, 150, 300 mL); contains benzyl alcohol
   Omeprazole and Syrspend SF Alka: 2 mg/mL (100 mL); sugar free and preservative free
   Compounded formulation: 2 mg/mL contains ≈ 0.5 mEq sodium bicarbonate per 1 mg drug
Granules for oral suspension (Prilosec): 2.5, 10 mg packets (30s)
In combination with sodium bicarbonate:
   Powder for oral suspension (Zegerid): 20, 40 mg packets (30s); each packet (regardless of
   strength) contains 1680 mg (20 mEq) sodium bicarbonate
   Caps, immediate-release (Zegerid): 20, 40 mg; each capsule (regardless of strength) contains
   1100 mg (13.1 mEq) sodium bicarbonate
   Chewable tabs (Zegerid): 20, 40 mg; each tab (regardless of strength) contains 600 mg (7.1
   mEq) sodium bicarbonate and 700 mg magnesium hydroxide

Child (≥1 yr):
   Esophagitis, GERD, or ulcers: Start at 1 mg/kg/24 hr PO ÷ once daily–BID (**max. dose:**
   20 mg/24 hr). Reported effective range: 0.2–3.5 mg/kg/24 hr. Children 1–6 yr may require
   higher doses because of enhanced drug clearance.

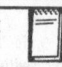

OMEPRAZOLE *continued*

Alternative dosing for patients ≥1 yr:
    5–<10 kg: 5 mg PO once daily
    10–<20 kg: 10 mg PO once daily
    ≥20 kg: 20 mg PO once daily

Adult:
    Duodenal ulcer or GERD: 20 mg/dose PO once daily × 4–8 wk; may give up to 12 wk for erosive esophagitis
    Gastric ulcer: 40 mg/24 hr PO ÷ once daily–BID × 4–8 wk.
    Pathologic hypersecretory conditions: Start with 60 mg/24 hr PO once daily. If needed, dose may be increased up to 120 mg/24 hr PO ÷ TID. Daily doses >80 mg should be administered in divided doses.

Common side effects: Headache, diarrhea, nausea, and vomiting. Allergic reactions including anaphylaxis have been reported. Has been associated with increased risk for *Clostridium difficile*–associated diarrhea.

Drug induces CYP 450 1A2 (decreases theophylline levels) and is also a substrate and inhibitor of CYP 2C19. Increases $T_{1/2}$ of citalopram, diazepam, phenytoin, and warfarin. May decrease effects of itraconazole, ketoconazole, clopidogrel, iron salts, and ampicillin esters. St. John's wort and rifampin may decrease omeprazole's effects. May be used in combination with clarithromycin and amoxicillin for *Helicobacter pylori* infections.

Bioavailability may be increased with hepatic dysfunction or in patients of Asian descent. Safety and efficacy for GERD in children <1 yr have **not** been established.

Administer all doses before meals. Administer 30 min before sucralfate. Capsules contain enteric-coated granules to ensure bioavailability. **Do not** chew or crush capsule. For doses unable to be divided by 10 mg, capsule may be opened and intact pellets may be administered in an acidic beverage (e.g., apple juice, cranberry juice) or applesauce. The extemporaneously compounded oral suspension product may be less bioavailable owing to loss of enteric coating.

ONDANSETRON
Zofran and generics
Antiemetic agent, 5-HT₃ antagonist

  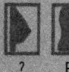
    Yes   No   ?   B

Injection: 2 mg/mL (2, 20 mL); may contain parabens; some preparations are preservative free.
Tabs: 4, 8, 24 mg
Tabs, orally disintegrating (ODT): 4, 8 mg; contains aspartame
Oral solution: 4 mg/5 mL (50 mL); contains sodium benzoate

Preventing nausea and vomiting associated with chemotherapy:
    Oral (give initial dose 30 min before chemotherapy):
        Child (≥2 yr and adolescent), dose based on body surface area:
            <0.3 m²: 1 mg TID PRN nausea
            0.3–0.6 m²: 2 mg TID PRN nausea
            0.6–1 m²: 3 mg TID PRN nausea
            >1 m²: 4–8 mg TID PRN nausea
        Dose based on age:
            <4 yr: Use dose based on body surface area from preceding dosages.
            4–11 yr: 4 mg TID PRN nausea
            >11 yr and adult: 8 mg TID or 24 mg once daily PRN nausea
    IV (child and adult):
        Moderately emetogenic drugs: 0.15 mg/kg/dose (**max. dose:** 8 mg/dose for child and 16 mg/dose adult) at 30 min before, 4 and 8 hr after emetogenic drugs. Then same dose Q4 hr PRN.

Continued

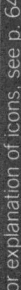
For explanation of icons, see p. 648

ONDANSETRON *continued*

IV (child and adult):

Highly emetogenic drugs: 0.15 mg/kg/dose (**max. dose:** 16 mg/dose) 30 min before, 4 and 8 hr after emetogenic drugs. Then 0.15 mg/kg/dose (**max. dose:** 16 mg/dose) Q4 hr PRN.

Preventing nausea and vomiting associated with surgery (additional doses for controlling nausea and vomiting may not provide any benefits):

IV/IM (administered before anesthesia over 2–5 min):

Child (2–12 yr):

≤**40 kg:** 0.1 mg/kg/dose × 1

>**40 kg:** 4 mg × 1

Adult: 4 mg × 1

PO:

Adult: 16 mg × 1, 1 hr before induction of anesthesia

Preventing nausea and vomiting associated with radiation therapy:

Child: Use above dosage for preventing nausea and vomiting associated with chemotherapy, and give initial dose 1–2 hr before radiation.

Adult:

Total body irradiation: 8 mg PO 1–2 hr before radiation once daily

Single high-dose fraction radiation to abdomen: 8 mg PO 1–2 hr before radiation, with subsequent doses Q8 hr after first dose × 1–2 days after completion of radiation

Daily fractionated radiation to abdomen: 8 mg PO 1–2 hr before radiation, with subsequent doses Q8 hr after first dose for each day radiation is given

Vomiting in acute gastroenteritis (PO route is preferred, use IV when PO is not possible):

PO (6 mo–10 yr and ≥8 kg; use oral disintegrating tablet):

8–15 kg: 2 mg × 1

>**15 and ≤30 kg:** 4 mg × 1

>**30 kg:** 8 mg × 1

IV (≥1 mo): 0.15–0.3 mg/kg/dose × 1; **max. dose:** mg/dose

Avoid use in congenital long QTc syndrome. Bronchospasm, tachycardia, hypokalemia, seizures, headaches, lightheadedness, constipation, diarrhea, and transient increases in AST, ALT, and bilirubin may occur. Transient blindness (resolution within a few min up to 48 hr), arthralgia, hepatic dysfunction, and rare/transient ECG changes (including QTc interval prolongation) have been reported. Data limited for use in children <3 yr.

ECG monitoring is recommended in patients with electrolyte abnormalities, CHF, or bradyarrhythmias. Drug clearance is higher for surgical and cancer patients <18 yr when compared with adults. Clearance is slower for children 1–4 mo old compared with children >4–24 mo.

Ondansetron is a substrate for CYP 450 1A2, 2D6, 2E1, and 3A3/4 drug-metabolizing enzymes. It is likely that the inhibition/loss of one of the previously listed enzymes will be compensated by others and may result in insignificant changes to ondansetron's elimination. Ondansetron's elimination may be affected by CYP 450 enzyme inducers. Follow theophylline, phenytoin, or warfarin levels closely if used in combination. Use with apomorphine may result in profound hypotension and loss of consciousness and is **contraindicated**.

OSELTAMIVIR PHOSPHATE
Tamiflu
Antiviral

No   Yes   2   C

Caps: 30, 45, 75 mg
Oral suspension: 6 mg/mL (60 mL); may contain saccharin and sodium benzoate
NOTE: Previous oral suspension concentration of 12 mg/mL has been replaced with a 6 mg/mL concentration so that both commercially available and compounded products are similar in concentration to prevent dosing errors.

Treatment of influenza (initiate therapy within 2 days of onset of symptoms):
Preterm neonate (24–37 weeks' gestation; based on pharmacokinetic data from 20 neonates): 1 mg/kg/dose PO BID
Full-term neonate:
   <14 days old: 3 mg/kg/dose PO once daily × 5 days
   ≥14 days old: 3 mg/kg/dose PO BID × 5 days
Child < 1 yr: See following table

Age (months)	Dosage for 5 days	Volume of Oral Suspension (6 mg/mL)
<3	12 mg PO BID	2 mL
3–5	20 mg PO BID	3.33 mL
6–11	25 mg PO BID	4.2 mL

Child ≥ 1–12 yr: See following table.

Weight (kg)	Dosage for 5 days	Volume of Oral Suspension (6 mg/mL)
≤15	30 mg PO BID	5 mL
>15–23	45 mg PO BID	7.5 mL
>23–40	60 mg PO BID	10 mL
>40	75 mg PO BID	12.5 mL

≥13 yr and adult: 75 mg PO BID × 5 days
Prophylaxis of influenza (initiate therapy within 2 days of exposure [see remarks]):
Child 3 mo–<1 yr: 3 mg/kg/dose PO once daily
   Alternative dosage based on age:
      3–5 mo: 20 mg PO once daily
      6–11 mo: 25 mg PO once daily
Child 1–12 yr:
   ≤15 kg: 30 mg PO once daily
   16–23 kg: 45 mg PO once daily
   24–40 kg: 60 mg PO once daily
   >40 kg: 75 mg PO once daily
≥13 yr and adult: 75 mg PO once daily for a minimum of 7 days and up to 6 wk; initiate therapy within 2 days of exposure.

Currently indicated for treatment of influenza A and B strains. Use in children <1 yr has not been recommended owing to concerns of excessive CNS penetration and fatalities in 7-day-old rats.
Nausea and vomiting (generally occurring within first 2 days) are most common adverse effects. Insomnia, vertigo, seizures, hypothermia, neuropsychiatric events (may result in fatal outcomes), arrhythmias, rash, and toxic epidermal necrolysis have also been reported. If GFR is 10–30 mL/min, reduce dosage to 75 mg PO once daily × 5 days for adults (see Chapter 31).
PROPHYLAXIS USE: Oseltamivir is not a substitute for annual flu vaccination. Safety and efficacy have been demonstrated for ≤6 wk of therapy; duration of protection lasts for as long as dosing is continued. Adjust prophylaxis dose if GFR is 10–30 mL/min by extending dosage interval to once every other day.

Continued

OSELTAMIVIR PHOSPHATE *continued*

Probenecid increases oseltamivir levels. Oseltamivir decreases efficacy of the nasal influenza vaccine (FluMist; discontinue oseltamivir 48 hr before and **do not** restart for at least 1–2 wk after FluMist administration).

Dosage adjustments in hepatic impairment, severe renal disease, and dialysis have not been established for either treatment or prophylaxis use. Safety and efficacy of repeated treatment or prophylaxis courses have not been evaluated. Doses may be administered with or without food.

OXACILLIN
Various generic brands
Antibiotic, penicillin (penicillinase resistant)

   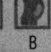

Yes   Yes   2   B

Injection: 1, 2, 10 g
Injection, premixed in iso-osmotic dextrose: 1 g/50 mL, 2 g/50 mL
Injectable products contain 2.8–3.1 mEq Na per 1 g drug

Neonate: IM/IV
  ≤7 days:
    <1.2 kg: 50 mg/kg/24 hr ÷ Q12 hr
    <1.2–2 kg: 50–100 mg/kg/24 hr ÷ Q12 hr
    ≥2 kg: 75–150 mg/kg/24 hr ÷ Q8 hr
  >7 days:
    <1.2 kg: 50 mg/kg/24 hr ÷ Q12 hr
    1.2–2 kg: 75–150 mg/kg/24 hr ÷ Q8 hr
    ≥2 kg: 100–200 mg/kg/24 hr ÷ Q6 hr
Infant and child (IM/IV): 100–200 mg/kg/24 hr ÷ Q4–6 hr (**max. dose:** 12 g/24 hr); use 200 mg/kg/24 hr for endocarditis and severe infections.
Adult (IM/IV): 250–2000 mg/dose Q4–6 hr; use higher dosage range for endocarditis or severe infections. **Max. dose:** 12 g/24 hr.

Rash and GI disturbances are common. Leukopenia, reversible hepatotoxicity, and acute interstitial nephritis has been reported. Hematuria and azotemia have occurred in neonates and infants with high doses. May cause false-positive urinary and serum proteins.

Probenecid increases serum oxacillin levels. Tetracyclines may antagonize the bactericidal effects of oxacillin.

CSF penetration is poor unless meninges are inflamed. Use the lower end of the usual dosage range for patients with creatinine clearances <10 mL/min. **Adjust dose in renal failure (see Chapter 31).**

OXCARBAZEPINE
Trileptal, Oxtellar, and generics
Anticonvulsant

   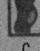

No   Yes   2   C

Tabs: 150, 300, 600 mg
Extended-release tabs (Oxtellar): 150, 300, 600 mg
Oral suspension: 300 mg/5 mL (250 mL); contains saccharin, ethanol, and propylene glycol

IMMEDIATE-RELEASE PRODUCT:
  Child (2–<4 yr):
    Adjunctive therapy: Start with 8–10 mg/kg/24 hr PO ÷ BID up to a **max. dose** of 600 mg/24 hr. For children <20 kg, may consider using a starting dose of 16–20 mg/kg/24 hr PO ÷ BID; gradually increase the dose over a 2–4-week period and **do not exceed** 60 mg/kg/24 hr ÷ BID.

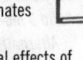

OXCARBAZEPINE *continued*

IMMEDIATE-RELEASE PRODUCT:

Child (4–16 yr [see remarks]):

Adjunctive therapy: Start with 8–10 mg/kg/24 hr PO ÷ BID up to a **max. dose** of 600 mg/24 hr. Then gradually increase dose over a 2-wk period to the following maintenance doses:

20–29 kg: 900 mg/24 hr PO ÷ BID

29.1–39 kg: 1200 mg/24 hr PO ÷ BID

>39 kg: 1800 mg/24 hr PO ÷ BID

Conversion to monotherapy: Start with 8–10 mg/kg/24 hr PO ÷ BID, and simultaneously initiate dosage reduction of concomitant AEDs and withdraw completely over 3–6 wk. Dose may be increased at weekly intervals (as clinically indicated) by a **max.** of 10 mg/kg/24 hr to achieve recommended monotherapy maintenance dose as described in the following table.

Initiation of monotherapy: Start with 8–10 mg/kg/24 hr PO ÷ BID. Then increase by 5 mg/kg/24 hr Q3 days up to recommended monotherapy maintenance dose as described in the following table:

Recommended Monotherapy Maintenance Doses for Children by Weight

Weight (kg)	Daily Oral Maintenance Dose (mg/24 hr) Divided BID
20–<25	600–900
25–<35	900–1200
35–<45	900–1500
45–<50	1200–1500
50–<60	1200–1800
60–<70	1200–2100
≥70	1500–2100

Adult:

Adjunctive therapy: Start with 600 mg/24 hr PO ÷ BID. Dose may be increased at weekly intervals (as clinically indicated) by a **max.** of 600 mg/24 hr. Usual maintenance dose is 1200 mg/24 hr PO ÷ BID. Doses ≥2400 mg/24 hr are generally not well tolerated owing to CNS side effects.

Conversion to monotherapy: Start with 600 mg/24 hr PO ÷ BID, and simultaneously initiate dosage reduction of concomitant AEDs. Dose may be increased at weekly intervals (as clinically indicated) by a **max.** of 600 mg/24 hr to achieve a dose of 2400 mg/24 hr PO ÷ BID. Concomitant AEDs should be terminated gradually over ≈ 3–6 wk.

Initiation of monotherapy: Start with 600 mg/24 hr PO ÷ BID. Then increase by 300 mg/24 hr Q3 days up to 1200 mg/24 hr PO ÷ BID.

EXTENDED-RELEASE TABS (Oxtellar [see remarks]):

Child 6–17 yr:

Adjunctive therapy: Start with 8–10 mg/kg/24 hr PO once daily up to a **max. dose** of 600 mg/24 hr. Then gradually increase at weekly intervals in 8–10 mg/kg/24 hr increments (**max. dosage increment:** 600 mg) to the following maintenance doses:

20–29 kg: 900 mg PO once daily

29.1–39 kg: 1200 mg PO once daily

≥39.1 kg: 1800 mg PO once daily

Adult:

Adjunctive therapy: Start with 600 mg PO once daily (consider using 900 mg if receiving concomitant enzyme-inducing antiepileptic drugs). Then gradually increase at weekly intervals in 600 mg/24 hr increments to the maintenance dose of 1200–2400 mg once daily.

Clinically significant hyponatremia may occur; generally seen within first 3 mo of therapy. May also cause headache, dizziness, drowsiness, ataxia, fatigue, nystagmus, urticaria, diplopia, abnormal gait, and GI discomfort. About 25% to 30% of patients with carbamazepine hypersensitivity will experience a cross-reaction with oxcarbazepine. Serious

Continued

For explanation of icons, see p. 648

OXCARBAZEPINE *continued*

dermatologic reactions (Stevens-Johnson syndrome and TEN), multiorgan hypersensitivity reactions, bone marrow depression, pancreatitis, folic acid deficiency, hypothyroidism, rare cases of anaphylaxis and angioedema, and suicidal behavior or ideation have been reported.

Inhibits CYP 450 2C19 and induces CYP 450 3A4/5 drug–metabolizing enzymes. Carbamazepine, cyclosporine, phenobarbital, phenytoin, valproic acid, and verapamil may decrease oxcarbazepine levels. Oxcarbazepine may increase phenobarbital and phenytoin levels. Oxcarbazepine can decrease effects of oral contraceptives, felodipine, and lamotrigine.

If GFR < 30 mL/min, adjust dosage by administering 50% of normal starting dose (**max. dose:** 300 mg/24 hr), followed by a slower-than-normal increase in dose if necessary (**see Chapter 31**). No dosage adjustment required in mild/moderate hepatic impairment. Use is **not recommended** in severe hepatic impairment owing to lack of information.

Extended-release and immediate-release products are not bioequivalent; higher doses of the extended-release product may be necessary. Doses may be administered with or without food.

OXYBUTYNIN CHLORIDE
Ditropan, Ditropan XL, Oxytrol, and generics
Anticholinergic agent, antispasmodic

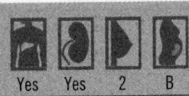

Yes   Yes   2   B

Tabs: 5 mg
Tabs, extended-release (Ditropan XL and generics): 5, 10, 15 mg
Syrup: 1 mg/mL (473 mL); contains parabens
Transdermal system (Oxytrol): Delivers 3.9 mg/24 hr (1, 2s, 4s, 8s); contains 36 mg per system

Child ≤ 5 yr:
 Immediate release: 0.2 mg/kg/dose BID–TID PO; **max. dose:** 15 mg/24 hr
Child > 5 yr:
 Immediate release: 5 mg/dose BID–TID PO; **max. dose:** 15 mg/24 hr
 Extended release (≥6 yr): Start with 5 mg/dose once daily PO; if needed, increase as tolerated by 5-mg increments up to a **max.** of 20 mg/24 hr.
Adult:
 Immediate release: 5 mg/dose BID–TID PO
 Extended release (Ditropan XL): 5–10 mg/dose once daily PO up to a **max. dose** of 30 mg/dose once daily PO
 Transdermal system: 1 patch (3.9 mg/24 hr) Q3–4 days (twice weekly)

Use with caution in hepatic or renal disease, hyperthyroidism, IBD, or cardiovascular disease. Anticholinergic side effects may occur, including drowsiness and hallucinations.
Contraindicated in glaucoma, GI obstruction, megacolon, myasthenia gravis, severe colitis, hypovolemia, and GU obstruction. Memory impairment, angioedema, and QT interval prolongation have been reported. Oxybutynin is a CYP 450 3A4 substrate; inhibitors and inducers of CYP 450 3A4 may increase and decrease effects of oxybutynin, respectively.

Dosage adjustments for extended-release dosage form are at weekly intervals. **Do not** crush, chew, or divide extended-release tablets. Apply transdermal system on dry intact skin on the abdomen, hip, or buttock by rotating the site and avoiding same site application within 7 days.

OXYCODONE
OxyContin, Roxicodone, and many others
Narcotic, analgesic

 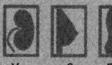

Yes   Yes   2   B/D

Solution: 1 mg/mL (5, 15, 500 mL); contains alcohol
Concentrated solution: 20 mg/mL (30 mL); may contain saccharin
Tabs: 5, 10, 15, 20, 30 mg
Controlled-release tabs (OxyContin and others): 10, 15, 20, 30, 40, 60, 80 mg (80-mg strength for opioid-tolerant patients only)
Caps: 5 mg

Opioid-naïve doses based on oxycodone salt:
  Child: 0.05–0.15 mg/kg/dose Q4–6 hr PRN up to 5 mg/dose PO
  Adolescent (≥50 kg) and adult: 5–10 mg Q4–6 hr PRN PO; see remarks for use of controlled-release tablets.

Abuse potential, CNS and respiratory depression, increased ICP, histamine release, constipation, and GI distress may occur. **Use with caution** in severe renal impairment (increases $T_{1/2}$) and mild/moderate hepatic dysfunction (use ⅓ to ½ of usual dose has been recommended). **Naloxone is the antidote.** See Chapter 6 for equianalgesic dosing. Check dosages of acetaminophen or aspirin when using combination products (e.g., Tylox, Percodan). Aspirin is **not recommended** in children due to concerns of Reye syndrome. Oxycodone is metabolized by the CYP 450 3A4 (major) and 2D6 (minor) isoenzyme.

When using controlled-released tablets (OxyContin), determine patient's total 24-hr requirements and divide by 2 to administer on a Q12-hr dosing interval. OxyContin 80-mg tablet is **USED ONLY** for opioid-tolerant patients; this strength can cause fatal respiratory depression in opioid-naïve patients. Controlled-release dosage form **should not be used** as a PRN analgesic and must be swallowed whole.

Pregnancy category changes to "D" if used for prolonged periods or in high doses at term.

OXYCODONE AND ACETAMINOPHEN
Endocet, Roxilox, Percocet, Roxicet, Roxicet 5/500, and many others
Combination analgesic with narcotic

Yes   Yes   2   C

Capsule or caplet (Roxilox 5/500): oxycodone HCl 5 mg + acetaminophen 500 mg
Tabs (Percocet, Endocet, and others):
  Most common strength: Oxycodone HCl 5 mg + acetaminophen 325 mg
  Other strengths:
    Oxycodone HCl 2.5 mg + acetaminophen 325 mg
    Oxycodone HCl 7.5 mg + acetaminophen 325 mg or 500 mg
    Oxycodone HCl 10 mg + acetaminophen 325 mg or 650 mg
  Oral solution (Roxicet): Oxycodone HCl 5 mg + acetaminophen 325 mg/5 mL (5, 500 mL); contains 0.4% alcohol and saccharin

Dose based on amount of oxycodone and acetaminophen. Do not exceed 4 g/24 hr of acetaminophen.

See *Oxycodone* and *Acetaminophen*. Check dosages of acetaminophen when using these combination products.

OXYCODONE AND ASPIRIN
Percodan, Endodan, and generics
Combination analgesic (narcotic and salicylate)

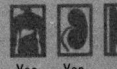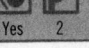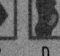
Yes Yes 2 D

Tabs: Oxycodone 4.8355 mg and aspirin 325 mg

Dose based on amount of oxycodone and aspirin. Do not exceed 4 g/24 hr of aspirin.

See *Oxycodone* and *Aspirin*. **Do not use** in children <16 yr because of risk for Reye syndrome. Check dosages of aspirin when using these combination products.

OXYMETAZOLINE
Nasal: Afrin 12 Hour, Duramist 12-Hr Nasal, Neo-Synephrine 12-Hour Nasal, Nostrilla, and many others
Ophthalmic: Visine LR
Nasal decongestant, vasoconstrictor

No No ? C

Nasal spray [OTC]: 0.05% (15, 30 mL); may contain benzalkonium chloride and propylene glycol
Ophthalmic drops [OTC]: 0.025% (15 mL); contains benzalkonium chloride and EDTA

Nasal decongestant (not to exceed 3 days in duration):
≥6 yr–adult: 2–3 sprays or 2–3 drops or 1–2 metered sprays (Nostrilla) in each nostril BID.
Do not exceed 2 doses/24 hr period.
Ophthalmic:
≥6 yr–adult: Instill 1–2 drops in affected eye(s) Q6 hr.

Contraindicated in patients on MAO inhibitor therapy. Rebound nasal congestion may occur with excessive use (>3 days) via nasal route. Systemic absorption may occur with either route of administration. Headache, dizziness, hypertension, transient burning, stinging, dryness, nasal mucosa ulceration, sneezing, blurred vision, and mydriasis have occurred. **Do not use** ophthalmic solution if it changes color or becomes cloudy.

Accidental ingestion of either dosage form in children <5 yr has been reported and required hospitalization for adverse events (nausea, vomiting, lethargy, tachycardia, respiratory depression, bradycardia, hypotension, hypertension, sedation, mydriasis, stupor, hypothermia, drooling, and coma).

PALIVIZUMAB
Synagis
Monoclonal antibody

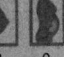
No No ? C

Injection, solution: 100 mg/mL (0.5, 1 mL; single use); contains glycine and histidine

RSV prophylaxis during RSV season for the following age and clinical criteria (see latest edition of AAP Red Book for most recent indications):
<3 mo of age, born at 32–<35 wk' gestation, and with either daycare attendance or >1 sibling (<5 yr old) living in the same household
<6 mo of age and born at 29–<32 wk' gestation
<12 mo of age and one of the following:
Born at ≤28 wk' gestation; OR

PALIVIZUMAB *continued*

> With congenital airway abnormalities or neuromuscular disorders that decrease ability to manage airway secretions
>
> **≤24 mo of age** and one of the following:
>
> With chronic lung disease requiring medical therapy within 6 mo before start of RSV season; OR
>
> With congenital heart disease and one of the following conditions: Cyanotic heart, moderate/severe pulmonary hypertension, or receiving CHF pharmacotherapy

DOSE: 15 mg/kg/dose IM Q monthly just before and during RSV season

RSV season typically November through April in Northern Hemisphere but may begin earlier or persist later in certain communities. IM is currently the only route of administration, so **use with caution** in patients with thrombocytopenia or any coagulation disorder. The following adverse effects have been reported at slightly higher incidences when compared with placebo: rhinitis, rash, pain, increased liver enzymes, pharyngitis, cough, wheeze, diarrhea, vomiting, conjunctivitis, and anemia. Rare acute hypersensitivity reactions have been reported (first or subsequent doses).

Does not interfere with response to routine childhood vaccines. May interfere with immunologic-based RSV diagnostic tests (some antigen detection–based assays and viral culture assays), but not with reverse transcriptase–PCR-based assays.

Palivizumab is currently indicated for RSV prophylaxis in high-risk infants only. Efficacy and safety have not been demonstrated for treatment of RSV.

Each dose should be administered IM in anterolateral aspect of thigh. It is recommended to divide doses with total injection volumes >1 mL. **Avoid** injection in gluteal muscle because of risk for damage to sciatic nerve.

PANCREATIC ENZYMES
See Chapter 30 for description and contents of lipase, protease, and amylase.

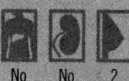

No   No   2   C

Initial doses (actual requirements are patient specific):
Enteric-coated microspheres and microtabs:
Infant: 2000–4000 U lipase per 120 mL (formula or breast milk)
Child < 4 yr: 1000 U lipase/kg/meal
Child ≥ 4 yr and adult: 500 U lipase/kg/meal
Max. dose (child–adult): 2500 U lipase/kg/meal, or 10,000 U lipase/kg/24 hr, or 4000 U lipase/g fat/24 hr

Total daily dose should include ≈ 3 meals and 2–3 snacks per day. Snack doses are ≈ half of meal doses, depending on amount of fat and food consumed.

May cause occult GI bleeding, allergic reactions to porcine proteins, hyperuricemia, and hyperuricosuria with high doses. Dose should be titrated to eliminate diarrhea and minimize steatorrhea. **Do not** chew microspheres or microtabs. Concurrent administration with H_2 antagonists or gastric acid pump inhibitors may enhance enzyme efficacy. Doses higher than 6000 U lipase/kg/meal have been associated with colonic strictures in children <12 yr. Powder dosage form is **not** preferred, owing to potential GI mucosal ulceration.

Avoid use of generic pancreatic enzyme products because they have been associated with treatment failures. Products not approved by the FDA are no longer allowed to be distributed in the United States.

PANCURONIUM BROMIDE
Various generic brands
Nondepolarizing neuromuscular blocking agent

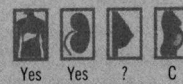

Yes   Yes   ?   C

Injection: 1 mg/mL (10 mL), 2 mg/mL (2, 5 mL); contains benzyl alcohol

Intermittent dosing (see remarks):
   Neonate:
      Initial: 0.02 mg/kg/dose IV
      Maintenance: 0.05–0.1 mg/kg/dose IV Q0.5–4 hr PRN
   1 mo–adult:
      Initial: 0.04–0.1 mg/kg/dose IV
      Maintenance: 0.015–0.1 mg/kg/dose IV Q30–60 min
Continuous IV infusion (see remarks):
   Neonate: 0.02–0.04 mg/kg/hr
   Child: 0.03–1 mg/kg/hr
   Adolescent and adult: 0.02–0.04 mg/kg/hr

Onset of action is 1–2 min. May cause tachycardia, salivation, and wheezing. Severe anaphylactic reactions have been reported; cross-reactivity between neuromuscular blocking agents has been reported.

Drug effects may be accentuated by hypothermia, acidosis, neonatal age, decreased renal function, halothane, succinylcholine, hypokalemia, hyponatremia, hypocalcemia, clindamycin, tetracycline, and aminoglycoside antibiotics. Drug effects may be antagonized by alkalosis, hypercalcemia, peripheral neuropathies, diabetes mellitus, demyelinating lesions, carbamazepine, phenytoin, theophylline, anticholinesterases (e.g., neostigmine, pyridostigmine), and azathioprine. For obese patients, use of lean body weight for dose calculation has been recommended to prevent intense block of long duration and possible overdose.

Antidote is neostigmine (with atropine or glycopyrrolate). **Avoid** use in severe renal impairment (<10 mL/min). Patients with cirrhosis may require a high initial dose to achieve adequate relaxation, but muscle paralysis will be prolonged.

PANTOPRAZOLE
Protonix and generics
Gastric acid pump inhibitor

Yes   No   2   B

Tab, delayed release, enteric coated: 20, 40 mg
Injection: 40 mg; contains edetate sodium
Oral suspension: 2 mg/mL; contains 0.25 mEq sodium bicarbonate per 1 mg drug
Powder for delayed-release oral suspension (Protonix): 40 mg (30s); contains polysorbate 80

Child (see remarks):
   GERD (limited data):
      Infant and < 5 yr: 1.2 mg/kg/24 hr PO once daily. **Note:** Pantoprazole did not significantly improve GERD symptom scores in an open-label trial in 128 infants (1–11 mo) receiving 1.2 mg/kg/24 hr PO once daily × 4 wk, followed by a 4-wk double-blinded placebo-controlled withdrawal phase.
      ≥5 yr and adolescent: 20 or 40 mg PO once daily
   GERD with erosive esophagitis:
      1–5 yr (limited data): 0.3, 0.6, or 1.2 mg/kg/24 hr PO once daily all improved GERD symptoms in an 8-wk multicenter randomized placebo-controlled trial for 60 subjects with GERD and histologic/erosive esophagitis.

PANTOPRAZOLE *continued*

GERD with erosive esophagitis:
≥5 yr (up to 8 wk of therapy):
15–<40 kg: 20 mg PO once daily
≥40 kg: 40 mg PO once daily
IV (data limited to pharmacokinetic trials): Some doses ranging from 0.32–1.88 mg/kg/dose have been reported from three separate trials (total N = 31; 0.01–16.4 yr). Patients with systemic inflammatory response syndrome (SIRS) cleared the drug more slowly, resulting in higher $T_{1/2}$ and AUC, than patients without. Despite limited data, doses of 1–2 mg/kg/24 hr ÷ Q12–24 hr have been used. Additional studies are needed.

Adult:
GERD with erosive esophagitis: 40 mg PO once daily × 8–16 wk or 40 mg IV once daily × 7–10 days
Peptic ulcer: 40–80 mg PO once daily × 4–8 wk
Hypersecretory conditions:
PO: 40 mg BID; dose may be increased as needed up to a **max. dose** of 240 mg/24 hr.
IV: 80 mg Q12 hr; dose may be increased as needed to Q8 hr (**max. dose:** 240 mg/24 hr). Therapy > 6 days at 240 mg/24 hr has not been evaluated.

Convert from IV to PO therapy as soon as patient is able to tolerate PO. Common side effects include diarrhea and headache. May cause transient elevation in LFTs. Like other PPIs, may increase risk for *C. difficile*–associated diarrhea. Hypomagnesemia has been reported with long-term use. Drug is a substrate for CYP 450 2C19 (major), 2D6 (minor), and 3A3/4 (minor) isoenzymes. May decrease absorption of itraconazole, ketoconazole, iron salts, and ampicillin esters. May increase effect/toxicity of methotrexate.

Children 1–2 yr of age have demonstrated more rapid clearance of pantoprazole in pharmacokinetic studies; this age group may require higher doses. All oral doses may be taken with or without food. **Do not** crush or chew tablets. Extemporaneously compounded oral suspension may be less bioavailable owing to loss of enteric coating. Powder for delayed-release oral suspension product may be mixed with 5 mL apple juice (administer immediately, followed by rinsing container with more apple juice) or sprinkled on 1 teaspoonful of applesauce (administer within 10 min); see package insert for NG administration.

For IV infusion, doses may be administered over 15 min at a concentration of 0.4–0.8 mg/mL or over 2 min at a concentration of 4 mg/mL. Midazolam and zinc are **not compatible** with the IV dosage form. Parenteral routes other than IV are **not recommended**.

PAROMOMYCIN SULFATE
Humatin and generics
Amebicide, antibiotic (aminoglycoside)

No   No   1   ?

Caps: 250 mg

Intestinal amebiasis (Entamoeba histolytica), Dientamoeba fragilis, and Giardia lamblia infection:
Child and adult: 25–35 mg/kg/24 hr PO ÷ Q8 hr × 7 days
Tapeworm (Taenia saginata, Taenia solium, Diphyllobothrium latum, and Dipylidium caninum):
Child: 11 mg/kg/dose PO Q15 min × 4 doses
Adult: 1 g PO Q15 min × 4 doses
Tapeworm (Hymenolepis nana):
Child and adult: 45 mg/kg/dose PO once daily × 5–7 days

Continued

PAROMOMYCIN SULFATE *continued*

Cryptosporidial diarrhea:
Adult: 1.5–2.25 g/24 hr PO ÷ 3–6 × daily. Duration varies from 10–14 days to 4–8 wk. Maintenance therapy has also been used. Alternatively, 1 g PO BID × 12 wk in conjunction with azithromycin 600 mg PO once daily × 4 wk has been used in patients with AIDS.

Contraindicated in intestinal obstruction. **Use with caution** in ulcerative bowel lesions to avoid renal toxicity via systemic absorption. Drug is generally poorly absorbed and therefore **not** indicated for sole treatment of extraintestinal amebiasis. Side effects include GI disturbance, hematuria, rash, ototoxicity, and hypocholesterolemia. Bacterial overgrowth of nonsusceptible organisms, including fungi, may occur. May decrease effects of digoxin.
Pregnancy category has not been formally assigned by the FDA.

PAROXETINE
Paxil, Pexeva, Paxil CR, Brisdelle, and generics
Antidepressant, selective serotonin reuptake inhibitor

 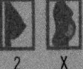

Yes	Yes	2	X

Tabs: 10, 20, 30, 40 mg
Caps (Brisdelle): 7.5 mg
Controlled-release tabs (Paxil CR and generics): 12.5, 25, 37.5 mg
Oral suspension: 10 mg/5 mL (250 mL); contains saccharin and parabens

Child:
Depression: Well-controlled clinical trials have failed to demonstrate efficacy in children. The FDA recommends paroxetine not be used for this indication.
Obsessive-compulsive disorder (limited data, based on a 10-wk randomized controlled trial in 207 children 7–17 yr; mean age 11.1 ± 3.03 yr): Start with 10 mg PO once daily. If needed, adjust upwards by increasing dose no more than 10 mg/24 hr, no more frequently than Q7 days, up to a **max. dose** of 50 mg/24 hr. Mean doses of 20.3 mg/24 hr (children) and 26.8 mg/24 hr (adolescents) were used.
Social anxiety disorder (8–17 yr): Start with 10 mg PO once daily. If needed, increase dose by 10 mg/24 hr no more frequently than Q7 days up to a **max. dose** of 50 mg/24 hr.
Adult:
Depression: Start with 20 mg PO QAM × 4 wk. If no clinical improvement, increase dose by 10 mg/24 hr Q7 days PRN up to a **max. dose** of 50 mg/24 hr.
  Paxil CR: Start with 25 mg PO QAM × 4 wk. If no improvement, increase dose by 12.5 mg/24 hr Q7 days PRN up to a **max. dose** of 62.5 mg/24 hr.
Obsessive compulsive disorder: Start with 20 mg PO once daily; increase dose by 10 mg/24 hr Q7 days PRN up to a **max. dose** of 60 mg/24 hr. Usual dose is 40 mg PO once daily.
Panic disorder: Start with 10 mg PO QAM; increase dose by 10 mg/24 hr Q7 days PRN up to a **max. dose** of 60 mg/24 hr.
  Paxil CR: Start with 12.5 mg PO QAM; increase dose by 12.5 mg/24 hr Q7 days PRN up to a **max. dose** of 75 mg/24 hr.

Contraindicated in patients taking MAOIs (within 14 days of discontinuing MAOIs), pimozide, or thioridazine. **Use with caution** in patients with history of seizures, renal or hepatic impairment, cardiac disease, suicidal concerns, mania/hypomania, and diuretic use. Patients with severe renal or hepatic impairment should initiate therapy at 10 mg/24 hr and increase dose as needed up to a **max. dose** of 40 mg/24 hr.
Common side effects include anxiety, nausea, anorexia, and decreased appetite. Monitor for clinical worsening of depression and suicidal ideation/behavior after initiation of therapy or after dose changes. Stevens-Johnson syndrome has been reported.

FORMULARY

PAROXETINE *continued*

Paroxetine is an inhibitor and substrate for CYP 450 2D6. May increase effects/toxicity of tricyclic antidepressants, theophylline, and warfarin. May decrease effects of tamoxifen. Cimetidine, ritonavir, MAOIs (fatal serotonin syndrome), dextromethorphan, phenothiazines, and type 1C antiarrhythmics may increase effect/toxicity of paroxetine. Weakness, hyperreflexia, and poor coordination have been reported when taken with sumatriptan.

Do not discontinue therapy abruptly; may cause sweating, dizziness, confusion, and tremor. May be taken with or without food.

PENICILLIN G PREPARATIONS—AQUEOUS POTASSIUM AND SODIUM
Pfizerpen and others
Antibiotic, aqueous penicillin

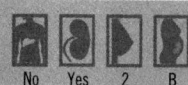

| No | Yes | 2 | B |

Injection (K⁺): 5, 20 million units (contains 1.7 mEq K and 0.3 mEq Na/1 million units penicillin G)
Premixed frozen injection (K⁺): 1 million units in 50 mL dextrose 4%; 2 million units in 50 mL dextrose 2.3%; 3 million units in 50 mL dextrose 0.7% (contains 1.7 mEq K and 0.3 mEq Na/1 million units penicillin G)
Injection (Na⁺): 5 million units (contains 2 mEq Na/1 million units penicillin G)
Conversion: 250 mg = 400,000 units

Neonate (IM/IV; use higher end of dosage range for meningitis and severe infections):
   ≤7 days:
      ≤2 kg: 50,000–100,000 units/kg/24 hr ÷ Q12 hr
      >2 kg: 75,000–150,000 units/kg/24 hr ÷ Q8 hr
   >7 days:
      <1.2 kg: 50,000–100,000 units/kg/24 hr ÷ Q12 hr
      1.2–2 kg: 75,000–150,000 units/kg/24 hr ÷ Q8 hr
      ≥2 kg: 100,000–200,000 units/kg/24 hr ÷ Q6 hr
   Group B streptococcal meningitis:
      ≤7 days: 250,000–450,000 units/kg/24 hr ÷ Q8 hr
      >7 days: 450,000–500,000 units/kg/24 hr ÷ Q4–6 hr
   Congenital syphilis (total of 10 days of therapy; if >1 day of therapy is missed, restart the entire course):
      ≤7 days: 100,000 units/kg/24 hr ÷ Q12 hr IV; increase to dosage below at day 8 of life
      >7 days: 150,000 units/kg/24 hr ÷ Q8 hr IV
Infant and child:
   IM/IV (use higher end of dosage range and Q4 hr interval for meningitis and severe infections):
   100,000–400,000 units/kg/24 hr ÷ Q4–6 hr; **max. dose:** 24 million units/24 hr
   Neurosyphilis: 200,000–300,000 units/kg/24 hr ÷ Q4–6 hr IV × 10–14 days; **max. dose:** 24 million units/24 hr
Adult:
   IM/IV: 4–24 million units/24 hr ÷ Q4–6 hr
   Neurosyphilis: 18–24 million units/24 hr ÷ Q4–6 hr IV × 10–14 days

---

Use penicillin V potassium for oral use. Side effects: anaphylaxis, urticaria, hemolytic anemia, interstitial nephritis, Jarisch-Herxheimer reaction (syphilis). Preparations containing potassium and/or sodium salts may alter serum electrolytes. $T_{1/2}$ = 30 min; may be prolonged by concurrent use of probenecid. For meningitis, use higher daily dose at shorter dosing intervals. For treatment of anthrax (*Bacillus anthracis*), see www.bt.cdc.gov for additional information. **Adjust dose in renal impairment (see Chapter 31).**
Tetracyclines, chloramphenicol, and erythromycin may antagonize penicillin's activity. Probenecid increases penicillin levels. May cause false-positive or -negative urinary glucose (Clinitest method), false-positive direct Coombs test, and false-positive urinary and/or serum proteins.

PENICILLIN G PREPARATIONS—BENZATHINE
Bicillin L-A
Antibiotic, penicillin (very long-acting IM)

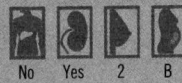

No   Yes   2   B

Injection: 600,000 units/mL (1, 2, 4 mL); contains parabens and povidone
Injection should be IM only.

Group A streptococci:
  Infant and child: 25,000–50,000 units/kg/dose IM × 1; **max. dose:** 1.2 million units/dose
    OR:
  >1 mo and <27 kg: 600,000 units/dose IM × 1
  ≥27 kg and adult: 1.2 million units/dose IM × 1
Rheumatic fever prophylaxis (Q3 wk administration recommended for high-risk situations):
  Infant and child (>1 mo and <27 kg): 600,000 units/dose IM Q3–4 wk
  Adult: 1.2 million units/dose IM Q3–4 wk
Syphilis (if >1 day of therapy is missed, restart the entire course; divided total dose into two injection sites):
  Infant and child:
    Primary, secondary, and early latent syphilis (<1 yr duration): 50,000 units/kg/dose × 1
    Late latent syphilis or latent syphilis of unknown duration: 50,000 units/kg/dose Q7 days × 3 doses
    Max. dose: 2.4 million units/dose
  Adult:
    Primary, secondary, and early latent syphilis: 2.4 million units/dose IM × 1
    Late latent syphilis or latent syphilis of unknown duration: 2.4 million units/dose IM Q7 days × 3 doses

Provides sustained levels for 2–4 wk. **Use with caution** in renal failure, asthma, and cephalosporin hypersensitivity. Side effects and drug interactions same as for *Penicillin G Preparations—Aqueous Potassium and Sodium.* Injection site reactions are common.
Deep IM administration only. Do not administer IV (cardiac arrest and death may occur) and **do not inject** into or near an artery or nerve (may result in permanent neurologic damage).

**PENICILLIN G PREPARATIONS—PENICILLIN G BENZATHINE
AND PENICILLIN G PROCAINE**
Bicillin C-R, Bicillin C-R 900/300
Antibiotic, penicillin (very long-acting IM)

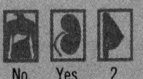

No   Yes   2   B

Bicillin CR: 300,000 units penicillin G procaine + 300,000 units penicillin G benzathine/mL to provide 600,000 units penicillin per 1 mL (2-mL Tubex syringe)
Bicillin CR (900/300): 150,000 units penicillin G procaine + 450,000 units penicillin G benzathine/mL (2-mL Tubex syringe)
All preparations contain parabens and povidone.
Injection should be for IM use only.

Dosage based on total amount of penicillin.
Group A streptococci:
  Child < 14 kg: 600,000 units/dose IM × 1
  Child 14–27 kg: 900,000–1,200,000 units/dose IM × 1
  Child > 27 kg and adult: 2,400,000 units/dose IM × 1

PENICILLIN G PREPARATIONS—PENICILLIN G BENZATHINE AND PENICILLIN
G PROCAINE *continued*

This preparation provides early peak levels in addition to prolonged levels of penicillin in the
blood. **Do not use this product to treat syphilis; treatment failure can occur**. Use with
caution in renal failure, asthma, significant allergies, and cephalosporin hypersensitivity.
Addition of procaine penicillin has not been shown more efficacious than benzathine alone,
but it may reduce injection discomfort.

Deep IM administration only. Do not administer IV (cardiac arrest and death may occur), and **do not
inject** into or near an artery or nerve (may result in permanent neurologic damage).

Side effects and drug interactions same as for *Penicillin G Preparations–Aqueous Potassium and
Sodium*. Immune hypersensitivity reaction has been reported.

PENICILLIN G PREPARATIONS—PROCAINE
Wycillin and generics
Antibiotic, penicillin (long-acting IM)

No   Yes   2   B

Injection: 600,000 units/mL (1, 2 mL); may contain parabens, phenol, povidone, and formaldehyde)
Contains 120 mg procaine per 300,000 units penicillin
Injection should be for IM use only.

Newborn (see remarks): 50,000 units/kg/24 hr IM once daily
Infant and child: 25,000–50,000 units/kg/24 hr ÷ Q12–24 hr IM; **max. dose:** 4.8 million
units/24 hr
Adult: 0.6–4.8 million units/24 hr ÷ Q12–24 hr IM
Congenital syphilis, syphilis (if >1 day of therapy is missed, restart the entire course):
  Neonate, infant, child: 50,000 units/kg/dose once daily IM × 10 days
Neurosyphilis:
  Adult: 2.4 million units IM once daily and Probenecid 500 mg Q6 hr PO × 10–14 days (both
  medications)
Inhaled anthrax: Postexposure prophylaxis (total duration of therapy with all forms of therapy is 60
days; switch to alternative form of therapy after 2 wk of procaine penicillin because of risk for
adverse effects):
  Child: 25,000 units/kg/dose (**max. dose:** 1.2 million units/dose) IM Q12 hr
  Adult: 1.2 million units IM Q12 hr

Provides sustained levels for 2–4 days. **Use with caution** in renal failure, asthma, significant
allergies, cephalosporin hypersensitivity, and in neonates (higher incidence of sterile abscess
at injection site and risk of procaine toxicity). Side effects and drug interactions similar to
Penicillin G Preparations–Aqueous Potassium and Sodium. In addition, may cause CNS
stimulation and seizures. Immune hypersensitivity reaction has been reported.

Deep IM administration only. Do not administer IV (cardiac arrest and death may occur) and **do not
inject** into or near an artery or nerve (may result in permanent neurologic damage). Large doses may
be administered in two injection sites. No longer recommended for empirical treatment of gonorrhea
due to resistant strains.

For explanation of icons, see p. 648

PENICILLIN V POTASSIUM
Veetids and generics
Antibiotic, penicillin

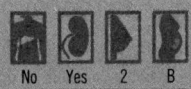

No   Yes   2   B

Tabs: 250, 500 mg
Oral solution: 125 mg/5 mL, 250 mg/5 mL (100, 200 mL); may contain saccharin
Contains 0.7 mEq potassium/250 mg drug
250 mg = 400,000 units

Child: 25–50 mg/kg/24 hr ÷ Q6–8 hr PO; **max. dose:** 3 g/24 hr
Adolescent and adult: 125–500 mg/dose PO Q6–8 hr
Acute group A streptococcal pharyngitis (use BID dosing regimen ONLY if good compliance is expected):
  Child < 27 kg: 250 mg PO BID–TID × 10 days
  ≥27 kg, adolescent and adult: 500 mg PO BID–TID × 10 days
Rheumatic fever prophylaxis and pneumococcal prophylaxis for sickle cell disease and functional or anatomic asplenia (regardless of immunization status):
  2 mo–<3 yr: 125 mg PO BID
  3–5 yr: 250 mg PO BID. For sickle cell and asplenia, use may be discontinued after age 5 if child received recommended pneumococcal immunizations and did not experience invasive pneumococcal infection.
Recurrent rheumatic fever prophylaxis:
  Child and adult: 250 mg PO BID

See *Penicillin G Preparations—Aqueous Potassium and Sodium* for side effects and drug interactions. GI absorption is better than penicillin G. **Note:** Must be taken 1 hr before or 2 hr after meals. Penicillin will prevent rheumatic fever if started within 9 days of the acute illness. **Adjust dose in renal failure (see Chapter 31).**

PENTAMIDINE ISETHIONATE
Pentam 300, NebuPent
Antibiotic, antiprotozoal

No   Yes   3   C

Injection (Pentam 300): 300 mg
Inhalation (NebuPent): 300 mg

Treatment:
  Pneumocystis jirovecii (carinii): 4 mg/kg/24 hr IM/IV once daily × 14–21 days
  (IV is the preferred route)
  Trypanosomiasis (Trypanosoma gambiense, T. rhodesiense): 4 mg/kg/24 hr IM once daily × 7 days
  Visceral leishmaniasis (Leishmania donovani, L. infantum, L. chagasi): 4 mg/kg/dose IM once daily, or once every other day × 15–30 doses
  Cutaneous leishmaniasis (Leishmania [Viannia] panamensis): 2–3 mg/kg/dose IM once daily or once every other day × 4–7 doses
Prophylaxis:
  Pneumocystis jirovecii (carinii):
    IM/IV: 4 mg/kg/dose Q2–4 wk
    Inhalation:
      ≥5 yr: 300 mg in 6 mL H₂O via inhalation Q month. Use with a Respigard II nebulizer.
  Max. single dose: 300 mg

FORMULARY

PENTAMIDINE ISETHIONATE *continued*

Use with caution in ventricular tachycardia, Stevens-Johnson syndrome, and daily doses >21 days. May cause hypoglycemia, hyperglycemia, hypotension (both IV and IM administration), nausea, vomiting, fever, mild hepatotoxicity, pancreatitis, megaloblastic anemia, nephrotoxicity, hypocalcemia, and granulocytopenia. Additive nephrotoxicity with aminoglycosides, amphotericin B, cisplatin, and vancomycin may occur. Aerosol administration may also cause bronchospasm, cough, oxygen desaturation, dyspnea, and loss of appetite. Infuse IV over 1–2 hr to reduce risk of hypotension. Sterile abscess may occur at IM injection site.
Adjust dose in renal impairment (see Chapter 31) with systemic use.

PENTOBARBITAL
Nembutal
Barbiturate

Yes   No   3   D

Injection: 50 mg/mL (20, 50 mL); contains propylene glycol and 10% alcohol

Hypnotic:
  Child:
    IM: 2–6 mg/kg/dose; **max. dose:** 100 mg
  Adult:
    IM: 150–200 mg
Preprocedure sedation:
  Child:
    IV/IM: 3–6 mg/kg/dose; **max. dose:** 150 mg
Barbiturate coma:
  Child and adult:
    IV, loading dose: 10–15 mg/kg given slowly over 1–2 hr
    Maintenance: Begin at 1 mg/kg/hr. Dose range: 1–3 mg/kg/hr as needed.

Contraindicated in liver failure and history of porphyria. **Use with caution** in hypovolemic shock, CHF, hypotension, and hepatic impairment. No advantage over phenobarbital for control of seizures. Adjunct in treatment of ICP. May cause drug-related isoelectric EEG. **Do not administer** for >2 wk in treatment of insomnia. May cause hypotension, arrhythmias, hypothermia, respiratory depression, and dependence.
Onset of action: IM, 10–15 min; IV, 1 min. Duration of action: IV, 15 min.
Administer IV at a rate of <50 mg/min.
Therapeutic serum levels: Sedation, 1–5 mg/L; hypnosis, 5–15 mg/L; coma, 20–40 mg/L (steady state is achieved after 4–5 days of continuous IV dosing).

PERMETHRIN
Elimite, Acticin, Nix, and generics
Scabicidal agent

No   No   2   B

Cream (Elimite, Acticin, and generics): 5% (60 g); contains 0.1% formaldehyde
Liquid cream rinse (Nix-OTC and generics): 1% (60 mL with comb); contains 20% isopropyl alcohol
Lotion [OTC]: 1% (60 mL with comb)
Additional permethrin products for use on bedding, furniture, and garments include:
  Liquid spray (Nix Lice Control Spray): 0.25% (150 mL)
  Solution (A200 Lice, Rid): 0.5% (170.1 g or 150 mL)

For explanation of icons, see p. 648.

Continued

PERMETHRIN *continued*

Pediculus humanus capitis, Phthirus pubis *(>2 mo)*:
  Head lice: Saturate hair and scalp with 1% cream rinse after shampooing, rinsing,
  and towel drying hair. Leave on for 10 min, then rinse. May repeat in 7 days. May be used for
  lice in other areas of the body (e.g., pubic lice) in same fashion. If the 1% cream rinse is resistant,
  the 5% cream may be used after shampooing, rinsing, and towel drying hair. Leave on for 8–14 hr
  overnight under a shower cap, then rinse off. May repeat in 7 days.
  Scabies: Apply 5% cream from neck to toe (head to toe for infants and toddlers); wash off with
  water in 8–14 hr. May repeat in 7 days. Use in infants <1 mo is safe and effective when applied for
  a 6-hr period.

Ovicidal activity generally makes single-dose regimen adequate, but resistance to permethrin
  has been reported. **Avoid** contact with eyes during application. Shake well before using. May
  cause pruritus, hypersensitivity, burning, stinging, erythema, and rash. For either lice or
  scabies, instruct patient to launder bedding and clothing. For lice, treat symptomatic
  contacts only. For scabies, treat all contacts even if asymptomatic. Topical cream dosage
  form contains formaldehyde. Dispense 60 g per 1 adult or 2 small children.

PHENAZOPYRIDINE HCL
Pyridium, Azo-Standard [OTC], and generics
Urinary analgesic

Yes	Yes	3	B

Tabs: 95 mg [OTC], 97.2 mg, 100 mg [OTC and Rx], 200 mg
Oral suspension: 10 mg/mL

UTI (use with an appropriate antibacterial agent):
  Child 6–12 yr: 12 mg/kg/24 hr ÷ TID PO until symptoms of lower urinary tract irritation are
  controlled or for 2 days
  Adult: 95–200 mg TID PO until symptoms are controlled or for 2 days

May cause pruritus, rash, GI distress, vertigo, and headache. Anaphylactoid-like reaction,
  methemoglobinemia, hemolytic anemia, and renal and hepatic toxicity have been reported,
  usually at overdosage levels. Colors urine orange; stains clothing. May also stain contact
  lenses and interfere with urinalysis tests based on spectrometry or color reactions. Give doses
  after meals.
**Avoid use use in moderate/severe renal impairment; adjust dose in mild renal impairment (see
  Chapter 31).**

PHENOBARBITAL
Luminal and generics
Barbiturate

Yes	Yes	2	D

Tabs: 15, 16.2, 30, 32.4, 60, 64.8, 97.2, 100 mg
Elixir or oral solution: 20 mg/5 mL; may contain alcohol
Injection: 65, 130 mg/mL; may contain 10% alcohol and propylene glycol

Status epilepticus:
  Loading dose, IV:
    Neonate, infant, and child: 15–20 mg/kg/dose (**max. loading dose:** 1000 mg) in a single or
    divided dose. May give additional 5-mg/kg doses Q15–30 min to a **max. total** of 40 mg/kg.

PHENOBARBITAL *continued*

> ***Maintenance dose, PO/IV:*** Monitor levels.
> > ***Neonate:*** 3–5 mg/kg/24 hr ÷ once daily–BID
> > ***Infant:*** 5–6 mg/kg/24 hr ÷ once daily–BID
> > ***Child 1–5 yr:*** 6–8 mg/kg/24 hr ÷ once daily–BID
> > ***Child 6–12 yr:*** 4–6 mg/kg/24 hr ÷ once daily–BID
> > ***>12 yr:*** 1–3 mg/kg/24 hr ÷ once daily–BID
>
> ***Hyperbilirubinemia (<12 yr):*** 3–8 mg/kg/24 hr PO ÷ BID–TID. Doses up to 12 mg/kg/24 hr have been used.
>
> ***Preoperative sedation (child):*** 1–3 mg/kg/dose IM/IV/PO × 1. Give 60–90 min before procedure.

Contraindicated in porphyria, severe respiratory disease with dyspnea, or obstruction.
Use with caution in hepatic or renal disease (reduce dose). IV administration may cause respiratory arrest or hypotension. Side effects include drowsiness, cognitive impairment, ataxia, hypotension, hepatitis, rash, respiratory depression, apnea, megaloblastic anemia, and anticonvulsant hypersensitivity syndrome. Paradoxical reaction in children (not dose related) may cause hyperactivity, irritability, insomnia. Induces several liver enzymes (CYP 450 1A2, 2B6, 2C8, 3A3/4, 3A5–7), thus decreases blood levels of many drugs (e.g., anticonvulsants). **IV push not to exceed 1 mg/kg/min.**

$T_{1/2}$ is variable with age: neonates, 45–100 hr; infants, 20–133 hr; children, 37–73 hr. Owing to long half-life, consider other agents for sedation for procedures.

Therapeutic levels: 15–40 mg/L. Recommended serum sampling time at steady state: trough level obtained within 30 minutes before next scheduled dose after 10–14 days of continuous dosing.
Adjust dose in renal failure (see Chapter 31).

PHENTOLAMINE MESYLATE
Regitine (previous brand name), OraVerse, and generics
Adrenergic blocking agent (alpha); antidote, extravasation

| No | No | ? | C |

Injection: 5 mg vial; may contain mannitol
Injection in solution: 5 mg/mL (1 mL)
Injection in solution for submucosal use:
> **OraVerse:** 0.4 mg/1.7 mL (1.7 mL in dental cartridges) (10s, 50s); contains edetate disodium

Treatment of α-adrenergic drug extravasation (most effective within 12 hr of extravasation):
All doses are 5 doses administered SC around site of extravasation within 12 hr of extravasation. See table below for weight-based dosing and recommended drug concentration.

Patient Weight	Drug Concentration (diluted with preservative-free NS)	Dose for each syringe \x 5 syringes	Total Dose from all 5 Syringes
<1 kg	0.2 mg/mL	0.05 mL	0.05 mg
1–< 2.5 kg	0.2 mg/mL	0.1 mL	0.1 mg
2.5–< 5 kg	0.2 mg/mL	0.25 mL	0.25 mg
5–< 10 kg	1 mg/mL	0.1 mL	0.5 mg
10–< 20 kg	1 mg/mL	0.2 mL	1 mg
20–< 30 kg	1 mg/mL	0.4 mL	2 mg
30–< 40 kg	1 mg/mL	0.6 mL	3 mg
40–< 50 kg	1 mg/mL	0.8 mL	4 mg
\ge 50 kg	1 mg/mL	1 mL	5 mg

For explanation of icons, see p. 648

Continued

PHENTOLAMINE MESYLATE *continued*

Max. total dose:
> *Neonate:* 2.5 mg; monitor BP when total dose exceeds 0.1 mg/kg.
> *Infant, child, adolescent, and adult:* 0.1–0.2 mg/kg/dose or 5 mg
> *Diagnosis of pheochromocytoma, IM/IV:*
>> *Child:* 0.05–0.1 mg/kg/dose up to a **max. dose** of 5 mg
>> *Adult:* 5 mg/dose
> *Hypertension, before surgery for pheochromocytoma, IM/IV:*
>> *Child:* 0.05–0.1 mg/kg/dose up to a **max. dose** of 5 mg 1–2 hr **before** surgery; repeat Q2–4 hr PRN.
>> *Adult:* 5 mg/dose 1–2 hr **before** surgery; repeat Q2–4 hr PRN.

Contraindicated in MI, coronary insufficiency and angina. **Use with caution** in hypotension, arrhythmias, and cerebral vascular spasm/occlusion.

For diagnosis of pheochromocytoma, patient should be resting in a supine position. A blood pressure reduction of >35 mmHg systolic and 24 mmHg diastolic is considered a positive test for pheochromocytoma. For treatment of extravasation, use 27- to 30-gauge needle with multiple small injections, and monitor site closely because repeat doses may be necessary.

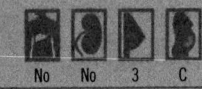

PHENYLEPHRINE HCL
Neo-Synephrine, many others, and generics
Adrenergic agonist

No   No   3   C

Injection: 10 mg/mL (1%) (1, 5, 10 mL); may contain bisulfites
Nasal spray [OTC]: 0.25, 0.5, 1% (15, 30 mL)
NOTE: For Neo-Synephrine 12-hr Nasal, see *Oxymetazoline*
Ophthalmic drops: 2.5% (2, 3, 5, 15 mL), 10% (5 mL)
Tabs (Medi-Pheny, Sudafed PE) [OTC]: 5, 10 mg
Oral solution [OTC]: 2.5 mg/5 mL (118 mL)
Oral drops [OTC]: 2.5 mg/1 mL (30 mL)

Hypotension:
NOTE: IV drip dosage units for children are in mcg/kg/min, compared with mcg/min for adults.
> To prepare infusion, see inside front cover.
> *Child:*
>> *IV bolus:* 5–20 mcg/kg/dose Q10–15 min PRN
>> *IV drip:* 0.1–0.5 mcg/kg/min; titrate to effect
>> *IM/SC:* 0.1 mcg/kg/dose Q1–2 hr PRN; **max. dose:** 5 mg
> *Adult:*
>> *IV bolus:* 0.1–0.5 mg/dose Q10–15 min PRN
>> *IV drip:* Initial rate at 100–180 mcg/min; titrate to effect. Usual maintenance dose: 40–60 mcg/min.
>> *IM/SC:* 2–5 mg/dose Q1–2 hr PRN; **max. initial dose:** 5 mg
Pupillary dilation (≥1 yr): 2.5% solution; 1 drop in each eye 15–30 min before examination
Nasal decongestant (in each nostril; give up to 3 days):
> *Child 6–12 yr:* 2–3 drops or 1–2 sprays of 0.25% solution Q4 hr PRN
> *>12 yr–adult:* 2–3 drops or 1–2 sprays of 0.25% or 0.5% solution Q4 hr PRN
Oral decongestant (see remarks):
> *4–<6 yr:*
>> *Oral drops (2.5 mg/mL):* 1 mL (2.5 mg) PO Q4 hr; **not to exceed** 6 doses (15 mg) in 24 hr
>> *Oral solution (2.5 mg/5 mL):* 5 mL (2.5 mg) PO Q4 hr, up to 30 mL (15 mg) per 24 hr
> *≥6–<12 yr:*
>> *Oral solution (2.5 mg/5 mL):* 10 mL (5 mg) PO Q4 hr up to 60 mL (30 mg) per 24 hr

PHENYLEPHRINE HCL *continued*

> **≥12 yr and adult:**
>> *Tabs:* 10–20 mg PO Q4 hr

Use with caution in presence of arrhythmias, hyperthyroidism, or hyperglycemia. May cause tremor, insomnia, palpitations. Metabolized by MAO. **Contraindicated** in pheochromocytoma and severe hypertension. Injectable product may contain sulfites.

Nasal decongestants may cause rebound congestion with excessive use (>3 days). The 1% nasal spray can be used in adults with extreme congestion.

Oral phenylephrine is found in a variety of combination cough and cold products and has replaced pseudoephedrine and phenylpropanolamine. Over-the-counter (nonprescription) use of this product is **not recommended** for children <age 6; reports of serious adverse effects (cardiac and respiratory distress, convulsions, and hallucinations) and fatalities (from unintentional overdosages, including combined use of other OTC products containing same active ingredients) have been made.

PHENYTOIN
Dilantin, Dilantin Infatab, Phenytek, and generics
Anticonvulsant, class Ib antiarrhythmic

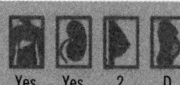

| Yes | Yes | 2 | D |

Chewable tabs (Dilantin Infatab and generics): 50 mg
Prompt-release caps: 100 mg
Extended-release caps: 30, 100, 200, 300 mg
Oral suspension: 125 mg/5 mL (240 mL); contains ≤0.6 % alcohol
Injection: 50 mg/mL (2, 5 mL); contains alcohol and propylene glycol

Status epilepticus: see Chapter 1.
  Loading dose (all ages): 15–20 mg/kg IV
  Max. dose: 1500 mg/24 hr
  Maintenance for seizure disorders (initiate 12 hr after administration of loading dose):
    Neonate: Start with 5 mg/kg/24 hr PO/IV ÷ Q12 hr. Usual range is 4–8 mg/kg/24 hr PO/IV ÷ Q8–12 hr.
    Infant/child: Start with 5 mg/kg/24 hr ÷ BID–TID PO/IV. Usual dose ranges are (doses divided BID–TID):
      6 mo–3 yr: 8–10 mg/kg/24 hr
      4–6 yr: 7.5–9 mg/kg/24 hr
      7–9 yr: 7–8 mg/kg/24 hr
      10–16 yr: 6–7 mg/kg/24 hr
    NOTE: Use once-daily–BID dosing with extended-release caps.
    Adult: Start with 100 mg/dose Q8 hr IV/PO and carefully titrate (if needed) by 100-mg increments Q2–4 wk to 300–600 mg/24 hr (or 6–7 mg/kg/24 hr) ÷ Q8–24 hr IV/PO.
Antiarrhythmic (secondary to digitalis intoxication):
  Loading dose (all ages): 1.25 mg/kg IV Q5 min up to a **total** of 15 mg/kg
  Maintenance:
    Child (IV/PO): 5–10 mg/kg/24 hr ÷ Q8–12 hr
    Adult: 250 mg PO QID × 1 day, then 250 mg PO Q12 hr × 2 days, then 300–400 mg/24 hr ÷ Q6–24 hr

Contraindicated in patients with heart block or sinus bradycardia, and those who are receiving delavirdine (decrease virologic response). IM administration is **not recommended** because of erratic absorption and pain at injection site; consider fosphenytoin. Side effects include gingival hyperplasia, hirsutism, dermatitis, blood dyscrasia, ataxia, lupus-like and Stevens-Johnson syndromes, lymphadenopathy, liver damage, and nystagmus. Suicidal

For explanation of icons, see p. 648

PHENYTOIN *continued*

behavior or ideation and multiorgan hypersensitivity (DRESS) have been reported. Increased risk for serious skin reactions (e.g., TEN, Stevens-syndrome) in patients with the HLA-B*1502 allele.

Many drug interactions: Levels may be increased by cimetidine, chloramphenicol, INH, sulfonamides, trimethoprim, etc. Levels may be decreased by some antineoplastic agents. Phenytoin induces hepatic microsomal enzymes (CYP 450 1A2, 2C8/9/19, and 3A3/4), leading to decreased effectiveness of oral contraceptives, fosamprenavir (used without ritonavir), quinidine, valproic acid, theophylline, and other substrates to the previously listed CYP 450 hepatic enzymes. May cause resistance to neuromuscular blocking action of nondepolarizing neuromuscular blocking agents (e.g., pancuronium, vecuronium, rocuronium, and cisatracurium).

Suggested dosing intervals for specific oral dosage forms: Extended-release caps, once daily–BID; chewable and immediate-release tablets and oral suspension, TID. Oral absorption reduced in neonates. $T_{1/2}$ is variable (7–42 hr) and dose dependent. Drug is highly protein bound; free fraction of drug will be increased in patients with hypoalbuminemia.

For seizure disorders, therapeutic levels are 10–20 mg/L (free and bound phenytoin) *OR* 1–2 mg/L (free only). Monitor free phenytoin levels in hypoalbuminemia or renal insufficiency. Recommended serum sampling times: trough level (PO/IV) within 30 min before next scheduled dose; peak or post-load level (IV) 1 hr after end of IV infusion. Steady state is usually achieved after 5–10 days of continuous dosing. For routine monitoring, measure trough.

IV push/infusion rate **not to exceed** 0.5 mg/kg/min in neonates, or 1 mg/kg/min in infants, children, and adults, with **max.** of 50 mg/min; may cause cardiovascular collapse. Consider fosphenytoin in situations of tenuous IV access and risk for extravasation.

PHOSPHORUS SUPPLEMENTS
K-PHOS Neutral, Phospha 250 Neutral, PHOS-NaK, Sodium Phosphate, Potassium Phosphate, and many generics for injection

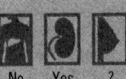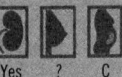
No   Yes   ?   C

Oral: (Reconstitute in 75 mL H_2O per tablet or packet of powder.)
Na and K phosphate:
  PHOS-NaK, powder [OTC]: 250 mg (8 mM) P, 6.96 mEq (160 mg) Na, 7.16 mEq (280 mg) K per packet of powder (100s)
  K-PHOS Neutral or Phospha 250 Neutral, tabs: 250 mg P (8 mM), 13 mEq Na, 1.1 mEq K
  K-PHOS No. 2, tabs: 250 mg P (8 mM), 5.8 mEq Na, 2.3 mEq K
Injection:
  Na phosphate: 3 mM (93 mg) P, 4 mEq Na/mL
  K phosphate: 3mM (93 mg) P, 4.4 mEq K/mL
Conversion: 31 mg P = 1 mM P

Acute hypophosphatemia: 0.16–0.32 mM/kg/dose (or 5–10 mg/kg/dose) IV over 6 hr
Maintenance/replacement:
  Child:
    IV: 0.5–1.5 mM/kg (or 15–45 mg/kg) over 24 hr
    PO: 30–90 mg/kg/24 hr (or 1–3 mM/kg/24 hr) ÷ TID–QID
  Adult:
    IV: 50–65 mM (or 1.5–2 g) over 24 hr
    PO: 3–4.5 g/24 hr (or 100–150 mM/24 hr) ÷ TID–QID

Recommended IV infusion rate: ≤0.1 mM/kg/hr (or 3.1 mg/kg/hr) of phosphate. When potassium salt is used, the rate will be limited by the **max.** potassium infusion rate. **Do not** co-infuse with calcium-containing products.

PHOSPHORUS SUPPLEMENTS *continued*

May cause tetany, hyperphosphatemia, hyperkalemia, hypocalcemia. **Use with caution** in patients with renal impairment. Be aware of sodium and/or potassium load when supplementing phosphate. IV administration of potassium-salt product may cause hypotension, renal failure, arrhythmias, heart block, or cardiac arrest. PO dosing may cause nausea, vomiting, abdominal pain, or diarrhea. See Chapter 21 for daily requirements and Chapter 11 for additional information on hypophosphatemia and hyperphosphatemia.

PHYSOSTIGMINE SALICYLATE
Antilirium (former brand name) and generics
Cholinergic agent

No   No   ?   ?

Injection: 1 mg/mL (2 mL); contains 2% benzyl alcohol and 0.1% sodium bisulfite

Reversal of toxic anticholinergic effects from antihistamine or anticholinergic agents:
   Child: 0.01–0.03 mg/kg/dose IV administered over 3–5 min. Dose may be repeated Q20 min if no response or return of anticholinergic symptoms up to a **max. total** of 2 mg.
   Adult: 0.5–2 mg IV (administered over 5 min)/IM/SC. If needed, repeat dose Q20 min until response is seen or when adverse effects occur.

Physostigmine antidote: Atropine always should be available. **Contraindicated** in asthma, gangrene, diabetes, cardiovascular disease, GI or GU tract obstruction, any vagotonic state, and patients receiving choline esters or depolarizing neuromuscular blocking agents (e.g., decamethonium, succinylcholine). May cause seizures, arrhythmias, bradycardia, GI symptoms, and other cholinergic effects. Rapid IV administration can cause bradycardia and hypersalivation leading to respiratory distress and seizures.
Pregnancy code not formally assigned by the FDA.

PHYTONADIONE/VITAMIN K₁
Mephyton and generics
Vitamin, fat soluble

No   No   2   C

Tabs (Mephyton): 5 mg
Oral suspension: 1 mg/mL
Injection, emulsion:
   2 mg/mL (0.5 mL); preservative free
   10 mg/mL (1 mL); contains 0.9% benzyl alcohol

Neonatal hemorrhagic disease (vitamin K deficiency bleeding):
   Prophylaxis: 0.5–1 mg IM × 1 within 1 hr after birth
   Treatment: 1–2 mg/24 hr IM/SC/IV
Oral anticoagulant (warfarin) overdose (see remarks):
   INR ≥ 5 and no serious bleeding:
      <40 kg: 30 mcg/kg PO/IV
      ≥40 kg: 1–2.5 mg PO/IV
      Suggested INR monitoring schedule:
         INR 5–8: Q12–24 hr
         INR ≥ 8: Q6–12 hr and repeat dose if necessary

For explanation of icons, see p. 648

Continued

PHYTONADIONE/VITAMIN K₁ *continued*

> ***Serious bleeding (any elevated INR):*** 2.5–5 mg PO/IV and monitor INR Q6 hr and repeat dose if necessary.
> ***Life-threatening bleeding (any elevated INR):*** 5–10 mg PO/IV and monitor INR Q2–4 hr and repeat dose if necessary. Consider the use of FFP.

> ***Vitamin K deficiency:***
> > ***Infant and child:***
> > > ***PO:*** 2.5–5 mg/24 hr
> > > ***IM/SC/IV:*** 1–2 mg/dose × 1
> > ***Adolescent and adult:***
> > > ***PO:*** 2.5–25 mg/24 hr
> > > ***IM/SC/IV:*** 2.5–10 mg/dose × 1

Monitor PT/PTT. Large doses (10–20 mg) in newborns may cause hyperbilirubinemia and severe hemolytic anemia. Blood coagulation factors increase within 6–12 hr after oral doses and within 1–2 hr after parenteral administration.

IV injection rate **not to exceed** 3 mg/m²/min or 1 mg/min. IV or IM doses may cause flushing, dizziness, cardiac/respiratory arrest, hypotension, and anaphylaxis. IV or IM administration is indicated only when other routes of administration are not feasible (or in emergency situations).

Concurrent administration of oral mineral oil may decrease GI absorption of oral vitamin K. Protect product from light. See Chapter 21 for multivitamin preparations.

PILOCARPINE HCL
Isopto Carpine, Salagen, Pilopine HS, and others
Cholinergic agent

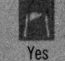

Yes No 3 C

Ophthalmic solution (Isopto Carpine and generics): 1% (15 mL), 2% (15 mL), 4% (15 mL); may contain benzalkonium chloride
Ophthalmic gel (Pilopine HS): 4% (4 g); contains benzalkonium chloride
Tab (Salagen and others): 5, 7.5 mg

For elevated intraocular pressure:
> *Child and adult:*
> > *Drops:* 1–2 drops in each eye 4–6 times a day; adjust concentration and frequency as needed.
> > *Gel:* 0.5-inch ribbon applied to lower conjunctival sac QHS. Adjust dose as needed.

Xerostomia:
> *Adult:* 5 mg/dose PO TID; dose may be titrated to 10 mg/dose PO TID in patients who do not respond to lower dose and who are able to tolerate the drug. 5 mg/dose PO QID has been used in Sjögren syndrome.

OPHTHALMIC USE: Contraindicated in acute iritis or anterior chamber inflammation and uncontrolled asthma. May cause stinging, burning, lacrimation, headache, and retinal detachment. **Use with caution** in patients with corneal abrasion or significant cardiovascular disease. Use with topical NSAIDs (e.g., ketorolac) may decrease topical pilocarpine effects.

ORAL USE: Sweating, nausea, rhinitis, chills, flushing, urinary frequency, dizziness, asthenia, and headaches have also been reported. Reduce oral dosing in the presence of mild hepatic insufficiency (Child-Pugh score of 5–6); use in severe hepatic insufficiency is **not recommended**.

PIMECROLIMUS
Elidel
Topical immunosuppressant

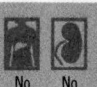 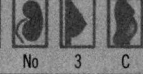

No   No   3   C

Cream: 1% (30, 60, 100 g); contains benzyl alcohol and propylene glycol

Atopic dermatitis (second-line therapy):
≥2 yr and adult (see remarks): Apply a thin layer to affected area BID and rub in gently and completely. Reevaluate patient in 6 wk if lesions are not healed.

Do not use in children <2 (higher rate of upper respiratory infections), immunocompromised patients, or with occlusive dressings (promotes systemic absorption). Approved as a second-line therapy for atopic dermatitis for patients who fail to respond or do not tolerate other approved therapies. Use medication for short periods of time by using the minimal amounts to control symptoms; long-term safety is unknown. **Avoid** contact with eyes, nose, mouth, and cut, infected, or scraped skin. Minimize and **avoid** exposure to natural and artificial sunlight, respectively.

Most common side effects include burning at application site, headache, viral infections, and pyrexia. Skin discoloration, skin flushing associated with alcohol use, anaphylactic reactions, ocular irritation after application to eyelids or near eyes, angioneurotic edema, and facial edema have been reported. Although risk is uncertain, the FDA has issued an alert about potential cancer risk with use of this product. See www.fda.gov/medwatch for latest information. Drug is a CYP 450 3A3/4 substrate.

PIPERACILLIN WITH TAZOBACTAM
Zosyn and generics
Antibiotic, penicillin (extended spectrum with β-lactamase inhibitor)

No   Yes   2   B

8:1 ratio of piperacillin to tazobactam:
Injection, powder: 2 g piperacillin and 0.25 g tazobactam; 3 g piperacillin and 0.375 g tazobactam; 4 g piperacillin and 0.5 g tazobactam; 36 g piperacillin and 4.5 g tazobactam
Injection, premixed in iso-osmotic dextrose: 2 g piperacillin and 0.25 g tazobactam in 50 mL; 3 g piperacillin and 0.375 g tazobactam in 50 mL; 4 g piperacillin and 0.5 g tazobactam in 100 mL
Contains 2.79 mEq Na/g piperacillin

All doses based on piperacillin component.
Neonate: 100 mg/kg/dose IV at the following intervals:
　<1 kg:
　　≤14 days old: Q12 hr
　　15–28 days old: Q8 hr
　≥1 kg:
　　≤7 days old: Q12 hr
　　8–28 days old: Q8 hr
Severe infections (IV; shortening the dosing interval to Q6 hr and lengthening the dose administration time (see remarks) may enhance the pharmacodynamic properties):
　<2 mo (currently undefined by manufacturer; extrapolated from piperacillin dosing): 300–400 mg/kg/24 hr ÷ Q6 hr
　2–9 mo: 240 mg/kg/24 hr ÷ Q8 hr
　>9 mo: 300 mg/kg/24 hr ÷ Q8 hr; **max. dose:** 16 g/24 hr

Continued

PIPERACILLIN WITH TAZOBACTAM *continued*

Appendicitis or peritonitis (IV route for 7–10 days; dosing interval may be shortened to Q6 hr to enhance pharmacodynamic properties):

2–9 mo: 240 mg/kg/24 hr ÷ Q8 hr

>9 mo–adolescent and ≤40 kg: 300 mg/kg/24 hr ÷ Q8 hr

>9 mo–adolescent and >40 kg: 3 g Q6 hr; **max. dose:** 16 g/24 hr

Adult:

Intraabdominal or soft-tissue infections: 3 g IV Q6 hr

Nosocomial pneumonia: 4 g IV Q6 hr

Cystic fibrosis (antipseudomonal): 350–600 mg/kg/24 hr IV ÷ Q4–6 hr; **max. dose:** 24 g/24 hr

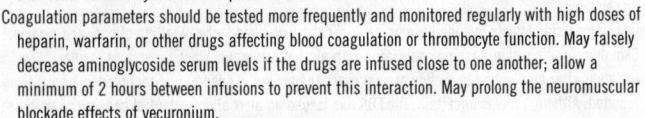

Tazobactam is a β-lactamase inhibitor, thus extending the spectrum of piperacillin. Like other penicillins, CSF penetration occurs only with inflamed meninges. GI disturbances, pruritus, rash, and headaches are common. Abnormal platelet aggregation and prolonged bleeding, serious skin reactions (e.g., Stevens-Johnson syndrome, TEN) have been reported in patients with renal failure. Cystic fibrosis patients have an increased risk for fever and rash.

Coagulation parameters should be tested more frequently and monitored regularly with high doses of heparin, warfarin, or other drugs affecting blood coagulation or thrombocyte function. May falsely decrease aminoglycoside serum levels if the drugs are infused close to one another; allow a minimum of 2 hours between infusions to prevent this interaction. May prolong the neuromuscular blockade effects of vecuronium.

Prolonging the dose administration time to 4 hr will maximize the pharmacokinetic/pharmacodynamic properties by prolonging the time of drug concentration above the MIC. **Adjust dose in renal impairment (see Chapter 31).**

POLYCITRA

See Citrate Mixtures

POLYETHYLENE GLYCOL—ELECTROLYTE SOLUTION
Bowel cleansing products: GoLYTELY, CoLyte, NuLYTELY, TriLyte, and generics
Laxative products: MiraLax, Dulcolax Balance, and generics
Bowel evacuant, osmotic laxative

No   No   ?   C

Powder for oral solution:

GoLYTELY and others: Polyethylene glycol 3350 236 g, Na sulfate 22.74 g, Na bicarbonate 6.74 g, NaCl 5.86 g, KCl 2.97 g (mixed with water to 4 L). Contents vary somewhat. See package insert for specific contents of other products.

MiraLax [OTC], Dulcolax Balance [OTC], and others: Polyethylene glycol 3350 (17, 119, 238, 250, 255, 500, 510, 527, 850 g)

Bowel cleansing (use products containing supplemental electrolytes for bowel cleansing, such as GoLYTELY, CoLyte, NuLYTELY, TriLyte and others; patients should be NPO 3–4 hr before dosing):

Child:

Oral/nasogastric: 25–40 mL/kg/hr until rectal effluent is clear (usually in 4–10 hr)

Adult:

Oral: 240 mL PO Q10 min up to 4 L or until rectal effluent is clear

Nasogastric: 20–30 mL/min (1.2–1.8 L/hr) up to 4 L

PHYTONADIONE/VITAMIN K₁ *continued*

Constipation (MiraLax, Dulcolax Balance, and others):
   Child (limited data in 20 children with chronic constipation, 18 mo–11yr; see remarks): A mean effective dose of 0.84 g/kg/24 hr PO ÷ BID for 8 wk (range, 0.25–1.42 g/kg/24 hr) was used to yield 2 soft stools per day. Do not exceed 17 g/24 hr. If patient > 20 kg, use adult dose.
   Adult: 17 g (one heaping tablespoonful) mixed in 240 mL of water, juice, soda, coffee, or tea PO once daily
Fecal impaction (MiraLax, Dulcolax Balance, and others):
   >3 yr: 1–1.5 g/kg/24 hr (**max. dose:** 100 g/24 hr) PO × 3 days

Contraindicated in polyethylene glycol hypersensitivity. Monitor electrolytes, BUN, serum glucose, and urine osmolality with prolonged administration. Seizures resulting from electrolyte abnormalities have been reported.
BOWEL CLEANSING: Contraindicated in toxic megacolon, gastric retention, colitis, and bowel perforation. **Use with caution** in patients prone to aspiration or with impaired gag reflex. Effect should occur within 1–2 hr. Solution generally more palatable if chilled.
CONSTIPATION (MiraLax and others): Contraindicated in bowel obstruction
   Child: Dilute powder using the ratio of 17 g powder to 240 mL of water, juice, or milk. Onset of action within 1 wk in 12 of 20 patients, with remaining 8 patients reporting improvement during second wk of therapy. Side effects reported in this trial included diarrhea, flatulence, and mild abdominal pain. (See *J Pediatr.* 2001;139:428-432 for additional information.)
   Adult: 2 to 4 days may be required to produce a bowel movement. Most common side effects include nausea, abdominal bloating, cramping, and flatulence. Use beyond 2 wk has not been studied.

POLYMYXIN B SULFATE AND BACITRACIN

See Bacitracin ± Polymyxin B

POLYMYXIN B SULFATE AND TRIMETHOPRIM SULFATE
Polytrim Ophthalmic Solution and various others
Topical antibiotic (ophthalmic preparations listed)

No   No   2   C

Ophthalmic solution: Polymyxin B sulfate 10,000 U, trimethoprim sulfate 1 mg/mL (10 mL); some preparations may contain 0.04 mg/mL benzalkonium chloride.

≥2 mo and adult: Instill 1 drop in affected eye(s) Q3 hr (**max. of 6 doses/24 hr**) × 7–10 days.

Active against susceptible strains of *Staphylococcus aureus, Staphylococcus epidermidis, Streptococcus pneumoniae, Streptococcus viridans, Haemophilus influenzae,* and *Pseudomonas aeruginosa.* **Not indicated** for prophylaxis or treatment of ophthalmia neonatorum. Local irritation consisting of redness, burning, stinging, and/or itching is common. Hypersensitivity reactions consisting of lid edema, itching, increased redness, tearing, and/or circumocular rash have been reported.
Apply finger pressure to lacrimal sac during for 1–2 min after dose application.

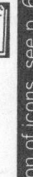

For explanation of icons, see p. 648

POLYMYXIN B SULFATE, NEOMYCIN SULFATE, HYDROCORTISONE
Cortisporin Otic, AK-Spore H.C. Otic, PediOtic, and generics
Topical antibiotic (otic and ophthalmic preparations listed)

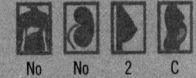

No   No   2   C

Otic solution or suspension: Polymyxin B sulfate 10,000 U, neomycin sulfate 5 mg (3.5 mg neomycin base), hydrocortisone 10 mg/mL (10 mL); some preparations may contain thimerosol and metabisulfite.
Ophthalmic suspension: Polymyxin B sulfate 10,000 U, neomycin sulfate 5 mg (3.5 mg neomycin base), hydrocortisone 10 mg/mL (7.5 mL); may contain thimerosol and propylene glycol.

Otitis externa:
≥2 yr–adult: 3–4 drops TID–QID × 7–10 days. If preferred, a cotton wick may be saturated and inserted into ear canal. Moisten wick with antibiotic Q4 hr. Change wick Q24 hr.
Ophthalmic:
  Child, adolescent and adult: Instill 1–2 drops into affected eye(s) Q3–4 hr.

Neomycin may cause sensitization. Prolonged treatment may result in overgrowth of nonsusceptible organisms and fungi. May cause cutaneous sensitization.
OTIC USE: Shake suspension well before use. **Contraindicated** in patients with active varicella and herpes simplex and in cases with perforated eardrum (possible ototoxicity). **Use with caution** in chronic otitis media and when integrity of tympanic membrane is in question. Metabisulfite-containing products may cause allergic reactions to susceptible individuals. Hypersensitivity (itching, skin rash, redness, swelling, or other sign of irritation in or around ear) may occur. Warm medication to body temperature befire use.
OPHTHALMIC USE: Use with caution in glaucoma. Blurred vision, burning, and stinging may occur. Increased intraocular pressure and mycosis may occur with prolonged use. Apply finger pressure to lacrimal sac during and for 1–2 min after dose application.

POLYTRIM OPHTHALMIC SOLUTION

See Polymixin B Sulfate and Trimethoprim Sulfate

POTASSIUM IODIDE
Iosat, SSKI, ThyroShield, ThyroSafe, and others
Antithyroid agent

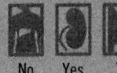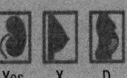

No   Yes   X   D

Tabs:
  Iosat [OTC]: 65 mg (50 mg iodine), 130 mg
  ThyroSafe [OTC]: 65 mg
Oral solution:
  ThyroShield [OTC]: 65 mg/mL (30 mL); contains parabens and saccharin
  Saturated solution (SSKI): 1000 mg/mL (30, 240 mL); 10 drops = 500 mg potassium iodide
  Potassium content is 6 mEq (234 mg) K^+/g potassium iodide.

Neonatal Grave's disease: 50–100 mg (about 1–2 drops of SSKI) PO once daily
Thyrotoxicosis:
  Child: 50–250 mg (about 1–5 drops of SSKI) PO TID
  Adult: 50–500 mg (1–10 drops of SSKI) PO TID

POTASSIUM IODIDE *continued*

Cutaneous or lymphocutaneous sporotrichosis (treat for 4–6 wk after lesions have completely healed; increase dose until either max. dose is achieved or signs of intolerance appear):
   Child and adult: Start with 250 mg PO TID. Doses may be gradually increased as tolerated to the following **max. doses:**
      Child max. dose: 1250–2000 mg PO TID
      Adult max. dose: 2000–2500 mg PO TID

Contraindicated in pregnancy, hyperkalemia, iodine-induced goiter, and hypothyroidism. **Use with caution** in cardiac disease and renal failure. GI disturbance, metallic taste, rash, salivary gland inflammation, headache, lacrimation, and rhinitis are symptoms of iodism. Give with milk or water after meals. Monitor thyroid function tests. Onset of antithyroid effects: 1–2 days.

Lithium carbonate and iodide-containing medications may have synergistic hypothyroid activity. Potassium-containing medications, potassium-sparing diuretics, and ACE inhibitors may increase serum potassium levels.

For use as a thyroid blocking agent in radiation emergencies, see www.fda.gov/cder/guidance/4825fnl.pdf.

PORACTANT ALFA

See Surfactant, pulmonary

POTASSIUM SUPPLEMENTS
Many brand names and generics
Electrolyte

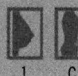

No   Yes   1   C

   Potassium chloride (40 mEq K = 3 g KCl):
      Sustained-release caps: 8, 10 mEq
      Sustained-release tabs: 8, 10, 15, 20 mEq
      Powder: 20, 25 mEq/packet
      Oral solution/liquid: 10% (6.7 mEq/5 mL), 20% (13.3 mEq/5 mL)
      Concentrated injection: 2 mEq/mL
   Potassium gluconate (40 mEq K = 9.4 g K gluconate):
      Tabs: 465 mg (2 mEq), 581 mg (2.5 mEq)
      Caps [OTC as K-99]: 595 mg (2.56 mEq)
   Potassium acetate (40 mEq K = 3.9 g K acetate):
      Concentrated injection: 2, 4 mEq/mL
   Potassium bicarbonate (10 mEq K = 1 g K bicarbonate):
      Caps: 99 mg
      Effervescent tab for oral solution: 25 mEq
   Potassium phosphate:
      See *Phosphorus Supplements.*

Normal daily requirements: **See Chapter 21.**
Replacement: Determine based on maintenance requirements, deficit, and ongoing losses. See Chapter 11.
Hypokalemia:
   Oral:
      Child: 1–4 mEq/kg/24 hr ÷ BID–QID. Monitor serum potassium.
      Adult: 40–100 mEq/24 hr ÷ BID–QID

Continued

POTASSIUM SUPPLEMENTS *continued*

Hypokalemia (cont.)
IV: CLOSELY MONITOR SERUM K.
   Child: 0.5–1 mEq/kg/dose given as an infusion of 0.5 mEq/kg/hr × 1–2 hr
     Max. IV infusion rate: 1 mEq/kg/hr. This may be used in critical situations (i.e., hypokalemia with arrhythmia).
   Adult:
     Serum K ≥ 2.5 mEq/L: Replete at rates up to 10 mEq/hr. **Total dosage not to exceed 200 mEq/24 hr.**
     Serum K < 2 mEq/L: Replete at rates up to 40 mEq/hr. **Total dosage not to exceed 400 mEq/24 hr.**
Max. peripheral IV solution concentration: 40 mEq/L
Max. concentration for central line administration: 150–200 mEq/L

PO administration may cause GI disturbance and ulceration. Oral liquid supplements should be diluted in water or fruit juice before administration. Sustained-release tablets must be swallowed whole and **NOT** dissolved in the mouth or chewed.

Do not administer IV potassium undiluted. IV administration may cause irritation, pain, and phlebitis at infusion site. **Rapid or central IV infusion may cause cardiac arrhythmias.** Patients receiving infusion > 0.5 mEq/kg/hr (>20 mEq/hr for adults) should be placed on ECG monitor.

PRALIDOXIME CHLORIDE
Protopam, 2-PAM, and generics
In combination with atropine: Duodote
Antidote, organophosphate poisoning

| No | Yes | ? | C |

Injection: 1000 mg
Injection for intramuscular injection, in auto-injector device: 600 mg/2 mL (2 mL); dispenses 600 mg; contains benzyl alcohol
In combination with atropine (Duodote): 600 mg/2 mL of pralidoxime and 2.1 mg/0.7 mL of atropine. Duodote must be administered by emergency medical services personnel who have had adequate training in recognition and treatment of nerve agent or insecticide intoxication.

Organophosphate poisoning (use with atropine):
Child:
   IV: 20–50 mg/kg/dose (**max. dose:** 2000 mg) × 1 IV. May repeat in 1–2 hr if muscle weakness is not relieved, then at Q10–12 hr PRN if cholinergic signs reappear.
   IV continuous infusion: Loading dose of 20–50 mg/kg/dose (**max. dose:** 2000 mg) IV over 15–30 min, followed by 10–20 mg/kg/hr.
   IM:
     <40 kg: 15 mg/kg/dose × 1 IM. May repeat Q15 min PRN up to a **max. total dose** of 45 mg/kg for mild symptoms. May repeat twice in rapid succession for severe symptoms (**max. total dose** of 45 mg/kg). For persistent symptoms, may repeat another **max.** 45 mg/kg series (in 3 divided doses) ≈ 1 hr after last injection.
     ≥40 kg: 600 mg × 1 IM. May repeat Q15 min PRN up to a **max. total dose** of 1800 mg for mild symptoms. May repeat twice in rapid succession for severe symptoms (**max. total dose** of 1800 mg). For persistent symptoms, may repeat another **max.** 1800 mg series (in 3 divided doses) ≈ 1 hr after last injection.

PRALIDOXIME CHLORIDE *continued*

Adult:

IV: 1–2 g/dose × 1 IV. May repeat in 1–2 hr if muscle weakness is not relieved, then at Q10–12 hr PRN if cholinergic signs reappear.

IM: Use ≥40 kg child IM dosage from above.

Contraindicated in poisonings due to phosphorus, inorganic phosphates, or organic phosphates without anticholinesterase activity. **Do not use** as an antidote for carbamate classes of pesticides. Removal of secretions and maintaining a patent airway is critical. May cause muscle rigidity, laryngospasm, and tachycardia after rapid IV infusion. Drug is generally ineffective if administered 36–48 hr after exposure. Additional doses may be necessary.

For IV administration, dilute to 50 mg/mL or less, and infuse over 15–30 min (**not to exceed** 200 mg/min). Reduce dosage in renal impairment, since 80%–90% of drug is excreted unchanged in urine 12 hr after administration.

PREDNISOLONE
Oral products:
Orapred, Orapred ODT, Prelone, Pediapred, Millipred, Veripred 20, and generics
Ophthalmic products:
Pred Forte, Pred Mild, Omnipred, and generics
Corticosteroid

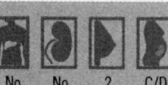

No   No   2   C/D

Tabs: 5 mg
Syrup (Prelone and generics): 15 mg/5 mL (240 mL); may contain alcohol and saccharin
Tablets, orally disintegrating (as Na phosphate) (Orapred ODT): 10, 15, 30 mg
Oral solution (as Na phosphate):
   Pediapred and generics: 5 mg/5 mL (120 mL); alcohol and dye free
   Orapred and generics: 15 mg/5 mL (237 mL); may contain 2% alcohol and is dye free
   Millipred: 10 mg/5 mL (237 mL); contains parabens and is dye free
   Veripred 20: 20 mg/5 mL (237 mL); alcohol and dye free; and contains parabens
Ophthalmic suspension (as acetate): 0.12% (5, 10 mL), 1% (5, 10, 15 mL); contains benzalkonium chloride and may contain bisulfites
Ophthalmic solution (as Na phosphate): 1% (10 mL); may contain benzalkonium chloride

See *Prednisone* (equivalent dosing).
Ophthalmic (consult ophthalmologist before use):
   Child and adult: Start with 1–2 drops Q1 hr during the day and Q2 hr during the night until favorable response, then reduce dose to 1 drop Q4 hr. Dose may be further reduced to 1 drop TID–QID.

See *Prednisone* for remarks. See Chapter 30 for relative steroid potencies. Pregnancy category changes to "D" if used in first trimester. Orapred oral solution product should be stored in refrigerator.

OPHTHALMIC USE: Contraindicated in viral (e.g., herpes simplex, vaccinia and varicella), fungal, and mycobacterial infections of cornea and conjunctiva. Increase in intraocular pressure, cataract formation, and delayed wound healing may occur.

For explanation of icons, see p. 648

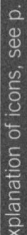

PREDNISONE
Orasone, Deltasone, Liquid Pred, Rayos, and generics
Corticosteroid

Yes   No   2   C/D

Tabs: 1, 2.5, 5, 10, 20, 50 mg
Delayed-release tabs (Rayos): 1, 2, 5 mg
Oral solution: 1 mg/mL (120, 500 mL); may contain 5% alcohol and saccharin
Concentrated solution: 5 mg/mL (30 mL); contains 30% alcohol

Antiinflammatory/immunosuppressive:
   Child: 0.5–2 mg/kg/24 hr PO ÷ once daily–BID
Acute asthma:
   Child: 2 mg/kg/24 hr PO ÷ once daily–BID × 5–7 days. **Max. dose:** 80 mg/24 hr. Patients may
   benefit from tapering if therapy exceeds 5–7 days.
Asthma exacerbations (2007 National Heart, Lung, and Blood Institute Guideline Recommendations;
   dose until peak expiratory flow reaches 70% of predicted or personal best):
   Child ≤ 12 yr: 1–2 mg/kg/24 hr PO ÷ Q12 hr (**max. dose:** 60 mg/24 hr)
   >12 yr and adult: 40–80 mg/24 hr PO ÷ Q12–24 hr
Outpatient asthma exacerbation burst therapy (longer durations may be necessary):
   Child ≤ 12 yr: 1–2 mg/kg/24 hr PO ÷ Q12–24 hr (**max. dose:** 60 mg/24 hr) × 3–10 days
   Child > 12 yr and adult: 40–60 mg/24 hr PO ÷ Q12–24 hr × 5–10 days
Nephrotic syndrome:
   Child: Starting dose of 2 mg/kg/24 hr PO (**max. dose:** 80 mg/24 hr) ÷ once daily–TID is
   recommended. Further treatment plans are individualized. Consult a nephrologist.

See Chapter 30 for physiologic replacement, relative steroid potencies, and doses based on
   body surface area. Methylprednisolone is preferable in hepatic disease, because prednisone
   must be converted to methylprednisolone in the liver.
Side effects may include mood changes, seizures, hyperglycemia, diarrhea, nausea, abdominal
   distension, GI bleeding, HPA axis suppression, osteopenia, cushingoid effects, and cataracts with
   prolonged use. Prednisone is a CYP 450 3A3/4 substrate and inducer. Barbiturates, carbamazepine,
   phenytoin, rifampin, and isoniazid may reduce effects of prednisone, whereas estrogens may
   enhance effects. Pregnancy category changes to "D" if used in first trimester.

PRIMAQUINE PHOSPHATE
Various generic brands
Antimalarial

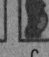

No   No   ?   C

Tabs: 26.3 mg (15 mg base)
Oral suspension: 10.52 mg (6 mg base)/5 mL

Doses expressed in mg of primaquine base.
Malaria:
   Prevention of relapses for Plasmodium vivax or Plasmodium ovale only (initiate therapy
   during last 2 wk of, or after a course of, suppression with chloroquine or comparable drug):
     Child: 0.5 mg/kg/dose (**max. dose:** 30 mg/dose) PO once daily × 14 days
     Adult: 30 mg PO once daily × 14 days
   Prevention of chloroquine-resistant strains (initiate 1 day before departure and continue until
   3–7 days after leaving endemic area):
     Child: 0.5 mg/kg/dose PO once daily; **max. dose:** 30 mg/24 hr
     Adult: 30 mg PO once daily

PRIMAQUINE PHOSPHATE *continued*

Pneumocystis jirovecii (carinii) *pneumonia (in combination with clindamycin):*
   Child: 0.3 mg/kg/dose (**max. dose:** 30 mg/dose) PO once daily × 21 days
   Adult: 30 mg PO once daily × 21 days

Contraindicated in granulocytopenia (e.g., rheumatoid arthritis, lupus erythematosus) and bone marrow suppression. **Avoid use** with quinacrine and other drugs that have a potential for causing hemolysis or bone marrow suppression. **Use with caution** in G6PD and NADH methemoglobin reductase–deficient patients; increased risk for hemolytic anemia and leukopenia, respectively. Use in pregnancy is **not recommended** by the AAP *Red Book*. Cross-sensitivity with iodoquinol.

May cause headache, visual disturbances, nausea, vomiting, and abdominal cramps. Hemolytic anemia, leukopenia, and methemoglobinemia have been reported. Administer all doses with food to mask bitter taste.

PRIMIDONE
Mysoline and generics
Anticonvulsant, barbiturate

| | Yes | Yes | 2 | D |

Tabs: 50, 250 mg

Neonate: 12–20 mg/kg/24 hr PO ÷ BID–QID. Initiate therapy at the lower dosage range and titrate upwards.
Child, adolescent, and adult:

Day of Therapy	<8 yr	≥8 yr and Adult
Days 1–3	50 mg PO QHS	100–125 mg PO QHS
Days 4–6	50 mg PO BID	100–125 mg PO BID
Days 7–9	100 mg PO BID	100–125 mg PO TID
Day 10 and thereafter	125–250 mg PO TID or 10–25 mg/kg/ 24 hr ÷ TID–QID	250 mg PO TID–QID; max. dose: 2 g/24 hr

Use with caution in renal or hepatic disease and pulmonary insufficiency. Primidone is metabolized to phenobarbital and has the same drug interactions and toxicities (see *Phenobarbital*). Additionally, primidone may cause vertigo, nausea, leukopenia, malignant lymphoma–like syndrome, diplopia, nystagmus, and systemic lupus–like syndrome. Monitor for suicidal behavior or ideation. Acetazolamide may decrease primidone absorption. **Adjust dose in renal failure (see Chapter 31).**

Follow both primidone and phenobarbital levels. Therapeutic levels: 5–12 mg/L of primidone and 15–40 mg/L of phenobarbital. Recommended serum sampling time at steady state: trough level obtained within 30 min before next scheduled dose after 1–4 days of continuous dosing.

PROBENECID
Various generic brands
Penicillin therapy adjuvant, uric acid–lowering agent

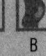
No   Yes   ?   B

Tabs: 500 mg

To prolong penicillin levels:
Child (2–14 yr): 25 mg/kg PO × 1, then 40 mg/kg/24 hr ÷ QID. **Max. single dose:**
500 mg/dose. Use adult dose if >50 kg.
Adult: 500 mg PO QID
Hyperuricemia:
Adult: 250 mg PO BID × 1 wk, then 500 mg PO BID. May increase by 500-mg increments Q4 wk PRN
up to a **max. dose** of 2–3 g/24 hr ÷ BID.
Gonorrhea, antibiotic adjunct (just before antibiotic):
≤45 kg: 23 mg/kg/dose PO × 1 just before antibiotic
>45 kg: 1 g PO × 1

Use with caution in patients with peptic ulcer disease. **Contraindicated** in children <2 yr
and patients with renal insufficiency. **Do not use** if GFR < 30 mL/min.
Increases uric acid excretion. Inhibits renal tubular secretion of acyclovir, ganciclovir,
ciprofloxacin, levofloxacin, nalidixic acid, moxifloxacin, organic acids, penicillins, cephalosporins,
AZT, dapsone, methotrexate, NSAIDs, and benzodiazepines. Salicylates may decrease probenecid's
activity. Alkalinize urine in patients with gout. May cause headache, GI symptoms, rash, anemia,
and hypersensitivity. False-positive glucosuria with Clinitest may occur.

PROCAINAMIDE
Various generic brands
Antiarrhythmic, class Ia

Yes   Yes   X   C

Injection: 500 mg/mL (2, 10 mL); may contain methylparabens and bisulfites

Child:
V. tach with poor perfusion: Consider 15 mg/kg/dose IV × 1 over 30–60 min if cardioversion
ineffective. Follow with continuous infusion if effective (see information that follows).
   IM: 20–30 mg/kg/24 hr ÷ Q4–6 hr; **max. dose:** 4 g/24 hr (peak effect in 1 hr)
   IV: Loading: 3–6 mg/kg/dose over 5 min (**max. dose:** 100 mg/dose). Repeat dose Q5–10 min
   PRN up to a **total max. dose** of 15 mg/kg. **Do not exceed** 500 mg in 30 min.
      Maintenance: 20–80 mcg/kg/min by continuous infusion; **max. dose:** 2 g/24 hr
Adult:
   IM: 50 mg/kg/24 hr ÷ Q3–6 hr
   IV: Loading: 50–100 mg/dose. Repeat dose Q5 min PRN to a **max. total dose** of 1000–1500 mg.
      Maintenance: 1–6 mg/min by continuous infusion
NOTE: IV infusion dosage units for adults are in mg/min, compared with mcg/kg/min for children.

Contraindicated in myasthenia gravis, complete heart block, SLE, and torsades de pointes.
Use with caution in asymptomatic PVCs, digitalis intoxication, CHF, renal or hepatic
dysfunction. **Adjust dose in renal failure (see Chapter 31).**
May cause lupus-like syndrome, positive Coombs test, thrombocytopenia, arrhythmias, GI complaints,
and confusion. Increased LFTs and liver failure have been reported. Monitor BP and ECG when using
IV. QRS widening by >0.02 sec suggests toxicity.

PROCAINAMIDE *continued*

Do not use with desipramine and other TCAs. Cimetidine, ranitidine, amiodarone, β-blockers, and trimethoprim may increase procainamide levels. Procainamide may enhance effects of skeletal muscle relaxants and anticholinergic agents. Therapeutic levels: 4–10 mg/L of procainamide or 10–30 mg/L of procainamide and NAPA levels combined.

Recommended serum sampling times:

IM intermittent dosing: Trough level within 30 min before next scheduled dose after 2 days of continuous dosing (steady state).

IV continuous infusion: 2 and 12 hr after start of infusion and at 24-hr intervals thereafter.

PROCHLORPERAZINE
Compazine and generics
Antiemetic, phenothiazine derivative

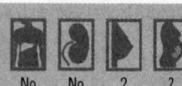

| No | No | 2 | ? |

Tabs (as maleate): 5, 10 mg
Suppository: 25 mg (12s)
Injection (as edisylate): 5 mg/mL (2, 10 mL); may contain bisulfites and benzyl alcohol

Antiemetic doses:
Child (>10 kg or > 2 yr):
   PO or PR: 0.4 mg/kg/24 hr ÷ TID–QID **OR** alternative dosing by weight:
      10–14 kg: 2.5 mg once daily–BID; **max. dose:** 7.5 mg/24 hr
      15–18 kg: 2.5 mg BID–TID; **max. dose:** 10 mg/24 hr
      19–39 kg: 2.5 mg TID or 5 mg BID; **max. dose:** 15 mg/24 hr
      >39 kg: Use adult dose.
   IM: 0.1–0.15 mg/kg/dose TID–QID; **max. dose:** 10 mg/single dose or 40 mg/24 hr
Adult:
   PO: 5–10 mg/dose TID–QID; **max. dose:** 40 mg/24 hr
   PR: 25 mg/dose BID
   IM: 5–10 mg/dose Q3–4 hr
   IV: 2.5–10 mg/dose; may repeat Q3–4 hr
   Max. IM/IV dose: 40 mg/24 hr
Psychoses:
Child 2–12 yr and >9 kg:
   PO: Start with 2.5 mg BID–TID with a **max. first day dose** of 10 mg/24 hr. Dose may be increased as needed to 20 mg/24 hr for children 2–5 yr and 25 mg/24 hr for 6–12 yr.
   IM: 0.13 mg/kg/dose × 1 and convert to PO immediately.
Adult:
   PO: 5–10 mg TID–QID; may be increased as needed to a **max. dose** of 150 mg/24 hr.
   IM: 10–20 mg Q2–4 hr PRN; convert to PO immediately.

Toxicity as for other phenothiazines (see *Chlorpromazine*). Extrapyramidal reactions (reversed by diphenhydramine) or orthostatic hypotension may occur. May mask signs and symptoms of overdosage of other drugs and may obscure diagnosis and treatment of conditions such as intestinal obstruction, brain tumor, and Reye syndrome. May cause false-positive test for phenylketonuria, urinary amylase, uroporphyrins, and urobilinogen. **Do not use** IV route in children. Use only in management of prolonged vomiting of known etiology.

For children 5–18 yr, a 0.15-mg/kg/dose IV over 10 min was effective in migraine headaches presenting in emergency departments (see *Ann Emerg Med.* 2004;43:256-262).

Pregnancy category has not been formally assigned by the FDA.

For explanation of icons, see p. 648

FORMULARY

PROMETHAZINE
Phenergan and generics
Antihistamine, antiemetic, phenothiazine derivative

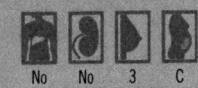

No   No   3   C

Tabs: 12.5, 25, 50 mg
Oral solution/syrup: 6.25 mg/5 mL (118, 473 mL); contains alcohol
Suppository: 12.5, 25, 50 mg (12s)
Injection: 25, 50 mg/mL (1 mL); may contain sulfites

Antihistaminic:
 Child ≥ 2 yr: 0.1 mg/kg/dose (**max. dose:** 12.5 mg/dose) Q6 hr PO during daytime hours
 and 0.5 mg/kg/dose (**max. dose:** 25 mg/dose) QHS PO PRN
 Adult: 6.25–12.5 mg PO/PR TID and 25 mg QHS
Nausea and vomiting PO/IM/IV/PR (see remarks):
 Child ≥ 2 yr: 0.25–1 mg/kg/dose Q4–6 hr PRN; **max. dose:** 25 mg/dose
 Adult: 12.5–25 mg Q4–6 hr PRN
Motion sickness: (1st dose 0.5–1 hr before departure):
 Child ≥ 2 yr: 0.5 mg/kg/dose Q12 hr PO/PR PRN; **max. dose:** 25 mg/dose
 Adult: 25 mg PO Q8–12 hr PRN

Avoid use in children <2 yr because of risk for fatal respiratory depression. Toxicity similar to
other phenothiazines (see *Chlorpromazine*). **Do not** administer SC or intraarterially because
of severe local reactions. IV route of administration is **not recommended** (IM preferred)
owing to severe tissue injury (tissue necrosis and gangrene). If using IV route, dilute 25 mg/
mL–strength product with 10–20 mL NS, and administer over 10–15 min; consider lower
initial doses, administer through a large-bore vein, check patency of line before
administering, administer through an IV line at the port farthest from the patient's vein,
and monitor for burning or pain during or after injection. Administer oral doses with meals
to decrease GI irritation.
May cause profound sedation, blurred vision, respiratory depression (use lowest effective dose in
children and **avoid** concomitant use of respiratory depressants), and dystonic reactions (reversed by
diphenhydramine). Cholestatic jaundice and neuroleptic malignant syndrome has been reported. May
interfere with pregnancy tests (immunologic reactions between hCG and anti-hCG). **For nausea and
vomiting, use only in management of prolonged vomiting of known etiology.**

PROPRANOLOL
Inderal, Inderal LA, and generics
Adrenergic blocking agent (beta), class II antiarrhythmic

Yes   Yes   1   C/D

Tabs: 10, 20, 40, 60, 80 mg
Extended-release caps (Inderal LA and others): 60, 80, 120, 160 mg
Oral solution: 20 mg/5 mL, 40 mg/5 mL; contains parabens and saccharin
Concentrated solution: 80 mg/mL; alcohol and dye free
Injection: 1 mg/mL (1 mL)

Arrhythmias:
 Child:
  IV: 0.01–0.1 mg/kg/dose IV push over 10 min, repeat Q6–8 hr PRN; **max. dose:**
  1 mg/dose for infant; 3 mg/dose for child
  PO: Start at 0.5–1 mg/kg/24 hr ÷ Q6–8 hr; increase dosage Q3–5 days PRN. Usual dosage range:
  2–4 mg/kg/24 hr ÷ Q6–8 hr; **max. dose:** 60 mg/24 hr or 16 mg/kg/24 hr

PROPRANOLOL *continued*

> **Adult:**
> > **IV:** 1 mg/dose Q5 min up to **total** 5 mg
> > **PO:** 10–20 mg/dose TID–QID; increase PRN. Usual range: 40–320 mg/24 hr ÷ TID–QID.
>
> **Hypertension:**
> > **Child:**
> > > **PO:** Initial: 0.5–1 mg/kg/24 hr ÷ Q6–12 hr. May increase dose Q5–7 days PRN to **max. dose** of 8 mg/kg/24 hr.
> >
> > **Adult:**
> > > **PO:** 40 mg/dose PO BID or 60–80 mg/dose (sustained-release capsule) PO once daily. May increase 10–20 mg/dose Q3–7 days; **max. dose:** 640 mg/24 hr
>
> **Migraine prophylaxis:**
> > **Child:**
> > > **<35 kg:** 10–20 mg PO TID
> > > **≥35 kg:** 20–40 mg PO TID
> >
> > **Adult:** 80 mg/24 hr ÷ Q6–8 hr PO; increase dose by 20–40 mg/dose Q3–4 wk PRN. Usual effective dose range: 160–240 mg/24 hr.
>
> **Tetralogy spells:**
> > **IV:** 0.15–0.25 mg/kg/dose slow IV push. May repeat in 15 min × 1. See Chapter 7.
> > **PO:** Start at 2–4 mg/kg/24 hr ÷ Q6 hr PRN. Usual dose range: 4–8 mg/kg/24 hr ÷ Q6 hr PRN. Doses as high as 15 mg/kg/24 hr have been used with careful monitoring.
>
> **Thyrotoxicosis:**
> > **Neonate:** 2 mg/kg/24 hr PO ÷ Q6–12 hr
> > **Adolescent and adult:**
> > > **IV:** 1–3 mg/dose over 10 min. May repeat in 4–6 hr.
> > > **PO:** 10–40 mg/dose PO Q6 hr
>
> **Infantile hemangioma (see remarks):**
> > Start at 1 mg/kg/24 hr ÷ Q8 hr PO. If tolerated after 1 day, increase dose to 2 mg/kg/24 hr ÷ Q8 hr PO.

Contraindicated in asthma, Raynaud syndrome, heart failure, and heart block. **Not indicated** for treatment of hypertensive emergencies. **Use with caution** in presence of obstructive lung disease, diabetes mellitus, renal or hepatic disease. May cause hypoglycemia, hypotension, nausea, vomiting, depression, weakness, impotence, bronchospasm, and heart block. Cutaneous reactions, including Stevens-Johnson syndrome, TEN, exfoliative dermatitis, erythema multiforme, and urticaria have been reported. Acute hypertension has occurred after insulin-induced hypoglycemia in patients on propranolol.

Therapeutic levels: 30–100 ng/mL. Drug is metabolized by CYP 450 1A2, 2C18, 2C19, and 2D6 isoenzymes. Concurrent administration with barbiturates, indomethacin, or rifampin may cause decreased activity of propranolol. Concurrent administration with cimetidine, hydralazine, flecainide, quinidine, chlorpromazine, or verapamil may lead to increased activity of propranolol. **Avoid** IV use of propranolol with calcium channel blockers; may increase effect of calcium channel blocker. Use with amiodarone may increase negative chronotropic effects.

For infantile hemangioma, monitor BP, HR, and blood glucose. Infants <6 mo must be fed Q4 hr. Successful use in infantile hepatic hemangiomas has also been reported.

Pregnancy category changes to "D" if used in second or third trimesters.

For explanation of icons, see p. 648

PROPYLTHIOURACIL
PTU and generics
Antithyroid agent

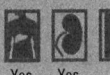

Yes   Yes   2   D

Tabs: 50 mg
Oral suspension: 5 mg/mL
100 mg PTU = 10 mg methimazole

Dosages should be adjusted as required to achieve and maintain T_4, TSH levels in normal ranges.

Neonate: 5–10 mg/kg/24 hr ÷ Q8 hr PO

Child:
  Initial: 5–7 mg/kg/24 hr ÷ Q8 hr PO, OR by age:
    6–10 yr: 50–150 mg/24 hr ÷ Q8 hr PO
    >10 yr: 150–300 mg/24 hr ÷ Q8 hr PO
  Maintenance: Generally begins after 2 mo. Usually ⅓–⅔ initial dose in divided doses (Q8–12 hr) when patient is euthyroid.

Adult:
  Initial: 300–400 mg/24 hr ÷ Q6–8 hr PO; some may require larger doses of 600–900 mg/24 hr.
  Maintenance: 100–150 mg/24 hr ÷ Q8 hr PO

May cause blood dyscrasias, fever, liver disease, dermatitis, urticaria, malaise, CNS stimulation or depression, and arthralgias. Glomerulonephritis, severe liver injury/failure, agranulocytosis, interstitial pneumonitis, exfoliative dermatitis, and erythema nodosum have also been reported. May decrease effectiveness of warfarin. Monitor thyroid function. A dose reduction of β-blocker may be necessary when hyperthyroid patient becomes euthyroid.

For neonates, crush tablets, weigh appropriate dose, and mix in formula/breast milk. **Adjust dose in renal failure (see Chapter 31).**

PROSTAGLANDIN E₁

See Alprostadil

PROTAMINE SULFATE
Various generic brands
Antidote, heparin

No   No   ?   C

Injection: 10 mg/mL (5, 25 mL); preservative free

Heparin antidote, IV:
1 mg protamine will neutralize 115 U porcine intestinal heparin, 90 U beef lung heparin, or 100 U (1 mg) low-molecular-weight heparin.

Consider time since last heparin dose:
  If < 0.5 hr: Give 100% of specified dose.
  If within 0.5–1 hr: Give 50%–75% of aforementioned dose.
  If within 1–2 hr: Give 37.5%–50% of aforementioned dose.
  If ≥ 2 hr: Give 25%–37.5% of aforementioned dose.
  Max. dose: 50 mg IV
  Max. infusion rate: 5 mg/min
  Max. IV concentration: 10 mg/mL

FORMULARY

PROTAMINE SULFATE *continued*

If heparin was administered by deep SC injection, give 1–1.5 mg protamine per 100 U heparin as
follows:
Load with 25–50 mg via slow IV infusion, followed by rest of calculated dose via continuous infusion
over 8–16 hr or expected duration of heparin absorption.

Enoxaparin overdosage, IV (see remarks): ≈ 1 mg protamine will neutralize 1 mg enoxaparin.
Consider time since last enoxaparin dose:
If < 8 hr: Give 100% of aforementioned dose.
If within 8–12 hr: Give 50% of aforementioned dose.
If > 12 hr: Protamine not required, but if serious bleeding is present, give 50% of aforementioned dose.
If APTT remains prolonged 2–4 hr after first protamine dose, a second infusion of 0.5 mg
protamine per 1 mg enoxaparin may be given.
Max. dose: 50 mg. See *Heparin* antidote IV dosage for **max.** administration concentration and rate.

Risk factors for protamine hypersensitivity include known hypersensitivity to fish and exposure
to protamine-containing insulin or prior protamine therapy.

May cause hypotension, bradycardia, dyspnea, and anaphylaxis. Monitor APTT or ACT.

Heparin rebound with bleeding has been reported to occur 8–18 hr later.

Use in enoxaparin overdose may not be complete despite using multiple doses of protamine.

PSEUDOEPHEDRINE
Sudafed, Sudafed 12 Hour, Sudafed 24 Hour, and generics
Sympathomimetic, nasal decongestant

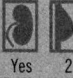

No   Yes   2   C

Tabs [OTC]: 30, 60 mg
Extended-release tab [OTC]:
Sudafed 12 Hour: 120 mg
Sudafed 24 Hour: 240 mg
Oral liquid [OTC]: 15 mg/5 mL, 30 mg/5 mL (120, 473 mL)
Oral syrup [OTC]: 30 mg/5 mL (473 mL); contains parabens
Purchases of OTC products are limited to behind the pharmacy counter sales, with monthly sale
limits because of the methamphetamine epidemic.

Child < 12 yr: 4 mg/kg/24 hr ÷ Q6 hr PO or by age:
<4 yr: 4 mg/kg/24 hr ÷ Q6 hr PO
4–5 yr: 15 mg/dose Q4–6 hr PO; **max. dose:** 60 mg/24 hr
6–12 yr: 30 mg/dose Q4–6 hr PO; **max. dose:** 120 mg/24 hr
Child ≥ 12 yr and adult:
Immediate release: 30–60 mg/dose Q4–6 hr PO; **max. dose:** 240 mg/24 hr
Sustained release:
Sudafed 12 Hour: 120 mg PO Q12 hr
Sudafed 24 Hour: 240 mg PO Q24 hr

Contraindicated with MAOI drugs and in severe hypertension and severe coronary artery
disease. **Use with caution** in mild/moderate hypertension, hyperglycemia, hyperthyroidism,
and cardiac disease. May cause dizziness, nervousness, restlessness, insomnia, and
arrhythmias. Pseudoephedrine is a common component of OTC cough and cold preparations
and is combined with several antihistamines; these products are not recommended for
children <6 yr. Because drug and active metabolite are primarily excreted renally, **doses**
should be adjusted in renal impairment. May cause false-positive test for amphetamines
(EMIT assay).

For explanation of icons, see p. 648

PSYLLIUM
Metamucil, Fiberall, Konsyl, Reguloid, and many others
Bulk-forming laxative

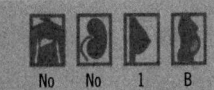

No   No   1   B

Granules [OTC]: 100% psyllium (Konsyl: 6 g/rounded teaspoon) (300 g); contains maltodextrin; sugar and gluten free
Powder [OTC]: 100% psyllium, some versions containing sucrose (sugar-free version available) (Metamucil: 3.4 g/rounded teaspoon). For other products, check label for amount of psyllium per unit of measurement.
Caps (Konsyl and Reguloid): 0.52 g
3.4 g psyllium hydrophilic mucilloid is equivalent to 2 g soluble fiber.

Constipation (granules or powder must be mixed with a full glass of water or juice):
<6 yr: 1.25–2.5 g/dose PO once daily–TID; **max. dose:** 7.5 g/24 hr
6–11 yr: 2.5–3.75 g/dose PO once daily–TID; **max. dose:** 15 g/24 hr
≥12 yr and adult: 2.5–7.5 g/dose PO once daily–TID; **max. dose:** 30 g/24 hr

Contraindicated in cases of fecal impaction or GI obstruction. **Use with caution** in patients with esophageal strictures and rectal bleeding. Phenylketonurics should be aware that certain preparations may contain aspartame. Should be taken with a full glass (240 mL) of liquid. Onset of action: 12–72 hr.

PYRANTEL PAMOATE
Reese's Pinworm, Pamix, Pin-Rid, Pin-X, and generics
Anthelmintic

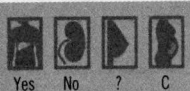

Yes   No   ?   C

Oral suspension [OTC]: 50 mg/mL pyrantel base (144 mg/mL pyrantel pamoate) (30, 60, 240 mL); may contain sodium benzoate, parabens, and saccharin
Tabs [OTC]: 62.5 mg pyrantel base (180 mg pyrantel pamoate)
Chewable tabs [OTC]: 250 mg pyrantel base (720.5 mg pyrantel pamoate); contains aspartame

All doses expressed in terms of pyrantel base.
Child (≥2 yr) and adult:
Ascaris *(roundworm)* and **Trichostrongylus:** 11 mg/kg/dose PO × 1
Enterobius *(pinworm):* 11 mg/kg/dose PO × 1. Repeat same dose 2 wk later.
Hookworm or eosinophilic enterocolitis: 11 mg/kg/dose PO once daily × 3 days
Moniliformis: 11 mg/kg/dose PO × 1. Repeat twice 2 weeks apart.
Max. dose (all indications): 1 g/dose

Use with caution in liver dysfunction. **Do not use** in combination with piperazine because of antagonism. May cause nausea, vomiting, anorexia, transient AST elevations, headaches, rash, and muscle weakness. Limited experience in children <2 yr. May increase theophylline levels. Drug may be mixed with milk or fruit juice and may be taken with food.

PYRAZINAMIDE
Pyrazinoic acid amide and generics
Antituberculous agent

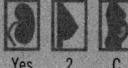
Yes   Yes   2   C

Tab: 500 mg
Oral suspension: 10, 100 mg/mL
In combination with isoniazid and rifampin (Rifater):
   Tab: 300 mg with 50 mg isoniazid and 120 mg rifampin; contains povidone and propylene glycol

Tuberculosis: Use as part of a multidrug regimen for tuberculosis. See latest edition
of AAP *Red Book* for recommended treatment for tuberculosis.
   Child:
      Daily dose: 30–40 mg/kg/24 hr PO ÷ once daily–BID; **max. dose:** 2 g/24 hr
      Twice-weekly dose: 50 mg/kg/dose PO 2 × per week; **max. dose:** 2 g/dose
   Adult:
      Daily dose: 15–30 mg/kg/24 hr PO ÷ once daily–QID; **max. dose:** 2 g/24 hr
      Twice-weekly dose: 50–70 mg/kg/dose PO 2 × per week; **max. dose:** 4 g/dose
Mycobacterium tuberculosis in HIV, prophylaxis to prevent first episode:
   Infant and child: Not recommended because of increased risk of severe/fatal hepatotoxicity
   Adolescent and adult: 15–20 mg/kg/24 hr PO once daily × 2 mo in combination with either 600 mg
   rifampin PO once daily × 2 mo or 300 mg rifabutin PO once daily × 2 mo

See latest edition of the AAP *Red Book* for recommended treatment for tuberculosis.
   Contraindicated in severe hepatic damage and acute gout. The CDC and ATS **do not**
   recommend the combination of pyrazinamide and rifampin for latent TB infections. **Use with**
   caution in patients with renal failure (dosage reduction has been recommended), gout, or
   diabetes mellitus. Monitor liver function tests (baseline and periodic) and serum uric acid.
Hepatotoxicity is most common dose-related side effect; doses ≤30 mg/kg/24 hr minimize effect.
Hyperuricemia, maculopapular rash, arthralgia, fever, acne, porphyria, dysuria, and photosensitivity
may occur. Severe hepatic toxicity may occur with rifampin use. May decrease isoniazid levels.

PYRETHRINS WITH PIPERONYL BUTOXIDE
Tisit, A-200, Pyrinyl, Pronto, RID, Licide, Klout, and others
Pediculicide

  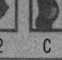
No   No   2   C

All products are available without a prescription.
   Lotion (Tisit): 0.3% pyrethrins and 2% piperonyl butoxide (59, 118 mL); contains petroleum
   distillate and equivalent to 1.6% ether
   Gel (Tisit): 0.3% pyrethrins and 3% piperonyl butoxide (30 mL)
   Shampoo (Tisit, RID, Pronto, Licide, Klout, A-200): 0.33% pyrethrins and 4% piperonyl butoxide
   (60, 120, 240 mL); may contain alcohol
   Mousse (RID): 0.33% pyrethrins and 4% piperonyl butoxide (165 mL); contains alcohol

Pediculosis: Apply to hair or affected body area for 10 min, then wash thoroughly and comb
with fine-tooth or nit-removing comb; repeat in 7–10 days.

Contraindicated in ragweed hypersensitivity; drug is derived from chrysanthemum flowers. For
topical use only. **Avoid** use in and around the eyes, mouth, nose, or vagina. **Avoid** repeat
applications in <24 hr. Low ovicidal activity requires repeat treatment. Dead nits require
mechanical removal. Wash bedding and clothing to eradicate infestation.
Local irritation, including erythema, pruritus, urticaria, edema, and eczema may occur.

For explanation of icons, see p. 648

PYRIDOSTIGMINE BROMIDE
Mestinon, Regonol, and generics
Cholinergic agent

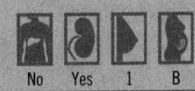

No   Yes   1   B

Oral syrup: 60 mg/5 mL (480 mL); contains 5% alcohol
Tabs: 60 mg
Sustained-release tab: 180 mg
Injection (Regonol): 5 mg/mL (2 mL); may contain 0.2% parabens and benzyl alcohol

Myasthenia gravis:
  Neonate:
    PO: 5 mg/dose Q4–6 hr
    IM/IV: 0.05–0.15 mg/kg/dose Q4–6 hr; **max. single IM/IV dose:** 10 mg
  Child:
    PO: 7 mg/kg/24 hr in 5–6 divided doses
    IM/IV: 0.05–0.15 mg/kg/dose Q4–6 hr; **max. single IM/IV dose:** 10 mg
  Adult:
    PO (immediate release): 60 mg TID; increase Q48 hr PRN. Usual effective dose:
    60–1500 mg/24 hr.
    PO (sustained release): 180–540 mg once daily–BID
    IM/IV (use when PO therapy is not practical): Give 1/30 of the usual PO.

Contraindicated in mechanical intestinal or urinary obstruction. **Use with caution** in patients with epilepsy, asthma, bradycardia, hyperthyroidism, arrhythmias, or peptic ulcer. May cause nausea, vomiting, diarrhea, rash, headache, and muscle cramps. Pyridostigmine is mainly excreted unchanged by the kidney. Therefore, lower doses titrated to effect in renal disease may be necessary.

Changes in oral dosages may take several days to show results. **Atropine is the antidote.**

PYRIDOXINE
Vitamin B$_6$, and various names, including generics
Vitamin, water soluble

No   No   1   A/C

Tabs (HCl) [OTC]: 25, 50, 100, 250, 500 mg
Oral solution (HCl): 1 mg/mL
Injection (HCl): 100 mg/mL (1 mL); some products may contain aluminum.

Deficiency, IM/IV/PO (PO preferred):
  Child: 5–25 mg/24 hr × 3 wk, followed by 2.5–5 mg/24 hr as maintenance therapy
  (via multivitamin preparation)
  Adolescent and adult: 10–20 mg/24 hr × 3 wk, followed by 2–5 mg/24 hr as maintenance therapy
  (via multivitamin preparation)
Drug-induced neuritis (PO):
  Prophylaxis:
    Child: 1 mg/kg/24 hr or 10–50 mg/24 hr
    Adolescent and adult: 25–50 mg/24 hr
  Treatment (optimal dose not established):
    Child: 50–200 mg/24 hr
    Adolescent and adult: 50–300 mg/24 hr

PYRIDOXINE *continued*

Pyridoxine-dependent seizures:
  Neonate and infant:
    Initial: 50–100 mg/dose IM or rapid IV × 1
    Maintenance: 50–100 mg/24 hr PO
Recommended daily allowance: See Chapter 21.

Use caution with concurrent levodopa therapy. Chronic administration has been associated with sensory neuropathy. Nausea, headache, increased AST, decreased serum folic acid level, and allergic reaction may occur. May lower phenobarbital and phenytoin levels. See Chapter 20 for management of neonatal seizures.

Pregnancy category changes to "C" if dosage exceeds U.S. RDA recommendation.

PYRIMETHAMINE
Daraprim
Antiparasitic agent

Yes   Yes   2   C

Tabs: 25 mg
Oral suspension: 2 mg/mL
Combination product with sulfadoxine (Fansidar) is no longer available in the United States.

Congenital toxoplasmosis (administer with sulfadiazine and leucovorin [see remarks]):
  Loading dose: 2 mg/kg/24 hr PO ÷ Q12 hr × 2 days
  Maintenance: 1 mg/kg/24 hr PO once daily × 2–6 mo, then 1 mg/kg/24 hr 3 × per wk
  to complete total 12 mo of therapy
Toxoplasmosis (administer with sulfadiazine or trisulfapyrimidines, and leucovorin):
  Child:
    Loading: 2 mg/kg/24 hr PO ÷ BID × 3 days; **max. dose:** 100 mg/24 hr
    Maintenance: 1 mg/kg/24 hr PO ÷ once daily–BID × 4 wk; **max. dose:** 25 mg/24 hr
  Adult: 50–75 mg/24 hr × 3–4 wk depending on response. After response, decrease dose by 50% and continue for an additional 4–5 wk.

Pyrimethamine is a folate antagonist. Supplementation with folinic acid leucovorin at 5–15 mg/24 hr is recommended. **Contraindicated** in megaloblastic anemia secondary to folate deficiency. **Use with caution** in G6PD deficiency, malabsorption syndromes, alcoholism, pregnancy, and renal or hepatic impairment. Pyrimethamine can cause glossitis, bone marrow suppression, seizures, rash, and photosensitivity. For congenital toxoplasmosis, see *Clin Infect Dis.* 1994;18:38-72. Zidovudine and methotrexate may increase risk for bone marrow suppression. Aurothioglucose, trimethoprim, and sulfamethoxazole may increase risk for blood dyscrasias. Administer doses with meals. Most cases of acquired toxoplasmosis **do not** require specific antimicrobial therapy.

QUINIDINE
Various generic brands
Class Ia antiarrhythmic

Yes   Yes   2   C

As gluconate (62% quinidine):
  Slow-release tabs: 324 mg
  Injection: 80 mg/mL (50 mg/mL quinidine) (10 mL); contains phenol
As sulfate (83% quinidine):

Continued

QUINIDINE *continued*

Tabs: 200, 300 mg
Slow-release tab: 300 mg
Oral suspension: 10 mg/mL
Equivalents: 200 mg sulfate = 267 mg gluconate

All doses expressed as salt forms.

Antiarrhythmic:

Child (give PO as sulfate; give IM/IV as gluconate):

Test dose: 2 mg/kg × 1 IM/PO; **max. dose:** 200 mg

Therapeutic dose:

IV (as gluconate): 2–10 mg/kg/dose Q3–6 hr PRN

PO (as sulfate): 15–60 mg/kg/24 hr ÷ Q6 hr

Adult (give PO as sulfate; give IM as gluconate):

Test dose: 200 mg × 1 IM/PO

Therapeutic dose:

As sulfate:

PO, immediate-release: 100–600 mg/dose Q4–6 hr. Begin at 200 mg/dose and titrate to desired effect.

PO, sustained release: 300–600 mg/dose Q 8–12 hr

As gluconate:

IM: 400 mg/dose Q4–6 hr

IV: 200–400 mg/dose, infused at a rate of ≤10 mg/min

PO: 324–972 mg Q8–12 hr

Malaria:

Child and adult (give IV as gluconate [see remarks]):

Loading dose: 10 mg/kg/dose (**max. dose:** 600 mg) IV over 1–2 hr, followed by maintenance dose. Omit or decrease load if patient has received quinine or mefloquine.

Maintenance dose: 0.02 mg/kg/min IV as continuous infusion until oral therapy can be initiated. If more than 48 hr of IV therapy is required, reduce dose by 30%–50%.

Test dose is given to assess for idiosyncratic reaction to quinidine. Toxicity indicated by increase of QRS interval by ≥0.02 sec (skip dose or stop drug). May cause GI symptoms, hypotension, tinnitus, TTP, rash, heart block, and blood dyscrasias. When used alone, may cause 1:1 conduction in atrial flutter, leading to ventricular fibrillation. May get idiosyncratic ventricular tachycardia with low levels, especially when initiating therapy.

Quinidine is a substrate of CYP 450 3A3/4 and 3A5–7 enzymes, and an inhibitor of CYP 450 2D6 and 3A3/4 enzymes. Can cause increase in digoxin levels. Quinidine potentiates effect of neuromuscular blocking agents, β-blockers, anticholinergics, and warfarin. Amiodarone, antacids, delavirdine, diltiazem, grapefruit juice, saquinavir, ritonavir, verapamil, or cimetidine may enhance drug's effect. Barbiturates, phenytoin, cholinergic drugs, nifedipine, sucralfate, or rifampin may reduce quinidine's effect. **Use with caution** in renal insufficiency (15%–25% of drug is eliminated unchanged in the urine), myocardial depression, sick sinus syndrome, G6PD deficiency, and hepatic dysfunction.

Therapeutic levels: 3–7 mg/L. Recommended serum sampling times at steady state: trough level obtained within 30 min before next scheduled dose after 1–2 days of continuous dosing (steady state).

MALARIA USE: Continuous monitoring of ECG, BP, and serum glucose are recommended, especially in pregnant women and young children.

QUINUPRISTIN AND DALFOPRISTIN
Synercid
Antibiotic, streptogramin

Yes   No   ?   B

Injection: 500 mg (150 mg quinupristin and 350 mg dalfopristin)

Doses expressed in mg of combined quinupristin and dalfopristin.
Vancomycin-resistant Enterococcus faecium (VREF):
  Child < 16 yr (limited data), ≥ *16 yr and adult:* 7.5 mg/kg/dose IV Q8 hr
Complicated skin infections:
  Child < 16 yr (limited data), ≥ *16 yr and adult:* 7.5 mg/kg/dose IV Q12 hr for at least 7 days
VREF endocarditis:
  Child and adult: 7.5 mg/kg/dose IV Q8 hr for at least 8 weeks

---

Not active against *Enterococcus faecalis.* **Use with caution** in hepatic impairment; dosage
reduction may be necessary. Most common side effects include pain, burning, inflammation
and edema at IV infusion site, thrombophlebitis and thrombosis, GI disturbances, rash,
arthralgia, myalgia, increased liver enzymes, hyperbilirubinemia, and headache. Dose-
frequency reductions (Q8 hr to Q12 hr) or discontinuation can improve severe cases of
arthralgia and myalgia. Use total body weight for obese patients when calculating dosages.
Drug is an inhibitor of CYP 450 3A4 isoenzyme. **Avoid use** with CYP 450 3A4 substrates, which can
prolong QTc interval (e.g., cisapride). May increase effects/toxicity of cyclosporine, tacrolimus,
sirolimus, delavirdine, nevirapine, indinavir, ritonavir, diazepam, midazolam, carbamazepine,
methylprednisolone, vinca alkaloids, docetaxel, paclitaxel, quinidine, and some calcium channel
blockers.
Pediatric pharmacokinetic studies have not been completed. Reduce dose for patients with hepatic
cirrhosis (Child-Pugh A or B).
Drug is compatible with D_5W and incompatible with saline and heparin. Infuse each dose over 1 hr
using the following **max. IV concentrations:** peripheral line, 2 mg/mL; central line, 5 mg/mL. If
injection site reaction occurs, dilute infusion to <1 mg/mL.

RANITIDINE HCL
Zantac, Zantac 75 [OTC], Zantac 150 Maximum Strength [OTC],
and many generics
Histamine-2-antagonist

Yes   Yes   1   B

Tabs: 75 [OTC], 150 [OTC and Rx], 300 mg
Caps: 150, 300 mg
Oral syrup: 15 mg/mL (480 mL); may contain 7.5% alcohol and parabens
Injection: 25 mg/mL (2, 6, 40 mL); may contain 0.5% phenol

Neonate:
  PO: 2–4 mg/kg/24 hr ÷ Q8–12 hr
  IV: 2 mg/kg/24 hr ÷ Q6–8 hr
≥*1 mo–16 yr:*
  Duodenal/gastric ulcer (see remarks):
    PO:
      Treatment: 4–8 mg/kg/24 hr ÷ Q12 hr; **max. dose:** 300 mg/24 hr
      Maintenance: 2–4 mg/kg/24 hr ÷ Q12 hr; **max. dose:** 150 mg/24 hr
    IV/IM: 2–4 mg/kg/24 hr ÷ Q6–8 hr; **max. dose:** 200 mg/24 hr

Continued

RANITIDINE HCL *continued*

> ### *GERD/erosive esophagitis:*
> **PO:** 5–10 mg/kg/24 hr ÷ Q8–12 hr. **GERD max. dose:** 300 mg/24 hr; **erosive esophagitis max. dose:** 600 mg/24 hr
> **IV/IM:** 2–4 mg/kg/24 hr ÷ Q6–8 hr; **max. dose:** 200 mg/24 hr
> ### *Adolescent and adult:*
> **PO:** 150 mg/dose BID or 300 mg/dose QHS
> **IM/IV:** 50 mg/dose Q6–8 hr; **max. dose:** 400 mg/24 hr
> ***Continuous infusion, all ages:*** Administer daily IV dosage over 24 hr (may be added to parenteral nutrition solutions).

May cause headache and GI disturbance, malaise, insomnia, sedation, arthralgia, and hepatotoxicity. May increase levels of nifedipine and midazolam. May decrease levels of ketoconazole, itraconazole, and delavirdine. May cause false-positive urine protein test (Multistix).

Duodenal/gastric ulcer doses for ≥1 mo–16 yr are extrapolated from clinical adult trials and pharmacokinetic data in children. Extemporaneously compounded carbohydrate-free oral solution dosage form is useful for patients receiving the ketogenic diet. The syrup dosage form has a peppermint flavor and may not be tolerated. **Adjust dose in renal failure (see Chapter 31).**

RASBURICASE
Elitek
Antihyperuricemic agent

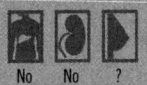

No   No   ?   C

Injection: 1.5, 7.5 mg; contains mannitol

Hyperuricemia: 0.1–0.2 mg/kg/dose (rounded down to nearest whole 1.5 mg multiple) IV over 30 min × 1. Patients generally respond to 1 dose, but if needed, dose may be repeated Q24 hr for up to 4 additional doses.

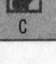

Contraindicated in G6PD deficiency or history of hypersensitivity, hemolytic reactions, or methemoglobinemia with rasburicase. **Use with caution** in asthma, allergies, hypersensitivity with other medications, and children <2 yr (decreased efficacy and increased risk for rash, vomiting, diarrhea, and fever).

Common side effects include nausea, vomiting, abdominal pain, discomfort, diarrhea, constipation, mucositis, fever, and rash.

During therapy, uric acid blood samples must be sent to the laboratory immediately. Blood should be collected in prechilled tubes containing heparin, and placed in an ice-water bath to avoid potential falsely low uric acid levels (degradation of plasma uric acid occurs in the presence of rasburicase at room temperature). Centrifugation in a precooled centrifuge (4°C) is indicated. Plasma samples must be assayed within 4 hr of sample collection.

RH₀(D) IMMUNE GLOBULIN INTRAVENOUS (HUMAN)
WinRho-SDF
Immune globulin

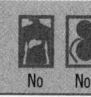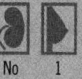

No   No   1   C

Injection: 1500 (1.3 mL), 2500 (2.2 mL), 5000 (4.4 mL), 15,000 IU (13 mL)
Conversion: 1 mcg = 5 IU

All doses based on international units (IU).
Immune thrombocytopenic purpura (nonsplenectomized Rh₀(D)-positive patients):
  Initial dose (may be given in two divided doses on separate days or as a single dose):
    Hemoglobin ≥ 10 mg/dL: 250 IU/kg/dose IV × 1
    Hemoglobin < 10 mg/dL: 125–200 IU/kg/dose IV × 1. See remarks for hemoglobin < 8 mg/dL.
  Additional doses:
    Responders to initial dose: 125–300 IU/kg/dose IV; actual dose and frequency of administration
    is determined by patient's response and subsequent hemoglobin level.
    Non-responders to initial dose:
      Hemoglobin < 8 g/dL: Alternative therapy should be used.
      Hemoglobin 8–10 g/dL: 125–200 IU/kg/dose IV × 1
      Hemoglobin > 10 g/dL: 250–300 IU/kg/dose × 1

WinRho SDF is currently the only Rh₀(D) immune globulin product indicated for ITP.
Contraindicated in IgA deficiency. **Use with extreme caution** in patients with a hemoglobin
<8 mg/dL and thrombocytopenia or bleeding disorders. Adverse events associated with ITP
include headache, chills, fever, and reduction in hemoglobin (due to destruction of Rh₀(D)
antigen–positive red cells). Intravascular hemolysis resulting in anemia and renal
insufficiency has been reported. May interfere with immune response to live virus vaccines
(e.g., MMR, varicella). Rh₀(D)-positive patients should be monitored for signs and symptoms
of intravascular hemolysis, anemia, and renal insufficiency. Administer IV doses over
3–5 min.

RIBAVIRIN
Oral: Rebetol, Copegus, Ribasphere, and other generics
Inhalation: Virazole
Antiviral agent

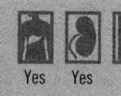

Yes   Yes   ?   X

Oral solution (Rebetol): 200 mg/5 mL (100 mL); contains sodium benzoate
Oral caps (Rebetol, Ribasphere): 200 mg
Tabs:
  Copegus: 200 mg
  Ribasphere: 200, 400, 600 mg
Aerosol (Virazole): 6 g

Hepatitis C (PO, see remarks):
  Child ≥ 3 yr (in combination with interferon alfa-2b at 3 million units 3 × per wk SC;
  use oral solution or capsule): 15 mg/kg/24 hr ÷ BID or by the following weight categories:
    25–36 kg: 200 mg BID
    37–49 kg: 200 mg QAM and 400 mg QPM
    50–61 kg: 400 mg BID
    >61–75 kg: 400 mg QAM and 600 mg QPM
    >75 kg: 600 mg BID

Continued

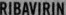

RIBAVIRIN *continued*

Duration of therapy:

    Genotype 1: 48 weeks. Consider discontinuing at 12 weeks if a 2-log decrease in viral load is achieved or if virus is still detectable at 24 weeks.

    Genotypes 2 and 3: 24 weeks

    Dosage modification for toxicity: See remarks.

Adult:

    Oral capsules in combination with interferon alfa-2b at 3 million units 3 × per week SC:

        ≤75 kg: 400 mg QAM and 600 mg QPM

        >75 kg: 600 mg BID

    Oral capsules in combination with peginterferon alfa-2b: 400 mg BID

    Oral tablets in combination with peginterferon alfa-2a for hepatitis C genotype 1, 4:

        ≤75 kg: 500 mg BID × 48 wk

        >75 kg: 600 mg BID × 48 wk

    Oral tablets in combination with peginterferon alfa-2a for genotype 2, 3: 400 mg BID × 24 wk

    Oral tablets in combination with peginterferon alfa-2a for HIV co-infected patient (regardless of hepatitis C genotype): 400 mg BID × 48 wk

    Dosage modification for toxicity: See remarks.

Inhalation:

    Continuous: Administer 6 g by aerosol over 12–18 hr once daily for 3–7 days. The 6-g ribavirin vial is diluted in 300 mL preservative-free sterile water to a final concentration of 20 mg/mL. Must be administered with Viratek Small Particle Aerosol Generator (SPAG-2).

    Intermittent (for nonventilated patients): Administer 2 g by aerosol over 2 hr TID for 3–7 days. The 6-g ribavirin vial is diluted in 100 mL preservative-free sterile water to a final concentration of 60 mg/mL. Intermittent use is not recommended in patients with endotracheal tubes.

ORAL RIBAVIRIN: Contraindicated in pregnancy, significant or unstable cardiac disease, autoimmune hepatitis, hepatic decompensation (Child-Pugh score > 6; class B or C), hemoglobinopathies, and creatinine clearance < 50 mL/min. **Use with caution** in preexisting cardiac disease, pulmonary disease, and sarcoidosis. Anemia (most common), insomnia, depression, irritability, and suicidal behavior (higher in adolescent and pediatric patients) have been reported with the oral route.

Tinnitus, hearing loss, vertigo, and severe hypertriglyceridemia have been reported in combination with interferon. Pancytopenia has been reported in combination with interferon and azathioprine. Increased risk for hepatic decompensation with cirrhotic chronic hepatitis C patients treated with alpha interferons or with HIV co-infection receiving HAART and interferon alfa-2a.

May decrease effects of zidovudine, stavudine; and increase risk for lactic acidosis with nucleoside analogs. **Reduce or discontinue dosage for toxicity as follows:**

Patient with no cardiac disease:

    Hgb < 10 g/dL and ≥ 8.5 g/dL:

        Child: 12 mg/kg/dose PO once daily; may further reduce to 8 mg/kg/dose PO once daily

        Adult: 600 mg PO once daily (capsules or solution) or 200 mg PO QAM and 400 mg PO QPM (tablets)

    Hgb < 8.5 g/dL: Discontinue therapy permanently.

Patient with cardiac disease:

    ≥2 mg/dL decrease in Hgb during any 4-wk period during therapy:

        Child: 12 mg/kg/dose PO once daily; may further reduce to 8 mg/kg/dose PO once daily (monitor weekly)

        Adult: 600 mg PO once daily (capsules or solution) or 200 mg PO QAM and 400 mg PO QPM (tablets)

    Hgb < 12 g/dL after 4 wk of reduced dose: Discontinue therapy permanently.

RIBAVIRIN *continued*

INHALED RIBAVIRIN: Use of ribavirin for RSV is controversial and **not** routinely indicated. Aerosol therapy may be considered for selected infants and young children at high risk for serious RSV disease (see most recent edition of AAP *Red Book*). Most effective if begun early in course of RSV infection, generally in first 3 days. May cause worsening respiratory distress, rash, conjunctivitis, mild bronchospasm, hypotension, anemia, and cardiac arrest. **Avoid** unnecessary occupational exposure to ribavirin owing to its teratogenic effects. Drug can precipitate in respiratory equipment.

RIBOFLAVIN
Vitamin B₂ and various brands and generics
Water-soluble vitamin

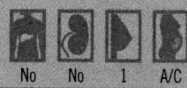

No	No	1	A/C

Tabs [OTC]: 25, 50, 100 mg
Caps [OTC]: 50 , 400 mg

Riboflavin deficiency:
  Child: 2.5–10 mg/24 hr ÷ once daily–BID PO
  Adult: 5–30 mg/24 hr ÷ once daily–BID PO
U.S. RDA requirements: see Chapter 21.

Hypersensitivity may occur. Administer with food. Causes yellow to orange discoloration of urine. For multivitamin information, see Chapter 21.
Pregnancy category changes to "C" if used in doses above the RDA.

RIFABUTIN
Mycobutin
Antituberculous agent

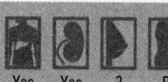

Yes	Yes	3	B

Caps: 150 mg
Oral suspension: 20 mg/mL

MAC prophylaxis for first episode and recurrence of opportunistic disease in HIV (see remarks for interactions and www.aidsinfo.nih.gov/guidelines):
  ≥6 yr and adult: 300 mg PO once daily. Doses may be administered as 150 mg PO BID if GI upset occurs.
MAC prophylaxis for recurrence of opportunistic disease in HIV (in combination with ethambutol and a macrolide antibiotic [clarithromycin or azithromycin]):
  Infant and child: 5 mg/kg/24 hr PO once daily; max. dose: 300 mg/24 hr
  Adolescent and adult: 300 mg PO once daily. Doses may be administered as 150 mg PO BID if GI upset occurs.
MAC treatment:
  Child: 10–20 mg/kg/24 hr PO once daily; max. dose: 300 mg/24 hr as part of a multidrug regimen for severe disease.
  Adult: 300 mg PO once daily; may be used in combination with azithromycin and ethambutol
    In combination with non-nucleoside reverse transcriptase inhibitors:
      With efavirenz and no concomitant protease inhibitor: 450 mg PO once daily or 600 mg PO 3 × per wk
      With nevirapine: 300 mg PO 3 × per wk

Continued

RIFABUTIN *continued*

MAC treatment (adult):
   In combination with protease inhibitors:
      With amprenavir, indinavir, or nelfinavir: 150 mg PO once daily or 300 mg PO 3 × per wk
      With ritonavir-boosted regimens (e.g., saquinavir/ritonavir, or lopinavir/ritonavir): 150 mg PO
      once every other day or 150 mg PO 3 × per week

Should not be used for MAC prophylaxis with active TB. May cause GI distress, discoloration of
skin and body fluids (brown-orange color), and marrow suppression. **Use with caution** in
renal and liver impairment. **Adjust dose in renal impairment (see Chapter 31).** May
permanently stain contact lenses. Uveitis can occur when using high doses (>300 mg/24 hr
in adults) in combination with macrolide antibiotics.

Rifabutin is an inducer of CYP 450 3A enzyme and is structurally similar to rifampin (similar drug
interactions, see *Rifampin*). Clarithromycin, fluconazole, itraconazole, nevirapine, and protease
inhibitors increase rifabutin levels. Efavirenz may decrease rifabutin levels. May decrease
effectiveness of dapsone, delavirdine, nevirapine, amprenavir, indinavir, nelfinavir, saquinavir,
itraconazole, warfarin, oral contraceptives, digoxin, cyclosporine, ketoconazole, and narcotics.

Doses may be administered with food if patient experiences GI intolerance.

RIFAMPIN
Rimactane, Rifadin and other generics
Antibiotic, antituberculous agent, rifamycin

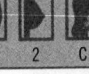

Yes   Yes   2   C

Caps: 150, 300 mg
Oral suspension: 10, 15, 25 mg/mL \Rx
Injection: 600 mg

Staphylococcus aureus *infections (as part of synergistic therapy with other anti-*
staphylococcal agents):
  0–1 mo:
    IV: 10–20 mg/kg/24 hr ÷ Q12 hr
    PO: 10–20 mg/kg/dose Q24 hr
  >1 mo: 10–20 mg/kg/24 hr ÷ Q12 hr IV/PO; **max. dose:** 600 mg/24 hr
    Prosthetic valve endocarditis: 15–20 mg/kg/24 hr IV/PO ÷ Q8 hr
  Adult: 300–600 mg Q12 hr IV/PO
    Prosthetic valve endocarditis: 300 mg Q8 hr IV/PO for a minimum of 6 wk in combination with
    antistaphylococcal penicillin with or without gentamicin
Tuberculosis *(see latest edition of the AAP* Red Book *for duration of therapy and combination*
therapy): Twice weekly therapy may be used after 1–2 months of daily therapy.
  Infant, child and adolescent:
    Daily therapy: 10–20 mg/kg/24 hr ÷ Q12–24 hr IV/PO
    Twice weekly therapy: 10–20 mg/kg/24 hr PO twice weekly
    Max. daily dose: 600 mg/24 hr
  Adult:
    Daily therapy: 10 mg/kg/24 hr once daily PO
    Twice weekly therapy: 10 mg/kg/24 hr once daily twice weekly
    Max. daily dose: 600 mg/24 hr
Prophylaxis for Neisseria meningitidis *(see latest edition of AAP* Red Book *for additional*
information):
  0–<1 mo: 10 mg/kg/24 hr ÷ Q12 hr PO × 2 days
  ≥1 mo: 20 mg/kg/24 hr ÷ Q12 hr PO × 2 days

RIFAMPIN *continued*

> ***Adult:*** 600 mg PO Q12 hr × 2 days
> **Max. dose (all ages):** 1200 mg/24 hr

Never use as monotherapy except when used for prophylaxis. Patients with latent tuberculosis infection should not be treated with rifampin and pyrazinamide because of risk of severe liver injury. Use is **not recommended** in porphyria. **Use with caution** in diabetes.

May cause GI irritation, allergy, headache, fatigue, ataxia, muscle weakness, confusion, fever, hepatitis, transient LFT abnormalities, blood dyscrasias, interstitial nephritis, and elevated BUN and uric acid. Causes red discoloration of body secretions, such as urine, saliva, and tears (which can permanently stain contact lenses). Induces hepatic enzymes (CYP 450 2C9, 2C19, and 3A4), which may decrease plasma concentration of digoxin, corticosteroids, buspirone, benzodiazepines, fentanyl, calcium channel blockers, β-blockers, cyclosporine, tacrolimus, itraconazole, ketoconazole, oral anticoagulants, barbiturates, and theophylline. May reduce effectiveness of oral contraceptives and antiretroviral agents (protease inhibitors and non-nucleoside reverse transcriptase inhibitors). Hepatotoxicity is a concern when used in combination with pyrazinamide and ritonavir-boosted saquinavir **(use is contraindicated).**

Adjust dose in renal failure (see Chapter 31). Reduce dose in hepatic impairment. Give 1 hr before or 2 hr after meals.

For *Haemophilus influenza* prophylaxis, see latest edition of AAP *Red Book.*

RIMANTADINE
Flumadine and generics
Antiviral agent

 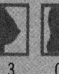

Yes	Yes	3	C

Tabs: 100 mg
Oral suspension: 10 mg/1 mL \Rx ✄

Influenza A prophylaxis (for at least 10 days after known exposure; usually for 6–8 wk during influenza A season or local outbreak):
Child:
> ***1–9 yr:*** 5 mg/kg/24 hr PO once daily–BID; **max. dose:** 150 mg/24 hr
> ***≥10 yr:***
> > ***<40 kg:*** 5 mg/kg/24 hr PO ÷ BID; **max. dose:** 150 mg/24 hr
> > ***≥40 kg:*** 100 mg/dose PO BID
>
> ***Adult:*** 100 mg PO BID

Influenza A treatment (within 48 hr of illness onset):
> Use the aforementioned prophylaxis dosage × 5–7 days.

Resistance to influenza A and recommendations against the use for treatment and prophylaxis have been reported by the CDC. Check with local microbiology laboratories and the CDC for seasonal susceptibility/resistance.

Preferred over amantadine for influenza; lower incidence of adverse events. Individuals immunized with live attenuated influenza vaccine (e.g., FluMist) should not receive rimantadine prophylaxis for 14 days after the vaccine. Chemoprophylaxis does not interfere with immune response to inactivated influenza vaccine.

May cause GI disturbance, xerostomia, dizziness, headache, and urinary retention. CNS disturbances are less than with amantadine. **Contraindicated** in amantadine hypersensitivity. **Use with caution** in renal or hepatic insufficiency; dosage reduction may be necessary. A dosage reduction of 50% has been recommended in severe hepatic or renal impairment. Subjects with severe renal impairment have been reported to have an 81% increase in systemic exposure.

For explanation of icons, see p. 648

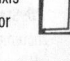

RISPERIDONE
Risperdal, Risperdal M-Tab, and Risperdal Consta
Atypical antipsychotic, serotonin (5-HT₂) and dopamine (D₂) antagonist

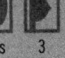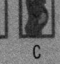

Yes   Yes   3   C

Tabs: 0.25, 0.5, 1, 2, 3, 4 mg
Oral solution: 1 mg/mL (30 mL); may contain benzoic acid
Orally disintegrating tabs (Risperdal M-Tab and generics): 0.5, 1, 2, 3, 4 mg; contains phenylalanine
Injection (Risperdal Consta): 12.5, 25, 37.5, 50 mg (prefilled syringe with 20G, 2-inch needle and 2 mL diluent); for IM administration only

Irritability associated with autistic disorder:
5–16 yr (PO daily doses may be administer once daily–BID; patients experiencing somnolence may benefit from QHS or BID dosing or dose reduction):
  Initial dose:
    <20 kg: 0.25 mg/24 hr PO for a minimum of 4 days; **use with caution** if < 15 kg (dosing recommendation is not established).
    ≥20 kg: 0.5 mg/24 hr PO for a minimum of 4 days
  Dose increment (if needed) after 4 days of initial dose:
    <20 kg: 0.5 mg/24 hr PO for a minimum of 14 days. If additional increments needed, increase dose by 0.25 mg/24 hr at intervals of at least 14 days.
    ≥20 kg: 1 mg/24 hr PO for a minimum of 14 days. If additional increments needed, increase dose by 0.5 mg/24 hr at intervals of at least 14 days.
  Max. daily dose for plateau of therapeutic effect (from one pivotal clinical trial):
    <20 kg: 1 mg/24 hr
    ≥20–45 kg: 2.5 mg/24 hr
    >45 kg: 3 mg/24 hr
Bipolar mania: Oral doses may be administered once daily–BID, and patients experiencing somnolence may benefit from QHS or BID dosing or dose reduction. Long-term use beyond 3 wk and doses (all ages) > 6 mg/24 hr have not been evaluated.
  Child (10–17 yr): Start with 0.5 mg/24 hr PO once daily (QAM or QHS). If needed, increase dose at intervals not <24 hr in increments of 0.5 or 1 mg/24 hr, as tolerated, up to a recommended dose of 2.5 mg/24 hr. Although efficacy has been demonstrated between 0.5–6 mg/24 hr, no additional benefit was seen above 2.5 mg/24 hr. Higher doses were associated with more adverse effects.
  Adult: Start with 2–3 mg PO once. Dosage increases or decreases of 1 mg/24 hr can be made at 24-hr intervals. Dosage range: 1–6 mg/24 hr.
Schizophrenia: Oral doses may be administered once daily–BID, and patients experiencing somnolence may benefit from BID dosing (see remarks).
  Adolescent (13–17 yr): No data are available to support long-term use of >8 wk.
    PO: Start with 0.5 mg once daily (QAM or QHS). If needed, increase dose at intervals not <24 hr in increments of 0.5 to 1 mg/24 hr, as tolerated, to a recommended dose of 3 mg/24 hr. Although efficacy has been demonstrated between 1–6 mg/24 hr, no additional benefit was seen above 3 mg/24 hr. Doses >6 mg/24 hr have not been studied.
  Adult:
    PO: Start with 1 mg BID on day 1; if tolerated, increase to 2 mg BID on day 2 and to 3 mg BID thereafter. Dosage increases or decreases of 1–2 mg can be made on a weekly basis if needed. Usual effective dose: 2–8 mg/24 hr. Doses above 16 mg/24 hr have not been evaluated.
    IM: Start with 25 mg Q2 wk; if no response, dose may be increased to 37.5 mg or 50 mg at 4-wk intervals. **Max. IM dose:** 50 mg Q2 wk.

RISPERIDONE *continued*

Use with caution in cardiovascular disorders, diabetes, renal or hepatic impairment (dose reduction necessary), hypothermia or hyperthermia, seizures, breast cancer or other prolactin-dependent tumors, and dysphagia. Common side effects include abdominal pain and other GI disturbances, arthralgia, anxiety, dizziness, headache, insomnia, somnolence (use QHS dosing), EPS, cough, fever, pharyngitis, rash, rhinitis, sexual dysfunction, tachycardia, and weight gain. Weight gain, somnolence, and fatigue were common side effects reported in the autism studies. Priapism, hypothermia, sleep apnea syndrome, urinary retention, diabetes mellitus, and hypoglycemia have been reported in postmarketing reports.

In the presence of severe renal or hepatic impairment or risk for hypotension, the following adult dosing has been recommended: Start with 0.5 mg PO BID. Increase dose, if needed and tolerated, in increments no more than 0.5 mg BID. Increases to doses >1.5 mg BID should occur at intervals of at least 1 wk; slower titration may be required in some patients.

Limited studies in pediatric-related Tourette syndrome, schizophrenia, and aggressive behavior in psychiatric disorders are reported. Autistic disorder safety and efficacy in children <5 yr have not been established. If therapy has been discontinued for a period of time, therapy should be reinitiated with the same initial titration regimen.

Drug is a CYP 450 2D6 and 3A4 isoenzyme substrate. Concurrent use of isoenzyme inhibitors (e.g., fluoxetine, paroxetine, sertraline, cimetidine) and inducers (e.g., carbamazepine, rifampin, phenobarbital, phenytoin) may increase and decrease effects of risperidone, respectively. Alcohol, CNS depressants, and St. John's wort may potentiate drug's side effects. Risperidone may enhance hypotensive effects of levodopa and dopamine agonists.

Oral dosage forms may be administered with or without food. Oral solution can be mixed in water, coffee, orange juice, or low-fat milk but is incompatible with cola or tea. **Do not** split or chew the orally disintegrating tablet. Use IM suspension preparation within 6 hr after reconstitution.

ROCURONIUM
Zemuron and generics
Nondepolarizing neuromuscular blocking agent

Yes   No   ?   C

Injection: 10 mg/mL (5, 10 mL)

Use of a peripheral nerve stimulator to monitor drug effect is recommended.
Infant:
> *IV:* 0.5 mg/kg/dose; may repeat Q20–30 min PRN

Child (3 mo–12 yr):
> *IV:* 0.6 mg/kg/dose × 1. If needed, give maintenance doses of 0.075–0.125 mg/kg/dose Q 20–30 min PRN when neuromuscular blockade returns to 25% of control. Alternatively, a maintenance continuous IV infusion may be used starting at 7–12 mcg/kg/min (use lower end for children 2–11 yr) when neuromuscular blockade returns to 10% of control.

Adolescent and adult:
> *IV:* Start with 0.6–1.2 mg/kg/dose × 1. If needed, maintenance doses at 0.1–0.2 mg/kg/dose Q20–30 min PRN. Alternatively, a maintenance continuous IV infusion may be used starting at 10–12 mcg/kg/min (range, 4–16 mcg/kg/min).

Use with caution in hepatic impairment and history of anaphylaxis with other neuromuscular blocking agents. Hypertension, hypotension, arrhythmia, tachycardia, nausea, vomiting, bronchospasm, wheezing, hiccups, rash, and edema at injection site may occur. Myopathy after long-term use in an ICU, and QT-interval prolongation in pediatric patients receiving general anesthetic agents have been reported. Increased neuromuscular blockade may occur

Continued

ROCURONIUM *continued*

with concomitant use of aminoglycosides, clindamycin, tetracycline, magnesium sulfate, quinine, quinidine, succinylcholine, and inhalation anesthetics (for continuous infusion, reduce infusion by 30%–50% at 45–60 min after intubating dose).

Caffeine, calcium, carbamazepine, phenytoin, phenylephrine, azathioprine, and theophylline may reduce neuromuscular blocking effects.

Use must be accompanied by adequate anesthesia or sedation. Peak effects occur in 0.5–1 min for children and in 1–3.7 min for adults. Duration of action: 30–40 min in children and 20–94 min in adults (longer in geriatrics). Recovery time in children 3 mo–1 yr is similar to adults. To prevent residual paralysis, extubate patient **only** after sufficiently recovered from neuromuscular blockade. In obese patients, use actual body weight for dosage calculation.

SALMETEROL
Serevent Diskus
β₂-Adrenergic agonist (long acting)

   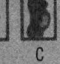

No   No   2   C

Dry powder inhalation (DPI; Diskus): 50 mcg/inhalation (28, 60 inhalations); contains lactose
In combination with fluticasone: See *Fluticasone Propionate and Salmeterol*

Persistent asthma (see remarks):
≥4 yr and adult: 1 inhalation (50 mcg) Q12 hr
Prevention of exercise-induced bronchospasm:
≥4 yr and adult: 1 inhalation 30–60 min before exercise. Additional does should not be used for another 12 hr. Patients who are already using Q12 hr dosing for persistent asthma should not use additional salmeterol doses for this indication and use alternative therapy (e.g., cromolyn) before exercise.

For long-term asthma control, should be used in combination with inhaled corticosteroids.
Should not be used to relieve symptoms of acute asthma. It is long acting and has its onset of action in 10–20 min, with a peak effect at 3 hr. May be used QHS (1 inhalation of the DPI) for nocturnal symptoms. Salmeterol is a chronic medication and is **not** used in similar fashion to short-acting β-agonists (e.g., albuterol). Patients already receiving salmeterol Q12 hr should not use additional doses for prevention of exercise-induced bronchospasm; consider alternative therapy. Asthma exacerbations or hospitalizations were reported to be lower when used with an inhaled corticosteroid.

WARNING: Long-acting β₂-agonists may increase risk of asthma-related death. A subgroup analysis suggested higher risk in African-American patients compared with Caucasians. Use salmeterol only as additional therapy for patients not adequately controlled on other asthma-controller medications (e.g., low- to medium-dose inhaled corticosteroids) or whose disease severity clearly requires initiation of treatment with two maintenance therapies.

Should not be used in conjunction with an inhaled long-acting β₂-agonist and is **not** a substitute for inhaled or systemic corticosteroid. Use with strong CYP 3A4 inhibitors (e.g., ketoconazole, HIV protease inhibitors, clarithromycin, itraconazole, nefazodone, and telithromycin) are not recommended owing to risk for cardiovascular adverse events (e.g., QTc prolongation, tachycardia). Salmeterol is a P450 3A4 substrate.

Proper patient education is essential. Side effects are similar to albuterol. Hypertension and arrhythmias have been reported. See Chapter 24 for recommendations for asthma controller therapy.

SCOPOLAMINE HYDROBROMIDE
Transderm Scop, Isopto Hyoscine, and generics
Anticholinergic agent

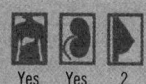

Yes   Yes   2   C

Injection: 0.4 mg/mL (1 mL); may contain alcohol
Transdermal (Transderm Scōp): 1.5 mg/patch (4s, 10s and 24s); delivers ≈ 1 mg over 3 days
Ophthalmic solution (Isopto Hyoscine): 0.25% (5 mL); contains benzalkonium chloride

Antiemetic (SC/IM/IV):
  Child: 6 mcg/kg/dose Q6–8 hr PRN; **max. dose:** 300 mcg/dose
  Adult: 0.32–0.65 mg/dose Q6–8 hr PRN
Transdermal (≥12 yr) (see remarks):
  Motion sickness: Apply patch behind the ear at least 4 hr before exposure to motion; remove after 72 hr.
  Antiemetic before surgery: Apply patch behind the ear the evening before surgery. Remove patch 24 hr after surgery.
  Antiemetic before cesarean section: Apply patch behind the ear 1 hr before surgery to minimize infant exposure. Remove patch 24 hr after surgery.
Ophthalmic (see remarks):
  Refraction:
    Child: 1 drop BID for 2 days before procedure
    Adult: 1–2 drop(s) 1 hr before procedure
  Iridocyclitis:
    Child: 1 drop up to TID
    Adult: 1–2 drop(s) up to TID

Toxicities similar to atropine. **Contraindicated** in urinary or GI obstruction and glaucoma. **Use with caution** in hepatic or renal dysfunction, cardiac disease, seizures, or psychoses. May cause dry mouth, drowsiness, and blurred vision.
Transdermal route should **NOT** be used in children <12 yr. Drug withdrawal symptoms (nausea, vomiting, headache, vertigo) have been reported after removal of transdermal patch in patients using patch for >3 days. For perioperative use, patch should be kept in place for 24 hr after surgery. Systemic effects have been reported with both transdermal and ophthalmic preparations. Compress nasolacrimal ducts to minimize systemic effects when using ophthalmic preparations.

SELENIUM SULFIDE
Selsun and others
Topical antiseborrheic agent

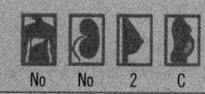

No   No   2   C

Lotion/Shampoo: 1% [OTC] (120, 210, 325, 400 mL); some shampoo products are available with conditioner.
Topical lotion: 2.5% (120 mL)
Topical aerosol foam: 2.25% (70 g)

≥2 yr and adult:
  Seborrhea/dandruff: Massage 5–10 mL of shampoo into wet scalp and leave on scalp for 2–3 min. Rinse thoroughly and repeat. Shampoo twice weekly × 2 weeks. Maintenance applications once every 1–4 wk.
  Tinea versicolor: Apply 2.5% lotion to affected areas of skin. Allow to remain on skin × 10 min. Rinse thoroughly. Repeat once daily × 7 days. Follow with monthly applications for 3 mo to prevent recurrences.

Continued

SELENIUM SULFIDE *continued*

Rinse hands and body well after treatment. May cause local irritation, hair loss, and hair discoloration. **Avoid** eyes, genital areas, and skin folds. Shampoo may be used for tinea capitis to reduce risk of transmission to others (does not eradicate tinea infection).

For tinea versicolor, 15%–25% sodium hyposulfite or thiosulfate (Tinver lotion) applied to affected areas BID × 2–4 wk is an alternative. Topical antifungals (e.g., clotrimazole, miconazole) may be used for small focal infections. **Do not use** for tinea versicolor during pregnancy.

SENNA/SENNOSIDES
Senokot, Senna-Gen, Lax-Pills, and many others
Laxative, stimulant

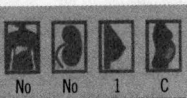

No   No   1   C

Based on mg of senna (all products are OTC):
    Granules: 326 mg/tsp
    Oral syrup: 176 mg/5 mL, 218 mg/5 mL (60 mL, 240 mL)
    Tabs: 187, 217, 374 mg
    187 mg senna extract is approximately 8.6 mg sennosides.
Based on mg of sennosides (all products are OTC):
    Granules: 15 mg/tsp, 20 mg/tsp
    Oral syrup: 8.8 mg/5 mL (60, 240 mL)
    Tabs: 8.6, 15, 17.2, 25 mg
    Chewable tabs: 15 mg
    8.6 mg sennosides is approximately 187 mg senna extract.

Constipation:
Dosing based on mg senna:
  Child:
    Oral: 10–20 mg/kg/dose PO QHS (to **max. dose** as shown below) or dosage by age:
      1 mo–1 yr: 55–109 mg PO QHS to **max. dose** of 218 mg/24 hr
      1–5 yr: 109–218 mg PO QHS to **max. dose** of 436 mg/24 hr
      5–15 yr: 218–436 mg PO QHS to **max. dose** of 872 mg/24 hr
  Adult:
    Granules: 326 mg (1 tsp) PO at bedtime; **max. dose:** 652 mg (2 tsp) BID
    Syrup: 436–654 mg PO at bedtime; **max.** 654 mg (15 mL) BID
    Tabs: 374 mg PO at bedtime; **max.** 748 mg BID
Dosing based on mg sennosides:
  Child:
    Syrup:
      1 mo–2 yr: 2.2–4.4 mg (1.25–2.5 mL) PO QHS to **max. dose** of 8.8 mg/24 hr
      2–5 yr: 4.4–6.6 mg (2.5–3.75 mL) PO QHS to **max. dose** of 6.6 mg BID
      6–12 yr: 8.8–13.2 mg (5–7.5 mL) PO QHS to **max. dose** of 13.2 mg BID
    Tabs:
      2–5 yr: 4.3 mg PO QHS to **max. dose** of 8.6 mg BID
      6–12 yr: 8.6 mg PO QHS to **max. dose** of 17.2 mg BID
  >12 yr and adult:
    Granules: 15 mg PO QHS to **max. dose** of 30 mg BID
    Syrup: 17.6–26.4 mg (10–15 mL) PO QHS to **max. dose** of 26.4 mg BID
    Tabs: 17.2 mg PO QHS to **max. dose** of 34.4 mg BID

Effects occur within 6–24 hr after oral administration. Prolonged use (>1 wk) should be **avoided**; may lead to dependency. May cause nausea, vomiting, diarrhea, abdominal cramps. Active metabolite stimulates Auerbach's plexus. Syrup may be administered with juice, milk, or mixed with ice cream. Granules may be sprinkled onto food or mixed with drinks.

SERTRALINE HCL
Zoloft and generics
Antidepressant (selective serotonin reuptake inhibitor)

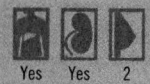

Yes | Yes | 2 | C

Tabs: 25, 50, 100 mg
Oral concentrate solution: 20 mg/mL (60 mL); contains alcohol and menthol

Depression:
  Child ≥ 6–12 yr (data limited in this age group): Start at 12.5–25 mg PO once daily.
  May increase dosage by 25 mg at 1-wk intervals up to a **max. dose** of 200 mg/24 hr.
  Child ≥ 13 yr and adult: Start at 25–50 mg PO once daily. May increase dosage by 50 mg at 1-wk
  intervals up to a **max. dose** of 200 mg/24 hr.
Obsessive-compulsive disorder:
  Child ≥ 6–12 yr: Start at 25 mg PO once daily. May increase dosage by 25 mg at 3–4 day intervals
  or by 50 mg at 7-day intervals up to a **max. dose** of 200 mg/24 hr.
  Child ≥ 13 yr and adult: Start at 50 mg PO once daily. May increase dosage by 50 mg at 1-wk
  intervals up to **max. dose** of 200 mg/24 hr.

Drug is **contraindicated** in combination (or within 14 days of discontinuing use) with an
MAOI (e.g., linezolid or IV methylene blue) or pimozide (increases adverse/toxic effects of
pimozide). **Use with caution** in patients with abnormal bleeding, SIADH, and hepatic or renal
impairment. Adverse effects include nausea, diarrhea, tremor, and increased sweating.
Hyponatremia, diabetes mellitus, and platelet dysfunction have been reported. Monitor for
clinical worsening of depression and suicidal ideation/behavior after initiation of therapy or
after dose changes. Use during late third trimester of pregnancy may increase risk for
newborn withdrawal symptoms and persistent pulmonary hypertension in the newborn.
Use with drugs that interfere with hemostasis (e.g., NSAIDs, aspirin, warfarin) may increase risk for GI
bleeds. Use with warfarin may increase PT. Inhibits the CYP 450 2D6 drug metabolizing enzyme.
Serotonin syndrome may occur when taken with SSRIs (e.g., amitriptyline, amphetamines, buspirone,
dihydroergotamine, sumatriptan, sympathomimetics).
Mix oral concentrate solution with 4 oz of water, ginger ale, lemon/lime soda, lemonade, or orange
juice. After mixing, a slight haze may appear; this is normal. This dosage form should be **used
cautiously** in patients with latex allergy; dropper contains dry natural rubber.

SILDENAFIL
Revatio, Viagra, and generics
Phosphodiesterase type 5 (PDE5) inhibitor

Yes | Yes | ? | B

Tabs:
  Revatio and generic: 20 mg
  Viagra: 25, 50, 100 mg
Oral suspension: 2.5 mg/mL
  Revatio: 10 mg/mL (112 mL)
Injection:
  Revatio: 0.8 mg/mL (12.5 mL)

Pulmonary hypertension:
Neonate (limited data from case reports and small clinical trials):
  PO: Several dosages have been reported and have ranged from 0.5–3 mg/kg/dose Q6–12 hr
  PO. A single ≈ 0.3 mg/kg/dose PO has been used in selected patients to facilitate weaning
  from inhaled nitric oxide.
  IV (case report from 4 neonates > 34 wk' gestation and < 72 hr old): Start with 0.4 mg/kg/dose
  IV over 3 hr, followed by a continuous infusion of 1.6 mg/kg/24 hr (0.067 mg/kg/hr) for up to 7 days.

Continued

SILDENAFIL *continued*

Infant and child:

PO: Several dosages have been reported. Start at 0.25–0.5 mg/kg/dose Q4–8 hr PO; if needed and tolerated, increase to 1 mg/kg/dose Q4–8 hr PO. Doses as high as 2 mg/kg/dose Q4 hr PO have been given in case reports. A single ≈ 0.4 mg/kg/dose PO has been used in selected patients to facilitate weaning from inhaled nitric oxide.

Child 1–17 yr (results from a 16-wk dose-ranging study in 235 treatment-naïve children ≥ 8 kg with pulmonary arterial hypertension [see remarks]):

PO:

≥*8–20 kg:* 10–20 mg TID
>*20–45 kg:* 20–40 mg TID
>*45 kg:* 40–80 mg TID

Pulmonary arterial hypertension:

Adult:

PO: 20 mg TID (taken at least 4–6 hr apart)
IV: 10 mg TID

Contraindicated with concurrent use of nitrates (e.g., nitroglycerin) and other nitric oxide donors; potentiates hypotensive effects. **Use with caution** in sepsis (high levels of cGMP may potentiate hypotension), hypotension, sickle cell (use not established), anemias, and with concurrent CYP 450 3A4–inhibiting medications (see discussion that follows) and antihypertensive medications. Hepatic insufficiency or severe renal impairment (GFR < 30 mL/min) significantly reduces sildenafil clearance.

Findings from the dose-ranging study in 1- to 17-year-olds with pulmonary arterial hypertension found an association of increased mortality risk with long-term use (>2 yr). Headache, pyrexia, URTIs, vomiting, and diarrhea were the most frequently reported side effects in this study. Optimal dosing based on age and body weight has yet to be determined.

In adults, a transient impairment of color discrimination may occur; this effect could increase risk of severe retinopathy of prematurity in neonates. Common side effects reported in adults have included flushing, rash, diarrhea, indigestion, headache, abnormal vision, and nasal congestion. Hearing loss has been reported.

Sildenafil is a substrate for CYP 450 3A4 (major) and 2C8/9 (minor). Azole antifungals, cimetidine, ciprofloxacin, clarithromycin, erythromycin, nicardipine, propofol, protease inhibitors, quinidine, verapamil, and grapefruit juice may increase effects/toxicity of sildenafil. Bosentan, efavirenz, carbamazepine, phenobarbital, phenytoin, rifampin, St. John's wort, and high-fat meals decrease sildenafil's effects.

SILVER SULFADIAZINE
Silvadene, Thermazene, SSD Cream, and generics
Topical antibiotic

Yes   Yes   3   B

Cream: 1% (20, 25, 50, 85, 400, 1000 g); contains methylparabens and propylene glycol

Child (≥2 mo) and adult: Cover affected areas completely once daily–BID. Apply cream to a thickness of 1/16 inch using sterile technique.

Contraindicated in premature infants and infants ≤ 2 mo of age owing to concerns of kernicterus; and pregnancy (approaching term). **Use with caution** in G6PD and renal and hepatic impairment. Discard product if cream has darkened. Significant systemic absorption may occur in severe burns. Adverse effects include pruritus, rash, bone marrow suppression, hemolytic anemia, and interstitial nephritis. **NOT** for ophthalmic use. Dressing may be used but is **not** necessary. See Chapter 4 for more information.

S

FORMULARY

SIMETHICONE
Mylicon, Phazyme, Mylanta Gas, Gas-X and generics
Antiflatulent

No   No   1   C

All dosage forms available OTC
Oral drops: 40 mg/0.6 mL (30 mL)
Caps: 125, 180 mg
Tabs: 60, 95 mg
Chewable tabs: 80, 125 mg
Strip, orally disintegrating: 40 mg (16s), 62.5 mg (18s, 30s); may contain alcohol

Infant and child < 2 yr: 20 mg PO QID PRN; **max. dose:** 240 mg/24 hr
2–12 yr: 40 mg PO QID PRN
>12 yr and adult: 40–250 mg PO QPC and QHS PRN; **max. dose:** 500 mg/24 hr

Efficacy has not been demonstrated for treating infant colic. **Avoid** carbonated beverages and gas-forming foods. Oral liquid may be mixed with water, infant formula, or other suitable liquids for ease of oral administration.

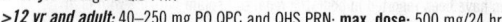

SIROLIMUS
Rapamune and generics
Immunosuppressant agent

Yes   Yes   3   C

Tabs: 0.5, 1, 2 mg
Oral solution: 1 mg/mL (60 mL); contains 1.5%–2.5% ethanol

Child ≥ 13 yr and < 40 kg: 3 mg/m^2/dose PO × 1 immediately after transplantation, followed by 1 mg/m^2/24 hr PO ÷ Q12–24 hr on the next day. Adjust dose to achieve desired trough blood levels.
Adult:
  Patients at low/moderate immunologic risk:
    In combination with cyclosporine (adjust dose to achieve desired trough blood levels):
      <40 kg: 3 mg/m^2/dose PO × 1 immediately after transplantation, followed by 1 mg/m^2/dose PO once daily on the next day
      ≥40 kg: 6 mg PO × 1 immediately after transplantation, followed by 2 mg PO once daily on the next day
  Patients at high immunologic risk:
    In combination with cyclosporine (withdrawal of cyclosporine is not recommended): 15 mg PO × 1 immediately after transplantation, followed by 5 mg PO once daily on the next day. Adjust dose to achieve desired trough blood levels.

Increased susceptibility to infection and development of lymphoma may result from immunosuppression. **Fatal** bronchial anastomotic dehiscence has been reported in lung transplantation. Excess mortality, graft loss, and hepatic artery thrombosis have been reported in liver transplantation when used with tacrolimus. Patients with the greatest amount of urinary protein excretion before sirolimus conversion were those whose protein excretion increased the most after conversion. Increased risk of BK virus–associated nephropathies have been reported. Increased mortality in stable liver transplant patients has been reported after conversion from a calcineurin inhibitor–based regimen to sirolimus.
Monitor whole blood trough levels (just before a dose at steady state), especially with pediatric patients, hepatic impairment, concurrent use of CYP 450 3A4 and/or P-gp inducers and inhibitors, and/or if cyclosporine dosage is markedly changed or discontinued. Steady state is generally

Continued

For explanation of icons, see p. 648

SIROLIMUS *continued*

achieved after 5–7 days of continuous dosing. **Interpretation will vary based on specific treatment protocol and assay methodology (HPLC vs. immunoassay vs. LC/MS/MS).** Younger children may exhibit faster sirolimus clearance compared with adolescents.

Sirolimus is a substrate for CYP 450 3A4 and P-gp. Cyclosporine, diltiazem, protease inhibitors, erythromycin, grapefruit juice, and other inhibitors of CYP 3A4 may increase toxicity of sirolimus. Phenobarbital, carbamazepine, phenytoin, and St. John's wort may decrease effects of sirolimus. Strong inhibitors (e.g., azole antifungals and clarithromycin) and strong inducers (e.g., rifamycins) are **not recommended**.

Hypertension, peripheral edema, increased serum creatinine, dyspnea, epistaxis, headache, anemia, thrombocytopenia, hyperlipidemia, hypercholesterolemia, and arthralgia may occur. Progressive multifocal leukoencephalopathy (PML), ovarian cysts, and menstrual disorders have been reported. Urinary tract infections have been reported in pediatric renal transplant patients with high immunologic risk.

Two mg of the oral solution has been demonstrated to be clinically equivalent to 2-mg tablets. However, it is not known whether they are still therapeutically equivalent at higher doses. Reduce maintenance dosage by ⅓ in the presence of hepatic function impairment. Administer doses consistently with or without food. When administered with cyclosporine, give dose 4 hr after cyclosporine. **Do not** crush or split tablets. Measure the oral liquid dosage form with an amber oral syringe and dilute in a cup with 60 mL of water or orange juice only. Take dose immediately after mixing, add/mix additional 120 mL diluent into the cup, and drink immediately after mixing.

SODIUM BICARBONATE
Neut and many generics
Alkalinizing agent, electrolyte

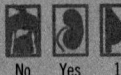

No   Yes   1   C

Injection: 4% (Neut) (0.48 mEq/mL) (5 mL), 4.2% (0.5 mEq/mL) (5, 10 mL), 7.5% (0.89 mEq/mL) (50 mL), 8.4% (1 mEq/mL) (10, 50 mL)
Tabs: 325 mg (3.8 mEq), 650 mg (7.6 mEq)
Powder: 120, 480 g; contains 30 mEq Na+ per ½ teaspoon
Each 1 mEq bicarbonate provides 1 mEq Na+.

Cardiac arrest: See inside cover.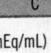

Correction of metabolic acidosis: Calculate patient's dose with the following formulas.

Neonate, infant and child:

HCO_3^- (mEq) = 0.3 × weight (kg) × base deficit (mEq/L), **OR**
HCO_3^- (mEq) = 0.5 × weight (kg) × [24 − serum HCO_3^- (mEq/L)]

Adult:

HCO_3^- (mEq) = 0.2 × weight (kg) × base deficit (mEq/L), **OR**
HCO_3^- (mEq) = 0.5 × weight (kg) × [24 − serum HCO_3^- (mEq/L)]

Urinary alkalinization (titrate dose accordingly to urine pH):

Child: 84–840 mg (1–10 mEq)/kg/24 hr PO ÷ QID
Adult: 4 g (48 mEq) × 1, followed by 1–2 g (12–24 mEq) PO Q4 hr. Doses up to 16 g (192 mEq)/24 hr have been used.

Contraindicated in respiratory alkalosis, hypochloremia, and inadequate ventilation during cardiac arrest. **Use with caution** in CHF, renal impairment, cirrhosis, hypocalcemia, hypertension, and concurrent corticosteroids. Maintain high urine output. Monitor acid-base balance and serum electrolytes. May cause hypernatremia (contains sodium), hypokalemia, hypomagnesemia, hypocalcemia, hyperreflexia, edema, and tissue necrosis (extravasation). Oral route of administration may cause GI discomfort and gastric rupture from gas production.

SODIUM BICARBONATE *continued*

For direct IV administration (cardiac arrest) in neonates and infants, use the 0.5 mEq/mL (4.2 %) concentration or dilute the 1 mEq/mL (8.4 %) concentration 1:1 with sterile water for injection and infuse at a rate **no greater than** 10 mEq/min. The 1 mEq/mL (8.4 %) concentration may be used in children and adults for direct IV administration.

For IV infusions (for all ages), dilute to a **max. concentration** of 0.5 mEq/mL in dextrose or sterile water for injection, and infuse over 2 hr using a **max. rate** of 1 mEq/kg/hr.

Sodium bicarbonate should **not** be mixed with or be in contact with calcium, norepinephrine, or dobutamine.

SODIUM CHLORIDE—INHALED PREPARATIONS
Hypersal, Simply Saline, Ocean, Ayr Saline, Rhinaris, and many other brands and generics
Electrolyte, inhalation

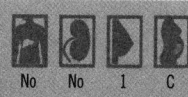

No   No   1   C

Nebulized solution: 0.9% (3, 5, 15 mL), 3% (4, 15 mL), 6% (4 mL), 7% (4 mL), 10% (4, 15 mL)
   Hypersal (preservative-free): 3.5% (4 mL), 7% (4 mL)
Nasal solution spray/drops/mist [OTC]: 0.125% (15 mL), 0.2% (30 mL), 0.65% (15, 30, 45 mL), 0.9% (45, 90 mL), 3% (44 mL)
Nasal gel: 0.2% (28.4 g), 0.65% (30 g), 3% (20 g)

Intranasal as moisturizer:
   Child and adult:
      Spray/Mist: 2–6 sprays into each nostril Q2 hr PRN
      Drops: 2–6 drops into each nostril Q2 hr PRN
      Nasal gel: Use PRN to relieve nasal discomfort. Use at bedtime helps in preventing drying and crusting.
Cystic fibrosis (pretreatment with albuterol is recommended to prevent bronchospasms [see remarks]):
   ≥6 yr and adult: Nebulize 4 mL of 7% solution once daily–BID. If unable to tolerate the 7% strength, lower strengths of 3%, 3.5%, or 5% may be used.
Acute viral bronchiolitis (for hospitalized patients only; pretreatment with albuterol is recommended to prevent bronchospasms [see remarks]):
   Infant (>34 week' gestation up to 18 mo old): Nebulize 4 mL of 3% solution Q2 hr × 3 doses, followed by Q4 hr × 5 doses, followed by Q6 hr until discharge.

INTRANASAL USE: May be used as a nasal wash for sinuses, restore moisture, thin nasal secretions, or relieve dry, crusted, and inflamed nasal membranes from colds, low humidity, allergies, nasal decongestant overuse, minor nose bleeds, and other irritations. Nasal administration instructions:
Nasal drops: Tilt head back and hold bottle upside down.
Nasal spray: Hold head in upright position and give short, firm squeezes into each nostril. Sniff deeply.
Nasal gel: Apply around nostrils, under nose, or in nostrils as needed to help relieve discomfort.
NEBULIZATION: Hypertonic solutions lowers sputum viscosity and enhances mucociliary clearance.
Cystic fibrosis: Improves FEV_1 and reduces pulmonary exacerbation frequency. May cause bronchospasm, cough, pharyngitis, hemoptysis, and acute decline in pulmonary function (administer first dose in a medical facility). It is recommended to withhold therapy in the presence of massive hemoptysis.
Acute viral bronchiolitis: Reduces length of hospitalization when compared to normal saline. May cause acute bronchospasm and local irritation.

For explanation of icons, see p. 648

SODIUM PHOSPHATE
Fleet Enema, Fleet Pedia-Lax, Fleet Enema Extra, Fleet
Phospho-Soda, OsmoPrep, and generics
Laxative, enema/oral

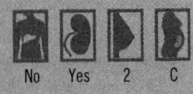

No   Yes   2   C

Enema [OTC]:
7 g dibasic sodium phosphate and 19 g monobasic sodium phosphate/118 mL; contains 4.4 g
sodium per 118 mL
>   **Pediatric size (Fleet Pedia-Lax):** 66 mL
>   **Adult size (Fleet Enema):** 133 mL

7 g dibasic sodium phosphate and 19 g monobasic sodium phosphate/197 mL; contains 4.4 g
sodium per 197 mL
>   **Fleet Enema Extra:** 230 mL

Oral solution (Fleet Phospho-Soda and generics) [OTC]: 2.4 g monobasic sodium phosphate and
0.9 g dibasic sodium phosphate/5 mL (45 mL); contains 96.4 mEq Na per 20 mL and 62.25 mEq
phosphate/5 mL

Oral tablets (OsmoPrep): 1.5 g

Not to be used for phosphorus supplementation (see *Phosphorus Supplements*).
Enema (see remarks):
>   **2–4 yr:** 33 mL enema (half of Fleet Pedia-Lax) × 1
>   **5–11 yr:** 66 mL enema (Fleet Pedia-Lax) × 1
>   **≥12 yr and adult:** 133 mL enema (Fleet Enema) *OR* 230 mL enema (Fleet enema Extra) × 1

Oral laxative (Fleet Phospho-Soda); mix with a full glass of water:
>   **5–9 yr:** 7.5 mL PO × 1
>   **10–11 yr:** 15 mL PO × 1
>   **≥12 yr and adult:** 15–45 mL PO × 1

Contraindicated in patients with severe renal failure, megacolon, bowel obstruction, and CHF. May
cause hyperphosphatemia, hypernatremia, hypocalcemia, hypotension, dehydration, and
acidosis. **Avoid** retention of enema solution and **do not exceed** recommended doses; may lead to
severe electrolyte disturbances due to enhanced systemic absorption. Colonic mucosal aphthous
ulceration should be considered when interpreting colonoscopy findings with use in patients with
known or suspected IBD. Rare but serious form of kidney failure (acute phosphate nephropathy)
has been reported with use of bowel-cleansing preparations such as Fleet Phospho-Soda.
Onset of action: PO, 3–6 hr; PR, 2–5 min

SODIUM POLYSTYRENE SULFONATE
Kayexalate, SPS, Kionex, and generics
Potassium-removing resin

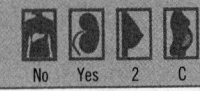

No   Yes   2   C

Powder: 454 g
Oral suspension: 15 g/60 mL (60, 120, 500 mL); contains 21.5 mL sorbitol per 60 mL and
0.1%–0.3% alcohol
Contains 4.1 mEq Na$^+$/g drug

NOTE: Suspension may be given PO or PR. Practical exchange ratio is 1 mEq K per 1 g resin. May
calculate dose according to desired exchange (see remarks).
Infant and child:
>   **PO:** 1 g/kg/dose Q6 hr
>   **PR:** 1 g/kg/dose Q2–6 hr. Dosing by practical exchange (1 mEq K per 1 g resin) has been
>   recommended for infants and smaller children.

SODIUM POLYSTYRENE SULFONATE *continued*

Adult:
  PO: 15 g once daily–QID
  PR: 30–50 g Q6 hr

Contraindicated in obstructive bowel disease, neonates with reduced gut motility, and oral administration in neonates. **Use cautiously** in presence of renal failure, CHF, hypertension, or severe edema. May cause hypokalemia, hypernatremia, hypomagnesemia, and hypocalcemia. Cases of colonic necrosis, GI bleeding, ischemic colitis, and perforation have been reported with concomitant use of sorbitol in patients with GI risk factors (prematurity, history of intestinal disease or surgery hypovolemia, and renal insufficiency/failure). Use in neonates generally **not recommended** owing to complication concerns for hypernatremia and NEC.
1 mEq Na delivered for each mEq K removed. **Do not administer** with antacids or laxatives containing Mg^{2+} or Al^{3+}; systemic alkalosis may result. Retain enema in colon for at least 30–60 min.

SPIRONOLACTONE
Aldactone and generics
Diuretic, potassium sparing

Yes   Yes   2   C/D

Tabs: 25, 50, 100 mg
Oral suspension: 1, 2, 2.5, 5, 10, 25 mg/mL

Diuretic:
  Neonate: 1–3 mg/kg/24 hr ÷ once daily–BID PO
  Child: 1–3.3 mg/kg/24 hr ÷ BID–QID PO; **max. dose:** 100 mg/24 hr
  Adult: 25–200 mg/24 hr ÷ once daily–BID PO (see remarks); **max.** 200 mg/24 hr
Diagnosis of primary aldosteronism:
  Child: 125–375 mg/m²/24 hr ÷ once daily–BID PO
  Adult: 400 mg once daily PO × 4 days (short test) or 3–4 wk (long test), then 100–400 mg once daily–BID maintenance
Hirsutism in women:
  Adult: 50–200 mg/24 hr ÷ once daily–BID PO

Contraindicated in Addison's disease, hyperkalemia, use with eplerenone, or **severe renal failure** (see Chapter 31). **Use with caution** in dehydration, hyponatremia, and renal or hepatic dysfunction. May cause hyperkalemia (especially with severe heart failure), GI distress, rash, lethargy, dizziness, and gynecomastia. May potentiate ganglionic blocking agents and other antihypertensives. Monitor potassium levels and be aware of other K^+ sources, K^+-sparing diuretics, and ACE inhibitors (all can increase K^+).
Do not use with other medications known to cause hyperkalemia (e.g., ACE inhibitors, angiotensin II antagonists, aldosterone blockers, and other potassium-sparing diuretics). Hyperkalemic metabolic acidosis has been reported with concurrent cholestyramine use. May cause false elevation in serum digoxin levels measured by radioimmunoassay.
Although TID–QID regimens have been recommended, data suggest once daily–BID dosing to be adequate. Pregnancy category changes to "D" if used in pregnancy-induced hypertension.

For explanation of icons, see p. 648

STREPTOMYCIN SULFATE
Various generics
Antibiotic, aminoglycoside; antituberculous agent

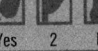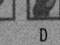

No   Yes   2   D

Powder for injection: 1 g

Tuberculosis: Use as part of multidrug regimen; see latest edition of AAP *Red Book*).
Infant, child, and adolescent:
 Daily therapy: 20–40 mg/kg/24 hr IM once daily; **max. daily dose:** 1 g/24 hr
 Twice-weekly therapy (under direct observation): 20–40 mg/kg/dose IM twice weekly; **max. daily dose:** 1.5 g/24 hr
Adult:
 Daily therapy: 15 mg/kg/24 hr IM once daily; **max. daily dose:** 1 g/24 hr
 Twice-weekly therapy (under direct observation): 25–30 mg/kg/dose IM twice weekly; **max. daily dose:** 1.5 g/24 hr
Brucellosis, tularemia, plague and rat bite fever: See latest edition of the *Red Book.*

Contraindicated with aminoglycoside and sulfite hypersensitivity. **Use with caution** in preexisting vertigo, tinnitus, hearing loss, and neuromuscular disorders. Drug is administered via deep IM injection **only**. Follow auditory status. May cause CNS depression, other neurologic problems, myocarditis, serum sickness, nephrotoxicity, and ototoxicity. Concomitant neurotoxic, ototoxic, or nephrotoxic drugs and dehydration may increase risk for toxicity.
Therapeutic levels: Peak 15–40 mg/L; trough: <5 mg/L. Recommended serum sampling time at steady state: trough within 30 min before third consecutive dose and peak 30–60 min after administration of third consecutive dose. Therapeutic levels are **not** achieved in CSF.
Adjust dose in renal failure (see Chapter 31).

SUCCIMER
Chemet, DMSA [dimercaptosuccinic acid]
Chelating agent

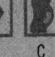

Yes   Yes   ?   C

Cap: 100 mg

Lead chelation, child:
 10 mg/kg/dose (or 350 mg/m²/dose) PO Q8 hr × 5 days, then 10 mg/kg/dose
 (or 350 mg/m²/dose) PO Q12 hr × 14 days
Manufacturer recommendation (see following table):

Weight (kg)	Dose (mg) Q8 hr × 5 Days, Followed by Same Dose Q12 hr × 14 Days
8–15	100
16–23	200
24–34	300
35–44	400
≥45	500

Use caution in patients with compromised renal or hepatic function. Repeated courses may be necessary. Follow serum lead levels. Allow minimum of 2 wk between courses unless blood levels require more aggressive management. Side effects: GI symptoms, increased LFTs (10%), rash, headaches, and dizziness. **Coadministration with other chelating agents is not recommended.** Treatment of iron deficiency is recommended, as well as environmental remediation. Contents of capsule may be sprinkled on food for those unable to swallow capsule.

SUCCINYLCHOLINE
Anectine, Quelicin, Quelicin-1000
Neuromuscular blocking agent

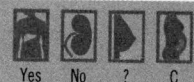

Yes   No   ?   C

Injection:

Anectine, Quelicin: 20 mg/mL (10 mL); contains parabens
Quelicin-1000: 100 mg/mL (10 mL); may contain parabens and/or benzyl alcohol

Paralysis for intubation (see remarks):
Infant and child:
Initial:
IV: 1–2 mg/kg/dose × 1
IM: 2.5–4 mg/kg/dose × 1
Max. dose: 150 mg/dose
Maintenance: 0.3–0.6 mg/kg/dose IV Q5–10 min PRN. Continuous infusion **not recommended** owing to risk of malignant hyperthermia.
Adult:
Initial:
IV: 0.3–1.1 mg/kg/dose × 1
IM: 2.5–4 mg/kg/dose × 1
Max. dose: 150 mg/dose
Maintenance: 0.04–0.07 mg/kg/dose IV Q5–10 min PRN. Continuous infusion **not recommended.**

Pretreatment with atropine is recommended to reduce incidence of bradycardia. For rapid sequence intubation, see Chapter 1.

Contraindicated after acute phase of an injury after major burns, multiple trauma, extensive denervation of skeletal muscle, or upper motor neuron injury, because severe hyperkalemia and subsequent **cardiac arrest** may occur.

Cardiac arrest has been reported in children and adolescents, primarily those with skeletal muscle myopathies (e.g., Duchenne muscular dystrophy). Identify developmental delays suggestive of a myopathy before use. Predose creatine kinase may be useful for identifying patients at risk. Monitoring of ECG for peaked T waves may be useful in detecting early signs of this adverse effect.

May cause malignant hyperthermia (use dantrolene to treat), bradycardia, hypotension, arrhythmia, and hyperkalemia. Severe anaphylactic reactions have been reported; **use caution** if previous anaphylactic reaction to other neuromuscular blocking agents. **Use with caution** in patients with severe burns, paraplegia, or crush injuries and in patients with preexisting hyperkalemia. Beware of prolonged depression in patients with liver disease, malnutrition, pseudocholinesterase deficiency, hypothermia, and those receiving aminoglycosides, phenothiazines, quinidine, β-blockers, amphotericin B, cyclophosphamide, diuretics, lithium, acetylcholine, and anticholinesterases. Diazepam may decrease neuromuscular blocking effects. Prior use of succinylcholine may enhance neuromuscular blocking effect of vecuronium and its duration of action.

Duration of action 4–6 min IV, 10–30 min IM. Must be prepared to intubate within 1 min.

For explanation of icons, see p. 648

SUCRALFATE
Carafate and many generics
Oral antiulcer agent

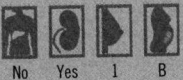

No   Yes   1   B

Tabs: 1 g
Oral suspension: 100 mg/mL (420 mL); contains sorbitol and parabens

Child:
Duodenal or gastric ulcer: 40–80 mg/kg/24 hr ÷ Q6 hr PO
Stomatitis: 5–10 mL (500–1000 mg of suspension), swish and spit or swish and swallow QID
Adult:
Duodenal ulcer:
Treatment: 1 g PO QID (1 hr before meals and QHS) or 2 g PO BID × 4–8 wk
Maintenance/prophylaxis: 1 g PO BID
Stress ulcer:
Treatment: 1 g PO Q4 hr
Prophylaxis: 1 g PO QID
Stomatitis: 10 mL (1000 mg of suspension), swish and spit or swish and swallow QID
Proctitis (use oral suspension as rectal enema): 20 mL (2 g) PR once daily–BID

May cause vertigo, constipation, and dry mouth. Hypersensitivity, including anaphylactic reaction, has been reported. Hyperglycemia has been reported in diabetic patients. Aluminum may accumulate in patients with renal failure. This may be augmented by the of aluminum-containing antacids. **Use with caution** in patients with dysphagia or other conditions that may alter gag or cough reflexes or diminish oropharyngeal coordination/motility in those receiving the oral tablet dosage form; cases of tablet aspiration with respiratory complications have been reported.

Decreases absorption of phenytoin, digoxin, theophylline, cimetidine, fat-soluble vitamins, ketoconazole, omeprazole, quinolones, and oral anticoagulants. Administer these drugs at least 2 hr before or after sucralfate doses.

Drug requires an acidic environment to form a protective polymer coating for damaged GI tract mucosa. Administer oral doses on an empty stomach (1 hr before meals and QHS).

SULFACETAMIDE SODIUM OPHTHALMIC
Bleph-10 and various generics
Ophthalmic antibiotic, sulfonamide derivative

No   No   ?   C

Ophthalmic solution: 10% (5, 15 mL); may contain methylparaben and propylparaben
Ophthalmic ointment: 10% (3.5 g); may contain phenylmercuric acetate

Ophthalmic (usual duration of therapy for ophthalmic use is 7–10 days):
>2 mo and adult:
Ointment: Apply 0.5-inch ribbon into conjunctival sac Q3–4 hr and QHS initially, and reduce the dosing frequency with adequate response.
Drops: 1–2 drops to affected eye(s) Q2–3 hr initially, and reduce the dosing frequency with adequate response.

Hypersensitivity reactions between different sulfonamides can occur regardless of route of administration. May cause local irritation, stinging, burning, conjunctival hyperemia, excessive tear production, and eye pain. Rare toxic epidermal necrolysis and Stevens-Johnson syndrome have been reported. Sulfacetamide preparations are incompatible with silver preparations.

To reduce risk of systemic absorption with ophthalmic solution, apply finger pressure to lacrimal sac during and 1–2 min after instillation.

SULFADIAZINE
Various generic products
Antibiotic, sulfonamide derivative

Yes   Yes   3   C/D

Tabs: 500 mg
Oral suspension: 100, 200 mg/mL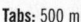

Infant ≥ 2 mo, child, and adolescent: 75 mg/kg/dose or 2000 mg/m^2/dose PO × 1, followed by
150 mg/kg/24 hr or 4000 mg/m^2/24 hr ÷ Q4–6 hr (**max. dose:** 6000 mg/24 hr).
Adult: 2–4 g/dose × 1, followed by 2–4 g/24 hr PO ÷ Q4–8 hr
*Congenital toxoplasmosis (administer with pyrimethamine and folinic acid; see pyrimethamine for
dosage information):*
Infant: 100 mg/kg/24 hr PO ÷ BID × 12 mo
*Toxoplasmosis (administer with pyrimethamine and folinic acid; see pyrimethamine for dosage
information):*
Infant ≥ 2 mo and child: 100–200 mg/kg/24 hr ÷ Q6 hr PO × 3–4 wk; **max. dose:** 6000 mg/24 hr.
Adult: 4–6 g/24 hr PO ÷ Q6 hr × 3–4 wk
Rheumatic fever prophylaxis:
≤27 kg: 500 mg PO once daily
>27 kg: 1000 mg PO once daily

Most cases of acquired toxoplasmosis do not require specific antimicrobial therapy.
Contraindicated in porphyria and hypersensitivity to sulfonamides. **Use with caution** in
premature infants and infants <2 mo because of risk of hyperbilirubinemia, and in hepatic or
renal dysfunction (30%–44% eliminated in urine). Maintain hydration. May cause fever,
rash, hepatitis, SLE-like syndrome, vasculitis, bone marrow suppression, and hemolysis in
patients with G6PD deficiency, and Stevens-Johnson syndrome.
May cause increased effects of warfarin, methotrexate, thiazide diuretics, uricosuric agents, and
sulfonylureas owing to drug displacement from protein-binding sites. Large quantities of vitamin C
or acidifying agents (e.g., cranberry juice) may cause crystalluria. Pregnancy category changes from
"C" to "D" if administered near term. Administer on an empty stomach with plenty of water.

SULFAMETHOXAZOLE AND TRIMETHOPRIM
Trimethoprim-sulfamethoxazole, Co-Trimoxazole, TMP-SMX;
Bactrim, Septra, Sulfatrim, and others
Antibiotic, sulfonamide derivative

Yes   Yes   2   D

Tabs (regular strength): 80 mg TMP/400 mg SMX
Tabs (double strength): 160 mg TMP/800 mg SMX
Oral suspension: 40 mg TMP/200 mg SMX per 5 mL (100, 480 mL)
Injection: 16 mg TMP/mL and 80 mg SMX/mL (5, 10, 30 mL); some preparations may contain
propylene glycol and benzyl alcohol.

Doses based on TMP component.
Minor/moderate infections (PO or IV):
Child: 8–12 mg/kg/24 hr ÷ BID
Adult (>40 kg): 160 mg/dose BID
Severe infections (PO or IV):
Child and adult: 20 mg/kg/24 hr ÷ Q6–8 hr
UTI prophylaxis:
Child: 2–4 mg/kg/24 hr PO once daily

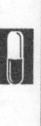

For explanation of icons, see p. 648

Continued

SULFAMETHOXAZOLE AND TRIMETHOPRIM *continued*

Pneumocystis jirovecii (carinii) *pneumonia* (PCP):

Treatment (PO or IV): 20 mg/kg/24 hr ÷ Q6–8 hr × 21 days

Prophylaxis (PO or IV):

≥*1 mo and child:* 150 mg/m²/24 hr ÷ BID for 3 consecutive days/wk; **max. dose:** 320 mg/24 hr

Adult: 160 mg once daily or 160 mg 3 days/wk

Not recommended for use with infants <2 mo (excluding PCP prophylaxis). **Contraindicated** in patients with sulfonamide or trimethoprim hypersensitivity, and megaloblastic anemia due to folate deficiency. May cause kernicterus in newborns. May cause blood dyscrasias, crystalluria, glossitis, renal or hepatic injury, GI irritation, rash, Stevens-Johnson syndrome, hemolysis in patients with G6PD deficiency. Severe hyponatremia may occur during treatment of PCP. Hyperkalemia may appear in HIV/AIDS patients. **Use with caution** in renal and hepatic impairment and G6PD deficiency. QT prolongation resulting in ventricular tachycardia has been reported.

Epidemiologic studies suggest use during pregnancy may be associated with increase risk of congenital malformations (particularly neural tube defects), cardiovascular malformations, urinary tract defects, oral clefts, and club foot.

Sulfamethoxazole is a CYP 450 2C9 substrate and inhibitor. Trimethoprim is a CYP 450 2C9, 3A4 substrate and 2C8/9 inhibitor. **Reduce dose in renal impairment (see Chapter 31). See Chapter 17 for PCP prophylaxis guidelines.**

SULFASALAZINE
Sulfazine, Sulfazine EC, Azulfidine, Azulfidine EN-tabs,
Salicylazosulfapyridine and generics
Antiinflammatory agent

Yes	Yes	2	B/D

Tabs: 500 mg
Delayed-release tabs (Azulfidine EN-tabs, Sulfazine EC): 500 mg
Oral suspension: 100 mg/mL

Inflammatory bowel disease:

Child ≥ 6 yr:

Initial dosing:

Mild: 40–50 mg/kg/24 hr ÷ Q6 hr PO

Moderate/severe: 50–75 mg/kg/24 hr ÷ Q4–6 hr PO

Max. initial dose: 4 g/24 hr

Maintenance: 30–70 mg/kg/24 hr ÷ Q4–8 hr PO; **max. dose:** 4 g/24 hr

Adult:

Initial: 3–4 g/24 hr ÷ Q4–8 hr PO

Maintenance: 2 g/24 hr ÷ Q6 hr PO

Max. dose: 6 g/24 hr

Juvenile idiopathic arthritis:

Child 6–16 yr: Start with 10 mg/kg/24 hr ÷ BID PO, and increase by 10 mg/kg/24 hr Q7 days until planned maintenance dose is achieved. Usual maintenance dose is 30–50 mg/kg/24 hr ÷ BID PO up to a **max.** of 2 g/24 hr.

Contraindicated in sulfa or salicylate hypersensitivity, porphyria, and GI or GU obstruction. **Use with caution** in renal impairment, blood dyscrasias, or asthma. Maintain hydration. May cause orange-yellow discoloration of urine and skin. May permanently stain contact lenses.

SULFASALAZINE *continued*

May cause photosensitivity, hypersensitivity, blood dyscrasias, CNS changes, nausea, vomiting, anorexia, diarrhea, and renal damage. Hepatotoxicity/hepatic failure, anaphylaxis, angioedema, severe drug rash with eosinophilia and systemic symptoms (DRESS), interstitial lung disease have been reported. May cause hemolysis in patients with G6PD deficiency. Decreases folic acid absorption and reduces serum digoxin and cyclosporine levels. Slow acetylators may require lower dosage owing to accumulation of active sulfapyridine metabolite.

Pregnancy category changes to "D" if administered near term. Bloody stools or diarrhea have been reported in breast-fed infants of mothers receiving sulfasalazine.

SUMATRIPTAN SUCCINATE
Imitrex, Alsuma, and generics
Antimigraine agent, selective serotonin agonist

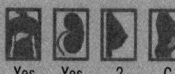
Yes   Yes   2   C

Injection for subcutaneous use: 8, 12 mg/mL (0.5 mL)
Tabs: 25, 50, 100 mg
Oral suspension: 5 mg/mL
Nasal spray (as a unit-dose spray device): 5 mg dose in 100 microliters (6 units per pack); 20 mg dose in 100 microliters (6 units per pack)

Adolescent and adult (see remarks):

PO: 25 mg as soon as possible after onset of headache. If no relief in 2 hr, give 25–100 mg Q2 hr up to a daily **max.** of 200 mg.
  Max. single dose: 100 mg/dose
  Max. daily dose: 200 mg/24 hr (with exclusive PO dosing or with an initial SC dose and subsequent PO dosing)
SC: 4–6 mg × 1 as soon as possible after onset of headache. If no response, may give an additional dose 1 hr later; **max. daily dose:** 12 mg/24 hr.
Nasal: 5–20 mg/dose into one nostril or divided into each nostril after onset of headache. Dose may be repeated in 2 hr up to a **max.** of 40 mg/24 hr.

Contraindicated with concomitant administration of ergotamine derivatives, MAOIs (and use within the past 2 wk) or other vasoconstrictive drugs. **Not** for migraine prophylaxis. **Use with caution** in renal or hepatic impairment. **A max. single dose** of 50 mg has been recommended in adults with hepatic dysfunction. Acts as selective agonist for serotonin receptor. Induration and swelling at injection site, flushing, dizziness, chest, jaw and neck tightness may occur with SC administration. Weakness, hyperreflexia, incoordination, and serotonin syndrome (may be life threatening) have been reported with use in combination with SSRIs (e.g., fluoxetine, fluvoxamine, paroxetine, sertraline).

May cause coronary vasospasm if administered IV. **Use injectable form SC only!** Onset of action is 10–120 min SC and 60–90 min PO. For nasal use, the safety of treating more than 4 headaches in a 30-day period has not been established.

Efficacy studies were not conclusive in clinical trials for children. Some **do not recommend** use in patients <18 yr owing to poor efficacy and reports of serious adverse events (e.g., stroke, visual loss, death) in both children and adults with all dosage forms.

To minimize infant exposure to sumatriptan, avoid breast-feeding for 12 hr after treatment.

For explanation of icons, see p. 648

SURFACTANT, PULMONARY/BERACTANT
Survanta
Bovine lung surfactant

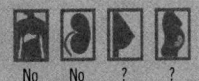

No   No   ?   ?

Suspension for inhalation: 25 mg/mL phospholipids (4, 8 mL); contains 0.5–1.75 mg triglycerides, 1.4–3.5 mg free fatty acids, and <1 mg protein per 1 mL drug

Prophylactic therapy: 4 mL/kg/dose intratracheally as soon as possible. Up to 4 doses may be given at intervals no shorter than Q6 hr during first 48 hr of life.

Rescue therapy (treatment): 4 mL/kg/dose intratracheally, immediately after diagnosis of respiratory distress syndrome (RDS). May repeat dose as needed Q6 hr to **max.** of 4 doses total.

Method of administration for previously listed therapies (see remarks): Suction infant before administration. Each dose is divided into 4 1-mL/kg aliquots; administer 1 mL/kg in each of 4 different positions (slight downward inclination with head turned to right, head turned to left; slight upward inclination with head turned to right, head turned to left).

Transient bradycardia, O_2 desaturation, pallor, vasoconstriction, hypotension, endotracheal tube blockage, hypercarbia, hypercapnia, apnea, and hypertension may occur during administration process. Other side effects may include pulmonary interstitial emphysema, pulmonary air leak, and posttreatment nosocomial sepsis. Monitor heart rate and transcutaneous O_2 saturation during dose administration. Monitor arterial blood gases for post-dose hyperoxia and hypocarbia after administration.

All doses are administered intratracheally via a 5 french feeding catheter. If suspension settles during storage, gently swirl contents—**do not shake**. Drug is stored in refrigerator, protected from light, and has to be warmed by standing at room temperature for at least 20 min or warmed in the hand for at least 8 min. Artificial warming methods should **NOT** be used.

SURFACTANT, PULMONARY/CALFACTANT
Infasurf
Bovine lung surfactant

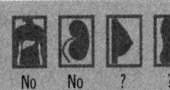

No   No   ?   ?

Intratracheal suspension: 35 mg/mL phospholipids (3, 6 mL); contains 26 mg phosphatidylcholine, 0.7 mg protein, and 0.26 mg surfactant protein B per 1 mL

Prophylactic therapy: 3 mL/kg/dose intratracheally as soon as possible. Up to a total of 3 doses may be given Q12 hr.

Rescue therapy (treatment [see remarks]): 3 mL/kg/dose intratracheally immediately after diagnosis of respiratory distress syndrome (RDS). May repeat dose as needed Q12 hr to **max.** of 3 doses total.

Method of administration for previously listed therapies (see remarks): Suction infant before administration. Manufacturer recommends administration through a side-port adapter into endotracheal tube with two attendants (one to instill drug and another to monitor and position patient). Each dose is divided into 2 1.5-mL/kg aliquots; administer 1.5 mL/kg in each of 2 different positions (infant positioned with either right or left side dependent). Drug is administered while ventilation is continued over 20–30 breaths for each aliquot, with small bursts timed only during inspiratory cycles. A pause followed by evaluation of respiratory status and repositioning should separate the 2 aliquots. Drug has also been administered by divided dose into 4 equal aliquots and administered with repositioning in prone, supine, right, and left lateral positions.

Common adverse effects include cyanosis, airway obstruction, bradycardia, reflux of surfactant into ET tube, requirement for manual ventilation, and reintubation. Monitor O_2 saturation and lung compliance after each dose such that oxygen therapy and ventilator pressure are adjusted as necessary.

SURFACTANT, PULMONARY/CALFACTANT *continued*

All doses administered intratracheally via a 5 french feeding catheter. If suspension settles during storage, gently swirl contents—**do not shake**. Drug is stored in refrigerator, protected from light, and does not have to be warmed before administration. Unopened vials that have been warmed to room temperature (once only) may be refrigerated within 24 hours and stored for future use.

For rescue therapy, repeat doses may be administered as early as 6 hr after previous dose for a total of up to 4 doses if infant is still intubated and requires at least 30% inspired oxygen to maintain a $Pao_2 \geq 80$ torr.

SURFACTANT, PULMONARY/LUCINACTANT
Surfaxin
Synthetic lung surfactant

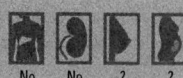

No   No   ?   ?

Suspension for inhalation: 30 mg/mL phospholipids (8.5 mL); contains 4.05 mg palmitic acid and 0.862 mg sinapultide per 1 mL drug

Prophylaxis therapy: 5.8 mL/kg/dose intratracheally as soon as possible; up to 4 doses may be given at intervals no shorter than 6 hr during first 48 hr of life.

Method of administration (see remarks): Suction infant before administration. Each dose is divided into 4 aliquots. Position infant in right lateral decubitus position with head and thorax inclined upward 30 degrees. Instill first aliquot (¼ of total dose) as a bolus while continuing positive-pressure mechanical ventilation and maintaining positive end-expiratory pressure of 4 to 5 cc H_2O (ventilator setting may be adjusted at clinician's discretion to maintain appropriate oxygenation and ventilation). Ventilate until infant is stable (at least 90% O_2 saturation and heart rate ≥ 120 beats/min), and repeat procedure and administer 2nd aliquot with infant in left decubitus position while maintaining adequate positive-pressure ventilation. Administer 3rd and 4th aliquots by repeating aforementioned procedures with infant in right and then left decubitus position, respectively. Remove catheter after administering 4th aliquot, and resume ventilator management and care with infant's head elevated at least 10 degrees for at least 1–2 hr. **Do not** suction infant during first hour unless significant airway obstruction.

Currently FDA approved for prophylaxis (prevention) of RDS. Bradycardia, oxygen desaturation, reflux of drug into ET tube, and airway/ET tube obstruction may occur (drug administration should be interrupted if any of these events occur). Suctioning of ET tube or reintubation may be necessary if airway obstruction persists or is severe.

All doses administered intratracheally via a 5 french catheter. Warm each vial for 15 min in a preheated dry block heater set at 44°C. Then shake vial vigorously until contents is a uniform and free-flowing suspension. If not immediately used after warming, vial can be stored at room temperature and protected from light for up to 2 hr. **Do not** return vial to refrigerator after warming. Single-use vials; discard unused portion if not used within 2 hr of warming.

For explanation of icons, see p. 648

SURFACTANT, PULMONARY/PORACTANT ALFA
Curosurf
Porcine lung surfactant

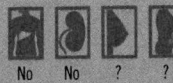

No   No   ?   ?

Intratracheal suspension: 80 mg/mL (1.5, 3 mL): contains 76 mg phospholipids, 1 mg and 0.45 mg surfactant protein B per 1 mL drug

Rescue therapy (treatment): 2.5 mL/kg/dose × 1 intratracheally immediately after diagnosis of respiratory distress syndrome (RDS). May administer 1.25 mL/kg/dose Q12 hr × 2 doses as needed up to a **max. total dose** of 5 mL/kg.

Method of administration (see remarks): Suction infant before administration. Each dose is divided into 2 aliquots, with each aliquot administered into 1 of the 2 main bronchi by positioning infant with either right or left side dependent. After first aliquot is administered, remove catheter from ET tube and manually ventilate infant with 100% oxygen at a rate of 40–60 breaths/min for 1 min. When infant is stable, reposition infant and administer second dose with same procedures. Then remove catheter **without** flushing.

Currently FDA approved for treatment (rescue therapy) of RDS. Transient episodes of bradycardia, decreased oxygen saturation, reflux of surfactant into ET tube, and airway obstruction have occurred during dose administration. Monitor O_2 saturation and lung compliance after each dose, and adjust oxygen therapy and ventilator pressure as necessary. Pulmonary hemorrhage has been reported.

All doses administered intratracheally via a 5 french feeding catheter. Suction infant before administration and 1 hr after surfactant instillation (unless signs of significant airway obstruction).

Drug is stored in refrigerator and protected from light. Each vial of drug should be slowly warmed to room temperature and gently turned upside down for uniform suspension (**do not shake**) before administration. Unopened vials that have been warmed to room temperature (once only) may be refrigerated within 24 hr and stored for future use.

TACROLIMUS
Astragraf XL, FK506, Hecoria, Prograf, Protopic, and generics
Immunosuppressant

Yes   Yes   2   C

Caps (Hecoria, Prograf, and generics): 0.5, 1, 5 mg
Extended-release caps (Astragraf XL): 0.5, 1, 5 mg (see remarks)

Oral suspension: 0.5, 1 mg/mL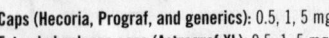
Injection (Prograf): 5 mg/mL (1 mL); contains alcohol, and polyoxyl 60 hydrogenated castor oil (cremophor)
Topical ointment (Protopic): 0.03%, 0.1% (30, 60, 100 g)

Child:
    Liver transplantation without preexisting renal or hepatic dysfunction (initial doses; titrate to therapeutic levels):
        IV: 0.03–0.05 mg/kg/24 hr by continuous infusion
        PO: 0.15–0.2 mg/kg/24 hr ÷ Q12 hr
Adult (initial doses; titrate to therapeutic levels):
    IV: 0.01–0.05 mg/kg/24 hr by continuous infusion
    PO: 0.075–0.2 mg/kg/24 hr ÷ Q12 hr
        Liver transplantation: 0.1–0.15 mg/kg/24 hr ÷ Q12 hr
        Kidney transplantation: 0.1–0.2 mg/kg/24 hr ÷ Q12 hr
        Cardiac transplantation: 0.075 mg/kg/24 hr ÷ Q12 hr

TACROLIMUS *continued*

Atopic dermatitis (continue treatment for 1 wk after clearing of signs and symptoms [see remarks]):

Child ≥ 2–15 yr old: Apply a thin layer of 0.03% ointment to affected skin areas BID and rub in gently and completely.

Adolescent ≥ 16 yr and adult: Apply a thin layer of 0.03% or 0.1% ointment to affected skin areas BID and rub in gently and completely.

Avoid use in patients with prolonged cardiac QT intervals. IV dosage form **contraindicated** in patients allergic to polyoxyl 60 hydrogenated castor oil (cremophor). Experience in pediatric kidney transplantation is limited. Pediatric patients have required higher mg/kg doses than adults. For BMT use (beginning 1 day before BMT), dose and therapeutic levels similar to those in liver transplantation have been used.

Major adverse events include tremor, headache, insomnia, diarrhea, constipation, hypertension, nausea, and renal dysfunction. Hypokalemia, hypomagnesemia, hyperglycemia, confusion, depression, infections, lymphoma, liver enzyme elevation, and coagulation disorders may also occur. GI perforation, agranulocytosis, and hemolytic anemia have been reported.

Tacrolimus is a substrate of the CYP 450 3A4 drug metabolizing enzyme. Calcium channel blockers, imidazole antifungals (ketoconazole, itraconazole, fluconazole, clotrimazole, posaconazole), macrolide antibiotics (erythromycin, clarithromycin, troleandomycin), cisapride, cimetidine, cyclosporine, danazol, methylprednisolone, and grapefruit juice can increase tacrolimus serum levels. In contrast, carbamazepine, caspofungin, phenobarbital, phenytoin, rifampin, rifabutin, and sirolimus may decrease levels. Use with sirolimus may increase risk for hepatic artery thrombosis. Use with other CYP 450 3A inhibitors and substrates have the potential to prolong cardiac QT interval. Reduce dose in renal or hepatic insufficiency.

Monitor trough levels (just before a dose at steady state). Steady state is generally achieved after 2–5 days of continuous dosing. Interpretation will vary based on treatment protocol and assay methodology (whole blood ELISA vs. MEIA vs. HPLC). Whole blood trough concentrations of 5–20 ng/mL have been recommended in liver transplantation at 1–12 mo. Trough levels of 7–20 ng/mL (whole blood) for the first 3 mo and 5–15 ng/mL after 3 mo have been recommended in renal transplantation.

Tacrolimus therapy generally should be initiated 6 hr or more after transplantation. PO is the preferred route of administration and should be administered on an empty stomach. Safety and efficacy of extended-release capsules have not been established for kidney transplant patients <16 yr old. IV infusions should be administered at concentrations between 0.004 and 0.02 mg/mL diluted with NS or D₅W.

TOPICAL USE: Not recommended for use in patients with skin conditions with a skin barrier defect with potential for systemic absorption. **Do not use** in children <2 yr, immunocompromised patients, or with occlusive dressings (promotes systemic absorption). Approved as second-line therapy for short-term and intermittent treatment of atopic dermatitis for patients who fail to respond or do not tolerate other approved therapies. Long-term safety is unknown. Skin burn sensation, pruritus, flulike symptoms, allergic reaction, skin erythema, headache, and skin infection are the most common side effects. Application site edema has been reported. Although the risk is uncertain, the FDA has issued an alert about potential cancer risk with use of this product. See www.fda.gov/medwatch for latest information.

For explanation of icons, see p. 648

TERBUTALINE
Various generics; previously available as Brethine
β₂-Adrenergic agonist

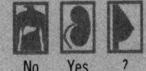

No   Yes   ?   C

Tabs: 2.5, 5 mg
Oral suspension: 1 mg/mL
Injection: 1 mg/mL (1 mL)

Oral:
≤12 yr: Initial: 0.05 mg/kg/dose Q8 hr; increase as required; **max. dose:** 0.15 mg/kg/dose Q8 hr or total of 5 mg/24 hr
>12 yr and adult: 2.5–5 mg/dose PO Q6–8 hr
   Max. dose:
     12–15 yr: 7.5 mg/24 hr
     >15 yr: 15 mg/24 hr
Nebulization:
  <2 yr: 0.5 mg in 2.5 mL NS Q4–6 hr PRN
  2–9 yr: 1 mg in 2.5 mL NS Q4–6 hr PRN
  >9 yr: 1.5–2.5 mg in 2.5 ml NS Q4–6 hr PRN
SC injection:
  ≤12 yr: 0.005–0.01 mg/kg/dose (**max. dose:** 0.4 mg/dose) Q15–20 min × 3 ; if needed, Q2–6 hr PRN
  >12 yr and adult: 0.25 mg/dose Q15–30 min PRN × 3; **max. total dose:** 0.75 mg
Continuous infusion, IV: 2–10 mcg/kg loading dose, followed by infusion of 0.1–0.4 mcg/kg/min. May titrate in increments of 0.1–0.2 mcg/kg/min Q30 min depending on clinical response. Doses as high as 10 mcg/kg/min have been used. **To prepare infusion,** see *IV Infusions* on page i.

Use of IV and PO routes should **not** be used for prevention or prolonged treatment of preterm labor; potential for serious maternal **cardiac events and even death**. Nervousness, tremor, headache, nausea, tachycardia, arrhythmias, and palpitations may occur. Paradoxical bronchoconstriction may occur with excessive use; if it occurs, discontinue drug immediately. Injectable product may be used for nebulization. For acute asthma, nebulizations may be given more frequently than Q4–6 hr. Use spacer device with inhaler to optimize drug delivery.
Monitor heart rate, blood pressure, respiratory rate, and serum potassium when using continuous IV infusion route of administration. **Adjust dose in renal failure (see Chapter 31).**

TETRACYCLINE HCL
Various generics; previously available as Sumycin
Antibiotic

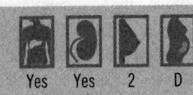

Yes   Yes   2   D

Caps: 250, 500 mg
Oral suspension: 25 mg/mL

Do not use in children <8 yr.
Child ≥ 8 yr: 25–50 mg/kg/24 hr PO ÷ Q6 hr; **max. dose:** 3 g/24 hr
Adult: 1–2 g/24 hr PO ÷ Q6–12 hr
  Acne vulgaris: 250 mg PO every other day to 500 mg PO once daily

Not recommended in patients <8 yr, owing to tooth staining and decreased bone growth. Also **not recommended** for use in pregnancy, because these side effects may occur in the fetus. Risk for these adverse effects are highest with long-term use. May cause nausea, GI upset,

TETRACYCLINE HCL *continued*

hepatotoxicity, stomatitis, rash, fever, and superinfection. Photosensitivity reaction may occur. Avoid prolonged exposure to sunlight.

Never use outdated tetracyclines; they may cause Fanconi-like syndrome. **Do not** give with dairy products or any divalent cations (i.e., Fe^{2+}, Ca^{2+}, Mg^{2+}). Give 1 hr before or 2 hr after meals.

May decrease effectiveness of oral contraceptives, increase serum digoxin levels, and increase effects of warfarin. Use with methoxyflurane increases risk for nephrotoxicity. Use with isotretinoin is associated with pseudotumor cerebri. **Adjust dose in renal failure (see Chapter 31).**

Short-term maternal use is not likely to cause harm to breast-feeding infant.

THEOPHYLLINE
Theo-24, Theochron, Elixophyllin, and generics
Bronchodilator, methylxanthine

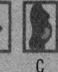

Yes No 2 C

Other dosage forms may exist.
Immediate release:
   Elixir (Elixophyllin): 80 mg/15 mL (473 mL); may contain up to 20% alcohol
Sustained/extended release (see remarks):
   Tabs:
      Q12 hr dosing, Theochron and generics: 100, 200, 300, 450 mg
      Q24 hr dosing, generics: 400, 600 mg
   Caps (Q24 hr dosing: Theo-24): 100, 200, 300, 400 mg
   Sustained-release forms should **not** be chewed or crushed. Capsules may be opened and contents sprinkled on food.

Dosing intervals are for immediate-release preparations.
For sustained-release preparations, divide daily dose >Q8–24 hr based on product.
Neonatal apnea:
   Loading dose: 5 mg/kg/dose PO × 1
   Maintenance: 3–6 mg/kg/24 hr PO ÷ Q6–8 hr
Bronchospasm; PO:
   Loading dose: 1 mg/kg/dose for each 2 mg/L desired increase in serum theophylline level
   Maintenance, infant (<1 yr):
      Preterm:
         <24 days old (postnatal): 1 mg/kg/dose PO Q12 hr
         ≥24 days old (postnatal): 1.5 mg/kg/dose PO Q12 hr
      Full term up to 1 yr old: Total daily dose (mg) = [(0.2 × age in weeks) + 5] × (kg body weight)
         ≤6 mo: Divide daily dose Q8 hr.
         >6 mo: Divide daily dose Q6 hr.
   Maintenance, child > 1 yr and adult without risk factors for altered clearance (see remarks):
      <45 kg: Begin therapy at 12–14 mg/kg/24 hr ÷ Q4–6 hr up to **max. dose** of 300 mg/24 hr. If needed (based on serum levels), gradually increase to 16–20 mg/kg/24 hr ÷ Q4–6 hr. **Max. dose:** 600 mg/24 hr.
      ≥45 kg: Begin therapy with 300 mg/24 hr ÷ Q6–8 hr. If needed (based on serum levels), gradually increase to 400–600 mg/24 hr ÷ Q6–8 hr.

Drug metabolism varies widely with age, drug formulation, and route of administration. Most common side effects and toxicities are nausea, vomiting, anorexia, abdominal pain, gastroesophageal reflux, nervousness, tachycardia, seizures, and arrhythmias.

Continued

THEOPHYLLINE *continued*

Serum levels should be monitored. Therapeutic levels: bronchospasm, 10–20 mg/L; apnea, 7–13 mg/L. Half-life is age dependent: 30 hr (newborns); 6.9 hr (infants); 3.4 hr (children); 8.1 hr (adults). See *Aminophylline* for guidelines for serum level determinations. Liver impairment, cardiac failure, and sustained high fever may increase theophylline levels. Theophylline is a substrate for CYP 450 1A2. Levels are increased with allopurinol, alcohol, ciprofloxacin, cimetidine, clarithromycin, disulfiram, erythromycin, estrogen, isoniazid, propranolol, thiabendazole, and verapamil. Levels are decreased with carbamazepine, isoproterenol, phenobarbital, phenytoin, and rifampin. May cause increased skeletal muscle activity, agitation, and hyperactivity when used with doxapram. May increase quinine levels/toxicity.

Because of poor distribution into body fat, use ideal body weight in obese patients when calculating dosage. Risk factors for increased clearance include smoking, cystic fibrosis, hyperthyroidism, and high-protein diet. Factors for decreased clearance include CHF, correction of hyperthyroidism, fever, viral illness, sepsis and high carbohydrate diet.

Suggested dosage intervals for sustained-released products (see following table):

Theophylline Sustained-Release Products

Trade Name	Available Strengths	Dosage Interval
CAPSULES		
Theo-24	100, 200, 300, 400 mg	Q24 hr
TABLETS		
Theocron	100, 200, 300, 450 mg	Q12–24 hr
Generic	400, 600 mg	Q24 hr

THIAMINE
Vitamin B$_1$, many generic products
Water-soluble vitamin

| No | No | 1 | A/C |

Tabs [OTC]: 50, 100, 250, 500 mg
Caps [OTC]: 50, 100, 500 mg
Injection: 100 mg/mL (2 mL); may contain benzyl alcohol

For US RDA, see Chapter 21.
Beriberi (thiamine deficiency):
  Child: 10–25 mg/dose IM/IV once daily (if critically ill) *OR* 10–50 mg/dose PO once daily × 2 wk, followed by 5–10 mg/dose once daily × 1 mo
  Adult: 5–30 mg/dose IM/IV TID (if critically ill) × 2 wk, followed by 5–30 mg/24 hr PO ÷ once daily or TID × 1 mo
Wernicke's encephalopathy syndrome:
  Adult: 100 mg IV × 1, then 50–100 mg IM/IV once daily until patient resumes a normal diet. (Administer thiamine before starting glucose infusion.)

Multivitamin preparations contain amounts meeting RDA requirements. Allergic reactions and anaphylaxis may occur, primarily with IV administration. Therapeutic range: 1.6–4 mg/dL. High-carbohydrate diets or IV dextrose solutions may increase thiamine requirements. Large doses may interfere with serum theophylline assay. Pregnancy category changes to "C" if used in doses above the RDA.

T

THIORIDAZINE
Various generic products, previously available as Mellaril
Antipsychotic, phenothiazine derivative

  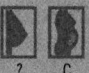

Yes No ? C

Tabs: 10, 25, 50, 100 mg

Child 2–12 yr: Start with 0.5 mg/kg/24 hr PO ÷ BID–TID; dosage range: 0.5–3 mg/kg/24 hr PO ÷ BID–TID. **Max. dose:** 3 mg/kg/24 hr.

>12 yr and adult: Start with 75–300 mg/24 hr PO ÷ TID. Then gradually increase PRN to **max. dose** of 800 mg/24 hr ÷ BID–QID.

Indicated for schizophrenia unresponsive to standard therapy. **Contraindicated** in severe CNS depression, brain damage, narrow-angle glaucoma, blood dyscrasias, and severe liver or cardiovascular disease. **DO NOT** coadminister with drugs that may inhibit CYP 450 2D6 isoenzymes (e.g., SSRIs [fluoxetine, fluvoxamine, paroxetine], β-blockers [propranolol, pindolol]), drugs that may widen QTc interval (e.g., disopyramide, procainamide, quinidine), or in patients with known reduced activity of CYP 450 2D6.

May cause drowsiness, extrapyramidal reactions, autonomic symptoms, ECG changes (QTc prolongation in a dose-dependent manner), arrhythmias, paradoxical reactions, and endocrine disturbances. Long-term use may cause tardive dyskinesia. Pigmentary retinopathy may occur with higher doses; a periodic eye examination is recommended. More autonomic symptoms and less extrapyramidal effects than chlorpromazine. Concurrent use with epinephrine can cause hypotension. Increased cardiac arrhythmias may occur with tricyclic antidepressants.

In an overdose situation, monitor ECG and avoid drugs that can widen QTc interval.

TIAGABINE
Gabitril and generics
Anticonvulsant

   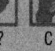

Yes No ? C

Tabs: 2, 4, 12, 16 mg
Oral suspension: 1 mg/mL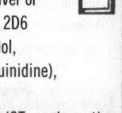

Adjunctive therapy for refractory seizures (see remarks):
Child ≥ 2 yr (limited data from a safety and tolerability study in 52 children 2–17 yr, mean 9.3 ± 4.1): Initial dose of 0.25 mg/kg/24 hr PO ÷ TID × 4 wk. Dosage was increased at 4-wk intervals to 0.5, 1, and 1.5 mg/kg/24 hr until an effective and well-tolerated dose was established. Criteria for dose increase required tolerance of the current dosage level and <50% reduction in seizures. Patients receiving enzyme-inducing antiepileptic drugs (AEDs) received a **max. daily dose** of 0.73 ± 0.44 mg/kg/24 hr, and patients receiving non–enzyme-inducing AEDs received a **max.** of 0.61 ± 0.32 mg/kg/24 hr.

Adjunctive therapy for partial seizures (dosage based on use with enzyme-inducing AEDs [see remarks]):
≥12 yr and adult: Start at 4 mg PO once daily × 7 days. If needed, increase dose to 8 mg/24 hr PO ÷ BID. Dosage may be increased further by 4–8 mg/24 hr at weekly intervals (daily doses may be divided BID–QID) until a clinical response is achieved or up to specified max. dose. **NOTE:** Patients receiving non–enzyme-inducing AEDs had tiagabine blood levels about 2 times higher than patients receiving enzyme-inducing AEDs.

Max. dose:
12–18 yr: 32 mg/24 hr
Adult: 56 mg/24 hr

Continued

TETRACYCLINE HCL *continued*

Use with caution in hepatic insufficiency (may have to reduce dose and/or increase dosing interval). Most common side effects include dizziness, somnolence, depression, confusion, and asthenia. Nervousness, tremor, nausea, abdominal pain, confusion, and difficulty in concentrating may also occur. Cognitive/neuropsychiatric symptoms resulting in nonconvulsive status epilepticus requiring subsequent dose reduction or drug discontinuation have been reported. Suicidal behavior or ideation has been reported. **Off-label use in patients WITHOUT epilepsy is discouraged** because of reports of seizures in these patients.

Tiagabine's clearance is increased by concurrent hepatic enzyme–inducing AEDs (e.g., phenytoin, carbamazepine, barbiturates). Lower doses or a slower titration for clinical response may be necessary for patients receiving non–enzyme-inducing drugs (e.g., valproate, gabapentin, lamotrigine). **Avoid** abrupt discontinuation of drug.

TID dosing schedule may be preferred because BID schedule may not be well tolerated. Doses should be administered with food.

TICARCILLIN AND CLAVULANATE
Timentin
Antibiotic, penicillin (extended spectrum with β-lactamase inhibitor)

   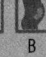
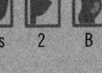

Yes   Yes   2   B

Injection: 3.1 g (3 g ticarcillin and 0.1 g clavulanate); contains 4.51 mEq Na$^+$ and 0.15 mEq K$^+$ per 1 g drug
Premixed injection: 3.1 g (3 g ticarcillin and 0.1 g clavulanate) in 100 mL; contains 18.7 mEq Na$^+$ and 0.5 mEq K$^+$ per 100 mL

All doses based on ticarcillin component.
Neonate (IV):

  ≤7 days:
    <2 kg: 150 mg/kg/24 hr ÷ Q12 hr
    ≥2 kg: 225 mg/kg/24 hr ÷ Q8 hr
  >7 days:
    <1.2 kg: 150 mg/kg/24 hr ÷ Q12 hr
    1.2–2 kg: 225 mg/kg/24 hr ÷ Q8 hr
    >2 kg: 300 mg/kg/24 hr ÷ Q8 hr
Term neonate and infant < 3 mo: 200–300 mg/kg/24 hr IV ÷ Q4–6 hr
Infant ≥ 3 mo and child < 60 kg:
  Mild/moderate infections: 200 mg/kg/24 hr IV ÷ Q6 hr
  Severe infections: 300 mg/kg/24 hr IV ÷ Q4–6 hr
  Max. dose: 18–24 mg/24 hr
Cystic fibrosis: 300–600 mg/kg/24 hr IV ÷ Q4–6 hr IV. **Max. dose:** 24 g/24 hr.
Adult: 3 g/dose IV Q4–6 hr IV
  UTI: 3 g/dose IV Q6–8 hr
  Max. dose: 18–24 g/24 hr

β-Lactamase inhibitor broadens spectrum to include *Staphylococcus aureus* and *Haemophilus influenzae*. Thrombophlebitis, rash, and immune hypersensitivity are common side effects. May also cause decreased platelet aggregation, bleeding diathesis, hypernatremia, hematuria, hypokalemia, hypocalcemia, allergy, and increased AST. Hemorrhagic cystitis has been reported. Use with caution with cephalosporin hypersensitivity and CHF (high sodium content). Like other penicillins, CSF penetration occurs only with inflamed meninges. May cause false-positive tests for urine protein and serum Coombs test.

Do not mix with aminoglycoside in same solution. Ticarcillin elimination is prolonged with impaired hepatic and/or renal function **(adjust dosage in renal impairment; see Chapter 31).**

TOBRAMYCIN
Bethkis, Nebcin, Tobrex, AKTob, TOBI, TOBI Podhaler, and generics
Antibiotic, aminoglycoside

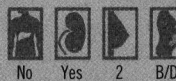

No   Yes   2   B/D

Injection: 10, 40 mg/mL; may contain phenol and bisulfites
Premixed injection: 80 mg in 100 mL NS
Powder for injection: 1.2 g; preservative free
Ophthalmic ointment (Tobrex, AKTob): 0.3% (3.5 g)
   In combination with dexamethasone (TobraDex): 0.3% tobramycin with 0.1% dexamethasone
   (3.5 g); contains 0.5% chlorbutanol
Ophthalmic solution (Tobrex): 0.3% (5 mL)
   In combination with dexamethasone: 0.3% tobramycin with 0.1% dexamethasone (2.5, 5, 10
   mL); contains 0.01% benzalkonium chloride and EDTA
Nebulizer solution:
   Bethkis: 300 mg/4 mL (56s); preservative free
   TOBI and generic: 300 mg/5 mL (56s); preservative free 170 mg/3.4 mL (mixed in 0.45% NS,
   preservative free, use with eFlow/Trio nebulizer)
Powder for inhalation:
   TOBI Podhaler: 28 mg capsules (224 capsules in 4 weekly packs with inhalation device)

Initial empirical dosage; patient-specific dosage defined by therapeutic drug monitoring
(see remarks):
Neonate/infant, IM/IV (see following table):

Postconceptional Age (wk)	Postnatal Age (Days)	Dose (mg/kg/dose)	Interval (hr)
≤29*	0–7	5	48
	8–28	4	36
	>28	4	24
30–33	0–7	4.5	36
	>7	4	24
34–37	0–7	4	24
	>7	4	18–24
≥38	0–7	4	24†
	>7	4	12–18

*Or significant asphyxia, PDA, indomethacin use, poor cardiac output, reduced renal function.
†Use Q36 hr interval for HIE patients receiving whole-body therapeutic cooling.

Child: 7.5 mg/kg/24 hr ÷ Q8 hr IV/IM
Cystic fibrosis (if available, use patient's previous therapeutic mg/kg dosage):
   Conventional Q8 hr dosing: 7.5–10.5 mg/kg/24 hr ÷ Q8 hr IV
   High-dose extended interval (once daily) dosing: 10–12 mg/kg/dose Q24 hr IV
Adult: 3–6 mg/kg/24 hr ÷ Q8 hr IV/IM
Ophthalmic:
   Tobramycin:
     Child and adult:
       Ophthalmic ointment: Apply 0.5-inch ribbon into conjunctival sac(s) BID–TID; for severe
       infections, apply Q3–4 hr.
       Ophthalmic drop: Instill 1–2 drops of solution to affected eye(s) Q4 hr; for severe infections,
       instill 2 drops Q30–60 min initially, then reduce dosing frequency.
   Tobramycin with dexamethasone:

Continued

TOBRAMYCIN *continued*

> **≥2 yr and adult:**
>> ***Ophthalmic ointment:*** Apply 0.5-inch ribbon of ointment into conjunctival sac(s) TID–QID.
>> ***Ophthalmic drop:*** Instill 1–2 drops of solution to affected eye(s) Q2 hr × 24–48 hr, then 1–2 drops Q4–6 hr.

Inhalation:
> **Cystic fibrosis prophylaxis therapy:**
>> **≥6 yr and adult:**
>>> ***Bethkis, TOBI, and generic product:*** 300 mg Q12 hr administered in repeated cycles of 28 days on drug, followed by 28 days off drug.
>>> ***Use with eFlow/Trio nebulizer:*** 170 mg Q12 hr administered in repeated cycles of 28 days on drug, followed by 28 days off drug.
>>> ***TOBI Podhaler:*** Four 28-mg capsules Q12 hr administered in repeated cycles of 28 days on drug, followed by 28 days off drug.

Use with caution in combination with neurotoxic, ototoxic, or nephrotoxic drugs; anesthetics or neuromuscular blocking agents; preexisting renal, vestibular, or auditory impairment; and in patients with neuromuscular disorders. May cause ototoxicity, nephrotoxicity, and neuromuscular blockade. Serious allergic reactions including anaphylaxis, and dermatologic reactions, including exfoliative dermatitis, toxic epidermal necrolysis, erythema multiforme, and Stevens-Johnson syndrome have been reported rarely. **Ototoxic effects synergistic with furosemide.**

Higher doses are recommended in patients with cystic fibrosis, neutropenia, or burns. **Adjust dose in renal failure (see Chapter 31).** Monitor peak and trough levels.

Therapeutic peak levels with conventional Q8 hr dosing:
   6–10 mg/L in general
   8–10 mg/L in pulmonary infections, neutropenia, osteomyelitis, and severe sepsis

Therapeutic trough levels with conventional Q8 hr dosing: <2 mg/L. Recommended serum sampling time at steady state: trough within 30 min before third consecutive dose and peak 30–60 min after administration of third consecutive dose.

Therapeutic peak and trough goals for high-dose extended-interval dosing for cystic fibrosis:
   Peak: 20–40 mg/L; recommended serum sampling time at 30–60 min after administration of first dose
   Trough: <1 mg/L; recommended serum sampling time within 30 min before second dose

Serum levels should be rechecked with changing renal function, poor clinical response, and at a minimum of once weekly for prolonged therapies.

To maximize bactericidal effects, an individualized peak concentration to target a peak/MIC ratio of 8–10:1 may be applied.

For initial dosing in obese patients, use an adjusted body weight (ABW). ABW = Ideal body weight + 0.4 (Total body weight − Ideal body weight).

INHALATIONAL USE: Transient voice alteration, bronchospasm, dyspnea, pharyngitis, and increased cough may occur. Transient tinnitus and hearing loss have been reported. If used with other medications in cystic fibrosis, use the following order of administration: bronchodilator first, chest physiotherapy, other inhaled medications (if indicated), and tobramycin last. For TOBI Podhaler, inhale entire contents of each capsule.

Pregnancy category is "D" for injection and inhalation routes of administration and "B" for ophthalmic route.

TOLNAFTATE
Tinactin and many generics
Antifungal agent
No No ? ?

Topical aerosol liquid [OTC]: 1% (128, 150 g); may contain 29% vol/vol or 41% wt/wt alcohol
Aerosol powder [OTC]: 1% (133 g); contains 11% vol/vol alcohol and talc
Cream [OTC]: 1% (15, 30, 114 g)
Topical powder [OTC]: 1% (45, 60, 108 g)
Topical solution [OTC]: 1% (10, 30 mL)

Child (≥2 yr) and adult:
Topical: Apply 1–3 drops of solution or small amount of liquid, cream, or powder to affected
areas BID–TID for 2–4 wk.

May cause mild irritation and sensitivity. Contact dermatitis has been reported. **Avoid** eye
contact. **Do not use** for nail or scalp infections. Discontinue use if sensitization develops.
Pregnancy category not formally assigned by FDA.

TOPIRAMATE
Topamax, Topiragen, Trokendi XR, and generics
Anticonvulsant
Yes Yes 2 D

Caps, sprinkle: 15, 25 mg
Tabs: 25, 50, 100, 200 mg
Extended-release caps (Trokendi XR; Q24 hr dosing): 25, 50, 100, 200 mg
Oral suspension: 6 mg/mL

Adjunctive therapy for partial onset seizures or Lennox-Gastaut syndrome:
Child 2–16 yr: Start with 1–3 mg/kg/dose (**max. dose:** 25 mg/dose) PO QHS × 7 days,
then increase by 1–3 mg/kg/24-hr increments at 1- to 2-wk intervals (divided daily dose BID)
to response. Usual maintenance dose is 5–9 mg/kg/24 hr PO ÷ BID.
≥17 yr and adult: Start with 25–50 mg PO QHS × 7 days, then increase by 25–50 mg/24 hr
increments at 1-wk intervals until adequate response. Doses >50 mg should be divided BID. Usual
maintenance dose: 100–200 mg/24 hr. Doses above 1600 mg/24 hr have not been studied.
Adjunctive therapy for primary generalized tonic-clonic seizures:
Child 2–16 yr: Use above initial dose and slower titration rate by reaching 6 mg/kg/24 hr by the end
of 8 weeks.
≥17 yr and adult: Use above initial dose and slower titration rate by reaching 200 mg BID by the
end of 8 weeks; **max. dose:** 1600 mg/24 hr.
Monotherapy for partial-onset seizures or primary generalized tonic-clonic seizures:
Child 2–<10 yr: Start with 25 mg PO QHS × 7 days. If needed and tolerated, may increase dose to
25 mg PO BID. May further increase by 25–50 mg/24 hr at weekly intervals over 5–7 weeks up to
lower end of the following daily target maintenance dosing range. (If needed and tolerated, increase
to higher end of dosing range by increasing by 25–50 mg/24 hr at weekly intervals.):
　　　≤11 kg: 150–250 mg/24 hr ÷ BID
　　　12–22 kg: 200–300 mg/24 hr ÷ BID
　　　23–31 kg: 200–350 mg/24 hr ÷ BID
　　　32–38 kg: 250–350 mg/24 hr ÷ BID
　　　>38 kg: 250–400 mg/24 hr ÷ BID
Child ≥ 10 yr and adult: Start with 25 mg PO BID × 7 days, then increase by 50 mg/24-hr increments
at 1-wk intervals up to a **max. dose** of 100 mg PO BID at wk 4. If needed, dose may be further
increased at weekly intervals by 100 mg/24 hr up to a recommended **max. dose** of 200 mg PO BID.
Continued

TOPIRAMATE *continued*

Use with caution in renal and hepatic dysfunction (decreased clearance) and sulfa
hypersensitivity. **Reduce dose by 50% when creatinine clearance is <70 mL/min.**
Common side effects (incidence lower in children) include ataxia, cognitive dysfunction,
dizziness, nystagmus, paresthesia, sedation, visual disturbances, nausea, dyspepsia, and
kidney stones. Secondary angle-closure glaucoma characterized by ocular pain, acute
myopia, and increased intraocular pressure has been reported and may lead to blindness if
left untreated. Patients should be instructed to seek immediate medical attention if they
experience blurred vision or periorbital pain. Oligohidrosis and hyperthermia have been
reported, primarily in children, and should be monitored, especially during hot weather and
with use of drugs that predispose patients to heat-related disorders (e.g., carbonic anhydrase
inhibitors, anticholinergics). Hyperchloremic non–anion gap metabolic acidosis has also been
reported. Suicidal behavior or ideation have been reported.

Drug is metabolized by and inhibits the CYP 450 2C19 isoenzyme. Phenytoin, valproic acid, and
carbamazepine may decrease topiramate levels. Topiramate may decrease valproic acid, digoxin,
and ethinyl estradiol (to decrease oral contraceptive efficacy) levels but may increase phenytoin
levels. Alcohol and CNS depressants may increase CNS side effects. Carbonic anhydrase inhibitors
(e.g., acetazolamide) may increase risk of metabolic acidosis, nephrolithiasis, or paresthesia. Use
with valproic acid may result in development of hyperammonemia.

Safety and efficacy in migraine prophylaxis in pediatrics have not been established; an increase in
serum creatinine has been reported in a clinical trial.

Doses may be administered with or without food. Capsule may be opened and sprinkled on small
amount of food (e.g., 1 teaspoonful of applesauce) and swallowed whole (**do not chew**). Maintain
adequate hydration to prevent kidney stone formation.

TRAZODONE
Many generics, previously available as Desyrel
Antidepressant, triazolopyridine derivative

   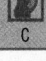

Yes   Yes   2   C

Tabs: 50, 100, 150, 300 mg

Depression (titrate to lowest effective dose [see remarks]):
  Child (6–18 yr): Start at 1.5–2 mg/kg/24 hr PO ÷ BID–TID. If needed, gradually increase
  dose Q3–4 days up to a **max. dose** of 6 mg/kg/24 hr ÷ TID.
    Alternative dosing for adolescent: Start at 25–50 mg/24 hr. If needed, increase to 100–150
    mg/24 hr in divided doses.
  Adult: Start at 150 mg/24 hr PO ÷ TID. If needed, increase by 50 mg/24 hr Q3–4 days up a **max.
  dose** of 600 mg/24 hr for hospitalized patients (400 mg/24 hr for ambulatory patients).
Insomnia with comorbid psychiatric disorders (limited data):
  18 mo–<3 yr: Start at 25 mg PO QHS. If needed, increase by 25 mg Q2 week up to a **max.** of 100
  mg/24 hr.
  3–5 yr: Start at 50 mg PO QHS. If needed, increase by 25 mg Q2 week up to a **max.** of 150 mg/24 hr.
  5 yr–adolescent: 25–50 mg PO QHS. If needed, increase by 25–50 mg Q2 week up to a **max.** of 200
  mg/24 hr. Daily dose may be divided BID–TID when used for palliative care.

Use with caution in preexisting cardiac disease, initial recovery phase of MI, in patients
receiving antihypertensive medications, renal and hepatic impairment (has not been
evaluated), and electroconvulsive therapy. Common side effects include dizziness,
drowsiness, dry mouth, and diarrhea. Seizures, tardive dyskinesia, EPS, arrhythmias,
priapism, blurred vision, neuromuscular weakness, anemia, orthostatic hypotension, and

TRAZODONE *continued*

rash have been reported. Monitor for clinical worsening of depression and suicidal ideation/behavior after initiation of therapy or after dose changes.

Trazodone is a CYP 450 3A4 isoenzyme substrate (may interact with inhibitors and inducers) and may increase digoxin levels and increase CNS effects of alcohol, barbiturates, and other CNS depressants. **Max. antidepressant effect is seen at 2–6 wk.**

TRETINOIN—TOPICAL PREPARATIONS
Retin-A, Retin-A Micro, Avita, Renova, and many others
Retinoic acid derivative, topical acne product

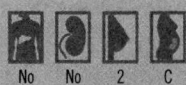

No   No   2   C

Cream: 0.02% (40, 60 g), 0.025% (20, 45 g), 0.05% (20, 40 g), 0.0375% (35 g), 0.07% (35 g); may contain parabens
Topical gel: 0.01% (15, 45 g), 0.025% (15, 20, 45 g), 0.04% (20, 45, 50 g), 0.05% (45 g), 0.1% (20, 45, 50 g); may contain 90% alcohol, benzyl alcohol, and propylene glycol

Topical:
Child > 12 yr and adult: Gently wash face with a mild soap, pat skin dry, and wait 20–30 min before use. Initiate therapy with either 0.02% or 0.025% cream or 0.01% gel, and apply a small pea-sized amount to affected areas of face QHS or on alternate days. See remarks.

Contraindicated in sunburns. **Avoid** excessive sun exposure. If stinging or irritation occurs, decrease frequency of administration to every other day. **Avoid** contact with eyes, ears, nostrils, mouth, or open wounds. Local adverse effects include irritation, erythema, excessive dryness, blistering, crusting, hyperpigmentation or hypopigmentation, and acne flare-ups. Concomitant use of other topical acne products may lead to significant skin irritation. Onset of therapeutic benefits may be experienced within 2–3 wk, with optimal effects in 6 wk. Gel dosage form is flammable and should not be exposed to heat or temperatures >120°F.

TRIAMCINOLONE
Aristospan, Kenalog, Nasacort AQ, Oralone, Trianex, Triderm, and generics
Corticosteroid

Yes   Yes   2   C/D

Nasal spray:
  Nasacort AQ and generics: 55 mcg/actuation (120 actuations per 16.5 g); contains benzalkonium chloride and EDTA
Cream:
  Triderm and generics: 0.1% (15, 28.4, 30, 85.2, 454 g)
  Generics: 0.025% (15, 80, 454 g), 0.5% (15 g)
Ointment:
  Trianex: 0.05% (17, 85 g)
  Generics: 0.025%, 0.1% (15, 80, 454 g), 0.5% (15 g)
Lotion: 0.025%, 0.1% (60 mL)
Topical aerosol (Kenalog): 0.2 mg/2-second spray (63, 100 g); contains 10.3% alcohol
Dental paste (Oralone and generics): 0.1% (5 g)
See Chapter 30 for potency rankings and sizes of topical preparations.
Injection as acetonide: 10 mg/mL (Kenalog-10) (5 mL), 40 mg/mL (Kenalog-40) (1, 5, 10 mL); contains benzyl alcohol
Injection as hexacetonide: 5 mg/mL (Aristospan Intralesional) (5 mL), 20 mg/mL (Aristospan Intraarticular) (1, 5 mL); contains benzyl alcohol

Continued

TRIAMCINOLONE *continued*

Intranasal (titrate to lowest effective dose after symptoms are controlled; discontinue use if no relief of symptoms after 3 wk of use):

Nasacort AQ:

Child 2–5 yr: 1 spray in each nostril once daily (110 mcg/24 hr; starting and **max. dose**).

Child 6–11 yr: Start with 1 spray in each nostril once daily (110 mcg/24 hr). If no benefit in 1 wk, dose may be increased to 2 sprays in each nostril once daily (220 mcg/24 hr). Decrease dose back to 1 spray in each nostril when symptoms are controlled.

≥12 yr and adult: 2 sprays in each nostril once daily (220 mcg/24 hr; starting and **max. dose**). Decrease dose to 1 spray in each nostril when symptoms are controlled.

Topical cream/ointment/lotion:

Child and adult: Apply a thin film to affected areas BID–TID for topical concentrations of 0.1% or 0.5%, and BID–QID for 0.025% or 0.05%.

Topical spray:

Child and adult: Spray to affected area TID–QID.

Intralesional:

≥12 yr and adult:

Acetonide salt (Kenalog-10; 10 mg/mL): Up to 1 mg/site at intervals of 1 wk or more. May give separate doses in sites >1 cm apart, **not to exceed** 30 mg.

Hexacetonide salt (Aristospan Intralesional; 5 mg/mL): Up to 0.5 mg/square inch of affected skin (initial dose range: 2–48 mg). Additional injections should be administered according to patient response.

Rare reports of bone mineral density loss and osteoporosis have been reported with prolonged use of inhaled dosage form. Nasal preparations may cause epistaxis, cough, fever, nausea, throat irritation, dyspepsia, and fungal infections (rarely). Topical preparations may cause dermal atrophy, telangiectasias, and hypopigmentation. Anaphylaxis has been reported with use of injectable dosage form. Topical steroids should be **used with caution** on the face and in intertriginous areas. See Chapter 8.

Dosage adjustment for hepatic failure with systemic use may be necessary. **Use with caution** in thyroid dysfunction, respiratory TB, ocular herpes simplex, peptic ulcer disease, osteoporosis, hypertension, CHF, myasthenia gravis, ulcerative colitis, and renal dysfunction. With systemic use, pregnancy category changes to "D" if used during first trimester. Pregnancy category is "D" with ophthalmic route.

Shake intranasal dosage forms before each use. **Avoid** SC and IV administration with injectable dosage forms. Injectable forms contain benzyl alcohol. Avoid spraying eyes or inhaling topical aerosol dosage form.

TRIAMTERENE
Dyrenium
Diuretic, potassium sparing

   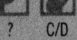

Yes	Yes	?	C/D

Caps: 50, 100 mg; may contain benzyl alcohol and povidone

Child: 1–2 mg/kg/24 hr ÷ BID PO. May increase up to a **max. dose** of 3–4 mg/kg/24 hr up to 300 mg/24 hr.

Adult: 50–100 mg/24 hr ÷ once daily–BID PO; **max. dose:** 300 mg/24 hr.

Do not use if GFR < 10 mL/hr. **Adjust dose in renal impairment (see Chapter 31)** and cirrhosis. Monitor serum electrolytes. May cause hyperkalemia, hyponatremia, hypomagnesemia, and metabolic acidosis. Interstitial nephritis, thrombocytopenia, and anaphylaxis have been reported.

TRIAMTERENE *continued*

Concurrent use of ACE inhibitors may increase serum potassium. **Use with caution** when administering medications with high potassium load (e.g., some penicillins) and in patients with hepatic impairment or on high potassium diets. Cimetidine may increase effects. This drug is also available as a combination product with hydrochlorothiazide; erythema multiforme and toxic epidermal necrolysis have been reported with this combination product. Administer doses with food to minimize GI upset. Pregnancy category changes to "D" if used in pregnancy-induced hypertension.

TRILISATE

See Choline Magnesium Trisalicylate

TRIMETHOBENZAMIDE HCL
Tigan and generics
Antiemetic

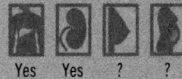
Yes   Yes   ?   ?

Caps: 300 mg
Injection: 100 mg/mL (2, 20 mL); may contain phenol or parabens

Child (PO): 15–20 mg/kg/24 hr ÷ TID–QID
  Alternative dosing:
    <13.6 kg: 100 mg TID–QID
    13.6–40 kg: 100–200 mg/dose TID–QID
    >40 kg: 300 mg/dose TID–QID
Adult:
  PO: 300 mg/dose TID–QID
  IM: 200 mg/dose TID–QID

Do not use in premature or newborn infants. **Avoid** use in patients with hepatotoxicity, acute vomiting, or allergic reaction. CNS disturbances are common in children (extrapyramidal symptoms, drowsiness, confusion, dizziness). Hypotension, especially with IM use, may occur. **IM not recommended in children.** Consider reducing dosage in the presence of renal impairment; significant amount of drug is excreted and eliminated by kidney.
FDA pregnancy category has not been formally assigned.

TRIMETHOPRIM AND SULFAMETHOXAZOLE

See Sulfamethoxazole and Trimethoprim

URSODIOL
Actigall, Urso 250, Urso Forte, and generics
Gallstone solubilizing agent, cholelitholytic agent

Yes   No   1   B

Oral suspension: 20, 25, 50, 60 mg/mL
Caps (Actigall and generics): 300 mg
Tabs:
  Urso 250 and generics: 250 mg
  Urso Forte and generics: 500 mg

Continued

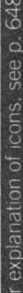

URSODIOL *continued*

Biliary atresia:
Infant (limited data): 10–15 mg/kg/24 hr once daily PO
TPN-induced cholestasis:
Infant and child (limited data from *Gastroenterology. 1996;111:716-719*): 30 mg/kg/24 hr ÷ TID PO
Gallstone dissolution:
Adult: 8–10 mg/kg/24 hr ÷ BID–TID PO
Cystic fibrosis (to improve fatty acid metabolism in liver disease):
Child: 15–30 mg/kg/24 hr ÷ BID–TID PO

Contraindicated in calcified cholesterol stones, radiopaque stones, bile pigment stones, or stones > 20 mm in diameter. **Use with caution** in patients with nonvisualizing gallbladder and chronic liver disease. May cause GI disturbance, rash, arthralgias, anxiety, headache, and elevated liver enzymes (elevated ALT, AST, alkaline phosphatase, bilirubin, GGT). Monitor LFTs Q mo for first 3 mo after initiating therapy and Q6 mo thereafter. Thrombocytopenia has been reported in clinical trials.

Aluminum-containing antacids, cholestyramine, and oral contraceptives decrease ursodiol effectiveness. Dissolution of stones may take several mo. Stone recurrence occurs in 30%–50% of patients within 5 yr.

VALACYCLOVIR
Valtrex and generics
Antiviral agent

Yes Yes 1 B

Tabs/Caplets: 500, 1000 mg
Oral suspension: 50 mg/mL

Child: Recommended dosages based on steady-state pharmacokinetic data in
immunocompromised children. Efficacy data are incomplete.
To mimic an IV acyclovir regimen of 250 mg/m²/dose or 10 mg/kg/dose TID:
30 mg/kg/dose PO TID OR alternatively by weight:
4–12 kg: 250 mg PO TID
13–21 kg: 500 mg PO TID
22–29 kg: 750 mg PO TID
≥30 kg: 1000 mg PO TID
To mimic a PO acyclovir regimen of 20 mg/kg/dose 4 or 5 times a day:
20 mg/kg/dose PO TID OR alternatively by weight:
6–19 kg: 250 mg PO TID
20–31 kg: 500 mg PO TID
≥32 kg: 750 mg PO TID
Chickenpox (immunocompetent patient; initiate therapy at earliest signs or symptoms within 24 hr of rash onset):
2–<18 yr: 20 mg/kg/dose PO TID × 5 days; **max. dose:** 1 g/dose TID
HSV treatment (immunocompetent):
3 mo–11 yr: 20 mg/kg/dose PO BID; **max. dose:** 1000 mg/dose
Herpes zoster (see remarks):
Adult (immunocompetent): 1 g/dose PO TID × 7 days within 48–72 hours of onset of rash
Genital herpes:
Adolescent and adult:
Initial episodes: 1 g/dose PO BID × 10 days

Continued

VALACYCLOVIR *continued*

Recurrent episodes: 500 mg/dose PO BID × 3 days
Suppressive therapy:
> ***Immunocompetent patient:*** 500–1000 mg/dose PO once daily × 1 year, then reassess
> for recurrences. Patients with <9 recurrences/yr may be dosed at 500 mg/dose PO once
> daily × 1 yr.

Herpes labialis (cold sores; initiated at earliest symptoms):
> **≥12 yr and adult:** 2 g/dose PO Q12 hr × 1 day

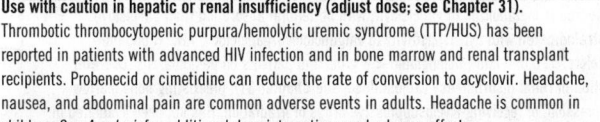

This prodrug is metabolized to acyclovir and L-valine, with better oral absorption than acyclovir.
Use with caution in hepatic or renal insufficiency (adjust dose; see Chapter 31).
Thrombotic thrombocytopenic purpura/hemolytic uremic syndrome (TTP/HUS) has been
reported in patients with advanced HIV infection and in bone marrow and renal transplant
recipients. Probenecid or cimetidine can reduce the rate of conversion to acyclovir. Headache,
nausea, and abdominal pain are common adverse events in adults. Headache is common in
children. See *Acyclovir* for additional drug interactions and adverse effects.

For initial episodes of genital herpes, therapy is most effective when initiated within 48 hr of symptom
onset. Therapy should be initiated immediately after onset of symptoms in recurrent episodes (no
efficacy data when initiating therapy >24 hr after onset of symptoms). Data unavailable for use as
suppressive therapy for periods >1 yr.

Valacyclovir **CANNOT** be substituted for acyclovir on a one-to-one basis. Doses may be administered
with or without food.

VALGANCICLOVIR
Valcyte
Antiviral agent

Yes Yes 3 C

Tabs: 450 mg
Oral solution: 50 mg/mL (88 mL); contains saccharin and sodium benzoate
Oral suspension: 60 mg/mL

Neonate and infant:
> ***Symptomatic congenital CMV (from pharmacokinetic [PK] data in 8 infants 4–90 days
> old (mean, 20 days) and 24 neonates 8–34 days old):*** 15–16 mg/kg/dose PO BID produced
> similar levels to IV ganciclovir 6 mg/kg/dose BID. Additional PK, safety, and efficacy studies are
> required.

Child (4 mo–16 yr):
> ***CMV prophylaxis in kidney or heart transplantation (once-daily PO dosage is calculated with the
> following equation):***
>> Daily mg dose (**max. dose:** 900 mg) = $7 \times BSA \times CrCl$. BSA is determined by the Mosteller
>> equation, and CrCl is determined by a modified Schwartz equation (**max. value:** 150 mL/
>> min/1.73m²).
>> **Mosteller BSA (m²) equation:** Square root of [(height (cm) × weight (kg)) ÷ 3600]
>> **Modified Schwartz (mL/min/1.73m²) equation (max. value: 150 mL/min/1.73m²):** k × height (cm)
>> ÷ serum creatinine (mg/dL), where k = 0.45 if patient is 4 mo to <2 yr old; k = 0.55 for boys
>> 2–<13 yr old and girls aged 2–16 yr old; or k = 0.7 if boys 13–16 yr old.
>
> ***CMV prophylaxis in liver transplantation (limited data based on a retrospective review in 10 patients,
> mean age 4.9 ± 5.6 yr):*** 15–18 mg/kg/dose PO once daily × 100 days after transplantation resulted in
> 1 case of asymptomatic CMV infection detected by CMV antigenemia at day 7 of therapy. This patient
> then received a higher dose of 15 mg/kg/dose BID until 3 consecutive negative CMV antigenemia tests
> were achieved. Dose was switched back to a prophylactic regimen at day 46 post transplant.

Continued

For explanation of icons, see p. 648

VALGANCICLOVIR *continued*

Adolescent (>16 yr) and adult:
   CMV retinitis:
      Induction therapy: 900 mg PO BID × 21 days with food
      Maintenance therapy: 900 mg PO once daily with food
   CMV prophylaxis in heart, kidney, and kidney-pancreas transplantation: 900 mg PO once daily, starting within 10 days of transplantation until 100 days post heart or kidney-pancreas transplantation, or until 200 days post kidney transplantation.

This prodrug is metabolized to ganciclovir, with better oral absorption than ganciclovir. **Contraindicated** with hypersensitivity to valganciclovir/ganciclovir, ANC < 500 mm³, platelets < 25,000 mm³, hemoglobin < 8 g/dL, and patients on hemodialysis. **Use with caution in renal insufficiency (adjust dose; see Chapter 31),** preexisting bone marrow suppression, or receiving myelosuppressive drugs or irradiation. Has not been evaluated in hepatic impairment. May cause headache, insomnia, peripheral neuropathy, diarrhea, vomiting, neutropenia, anemia, and thrombocytopenia. Use effective contraception during and for at least 90 days after therapy; may impair fertility in men and women. See *Ganciclovir* for drug interactions and additional adverse effects.

Valganciclovir **CANNOT** be substituted for ganciclovir on a one-to-one basis. All doses are administered with food. **Avoid** direct skin or mucous membrane contact with broken or crushed tablets.

VALPROIC ACID
Depakene, Depacon, Stavzor, and various generics
[Depakote: See Divalproex Sodium]
Anticonvulsant

Yes   No   2   D/X

Caps: 250 mg
Delayed-release caps (Stavzor): 125, 250, 500 mg
Syrup: 250 mg/5 mL (473 mL); may contain parabens
Injection (Depacon): 100 mg/mL (5mL)

Oral:
   Initial: 10–15 mg/kg/24 hr ÷ once daily–TID
   Increment: 5–10 mg/kg/24 hr at weekly intervals to **max. dose** of 60 mg/kg/24 hr
   Maintenance: 30–60 mg/kg/24 hr ÷ BID–TID. Owing to drug interactions, higher doses may be required in children on other anticonvulsants. If using divalproex sodium, administer BID.
IV (use only when PO is not possible):
   Use same PO daily dose ÷ Q6 hr. Convert back to PO as soon as possible.
Rectal (use syrup diluted 1:1 with water, given PR as a retention enema):
   Loading dose: 20 mg/kg/dose
   Maintenance: 10–15 mg/kg/dose Q8 hr
Migraine prophylaxis:
   Child (limited data): 15–30 mg/kg/24 hr PO ÷ BID; alternative dosing for children ≥12 yr is 250 mg PO BID (**max. dose:** 1000 mg/24 hr).
   Adult: Start with 500 mg/24 hr ÷ PO BID. Dose may be increased to a **max.** of 1000 mg/24 hr ÷ PO BID. If using divalproex sodium extended-release tablets, administer daily dose once daily.

Contraindicated in hepatic disease, pregnancy (for migraine indication), mitochondrial disorders with mutations in DNA polymerase gamma (e.g., Alpers-Huttenlocher syndrome), and children <2 yr suspected of the aforementioned mitochondrial disorder. May cause GI, liver, blood, and CNS toxicity. May also cause weight gain, transient alopecia, pancreatitis

Continued

VALPROIC ACID *continued*

(potentially life threatening), nausea, sedation, vomiting. headache, thrombocytopenia, platelet dysfunction, rash (especially with lamotrigine), and hyperammonemia. Hepatic failure has occurred, especially in children <2 yr (especially those receiving multiple anticonvulsants or with congenital metabolic disorders, severe seizure disorders with mental retardation, and organic brain disease). Idiosyncratic life-threatening pancreatitis has been reported in children and adults. Hyperammonemic encephalopathy has been reported in patients with urea cycle disorders. Suicidal behavior or ideation have been reported.

Valproic acid is a substrate for CYP 450 2C19 isoenzyme and an inhibitor of CYP 450 2C9, 2D6, and 3A3/4 (weak). It increases amitriptyline/nortriptyline, phenytoin, diazepam, and phenobarbital levels. Concomitant phenytoin, phenobarbital, topiramate, meropenem, and carbamazepine may decrease valproic acid levels. Amitriptyline or nortriptyline may increase valproic acid levels. May interfere with urine ketone and thyroid tests.

Do not give syrup with carbonated beverages. Use of IV route has not been evaluated for > 14 days of continuous use. Infuse IV over 1 hr up to a **max. rate** of 20 mg/min. Depakote and Depakote ER are **NOT** bioequivalent; see package insert for dose conversion.

Therapeutic levels: 50–100 mg/L. Recommendations for serum sampling at steady state: Obtain trough level within 30 min before next scheduled dose after 2–3 days of continuous dosing. Levels of 50–60 mg/L and as high as 85 mg/L have been recommended for bipolar disorders. Monitor CBC and LFTs before and during therapy.

Valproic acid and divalproex should not be used in pregnant women. Increased risk of neural tube defects, decreased child IQ scores, craniofacial defects, and cardiovascular malformations have been reported in babies exposed to valproic acid and divalproex sodium.

Pregnancy category is "X" when used for migraine prophylaxis and "D" for all other indications.

VALSARTAN
Diovan
Angiotensin II receptor blocker, antihypertensive agent

Yes   Yes   ?   D

Tabs: 40, 80, 160, 320 mg
Oral suspension: 4 mg/mL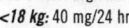

Hypertension (see remarks):
Child 1–5 yr (≥8 kg, limited data): a reported range of 0.4–3.4 mg/kg/dose PO once daily, with the following maximum doses:
    <18 kg: 40 mg/24 hr
    ≥18 kg: 80 mg/24 hr
Child 6–16 yr: Start at 1.3 mg/kg/dose (**max. dose:** 40 mg) PO once daily. Dose may be increased up to 2.7 mg/kg/dose up to 160 mg; doses greater than this have not been studied.
Adolescent ≥ 17 yr and adult (non–volume-depleted status): Start at 80 or 160 mg PO once daily; usual dose range is 80–320 mg once daily. **Max. dose:** 320 mg/24 hr.

Contraindicated with aliskiren use in diabetic patients. Discontinue use immediately after pregnancy is detected. **Use with caution** in renal and liver insufficiency (no data available), heart failure, post MI, renal artery stenosis, renal function changes, and volume depletion.

Hypotension, dizziness, headache, cough, and increases in BUN and SCr are common side effects. Hyperkalemia, angioedema, acute renal failure, and dysgeusia have been reported.

Onset of initial antihypertensive effects is 2 hr, with max. effects after 2–4 wk of chronic use. Patients may require higher doses of oral tablet dosage form than oral suspension (increased bioavailability with oral suspension).

For explanation of icons, see p. 648

VANCOMYCIN
Vancocin and generics
Antibiotic, glycopeptide

   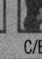

No Yes 2 C/B

Injection: 0.5, 0.75, 1, 5, 10 g
Premixed injection: 500 mg/100 mL in dextrose, 750 mg/150 mL in dextrose, 1000 mg/200 mL in dextrose (iso-osmotic solutions)
Caps: 125, 250 mg
Oral solution: 25 mg/mL

Initial empirical dosage; patient-specific dosage defined by therapeutic drug monitoring (see remarks).

Neonate, IV (see following table for dosage interval):
Bacteremia: 10 mg/kg/dose
Meningitis, pneumonia: 15 mg/kg/dose

Postmenstrual Age (wk)*	Postnatal Age (days)	Dosage Interval (hr)
≤29	0–14	18
	>14	12
30–36	0–14	12
	>14	8
37–44	0–7	12
	>7	8
≥45	All	6

*Postmenstrual age = gestational age + postnatal age.

Infant, child, adolescent, and adult, IV:

Age	General Dosage	CNS Infections, Endocarditis, Osteomyelitis, Pneumonia, and MRSA Bacteremia
1 mo–12 yr	15 mg/kg Q6 hr	20 mg/kg Q6 hr
Adolescent	15 mg/kg Q6–8 hr	20 mg/kg Q6–8 hr
Adult	15 mg/kg Q8–12 hr	20 mg/kg Q8–12 hr

Clostridium difficile *colitis*:
Child: 40–50 mg/kg/24 hr ÷ Q6 hr PO × 7–10 days
Max. dose: 500 mg/24 hr; higher max. of 2 g/24 hr has also been used.
Adult: 125 mg/dose PO Q6 hr × 7–10 days; dosages as high as 2 g/24 hr ÷ Q6–8 hr have also been used.
Endocarditis prophylaxis for GU or GI (excluding esophageal) procedures (complete all antibiotic dose infusion[s] within 30 min of starting procedure):
Moderate-risk patients allergic to ampicillin or amoxicillin:
Child: 20 mg/kg/dose IV over 1–2 hr × 1
Adult: 1 g/dose IV over 1–2 hr × 1
High-risk patients allergic to ampicillin or amoxicillin:
Child and adult: Same dose as moderate-risk patients plus gentamicin 1.5 mg/kg/dose (**max. dose:** 120 mg/dose) IV/IM × 1

Ototoxicity and nephrotoxicity may occur and may be exacerbated with concurrent aminoglycoside use. Greater nephrotoxicity risk has been associated with higher therapeutic serum trough concentrations (≥15 mg/mL) and receiving furosemide in the ICU. **Adjust dose in renal failure (see Chapter 31).** Use total body weight for obese patients when calculating dosages. Low concentrations of the drug may appear in CSF with inflamed meninges. Nausea,

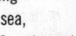

Continued

VANCOMYCIN *continued*

vomiting, and drug-induced erythroderma are common with IV use. "Red man syndrome" associated with rapid IV infusion may occur. Infuse over 60 min (may infuse over 120 min if 60-min infusion is not tolerated). **NOTE:** Diphenhydramine is used to reverse red man syndrome. Allergic reactions (including drug rash with eosinophilia and systemic symptoms [DRESS]), neutropenia, and immune-mediated thrombocytopenia have been reported.

Although current extrapolated adult guidelines suggest measuring only trough levels, an additional post-distributional level may be useful in characterizing enhanced/altered drug clearance for quicker dosage modification to attain target levels. This may be useful for infants with known faster clearance and patients in renal compromise. Consult a pharmacist.

The following therapeutic trough level recommendations are based on the assumption that the pathogen's vancomycin MIC is ≤1 mg/L.

Indication	Goal Trough Level
Uncomplicated skin and soft tissue infection, non-MRSA bacteremia, febrile neutropenia	10–15 mg/L
CNS infections, endocarditis, pneumonia, osteomyelitis, MRSA bacteremia	15–20 mg/L

Peak level measurement (20–50 mg/L) has also been recommended for patients with burns, clinically nonresponsive in 72 hr of therapy, persistent positive cultures, and CNS infections (≥30 mg/L).

Recommended serum sampling time at steady state: Trough within 30 min before fourth consecutive dose and peak 60 min after administration of fourth consecutive dose. Infants with faster elimination (shorter $T_{1/2}$) may be sampled around third consecutive dose.

ORAL USE: Metronidazole (PO) is the drug of choice for *C. difficile* colitis; vancomycin should be avoided owing to emergence of vancomycin-resistant enterococcus. Common adverse effects with oral vancomycin capsules in adults include nausea, abdominal pain, and hypokalemia.

Pregnancy category "B" is assigned with the oral route of administration.

VARICELLA-ZOSTER IMMUNE GLOBULIN (HUMAN)
VariZig, VZIG
Hyperimmune globulin, varicella-zoster

No   No   2   C

Injection: 125 U; contains 60–200 mg human immunoglobulin (Ig)G, 0.1 M glycine, 0.04 M sodium chloride, and 0.01% polysorbate 80. A vial of 8.5 mL sterile diluent is provided.

Dose should be given within 48 hr of varicella exposure and no later than 96 hr post exposure. IM (preferred route) or IV (see remarks):
  <2 kg: 62.5 U
  2.1–10 kg: 125 U
  10.1–20 kg: 250 U
  20.1–30 kg: 375 U
  30.1–40 kg: 500 U
  >40 kg: 625 U
  Max. dose: 625 U/dose
If patient is high risk and reexposed to varicella for >3 weeks after a prior dose, another full dose may be given.

Contraindicated in severe thrombocytopenia (risk with IM injection), IgA deficiency (anaphylactic reactions may occur), and known immunity to varicella-zoster virus. See Chapter 16 for indications. Local discomfort, redness, and swelling at injection site and headache may occur.

Continued

VARICELLA-ZOSTER IMMUNE GLOBULIN (HUMAN) *continued*

Hyperviscosity of blood may increase risk for thrombotic events. IM route is preferred over IV in patients with preexisting respiratory conditions. Interferes with immune response to live virus vaccines such as measles, mumps, and rubella; defer administration of live vaccines 6 mo or longer after VZIG dose. See latest AAP *Red Book* for additional information.

IM route is the preferred route by diluting each vial with 1.25 mL of diluent for a 100 U/mL concentration. **Avoid** IM injection into the gluteal region (risk for sciatic nerve damage), and **do not exceed** age-specific **single max. IM injection** volume. For IV administration, dilute each vial with 2.5 mL of diluent for a 50 U/mL concentration. IV doses are administered over 3–5 min.

VASOPRESSIN
Pitressin and various generics, 8-Arginine Vasopressin
Antidiuretic hormone analog

Yes   No   2   C

Injection: 20 U/mL (aqueous) (0.5, 1, 10 mL); may contain 0.5% chlorobutanol

Diabetes insipidus: Titrate dose to effect.
  SC/IM:
    Child: 2.5–10 U BID–QID
    Adult: 5–10 U BID–QID
  Continuous infusion (adult and child): Start at 0.5 mU/kg/hr (0.0005 U/kg/hr). Double dosage every 30 min PRN up to **max. dose** of 10 mU/kg/hr (0.01 U/kg/hr).
Growth hormone and corticotropin provocative tests:
    Child: 0.3 U/kg IM; **max. dose:** 10 U
    Adult: 10 U IM
GI hemorrhage (IV; NOTE: dosage metric is U/kg/min for children and U/min for adults):
    Child: Start at 0.002–0.005 U/kg/min. Increase dose as needed to **max. dose** of 0.01 U/kg/min.
    Adult: Start at 0.2–0.4 U/min. Increase dose as needed to **max. dose** of 0.8 U/min.
Cardiac arrest, ventricular fibrillation, and pulseless ventricular tachycardia:
    Child (use after 2 doses of epinephrine; limited data): 0.4 U/kg IV × 1
    Adult: 40 U IV or IO × 1
Vasodilatory shock with hypotension (unresponsive to fluids and pressors. NOTE: dosage metric is U/kg/min for children and U/min for adults):
    Infant, child, adolescent (various reports): 0.00017–0.008 U/kg/min via continuous IV infusion in combination with pressors.
    Adult: 0.01–0.04 U/min via continuous IV infusion in combination with pressors.

Use with caution in seizures, migraine, asthma, and renal, cardiac, or vascular diseases. Side effects include tremor, sweating, vertigo, abdominal discomfort, nausea, vomiting, urticaria, anaphylaxis, hypertension, and bradycardia. May cause vasoconstriction, water intoxication, and bronchoconstriction. Drug interactions: lithium, demeclocycline, heparin, and alcohol reduce activity; carbamazepine, tricyclic antidepressants, fludrocortisone, and chlorpropamide increase activity.
Do not abruptly discontinue IV infusion (taper dose). Patients with variceal hemorrhage and hepatic insufficiency may respond to lower dosages. Monitor fluid intake and output, urine specific gravity, urine and serum osmolality, and sodium.

VECURONIUM BROMIDE
Various generics; previously available as Norcuron
Nondepolarizing neuromuscular blocking agent

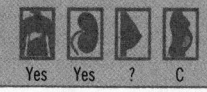

Yes   Yes   ?   C

Injection: 10, 20 mg; diluent for reconstitution may contain benzyl alcohol.

Neonate:
Initial: 0.1 mg/kg/dose IV
Maintenance: 0.03–0.15 mg/kg/dose IV Q1–2 hr PRN
Infants (>7 wk–1 yr) (see remarks):
Initial: 0.08–0.1 mg/kg/dose IV
Maintenance: 0.05–0.1 mg/kg/dose IV Q1 hr PRN; may administer via continuous infusion
at 0.06–0.09 mg/kg/hr IV.
>1 yr–adult (see remarks):
Initial: 0.08–0.1 mg/kg/dose IV
Maintenance: 0.05–0.1 mg/kg/dose IV Q1 hr PRN; may administer via continuous infusion
at 0.09–0.15 mg/kg/hr IV.

Use with caution in patients with neuromuscular disease and renal or hepatic impairment.
Dose reduction may be necessary in hepatic insufficiency. Infants (7 wk–1 yr) are more
sensitive to the drug and may have a longer recovery time. Children (1–10 yr) may require
higher doses and more frequent supplementation than adults. Enflurane, isoflurane,
aminoglycosides, β-blockers, calcium channel blockers, clindamycin, furosemide, magnesium
salts, quinidine, procainamide, and cyclosporine may increase potency and duration of
neuromuscular blockade. Calcium, caffeine, carbamazepine, phenytoin, steroids (chronic
use), acetylcholinesterases, and azathioprine may decrease effects. May cause arrhythmias,
rash, and bronchospasm. Severe anaphylactic reactions have been reported.
Neostigmine, pyridostigmine, or edrophonium are antidotes. Onset of action within 1–3 min.
Duration is 30–40 min. **See Chapter 1 for rapid sequence intubation.**

VERAPAMIL
Calan, Calan SR, Isoptin SR, Verelan, Verelan PM, and generics
Calcium channel blocker

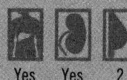

Yes   Yes   2   C

Tabs: 40, 80, 120 mg
Extended/sustained-release tabs: 120, 180, 240 mg
Extended/sustained-release caps (for Q24 hr dosing): 100, 120, 180, 200, 240, 300, 360 mg
Injection: 2.5 mg/mL (2, 4 mL)
Oral suspension: 50 mg/mL

IV for dysrhythmias: Give over 2–3 min. May repeat once after 30 min.
1–16 yr, for PSVT: 0.1–0.3 mg/kg/dose × 1; may repeat dose in 30 min; **max. dose:** 5 mg first
dose, 10 mg second dose
Adult, for SVT: 5–10 mg (0.075–0.15 mg/kg) × 1; may administer second dose of 10 mg (0.15 mg/
kg) 15–30 min later
PO for hypertension:
Child: 4–8 mg/kg/24 hr ÷ TID or by age:
  1–5 yr: 40–80 mg Q8 hr
  >5 yr: 80 mg Q6–8 hr
Adult: 240–480 mg/24 hr ÷ TID–QID, or divide once daily–BID for sustained-release preparations

Continued

VERAPAMIL *continued*

Contraindications include hypersensitivity, cardiogenic shock, severe CHF, sick sinus syndrome, or AV block. **Use with caution** in hepatic and renal impairment (**reduce dose in renal insufficiency [see Chapter 31]**). Owing to negative inotropic effects, verapamil should not be used to treat SVT in an emergency setting in infants. Avoid IV use in neonates and young infants; may cause apnea, bradycardia, and hypotension. May cause constipation, headache, dizziness, edema, and hypotension. EPS has been reported.

Monitor ECG. **Have calcium and isoproterenol available to reverse myocardial depression.** May decrease neuromuscular transmission in patients with Duchenne muscular dystrophy and worsen myasthenia gravis.

Drug is a substrate of CYP 450 1A2 and 3A3/4, and an inhibitor of CYP 3A4 and P-gp transporter. Barbiturates, sulfinpyrazone, phenytoin, vitamin D, and rifampin may decrease serum levels/effects of verapamil; quinidine and grapefruit juice may increase serum levels/effects. Verapamil may increase effects/toxicity of β-blockers (severe myocardial depression), carbamazepine, cyclosporine, digoxin, ethanol, fentanyl, lithium, nondepolarizing muscle relaxants, prazosin, and tizanidine. Use with telithromycin has resulted in hypotension, bradyarrhythmias, and lactic acidosis. Bradycardia has been reported with concurrent use of clonidine, and increased bleeding times have been reported when used with aspirin.

VIGABATRIN
Sabril
Anticonvulsant

 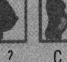

Yes   Yes   ?   C

Tabs: 500 mg
Powder for oral solution: 500 mg per packet to be dissolved in 10 mL water (50s)

Infantile spams (1 mo–2 yr; see remarks for discontinuation of therapy): Start at 50 mg/kg/24 hr ÷ BID PO. If needed and tolerated, may titrate dosage upwards by 25–50 mg/kg/24 hr increments Q3 days up to a **max.** of 150 mg/kg/24 hr ÷ BID.

Adjunctive therapy for refractory complex partial seizures (see remarks for discontinuation of therapy):
Child (≥10 kg): Start at 40 mg/kg/24 hr ÷ BID PO. If needed and tolerated, adjust dose to the following maintenance dose:
   10–15 kg: 500–1000 mg/24 hr ÷ BID
   16–30 kg: 1000–1500 mg/24 hr ÷ BID
   31–50 kg: 1500–3000 mg/24 hr ÷ BID
   >50 kg: 2000–3000 mg/24 hr ÷ BID
Adolescent (≥16 yr) and adult (see remarks for discontinuation of therapy): Start at 500 mg BID PO. If needed and tolerated, increase daily dose by 500-mg increments at 7-day intervals. Usual dose: 1500 mg BID. **Max. dose:** 6000 mg/24 hr. Doses >3 g/24 hr have not been shown to provide additional benefit and are associated with more side effects.

Use with caution in renal impairment (reduce dose [see Chapter 31]) and with other CNS depressants (enhanced effects). Can cause progressive and permanent vision loss (risk increases with dose and duration); periodic vision testing is required. Common side effects include rash, weight gain, GI disturbances, arthralgia, visual disturbances, vertigo, sedation, headache, confusion, and URI. Liver failure, anemia, psychotic disorder, angioedema, Stevens-Johnson syndrome, and suicidal ideation have been reported. Dose-dependent abnormal MRIs have been reported in infants treated for infantile spasms.

Ketorolac, naproxen, and mefloquine may decrease effect of vigabatrin. Vigabatrin may decrease effects/levels of phenytoin but increase levels/toxicity of carbamazepine.

Continued

VIGABATRIN *continued*

DO NOT rapidly withdraw therapy. Dosage must be tapered when discontinuing therapy to minimize increased seizure frequency. The following tapering guidelines have been recommended:

Infant and child: Decrease by 25–50 mg/kg every 3–4 days.

Adult: Decrease by 1 g/24 hr every 7 days.

Doses may be administered with or without food. Access to this medication is restricted to prescribers and pharmacies registered under a special restricted distribution program (SHARE) in the United States. Call 888–45-SHARE for more information.

VITAMIN A
Aquasol A and many generics
Vitamin, fat-soluble

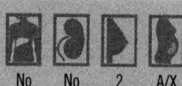

No   No   2   A/X

Caps [OTC]: 8,000, 10,000, 25,000 IU
Tabs [OTC]: 5,000, 10,000 IU
Injection (Aquasol A): 50,000 IU/mL (2 mL); contains polysorbate 80 and chlorobutanol

U.S. RDA: See Chapter 21.
Supplementation in measles (see remarks):
  <6 mo: 50,000 IU/dose once daily PO × 2 days. Repeat 1 dose at 4 wk.
  6 mo–1 yr: 100,000 IU/dose once daily PO × 2 days. Repeat 1 dose at 4 wk.
  1–2 yr: 200,000 IU/dose once daily PO × 2 days. Repeat 1 dose at 4 wk.
Malabsorption syndrome prophylaxis:
  Child > 8 yr and adult: 10,000–50,000 IU/dose once daily PO of water-miscible product

High doses above the U.S. RDA are teratogenic (category X). Use of vitamin A in measles is recommended in children 6 mo–2 yr of age who are either hospitalized or have any of the following risk factors: immunodeficiency, ophthalmologic evidence of vitamin A deficiency, impaired GI absorption, moderate to severe malnutrition, and recent immigration from areas with high measles mortality. May cause GI disturbance, rash, headache, increased ICP (pseudotumor cerebri), papilledema, and irritability. Large doses may increase effects of warfarin. Mineral oil, cholestyramine, and neomycin will reduce vitamin A absorption. Do not access vitamin A levels during an acute inflammatory condition as falsely low levels have been reported. **See Chapter 21 for multivitamin preparations.**

VITAMIN B₁

See *Thiamine*

VITAMIN B₂

See *Ribovlavin*

VITAMIN B₃

See *Niacin*

VITAMIN B₆

See *Pyridoxine*

VITAMIN B₁₂

See *Cyanocobalamin*

VITAMIN C

See *Ascorbic Acid*

VITAMIN D₂

See *Ergocalciferol*

VITAMIN D₃

See *Cholecalciferol*

VITAMIN E/α-TOCOPHEROL
Aquasol E, Aquavit-E, Nutr-E-Sol, and others
Vitamin, fat soluble

No   No   2   A/C

Tabs [OTC]: 100, 200, 400 IU
Caps [OTC]: 100, 200, 400, 600, 1000 IU
Oral solution (Aquasol E, Aquavit-E) [OTC]: 50 IU/mL (12, 30 mL); may contain propylene glycol, polysorbate 80, and saccharin
Oral liquid (Nutr-E-Sol) [OTC]: 400 IU/15 mL (473 mL)

U.S. RDA: See Chapter 21.
Vitamin E deficiency, PO: Follow levels.
   Use water-miscible form with malabsorption.
   Neonate: 25–50 IU/24 hr × 1 week, followed by recommended dietary intake
   Child: 1 IU/kg/24 hr
   Adult: 60–75 IU/24 hr
Cystic fibrosis (use water-miscible form): 5–10 IU/kg/24 hr PO once daily. **Max. dose:** 400 IU/24 hr.

Adverse reactions include GI distress, rash, headache, gonadal dysfunction, decreased serum thyroxine and triiodothyronine, and blurred vision. Necrotizing enterocolitis has been associated with large doses (>200 units/24 hr) of a hyperosmolar product administered to low-birth-weight infants. May increase hypoprothrombinemic response of oral anticoagulants (e.g., warfarin), especially in doses >400 IU/24 hr.
One unit of vitamin E = 1 mg of dl-α-tocopherol acetate. In malabsorption, water-miscible preparations are better absorbed. Therapeutic levels: 6–14 mg/L.
Pregnancy category changes to "C" if used in doses above the RDA. **See Chapter 21 for multivitamin preparations.**

VITAMIN K

See *Phytonadione*

VORICONAZOLE
Vfend and generics
Antifungal, triazole

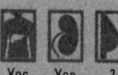

Yes   Yes   ?   D

Tabs: 50, 200 mg; contains povidone
Oral suspension: 40 mg/mL (75 mL); may contain sodium benzoate
Injection: 200 mg; contains 3200 mg sulfobutyl ether β-cyclodextrin (SBECD)

*Empirical doses. Between-patient and inter-occasion pharmacokinetic variability is high.
Monitor trough level, and adjust dose accordingly.* See www.clinicaltrials.gov for updated
dosing information.

<2 yr (limited data): 9 mg/kg/dose IV/PO Q12 hr

2–11 yr (limited data [see remarks]): 7–9 mg/kg/dose IV/PO Q12 hr. **Max. initial dose:** 350 mg/dose.
Invasive aspergillosis, invasive candidiasis, or other rare molds (e.g., **Scedosporium** *and*
Fusarium*)—including 12–14-yr-olds weighing <50 kg; dosing based on a previous clinical trial
that was terminated because of slow enrollment:* 9 mg/kg/dose IV Q12 hr × 2 doses, followed by 8
mg/kg/dose IV Q12 hr. Convert to oral therapy when significant clinical improvement after 1 week of
IV therapy at a dose of 9 mg/kg/dose PO Q12 hr (**max. dose:** 350 mg Q12 hr).
*Esophageal candidiasis—including 12–14-yr-olds weighing <50 kg; dosing based on a previous
clinical trial that was terminated because of slow enrollment:*
   IV: 4 mg/kg/dose Q12 hr
   PO: 9 mg/kg/dose Q12 hr; **max. dose:** 350 mg Q12 hr
Prophylaxis in pediatric acute leukemia (regimen currently being evaluated): 6 mg/kg/dose PO
Q12 hr × 2 doses, followed by 4 mg/kg/dose PO Q12 hr

≥12 yr and adolescent:
Invasive aspergillosis, invasive candidiasis, or other rare molds (e.g., **Scedosporium** *and*
Fusarium*)—excluding 12–14-yr-olds weighing <50 kg; dosing based on a previous clinical trial
that was terminated because of slow enrollment:* 6 mg/kg/dose IV Q12 hr × 2 doses, followed by
4 mg/kg/dose IV Q12 hr. Convert to oral therapy when significant clinical improvement after 1 week
of IV therapy at a dose of 200 mg PO Q12 hr. For patients weighing <50 kg, use 2–11-yr dosing
regimen. Alternatively, use adult PO dosage.
*Esophageal candidiasis—excluding 12–14-yr-olds weighing <50 kg; use 2–11-yr dosing regimen
for patients <50 kg); dosing based on a previous clinical trial that was terminated because of slow
enrollment:*
   IV: 3 mg/kg/dose Q12 hr
   PO: 200 mg Q12 hr; alternatively, use adult PO dosage.
Prophylaxis in pediatric acute leukemia (up to 15 yr old); regimen currently being evaluated:
6 mg/kg/dose PO Q12 hr × 2 doses, followed by 4 mg/kg/dose PO Q12 hr

Adult:
Invasive aspergillosis, candidemia, Fusarium/scedosporiosis, *or other serious fungal infections:*
   Loading dose: 6 mg/kg/dose IV Q12 hr x 2 doses
   Maintenance dose:
      Candidemia: 3–4 mg/kg/dose IV Q12 hr
      Invasive aspergillosis, Fusarium/scedosporiosis, *or other serious fungal infections:* 4 mg/kg/
      dose IV Q12 hr. If patient unable to tolerate, reduce dose to 3 mg/kg/dose IV Q12 hr.

Continued

For explanation of icons, see p. 648

VORICONAZOLE *continued*

PO maintenance dose: Initial dose may be increased to max. dose when response is inadequate. If dose is not tolerated, reduce dose by 50-mg increments until tolerated, with minimum of initial recommended dose.

<40 kg: 100 mg Q12 hr; **max. dose:** 300 mg/24 hr

≥40 kg: 200 mg Q12 hr; **max. dose:** 600 mg/24 hr

Esophageal candidiasis (treat for a minimum of 14 days and until 7 days after resolution of symptoms): Initial dose may be increased to max. dose when response is inadequate. If dose is not tolerated, reduce dose by 50-mg increments until tolerated, with minimum of initial recommended dose.

<40 kg: 100 mg Q12 hr; **max. dose:** 300 mg/24 hr

≥40 kg: 200 mg Q12 hr; **max. dose:** 600 mg/24 hr

Contraindicated with concomitant administration of CYP 450 3A4 substrates that can lead to prolonged QTc interval (e.g., cisapride, pimozide, quinidine); concomitant administration of rifampin, carbamazepine, barbiturates, ritonavir, efavirenz, rifabutin, and St. John's wort (decreases voriconazole levels); and concomitant administration of sirolimus, efavirenz, rifabutin, and ergot alkaloids (voriconazole increases levels of these drugs). Drug is a substrate and inhibitor of CYP 450 2C9, 2C19 (major substrate), and 3A4 isoenzymes. **Use with caution** in severe hepatic disease and galactose intolerance.

Currently approved for use in invasive aspergillosis, candidal esophagitis, and *Fusarium* and *Scedosporium apiospermum* infections. Common side effects include GI disturbances, fever, headache, hepatic abnormalities, photosensitivity (avoid direct sunlight), rash (6%), and visual disturbances (30%). Serious but rare side effects include anaphylaxis, liver or renal failure, and Stevens-Johnsons syndrome. Pancreatitis has been reported in children.

Adjust dose in hepatic impairment by decreasing only the maintenance dose by 50% for patients with a Child-Pugh class A or B. **Do not use** IV dosage form for patients with GFR <50 mL/min because of accumulation of the cyclodextrin excipient; switch to oral therapy if possible. Patients receiving concurrent phenytoin should increase their voriconazole maintenance doses (IV: 5 mg/kg/dose Q12 hr; PO: double the usual dose).

See www.clinicaltrials.gov for updated pediatric clinical trial information. Inter-occasion pharmacokinetic variability is high, requiring serum level monitoring. Therapeutic levels: trough, 1–5.5 mg/L. Levels <1 mg/L have resulted in treatment failures, and levels >5.5 mg/L have resulted in neurotoxicity (e.g., encephalopathy). Recommended serum sampling time: Obtain trough within 30 min before a dose. Steady state is typically achieved 5–7 days after initiating therapy.

Administer IV over 1–2 hr, with a **max. rate** of 3 mg/kg/hr at a concentration ≤5 mg/mL. Administer oral doses 1 hr before and after meals.

WARFARIN
Coumadin, Jantoven, and generics
Anticoagulant

Yes | Yes | 1 | X

Tabs: 1, 2, 2.5, 3, 4, 5, 6, 7.5, 10 mg
Injection: 5 mg

Infant and child (see remarks), to achieve an INR between 2 and 3:

Loading dose on day 1:

Baseline INR ≤ 1.3: 0.2 mg/kg/dose PO; **max. dose:** 7.5 mg/dose

Liver dysfunction, baseline INR > 1.3, undergone Fontan procedure, NPO status/poor nutrition, receiving broad-spectrum antibiotics, receiving medications that significantly inhibit CYP 450 2C9 or slow metabolizers of warfarin (see remarks): 0.1 mg/kg/dose PO; **max. dose:** 5 mg/dose

Continued

WARFARIN *continued*

Loading dose on days 2–4:
If INR 1.1–1.3: Repeat day 1 loading dose.
If INR 1.4–1.9: Decrease day 1 loading dose by 50%.
If INR 2–3: Decrease day 1 loading dose by 50%.
If INR 3.1–3.5: Decrease day 1 loading dose by 75%.
If INR > 3.5: Hold doses until INR < 3.5, and restart at 50% of previous dose.

Maintenance dose (therapy day ≥ 5):
If INR 1.1–1.4: Increase previous dose by 20%.
If INR 1.5–1.9: Increase previous dose by 10%.
If INR 2–3: No change.
If INR 3.1–3.5: Decrease previous dose by 10%.
If INR > 3.5: Hold doses until INR < 3.5, and restart at 20% less than the last dose.
Usual maintenance dose: ≈0.1 mg/kg/24 hr PO once daily; range, 0.05–0.34 mg/kg/24 hr. (See remarks.)

Adult (see remarks): 5–10 mg PO once daily × 2–5 days. Adjust dose to achieve the desired INR or PT.
Maintenance dose range: 2–10 mg/24 hr PO once daily

Contraindicated in severe liver or kidney disease, uncontrolled bleeding, GI ulcers, and malignant hypertension. Acts on vitamin K–dependent coagulation factors II, VII, IX, and X. Side effects include fever, skin lesions, skin necrosis (especially in protein C deficiency), anorexia, nausea, vomiting, diarrhea, hemorrhage, and hemoptysis.

Warfarin is a substrate for CYP 450 1A2, 2C8, 2C9, 2C18, 2C19, and 3A3/4. Chloramphenicol, chloral hydrate, cimetidine, delavirdine, fluconazole, fluoxetine, metronidazole, indomethacin, large doses of vitamins A or E, NSAIDs, omeprazole, oxandrolone, quinidine, salicylates, SSRIs (e.g., fluoxetine, paroxetine, sertraline), sulfonamides, and zafirlukast may increase warfarin's effect. Ascorbic acid, barbiturates, carbamazepine, cholestyramine, dicloxacillin, griseofulvin, oral contraceptives, rifampin, spironolactone, sucralfate, and vitamin K (including foods with high content) may decrease warfarin's effect.

Younger children generally require higher doses to achieve desired effect. A cohort study of 319 children found that infants <1 yr required an average daily dose of 0.33 mg/kg, and teenagers 11–18 yr required 0.09 mg/kg to maintain a target INR of 2–3. Children receiving Fontan cardiac surgery may require smaller doses than children with either congenital heart disease (without Fontan) or no congenital heart disease. (See *Chest.* 2004;126:645-687S and *Blood.* 1999;94:3007-3014 for additional information.)

Lower initial doses should be considered for patients with pharmacogenetic variations in CYP 2C9 (e.g., *2 and *3 alleles) and VKORC1 (e.g., 1639G>A allele) enzymes, elderly and/or debilitated patients, and patients with a potential to exhibit greater than expected PT/INR response to warfarin.

The INR (international normalized ratio) is the recommended test to monitor warfarin anticoagulant effect. It takes 5–7 days for an INR to reach steady state on a consistent dosing schedule. The particular INR desired is based upon the indication and has been extrapolated from adults. An INR of 2–3 has been recommended for prophylaxis and treatment of DVT, pulmonary emboli, and bioprosthetic heart valves. An INR of 2.5–3.5 has been recommended for mechanical prosthetic heart valves and prevention of recurrent systemic emboli. If PT is monitored, it should be 1.5–2 times the control. Patients at high risk for bleeding may benefit from more frequent INR monitoring.

Onset of action occurs within 36–72 hr, and peak effects occur within 5–7 days. IV dosing is equivalent to PO doses and is used in situations where oral dosing is not possible. **The antidote is vitamin K and fresh frozen plasma.**

For explanation of icons, see p. 648

ZAFIRLUKAST
Accolate and generics
Anti-asthmatic, leukotriene receptor antagonist

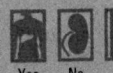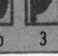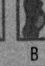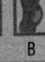

Yes | No | 3 | B

Tabs: 10, 20 mg

Asthma:
Child 5–11 yr: 10 mg PO BID
Child ≥ 12 yr and adult: 20 mg PO BID

Contraindicated in hepatic impairment, including hepatic cirrhosis. May cause headache, dizziness, nausea, diarrhea, abdominal pain, vomiting, generalized pain, asthenia, myalgia, fever, LFT elevation, and dyspepsia. Eosinophilia, vasculitic rash, worsening pulmonary symptoms, cardiac complications, and/or neuropathy have been reported, primarily in patients with oral steroid dose reduction. Hepatitis, hyperbilirubinemia, hepatic failure, hypersensitivity reactions (e.g., urticaria, angioedema and rashes), and neuropsychiatric events (e.g., aggression, anxiety, dream abnormalities, hallucinations, depression, suicidal behavior, insomnia) have also been reported.

Drug is a substrate for CYP 450 2C9 and inhibits CYP 450 2C9 and 3A4 isoenzymes. Erythromycin, terfenadine, and theophylline decrease zafirlukast levels; aspirin increases levels. Zafirlukast may increase effects of warfarin. Administer doses on an empty stomach, at least 1 hr before or 2 hr after eating.

ZIDOVUDINE
Retrovir, AZT, and generics
Antiviral agent, nucleoside analog reverse transcriptase inhibitor

Yes | Yes | 3 | C

Caps: 100 mg
Tabs: 300 mg
Oral syrup: 50 mg/5 mL (240 mL); contains 0.2% sodium benzoate
Injection: 10 mg/mL (20 mL); preservative free
In combination with lamivudine (3TC) as Combivir:
    Tabs: 300 mg zidovudine + 150 mg lamivudine
In combination with abacavir and lamivudine (3TC) as Trizivir:
    Tabs: 300 mg zidovudine + 300 mg abacavir + 150 mg lamivudine

HIV: See www.aidsinfo.nih.gov/guidelines.
Prevention of vertical transmission:
    14–34 weeks of pregnancy (maternal dosing):
        Until labor: 600 mg/24 hr PO ÷ BID–TID
    During labor: 2 mg/kg/dose IV over 1 hr, followed by 1 mg/kg/hr IV infusion until umbilical cord clamped
    Term neonate and infant < 6 wk (initiate therapy within 12 hr of birth and continue until 6 wk' of age):
        PO: 2 mg/kg/dose Q6 hr or 4 mg/kg/dose Q12 hr
        IV: 1.5 mg/kg/dose Q6 hr or 3 mg/kg/dose Q12 hr, administered over 60 min

ZIDOVUDINE *continued*

Premature infant:

Gestational Age (wk)	Oral (PO) Dosage	Intravenous (IV) Dosage*
<30	2 mg/kg/dose Q12 hr; increase to 3 mg/kg/dose Q12 hr at 4 wk of age	1.5 mg/kg/dose Q12 hr; increase to 2.3 mg/kg/dose Q12 hr at 4 wk of age
30–34	2 mg/kg/dose Q12 hr; increase to 3 mg/kg/dose Q12 hr at postnatal age of 15 days	1.5 mg/kg/dose Q12 hr; increase to 2.3 mg/kg/dose Q12 hr at postnatal age of 15 days
≥35	4 mg/kg/dose Q12 hr	3 mg/kg/dose Q12 hr

*Convert to PO route when possible.

HIV postexposure prophylaxis (all therapies to begin within 2 hr of exposure if possible):
≥*12 yr and adult:* 200 mg/dose PO TID or 300 mg/dose PO BID × 28 days. Use in combination with lamivudine or emtricitabine and with either one of the following: lopinavir/ritonavir, atazanavir/ritonavir, darunavir/ritonavir, raltegravir, etravirine, or etravirine × 28 days. Many other regimens exist; see www.aidsinfo.nih.gov/guidelines for the most recent information.

See www. aidsinfo.nih.gov/guidelines for additional remarks.

Use with caution in patients with impaired renal or hepatic function. Dosage reduction is recommended in severe renal impairment and may be necessary in hepatic dysfunction. Drug penetrates well into CNS. Most common side effects include anemia, granulocytopenia, nausea, and headache (dosage reduction, erythropoietin, filgrastim/GCSF, or discontinuance may be required, depending on event). Seizures, confusion, rash, myositis, myopathy (use > 1 yr), hepatitis, and elevated liver enzymes have been reported. Macrocytosis is noted after 4 wk of therapy and can be used as an indicator of compliance. Lactic acidosis and severe hepatomegaly with steatosis, including fatal cases, have been reported.

Do not use in combination with stavudine because of poor antiretroviral effect. Effects of interacting drugs include increased toxicity (acyclovir, trimethoprim-sulfamethoxazole), increased hematologic toxicity (ganciclovir, interferon-α, marrow-suppressive drugs), and granulocytopenia (drugs that affect glucuronidation). Methadone, atovaquone, cimetidine, valproic acid, probenecid, and fluconazole may increase levels of zidovudine. Rifampin, rifabutin, and clarithromycin may decrease levels.

Do not administer IM. IV form is incompatible with blood product infusions and should be infused over 1 hr (intermittent IV dosing). Despite manufacturer recommendations of administering oral doses 30 min before or 1 hr after meals, doses may be administered with food.

ZINC SALTS, SYSTEMIC
Galzin, Orazinc, and other generics
Trace mineral

No	No	3	A/C

Tabs as sulfate (Orazinc and generics) [OTC], 23% elemental: 50, 66, 110, 220 mg
Caps as sulfate (Orazinc, and generics) [OTC], 23% elemental: 220 mg
Caps as acetate (Galzin): 25, 50 mg elemental per capsule
Liquid as acetate: 5 mg elemental Zn/mL
Liquid as sulfate: 10 mg elemental Zn/mL
Injection as sulfate: 1 mg elemental Zn/mL (10 mL), 5 mg elemental Zn/mL (5 mL); may contain benzyl alcohol
Injection as chloride: 1 mg elemental Zn/mL (10 mL)

Continued

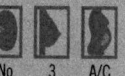
For explanation of icons, see p. 648

ZINC SALTS, SYSTEMIC *continued*

Zinc deficiency (see remarks):
   Infant and child: 0.5–1 mg elemental Zn/kg/24 hr PO ÷ once daily–TID
   Adult: 25–50 mg elemental Zn/dose (100–220 mg Zn sulfate/dose) PO TID
Wilson disease:
   Child (≥10 yr): 75 mg/24 hr elemental Zn PO ÷ TID. If needed, may increase to 150 mg/24 hr elemental Zn PO ÷ TID.
U.S. RDA: See Chapter 21.
For supplementation in parenteral nutrition, see Chapter 21.

Nausea, vomiting, GI disturbances, leukopenia, and diaphoresis may occur. Gastric ulcers, hypotension, and tachycardia may occur at high doses. Patients with excessive losses (burns) or impaired absorption require higher doses. Therapeutic levels: 70–130 mcg/dL.

May decrease absorption of penicillamine, tetracycline, and fluoroquinolones (e.g., ciprofloxacin). Drugs that increase gastric pH (e.g., H2 antagonists and proton pump inhibitors) can reduce zinc absorption. Excessive zinc administration can cause copper deficiency.

Approximately 20%–30% of oral dose is absorbed. Oral doses may be administered with food if GI upset occurs. Pregnancy category is "A" for zinc acetate and "C" for all other salt forms.

ZONISAMIDE
Zonegran and generics
Anticonvulsant

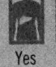
Yes   Yes   2   C

Caps: 25, 50, 100 mg
Oral syrup: 10 mg/mL

Infant and child (data incomplete):
   Suggested dosing from a review of Japanese open-label studies for partial and generalized seizures: Start with 1–2 mg/kg/24 hr PO ÷ BID. Increase dosage by 0.5–1 mg/kg/24 hr Q2 wk to usual dosage range of 5–8 mg/kg/24 hr PO ÷ BID.
   Recommended higher alternative dosing: Start with 2–4 mg/kg/24 hr PO ÷ BID–TID. Gradually increase dosage at 1- to 2-wk intervals to 4–8 mg/kg/24 hr. **Max. dose:** 12 mg/kg/24 hr.
   Infantile spasms (regimen that was effective in a small study from Japan; additional studies are needed): Start with 2–4 mg/kg/24 hr PO ÷ BID. Then increase by 2–5 mg/kg/24 hr every 2–4 day until seizures disappear, up to a **max.** of 20 mg/kg/24 hr.
>16 yr–adult:
   Adjunctive therapy for partial seizures: 100 mg PO once daily × 2 wk. Dose may be increased to 200 mg PO once daily × 2 wk. Additional dosage increments of 100 mg/24 hr can be made at 2-wk intervals to allow attainment of steady-state levels. Effective doses have ranged from 100–600 mg/24 hr ÷ once daily–BID (BID dosing may provide better efficacy). No additional benefit has been shown for doses >400 mg/24 hr.

Because zonisamide is a sulfonamide, it is **contraindicated** in patients allergic to sulfonamides (may result in Stevens-Johnson syndrome or TEN). Common side effects of drowsiness, ataxia, anorexia, GI discomfort, headache, rash, and pruritus usually occur early in therapy and can be minimized with slow dose titration. Urolithiasis and metabolic acidosis (more frequent and severe in younger patients) have been reported. Children are at increased risk for hyperthermia and oligohidrosis, especially in warm or hot weather. Suicidal behavior or ideation, acute pancreatitis, rhabdomyolysis, and elevated creatinine phosphokinase have been reported.

Continued

ZONISAMIDE *continued*

Although not fully delineated, therapeutic serum levels of 20–30 mg/L have been suggested because higher rates of adverse reactions have been seen at levels >30 mg/L.

Zonisamide is a CYP P450 3A4 substrate. Phenytoin, carbamazepine, and phenobarbital can decrease levels of zonisamide.

Use with caution in renal or hepatic impairment; slower dose titration and more frequent monitoring is recommended. **Do not use** if GFR is <50 mL/min. **Avoid** abrupt discontinuation or radical dose reductions. Swallow capsules whole, and **do not** crush or chew.

Bibliography

1. Daily Med: Current Medication Information. National Library of Medicine. National Institutes of Health. Bethesda, MD. http://dailymed.nlm.nih.gov/dailymed.
2. Drugs and Lactation Database (LactMed). National Library of Medicine, Toxicology Data Network. http://toxnet.nlm.nih.gov/cgi-bin/sis/htmlgen?LACT
3. Pickering LK, ed. *Red Book: 2012 Report of the Committee on Infectious Diseases.* 29th ed. Elk Grove Village, IL: American Academy of Pediatrics; 2012. http://aapredbook.aappublications.org.
4. AIDSinfo: Information on HIV/AIDS Treatment, Prevention, and Research. U.S. Department of Health and Human Services. www.aidsinfo.nih.gov.
5. Young TE, Mangum OB. *Pediatrics and Neofax electronic version.* New York, NY: Thomson Healthcare, USA. http://neofax.thomsonhc.com/neofax/neofax.php.
6. Field JM, Hazinski MF, Gilmore D, ed. *Handbook of Emergency Cardiovascular Care for Healthcare Providers: Guidelines CPR ECC 2005.* American Heart Association; 2005.
7. McEvoy GK, Snow EK, eds. *AHFS Drug Information. Stat!Ref electronic version.* Bethesda, MD: American Society of Health-System Pharmacists. www.ahfsdruginformation.com.
8. Micromedex Healthcare Series 2.0. electronic database. New York, NY: Thomson Healthcare, USA. Updated periodically. www.thomsonhc.com/micromedex2/librarian.
9. Takemoto CK, Hodding JH, Kraus DM. *Pediatric Dosage Handbook, electronic intranet database.* Hudson, OH: Lexi-Comp, Inc. Updated periodically. www.crlonline.com/crlsql/servlet/crlonline
10. National Institutes of Health: National Heart, Lung and Blood Institute–Expert Panel. Clinical practice guidelines: Guidelines for the diagnosis and management of asthma. http://www.nhlbi.nih.gov/guidelines/asthma/asthsumm.htm.
11. Bradley JS, Byington CL, Shah SS, et al. The management of community-acquired pneumonia in infants and children older than 3 months of age: Clinical practice guidelines by the Pediatric Infectious Disease Society and the Infectious Diseases Society of America. *Clin Infect Dis.* 2011;53:617-630.
12. National High Blood Pressure Education Program Working Group on High Blood Pressure in Children and Adolescents. The fourth report on the diagnosis, evaluation, and treatment of high blood pressure in children and adolescents. *Pediatrics.* 2004;114:555-576.

For explanation of icons, see p. 648

13. Flynn JT, Daniels SR. Pharmacologic treatment of hypertension in children and adolescents. *J Pediatr*. 2006;149:746-754.
14. Lande MB, Flynn JT. Treatment of hypertension in children and adolescents. *Pediatr Nephrol*. 2009:1939-1949.
15. Monagle P, Chalmers E, Chan A, et al. Antithrombotic therapy in neonates and children: American College of Chest Physicians evidence-based clinical practice guidelines 8th ed. *Chest*. 2008;133:887-968.
16. Yin T, Miyata T. Warfarin dose and the pharmacogenomics of CYP2C9 and VKORC1–Rationale and perspectives. *Thromb Res*. 2007;120:1-10.
17. American Thoracic Society. Targeted tuberculin testing and treatment of latent tuberculosis infection. *Am J Respir Crit Care Med*. 2000;161:1376-1395.
18. Food and Drug Administration Drug Safety Labeling Changes. www.fda.gov/Safety /MedWatch/SafetyInformation/Safety-RelatedDrugLabelingChanges/default.htm
19. Wagner CL, Greer FR. the Section on Breastfeeding and Committee on Nutrition. Prevention of rickets and vitamin D deficiency in infants, children, and adolescents. *Pediatrics*. 2008;122:1142-1152.
20. Committee to Review Reference Intakes for Vitamin D and Calcium. Ross AC (Chair). Institute of Medicine of the National Academies. Brief report: Dietary reference intakes for calcium and vitamin D. November 2010. www.iom.edu/ vitamind.
21. Registry and results database of publicly and privately supported clinical studies of human participants conducted around the world. U.S. National Institutes of Health. www.clinicaltrials.gov.
22. New Pediatric Drug Labeling Database. U.S. Food and Drug Administration. Silver Spring, MD. www.fda.gov/NewPedLabeling.

Chapter 30

Formulary Adjunct

Sara Mixter, MD, MPH, and
J. Deanna Wilson, MD

Special thanks go to the following people who provided guidance in preparing the elements of Chapter 30 in past editions: Sande Okelo, MD; Allison Kirk, MD; Bernard Cohen, MD; Katherine Puttgen, MD; Amy Schwartz, RD; Michael Repka, MD; Elizabeth Shumann, MD; Alix Dabb, Pharm D.

I. WEBSITES

Physician's Desk Reference: http://www.pdr.net/Default.aspx
Lexi-Comp Drug Reference: http://online.lexi.com
G6PD Deficiency: http://g6pddeficiency.org/index.php?cmd=contraindicated

II. SYSTEMIC CORTICOSTEROIDS

A. Body surface area nomogram and equation for calculating steroid dose (Fig. 30-1)

B. Potency of various therapeutic steroids content moved to Chapter 10, Endocrinology

III. INHALED CORTICOSTEROIDS FOR AIRWAY INFLAMMATION

Content moved to Chapter 24, Pulmonology

IV. TOPICAL CORTICOSTEROIDS

Content moved to Chapter 8, Dermatology

V. COMMON INSULIN FORMULATIONS

Content moved to Chapter 10, Endocrinology

VI. PANCREATIC ENZYME SUPPLEMENTS

See Table 30-1

VII. COMMON INDUCERS AND INHIBITORS OF THE CYTOCHROME P450 SYSTEM

Table 30-2 is meant to give some common pediatric examples of inducers/inhibitors. Other resources have more complete listings.[1]

VIII. OPHTHALMIC DRUGS

A. See Table 30-3
B. Content on treating allergic conjunctivitis moved to Chapter 15, Immunology and Allergy

30

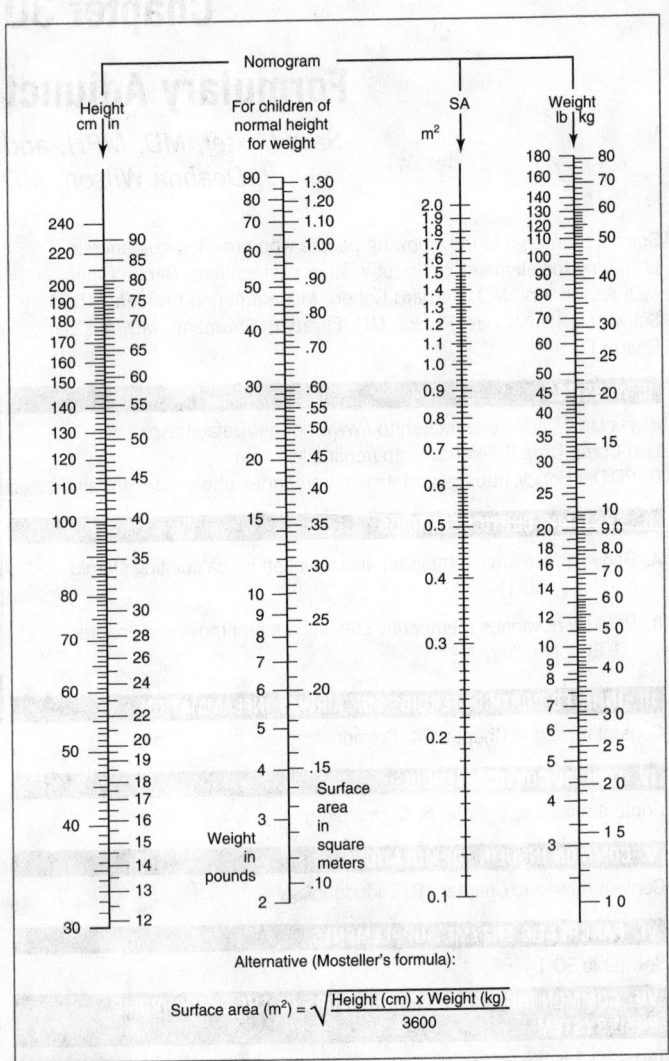

— Nomogram —

Height cm | in	For children of normal height for weight	SA m²	Weight lb | kg

Alternative (Mosteller's formula):

$$\text{Surface area (m}^2) = \sqrt{\frac{\text{Height (cm)} \times \text{Weight (kg)}}{3600}}$$

FIGURE 30-1

Body surface area nomogram and equation. *(From Briars GL, Bailey BJ. Surface area estimation: pocket calculator V nomogram. Arch Dis Child. 1994;70:246-247.)*

TABLE 30-1
PANCRELIPASE*

Product	Lipase (USP) Units	Amylase (USP) Units	Protease (USP) Units
Creon			
6	6000	30,000	19,000
12	12,000	60,000	38,000
24	24,000	120,000	76,000
Pancreaze MT			
4	4200	17,500	10,000
10	10,500	43,750	25,000
16	16,800	70,000	40,000
20	21,000	61,000	37,000
Zenpep			
5	5000	27,000	17,000
10	10,000	55,000	34,000
15	15,000	82,000	51,000
20	20,000	109,000	68,000

*See Formulary for side effects associated with administration. As of April 12, 2010, these are the only three products approved by the U.S. Food and Drug Administration (FDA). Many were recently removed from the market. Products are all supplied as delayed-release capsules.

http://www.zenpep.com/site/cfpatient.aspx

http://newdrugreview.com/index.php/gastrointestinal-drugs/pancreaze-3-dosage-forms-and-strengths

U.S. Food and Drug Administration: Updated questions and answers for healthcare professionals and the public: use an approved pancreatic enzyme product (PEP). Accessed August 11, 2010.

http://www.fda.gov/Drugs/DrugSafety/PostmarketDrugSafetyInformationforPatientsandProviders/ucm204745.htm

Data from http://www.creon-us.com/Healthcare-Professional/default.htm.

TABLE 30-2
EXAMPLES OF INDUCERS AND INHIBITORS OF CYTOCHROME P450 SYSTEM

Isoenzyme	Substrates (Drugs Metabolized by Isoenzyme)	Inhibitors*	Inducers
CYP1A2	Caffeine, theophylline, estradiol, propranolol	Cimetidine, quinolones, fluvoxamine, ketoconazole, lidocaine	Carbamazepine, smoking, phenobarbital, rifampin
CYP2B6	Cyclophosphamide, efavirenz, propofol	Paroxetine, sertraline	Carbamazepine, (fos)phenytoin, phenobarbital, rifampin
CYP2C9/10	Warfarin, phenytoin, tolbutamide, fluoxetine, sulfamethoxazole, fosphenytoin	Amiodarone, fluconazole, ibuprofen, indomethacin, nicardipine	Carbamazepine, (fos)phenytoin, rifampin, phenobarbital
CYP2C19	Diazepam, PPIs, phenytoin, desogestrel, ifosfamide, phenobarbital, sertraline	Cimetidine fluvoxamine, fluconazole, isoniazid, PPIs, sertraline	Carbamazepine, (fos)phenytoin, rifampin

Continued

TABLE 30-2

EXAMPLES OF INDUCERS AND INHIBITORS OF CYTOCHROME P450 SYSTEM (Continued)

Isoenzyme	Substrates (Drugs Metabolized by Isoenzyme)	Inhibitors*	Inducers
CYP2D6	Captopril, codeine, haloperidol, dextromethorphan, tricyclic antidepressants, hydrocodone, oxycodone, phenothiazines, metoprolol, propranolol, paroxetine, venlafaxine, risperidone, flecainide, sertraline, aripiprazole, fluoxetine, lidocaine, fosphenytoin, ritonavir	Chlorpromazine, cinacalcet, dexmedetomidine, cocaine, cimetidine, quinidine, ritonavir, fluoxetine, sertraline, amiodarone	None known
CYP2E1	Acetaminophen, alcohol, isoniazid, theophylline, isoflurane	Disulfiram	Alcohol
CYP3A4	Amlodipine, aripiprazole, budesonide, cocaine, clonazepam, diltiazem, efavirenz, erythromycin, estradiol, fentanyl, fluticasone, nifedipine, verapamil, cyclosporine, carbamazepine, cisapride, tacrolimus, midazolam, alfentanil, diazepam, ifosfamide, imatinib, itraconazole, ketoconazole, cyclophosphamide, PPIs, haloperidol, lidocaine, medroxyprogesterone, methadone, methylprednisolone, salmeterol, theophylline, quetiapine, ritonavir, indinavir, sildenafil	Erythromycin, cimetidine, clarithromycin, isoniazid, ketoconazole, itraconazole, metronidazole, sertraline, ritonavir, indinavir, imatinib, nicardipine, propofol, quinidine	Rifampin, (fos)phenytoin, phenobarbital, carbamazepine, dexamethasone

*Only strong and some moderate inhibitors are listed here. Weak inhibitors also exist.

NOTE: The cytochrome P450 enzyme system is composed of different isoenzymes. Each isoenzyme metabolizes a unique group of drugs or substrates. When an *inhibitor* of a particular isoenzyme is introduced, the serum concentration of any drug or *substrate* metabolized by that particular isoenzyme will *increase*. When an *inducer* of a particular isoenzyme is introduced, the serum concentration of drugs or *substrates* metabolized by that particular isoenzyme will *decrease*.

CYP, Cytochrome P450; PPI, proton pump inhibitor.

Data from Taketomo CK, Hodding JH, Kraus DM. *American Pharmaceutical Association Pediatric Dosage Handbook.* 16th ed. Hudson, OH: Lexi-Comp, 2009; Zevin S, Benowitz NL. Drug interactions with tobacco smoking. An update. *Clin Pharmacokinet.* 1999;36:425-438; Cupp MJ, Tracy TS. Cytochrome P450: new nomenclature and clinical implications. *Am Fam Physician.* 1998;57:107-116.

TABLE 30-3

OPHTHALMIC DRUGS

Brand Name	Ingredient	Indication	Dose
Alomide (>2 yr) Sol: 10 mL	Lodoxamide tromethamine 0.1% (mast cell stabilizer)	Vernal conjunctivitis and keratitis, keratoconjunctivitis	1–2 gtt QID up to 3 mo
Azasite (≥1 yr) Sol: 2.5 mL	Azithromycin 1% (contains benzalkonium chloride)	Conjunctivitis	1 gtt BID × 2 days, then Q day × 5 days
Bleph-10 (>2 mo) Sol: 2.5 mL, 5 mL, 15 mL Oint: 3.5 g	Sulfacetamide sodium 10% Sol: Benzalkonium chloride Oint: phenylmercuric acetate	Conjunctivitis Ophthalmic solution used as adjunct in trachoma	1–2 gtt Q2–3 hr or small amount of oint Q3–4 hr for 7–10 days Trachoma: 2 gtt Q2 hr w/systemic therapy
Cortisporin Oph susp: 7.5 mL Oph oint: 3.5 g	Susp (per mL): Polymyxin B sulfate (10,000 U), neomycin sulfate (0.35%), hydrocortisone (1%) Oint (per g): Polymyxin B sulfate (10,000 U), neomycin sulfate (0.35%), bacitracin zinc (400 U), hydrocortisone (1%)	Ocular inflammation associated with infection **Contraindicated in fungal, viral, or mycobacterial infection** Use with caution in glaucoma or in corneal or scleral thinning	1–2 gtt or small amount of oint TID–QID
Erythromycin Oint: 1, 3.5 g	Erythromycin (5 mg/g)	Conjunctivitis Prophylaxis of ophthalmia neonatorum	Small amount up to 6 times daily 0.5–1 cm to each conjunctival sac
Neosporin Oint: 3.75 g Sol: 10 mL	Oint (per g): Polymyxin B sulfate (10,000 U), bacitracin zinc (400 U), neomycin sulfate (3.5 mg) Sol (per mL): Polymyxin B sulfate (10,000 U), neomycin sulfate (1.75 mg), gramicidin (0.025 mg), 0.5% alcohol	Conjunctivitis	1–2 gtt or small amount of oint Q4 hr for 7–10 days For acute infections, 1–2 gtt 2–4 × Q1 hr initially
Ocuflox (>1 yr) Sol: 5 mL, 10 mL	Ofloxacin 0.3%, benzalkonium chloride	Conjunctivitis Corneal ulcer	1–2 gtt Q2–4 hr × 2 days, then QID × 5 days 1–2 gtt Q30 min while awake; at 4 hr and 6 hr during sleep × 2 days; then 1–2 gtt Q1 hr while awake × 5–7 days, then QID until treatment completion

30

Continued

TABLE 30-3

OPHTHALMIC DRUGS (Continued)

Brand Name	Ingredient	Indication	Dose
Poly-Pred Susp: 5 mL, 10 mL	Susp (per mL): Prednisolone acetate (0.5%), neomycin sulfate (0.35%), polymyxin B sulfate (10,000 U)	Ocular inflammation associated with infection **Contraindicated in fungal, viral, or mycobacterial infections** Use with caution in glaucoma or in corneal or scleral thinning	1–2 gtt Q3–4 hr
Polysporin Oint: 3.5 g	Oint (per g): Polymyxin B sulfate (10,000 U), bacitracin zinc (500 U)	Conjunctivitis	1–2 gtt Q3–4 hr; do not use >7 days
Polytrim (>2 mo) Sol: 10 mL	Trimethoprim sulfate (1 mg), polymyxin B sulfate (10,000 U/mL), benzalkonium chloride	Conjunctivitis	1 gtt Q3 hr × 7–10 days
Pred-Forte Sol: 1, 5, 10, 15 mL Pred-Mild Sol: 5, 10 mL	Prednisolone acetate 1% Prednisolone acetate 0.12%	Ocular/conjunctival inflammation. **Contraindicated in fungal, viral, or mycobacterial infections** Prolonged use may cause glaucoma, corneal/scleral thinning	1–2 gtt 2–4 × per day Safety and efficacy not established in children
Tobrex Sol: 5 mL Oint: 3.5 g	Sol: Tobramycin 0.3%, benzalkonium chloride Oint: Tobramycin 0.3%, chlorobutanol	Conjunctivitis	Severe infections: 2 gtt Q1 hr or ½ inch of ointment Q3–4 hr Mild–moderate infections: 1–2 gtt Q4 hr or ½ inch of ointment BID–TID
Vigamox (≥1 yr) Sol: 3 mL	Moxifloxacin hydrochloride 0.5% (fluoroquinolone)	Bacterial conjunctivitis	1 gtt TID × 7 days
Viroptic (>6 yr) Sol: 7.5 mL	Trifluridine 1%, contains thimerosal	Primary keratoconjunctivitis, recurrent epithelial keratitis due to herpes simplex virus 1 and 2	1 gtt Q2 hr while awake (maximum 9 gtt/day) 1 gtt Q4 hr × 7 days after re-epithelialization (maximum 21 days)
Zymar (≥1 yr) Sol: 5 mL	Gatifloxacin 0.3% (fluoroquinolone)	Bacterial conjunctivitis	1 gtt Q2 hr while awake, up to 8 times/day × 2 days; then 1 gtt up to QID × 5 days

Modified from *Physician's Desk Reference*. 64th ed. Montvale, NJ: Medical Economics, 2010.

IX. PSYCHIATRIC DRUG FORMULARY

Content moved to Chapter 9, Development, Behavior, and Mental Health

X. CHEMOTHERAPEUTIC AGENTS

Content moved to Chapter 22, Oncology

XI. OXIDIZING AGENTS AND GLUCOSE-6-PHOSPHATE DEHYDROGENASE (G6PD) DEFICIENCY

A comprehensive listing of relevant drugs is available at:
http://g6pddeficiency.org/index.php?cmd=contraindicated

REFERENCE

1. Taketomo CK, Hodding JH, Kraus DM. *American Pharmaceutical Association Pediatric Dosage Handbook*. 16th ed. Hudson, OH: Lexi-Comp, 2009.

Chapter 31

Drugs in Renal Failure

Monica C. Mix, MD, and Branden Engorn, MD

I. DOSE ADJUSTMENT METHODS

A. Maintenance Dose

In patients with renal insufficiency, the dose may be adjusted using the following methods:

1. **Interval extension (I):** Lengthen intervals between individual doses, keeping dose size normal. For this method, suggested interval is shown.
2. **Dose reduction (D):** Reduce amount of individual doses, keeping interval between doses normal; recommended when a relatively constant blood level of drug is desired. For this method, percentage of usual dose is shown.
3. **Interval extension and dose reduction (DI):** Both lengthen interval and reduce dose.
4. **Interval extension or dose reduction (D, I):** In some instances, either dose or interval can be changed.

   NOTE: These dose adjustment methods apply only to patients beyond the neonatal period. For neonatal renal dosing, please consult a neonatal dosage reference. Dose modifications given are only approximations. **Each patient must be monitored closely for signs of drug toxicity, and serum levels must be measured when available; drug dose and interval should be adjusted accordingly**. When in doubt, always consult a nephrologist or pharmacist who has expertise in renal dosing.

B. Dialysis

Quantitative effects of hemodialysis (He) and peritoneal dialysis (P) on drug removal are shown. "*Y*" indicates necessity for a supplemental dose with dialysis (in some cases, supplemental dose may not be a full dose). "*N*" indicates no need for adjustment. The designation "*No*" does not preclude use of dialysis or hemoperfusion for drug overdose. The "*?*" indicates insufficient data available. **Please consult with a nephrologist or pharmacist who is very familiar with renal dosing in dialysis.**

II. ANTIMICROBIALS REQUIRING ADJUSTMENT IN RENAL FAILURE (TABLE 31-1)

III. NON-ANTIMICROBIALS REQUIRING ADJUSTMENT IN RENAL FAILURE (TABLE 31-2)

TABLE 31-1

ANTIMICROBIALS REQUIRING ADJUSTMENT IN RENAL FAILURE[1-4]

Drug	Pharmacokinetics			Adjustments in Renal Failure				Supplemental Dose for Dialysis
	Route of Excretion*	Normal $t_{1/2}$ (hr)	Normal Dose Interval	Method	CrCl (mL/min)	Dose	Interval	
Acyclovir (IV)	Renal	2–4	Q8 hr	D, I	25–50	NI	Q12 hr	Y (He)
					10–25	NI	Q24 hr	N (P)
					<10	50% ↓	Q24 hr	
Amantadine†	Renal	10–28	Q12–24 hr	D, I	30–50	50% ↓	Q24 hr	N (He)α
					15–29	50% ↓	Q48 hr	N (P)
					<15	NI daily dose	Q7 days	
Amikacin	Renal	1.5–3	Q8–12 hr	I	Loading dose 5–7.5 mg/kg; subsequent doses are best determined by serum levels and assessment of renal insufficiency.[1]			Y (He)
								Y (P)
Amoxicillin‡	Renal	0.7–2	Q8–12 hr	I	10–50	NI	Q12 hr	Y (He)
					<10	NI	Q24 hr	N (P)
Amoxicillin/clavulanate‡	Renal	1	Q8–12 hr	I	10–30	NI	Q12 hr	Y (He)
					<10	NI	Q24 hr	N (P)
Amphotericin B	Renal (40% over 7 days)	Initial 15–48 hr Terminal 15 days	Q24 hr	D, I	Dosage adjustments are unnecessary with preexisting renal impairment. If decreased renal function is due to amphotericin B, daily dose can be decreased by 50%, or dose given every other day.[1]			N (He)
								N (P)
Amphotericin B lipid complex (Abelcet)	Renal (1%)	173	Q24 hr		No guidelines established.			N (He)
								N (P)
Amphotericin B, liposomal (AmBisome)	Renal (≤10%)	100–153	Q24 hr		No guidelines established.			N (He)
								N (P)
Ampicillin†	Renal	1–4	Q6–12 hr	I	10–50	NI	Q6–12 hr	Y (He)
					<10	NI	Q12 hr	? (P)

Continued

31

TABLE 31-1
ANTIMICROBIALS REQUIRING ADJUSTMENT IN RENAL FAILURE (Continued)

Drug	Pharmacokinetics			Adjustments in Renal Failure				Supplemental Dose for Dialysis
	Route of Excretion*	Normal $t_{1/2}$ (hr)	Normal Dose Interval	Method	CrCl (mL/min)	Dose	Interval	
Ampicillin/ sulbactam	Renal	1–1.8	Q4–6 hr	I	15–29	NI	Q12 hr	Y (He)
					<15	NI	Q24 hr	? (P)
Aztreonam	Renal (hepatic)	1.3–2.2	Q6–12 hr	D	10–30	50% ↓	NI	Y (He)
					<10	75% ↓	NI	Y (P)
Cefaclor	Renal	0.5–1	Q8–12 hr	D	<10	50% ↓	NI	Y (He)
								? (P)
Cefadroxil	Renal	1–2	Q12 hr	I	10–50	NI	Q24 hr	Y (He)
					<10	NI	Q36 hr	Y (P)
Cefazolin	Renal	1.5–2.5	Q6–8 hr	D, I	35–54	NI	Q8 hr	Y (He)
Note: Give initial loading dose, then adjust subsequent doses for renal function.					11–34	50% ↓$^\Sigma$	Q12 hr	N (P)
					<10	50% ↓$^\Sigma$	Q18–24 hr	
Cefdinir	Renal	1.1–2.3	Q12–24 hr	D, I	<30	7 mg/kg/dose (children; max 300 mg)	Q24 hr	Y (He)$^\Omega$
						He		? (P)
						NI	Q48 hr	
Cefepime†	Renal	1.8–2	Q8–12 hr	D, I	10–50	NI	Q24 hr	Y (He)
					<10	50% ↓	Q24 hr	? (P)

TABLE 31-1

ANTIMICROBIALS REQUIRING ADJUSTMENT IN RENAL FAILURE (Continued)

		Pharmacokinetics			Adjustments in Renal Failure			
Drug	Route of Excretion*	Normal t$_{1/2}$ (hr)	Normal Dose Interval	Method	CrCl (mL/min)	Dose	Interval	Supplemental Dose for Dialysis
Cefixime	Renal (hepatic)	3–4	Q12–24 hr	D	21–60	25% ↓	NI	Y (He)
					<20	50% ↓	NI	? (P)
Cefotaxime	Renal	1–3.5	Q6–12 hr	D	<20	50% ↓	NI	Y (He)
								? (P)
Cefotetan	Renal (hepatic)	3.5	Q12 hr	I	10–30	NI	Q24 hr	Y (He)
					<10	NI	Q48 hr	? (P)
Cefoxitin	Renal	0.75–1.5	Q4–8 hr	I	30–50	NI	Q8–12 hr	Y (He)
					10–30	NI	Q12–24 hr	? (P)
					<10	NI	Q24–48 hr	
Cefpodoxime	Renal	2.2	Q12 hr	I	<30	NI	Q24 hr	Y (He)§
								N (P)
Cefprozil	Renal	1.3	Q12–24 hr	D	<30	50% ↓	NI	Y (He)
								? (P)
Ceftazidime	Renal	1–2	Q8–12 hr	I	30–50	NI	Q12 hr	Y (He)
					10–30	NI	Q24 hr	? (P)
					<10	NI	Q24–48 hr	
Ceftibuten	Renal	1.5–2.5	Q24 hr	D	30–49	50% ↓	NI	Y (He)ααα
					5–29	75% ↓	NI	? (P)
Cefuroxime (IV)	Renal	1.6–2.2	Q8–12 hr	I	10–20	NI	Q12 hr	Y (He)
					<10	NI	Q24 hr	? (P)
Cephalexin	Renal	0.5–1.2	Q6–8 hr	I	10–40	NI	Q8–12 hr	Y (He)
					<10	NI	Q12–24 hr	? (P)

Continued

31

TABLE 31-1

ANTIMICROBIALS REQUIRING ADJUSTMENT IN RENAL FAILURE (Continued)

Drug	Pharmacokinetics			Adjustments in Renal Failure				Supplemental Dose for Dialysis
	Route of Excretion*	Normal t₁/₂ (hr)	Normal Dose Interval	Method	CrCl (mL/min)	Dose	Interval	
Ciprofloxacin†	Renal (hepatic)	1.2–5	Q8–12 hr	D, I	<30 (IV)	200–400 mg†	Q18–24 hr	Y (He)
					30–50 (PO)	250–500 mg†	Q12 hr	? (P)
					<30 (PO)	250–500 mg†	Q18 hr	
Clarithromycin	Renal (hepatic)	3–7	Q12 hr	D, I	<30	50% ↓	Q12–24 hr	? (He)
								? (P)
Ertapenem†	Renal (hepatic)	4	Q12–24 hr	D	≤30	50% ↓	NI	Y (He)
								? (P)
Erythromycin	Hepatic (renal)	1.5–2	Q6–12 hr	D	<10	25%–50%↓	NI	N (He)
								N (P)
Ethambutol	Renal (hepatic)	2.5–3.6	Q24 hr	I	10–50	NI	Q24–36 hr	Y (He)
					<10	NI	Q48 hr	? (P)
Famciclovir†	Renal (hepatic)	2–3	Q8 hr	D, I	**Herpes Zoster Treatment†,***			Y (He)
					40–59	500 mg	Q12 hr	? (P)
					20–39	500 mg	Q24 hr	
					<20	250 mg	Q24 hr	
					Recurrent Genital Herpes Treatment†,***			
					40–59	500 mg	Q12 hr × 1 day	
					20–39	500 mg	Single dose	
					<20	250 mg	Single dose	
					Recurrent Genital Herpes Suppression†,ΣΣ			
					>40	250 mg	Q12 hr	
					20–39	125 mg	Q12 hr	
					<20	125 mg	Q24 hr	

TABLE 31-1

ANTIMICROBIALS REQUIRING ADJUSTMENT IN RENAL FAILURE (Continued)

Drug	Pharmacokinetics			Adjustments in Renal Failure			Supplemental Dose for Dialysis
	Route of Excretion*	Normal t$_{1/2}$ (hr)	Normal Dose Interval	Method	CrCl (mL/min)	Dose	Interval	
					Recurrent Herpes Labialis—Single Dose Regimen†,***			
					>60	1500 mg as single dose		
					40–59	750 mg as single dose		
					20–39	500 mg as single dose		
					<20	250 mg as single dose		
					Recurrent Orolabial or Genital Herpes in HIV-Infected Patients†,***			
					40–59	500 mg	Q12 hr	
					20–39	500 mg	Q12 hr	
					<20	250 mg	Q24 hr	
Fluconazole†	Renal	19–25	Q24 hr	D	<50	50% ↓	NI	Y (He) ΣΣΣ ? (P)
Flucytosine	Renal	3–8	Q6 hr	I	20–40	NI	Q12 hr	Y (He)
					10–20	NI	Q24 hr	Y(P)
					<10	NI	Q24–48 hr	
Foscarnet	Renal	2–4.5	Induct: Q8 hr Maint: Q24 hr	D	See package insert for adjustments for induction and maintenance.			? (He) ? (P)
Ganciclovir	Renal	2.5–3.6	Induct: Q12 hr IV Maint: Q24 hr IV/PO OR Q8 hr	D, I	**Induction IV**			Y (He)§ N (P)
					50–69	2.5 mg/kg	Q12 hr	
					25–49	2.5 mg/kg	Q24 hr	
					10–24	1.25 mg/kg	Q24 hr	
					<10	1.25 mg/kg	3 times/wk after He	

Continued

TABLE 31-1
ANTIMICROBIALS REQUIRING ADJUSTMENT IN RENAL FAILURE (Continued)

Drug	Route of Excretion*	Normal t₁/₂ (hr)	Normal Dose Interval	Method	CrCl (mL/min)	Dose	Interval	Supplemental Dose for Dialysis
		Pharmacokinetics			Adjustments in Renal Failure			
					Maintenance IV			
					50–69	2.5 mg/kg	Q24 hr	
					25–49	1.25 mg/kg	Q24 hr	
					10–24	0.625 mg/kg	Q24 hr	
					<10	0.625 mg/kg	3 times/wk after He	
					Maintenance PO†			
					50–69	1500 mg *OR* 500 mg	Q24 hr Q8 hr	
					25–49	1000 mg *OR* 500 mg	Q24 hr Q12 hr	
					10–24	500 mg	Q24 hr	
					<10	500 mg	3 times/wk after He	
Gentamicin¶	Renal	1.5–3	Q8–12 hr	I	>50	NI	NI	Y (He)
					<50	Give usual initial dose and monitor levels.		Y (P)¶

TABLE 31-1

ANTIMICROBIALS REQUIRING ADJUSTMENT IN RENAL FAILURE (Continued)

	Pharmacokinetics			Adjustments in Renal Failure			
Drug	Route of Excretion*	Normal t₁/₂ (hr)	Normal Dose Interval	Method	CrCl (mL/min)	Dose	Interval	Supplemental Dose for Dialysis

Drug	Route of Excretion*	Normal $t_{1/2}$ (hr)	Normal Dose Interval	Method	CrCl (mL/min)	Dose	Interval	Supplemental Dose for Dialysis
Imipenem/ cilastatin	Renal	1–1.4	Q6–8 hr	D, I	41–70	50% ↓	Q6 hr	Y (He) ? (P)
					21–40	63% ↓	Q8 hr	
					6–20	75% ↓ in max daily dose	Q12 hr	
					≤5	Should not receive imipenem unless on hemodialysis		
Kanamycin	Renal	2–3	Q8 hr	I	>50	NI	Q12 hr	Y (He) Y (P)
					10–50	NI	Q12–18 hr	
					<10	NI	Q24–48 hr	
Lamivudine†,**	Renal	1.7–2.5	Q12 hr	D, I	30–49	NI	Q24 hr	N (He) N (P)
					15–29	First dose 100%, then 66%	Q24 hr	
					5–14	First dose 100%, then 33%	Q24 hr	
					<5	First dose 33%, then 17%	Q24 hr	

Continued

TABLE 31-1

ANTIMICROBIALS REQUIRING ADJUSTMENT IN RENAL FAILURE (Continued)

Drug	Route of Excretion*	Normal $t_{1/2}$ (hr)	Normal Dose Interval	Method	CrCl (mL/min)	Dose	Interval	Supplemental Dose for Dialysis
		Pharmacokinetics			Adjustments in Renal Failure			
Levofloxacin†	Renal (hepatic)	6-8	Q12-24 hr	D, I	500-mg Q24-hr Regimen			N (He) N (P)
					20-49	First dose 500 mg, then 250 mg	Q24 hr	
					10-19	First dose 250-500 mg, then 250 mg	Q48 hr	
					750-mg Q24-hr Regimen			
					20-49	750 mg	Q48 hr	
					10-19	500 mg	Q48 hr	
					250-mg Q24-hr Regimen			
					10-19	250 mg	Q48 hr	
Meropenem	Renal	1-1.5	Q8 hr	D, I	26-50	NI	Q12 hr	Y (He) ? (P)
					10-25	50% ↓	Q12 hr	
					<10	50% ↓	Q24 hr	
Metronidazole	Hepatic (renal)	6-12	Q6-12 hr	D	<10	50% ↓	NI	Y (He) Y (P)

TABLE 31-1

ANTIMICROBIALS REQUIRING ADJUSTMENT IN RENAL FAILURE (Continued)

Drug	Pharmacokinetics				Adjustments in Renal Failure			Supplemental Dose for Dialysis
	Route of Excretion*	Normal t$_{1/2}$ (hr)	Normal Dose Interval	Method	CrCl (mL/min)	Dose	Interval	
Norfloxacin	Hepatic (renal)	3–4	Q12 hr	I	10–50	NI	Q12–24 hr	N (He)
					<10	NI	Q24 hr	N (P)
Oseltamivir†	Renal	1–10	Q12–24 hr	I	**Influenza Treatment**			
					10–30	NI	Q24 hr	Y (He)
					<10	No recommended dosage regimen.		? (P)
					Influenza Prophylaxis			
					10–30	NI	Q48 hr	
					<10	No recommended dosage regimen.		
Oxacillin	Renal (hepatic)	23–45 min	Q4–12 hr	D	<10	Use lower range of usual dose.	NI	N (He)
								N (P)
Penicillin G— and aqueous K⁺Na⁺ (IV)	Renal (hepatic)	20–50 min	Q4–6 hr	D	10–50	25% ↓	NI	Y (He)
					<10	50%–80% ↓	NI	? (P)
Penicillin V K⁺ (PO)	Renal (hepatic)	30–40 min	Q6–8 hr	I	<10	NI	Q8 hr	Y (He)
								? (P)
Pentamidine	Renal	6.4–9	Q24 hr	I	10–30	NI	Q36 hr	N (He)
					<10	NI	Q48 hr	N (P)

Continued

31

TABLE 31-1

ANTIMICROBIALS REQUIRING ADJUSTMENT IN RENAL FAILURE (Continued)

Drug	Route of Excretion*	Normal $t_{1/2}$ (hr)	Normal Dose Interval	Method	CrCl (mL/min)	Dose	Interval	Supplemental Dose for Dialysis
Piperacillin	Renal (hepatic)	0.5–1.5	Q4–6 hr	I	20–40 / <20	NI / NI	Q8 hr / Q12 hr	Y (He) / ? (P)
Piperacillin/tazobactam	Renal	Piperacillin: 0.5–1.5 Tazobactam: 0.7–1.6	Q6–8 hr	D, I	20–40 / <20	30%↓ / 30%↓	Q6 hr / Q8 hr	? (He) / ? (P)
Rifabutin†	Renal (hepatic)	36–45	Q12–24 hr	D	<30	50%↓	NI	? (He) / ? (P)
Rifampin	Hepatic (renal)	1.5–5	Q12–24 hr	D	10–50 / <10	50%↓ / 50%↓	NI / NI	N (He) / Y (P)
Streptomycin sulfate	Renal	2.5	Q24 hr	D, I	50–80 / 10–50 / <10	50%↓ / 50%↓ / 50%↓	Q24 hr / Q24–72 hr / Q72–96 hr	? (He) / ? (P)
Sulfamethoxazole/trimethoprim	Sulfamethoxazole: hepatic (renal) Trimethoprim: renal (hepatic)	Sulfamethoxazole: 9–12 Trimethoprim: 6–11	Q12 hr	D	15–30 / <15	50%↓ / Not recommended	NI	Y (He) / ? (P)
Sulfisoxazole	Renal	4–8	Q6–12 hr	I	10–50 / <10	NI / NI	Q8–12 hr / Q12–24 hr	Y (He) / Y (P)

TABLE 31-1

ANTIMICROBIALS REQUIRING ADJUSTMENT IN RENAL FAILURE (Continued)

	Pharmacokinetics			Adjustments in Renal Failure			
Drug	Route of Excretion*	Normal t$_{1/2}$ (hr)	Normal Dose Interval	Method	CrCl (mL/min)	Dose	Interval	Supplemental Dose for Dialysis
Tetracycline	Renal (hepatic)	8–10	Q6 hr	I	50–80	NI	Q8–12 hr	N (He)
					10–50	NI	Q12–24 hr	N (P)
					<10	NI	Q24 hr	
Ticarcillin††	Renal	0.9–1.3	Q4–6 hr IV	I	10–30	NI	Q8 hr	Y (He)
			Q6–8 hr IM		<10	NI	Q12 hr	? (P)
Ticarcillin/ clavulanate††	Renal	Ticarcillin: 0.9–1.3 Clavulanate: 1–1.5	Q4–6 hr	I	10–30	NI	Q8 hr	Y (He)
					<10	NI	Q12 hr	? (P)
					<10 *AND* hepatic impairment	NI	Q24 hr	
Tobramycin ‖	Renal	1.5–3	Q8–12 hr	I	Any degree of renal insufficiency.	Give usual initial dose and then monitor levels.		Y (He) Y (P)¶
Valacyclovir†	88% as acyclovir in urine	Valacyclovir: ≈ 30 min Acyclovir: 2–3	Q12–24 hr	D, I	**Herpes Zoster (Adults)**			Y (He) ? (P)
					30–49	NI	Q12 hr	
					10–29	NI	Q24 hr	
					<10	50% ↓	Q24 hr	
					Genital Herpes (Adol/Adults): Initial Episode			
					10–29	NI	Q24 hr	
					<10	50% ↓	Q24 hr	

Continued

31

TABLE 31-1

ANTIMICROBIALS REQUIRING ADJUSTMENT IN RENAL FAILURE (Continued)

Drug	Route of Excretion*	Pharmacokinetics Normal t₁/₂ (hr)	Normal Dose Interval	Method	CrCl (mL/min)	Dose	Interval	Supplemental Dose for Dialysis
					Genital Herpes (Adol/Adults): Recurrent Episode			
					<30	NI	Q24 hr	
					Genital Herpes (Adol/Adults): Suppressive			
					<10	500 mg	Q24 hr (for usual dose of 1 g Q24 hr)	
						OR		
						500 mg	Q48 hr (for usual dose of 500 mg Q24 hr)	
					Herpes Labialis (Adol/Adults)			
					30–49	1 g	Q12 hr × 2 doses	
					10–29	500 mg	Q12 hr × 2 doses	
					<10	500 mg	Single dose	
Valganciclovir (see ganciclovir)								

ANTIMICROBIALS REQUIRING ADJUSTMENT IN RENAL FAILURE (Continued)

| Drug | Pharmacokinetics | | | Adjustments in Renal Failure | | | Supplemental |
	Route of Excretion*	Normal $t_{1/2}$ (hr)	Normal Dose Interval	Method	CrCl (mL/min)	Dose	Interval	Dose for Dialysis
Vancomycin ‖	Renal	2.2–8	Q6–12 hr	I	>90	NI	Q6 hr	N (He)††
Note: Alternative					70–89	NI	Q8 hr	N (P)
would be to give					46–69	NI	Q12 hr	
single dose and					30–45	NI	Q18 hr	
then check a					15–29	NI	Q24 hr	
trough level.					<15	10–20 mg/kg	Subsequent doses best determined by levels.	

*Route in parentheses indicates secondary route of excretion.

†In adults; guidelines not established in children.

ΦOn day 1, normal dose should be given, then decreased for subsequent doses based on renal insufficiency.

ΣAfter initial loading dose is administered, decrease dose based on renal insufficiency.

φPatients on hemodialysis should have a dose of 300 mg or 7 mg/kg/dose at conclusion of each hemodialysis session, with subsequent doses Q48 hr.

∞With hemodialysis, administer 9 mg/kg (max dose 400 mg) after hemodialysis.

***For patients on hemodialysis, administer 250 mg after each dialysis session.

ΣΣFor patients on hemodialysis, administer 125 mg after each dialysis session.

ΣΣΣFor patients on hemodialysis: administer 100% of recommended dose after each dialysis session.

‡Should not use 875-mg tablet or extended-release tablets in patients with CrCl <30 mL/min.

§For patients on hemodialysis, administer 3 times a week.

‖Subsequent doses best determined by measurement of serum levels and assessment of renal insufficiency.

*May add to peritoneal dialysate to obtain adequate serum levels.

**GFR ≥ 5 mL/min, give full dose as first dose; GFR < 5 mL/min, give 33% of full dose as first dose.

††May inactivate aminoglycosides in patients with renal impairment.

‡‡Rate of acetylation of isoniazid.

Adol, Adolescents; CrCl, creatinine clearance; D, dose reduction; GFR, glomerular filtration rate; He, hemodialysis; I, interval extension; IM, intramuscular; Induct, induction; IV, intravenous; K⁺, potassium; Maint, maintenance; Na⁺, sodium; NI, normal; P, peritoneal dialysis; PO, oral; $t_{1/2}$, half-life with normal renal function.

31

TABLE 31-2

NON-ANTIMICROBIALS REQUIRING ADJUSTMENT IN RENAL FAILURE[1-4]

Drug	Pharmacokinetics			Adjustments in Renal Failure				
	Route of Excretion*	Normal $t_{1/2}$ (hr)	Normal Dose Interval	Method	CrCl (mL/min)	Dose	Interval	Supplemental Dose for Dialysis
Acetaminophen	Hepatic	2–4	Q4–6 hr	I	10–50	NI	Q6 hr	N (He)
					<10	NI	Q8 hr	N (P)
Acetazolamide	Renal	2.4–5.8	Q6–24 hr	I	10–50	NI	Q12 hr	Y (He)
					<10	Avoid use		? (P)
Allopurinol	Renal	1–3	Q6–12 hr	D	10–50	50% ↓	NI	? (He)
					<10	70% ↓	NI	? (P)
Aminocaproic Acid	Renal	1–2	Q4–6 hr	D	Oliguria/ESRD	75% ↓	NI	? (He)
								? (P)
Aspirin†	Hepatic (renal)	3–10	Q4 hr	I	10–50	NI	Q4–6 hr	Y (He)
					<10	Avoid use		N (P)
Atenolol	Renal (GI)	3.5–7	Q24 hr	D, I	15–35	1 mg/kg OR 50 mg	Q24 hr	Y (He)
					<15	1 mg/kg OR 50 mg	Q48 hr	N (P)
Azathioprine‡	Hepatic (renal)	0.7–3	Q24 hr	D	10–50	25% ↓	NI	Y (He)
					<10	50% ↓	NI	? (P)
Bismuth subsalicylate	Hepatic (renal)	Salicylate: 2–5 Bismuth: 21–72 days	Q3–4 hr	D	Avoid use in patients with renal failure.			NA
Calcium supplements	GI	Variable	Variable		<25	May require dosage adjustment depending on calcium level.		
Captopril	Renal (hepatic)	1–12.5	Q6–24 hr	D	10–50	25% ↓	NI	Y (He)
					<10	50% ↓	NI	N (P)

TABLE 31-2

NON-ANTIMICROBIALS REQUIRING ADJUSTMENT IN RENAL FAILURE (Continued)

Drug	Route of Excretion*	Pharmacokinetics Normal t₁/₂ (hr)	Normal Dose Interval	Method	CrCl (mL/min)	Dose	Interval	Supplemental Dose for Dialysis
Carbamazepine	Hepatic (renal)	Initial: 25–65 Subsequent: 8–17	Q6–24 hr	D	<10	25% ↓ (monitor serum levels)	NI	? (He) ? (P)
Cetirizine	Renal (hepatic)	6.2–9	Q12–24 hr	D	**<6 yr with Renal Impairment** Use not recommended. **6–11 yr**			? (He) ? (P)
					Any degree of insufficiency.	<2.5 mg	Q24 hr	
					≥12 yr			
					11–30	15 mg	Q24 hr	
					<11	Use not recommended.		
Chloral hydrate	Renal	8–11	Q6–8 hr	NA	<50	Avoid use.		NA
Chloroquine	Renal (hepatic)	3–5 days	Q6 hr–7 days	D	<10	50% ↓	NI	N (He) N (P)
Chlorothiazide	Renal	0.75–2	Q12–24 hr	NA	<30	May be ineffective. Use not recommended.		NA
Cimetidine	Renal (hepatic)	1.4–2	Q6–12 hr	D, I	>40	NI	Q6 hr	Y (He) ? (P)
					20–40	NI	Q8 hr	
						OR 25% ↓	NI	
					<20	NI	Q12 hr	
						OR 50% ↓	NI	

Continued

31

TABLE 31-2

NON-ANTIMICROBIALS REQUIRING ADJUSTMENT IN RENAL FAILURE (Continued)

	Pharmacokinetics		Adjustments in Renal Failure			
Drug	Route of Excretion*	Normal t₁/₂ (hr)	Normal Dose Interval	Method	CrCl (mL/min)	Dose	Interval	Supplemental Dose for Dialysis

Drug	Route of Excretion*	Normal $t_{1/2}$ (hr)	Normal Dose Interval	Method	CrCl (mL/min)	Dose	Interval	Supplemental Dose for Dialysis
Clobazam	Renal (GI)	Children: 16 Adults: 36–42	Q12–24 hr	D	<30	Use with caution; has not been studied.	NI	? (He, P)
Desloratadine	Renal (GI)	27	Q24 hr	I	Any degree of renal impairment	NI	Q48 hr	? (He) ? (P)
Digoxin§	Renal	18–48	Q12–24 hr	D, I	**Digitalizing Dose** ESRD	50% ↓	NA	N (He) N (P)
					Maintenance Dose 10–50	25%–75% ↓ *OR* NI	NI Q36 hr	
					<10	75%–90% ↓ *OR* NI	NI Q48 hr	
Diphenhydr-amine	Hepatic	2–8	Q4–8 hr	I	10–50 <10	NI NI	Q6–8 hr Q6–12 hr	? (He) ? (P)
Disopyramide ‖	Renal (GI)	3.15–10	Q6 hr	I	30–40 15–30 <15	NI NI NI	Q8 hr Q12 hr Q24 hr	? (He) ? (P)
EDTA calcium chloride ‖	Renal	1.5 (IM) 0.3 (IV)	Q4 hr IM Q12 hr IV	D, I	**Serum Creatinine: IV Dose** ≤2 mg/dL 2–3 mg/dL 3–4 mg/dL >4 mg/dL	1 g/m² 500 mg/m² 500 mg/m² 500 mg/m²	Q24 hr × 5 days Q24 hr × 5 days Q48 hr × 3 doses Once weekly	? (He) ? (P)

TABLE 31-2
NON-ANTIMICROBIALS REQUIRING ADJUSTMENT IN RENAL FAILURE (Continued)

Drug	Route of Excretion*	Pharmacokinetics Normal t₁/₂ (hr)	Normal Dose Interval	Method	Adjustments in Renal Failure CrCl (mL/min)	Dose	Interval	Supplemental Dose for Dialysis
Enalapril (IV: enalaprilat)	Renal (hepatic)	1.3–6.3 (PO) 5.1–38 (IV)	Q6–24 hr	D	10–50 <10 Use not recommended in infants and children ≤16 yr with GFR. <30 mL/min/1.73 m².	0%–25% ↓ 50% ↓	NI NI	? (He) N (P)
Enoxaparin ‖,¶	Renal	4.5–7	Q12 hr	I	<30	NI	Q24 hr	? (He) ? (P)
Famotidine	Renal	0.8–5	Q8–12 hr	D, I	10–50 <10	50% ↓ *OR* NI NI	NI Q24 hr Q36–48 hr	? (He) ? (He) ? (P)
Felbamate ‖	Renal	20–30	Q6–8 hr	D	Any degree of renal impairment.	50% ↓	NI	? (He) ? (P)
Fentanyl	Renal (hepatic)	2–4	Q30 min–1 hr	D	10–50 <10	25% ↓ 50% ↓	NI NI	? (He) ? (P)
Fexofenadine	GI (renal)	14–18	Q12 hr	I	Any degree of renal impairment.	NI	Q24 hr	? (He) ? (P)
Flecainide	Renal/hepatic	8–27	Q8–12 hr	D	<20	25%–50% ↓	NI	? (He) ? (P)
Furosemide	Renal (hepatic)	0.5	Q6–24 hr PO Q6–12 hr IV		Avoid use in oliguric states.			N (He) N (P)

Continued

TABLE 31-2

NON-ANTIMICROBIALS REQUIRING ADJUSTMENT IN RENAL FAILURE (Continued)

		Pharmacokinetics			Adjustments in Renal Failure			
Drug	Route of Excretion*	Normal t₁/₂ (hr)	Normal Dose Interval	Method	CrCl (mL/min)	Dose	Interval	Supplemental Dose for Dialysis
Gabapentin ‖	Renal (hepatic)	4.7–9	Q8 hr	D, I	30–59	200–700 mg	Q12 hr	Y (He)
					15–29	200–700 mg	Q24 hr	N (P)
					<15	100–300 mg	Q24 hr	
Hydralazine#	Hepatic (renal)	2–8	Q4–6 hr (IV)	I	10–50	NI	Q8 hr (fast acetylator)	? (He)
			Q6–12 hr (PO)		<10	NI	Q8–16 hr (slow acetylator)	? (P)
							Q12–24 hr	
Insulin (regular)**	Hepatic (renal)	1.5	Variable	D	10–50	25% ↓	NI	N (He)
					<10	50%–75% ↓	NI	N (P)
Lacosamide	Renal (GI)	13	Q12 hr	D	<30	Maximum dose 300 mg/24-hr period	NI	Y (He); give 50% dose supplementation after 4-hr He session.
Levetiracetam ‖	Renal	5–8	Q12 hr	D	**Children**			Y (He)
					<50	50% ↓	NI	N (P)
					Adults			
					50–80	500–1000 mg	NI	
					30–50	250–750 mg	NI	
					<30	250–500 mg	NI	
					ESRD on dialysis	500–1000 mg	Q24 hr	

TABLE 31-2
NON-ANTIMICROBIALS REQUIRING ADJUSTMENT IN RENAL FAILURE (Continued)

Drug	Route of Excretion*	Normal t₁/₂ (hr)	Normal Dose Interval	Method	CrCl (mL/min)	Dose	Interval	Supplemental Dose for Dialysis
Lisinopril	Renal	11–13	Q24 hr	D	10–30	50% ↓	NI	Y (He)
					<10	75% ↓	NI	N (P)
Lithium	Renal	18–24	Q6–8 hr		Use not recommended for children with CrCl <30 mL/min/1.73 m².			
				D	10–50	25%–50% ↓	NI	Y (He)
					<10	50%–75% ↓	NI	N (P)
Loratadine	Renal/hepatic	Loratadine: 8.4 Metabolite: 28	Q24 hr	I	<30	NI	Q48 hr	? (He) ? (P)
Meperidine	Renal (hepatic) (normeperidine, renal)	2.3–4	Q3–4 hr	D	10–50	25% ↓	NI	? (He)
					<10	50% ↓	NI	? (P)
Methadone	Hepatic (renal)	4–87	Q3–12 hr	D	<10	25%–50% ↓	NI	N (He) N (P)
Methyldopa	Hepatic (renal)	1–3	Q6–12 hr PO Q6–8 hr IV	I	>50	NI	Q8 hr	Y (He)
					10–50	NI	Q8–12 hr	? (P)
					<10	NI	Q12–24 hr	
Metoclopramide	Renal	2.5–6	Q6 hr PO Q6–8 hr IV	D	40–50	25% ↓	NI	? (He)
					10–40	50% ↓	NI	? (P)
					<10	50%–75% ↓	NI	
Midazolam	Hepatic (renal)	2.2–6.8	Variable	D	10–29	25% ↓	NI	NA
					<10	50% ↓	NI	

Continued

31

TABLE 31-2

NON-ANTIMICROBIALS REQUIRING ADJUSTMENT IN RENAL FAILURE (Continued)

Drug	Route of Excretion*	Normal $t_{1/2}$ (hr)	Normal Dose Interval	Method	CrCl (mL/min)	Dose	Interval	Supplemental Dose for Dialysis
Milrinone	Renal	1.5–3.8	Continuous infusion	D	50 mL/min/1.73 m²		0.43 mcg/kg/min	NA
					40 mL/min/1.73 m²		0.38 mcg/kg/min	
					30 mL/min/1.73 m²		0.33 mcg/kg/min	
					20 mL/min/1.73 m²		0.28 mcg/kg/min	
					10 mL/min/1.73 m²		0.23 mcg/kg/min	
					5 mL/min/1.73 m²		0.2 mcg/kg/min	
Morphine	Hepatic (renal)	1–67.8	Variable	D	10–50	25% ↓	NI	? (He)
					<10	50% ↓	NI	? (P)
Neostigmine	Hepatic (renal)	0.5–2.1	Variable	D	10–50	50% ↓	NI	? (He)
					<10	75% ↓	NI	? (P)
Oxcarbazepine	Renal	Oxcarbazepine: 2 MHD: 9	Q12 hr	D	<30	50% ↓ in initial dose and slower titration	NI	? (He) ? (P)
Pancuronium bromide	Renal (hepatic)	1.8	Q30–60 min *OR* continuous infusion	D	10–50	50% ↓	NI	? (He) ? (P)
					<10	Avoid use.		
Phenazopyridine	Renal (hepatic)	?	Q8 hr for 2 days	I	50–80	NI	Q8–16 hr	NA
					<50	Avoid use.		
Phenobarbital	Hepatic (renal, 30%)	37–140	Q8–12 hr	I	<10	NI	Q24 hr	Y (He) Y (P)

TABLE 31-2

NON-ANTIMICROBIALS REQUIRING ADJUSTMENT IN RENAL FAILURE (Continued)

Drug	Route of Excretion*	Normal t₁/₂ (hr)	Normal Dose Interval	Method	CrCl (mL/min)	Dose	Interval	Supplemental Dose for Dialysis
Primidone	Hepatic (renal, 20%)	Primidone: 10–12 Metabolite: 16	Q6–12 hr	I	>50	NI	Q12 hr	Y (He)
					10–50	NI	Q12–24 hr	? (P)
					<10	NI	Q24 hr	
Procainamide	Hepatic (renal)	Procainamide: 1.7–4.7	Q4–6 hr	D	**IV (Adult) Maintenance**			Y (He)
					10–50	33% ↓	NI	N (P)
					<10	67% ↓	NI	
					IV (Adult) Loading Dose			
					<10	12 mg/kg	NA	
Quinidine	Renal	2.5–8	Q4–12 hr	D	<10	25% ↓	NI	Y (He)
								N (P)
Ranitidine	Renal (hepatic)	1.8–2.5	Q12 hr PO Q6–8 hr IV/IM	D	10–50	50% ↓	NI	N (He)††
					<10	75% ↓	NI	? (P)
Spironolactone	Renal (hepatic)	Spironolactone: 1.3–1.4	Q6–24 hr	I	10–50	NI	Q12–24 hr	NA
					<10	Avoid use		

Continued

TABLE 31-2

NON-ANTIMICROBIALS REQUIRING ADJUSTMENT IN RENAL FAILURE (Continued)

Drug	Route of Excretion*	Pharmacokinetics Normal t$_{1/2}$ (hr)	Normal Dose Interval	Method	CrCl (mL/min)	Adjustments in Renal Failure Dose	Interval	Supplemental Dose for Dialysis
Terbutaline	Renal (hepatic)	2.9–14	Variable	D	<50 / <10 use not recommended	50% ↓	NI	? (He) / ? (P)
Thiopental	Hepatic (renal)	3–11.5	One-time dose	D	<10	25% ↓	NI	NA
Triamterene	Hepatic (renal)	1.6–2.5	Q12–24 hr	I	>50 / <50	NI / Avoid use	Q12 hr	NA
Verapamil	Renal (hepatic)	2–8	Variable	D	<10 Use caution and closely monitor ECG for PR prolongation, BP, and other signs of overdose.	NI	NI	N (He) / N (P)
Vigabatrin (Sabril)	Renal	5–8	Q12 hr	D	50–80 / 30–50 / 10–30	25% ↓ / 50% ↓ / 75% ↓	NI / NI / NI	? (He) / ? (P)

*Route in parentheses indicates secondary route of excretion.

†With large doses, t$_{1/2}$ is prolonged up to 30 hours.

‡Azathioprine rapidly converted to mercaptopurine (t$_{1/2}$ = 0.5–4 hours).

§Decrease loading dose by 50% in end-stage renal disease because of decreased volume of distribution.

‖Guidelines for adults; guidelines not established for children.

¶Closely monitor antifactor Xa.

#Dose interval varies for rapid and slow acetylators with normal and impaired renal function.

**Renal failure may cause hyposensitivity or hypersensitivity to insulin; adjust to clinical response and blood glucose.

†††Adjust dose schedule to administer dose at end of dialysis.

BP, Blood pressure; CrCl, creatinine clearance; D, dose reduction; EDTA, ethylenediaminetetraacetic acid; ECG, electrocardiogram; ESRD, end-stage renal disease; GFR, glomerular filtration rate; GI, gastrointestinal; He, hemodialysis; I, interval extension; IM, intramuscular; IV, intravenous; MHD, 10-monohydroxy metabolite; N, normal; NA, not applicable; NI, normal; P, peritoneal dialysis; PO, oral; t$_{1/2}$, half life.

REFERENCES

1. Taketomo CK, Hodding JH, Kraus DM. Pediatric Dosage Handbook. Electronic database. Hudson, OH: Lexi-Comp Updated periodically. Avaliable at www.crlonline.com/crlsql/servelet/crloneline.
2. Aronoff GR, Bennett WM, Berns JS, et al. *Drug Prescribing in Renal Failure: Dosing Guidelines for Adults.* 5th ed. Philadelphia: American College of Physicians, 2007.
3. Veltri M, Neu AM, Fivush BA, et al. Dosing during intermittent hemodialysis and continuous renal replacement therapy: special considerations in pediatric patients. *Paediatr Drugs.* 2004;6:45-66.
4. Micromedex Healthcare Series 2.0. Electronic database. New York: Thomson Healthcare USA. Updated periodically. Last accessed Feburary 24, 2013. Available at http://www.thomsonhc.com.

31

Index

A

α. *See* Significance level of statistical tests
A-200. *See* Pyrethrins
A-a gradient. *See* Alveolar-arterial oxygen gradient
Abatacept, for arthritis, 608
Abbreviations, Joint Commission do not use list for, 646, 646t–647t
A-B-C pathway, 3, 61
Abdomen
  imaging of
    biliary atresia, 589
    bowel obstruction, 586–588
    esophageal atresia and tracheoesophageal fistula, 584, 585f
    high intestinal obstruction, 584–586, 586f
    intussusception, 588, 588f
    Meckel diverticulum, 588
    ND tube placement, 589
    neonatal enterocolitis, 584
    pyloric stenosis, 586, 587f
    trauma, 589
    after UTI, 444
  trauma to
    blunt, 65–66
    imaging of, 589
    penetrating, 66
    secondary survey of, 62t
Abdominal pain, acute, 269–270, 270t
Abdominal wall defects, 431.e1t, 431
Abelcet. *See* Amphotericin B lipid complex
ABG. *See* Arterial blood gas
Abilify. *See* Aripiprazole
ABLC. *See* Amphotericin B lipid complex
Absence seizures, 476t–477t, 478b
Absolute neutrophil count (ANC), 313, 314t
Absolute risk reduction (ARR), 640
Absorica. *See* Isotretinoin
Abstinence syndrome, neonatal, 432, 433b
Abstral. *See* Fentanyl

Abuse. *See* Child abuse
Abusive head trauma (AHT), 84
AC. *See* Assist control ventilation
Acanya. *See* Benzoyl peroxide and clindamycin
Accolate. *See* Zafirlukast
AccuNeb. *See* Albuterol
Accutane. *See* Isotretinoin
ACE inhibitors. *See* Angiotensin-converting enzyme inhibitors
Acetadote. *See* Acetylcysteine
Acetaminophen (Tylenol, Tempra, Panadol, Feverall, Aspirin Free Anacin, Paracetamol, Ofirmev)
  analgesic properties of, 112, 113.e1t
  formulary entry for, 667–668
  liver failure due to, 277
  for migraine headaches, 472
  poisoning/overdose of, 19, 23, 24f, 669
  renal failure dosage adjustments for, 1008t–1016t
Acetazolamide (Diamox)
  formulary entry for, 668–669
  for hydrocephalus, 480, 668–669
  renal failure dosage adjustments for, 1008t–1016t
Acetylcysteine (Mucomyst, Mucosol, Acetadote)
  for acetaminophen poisoning, 23, 669
  formulary entry for, 669
ACHES, for clotting symptoms, 100
Achondroplasia, growth charts for, 497
Acid-base disturbances, 264
  determination of primary, 264
  etiology of, 264, 265f–266f
  gas exchange evaluation with, 551, 552f, 552t
Acidemias, organic, 291
Acidification, urine, 447
Acidosis, 264
  arterial blood gas interpretation and, 552f
  compensatory responses to, 552t
  determination of, 264

Note: Page numbers with "*f*" denote figures; "*t*" tables; "*b*" boxes; "*e*" online content; "*cp*" color plates.

Acidosis *(Continued)*
etiology of, 265f–266f
evaluation of, 285, 289f
renal tubular, 456–458, 457t
Acid-suppressant therapy
for burns, 82
for GERD, 275
for GI bleeding, 269, 675
for prolonged NSAID use, 113
Acinetobacter spp., antibiotic sensitivity
of, 383t–384t
Aclovate. *See* Alclometasone dipropionate
Acne vulgaris
classification of, 187
clinical presentation of, 187
neonatal, 190, 191f
pathogenesis of, 186
treatment of, 187–188, 188t–189t
Acquired heart disease
endocarditis, 161–162
prophylaxis for, 162, 162t, 163b,
694–695
myocardial
dilated cardiomyopathy, 162–163
hypertrophic cardiomyopathy,
163–164
myocarditis, 164
restrictive cardiomyopathy, 164
pericardial
cardiac tamponade, 47, 48f–50f, 165
Kawasaki disease, 167.e1t,
166–168, 167f
Lyme disease, 168
pericardial effusion, 165
pericarditis, 164–165
rheumatic heart disease, 168, 169b
ACR. *See* American College of
Rheumatology
Acronyms, Joint Commission do not use
list for, 667, 667t–668t
ACT. *See* Airway clearance therapy
ACTH stimulation test, 226–227, 229
Acthar HP. *See* Corticotropin
ActHIB, 366
Acticin. *See* Permethrin
Actigall. *See* Ursodiol
Actinomycin D. *See* Dactinomycin
Actiq. *See* Fentanyl
Activase. *See* Alteplase
Activated partial thromboplastin time
(aPTT), 316
age-specific values for, 317t–318t

Activated protein C resistance, 319b
Acular. *See* Ketorolac
Acute abdominal pain, 269–270, 270t
Acute adrenal crisis, 230–231
Acute chest syndrome, in sickle cell
disease, 311t–312t
Acute graft-*versus*-host disease
(aGVHD), 534.e1t, 534
Acute headache, 470b
Acute hemolytic reaction, 331
Acute kidney injury (AKI), 448
ATN, 448–449
clinical presentation of, 449, 449t
complications of, 449
dialysis for, 450
etiology of, 448, 448t
treatment considerations for, 449
Acute liver failure (ALF), 276
etiologies of, 276–277
evaluation of, 277–278, 278t
presentation of, 277
Acute lymphocytic leukemia (ALL)
hyperleukocytosis/leukostasis in, 529
signs and symptoms of, 523t–524t
Acute myeloid leukemia (AML)
hyperleukocytosis/leukostasis in, 529
signs and symptoms of, 523t–524t
Acute nephritic syndrome, 451
Acute pancreatitis
conditions associated with, 280t
diagnosis/evaluation of, 279–280
management of, 280
presentation of, 278–279, 280t
Acute phase reactants
CRP, 602–603, 621t–623t
ESR, 602, 621t–623t
Acute transfusion reactions, 331–332
Acute tubular necrosis (ATN), 448–449
Acuvail. *See* Ketorolac
Acyanotic congenital heart disease, 156,
157t–158t
Acyclovir (Zovirax)
for cancer patients, 538t
for eczema herpeticum
superinfection, 183
formulary entry for, 670–671
for genital herpes, 106t–107t
for HSV, 389t–390t
for neonates, 435
renal failure dosage adjustments for,
995t–1007t
for varicella, 377, 389t–390t

Aczone. *See* Dapsone
Adacel. *See* Tetanus and diphtheria
        toxoids and acellular pertussis
        vaccine
Adalat CC. *See* Nifedipine
Adalimumab, for arthritis, 608
Adams forward bend test, 95.e1, 95.e2f
Adaptive skills, 196
    developmental milestones in,
        197t–198t
Adderall. *See* Dextroamphetamine and
        amphetamine
Addison disease, 229
    evaluation of, 226–227, 227t
    management of, 229–230, 229t
Adenocard. *See* Adenosine
Adenomas, hyperparathyroidism caused
        by, 225.e1b, 225
Adenosine (Adenocard)
    formulary entry for, 671
    for neonates, 435
Adequate intake (AI), 500
    fats, 501t
    fiber, 509t
ADH. *See* Antidiuretic hormone
ADHD. *See* Attention deficit/
        hyperactivity disorder
Adhesives, tissue, 57
Adjuncts
    for opioid tapering, 118
    for RSI, 6t–7t
Adolescents
    adult care transitioning for, 108–109
    eczema in, 180
    health maintenance for
        Bright Futures Guidelines for,
            94.e1b, 94
        chief complaint, 94
        confidentiality, 94
        family history, 94
        physical examination, 94–95,
            95.e2f
        review of systems, 94
        screening laboratory tests and
            procedures, 95–97, 97.e1t
    HIV testing for, 96, 402
    mental health of
        anxiety, depression, and bipolar
            disorder, 104
        school problems, 108
        substance use, 93b–94b, 108
        suicidality, 93b, 104–108

Adolescents (*Continued*)
    pain assessment for, 111
    PPE for, 97–98, 98.e1f
    psychosocial and medicosocial history
        for, 93.e1b, 93, 93b–94b
    psychosocial development of, 91,
        92.e1t
    pubertal development of, 91, 92f,
        92t–93t
    screening of, 95–97, 97.e1t, 402
    sexual health of
        contraception use, 98–104, 99f, 101f
        follow-up recommendations, 104
        gender identity, 98
        orientation, 98
        STIs, 93.e1b, 93b, 96, 104
        vaginal infections, genital ulcers,
            and warts, 104, 105t–107t
    websites for, 91
Adoxa. *See* Doxycycline
Adrenal crisis, 230–231
Adrenal gland function
    insufficiency
        acute adrenal crisis, 230–231
        congenital adrenal hyperplasia,
            227–229, 227f, 228t
        Cushing syndrome, 231, 236
        etiology of, 226
        evaluation of, 226–227, 227t
        management of, 229–230, 229t
        primary, 229
    pheochromocytoma, 231
Adrenalin. *See* Epinephrine HCl
Adrenocorticotropic hormone, 743
Adriamycin. *See* Doxorubicin
Adrucil. *See* Fluorouracil
Adult care, adolescent transition to,
        108–109
Adult formulas, nutrition components in,
        511t–517t
Advair. *See* Fluticasone propionate and
        salmeterol
Advance directive, 542
Adverse reactions
    to IMIG, 344
    to IVIG, 343
    to subcutaneous immunoglobulin, 344
Advil. *See* Ibuprofen
AED. *See* Automated external
        defibrillator
Aerobic bacteria, algorithm for
        identification of, 381f–382f

Aerospan. *See* Flunisolide

Aerospan MDI, dosage recommendations for, 558.e1t–558.e2t

AFI. *See* Amniotic fluid index

Afrin. *See* Oxymetazoline

AG. *See* Anion gap

Ages and Stages Questionnaire (ASQ), 201t, 202

Aggression, age-appropriate, 199t–200t

aGVHD. *See* Acute graft-*versus*-host disease

AHA. *See* American Heart Association

AHT. *See* Abusive head trauma

AI. *See* Adequate intake

AIDS. *See* Human immunodeficiency virus/acquired immunodeficiency syndrome

Airway
assessment of, 3
in burn patients, 78–80
emergency management of, 11–13
croup, 12
epiglottitis, 12
foreign-body aspiration, 13, 14f
imaging of
foreign bodies, 576
lateral radiographs, 576, 576t, 577f–578f
vascular rings, 576
management of, 3–7, 5f, 6t–7t
monitoring of, during procedural sedation, 121
obstructive disease of, 553, 554f–555f, 555t
restrictive disease of, 553, 554f–555f, 555t

Airway clearance therapy (ACT), 567–568

AKI. *See* Acute kidney injury

AK-Poly-Bac Ophthalmic. *See* Bacitracin and polymyxin B

AK-Spore H.C. Otic. *See* Polymyxin B sulfate, neomycin sulfate, hydrocortisone

AKTob. *See* Tobramycin

AK-Tracin Ophthalmic. *See* Bacitracin

Alanine aminotransferase (ALT)
liver function testing with, 277t
reference values for, 621t–623t

Alavert. *See* Loratadine and pseudoephedrine

Albumin (Albuminar, Albutein, Buminate, Plasbumin, Normal serum albumin, Human albumin)
formulary entry for, 672
neonate dosages of, 435
reference values for, 621t–623t

Albuterol (AccuNeb, ProAir HFA, Proventil, Ventolin HFA, VoSpire ER)
for anaphylaxis, 10
for asthma, 10, 672–673
formulary entry for, 672–673
for hyperkalemia, 260f
poisoning with, 20t–22t

Alclometasone dipropionate (Aclovate), for atopic dermatitis, 182t–183t

Alcohol abuse. *See* Substance abuse disorder

Aldactone. *See* Spironolactone

Aldolase, reference values for, 621t–623t

Aldosterone
biosynthesis of, 227f
potency of, 229t

Aleve. *See* Naproxen

ALF. *See* Acute liver failure

Alimentum, 511t–517t

Alkaline phosphatase
liver function testing with, 277t
reference values for, 621t–623t

Alkalinizing agents. *See also* Sodium bicarbonate.
citrate mixtures, 737

Alkalosis, 264
arginine chloride for, 688
arterial blood gas interpretation and, 552f
compensatory responses to, 552t
determination of, 264
etiology of, 265f–266f
in PPHN, 425

Alkeran. *See* Melphalan

ALL. *See* Acute lymphocytic leukemia

Allegra. *See* Fexofenadine and pseudoephedrine

Allergen avoidance
for allergic rhinitis, 335
for food allergies, 339

Allergen Ear Drops. *See* Antipyrine and benzocaine

Allergen-specific IgE, 334, 338–339

Allergic conjunctivitis, 336, 336t
Allergic contact dermatitis, CP10, 194
Allergic emergencies. *See* Anaphylaxis
Allergic eosinophilic esophagitis, 337
Allergic eosinophilic gastroenteritis, 337
Allergic reactions
   dermatitis, CP10, 194
   drug, 339–341, 340f
   food, 336–339, 338f, 518t–519t
   rhinitis, 334–336, 336t, 693–694
Allergic rhinitis
   diagnosis of, 334–335
   epidemiology of, 334
   treatment of, 335–336, 336t,
     693–694
Allogeneic HSCT, 532
Allopurinol (Alloprim, Zyloprim)
   formulary entry for, 673
   for GSD, 294–295
   for hyperleukocytosis/leukostasis, 529
   renal failure dosage adjustments for,
     1008t–1016t
   for tumor lysis syndrome, 529, 673
Almacone. *See* Aluminum hydroxide
   with magnesium hydroxide
Almotriptan (Axert), for migraine
   headaches, 473t
Alocril. *See* Nedocromil sodium 2%,
   benzalkonium chloride
Alomide. *See* Lodoxamide tromethamine
   ophthalmic
Alopecia. *See* Hair loss
Alopecia areata, CP8, 185–186
Alpha agonists
   clonidine as, 741
   dexmedetomidine as, 753–754
   guanfacine as, 804–805
   for hypertension, 463t–464t
   isoproterenol as, 821
   for opioid tapering, 118
Alpha blockers
   carvedilol as, 716
   for hypertension, 463t–464t
   labetalol as, 826
   methyldopa as, 852
   phentolamine mesylate as, 901–902
Alpha-fetoprotein, maternal, assessment
   of, 415.e1, 415.e1b
Alpha-tocopherol. *See* Vitamin E
Alprostadil (PGE$_1$, Prostaglandin E$_1$,
   Prostin VR Pediatric), formulary
   entry for, 674

ALT. *See* Alanine aminotransferase
ALTE. *See* Apparent-life-threatening
   event
Alteplase (Activase, Cathflo Activase),
   formulary entry for, 674–675
Altered states of consciousness, 13–15,
   14b, 15t
Aluminum hydroxide (AlternaGEL,
   Amphojel, Alu-Cap, Dialume)
   formulary entry for, 675
   for hyperphosphatemia, 263, 675
Aluminum hydroxide with magnesium
   hydroxide (Almacone, Maalox,
   Mylanta, Rulox), formulary entry
   for, 675–676
Alveolar gas equation, 76
Alveolar-arterial oxygen gradient
   (A-a gradient), 76
Alvesco. *See* Ciclesonide
Amantadine hydrochloride (Symmetrel)
   formulary entry for, 676
   for influenza chemoprophylaxis,
     369–370, 676
   renal failure dosage adjustments for,
     995t–1007t
Ambiguous genitalia, 239–242
AmBisome. *See* Amphotericin B liposomal
Amebicides
   chloroquine phosphate as,
     728–729
   paromomycin sulfate as, 893–894
Amerge. *See* Naratriptan
American College of Rheumatology
   (ACR), SLE classification criteria
   of, 609, 610t
American Heart Association (AHA),
   recommendations for
   participation cardiovascular
   screening of competitive athletes,
   170.e1b, 170
American Society of Anesthesiologists,
   Physical Status Classification of,
   120.e1t, 120
America's Store Brand Soy, 511t–517t
Amethopterin. *See* Methotrexate
Amicar. *See* Aminocaproic acid
Amifostine, toxicity of, 525t–528t
Amikacin sulfate (Amikin)
   formulary entry for, 677
   renal failure dosage adjustments for,
     995t–1007t
   sensitivity-based selection of, 385t

Amiloride, for hypertension, 463t–464t
Amino acid based formulas, nutrition
    components in, 511t–517t
Aminocaproic acid (Amicar)
    formulary entry for, 678
    renal failure dosage adjustments for,
        1008t–1016t
    for von Willebrand disease, 327t–328t
Aminoglycosides
    amikacin as, 677
    gentamicin as, 801
    kanamycin as, 823
    neomycin sulfate as, 871
    paromomycin sulfate as, 893–894
    sensitivity-based selection of, 385t
    streptomycin sulfate as, 946
    tobramycin as, 961–962
Aminophylline, formulary entry for,
        678–679
5-Aminosalicylates, for IBD, 274
5-Aminosalicylic acid. See Mesalamine
Amiodarone HCl (Cordarone, Nexterone,
        Pacerone), formulary entry for,
        679–680
Amitriptyline (Elavil)
    formulary entry for, 680–681
    for migraine headaches, 473t
AML. See Acute myeloid leukemia
Amlodipine (Norvasc)
    formulary entry for, 681
    for hypertension, 463t–464t, 681
Ammonia (NH$_3$)
    liver function testing with, 277t
    reference values for, 621t–623t
Ammonium chloride, formulary entry
        for, 682
Ammonium detoxicants
    lactulose as, 827
    neomycin sulfate as, 871
Amnesteem. See Isotretinoin
Amniocentesis, 415.e1
Amniotic fluid index (AFI), 415.e1,
        415.e2b
Amniotic fluid volume estimation,
        415.e1, 415.e2b
Amoclan. See Amoxicillin–clavulanic
        acid
Amoxicillin (Amoxil, Moxatag, Polymox,
        Trimox, Wymox)
    for chlamydia, 400t–401t
    for endocarditis prophylaxis, 162t
    formulary entry for, 682

Amoxicillin (Continued)
    for gastroenteritis, 393t–399t
    for Lyme disease, 409, 682
    for otitis media, 393t–399t, 682
    for pharyngitis, 393t–399t, 682
    for pneumonia, 393t–399t
    renal failure dosage adjustments for,
        995t–1007t
    sensitivity-based selection of,
        383t–384t
    for septic arthritis, 393t–399t
Amoxicillin–clavulanic acid (Amoclan,
        Augmentin)
    for bite infections, 393t–399t
    for cellulitis, 393t–399t
    for dental abscess, 393t–399t
    formulary entry for, 683
    for lymphadenitis, 393t–399t
    for otitis media, 393t–399t
    for parotitis, 393t–399t
    renal failure dosage adjustments for,
        995t–1007t
    sensitivity-based selection of,
        383t–384t
    for sinusitis, 393t–399t
Amoxil. See Amoxicillin
Amphadase. See Hyaluronidase
Amphetamines, poisoning with, 19,
        20t–22t
Amphocin. See Amphotericin B
Amphojel. See Aluminum hydroxide
Amphotericin B (Amphocin, Fungizone)
    formulary entry for, 684
    neonate dosages of, 435
    renal failure dosage adjustments for,
        995t–1007t
    for sinusitis, 393t–399t
Amphotericin B lipid complex (Abelcet,
        ABLC)
    formulary entry for, 684–685
    renal failure dosage adjustments for,
        995t–1007t
Amphotericin B liposomal (AmBisome)
    formulary entry for, 685
    renal failure dosage adjustments for,
        995t–1007t
Ampicillin (Omnipen, Principen,
        Totacillin)
    for endocarditis prophylaxis, 162t
    formulary entry for, 686
    for gastroenteritis, 393t–399t
    for maternal GBS prophylaxis, 386

Ampicillin *(Continued)*
  for neonatal meningitis, 392t
  for neonatal pneumonia, 392t
  for neonatal septic arthritis, 392t
  neonate dosages of, 435t
  for pneumonia, 393t–399t
  renal failure dosage adjustments for, 995t–1007t
  sensitivity-based selection of, 383t–384t
  for UTI, 393t–399t
Ampicillin/sulbactam (Unasyn)
  for bite infections, 393t–399t
  for cellulitis, 393t–399t
  formulary entry for, 687
  renal failure dosage adjustments for, 995t–1007t
  sensitivity-based selection of, 383t–384t
AMPLE history, 61
Amylase
  reference values for, 621t–623t
  supplementation of, 989t
ANA. *See* Antinuclear antibody
Anacin. *See* Aspirin
Anakinra, for arthritis, 608
Analgesia
  example protocols for, 125t
  local anesthetics for, 113.e1t, 113–116, 115t
  nonopioid agents for, 111–113, 113.e1t
  nonpharmacologic measures of, 116
  opioid agents for, 113.e1t, 113, 114t, 125t
  opioid tapering in, 117–118, 118t, 119b
  pain assessment for, 111, 112t, 113f
  patient-controlled, 116–118, 117t, 119b
  quick reference for, 113.e1t
  risks of, 27
  for sickle cell disease, 311t–312t
  websites for, 111
Anaphylactic shock, 71.e1t, 71
Anaphylaxis, 9
  food allergies causing, 336, 339
  initial management of, 9–10
Anaplasmosis, 410
Anaprox. *See* Naproxen
ANC. *See* Absolute neutrophil count
Ancef. *See* Cefazolin
Ancobon. *See* Flucytosine
Androstenedione, normal values of, 243.e3t, 243

Anectine. *See* Succinylcholine
Anemia. *See also* Sickle cell anemia.
  cancer patients with, 536
  causes of, 305–309
  classification of, 308t
  darbepoetin alfa for, 748–750
  diagnosis of, 305, 308t
  epoetin alfa for, 772–773
  general evaluation of, 305, 306t, 307f
  microangiopathic hemolytic, CP12, 315
Anemia of chronic inflammation, 309
Anesthesia. *See also* Procedural sedation.
  general
    ketamine for, 824
    for status epilepticus, 16t
  local
    lidocaine and prilocaine for, 115t, 125t
    lidocaine for, 835–836
Angioedema, food allergies causing, 336, 339
Angiotensin receptor blockers (ARBs)
  for hypertension, 463t–464t
  losartan as, 843
  for Marfan syndrome, 302
  valsartan as, 971
Angiotensin-converting enzyme (ACE) inhibitors
  captopril as, 712–713
  enalapril and enalaprilat as, 768–769
  for GSD, 294–295
  for hypertension, 463t–464t
  lisinopril as, 839–840
Animal bites
  management of, 77–78, 393t–399t
  wound considerations for, 76–77, 77t
Anion gap (AG), 264
Anion gap metabolic acidosis
  etiology of, 265f–266f
  evaluation of, 285, 289f
  poisoning diagnosis and, 20.e1t–20.e3t
Ankle, splinting of, 59
Antacids
  aluminum hydroxide as, 675
  aluminum hydroxide with magnesium hydroxide as, 675–676
  for burns, 82
  calcium carbonate as, 709
  magnesium hydroxide as, 844
Anteroposterior (AP) chest radiograph, normal anatomy on, 579f–580f

Anthralin, for alopecia areata, 186
Anthropometric measurements, 485
Anti-androgens, for acne vulgaris, 189t
Antiarrhythmics
  adenosine as, 671
  amiodarone as, 679–680
  digoxin as, 758
  esmolol HCl as, 777–778
  flecainide acetate as, 785–786
  lidocaine as, 835–836
  metoprolol as, 856–857
  phenytoin as, 903–904
  procainamide as, 916–917
  propranolol as, 918–919
  quinidine as, 925–926
Antibiotics. *See also specific antibiotic agents*
  for acne vulgaris, 187, 188t–189t
  for animal bites, 78
  for bacterial superinfection in atopic dermatitis, 183
  for burns, 83.e1b, 83
  for cancer patients
    infection treatment, 531–532, 533f
    prophylaxis, 538, 538t
  for CF, 568
  for endocarditis prophylaxis, 162, 162t, 163b
  for IBD, 274
  for impetigo, 192
  neonate dosages of, 435t
  for PPHN, 425
  sensitivity-based selection of, 380
    aminoglycosides, 385t
    beta-lactams, 383t–384t
    fluoroquinolones, 385t
    macrolides, 385t
    single drug class, 386t
    tetracyclines, 385t
  for shock, 71.e1t, 73f
  for sickle cell disease, 311t–312t
  for UTIs, 442
  for VUR prophylaxis, 444
Antibody deficiency
  evaluation for, 342t–343t
  IVIG for, 341
  subcutaneous immunoglobulin for, 344
Antibody-deficient disorders, IVIG for, 341
Anti-CCP antibodies. *See* Anti–cyclic citrullinated peptide antibodies

Anticholinergics
  for allergic rhinitis, 336
  atropine sulfate as, 691–692
  benztropine mesylate as, 700
  cyclopentolate as, 745
  cyclopentolate with phenylephrine as, 745
  glycopyrrolate as, 802–803
  ipratropium bromide as, 817–818
  oxybutynin chloride as, 888
  poisoning with, 21t
  scopolamine hydrobromide as, 937
  toxidrome of, 20t–22t
Anticholinesterase agents
  edrophonium chloride as, 768
  neostigmine as, 872–873
  poisoning with, 21t, 691–692
Anticoagulation
  coagulation tests and, 322–324
  enoxaparin for, 769–770
  heparin sodium for, 806–807
  for hypercoagulable states, 320–324, 321t–324t, 325b
  for Kawasaki disease, 167.e1t
  for stroke, 482–483, 531
  warfarin for, 980–981
Anticonvulsants
  carbamazepine as, 713–714
  clobazam as, 739–740
  clonazepam as, 740
  diazepam as, 756–757
  divalproex sodium as, 762
  ethosuximide as, 780
  felbamate as, 782–783
  fosphenytoin as, 797
  gabapentin as, 798–799
  lacosamide as, 826–827
  lamotrigine as, 828–831
  levetiracetam as, 832–833
  liver failure due to, 277
  lorazepam as, 842
  for migraine headaches, 473t
  oxcarbazepine as, 886–888
  phenytoin as, 903–904
  primidone as, 915
  for seizures, 479t
  tiagabine as, 959–960
  topiramate as, 963–964
  valproic acid as, 970–971
  vigabatrin as, 976–977
  zonisamide as, 984–985

Anti–cyclic citrullinated peptide (Anti-CCP) antibodies, 603t, 604
Antidepressants. *See also specific antidepressant classes*
  for depressive disorders, 209t, 210
  for mental health disorders, 209t
  for migraine headaches, 473t, 680–681
Antidiarrheal agents, 271
  bismuth subsalicylate as, 702–703
  loperamide as, 841
Antidiuretic hormone (ADH)
  conditions increasing release of, 246.e1b, 246
  vasopressin as analog of, 974
Antidotes
  for drug poisonings, 20–23, 21t
  methylene blue as, 852
  phentolamine mesylate as, 901–902
  pralidoxime chloride as, 912–913
  protamine sulfate as, 920–921
Antiemetics
  chlorpromazine as, 730–731
  dimenhydrinate as, 760
  dolasetron as, 763
  dronabinol as, 766
  droperidol as, 767
  granisetron as, 803
  hydroxyzine as, 811
  metoclopramide as, 855
  for migraine headaches, 472
  ondansetron as, 883–884
  prochlorperazine as, 917
  promethazine as, 918
  trimethobenzamide HCl as, 967
Antifungals
  amphotericin B as, 684
  amphotericin B lipid complex as, 684–685
  amphotericin B liposomal as, 685
  caspofungin as, 716–717
  clotrimazole as, 742
  fluconazole as, 786–787
  flucytosine as, 787
  griseofulvin as, 804
  itraconazole as, 822–823
  ketoconazole as, 824–825
  micafungin sodium as, 859
  miconazole as, 860
  nystatin as, 879–880
  for tinea infections, 184, 411t

Antifungals *(Continued)*
  tolnaftate as, 963
  voriconazole as, 979–980
Antihistamines
  for allergic rhinitis, 335
  for atopic dermatitis, 180
  azelastine as, 693–694
  brompheniramine with phenylephrine as, 703–704
  carbinoxamine as, 715
  cetirizine as, 726–727
  chlorpheniramine maleate as, 730
  cyproheptadine as, 746–747
  dimenhydrinate as, 760
  diphenhydramine as, 761
  fexofenadine and pseudoephedrine as, 784–785
  for food allergies, 339
  hydroxyzine as, 811
  loratadine and pseudoephedrine as, 841–842
  for migraine headaches, 473t
  olopatadine as, 881
  poisoning with, 20t–22t
  procedural sedation with, 121b–122b
  promethazine as, 918
Antihypertensives
  amlodipine as, 681
  captopril as, 712–713
  carvedilol as, 716
  for chronic hypertension, 462, 463t–464t, 681
  clonidine as, 741
  diazoxide as, 757
  diltiazem as, 759–760
  enalapril and enalaprilat as, 768–769
  esmolol HCl as, 777–778
  hydralazine hydrochloride as, 807–808
  labetalol as, 826
  lisinopril as, 839–840
  methyldopa as, 852
  minoxidil as, 863
  nicardipine as, 874–875
  nifedipine as, 875–876
  nitroglycerin as, 876–877
  nitroprusside as, 877
  valsartan as, 971
Antihyperuricemic agents. *See* Rasburicase

Antihypoglycemic agents
  diazoxide as, 757
  glucagon HCl as, 802
Anti-inflammatory drugs. *See also*
    Nonsteroidal antiinflammatory
    drugs
  aspirin as, 689
  mesalamine as, 849
  olsalazine as, 882
  sulfasalazine as, 950–951
Antilirium. *See* Physostigmine salicylate
Antimalarials
  chloroquine phosphate as, 728–729
  hydroxychloroquine as, 810
  mefloquine HCl as, 847–848
  primaquine phosphate as,
      914–915
  quinidine as, 925–926
Antimicrobial prophylaxis, 538, 538t
Antinuclear antibody (ANA), 603, 603t
  reference values for, 621t–623t
Antiparasitic agents
  metronidazole as, 857–858
  pyrimethamine as, 925
Antiparkinsonian agent, benztropine
      mesylate, 700
Antiphospholipid antibodies,
      hypercoagulable state caused
      by, 319b
Antiplatelet therapy
  aspirin as, 689
  for stroke, 482–483
Antiprotozoals
  atovaquone as, 691
  metronidazole as, 857–858
  pentamidine isethionate as, 898–899
Antipsychotics
  chlorpromazine as, 730–731
  haloperidol as, 805–806
  lithium as, 840
  for mental health disorders, 209t
  risperidone as, 934–935
  thioridazine as, 959
Antipyretics
  acetaminophen as, 667–668
  aspirin as, 689
  ibuprofen as, 811–812
Antipyrine and benzocaine (Allergen
      Ear Drops, Antipyrine and
      Benzocaine Otic, Aurodex,
      Auroguard Otic, Auralgan),
      formulary entry for, 687

Antiretroviral therapy (ART)
  for HIV management, 403t–404t,
      405–406
  lamivudine as, 828
  nevirapine as, 873
  for PEP, 412
  for perinatal HIV exposure, 402–405,
      403t–404t
  zidovudine as, 982–983
Antispasmodic agent, oxybutynin
      chloride, 888
Antistreptolysin O titer, reference values
      for, 621t–623t
Antithrombin III deficiency, 319b
Antithymocyte globulin, for GVHD
      prevention, 534
Antithyroid agents
  methimazole as, 851
  potassium iodide as, 910–911
  propylthiouracil as, 920
Anti-TNF agents. *See* Tumor necrosis
      factor inhibitors
Antituberculosis drugs
  ethambutol HCl as, 780
  isoniazid as, 820–821
  pyrazinamide as, 923
  rifabutin as, 931–932
  rifampin as, 932–933
  streptomycin sulfate as, 946
Antivirals. *See also* Antiretroviral therapy
  acyclovir as, 670–671
  amantadine hydrochloride as, 676
  cidofovir as, 734
  famciclovir as, 781
  foscarnet as, 796–797
  ganciclovir as, 800
  nevirapine as, 873
  oseltamivir phosphate as, 885–886
  ribavirin as, 929–931
  rimantadine as, 933
  valacyclovir as, 968–969
  valganciclovir as, 969–970
Antizol. *See* Fomepizole
Anxiety
  in adolescents, 104
  stranger/separation, 199t–200t
Anxiety disorders
  assessment of, 209–210
  categories of, 210
  epidemiology of, 209
  treatment of, 209t, 210
Anxiolysis, 118

Anxiolytics
diazepam as, 756–757
hydroxyzine as, 811
lorazepam as as, 842
for mental health disorders, 209t
Anzemet. *See* Dolasetron
Aorta, coarctation of, 157t–158t
Aortic stenosis (AS), 157t–158t
AP chest radiograph. *See*
Anteroposterior chest radiograph
Apidra. *See* Glulisine insulin
Aplastic anemia, 309
Aplastic crisis, in sickle cell disease,
311t–312t
Apnea
aminophylline for, 678–679
in newborns, 426–427, 426f
Apparent-life-threatening event (ALTE),
556
differential diagnosis of, 556,
556b–557b
workup for, 557
Aprepitant, for nausea and vomiting,
537
Apresoline. *See* Hydralazine
hydrochloride
aPTT. *See* Activated partial
thromboplastin time
Aquachloral Supprettes. *See* Chloral
hydrate
AquADEKs, 504t–506t
Aquasol A. *See* Vitamin A
Aquasol E. *See* Vitamin E
Aquavit-E. *See* Vitamin E
Ara-C. *See* Cytarabine
Aralen. *See* Chloroquine phosphate
Aranesp. *See* Darbepoetin alfa
Arbinoxa. *See* Carbinoxamine
ARBs. *See* Angiotensin receptor
blockers
Arestin. *See* Minocycline
Arginine
for metabolic crisis, 290
for urea cycle defects, 292
Arginine chloride (R-Gene 10),
formulary entry for, 688
8-Arginine Vasopressin. *See* Vasopressin
Aridol. *See* Mannitol
Aripiprazole (Abilify), for mental health
disorders, 209t
Aristospan. *See* Triamcinolone

Arms. *See* Extremities
ARR. *See* Absolute risk reduction
Arrhythmias. *See also* Antiarrhythmics
ECG of, 144, 145t–146t, 147f–148f,
148t
ART. *See* Antiretroviral therapy
Arterial blood gas (ABG)
gas exchange evaluation with, 550,
552f
reference values for, 621t–623t
Arterial switch procedure, 161
Arteries
dorsalis pedis, puncture of, 31
femoral, puncture of, 29–30, 29f
posterior tibial, puncture of, 31
radial, puncture of, 30–31
umbilical, catheterization of, 38–42,
39f, 41f
Arteriovenous O_2 difference (AVD$_{O_2}$),
76.e1
Arthritis
differential diagnosis of, 609, 609t
JIA, 606
autoantibodies associated with,
603t
classical divisions of, 607t
JRA, 606
autoantibodies associated with,
603t
joint fluid analysis for, 605f
management of
health maintenance, 608–609
pharmacologic agents, 608.e1t,
608
psoriatic, 606–607
reactive, 607–608
joint fluid analysis for, 605f
septic
joint fluid analysis for, 605f
management of, 393t–399t
neonatal, 392t
AS. *See* Aortic stenosis
ASA. *See* Aspirin
5-ASA. *See* Mesalamine
Asacol. *See* Mesalamine
Ascorbic acid (Vitamin C, Sunkist
Vitamin C)
DRIs for, 502t–503t
formulary entry for, 688
reference values for, 621t–623t
ASD. *See* Atrial septal defect
ASDs. *See* Autism spectrum disorders

Asmanex Twisthaler. *See* Mometasone

Asparaginase (L-Asp, PEG-Asp, Elspar, Erwinia), toxicity of, 525t–528t

Aspart insulin (Novo Log), 218t

Aspartate aminotransferase (AST)
  in hemolytic anemia, 307
  liver function testing with, 277t
  reference values for, 621t–623t

Aspiration
  foreign-body
    emergency management of, 13, 14f
    imaging of, 576
  procedural sedation risk for, 119.e1f
  soft tissue, 51–53
  suprapubic bladder, 51, 52f–53f

Aspirin (ASA, Anacin, Bufferin)
  analgesic properties of, 112, 689
  formulary entry for, 689
  for Kawasaki disease, 167.e1t, 168
  poisoning with, 19
  renal failure dosage adjustments for, 1008t–1016t
  for stroke, 482–483

Aspirin Free Anacin. *See* Acetaminophen

Asplenia, 361

ASQ. *See* Ages and Stages Questionnaire

Assist control ventilation (AC), 74

AST. *See* Aspartate aminotransferase

Astagraf XL. *See* Tacrolimus

Astelin. *See* Azelastine

Astepro. *See* Azelastine

Asthma
  clinical manifestations of, 558
  exacerbation prevention in, 558
  management of, 558, 559f–564f, 672–673, 678–679
    emergency, 10–11
    inhaled corticosteroid dosages, 558.e1t–558.e2t
  severity classification of, 559f–561f

Asymptomatic bacteriuria, 444

Ataxia, 480
  differential diagnosis of, 481b
  evaluation of, 481b
  poisoning diagnosis and, 20.e1t–20.e3t

Atelectasis, imaging of, 579–580

Atenolol (Tenormin)
  formulary entry for, 689–690
  for hypertension, 463t–464t

Atenolol *(Continued)*
  for Marfan syndrome, 302
  renal failure dosage adjustments for, 1008t–1016t

Athletes. *See* Sports participation

Ativan. *See* Lorazepam

ATN. *See* Acute tubular necrosis

Atomoxetine (Strattera), formulary entry for, 690

Atonic seizures, 478b

Atopic dermatitis
  clinical presentation of, CP6, CP7, 180
  complications of, 183
  epidemiology of, 180
  food allergies causing, 337, 339
  pathogenesis of, 180
  treatment of, 180, 182t–183t

Atovaquone (Mepron)
  for cancer patients, 538t
  formulary entry for, 691
  for perinatal HIV exposure, 403t–404t
  for *Pneumocystis jiroveci* pneumonia, 405.e1t–405.e2t, 691
  for *Toxoplasma gondii* infection, 405.e1t–405.e2t, 691

Atrial enlargement, 144, 144f

Atrial fibrillation, 145t–146t, 147f

Atrial flutter, 145t–146t, 147f

Atrial septal defect (ASD), 157t–158t

Atrial septostomy, 160

Atrioventricular septal defects, 157t–158t

Atropine sulfate (Sal-Tropine, AtroPen)
  for anticholinesterase poisoning, 21t, 691–692
  formulary entry for, 691–692
  for neonates, 435
  for organophosphate poisoning, 21t, 691–692
  procedural sedation with, 125t
  for RSI, 5f, 6t–7t, 691–692

Atrovent. *See* Ipratropium bromide

Attention deficit/hyperactivity disorder (ADHD)
  assessment of, 201t, 208–209
  cardiovascular screening in, 170
  epidemiology of, 208
  treatment for, 209, 209t, 690

Audiologic testing, 203

Augmentin. *See* Amoxicillin–clavulanic acid

Aura, 472

Auralgan. *See* Antipyrine and benzocaine

Auro Ear Drops. *See* Carbamide peroxide

Aurodex. *See* Antipyrine and benzocaine

Auroguard Otic. *See* Antipyrine and benzocaine

Auscultation, respiratory, 550t

Autism spectrum disorders (ASDs)
  developmental and mental health screening tools for, 201t
  as developmental disorders, 207–208

Autoantibodies
  laboratory studies of
    ANA, 603, 603t
    anti-CCP antibodies, 603t, 604
    RF, 603–604, 603t
  in SLE, 603t, 611

Autoimmune bullous diseases, CP10, 193

Autologous HSCT, 532

Automated external defibrillator (AED), 8

Autopsy consent, 547

AV reentrant SVT, 145t–146t, 147f

Avastin. *See* Bevacizumab

AVD$_{O2}$. *See* Arteriovenous O_2 difference

Avinza. *See* Morphine sulfate

Avita. *See* Tretinoin

Axert. *See* Almotriptan

Ayr Saline. *See* Sodium chloride, inhaled preparations

Azactam. *See* Aztreonam

Azasan. *See* Azathioprine

AzaSite. *See* Azithromycin

Azathioprine (Imuran, Azasan)
  for arthritis, 608.e1t
  for Behçet disease, 616.e2
  formulary entry for, 693
  for HSP, 614
  renal failure dosage adjustments for, 1008t–1016t

Azelaic acid, for acne vulgaris, 187, 188t–189t

Azelastine (Astelin, Astepro, Optivar)
  for allergic rhinitis, 335
  drug formulary for, 693–694

Azithromycin (AzaSite, Zithromax, Zmax)
  for chancroid, 106t–107t
  for chlamydia, 400t–401t, 694–695
  drug formulary for, 694–695

Azithromycin *(Continued)*
  for endocarditis prophylaxis, 162t
  for gastroenteritis, 393t–399t
  for gonorrhea, 400t–401t, 694–695
  for *Mycobacterium avium* complex infection, 405.e1t–405.e2t, 694–695
  for neonatal conjunctivitis, 392t
  for neonatal pneumonia, 392t
  ophthalmic, 991t–992t
  for otitis media, 393t–399t, 694–695
  for pertussis, 366, 393t–399t, 694–695
  for pneumonia, 393t–399t, 694–695
  sensitivity-based selection of, 385t

Azo-Standard. *See* Phenazopyridine HCl

AZT. *See* Zidovudine

Aztreonam (Azactam, Cayston)
  formulary entry for, 696
  renal failure dosage adjustments for, 995t–1007t
  sensitivity-based selection of, 383t–384t

Azulfidine. *See* Sulfasalazine

B

B cell count, reference values for, 347t

Baciguent Topical. *See* Bacitracin

Bacillus spp., antibiotic sensitivity of, 385t

Bacitracin (AK-Tracin Ophthalmic, Baciguent Topical)
  for burns, 83.e1b
  formulary entry for, 696–697

Bacitracin and polymyxin B
  (AK-Poly-Bac Ophthalmic, Polysporin Ophthalmic, Polysporin Topical), 991t–992t
  for conjunctivitis, 393t–399t
  formulary entry for, 696–697

Back trauma, secondary survey of, 62t

Baclofen (Gablofen, Kemstro, Lioresal), formulary entry for, 697–698

Bacteria, algorithm for identification of, 381f–382f

Bacterial endocarditis, 161–162
  prophylaxis for, 162, 162t, 163b, 694–695

Bacterial vaginosis
  in adolescents, 105t
  management of, 393t–399t

Bacteriuria, asymptomatic, 444

Bacteroides spp., antibiotic sensitivity of, 386t
Bactrim. *See* Trimethoprim-sulfamethoxazole
Bactroban. *See* Mupirocin
Bag-mask ventilation, 3, 8
BAL. *See* Dimercaprol
Banzel. *See* Rufinamide
Barbiturates
  pentobarbital as, 899
  phenobarbital as, 900–901
  poisoning with, 19, 20t–22t
  primidone as, 915
  procedural sedation with, 121b–122b, 123t
Bartonella spp., antibiotic sensitivity of, 385t–386t
Basal calorie method, maintenance fluid volume calculation with, 247
Basal energy expenditure (BEE), 497–499
Basal metabolic rate (BMR), 497
Basophilic stippling, blood smear demonstrating, CP11
BBB. *See* Bundle-branch block
BCNU. *See* Carmustine
Beclomethasone dipropionate (QVAR, Beconase AQ, Qnasl)
  for asthma, 558.e1t–558.e2t
  dosage recommendations for, 558.e1t–558.e2t
  formulary entry for, 698
BECTS. *See* Benign epilepsy of childhood with centrotemporal spikes
BEE. *See* Basal energy expenditure
Behavior, 195–196. *See also* Developmental disorders; Mental health disorders.
  characterization of, 195
  normal, guidelines for
    age-appropriate issues in infancy and early childhood, 196, 199t–200t
    developmental milestones, 196, 197t–198t
    Reach Out and Read milestones of early literacy, 196, 198t
  screening and evaluation of
    guidelines for, 200
    tools used for, 200–202, 201t, 202.e1b–202.e2b, 203f–204f
  websites for, 195

Behçet disease, 616.e2
Benazepril, for hypertension, 463t–464t
Benign epilepsy of childhood with centrotemporal spikes (BECTS), 476t–477t
Benign rolandic epilepsy, 476t–477t
Benzac AC. *See* Benzoyl peroxide
BenzaClin. *See* Benzoyl peroxide and clindamycin
Benzalkonium chloride, for allergic conjunctivitis, 336t
Benzamycin. *See* Benzoyl peroxide and erythromycin
Benzathine penicillin G (Bicillin L-A)
  formulary entry for, 896
  for pharyngitis, 393t–399t
  for syphilis, 388t, 400t–401t
Benzathine penicillin G and penicillin G procaine (Bicillin C-R), formulary entry for, 896–897
Benzocaine. *See* Antipyrine and benzocaine
Benzodiazepines
  antidote for, 21t, 788
  clobazam as, 739–740
  clonazepam as, 740
  diazepam as, 756–757
  lorazepam as, 842
  midazolam as, 860–861
  for nausea and vomiting, 537
  poisoning with, 20t–22t
  procedural sedation with, 121b–122b, 123t
Benzoyl peroxide (Benzac AC, BPO, Brevoxyl Creamy Wash, Desquam-E, NeoBenz Micro, Oxy-5, Oxy-10)
  for acne vulgaris, 187, 188t–189t
  formulary entry for, 699
Benzoyl peroxide and clindamycin (BenzaClin, Duac, Acanya), formulary entry for, 699
Benzoyl peroxide and erythromycin (Benzamycin), formulary entry for, 699
Benztropine mesylate (Cogentin), formulary entry for, 700
Bereavement
  etiquette for, 547
  services for, 547

Beta blockers
  atenolol as, 689–690
  carvedilol as, 716
  esmolol HCl as, 777–778
  for hypertension, 463t–464t
  labetalol as, 826
  for long QT, 150
  for Marfan syndrome, 302
  metoprolol as, 856–857
  for migraine headaches, 473t
  poisoning with, 21t
  propranolol as, 918–919
Beta-2 adrenergic agonists
  albuterol as, 672–673
  for asthma, 10, 562f–564f
  fluticasone propionate and salmeterol
      as, 792–793
  formoterol as, 705, 795–796
  isoproterenol as, 821
  levalbuterol as, 832
  salmeterol as, 936
  terbutaline as, 956
Beta-lactamase inhibitors
  amoxicillin–clavulanic acid as, 683
  ampicillin/sulbactam as, 687
Beta-lactams, sensitivity-based selection
      of, 383t–384t
Betamethasone (Beta-Val, Celestone,
      Celestone Soluspan, Diprolene,
      Diprosone, Luxiq, Maxivate)
  for atopic dermatitis, 182t–183t
  formulary entry for, 700–701
  potency of, 229t
Bethanechol chloride (Urecholine)
  formulary entry for, 701–702
  for GERD, 275
Bethkis. See Tobramycin
Bevacizumab (Avastin), toxicity of,
      525t–528t
Biaxin. See Clarithromycin
Bicarbonate. See also Sodium
      bicarbonate.
  reference values for, 621t–623t
Bicarbonate reabsorption, 447, 457t
Bicillin C-R. See Benzathine penicillin G
      and penicillin G procaine
Bicillin L-A. See Benzathine penicillin G
BiCNU. See Carmustine
Biguanides, metformin as, 850
Bile acid sequestrants, 170
Bilevel positive airway pressure
      (BiPAP), 74

Biliary atresia, 589
Bilious emesis, 431.e1t, 431
Bilirubin. See also Hyperbilirubinemia
  reference values for, 621t–623t
  in urine, 439, 440t
Biocef. See Cephalexin
Biologic immunomodulators
  for arthritis, 608.e1t, 608
  for SLE, 611
Biological response modifier therapy,
      immunoprophylaxis for patients
      on, 363
Biophysical profile, fetal assessment
      with, 415.e1, 415.e2t
Bio-Statin. See Nystatin
Biostatistics
  disease occurrence and treatment
      effect measurements,
      638t–639t
    absolute risk reduction, 640
    incidence, 639
    number needed to treat, 640
    odds ratio, 640
    prevalence, 639
    relative risk, 639
    relative risk reduction, 640
  statistical tests, 635–638, 636t
    confidence interval and, 637
    confounding variables and, 638
    effect modification and, 638
    power of, 637
    sample size and, 637
    significance level of, 637
  study design comparison,
      638t–639t
  test validity and reliability
      measurements, 641t
    likelihood ratio, 641
    negative predictive value, 641
    positive predictive value, 641
    sensitivity, 640
    specificity, 640
  websites for, 634
Biotin, DRIs for, 502t–503t
BiPAP. See Bilevel positive airway
      pressure
Bipolar disorder, 104
Birth, preventing HIV transmission
      during, 405
Birth control. See Contraception
Birth control pills. See Oral
      contraceptive pills

Birth trauma
brachial plexus injuries, 419
extradural fluid collections, 416, 419f,
419t
fractured clavicle, 419
Birth weight
assessment of, 415
expected weight by gestational age,
415.e2, 416t
Bisacodyl (Dulcolax, Fleet Laxative,
Fleet Bisacodyl, Doxidan)
for constipation, 272
formulary entry for, 702
Bischloronitrosourea. *See* Carmustine
Bismuth subsalicylate (Pepto-Bismol,
Kaopectate, Kao-Tin, Stomach
Relief)
formulary entry for, 702–703
renal failure dosage adjustments for,
1008t–1016t
Bisphosphates
for hypercalcemia, 261
for hyperparathyroidism, 225
Bites
animal
management of, 77–78,
393t–399t
wound considerations for,
76–77, 77t
human, 77t
in child abuse patients, 84
HIV transmission through, 412
management of, 393t–399t
Black dot tinea capitis, 185
Bladder, imaging of, 443–444, 443f
Blalock-Taussig shunt, 160f, 161
Bleeding
in child abuse patients, 84
GI, 268–269, 268t, 675
Bleeding disorders, 325, 326f, 327b,
327t–328t
Bleeding time, 319
age-specific values for,
317t–318t
Bleomycin (Blenoxane)
late effects of, 538.e1t
toxicity of, 525t–528t
Bleph 10. *See* Sulfacetamide sodium
ophthalmic
Block skills. *See* Gesell block skills
Blood, occult, 281
Blood cell indices, age-specific, 306t

Blood chemistries, reference values
for, 621
ABG, 621t–623t
albumin, 621t–623t
aldolase, 621t–623t
alkaline phosphatase, 621t–623t
ALT, 621t–623t
ammonia, 621t–623t
amylase, 621t–623t
ANA, 621t–623t
antistreptolysin O titer, 621t–623t
AST, 621t–623t
bicarbonate, 621t–623t
bilirubin, 621t–623t
blood gas, 621t–623t
calcium, 621t–623t
carbon dioxide, 621t–623t
carbon monoxide, 621t–623t
chloride, 621t–623t
cholesterol, 621t–623t
creatine kinase, 621t–623t
creatinine, 621t–623t
CRP, 621t–623t
ESR, 621t–623t
ferritin, 621t–623t
fibrinogen, 621t–623t
folate, 621t–623t
galactose, 621t–623t
GGT, 621t–623t
glucose, 621t–623t
haptoglobin, 621t–623t
HbA$_{1c}$, 621t–623t
hemoglobin F, 621t–623t
iron, 621t–623t
lactate, 621t–623t
LDH, 621t–623t
lead, 621t–623t
lipase, 621t–623t
lipids, 621t–623t
magnesium, 621t–623t
methemoglobin, 621t–623t
osmolality, 621t–623t
phenylalanine, 621t–623t
phosphorus, 621t–623t
porcelain, 621t–623t
potassium, 621t–623t
prealbumin, 621t–623t
protein electrophoresis, 621t–623t
pyruvate, 621t–623t
RF, 621t–623t
sodium, 621t–623t
TIBC, 621t–623t

Blood chemistries, reference values
        for (Continued)
    total protein, 621t–623t
    total triglyceride, 621t–623t
    transferrin, 621t–623t
    troponin-I, 621t–623t
    urea nitrogen, 621t–623t
    uric acid, 621t–623t
    vitamin A, 621t–623t
    vitamin B_1, 621t–623t
    vitamin B_2, 621t–623t
    vitamin B_{12}, 621t–623t
    vitamin C, 621t–623t
    vitamin D, 621t–623t
    vitamin E, 621t–623t
    zinc, 621t–623t
Blood component replacement
    blood product components
        cryoprecipitate, 331
        FFP, 330
        monoclonal factor VIII, 331
        platelets, 330
        RBCs/PRBCs, 325–330
        recombinant factor VIII or IX, 331
    blood volume, 325, 329t
    for cancer patients, 536
    complications of, 331–332
    direct donors for, 332
    for hyperleukocytosis/leukostasis, 529
    immunoprophylaxis for patients
        treated with, 363.e1t, 363
    PRBC exchange transfusion, 331
Blood culture, specimen collection for,
        380
Blood flow, imaging of, 583
Blood gases
    gas exchange evaluation with,
        550–551, 552f
    reference values for, 621t–623t
Blood glucose levels
    diabetes diagnosis/screening with,
        214, 219
    monitoring of, 219
    reference values for, 621t–623t
Blood pressure (BP)
    abnormalities in, 128
    assessment of, 128.e1t, 8, 128,
        129t–135t, 136f–138f
    definition of normal, 460
    linear regression by postconceptional
        age, 138f
    measurement of, 68, 460

Blood pressure (Continued)
    percentiles
        for boys 1-17 years by height,
            133t–135t
        for boys from birth to 12 months,
            136f
        for girls 1-17 years by height,
            129t–132t
        for girls from birth to 12 months,
            137f
        for infants 26-44 weeks
            postconceptional age, 128.e1t
    in PPHN, 425
Blood products
    cryoprecipitate, 331
    FFP, 330
    immunoprophylaxis for patients
        treated with, 363.e1t, 363
    monoclonal factor VIII, 331
    platelets, 330
    RBCs/PRBCs, 325–330
    recombinant factor VIII or IX, 331
Blood sampling
    dorsalis pedis artery puncture, 31
    external jugular puncture, 28–29, 28f
    femoral artery/vein punctures, 29–30,
        29f
    heelstick and fingerstick, 27–28
    posterior tibial artery puncture, 31
    radial artery puncture and
        catheterization, 30–31
Blood smears, CP11, CP12, 332–333
Blood urea nitrogen/creatinine (BUN/Cr)
        ratio, 449
Blood volume, estimated, 329t
Bloodborne pathogens, exposure to
    HBV prophylaxis after, 368t, 412–413
    HCV prophylaxis after, 413
    HIV prophylaxis after, 411–412
Bloodstream infections, catheter-related,
        393t–399t
Bloxiverz. See Neostigmine
Blunt abdominal trauma, 65–66
Blunt thoracic trauma, 65–66
BMI. See Body mass index
BMR. See Basal metabolic rate
Body fluids
    electrolyte composition of, 256t
    evaluation of
        CSF, 631t
        synovial fluid, 605, 605f, 632t
        transudate vs. exudate, 630t

Body fluids *(Continued)*
 sampling of
  chest tube placement and
   thoracentesis, 44–47, 45f–46f
  lumbar puncture, 42–44, 43f
  paracentesis, 47–49
  pericardiocentesis, 47, 48f–50f
  soft tissue aspiration, 51–53
  suprapubic bladder aspiration, 51,
   52f–53f
  urinary bladder catheterization,
   50–51
Body mass index (BMI)
 growth charts for
  boys, 494f
  girls, 492f
 as indicator of nutritional status, 486
Body surface area (BSA)
 corticosteroid dosing based on, 988f
 maintenance fluid volume calculation
  with, 248, 248t
Bone lesions
 imaging of
  Ewing sarcoma, 597, 598f
  fibroma, 590, 595f
  osteochondroma, 590, 594f
  osteoma, 590, 595f
  osteosarcoma, 590, 596f–597f
  unicameral bone cyst, 590, 594f
 sarcoma signs and symptoms,
  523t–524t
Bone marrow transplantation
 complications of
  aGVHD, 534.e1t, 534
  cGVHD, 534–535
  hemorrhagic cystitis, 536
  mucositis, 536
  thrombotic microangiopathy, 535
  veno-occlusive disease, 535
 goal of, 532
 immunoprophylaxis after, 362.e1t,
  361–362
 IVIG for, 341
 types of, 532
 vaccination after, 538.e2
Bones. *See also* Fractures
 age of, 597
Boost, 511t–517t
Boost Glucose Control, 511t–517t
Boost High Protein, 511t–517t
Boost Kid Essentials, 511t–517t
Boost Plus, 511t–517t

Boostrix. *See* Tetanus and diphtheria
  toxoids and acellular pertussis
  vaccine
Bordetella pertussis, antibiotic sensitivity
  of, 385t
Borrelia burgdorferi, antibiotic sensitivity
  of, 383t–385t
Bowel obstruction, 586–588
BP. *See* Blood pressure
BPD. *See* Bronchopulmonary dysplasia
BPO. *See* Benzoyl peroxide
Brachial plexus injuries, 419
Bradycardia
 atropine sulfate for, 691–692
 in newborns, 427
 poisoning diagnosis and, 20.e1t–20.e3t
Bradypnea, poisoning diagnosis and,
  20.e1t–20.e3t
Brain tumors, 523t–524t
Breastfeeding
 DRIs for, 501t–503t, 507t–509t
 drug categories for, 648
 EER for, 498
 HIV transmission through, 412
Breasts, adolescent
 development of, 91, 92f
 gynecomastia of, 91
 physical examination of, 95
Breath-holding spells, 474t
Breathing
 assessment of, 7
 in burn patients, 80–82
 management of, 8
Brethine. *See* Terbutaline
Brevibloc. *See* Esmolol HCl
Brevoxyl Creamy Wash. *See* Benzoyl
  peroxide
Bright Beginnings Soy Pediatric Drink,
  511t–517t
Bright Futures Guidelines, 94.e1b, 94
Brisdelle. *See* Paroxetine
British Anti-Lewisite. *See* Dimercaprol
Brompheniramine with phenylephrine
  (Dimetapp), formulary entry for,
  703–704
Bronchiolitis
 clinical manifestations of, 565
 clinical pearls for, 565
 treatment of, 565
Bronchodilators
 aminophylline as, 678–679
 for bronchiolitis, 565

Bronchodilators (Continued)
  for inhalation injury, 82
  theophylline as, 956–957
Bronchopulmonary dysplasia (BPD), 566
Bronchospasm, 691–692
Bruises, in child abuse patients, CP1, CP2, 84
BSA. See Body surface area
Budesonide (Entocort EC, Pulmicort, Rhinocort, Uceris)
  for allergic rhinitis, 335
  for asthma, 558.e1t–558.e2t
  for croup, 12
  for EE, 275
  formulary entry for, 704–705
Budesonide and formoterol (Symbicort)
  for asthma, 558.e1t–558.e2t
  formulary entry for, 705
Bufferin. See Aspirin
Bulla, 172, 173f–174f
Bullous lesions
  autoimmune bullous diseases, CP10, 193
  contact dermatitis, CP10, 193–194
  impetigo, 192
Bullous pemphigoid, 193
Bumetanide (Bumex)
  formulary entry for, 706
  for hypertension, 463t–464t
Buminate. See Albumin
BUN/Cr ratio. See Blood urea nitrogen/creatinine ratio
Bundle-branch block (BBB), 150t
Bupivacaine, analgesic properties of, 115t, 116
Burns
  in child abuse patients, CP1, CP2, 84
  classification of, 79t
  emergency management of, 78–83, 81f
  evaluation of, 78, 79t
  further management of, 83.e1b, 83
  mapping of, 78, 80f
  types of, 79t
Busulfan (Myleran)
  late effects of, 538.e1t
  toxicity of, 525t–528t
Butorphanol (Stadol), formulary entry for, 706

C
C3
  laboratory studies of, 604
  reference values for, 347t
C4
  laboratory studies of, 604
  reference values for, 347t
C-A-B pathway, 3, 61
Ca/Cr ratio. See Calcium/creatinine ratio
Cafcit. See Caffeine citrate
Cafergot. See Ergotamine tartrate with caffeine
Caffeine citrate (Cafcit)
  formulary entry for, 707
  for migraine headaches, 472
  neonate dosages of, 435
CAH. See Congenital adrenal hyperplasia
Calan. See Verapamil
Calcidol. See Ergocalciferol
Calciferol. See Ergocalciferol
Calcijex. See Calcitriol
Calcineurin inhibitors
  for atopic dermatitis, 180
  for nephrotic syndrome, 456
Calcionate. See Calcium glubionate
Calciquid. See Calcium glubionate
Calcitonin
  for hypercalcemia, 261
  for hyperparathyroidism, 225
Calcitonin–salmon (Miacalcin, Fortical Nasal Spray), formulary entry for, 707
Cal-Citrate. See Calcium citrate
Calcitriol (Rocaltrol, Calcijex)
  formulary entry for, 708
  for hypoparathyroidism, 225
Calcium. See also Hypercalcemia; Hypocalcemia
  DRIs for, 507t–508t
  formulas lower in, 518t–519t
  for hypermagnesemia, 262
  reference values for, 621t–623t
  serum disturbances in, 259–261, 261b
  supplementation of
    for hypoparathyroidism, 225
    renal failure dosage adjustments for, 1008t–1016t
  urine, 447, 447t

Calcium acetate (PhosLo, Calphron, Eliphos, Phoslyra), formulary entry for, 708
Calcium carbonate (Tums, Os-Cal, Children's Pepto)
   formulary entry for, 709
   for hyperphosphatemia, 263
Calcium channel blockers
   amlodipine as, 681
   diltiazem as, 759–760
   for hypertension, 463t–464t, 681
   for migraine headaches, 473t
   nicardipine as, 874–875
   nifedipine as, 875–876
   poisoning with, 21t
   verapamil as, 975–976
Calcium chloride
   for calcium channel blocker poisoning, 21t
   formulary entry for, 709
Calcium citrate (Cal-Citrate, Citracal), formulary entry for, 710
Calcium disodium versenate. See Edetate calcium disodium
Calcium glubionate (Calcionate, Calciquid), formulary entry for, 710
Calcium gluconate (Cal-Glu)
   for calcium channel blocker poisoning, 21t
   formulary entry for, 711
   for hyperkalemia, 260f
   neonate dosages of, 435
Calcium lactate (Cal-Lac), formulary entry for, 711–712
Calcium phosphate, tribasic (Posture-D), formulary entry for, 712
Calcium/creatinine (Ca/Cr) ratio, 447, 447t
Caldolor. See Ibuprofen
Cal-Glu. See Calcium gluconate
Cal-Lac. See Calcium lactate
Caloric calculations, of maintenance fluid volume, 247–248, 248b, 248t
Caloric modulars, 509, 510t
Calories
   formulas high in, 518t–519t
   newborn requirements for, 423
Calphron. See Calcium acetate
Camptosar. See Irinotecan
Campylobacter infection, gastroenteritis caused by, 393t–399t

Campylobacter jejuni, antibiotic sensitivity of, 386t
Canakinumab, for arthritis, 608
Canasa. See Mesalamine
Cancer
   chemotherapeutic drugs commonly used for, 525t–528t
   complications of bone marrow transplantation for
      aGVHD, 534.e1t, 534
      cGVHD, 534–535
      hemorrhagic cystitis, 536
      mucositis, 536
      thrombotic microangiopathy, 535
      veno-occlusive disease, 535
   darbepoetin alfa dose adjustment in, 748–750
   hematologic care and complications in, 536
      anemia, 536
      neutropenia, 537
      thrombocytopenia, 536–537
   HSCT for, 532–534
      immunoprophylaxis after, 361–362, 362.e1t
      vaccination after, 538.e2
   immunoprophylaxis for children with, 361–362, 362.e1t, 362t
   lymphadenopathy evaluation for, 524–525
   nausea treatment in, 537–538
   oncologic emergencies in
      cerebrovascular accident, 530–531
      fever and neutropenia, 531–532, 533f
      hyperleukocytosis/leukostasis, 529
      increased ICP, 530
      respiratory distress and superior vena cava syndrome, 531
      spinal cord compression, 530
      tumor lysis syndrome, 529–530, 673
      typhilitis, 531
   signs and symptoms of, 523, 523t–524t
   survivors of
      late effects in, 538.e1t, 538
      understanding treatment regimen used for, 538
   websites for, 523
Cancidas. See Caspofungin

Candidiasis
  diaper, CP10, 192
  intertriginous, 411t
  oral, 411t
Cannabinoids, for nausea and vomiting, 537
Ca$_{O_2}$. *See* Oxygen content
Capex. *See* Fluocinolone acetonide
Capillary blood gas (CBG), gas exchange evaluation with, 551
Capnography, gas exchange evaluation with, 550
Captopril (Capoten)
  formulary entry for, 712–713
  for hypertension, 463t–464t, 712–713
  renal failure dosage adjustments for, 1008t–1016t
Caput succedaneum, 419f, 419t
Capute Scales, 201t, 202
Carafate. *See* Sucralfate
Carbamazepine (Epitol, Tegretol, Carbatrol)
  formulary entry for, 713–714
  renal failure dosage adjustments for, 1008t–1016t
  for seizures, 476t–477t, 479t
Carbamide peroxide (Auro Ear Drops, Debrox, Murine Ear, Thera-Ear Gly-Oxide), formulary entry for, 714
Carbapenems
  ertapenem as, 775
  imipenem and cilastin as, 812–813
  meropenem as, 848
  sensitivity-based selection of, 383t–384t
Carbatrol. *See* Carbamazepine
Carbinoxamine (Arbinoxa, Palgic), formulary entry for, 715
Carbohydrate intolerance, 518t–519t
Carbohydrate metabolism disorders, 293–294
Carbon dioxide, reference values for, 621t–623t
Carbon monoxide
  poisoning with, 80–82
  reference values for, 621t–623t
Carbonic anhydrase inhibitors, acetazolamide as, 668–669
Carboplatin (CBDCA, Paraplatin), toxicity of, 525t–528t
Carboxyhemoglobin, reference values for, 621t–623t

Cardene. *See* Nicardipine
Cardiac arrest, 3
Cardiac catheterization, cardiology imaging with, 155.e1f, 155
Cardiac cycle, 127, 127f
Cardiac shunts, 160f, 161
Cardiac tamponade, 165
  pericardiocentesis for, 47, 48f–50f
Cardiogenic shock, 71.e1t, 71
Cardiology. *See also* Electrocardiography.
  acquired heart disease
    cardiac tamponade, 47, 48f–50f, 165
    dilated cardiomyopathy, 162–163
    endocarditis, 161–162, 162t, 163b
    hypertrophic cardiomyopathy, 163–164
    Kawasaki disease, 167.e1t, 166–168, 167f
    Lyme disease, 168
    myocarditis, 164
    pericardial effusion, 165
    pericarditis, 164–165
    restrictive cardiomyopathy, 164
    rheumatic heart disease, 168, 169b
  cardiac cycle, 127, 127f
  cardiovascular screening
    for ADHD patients, 170
    for sports, 170.e1b, 170
  congenital heart disease
    acyanotic, 156, 157t–158t
    cyanotic, 156.e1t, 156, 158t–160t
    exercise recommendations for, 168.e1t, 168
    imaging of, 583, 584f
    pulse oximetry screening for, 155–156
    surgeries and interventions for, 160–161, 160f
    syndromes associated with, 156, 156t
  imaging for
    blood flow, 583
    cardiac catheterization, 155.e1f, 155
    chest radiograph, 154–155, 154f, 157t–159t
    congenital heart disease, 583, 584f
    echocardiography, 155, 583
    vessel abnormalities, 584

Cardiology *(Continued)*
lipid monitoring recommendations for
goals for levels in childhood, 169
hyperlipidemia management, 170
screening of children and
adolescents, 168–169
newborn cardiac diseases, 427–428
physical examination for
blood pressure, 128.e1t, 128,
129t–135t, 136f–138f
heart murmurs, 128–139,
139b–140b, 139t
heart rate, 128, 142t
heart sounds, 128
websites for, 127
Cardiomyopathy
dilated, 162–163
hypertrophic, 163–164
restrictive, 164
Cardiopulmonary resuscitation. *See*
Resuscitation
Cardiovascular disturbances, poisoning
diagnosis and, 20.e1t–20.e3t
Cardiovascular screening
for ADHD patients, 170
for sports, 170.e1b, 170
Cardizem. *See* Diltiazem
Carimune NF. *See* Intravenous
immunoglobulin
Carmustine (Bischloronitrosourea,
BCNU, BiCNU), toxicity of,
525t–528t
Carnation Instant Breakfast Essentials,
511t–517t
Carnation Instant Breakfast Lactose
Free, 511t–517t
Carnitine (Levocarnitine, Carnitor,
L-Carnitine)
for FAO disorders, 291
formulary entry for, 715
for metabolic crisis, 290
for organic acidemias, 291
Carotid bruit, 139t
CARS. *See* Childhood Autism Rating
Scale
Carvedilol (Coreg)
formulary entry for, 716
for hypertension, 463t–464t
Case-control study design, 638t–639t
Casein formulas, 511t–517t
Caspofungin (Cancidas), formulary entry
for, 716–717

CAT. *See* Clinical Adaptive Test
Cat bites, 77t, 393t–399t
Catapres. *See* Clonidine
Catch clinical decision rule, 63b
Catch-up growth, energy requirements
for, 499–500, 500b
Catch-up immunization schedule, 350,
352f–358f
Catecholamines, normal values of,
243.e1t, 243
Catheterization
central venous, 28f, 31–37, 32f,
34f–36f, 582, 582f–583f
radial artery, 30–31
UA and UV, 38–42, 39f–41f
urinary bladder, 50–51
Catheter-related bloodstream infections,
393t–399t
Cathflo Activase. *See* Alteplase
CAVH/D. *See* Continuous arteriovenous
hemofiltration/hemodialysis
Cayston. *See* Aztreonam
CBDCA. *See* Carboplatin
CBG. *See* Capillary blood gas
CCNU. *See* Lomustine
CCr. *See* Creatinine clearance
CD3 count, reference values for, 347t
CD4 count, reference values for, 347t
CD8 count, reference values for, 347t
CD19 count, reference values for,
347t
2-CdA. *See* Cladribine
CDDP. *See* Cisplatin
Ceclor. *See* Cefaclor
Cedax. *See* Ceftibuten
Cefaclor (Ceclor, Raniclor)
formulary entry for, 717
renal failure dosage adjustments for,
995t–1007t
Cefadroxil (Duricef)
formulary entry for, 718
renal failure dosage adjustments for,
995t–1007t
Cefazolin (Ancef, Zolicef)
for endocarditis prophylaxis, 162t
formulary entry for, 718
for lymphadenitis, 393t–399t
for maternal GBS prophylaxis, 386
renal failure dosage adjustments for,
995t–1007t
sensitivity-based selection of,
383t–384t

Cefdinir (Omnicef)
  formulary entry for, 719
  renal failure dosage adjustments for,
    995t–1007t
  sensitivity-based selection of,
    383t–384t
  for sinusitis, 393t–399t
Cefepime (Maxipime)
  for catheter-related bloodstream
    infections, 393t–399t
  formulary entry for, 719
  for intraabdominal infections,
    393t–399t
  renal failure dosage adjustments for,
    995t–1007t
  sensitivity-based selection of,
    383t–384t
  for sinusitis, 393t–399t
  for tracheitis, 393t–399t
  for ventriculoperitoneal shunt
    infection, 393t–399t
Cefixime (Suprax)
  formulary entry for, 720
  renal failure dosage adjustments for,
    995t–1007t
  sensitivity-based selection of,
    383t–384t
  for sinusitis, 393t–399t
  for UTI, 393t–399t
Cefotan. *See* Cefotetan
Cefotaxime (Claforan)
  for cellulitis, 393t–399t
  formulary entry for, 720–721
  for gastroenteritis, 393t–399t
  for gonorrhea, 400t–401t
  for neonatal meningitis, 392t
  for neonatal septic arthritis, 392t
  neonate dosages of, 435t
  for pneumonia, 393t–399t
  renal failure dosage adjustments for,
    995t–1007t
  sensitivity-based selection of,
    383t–384t
  for UTI, 393t–399t
Cefotetan (Cefotan)
  formulary entry for, 721
  for pelvic inflammatory disease,
    400t–401t
  renal failure dosage adjustments for,
    995t–1007t
  sensitivity-based selection of,
    383t–384t

Cefoxitin (Mefoxin)
  formulary entry for, 721
  for pelvic inflammatory disease,
    400t–401t
  renal failure dosage adjustments for,
    995t–1007t
  sensitivity-based selection of,
    383t–384t
Cefpodoxime proxetil (Vantin)
  formulary entry for, 722
  renal failure dosage adjustments for,
    995t–1007t
  sensitivity-based selection of,
    383t–384t
  for sinusitis, 393t–399t
Cefprozil (Cefzil)
  formulary entry for, 722
  renal failure dosage adjustments for,
    995t–1007t
Ceftazidime (Fortaz, Tazidime, Tazicef,
    Ceptaz)
  formulary entry for, 723
  for osteomyelitis, 393t–399t
  renal failure dosage adjustments for,
    995t–1007t
  sensitivity-based selection of,
    383t–384t
  for UTI, 393t–399t
Ceftibuten (Cedax)
  formulary entry for, 723
  renal failure dosage adjustments for,
    995t–1007t
Ceftin. *See* Cefuroxime axetil
Ceftriaxone (Rocephin)
  for cellulitis, 393t–399t
  for chlamydia, 400t–401t
  for conjunctivitis, 393t–399t
  for endocarditis prophylaxis, 162t
  formulary entry for, 724
  for gastroenteritis, 393t–399t
  for gonorrhea, 400t–401t
  for intraabdominal infections,
    393t–399t
  for Lyme disease, 409
  for meningitis, 393t–399t
  for meningococcal exposure, 372
  for neonatal conjunctivitis, 392t
  for osteomyelitis, 393t–399t
  for otitis media, 393t–399t
  for pelvic inflammatory disease,
    400t–401t
  for pneumonia, 393t–399t

Ceftriaxone *(Continued)*
  sensitivity-based selection of,
      383t–384t
  for septic arthritis, 393t–399t
  for tracheitis, 393t–399t
  for UTI, 393t–399t
Cefuroxime (Zinacef)
  formulary entry for, 725
  for Lyme disease, 409
  for otitis media, 393t–399t
  renal failure dosage adjustments for,
      995t–1007t
  sensitivity-based selection of,
      383t–384t
  for sinusitis, 393t–399t
Cefuroxime axetil (Ceftin), formulary
      entry for, 725
Cefzil. *See* Cefprozil
Celestone. *See* Betamethasone
Celestone Soluspan. *See*
      Betamethasone
Celiac disease, 276
CellCept. *See* Mycophenolate mofetil
Cell-mediated immunity abnormalities,
      342t–343t
Cellulitis
  management of, 393t–399t
  orbital, 573, 574f
Celsius, conversion formulas for, 633
Center for Epidemiological Studies
      Depression Scale for Children
      (CES-DC), 201t
Centimeters, conversion formulas for, 633
Central alpha agonists
  clonidine as, 741
  for hypertension, 463t–464t
Central alpha blockers, methyldopa
      as, 852
Central DI, 232–233
Central hypothyroidism, 220t
Central hypotonia, 295, 296f–297f
Central line placement, imaging of, 582,
      582f–583f
Central precocious puberty, 238
Central venous catheter placement,
      28f, 31–37, 32f, 34f–36f, 582,
      582f–583f
Centrum Kids Complete, 505t–506t
Centrum Tablet, 505t–506t
Cephalexin (Keflex, Biocef)
  for cellulitis, 393t–399t
  for dacryocystitis, 393t–399t

Cephalexin *(Continued)*
  for endocarditis prophylaxis, 162t
  formulary entry for, 726
  for impetigo, 192
  for lymphadenitis, 393t–399t
  for pharyngitis, 393t–399t
  renal failure dosage adjustments for,
      995t–1007t
  sensitivity-based selection of,
      383t–384t
Cephalohematoma, 419f, 419t
Cephalosporins
  cefaclor as, 717
  cefadroxil as, 718
  cefazolin as, 718
  cefdinir as, 719
  cefepime as, 719
  cefixime as, 720
  cefotaxime as, 720–721
  cefotetan as, 721
  cefoxitin as, 721
  cefpodoxime proxetil as, 722
  cefprozil as, 722
  ceftazidime as, 723
  ceftibuten as, 723
  ceftriaxone as, 724
  cefuroxime as, 725
  cephalexin as, 726
  sensitivity-based selection of,
      383t–384t
Cephulac. *See* Lactulose
Ceptaz. *See* Ceftazidime
CeraLyte solutions, 519t
Cerebral edema, in diabetic
      ketoacidosis, 216
Cerebral palsy (CP), 207, 208t
Cerebrospinal fluid (CSF), evaluation
      of, 631t
Cerebrovascular accident. *See* Stroke
Cerebyx. *See* Fosphenytoin
Cerumenolytics
  antipyrine and benzocaine as, 687
  carbamide peroxide as, 714
Cervarix. *See* Human papilloma virus
      vaccine
Cervical cancer, adolescent screening
      for, 97.e1t, 97
Cervical spine (C-spine)
  in burn patients, 78–80
  clinical clearing of, 65
  imaging of, 573–574, 575f
  immobilization of, 65

Cervical spine (Continued)
  radiography of, 65
  trauma to, 65
    imaging of, 573
    secondary survey of, 62t
CES-DC. See Center for Epidemiological
    Studies Depression Scale for
    Children
Cetacort. See Hydrocortisone
Cetirizine (Zyrtec, Children's Zyrtec)
  for allergic rhinitis, 335
  formulary entry for, 726–727
  renal failure dosage adjustments for,
    1008t–1016t
Cetirizine and pseudoephedrine
    (Zyrtec-D 12 Hour), formulary
    entry for, 726–727
Cetraxal. See Ciprofloxacin
CF. See Cystic fibrosis
CGD. See Constitutional growth delay
cGVHD. See Chronic graft-versus-host
    disease
CH₅₀. See Total hemolytic complement
    level
Chancroid, 106t–107t
CHARGE syndrome, 420
Chédiak-Higashi syndrome, 342t–343t
Chelating agents
  deferoxamine mesylate as,
    750–751
  dimercaprol as, 761
  EDTA calcium disodium as, 767
  for lead poisoning, 23, 25t
  succimer as, 946
Chemet. See Succimer
Chemical burns, 79t, 83
Chemistry studies. See Blood
    chemistries
Chemotherapeutic drugs
  darbepoetin alfa dose adjustment
    with, 748–750
  late effects of, 538.e1t, 538
  nausea treatment used with,
    537–538
  toxicities of, 525t–528t
  vaccination after, 538.e2
Chest, imaging of
  atelectasis, 579–580
  cardiology radiography, 154–155,
    154f, 157t–159t
  central line placement, 582,
    582f–583f

Chest, imaging of (Continued)
    ETT placement, 583
    infiltrate, 580
    mediastinal masses, 580
    parapneumonic effusions and
      empyema, 580
    parenchymal findings, 580
    for pneumonia, 577
    posteroanterior and lateral
      radiographs, 577, 579f–582f
Chest compressions, 8
Chest radiography
  atelectasis, 579–580
  cardiology imaging with
    heart evaluation, 154, 154f
    lung field evaluation, 154–155,
      157t–159t
    skeletal evaluation, 155
    trachea evaluation, 155
  central line placement with, 582,
    582f–583f
  esophageal atresia and
    tracheoesophageal fistula on,
    584, 585f
  ETT placement with, 583
  infiltrate, 580
  mediastinal masses, 580
  parapneumonic effusions and
    empyema, 580
  parenchymal findings, 580
  for pneumonia, 577
  posteroanterior and lateral views, 577,
    579f–582f
Chest trauma
  blunt, 65–66
  secondary survey of, 62t
Chest tube placement, 44–47,
    45f–46f
CHF. See Congestive heart failure
Chief complaint, 94
Child abuse, CP1, CP2, 83–86, 85f
  skeletal survey for, 597, 599f–600f
Childhood Autism Rating Scale (CARS),
    201t, 207–208
Childhood eczema, CP6, CP7, 180
Childhood immunization schedule, 350,
    351f, 353f–358f
Children's Advil. See Ibuprofen
Children's Motrin. See Ibuprofen
Children's Pepto. See Calcium
    carbonate
Children's Zyrtec. See Cetirizine

Chlamydia
  adolescent screening for, 96
  management of, 400t–401t,
    694–695
  perinatal, 392t
Chlamydia spp., antibiotic sensitivity of,
    383t–386t
Chloral hydrate (Aquachloral
    Supprettes)
  formulary entry for, 727
  renal failure dosage adjustments for,
    1008t–1016t
Chlorambucil, for Behçet disease,
    616.e2
Chloramphenicol (Chloromycetin)
  formulary entry for, 728
  for meningitis, 393t–399t
Chloride, reference values for,
    621t–623t
Chloromycetin. See Chloramphenicol
Chloroquine phosphate (Aralen)
  formulary entry for, 728–729
  renal failure dosage adjustments for,
    1008t–1016t
Chlorothiazide (Diuril, Diurigen)
  formulary entry for, 729
  neonate dosages of, 435
  renal failure dosage adjustments for,
    1008t–1016t
Chlorpheniramine maleate (Chlor-
    Trimeton), formulary entry for,
    730
Chlorpromazine (Thorazine)
  formulary entry for, 730–731
  for nausea and vomiting, 537
Chlorthalidone, for hypertension,
    463t–464t
Chlor-Trimeton. See Chlorpheniramine
    maleate
Cholecalciferol (D-3, D Drops, Enfamil
    D-Vi-Sol, Vitamin D₃), formulary
    entry for, 731–732
Cholestasis, 276, 277t
Cholesterol. See Lipids
Cholestyramine (Questran, Prevalite),
    formulary entry for, 732
Choline, DRIs for, 502t–503t
Choline magnesium trisalicylate
    (Trilisate)
  analgesic properties of, 113
  formulary entry for, 733

Cholinergics
  bethanechol chloride as, 701–702
  neostigmine as, 872–873
  physostigmine salicylate as, 905
  pilocarpine HCl as, 906
  pyridostigmine bromide as, 924
  toxidrome of, 20t–22t
Chorionic villus sampling, 415.e1
Christmas disease, 326f, 327t–328t
Chromium, DRIs for, 507t–508t
Chromosome microarray, 299
Chronic graft-*versus*-host disease
    (cGVHD), 534–535
Chronic granulomatous disease,
    342t–343t
Chronic headache, differential diagnosis
    for, 470b
Chronic hypertension, 460
  antihypertensive drugs for (See
    Antihypertensives)
  classification of, 461, 462t
  etiologies of, 460, 461t
  evaluation of, 460–461
  treatment of, 461, 681
Chronic inflammation, anemia of, 309
Chronic kidney disease (CKD)
  clinical manifestations of, 458–460,
    459t
  etiology of, 458
Chronic Kidney Disease in Children
    (CKiD) equation, 445–446
Chronic lung disease of infancy. See
    Bronchopulmonary dysplasia
Chronic lung disease of prematurity. See
    Bronchopulmonary dysplasia
Chronic pancreatitis, 280–281,
    281.e1t
Chronulac. See Lactulose
CHT. See Closed head trauma
Churg-Strauss syndrome, 613t
Chvostek sign, poisoning diagnosis and,
    20.e1t–20.e3t
Chylothorax, 518t–519t
Ciclesonide (Alvesco, Omnaris,
    Zetonna)
  for allergic rhinitis, 335
  for asthma, 558.e1t–558.e2t
  formulary entry for, 733–734
Cidofovir (Vistide), formulary entry for,
    734
Ciloxan ophthalmic. See Ciprofloxacin

Cimetidine (Tagamet)
  formulary entry for, 735
  renal failure dosage adjustments for, 1008t–1016t
Ciprofloxacin (Cipro, Ciloxan ophthalmic, Cetraxal, Ciprodex)
  formulary entry for, 735–736
  for gastroenteritis, 393t–399t
  for meningococcal exposure, 372
  for otitis externa, 393t–399t
  renal failure dosage adjustments for, 995t–1007t
  sensitivity-based selection of, 385t
  for UTI, 393t–399t
Circulation
  assessment of, 3, 8
  management of, 8–9, 9t
Cisplatin (cis-platinum, CDDP, Platinol)
  late effects of, 538.e1t
  toxicity of, 525t–528t
Citracal. See Calcium citrate
Citrate mixtures
  formulary entry for, 737
  for GSD, 294–295
Citrulline, for urea cycle defects, 292
CKD. See Chronic kidney disease
CKiD equation. See Chronic Kidney Disease in Children equation
Cladribine (2-CdA, Leustatin), toxicity of, 525t–528t
Claforan. See Cefotaxime
CLAMS. See Clinical Linguistic and Auditory Milestone Scale
Claravis. See Isotretinoin
Clarithromycin (Biaxin)
  for endocarditis prophylaxis, 162t
  formulary entry for, 737–738
  for Mycobacterium avium complex infection, 405.e1t–405.e2t
  for pertussis, 366, 393t–399t
  renal failure dosage adjustments for, 995t–1007t
  sensitivity-based selection of, 385t
Claritin. See Loratadine and pseudoephedrine
Classic vibratory murmur, 139t
Clavicle fracture, birth trauma causing, 419
Clavulanic acid.
    See Amoxicillin–clavulanic acid
Clear liquid diet, 518t–519t

Clindamycin (Cleocin)
  for acne vulgaris, 187, 188t
  for bacterial vaginosis, 105t, 393t–399t
  for bite infections, 393t–399t
  for cellulitis, 393t–399t
  for dental abscess, 393t–399t
  for endocarditis prophylaxis, 162t
  formulary entry for, 738–739
  for impetigo, 192
  for lymphadenitis, 393t–399t
  for osteomyelitis, 393t–399t
  for parotitis, 393t–399t
  for pelvic inflammatory disease, 400t–401t
  for pharyngitis, 393t–399t
  for pneumonia, 393t–399t
  sensitivity-based selection of, 386t
  for septic arthritis, 393t–399t
  for tracheitis, 393t–399t
Clinical Adaptive Test (CAT), 201t, 202
Clinical Linguistic and Auditory Milestone Scale (CLAMS), 201t, 202
Clinical question
  applying evidence to, 635
  formulation of, 634
Clinical trial, 638t–639t
Clobazam (Onfi)
  formulary entry for, 739–740
  renal failure dosage adjustments for, 1008t–1016t
  for seizures, 479t
Clobetasol propionate (Clobex, Cormax, Olux, Temovate), for atopic dermatitis, 182t–183t
Clofarabine (Clolar), toxicity of, 525t–528t
Clonazepam (Klonopin)
  formulary entry for, 740
  for seizures, 479t
Clonic seizures, 478b
Clonidine (Catapres, Duraclon, Kapvay, Nexiclon)
  formulary entry for, 741
  for hypertension, 463t–464t
  for opioid tapering, 118
  poisoning with, 21t
Closed comedo, 187
Closed head trauma (CHT), 61–64, 62t, 63b

Clostridium difficile infection, 393t–399t

Clostridium spp., antibiotic sensitivity of, 383t–384t, 386t

Clotrimazole (Lotrimin AF, Gyne-Lotrimin)
  for candidiasis, 192, 411t
  formulary entry for, 742
  for tinea infections, 411t

CMV. *See* Cytomegalovirus

CMV-negative blood, 330

Coagulation
  age-specific values for, 317t–318t
  bleeding disorders, 325, 326f, 327b, 327t–328t
  cascade, 316f
  hypercoagulable states, 319b
    laboratory evaluation for, 319–320, 320b
    treatment of, 320–324, 321t–324t, 325b
  tests of, 316–319, 317t–318t, 322–324

Coarctation of aorta, 157t–158t

Cobalamin (Vitamin B₁₂)
  DRIs for, 502t–503t
  formulary entry for, 744
  reference values for, 621t–623t

Cobb angle, 95.e1, 95.e2f

Cocaine, poisoning with, 19, 20t–22t

Codeine
  analgesic properties of, 114t
  formulary entry for, 742

Cogentin. *See* Benztropine mesylate

Cognitive skills
  developmental and mental health screening tools for, 201t
  for early literacy, 198t

Cohort study design, 638t–639t

Colace. *See* Docusate

Colchicine
  for Behçet disease, 616.e2
  for scleroderma, 616.e2

Cold injury, 79t

Colic, 199t–200t

Colocort. *See* Hydrocortisone

Colony-stimulating factors, filgrastim as, 785

Color Doppler flow imaging, 583

Colposcopy, 97.e1t

Colyte. *See* Polyethylene glycol, electrolyte solution

Coma
  emergency management of, 13–15
  minor CHT with, 63
  poisoning diagnosis and, 20.e1t–20.e3t
  scales for assessment of, 15t

Combined hormonal contraception. *See also* Oral contraceptive pills
  clotting symptoms with, 100
  for EC, 102–103
  for PCOS management, 236

Combined hypotonia, 295, 298f

Combined proximal and distal RTA, 458

Comedones, 187

Common variable immunodeficiency, 342t–343t

Common warts, 177

Communication, in palliative care
  advance directive, 542
  child participation, 542, 542t
  decision-making tools, 541
  family meetings, 541–542

Communication disorders, 205

Compartment syndrome, 66

Compazine. *See* Prochlorperazine

Compensated shock, 71, 72t

Compleat, 511t–517t

Compleat Pediatric, 511t–517t

Complement
  decreased levels of, 604
  deficiency of, 342t–343t
  increased levels of, 604
  laboratory studies of, 604
  reference values for, 347t

Complement pathway, 348f

Complete Amino Acid Mix, 510t

Complete heart block, 149f, 149t

Complete precocious puberty (CPP), 238

Complex febrile seizure, 475

Complex partial seizures, 478b

Computed tomography (CT)
  for blunt thoracic and abdominal trauma, 65
  of eyes, 573, 574f
  head imaging with, 572–573
  judicious use of, 572
  for minor CHT, 63, 63b
  for seizures, 475

Comvax, 378

Concentration, urine, 447

Concerta. *See* Methylphenidate HCl

Concussion, 64

Conduction disturbances, 144, 149f, 149t–150t
Confidence intervals, 637
Confidentiality, 94
Confounding variables, 638
Congenital adrenal hyperplasia (CAH), 227–229, 227f, 228t
  evaluation of, 226–227, 227t
  management of, 229–230, 229t
Congenital heart disease
  acyanotic, 156, 157t–158t
  cyanotic, 156.e1t, 156, 158t–160t
  exercise recommendations for, 168.e1t, 168
  imaging of, 583, 584f
  pulse oximetry screening for, 155–156
  surgeries and interventions for, 160–161, 160f
  syndromes associated with, 156, 156t
Congenital immunodeficiency disorders, immunoprophylaxis for children with, 361
Congenital infections, 386.e1t, 382, 388t, 572–573
Congenital malformations. See also Dysmorphology.
  imaging of, 572
Congenital red cell aplasias, 309
Congestive heart failure (CHF), 155, 157t–159t
Conjugated bilirubin, reference values for, 621t–623t
Conjugated hyperbilirubinemia, 429–430
Conjunctivitis
  allergic, 336, 336t
  management of, 393t–399t
  neonatal, 392t
Connective tissue diseases, 301–302, 603t
Conscious sedation. See Moderate sedation
Consciousness, altered states of, 13–15, 14b, 15t
Consent, 27
  for autopsy, 547
  for immunization, 350
  for procedural sedation, 119
Constipation, 272–273
  diagnosis and evaluation of, 272, 273t
  treatment of, 272–273

Constitutional growth delay (CGD), 233–235, 234f
Contact burns, 79t
Contact dermatitis, CP10, 193–194
Continuous arteriovenous hemofiltration/hemodialysis (CAVH/D), 450
Continuous positive airway pressure (CPAP), 74
Continuous venovenous hemofiltration/hemodialysis (CVVH/D), 450
Contraception. See also Combined hormonal contraception.
  adolescent use of, 98–104, 99f, 101f
  medroxyprogesterone for, 846–847
  for PCOS management, 236
Conversion formulas
  length and weight, 633
  temperature, 633
Cooley's anemia, 313
Coombs test, 307
Coordination, examination of, 468
Copegus. See Ribavirin
Copper, DRIs for, 507t–508t
Copper IUD, 103
Cordarone. See Amiodarone HCl
Cordran. See Flurandrenolide
Coreg. See Carvedilol
Cormax. See Clobetasol propionate
Cornstarch, for GSD, 294–295
Corrected reticulocyte count (CRC), 307
Correlation, 637
Cortaid. See Hydrocortisone
Cortef. See Hydrocortisone
Cortenema. See Hydrocortisone
Corticosteroids
  for adrenal crisis, 230–231
  for adrenal insufficiency, 229–230, 229t
  adrenal insufficiency caused by, 226
  for allergic rhinitis, 335
  for anaphylaxis, 10
  for arthritis, 608
  for asthma, 10, 559f–564f
    dosages for inhaled steroids, 558.e1t–558.e2t
  beclomethasone dipropionate as, 698
  for Behçet disease, 616.e2
  betamethasone as, 700–701
  body surface area nomogram for dosing of, 988f
  budesonide as, 704–705

Corticosteroids *(Continued)*
ciclesonide as, 733–734
cortisone acetate as, 743
for croup, 12
dexamethasone as, 752–753
fludrocortisone acetate as,
787–788
flunisolide as, 788–789
fluticasone propionate and salmeterol
as, 792–793
fluticasone propionate as,
791–792
for food allergies, 339
for GVHD prevention, 534
for hemangioma, 177
for HSP, 614
hydrocortisone as, 808–809
for IBD, 274
immunoprophylaxis for patients on,
362, 362t
for increased ICP, 70, 530
for inhalation injury, 82
late effects of, 538.e1t
methylprednisolone as, 854–855
mometasone furoate as, 864–865
for nausea and vomiting, 537
for nephrotic syndrome, 455–456
for pemphigus vulgaris, 193
potency of, 229t
prednisolone as, 913
prednisone as, 914
for sarcoidosis, 616
for scleroderma, 616.e1
for shock, 73f
for Sjögren syndrome, 616.e3
for SLE, 611
for spinal cord compression, 530
for thrombocytopenia, 315
triamcinolone as, 965–966
Corticotropin (Acthar HP), formulary
entry for, 743
Cortifoam. *See* Hydrocortisone
Cortisol. *See also* Hydrocortisone
adrenal insufficiency evaluation using,
226, 227t
biosynthesis of, 227, 227f
Cushing syndrome diagnosis with,
231
Cortisone acetate
for adrenal crisis, 231
formulary entry for, 743
potency of, 229t

Cortisporin. *See* Polymyxin B sulfate,
neomycin sulfate, hydrocortisone
ophthalmic
Cortisporin Otic. *See* Polymyxin B sulfate,
neomycin sulfate, hydrocortisone
Co-trimoxazole. *See*
Trimethoprim-sulfamethoxazole
Coumadin. *See* Warfarin
Cow's milk
formulas based on, 511t–517t
formulas for allergies to, 518t–519t
nutrition components in, 511t–517t
Cozaar. *See* Losartan
CP. *See* Cerebral palsy
CPAP. *See* Continuous positive airway
pressure
C-peptide, 215
CPP. *See* Complete precocious puberty
Crackles, auscultation of, 550t
Cradle cap, CP10, 190
CRAFFT questionnaire, 94b, 108, 211,
211b
Cranial nerves, examination of, 468t
Craniosynostosis, 573
CRC. *See* Corrected reticulocyte count
C-reactive protein (CRP), 602–603
reference values for, 621t–623t
Creatine kinase, reference values for,
621t–623t
Creatinine, reference values for,
621t–623t
Creatinine clearance (CCr), 445
Cricothyrotomy, percutaneous (needle),
13, 14f
Critical care emergencies
acute hypertension, 68, 69t
increased ICP, 69–70
reference data for, 75–76
respiratory failure, 71–75, 75t
shock, 71.e1t, 71, 72t, 73f
Crohn's disease, 274
Cromolyn (Crolom, Intal, Gastrocrom,
NasalCrom, Opticrom)
for allergic rhinitis, 335
for asthma, 562f–564f
formulary entry for, 743–744
Cross-sectional study design, 638t–639t
Croup, 12
CRP. *See* C-reactive protein
Crucial, 511t–517t
Crust, on skin, 172, 173f–174f
Cryoprecipitate, 331

Cryptococcal infection, 685
Cryptorchidism, 241–242
CSF. *See* Cerebrospinal fluid
C-spine. *See* Cervical spine
CT. *See* Computed tomography
CTX. *See* Cyclophosphamide
Culture
    blood, 380
    urine, 442
Curosurf. *See* Surfactant, pulmonary/
        poractant alfa
Cushing syndrome, 231, 236
Cutivate. *See* Fluticasone propionate
Cuvposa. *See* Glycopyrrolate
CVVH/D. *See* Continuous venovenous
        hemofiltration/hemodialysis
Cyanide poisoning, 852
Cyanocobalamin (Cyanoject, Cyomin,
        Nascobal). *See also* Cobalamin
    formulary entry for, 744
Cyanosis
    in newborns
        differential diagnosis of, 423
        evaluation of, 423
    poisoning diagnosis and, 20.e1t–20.e3t
Cyanotic congenital heart disease,
        156.e1t, 156, 158t–160t
Cyclopentolate (Cyclogyl), formulary
        entry for, 745
Cyclopentolate with phenylephrine
        (Cyclomydril), formulary entry
        for, 745
Cyclophosphamide (CTX, Cytoxan)
    for arthritis, 608.e1t
    for HSP, 614
    late effects of, 538.e1t
    for nephrotic syndrome, 456
    for SLE, 611
    toxicity of, 525t–528t
Cyclosporine (Sandimmune)
    for arthritis, 608.e1t, 608
    for Behçet disease, 616.e2
    formulary entry for, 745–746
    for GVHD prevention, 534
    for IBD, 274
    for SLE, 611
Cyclosporine microemulsion (Neoral),
        formulary entry for, 745–746
Cyclosporine modified (Gengraf,
        Restasis), formulary entry for,
        745–746
Cyomin. *See* Cyanocobalamin

Cyproheptadine (Periactin)
    formulary entry for, 746–747
    for migraine headaches, 473t
    for nausea and vomiting, 537
    for serotonin syndrome, 21t
Cystic fibrosis (CF)
    clinical manifestations of, 567t
    diagnosis of, 566–567
    formula for, 518t–519t
    management of complications of, 568
    pulmonary therapies for, 567–568
Cystitis, 442
    after bone marrow transplantation,
        536
    management of, 393t–399t
Cystourethrogram, after UTI, 443–444,
        589
Cysts, bone, 590, 594f
Cytarabine (Ara-C), toxicity of,
        525t–528t
Cytochrome P450 system, inducers/
        inhibitors of, 989t–990t
Cytokine inhibitors, immunoprophylaxis
        for patients on, 363
Cytomegalovirus (CMV)
    congenital, 388t
    in HIV/AIDS patients,
        405.e1t–405.e2t
Cytovene. *See* Ganciclovir
Cytoxan. *See* Cyclophosphamide

D
D Drops. *See* Cholecalciferol
D Vi-Sol, 504t
D-3. *See* Cholecalciferol
Dacarbazine (DIC, DTIC, Imidazole
        carboxamide, DTIC-Dome),
        toxicity of, 525t–528t
Dacryocystitis, 393t–399t
Dactinomycin (Actinomycin D)
    late effects of, 538.e1t
    toxicity of, 525t–528t
Dantrolene (Dantrium, Revonto),
        formulary entry for, 747
Dapsone (Aczone,
        Diaminodiphenylsulfone, DDS)
    for acne vulgaris, 187
    for cancer patients, 538t
    for dermatitis herpetiformis, 193
    formulary entry for, 748
    for perinatal HIV exposure,
        403t–404t

Dapsone (Continued)
for Pneumocystis jiroveci pneumonia, 405.e1t–405.e2t
for Toxoplasma gondii infection, 405.e1t–405.e2t
Daraprim. See Pyrimethamine
Darbepoetin alfa (Aranesp), formulary entry for, 748–750
Daunorubicin (Daunomycin), toxicity of, 525t–528t
Daytrana. See Methylphenidate HCl
DBP. See Diastolic blood pressure
DCSS. See Diffuse cutaneous systemic scleroderma
DDAVP. See Desmopressin acetate
DDS. See Dapsone
Death
autopsy consent after, 547
bereavement after, 547
certificate for, 547
changes accompanying approach of, 544–545
children's conceptualization of, 542t
documentation of, 546
medication and management during last hours, 546t
pronouncement of, 545–547
Death certificate, 547
Debrox. See Carbamide peroxide
Decadron. See Dexamethasone
Decision making, in palliative care
advance directive, 542
child participation, 542, 542t
decision-making tools, 541
family meetings, 541–542
Decision-making tools (DMTs), 541
Decompensated shock, 71, 72t
Decongestants
brompheniramine with phenylephrine as, 703–704
fexofenadine and pseudoephedrine as, 784–785
loratadine and pseudoephedrine as, 841–842
oxymetazoline as, 890
pseudoephedrine as, 921
Deep partial thickness burns, 79t
Deep sedation, 119
Deferoxamine mesylate (Desferal)
formulary entry for, 750–751
for iron poisoning, 21t

Defibrotide, for veno-occlusive disease, 535
Dehydration
clinical observations in, 251t
deficit repletion in
based on FWD, 252
based on SFD, 252–253
calculation of appropriate fluids for, 253–256, 254t–255t
replacement strategy for, 253.e1t–253.e3t, 250f, 253
solute based on excess electrolyte deficits, 252
solute based on solute fluid deficit, 249–252, 251t
water volume, 249, 251t
ongoing losses in, 256, 256t
in preterm infants, 420, 421t
Dehydroepiandrosterone (DHEA)
normal levels of, 240t
in precocious puberty, 239, 240t
Dehydroepiandrosterone sulfate (DHEA-S)
normal levels of, 241t
in precocious puberty, 239, 241t
Delay, developmental, 196
Delayed puberty, 91, 236–237, 237t, 238f
Delayed transfusion reactions, 332
Delirium, poisoning diagnosis and, 20.e1t–20.e3t
Deltasone. See Prednisone
Dental abscesses, 393t–399t
Dental procedures, endocarditis prophylaxis for, 162, 162t, 163b, 694–695
Denver II Developmental Screening Test, 201t, 202
Deoxycorticosterone (DOC) acetate, 229t
Depacon. See Valproic acid
Depakene. See Valproic acid
Depakote. See Divalproex sodium
Depo-Medrol. See Methylprednisolone
Depo-Provera. See Medroxyprogesterone
Depo-Sub Q Provera 104. See Medroxyprogesterone
Depression
adolescent, 93b, 104
amitriptyline for, 680–681
poisoning diagnosis and, 20.e1t–20.e3t

Depressive disorders
assessment of, 210
developmental and mental health
screening tools for, 201t
epidemiology of, 210
treatment of, 209t, 210–211
Derm Atop. *See* Prednicarbate
Derma-Smoothe. *See* Fluocinolone
acetonide
Dermatitis herpetiformis, 193
Dermatology
acne vulgaris in
classification of, 187
clinical presentation of, 187
neonatal, CP9, 190
pathogenesis of, 186
treatment of, 187–188, 188t–189t
bullous lesions in
autoimmune bullous diseases,
CP10, 193
contact dermatitis, CP10, 193–194
impetigo, 192
evaluation and clinical descriptions of
findings in
primary skin lesions, 172,
173f–174f
secondary skin lesions, 172,
173f–174f
hair loss in
alopecia areata, CP8, 185–186
telogen effluvium, CP8, 186
tinea capitis, CP8, 185
traction alopecia, CP8, 186
trichotillomania, 186
neonatal conditions in
acne, CP9, 190
diaper candidiasis, CP10, 192
ETN, CP9, 190
evaluation algorithm for, 191f
milia, CP9, 190
miliaria, CP9, 190
Mongolian spots, 190–192
seborrheic dermatitis, CP10, 190
transient neonatal pustular
melanosis, CP9, 190
papulosquamous lesions in
atopic dermatitis, CP6, CP7,
180–183, 182t–183t, 337, 339
diagnosis algorithm, 181f
ichthyosis, CP7, 184
keratosis pilaris, CP5
papular urticaria, CP6, 183–184

Dermatology *(Continued)*
pityriasis alba, CP6
pityriasis rosea, CP5
post inflammatory
hyperpigmentation, CP6
psoriasis, CP5
tinea corporis, CP5, 184
tinea pedis, CP5
tinea versicolor, CP7, 184
poisoning diagnosis and, 20.e1t–20.e3t
skin lumps in
hemangiomas, CP3, 172–177
molluscum contagiosum, CP3,
177–178
pyogenic granuloma, CP3, 178
reactive erythema, CP3, CP4, 178,
179f
scabies, CP3, 178
warts, 177
websites for, 172
Dermatomes, 469f
Dermatomyositis, 603t, 614–615
Des Owen. *See* Desonide
Desensitization, for drug allergy
management, 340f, 341
Desferal. *See* Deferoxamine mesylate
Desloratadine
for allergic rhinitis, 335
renal failure dosage adjustments for,
1008t–1016t
Desmopressin acetate (DDAVP, Stimate)
for DI, 233
formulary entry for, 751–752
for von Willebrand disease, 327t–328t
Desonide (Des Owen, Desonate Gel,
Verdeso Foam), for atopic
dermatitis, 182t–183t
Desoximetasone (Topicort), for atopic
dermatitis, 182t–183t
Desquam-E. *See* Benzoyl peroxide
Desyrel. *See* Trazodone
Detemir insulin (Levemir), 218t
Detoxification, for adolescents, 108
Development, 195–196
characterization of, 195
normal, guidelines for
age-appropriate behavioral issues,
196, 199t–200t
developmental milestones, 196,
197t–198t
Reach Out and Read milestones of
early literacy, 196, 198t

Development *(Continued)*
  screening and evaluation of
    guidelines for, 200
    tools used for, 200–202, 201t,
      202.e1b–202.e2b, 203f–204f
Developmental disorders
  autism spectrum disorders, 201t,
    207–208
  cerebral palsy, 207, 208t
  communication disorders, 205
  evaluation of
    history, 202
    laboratory investigations, imaging,
      and other tests, 203–205
    physical examination, 202–203,
      203.e1t–203.e2t
  intellectual disability, 205, 206t–207t
  learning disabilities, 205–207
  referral and intervention for, 212
  websites for, 195
Developmental hip dysplasia,
    590, 591f
Developmental quotient (DQ), 195
Deviancy, 196
Dexamethasone (Decadron, Dexpak
    Taperpak, Hexadrol, Maxidex)
  for croup, 12
  formulary entry for, 752–753
  for increased ICP, 70, 530
  for nausea and vomiting, 537
  potency of, 229t
  for sickle cell disease, 311t–312t
  for spinal cord compression, 530
Dexamethasone suppression test, 231
Dexchlorpheniramine maleate,
    formulary entry for, 730
Dexedrine. *See* Dextroamphetamine
DexFerrum. *See* Iron, injectable
    preparations
Dexmedetomidine (Precedex)
  analgesic properties of, 113.e1t
  formulary entry for, 753–754
  for opioid tapering, 118
  procedural sedation with,
    121b–122b
Dexmethylphenidate (Focalin),
    formulary entry for, 754–755
Dexpak Taperpak. *See* Dexamethasone
Dexrazoxane, toxicity of, 525t–528t
Dextroamphetamine (Dexedrine,
    ProCentra, Zenzedi), formulary
    entry for, 755–756

Dextroamphetamine and amphetamine
    (Adderall), formulary entry for,
    755–756
Dextrose. *See also* Insulin/dextrose
  for hypoglycemia, 421t
  for metabolic crisis, 290
  for status epilepticus, 16t
  for sulfonylurea poisoning, 21t
DHEA. *See* Dehydroepiandrosterone
DHEA-S. *See* Dehydroepiandrosterone
    sulfate
DHT. *See* Dihydrotestosterone
DI. *See* Diabetes insipidus
Di-5-ASA. *See* Olsalazine
Diabetes
  classification of, 215–216, 215t
  DKA in, 216, 217f, 218t
  evaluation and diagnosis of, 214–215
  monitoring in, 219
  newborns of mothers with, 420
  type II, 215–219, 215t, 220f
Diabetes insipidus (DI)
  nephrogenic, 232–233, 458
  posterior pituitary gland/vasopressin
    function in, 232–233
Diabetic ketoacidosis (DKA), 216
  assessment of, 216, 217f
  cerebral edema caused by, 216
  insulin requirements after, 216, 218t
  management of, 216, 217f
Dialume. *See* Aluminum hydroxide
Dialysis
  for AKI, 450
  drug dosage adjustments for, 994
  formula used with, 518t–519t
Diaminodiphenylsulfone. *See* Dapsone
Diamond-Blackfan anemia, 309
Diamox. *See* Acetazolamide
Diaper candidiasis, CP10, 192
Diarrhea, 270
  diagnosis/evaluation of, 270–271
  etiology of, 271
  management of, 271–272
Diastat. *See* Diazepam
Diastat AcuDial. *See* Diazepam
Diastolic blood pressure (DBP)
  assessment of, 128.e1t, 128,
    129t–135t, 136f–138f
  definition of normal, 460
  percentiles
    for boys 1-17 years by height,
      133t–135t

Diastolic blood pressure *(Continued)*
    for boys from birth to 12 months, 136f
    for girls 1-17 years by height, 129t–132t
    for girls from birth to 12 months, 137f
    for infants 26-44 weeks postconceptional age, 128.e1t
Diastolic heart murmurs, 139, 139b–140b
Diastolic heart sounds, 128
Diastolic opening snap, 138b
Diazepam (Valium, Diastat, Diastat AcuDial)
    analgesic properties of, 113.e1t
    formulary entry for, 756–757
    palliative care with, 546t
    procedural sedation with, 123t
    for serotonin syndrome, 21t
    for status epilepticus, 16t
Diazoxide (Proglycem)
    formulary entry for, 757
    for hypertensive emergency, 69t
DIC. *See* Dacarbazine; Disseminated intravascular coagulation
Dicloxacillin sodium (Dycill, Pathocil)
    formulary entry for, 757
    for impetigo, 192
    for lymphadenitis, 393t–399t
    sensitivity-based selection of, 383t–384t
Diet. *See also* Nutrition
    special, clinical conditions requiring, 509, 518t–519t
Dietary reference intakes (DRIs)
    fat, 501t
    fiber, 509t
    measurement of, 500–501
    minerals, 504–509, 507t–508t
    in multivitamin examples, 504t–506t
    protein, 501t
    vitamins, 501–504, 502t–503t
Diethylene triamine pentaacetic acid (DTPA), 444
Diffuse cutaneous systemic scleroderma (DCSS), 616.e1–616.e2
Diflorasone diacetate (Florone, Psorcon), 182t–183t
Diflucan. *See* Fluconazole
DiGeorge syndrome, 302–303, 342t–343t
DigiFab. *See* Digoxin immune Fab (ovine)
Digitalis, ECG effects of, 151t–152t
Digoxin (Lanoxin)
    formulary entry for, 758
    for hyperthyroidism, 224
    renal failure dosage adjustments for, 1008t–1016t
Digoxin immune Fab (ovine) (DigiFab), formulary entry for, 759
Dihydrotestosterone (DHT), normal values of, 243.e1t, 243
Dihydroxyanthracenedione dihydrochloride. *See* Mitoxantrone
1,25-Dihydroxycholecalciferol. *See* Calcitriol
Dilacor. *See* Diltiazem
Dilantin. *See* Phenytoin
Dilantin Infatab. *See* Phenytoin
Dilated cardiomyopathy, 162–163
Dilated funduscopic exam, for ROP, 433
Dilaudid. *See* Hydromorphone HCl
Diltiazem (Cardizem, Dilacor, Matzim, Tiazac), formulary entry for, 759–760
Dimenhydrinate (Dramamine), formulary entry for, 760
Dimercaprol (British Anti-Lewisite, BAL)
    formulary entry for, 761
    for lead poisoning, 23
Dimercaptosuccinic acid. *See* Succimer
Dimercaptosuccinic acid (DMSA) scan, after UTI, 444, 589
Di-mesalazine. *See* Olsalazine
Dimetapp. *See* Brompheniramine with phenylephrine
Diovan. *See* Valsartan
Dipentum. *See* Olsalazine
Diphenhydramine (Benadryl)
    for allergic rhinitis, 335
    analgesic properties of, 113.e1t
    for anaphylaxis, 10
    formulary entry for, 761
    for nausea and vomiting, 537
    palliative care with, 546t
    procedural sedation with, 121b–122b
    renal failure dosage adjustments for, 1008t–1016t
Diphtheria, immunoprophylaxis for, 351f–358f, 362.e1t, 362t, 363

Diphtheria and tetanus toxoids and
acellular pertussis (DTaP)
vaccine, 363–366, 366t
for oncology patients, 362.e1t, 362t
recommended schedules for, 351f–358f
side effects of, 365
Diphtheria and tetanus toxoids (DT)
vaccine, 363–366, 366t
Diprolene. *See* Betamethasone
Diprosone. *See* Betamethasone
Dipstick tests. *See* Urinalysis
Dipyridamole, for Kawasaki disease, 168
Direct Coombs test, 307
Direct donors, for blood component
replacement, 332
Disease occurrence, measurements of,
638t–639t, 639–640
Disease-modifying antirheumatic drugs
(DMARDs)
for arthritis, 608.e1t, 608
for SLE, 611
Disopyramide, renal failure dosage
adjustments for, 1008t–1016t
Disseminated intravascular coagulation
(DIC), 315, 326f, 327b
Dissociation, 196
Dissociative sedation, 119
Distal tubule function tests, 447, 447t
Distributive shock, 71.e1t, 71
Ditropan. *See* Oxybutynin chloride
Diuretics
acetazolamide as, 668–669
ammonium chloride as, 682
bumetanide as, 706
chlorothiazide as, 729
furosemide as, 798
HCTZ as, 808
for hydrocephalus, 480,
668–669
for hypercalcemia, 261
for hypermagnesemia, 262
for hypertension, 463t–464t
mannitol as, 845–846
metolazone as, 856
spironolactone as, 945
triamterene as, 966–967
Diurigen. *See* Chlorothiazide
Diuril. *See* Chlorothiazide
Divalproex sodium (Depakote)
formulary entry for, 762
for migraine headaches, 473t
DKA. *See* Diabetic ketoacidosis

DMARDs. *See* Disease-modifying
antirheumatic drugs
DMPA. *See* Medroxyprogesterone
DMSA. *See* Succimer
DMSA scan. *See* Dimercaptosuccinic
acid scan
DMTs. *See* Decision-making tools
DNAR. *See* Do not attempt resuscitation
DNAse. *See* Dornase alfa
Do not attempt resuscitation (DNAR),
543–544, 543b
Dobutamine (Dobutrex)
formulary entry for, 762
for shock, 71.e1t
DOC acetate. *See* Deoxycorticosterone
acetate
Documentation
of child abuse, 85
of death, 546
Docusate (Colace, Kao-Tin, Sur-Q-Lax,
Enemeez), formulary entry for,
762–763
Dog bites, 77t, 393t–399t
Dolasetron (Anzemet)
formulary entry for, 763
for nausea and vomiting, 537
Dolophine. *See* Methadone HCl
Domperidone, for GERD, 275
Donepezil, poisoning with, 21t
Dopamine (Intropin)
formulary entry for, 764
normal values of, 243.e1t
for shock, 71.e1t, 73f
Doppler echocardiography, 155.e1, 583
Dopram. *See* Doxapram HCL
Dornase alfa (DNAse, Pulmozyme)
for CF, 568
formulary entry for, 764
Dorsalis pedis artery puncture, 31
Doryx. *See* Doxycycline
Dosage, drug. *See* Drug dosage
Down syndrome. *See* Trisomy 21
Doxapram HCL (Dopram), formulary
entry for, 765
Doxazosin, for hypertension, 463t–464t
Doxidan. *See* Bisacodyl
Doxorubicin (Adriamycin), toxicity of,
525t–528t
Doxycycline (Adoxa, Doryx, Periostat,
Vibramycin)
for acne vulgaris, 187, 188t
for chlamydia, 400t–401t

Doxycycline *(Continued)*
  for ehrlichiosis, 410
  formulary entry for, 765–766
  for gonorrhea, 400t–401t
  for Lyme disease, 409
  for pelvic inflammatory disease,
    400t–401t
  for Rocky Mountain spotted fever,
    409
  sensitivity-based selection of, 385t
  for syphilis, 400t–401t
D-penicillamine
  for lead poisoning, 23
  for scleroderma, 616.e2
DQ. *See* Developmental quotient
Dramamine. *See* Dimenhydrinate
DRIs. *See* Dietary reference intakes
Drisdol. *See* Ergocalciferol
Dronabinol (Marinol,
    Tetrahydrocannabinol, THC)
  formulary entry for, 766
  for nausea and vomiting, 537
Droperidol (Inapsine), formulary entry
    for, 767
Drug abuse. *See* Substance abuse
    disorder
Drug allergies
  diagnosis of, 340–341
  epidemiology of, 339–340
  management of, 340f, 341
Drug dosage
  adjustments for renal failure
    antimicrobials requiring,
      995t–1007t
    darbepoetin alfa, 748–750
    methods of, 994
    nonantimicrobials requiring,
      1008t–1016t
  breastfeeding categories, 648
  information data sources for,
    667–668
  Joint Commission do not use list,
    667, 667t–668t
  for neonates/newborns, 435,
    435t
  pregnancy categories, 648
  sample formulary entry, 647
  trade and generic name index,
    648–666
Drug intolerance, 340
Drug use, 93b–94b, 108
Drug-induced SLE, 603t, 611

Drugs. *See also* specific drugs
  administration of
    by intramuscular injection, 54
    by subcutaneous injection, 53
  ECG effects of, 150, 151t–152t
  poisoning caused by, 20–23, 21t
  trade and generic names for, 648–666
DT vaccine. *See* Diphtheria and tetanus
    toxoids vaccine
DTaP vaccine. *See* Diphtheria and
    tetanus toxoids and acellular
    pertussis vaccine
DTIC. *See* Dacarbazine
DTIC-Dome. *See* Dacarbazine
DTPA. *See* Diethylene triamine
    pentaacetic acid
Duac. *See* Benzoyl peroxide and
    clindamycin
Dulcolax. *See* Bisacodyl
Dulcolax Balance. *See* Polyethylene
    glycol, electrolyte solution
Dulera. *See* Mometasone furoate and
    formoterol fumarate
Duocal, 510t
Duodenal hematomas, 84
DuoDote. *See* Pralidoxime chloride with
    atropine
Duraclon. *See* Clonidine
Duragesic. *See* Fentanyl
Duramist. *See* Oxymetazoline
Duricef. *See* Cefadroxil
Dycill. *See* Dicloxacillin sodium
Dynacin. *See* Minocycline
Dyrenium. *See* Triamterene
Dysmorphology
  genetic disorders with
    chromosome microarray for, 299
    connective tissue diseases,
      301–302
    FISH for, 299
    fragile X syndrome, 303
    gene testing for, 299
    history for, 295
    imaging for, 295
    karyotyping for, 299
    NF1, 302
    physical examination for, 295
    trisomy 13, 300–301
    trisomy 18, 300
    trisomy 21, 299–300
    Turner syndrome, 301
    22q11 syndrome, 302–303

Dysmorphology *(Continued)*
    whole-exome sequencing for, 299
    workup for, 295–299
  imaging of, 572
Dysraphism, spinal, 574

E

EAR. *See* Estimated average
    requirement
Ear infections, 393t–399t, 682,
    694–695
Early childhood, age-appropriate
    behavioral issues in, 196,
    199t–200t
EBV. *See* Estimated blood volume
EC. *See* Emergency contraception
ECF deficit. *See* Extracellular fluid deficit
ECG. *See* Electrocardiography
Echocardiography
  blood flow imaging with, 583
  cardiology imaging with, 155
ECMO. *See* Extracorporeal membrane
    oxygenation
EC-Naprosyn. *See* Naproxen
Ecstasy, poisoning with, 21t
Ectopic atrial SVT, 145t–146t
Eczema. *See* Atopic dermatitis
Eczema herpeticum superinfection, 183
Edema
  CKD with, 458–460
  in DKA, 216
Edetate (EDTA), for lead poisoning, 24
Edetate calcium chloride, renal
    failure dosage adjustments for,
    1008t–1016t
Edetate calcium disodium (Calcium
    disodium versenate), formulary
    entry for, 767
Edrophonium chloride (Enlon, Tensilon),
    formulary entry for, 768
EDTA. *See* Edetate
EE. *See* Eosinophilic esophagitis
EEG. *See* Electroencephalogram
EER. *See* Estimated energy requirement
EES. *See* Erythromycin preparations
Efavirenz, for PEP, 412
Effect modification, 638
eGFR. *See* Estimated GFR
Ehrlichiosis, 409–410
Ejection click, 138b
Elavil. *See* Amitriptyline
ELBW. *See* Extremely low birth weight

EleCare, 511t–517t
Electrical injury, 79t, 82
Electrocardiography (ECG)
  of arrhythmias, 144, 145t–146t,
    147f–148f, 148t
  complexes, 127f, 140
  of conduction disturbances, 144,
    149f, 149t–150t
  of electrolyte disturbances,
    medications, and systemic
    illnesses, 150, 151t–152t
  of heart murmurs, 137
  of hyperkalemia, 151t–152t, 153,
    259, 260f
  lead placement for, 140, 141f
  of long QT, 150–153
  of MI in children, 153–154, 153f
  systematic evaluation approach to,
    140–144, 142t
    axis, 141, 142t, 143f
    hypertrophy/enlargement, 142t,
      144, 144f, 145b
    intervals, 141, 142t
    P waves, 141
    Q waves, 141
    R waves, 141, 142t
    rate, 140, 142t
    rhythm, 140–141
    ST-segment, 143, 143t
    T waves, 143, 143t, 144f
Electroencephalogram (EEG)
  for developmental disorder evaluation,
    205
  for seizures, 475
Electrolyte disturbances
  calcium, 259–261, 261b
  ECG of, 150, 151t–152t
  magnesium, 262, 262b
  phosphate, 263, 263b
  poisoning diagnosis and,
    20.e1t–20.e3t
  potassium, 257–259, 258t–259t, 260f
  sodium, 256–257, 257t–258t
Electrolyte management. *See* Fluid and
    electrolyte management
Electrophoresis
  Hb, 309, 310t
  protein, reference values for,
    621t–623t
Elements, DRIs for, 504–509, 507t–508t
Eletriptan (Relpax), for migraine
    headaches, 473t

Elidel. *See* Pimecrolimus

Elimination diet, food allergy evaluation with, 339

Elimite. *See* Permethrin

Eliphos. *See* Calcium acetate

Elitek. *See* Rasburicase

Elixophyllin. *See* Theophylline

Elocon. *See* Mometasone; Mometasone furoate

Elspar. *See* Asparaginase

Emergency contraception (EC), 102–104

Emergency management
  airway, 3–7, 5f, 6t–7t
  for anaphylaxis, 9–10
  breathing, 7–8
  circulation, 8–9, 9t
  for gastrointestinal conditions, 268–270, 268t, 270t
  initial assessment, 3
  for neurologic conditions, 13–17, 14b, 15t–16t
  for respiratory conditions, 10–13, 14f

Emergency plan, for procedural sedation, 120

Emesis. *See also* Nausea and vomiting
  in newborns, 431.e1t, 431

EMLA. *See* Eutectic mixture of local anesthetics

Emotion, as death approaches, 545

Empyema, 580

E-Mycin. *See* Erythromycin preparations

Enalapril maleate (Epaned, Vasotec)
  formulary entry for, 768–769
  for hypertension, 463t–464t
  for hypertensive urgency, 69t
  renal failure dosage adjustments for, 1008t–1016t

Enalaprilat (Vasotec)
  formulary entry for, 768–769
  renal failure dosage adjustments for, 1008t–1016t

Enbrel. *See* Etanercept

Encephalitis, 15

Encopresis, 272–273, 273t

Endocarditis, 161–162
  prophylaxis for, 162, 162t, 163b, 694–695

Endocet. *See* Oxycodone and acetaminophen

Endocrinology
  adrenal gland function in
    insufficiency, 226–231, 227f, 227t–229t
    pheochromocytoma, 231
  diabetes in
    classification of, 215–216, 215t
    DKA in, 216, 217f, 218t
    evaluation and diagnosis of, 214–215
    monitoring in, 219
    type II, 215–219, 215t, 220f
  growth in, 233–236, 234f, 235t
  neonatal hypoglycemia evaluation in, 242–243
  normal values in
    androstenedione, 243.e3t, 243
    catecholamines, 243.e1t, 243
    DHEA, 240t
    DHEA-S, 241t
    DHT, 243.e1t, 243
    estradiol, 239t
    FSH, 237t
    IGF-1, 235t
    IGF-BP3, 243.e2t, 243
    LH, 237t
    mean stretched penile length, 243.e3t, 243
    T_3, 221t
    T_4, 221t
    TBG, 221t
    testicle size and volume, 241t
    testosterone, 240t
    TSH, 221t
  parathyroid gland function in, 225.e1b, 224–225
  pituitary gland function in, 231–233
  sexual development in, 236–242, 237t, 238f, 239t–241t
  thyroid function in
    hyperthyroidism, 220t, 223–224
    hypothyroidism, 219–223, 220t, 222t
    tests of, 219, 220t–221t
  vitamin D deficiency in, 225–226, 225t–226t
  websites for, 214

Endodan. *See* Oxycodone and aspirin

Endothelial damage, 319b

Endotracheal tube (ETT), 4
  imaging of, 583
  for newborns, 415, 416t

Enemas
  for constipation, 272
  sodium phosphate as, 944
Enemeez. *See* Docusate
Energy deposition, 497
Energy needs, 497, 498t
  for catch-up growth, 499–500, 500b
  estimation of, 497–498, 499t
  in stressed conditions, 498–499
Enfacare LIPIL, 511t–517t
Enfagrow Premium Next Step,
    511t–517t
Enfagrow Soy Next Step, 511t–517t
Enfalyte, 519t
Enfamil A.R. LIPIL, 511t–517t
Enfamil D-Vi-Sol. *See* Cholecalciferol
Enfamil Gentlease, 511t–517t
Enfamil HMF with preterm human milk,
    511t–517t
Enfamil LactoFree LIPIL, 511t–517t
Enfamil LIPIL, 511t–517t
Enfamil Premature LIPIL, 511t–517t
Enfamil Premium LIPIL, 511t–517t
Enfamil Prosobee LIPIL, 511t–517t
Enfamil RestFull, 511t–517t
Enfaport LIPIL, 511t–517t
Engerix-B, 367
Engraftment HSCT, 532
Enlive, 511t–517t
Enlon. *See* Edrophonium chloride
Enoxaparin (Lovenox)
  antidote for, 920–921
  formulary entry for, 769–770
  renal failure dosage adjustments for,
    1008t–1016t
Ensure, 511t–517t
Ensure Plus, 511t–517t
Entamoeba histolytica, antibiotic
    sensitivity of, 386t
Enteral nutrition
  caloric modulars, 509, 510t
  formulas
    clinical conditions requiring, 509,
      518t–519t
    mixing instructions for, 510t
    nutrition components of, 509
    for special clinical circumstances,
      518t–519t
    websites for, 485
  oral rehydration solutions, 509, 519t
Enterobacter spp., antibiotic sensitivity
    of, 383t–384t

Enterococcus spp., antibiotic sensitivity
    of, 383t–386t
Enterocolitis
  food-induced, 337
  neutropenic, 531
  in newborns, 431.e1t, 431, 584
Enterovirus, perinatal, 389t–390t
Entocort EC. *See* Budesonide
Enulose. *See* Lactulose
EO28 Splash, 511t–517t
Eosinophilic esophagitis (EE), 275
Eosinophils, age-specific values of, 314t
Epaned. *See* Enalapril maleate
Epiglottitis, 12
Epilepsy, 475, 476t–477t. *See also* Seizure
  classification of, 478b
  differential diagnosis of events
    mimicking, 474t
  formula for, 518t–519t
Epinephrine, racemic (S-2 Inhalant)
  for anaphylaxis, 10
  for croup, 12
  formulary entry for, 772
Epinephrine HCl (Adrenalin, EpiPen)
  for anaphylaxis, 10
  for asthma, 10
  for croup, 12
  for food allergies, 339
  formulary entry for, 771–772
  for increased ICP, 70
  local anesthetic use with, 115t, 116
  neonate dosages of, 435
  normal values of, 243.e1t
  for shock, 71.e1t, 73f
Episodic rhinitis, 335
Epithelial cells, in urine, 440
Epitol. *See* Carbamazepine
Epivir. *See* Lamivudine
Epoetin alfa (Epogen, Procrit)
  darbepoetin alfa conversions for,
    748–750
  formulary entry for, 772–773
Epsom salts. *See* Magnesium sulfate
Erb-Duchenne palsy, 433t
Ergocalciferol (Drisdol, Calcidol,
    Calciferol, Vitamin D₂), formulary
    entry for, 774
Ergotamine tartrate (Ergomar), formulary
    entry for, 775
Ergotamine tartrate with caffeine
    (Cafergot, Migergot), formulary
    entry for, 775

Ertapenem (Invanz)
  formulary entry for, 775
  renal failure dosage adjustments for, 995t–1007t
  sensitivity-based selection of, 383t–384t
Erwinia. *See* Asparaginase
Ery-Ped. *See* Erythromycin preparations
Erythema, reactive, CP3, CP4, 178, 179f
Erythema toxicum neonatorum (ETN), CP9, 190
Erythrocin. *See* Erythromycin preparations
Erythrocyte sedimentation rate (ESR), 602
  reference values for, 621t–623t
Erythromycin ethylsuccinate and acetylsulfisoxazole (Pediazole, ESP), formulary entry for, 776
Erythromycin preparations (EES, E-Mycin, Ery-Ped, Erythrocin, Ilotycin, Pediamycin, Romycin)
  for acne vulgaris, 187, 188t
  for chlamydia, 400t–401t
  for conjunctivitis, 393t–399t
  formulary entry for, 776–777
  for gastroenteritis, 393t–399t
  for GERD, 275
  for neonatal conjunctivitis, 392t
  for neonatal pneumonia, 392t
  neonate dosages of, 435
  ophthalmic, 991t–992t
  for pertussis, 366, 393t–399t
  renal failure dosage adjustments for, 995t–1007t
  sensitivity-based selection of, 385t
Erythropoietin, recombinant human. *See* Epoetin alfa
Escherichia coli
  antibiotic sensitivity of, 383t–384t
  gastroenteritis caused by, 393t–399t
  perinatal infection with, 392t
Escitalopram (Lexapro), for mental health disorders, 209t
Eskalith. *See* Lithium
Esmolol HCl (Brevibloc), formulary entry for, 777–778
Esomeprazole (Nexium), formulary entry for, 778–779
Esophageal atresia, 584, 585f
Esophageal foreign bodies, 576
Esophagitis, 275, 337
ESP. *See* Erythromycin ethylsuccinate and acetylsulfisoxazole

ESR. *See* Erythrocyte sedimentation rate
Estimated average requirement (EAR), 500
Estimated blood volume (EBV), 329t
Estimated energy requirement (EER), 497–498
  equations for, 498
  for healthy boys and girls of median weight, 498, 499t
  under stressed conditions, 498–499
Estimated GFR (eGFR), 445
Estradiol
  normal levels of, 239t
  in precocious puberty, 239, 239t
Etanercept (Enbrel)
  for arthritis, 608
  formulary entry for, 779
Ethambutol HCl (Myambutol)
  formulary entry for, 780
  renal failure dosage adjustments for, 995t–1007t
  for tuberculosis, 407.e1t
Ethanol
  adolescent use of, 93b–94b, 108
  for ethylene glycol/methanol poisoning, 21t
  poisoning with, 19, 20t–21t
Ethinyl estradiol, for EC, 102–103
Ethionamide, for tuberculosis, 407.e1t
Ethosuximide (Zarontin)
  formulary entry for, 780
  for seizure, 476t–477t, 479t
Ethylene glycol, poisoning with, 21t, 795
ETN. *See* Erythema toxicum neonatorum
Etomidate
  procedural sedation with, 119
  for RSI, 5f, 6t–7t
Etoposide (VP-16, VePesid), toxicity of, 525t–528t
ETT. *See* Endotracheal tube
Eutectic mixture of local anesthetics (EMLA)
  analgesic properties of, 115t, 125t
  formulary entry for, 836–837
Evaporated milk, 511t–517t
Evidence-based medicine
  applying evidence to clinical question in, 635
  clinical question formulation in, 634
  evidence appraisal in, 635
  evidence searches in, 634
  websites for, 634

Ewing sarcoma, 597, 598f

Exalgo. See Hydromorphone HCl

Exchange transfusion, 428–429, 428t, 430f

Excitation, poisoning diagnosis and, 20.e1t–20.e3t

Excoriation, on skin, 172, 173f–174f

Exercise recommendations, for congenital heart disease, 168.e1t, 168

Extina. See Ketoconazole

External jugular vein
  catheter placement in, 28f, 31, 33
  puncture of, 28–29, 28f

Extracellular fluid (ECF) deficit, electrolyte replacement based on, 249–252, 251t

Extracorporeal membrane oxygenation (ECMO), for PPHN, 425–426

Extradural fluid collections, in newborn, 416, 419f, 419t

Extraglomerular hematuria, 450, 453

Extrapyramidal CP, 208t

Extremely low birth weight (ELBW), 415

Extremities
  imaging of
    bone age, 597
    bone lesions, 590–597, 594f–598f
    hip disorders, 590, 591f–593f
    osteomyelitis, 590
    skeletal survey for suspected child abuse, 597, 599f–600f
    stress fractures, 590
    trauma, 589
  pain in, 609t
  trauma to, 66, 67f, 67t
    in child abuse patients, 84, 85t
    imaging of, 589
    secondary survey of, 62t

Exudate, 630t

Eye
  burns of, 82
  imaging of, 573, 574f

F

Faces pain rating scale, 111, 113f

Factor IX deficiency, 326f, 327t–328t

Factor replacement, for bleeding disorders, 327t–328t

Factor V Leiden, 319b

Factor VIII deficiency, 326f, 327t–328t

Fahrenheit, conversion formulas for, 633

Failure to thrive, 499–500

Famciclovir (Famvir)
  formulary entry for, 781
  for genital herpes, 106t–107t
  renal failure dosage adjustments for, 995t–1007t

Familial short stature (FSS), 233–235, 234f

Family history, of adolescents, 94

Family meetings, in palliative care, 541–542

Family planning, for adolescents, 98–104, 99f, 101f

Famotidine (Pepcid)
  formulary entry for, 781–782
  renal failure dosage adjustments for, 1008t–1016t

Famvir. See Famciclovir

Fanconi anemia, 309

Fanconi syndrome, 458

FAO disorders. See Fatty acid oxidation disorders

FAS. See Fetal alcohol syndrome

Fasting blood glucose (FPG), 214, 219

Fasting recommendations, for procedural sedation, 119.e1f, 119, 120t

Fats
  DRIs for, 501t
  malabsorption of, formula for, 518t–519t

Fatty acid oxidation (FAO) disorders, 290–291

5-FC. See Flucytosine

Febrile illness–associated seizures, 475

Febrile neutropenia, 685

Febrile nonhemolytic reaction, 331

Fecal fat test, 281

FEF$_{25-75}$. See Forced expiratory flow between 25% and 75% of FVC

FeHCO$_3$. See Fractional excretion of bicarbonate

Felbamate (Felbatol)
  formulary entry for, 782–783
  renal failure dosage adjustments for, 1008t–1016t
  for seizures, 479t

Felodipine, for hypertension, 463t–464t

Femoral artery, puncture of, 29–30, 29f

Femoral vein
  catheter placement in, 31, 33–37, 36f
  puncture of, 29–30, 29f

FENa. See Fractional excretion of sodium

Fentanyl (Abstral, Actiq, Duragesic,
        Fentora, Lazanda, Sublimate)
    analgesic properties of, 113.e1t, 114t,
        125t
    formulary entry for, 783–784
    neonate dosages of, 435
    palliative care with, 546t
    PCA with, 117t
    procedural sedation with, 125t
    renal failure dosage adjustments for,
        1008t–1016t
    for RSI, 5f, 6t–7t
    tapering of, 118t, 119b
Feosol. See Iron, oral preparations
Fergon. See Iron, oral preparations
Fer-In-Sol. See Iron, oral preparations
Ferric gluconate. See Iron, injectable
        preparations
Ferritin, reference values for, 621t–623t
Ferrlecit. See Iron, injectable
        preparations
Ferrous bis-glycinate chelate.
        See Iron, oral preparations
Ferrous fumarate. See Iron, oral
        preparations
Ferrous gluconate. See Iron, oral
        preparations
Ferrous sulfate. See Iron, oral
        preparations
Fetal alcohol syndrome (FAS), 420
Fetal assessment
    anomaly screening, 415.e1
    expected birth weight by gestational
        age, 415.e2, 416t
    FHR monitoring, 415.e2–415.e3
    gestational age estimation, 415.e1
Fetal heart rate (FHR) monitoring,
    415.e2–415.e3
FEurea. See Fractional excretion of urea
FEV$_1$. See Forced expiratory volume in
    1 second
Fever
    without localizing source, 380–382,
        387f
    as oncologic emergency, 531–532,
        533f
    in sickle cell disease, 311t–312t
Feverall. See Acetaminophen
Fexofenadine
    for allergic rhinitis, 335
    renal failure dosage adjustments for,
        1008t–1016t

Fexofenadine and pseudoephedrine
        (Allegra), formulary entry for,
        784–785
FFP. See Fresh frozen plasma
FHR monitoring. See Fetal heart rate
        monitoring
Fiber, DRIs for, 509t
Fiberall. See Psyllium
Fibersource HN, 511t–517t
Fibrinogen, age-specific values for,
        317t–318t
Fibroma, 590, 595f
Fifth disease, CP4
Filgrastim (Neupogen, G-CSF)
    formulary entry for, 785
    for GSD, 294–295
Filtered RBCs, 329
Fine-motor skills, 196, 197t–198t
Fingerstick, 27–28
Fi$_{O2}$. See Inspired oxygen concentration
First-degree heart block, 149f, 149t
First-Lansoprazole. See Lansoprazole
First-Omeprazole. See Omeprazole
FISH. See Fluorescence in situ
        hybridization
Fissure, on skin, 172, 173f–174f
Fixed proteinuria, 454
FK506. See Tacrolimus
FLACC pain assessment scale, 111,
        112t
Flagyl. See Metronidazole
Flame burns, 79t
Flat warts, 177
Flebogamma DIF. See Intravenous
        immunoglobulin
Flecainide acetate (Tambocor)
    formulary entry for, 785–786
    renal failure dosage adjustments for,
        1008t–1016t
Fleet Bisacodyl. See Bisacodyl
Fleet Enema. See Sodium phosphate
Fleet Laxative. See Bisacodyl
Fleet Liquid Supp. See Glycerin
Fleet Mineral Oil. See Mineral oil
Fleet Pedia-Lax. See Sodium phosphate
Fleet Phospho-Soda. See Sodium
        phosphate
Flintstones Complete, 505t–506t
Flintstones Sour Gummies, 505t–506t
Flonase HFA. See Fluticasone
        propionate
Florinef. See Fludrocortisone acetate

Florone. *See* Diflorasone diacetate

Flovent Diskus. *See* Fluticasone
propionate

Flow-volume curve, normal, 554f

Floxin. *See* Ofloxacin

Fluconazole (Diflucan)
for cancer patients, 538t
formulary entry for, 786–787
renal failure dosage adjustments for,
995t–1007t
for tinea infections, 411t
for yeast infections, 105t

Flucytosine (Ancobon, 5-Fluorocytosine,
5-FC)
formulary entry for, 787
renal failure dosage adjustments for,
995t–1007t

Fludarabine (Fludara), toxicity of,
525t–528t

Fludrocortisone acetate
(Florinef, Fluohydrisone,
9-Fluorohydrocortisone)
for adrenal insufficiency, 229t, 230
formulary entry for, 787–788
potency of, 229t

Fluid and electrolyte management
for acid-base/osmolar gap
disturbances, 264
etiology of acid-base disturbances
and, 264, 265f–266f
primary acid-base disorder
determination for, 264
ADH release and, 246.e1b, 246
deficit repletion for
based on excess electrolyte deficits,
252
based on FWD, 252
based on SFD, 252–253
based on solute fluid deficit,
249–252, 251t
calculation of appropriate fluids for,
253–256, 254t–255t
replacement strategy for, 250f,
253.e1t–253.e3t, 253
water volume, 249, 251t
goals for, 246
maintenance requirements for,
246, 247f
fluid volume, 247–248, 248t, 248b
solute, 248–249, 248t, 256t
for newborns, 420, 421t–422t
for ongoing losses, 256, 256t

Fluid and electrolyte
management *(Continued)*
for serum electrolyte disturbances
calcium, 259–261, 261b
magnesium, 262, 262b
phosphate, 263, 263b
potassium, 257–259, 258t–259t,
260f
sodium, 256–257, 257t–258t

Fluid therapy
for burns, 78, 81f
for diabetic ketoacidosis, 217f
for GI bleeding, 269
ORT
common solutions for, 509, 519t
composition of fluids for,
254t–255t, 256
for diarrhea, 509
for shock, 71.e1t, 73f

Flumadine. *See* Rimantadine

Flumazenil (Romazicon)
for benzodiazepine poisoning, 21t, 788
formulary entry for, 788
for procedural sedation reversal, 120,
121b–122b, 122

Flunarizine, for migraine headaches, 473t

Flunisolide (Nasarel, Aerospan)
for allergic rhinitis, 335
for asthma, 558.e1t–558.e2t
formulary entry for, 788–789

Fluocinolone acetonide (Capex,
Derma-Smoothe, Synalar), for
atopic dermatitis, 182t–183t

Fluocinonide (Lidex, Vanos), for atopic
dermatitis, 182t–183t

Fluohydrisone. *See* Fludrocortisone
acetate

Fluorescence in situ hybridization
(FISH), for dysmorphology, 299

Fluoride (Luride, Fluoritab, Pediaflor)
DRIs for, 507t–508t
formulary entry for, 789
supplementation of, 504–509

9-αFluorocortisone. *See* Fludrocortisone

5-Fluorocytosine. *See* Flucytosine

9-Fluorohydrocortisone. *See*
Fludrocortisone acetate

Fluoroquinolones
for chlamydia, 400t–401t
for gastroenteritis, 393t–399t
sensitivity-based selection of, 385t
for sinusitis, 393t–399t

Fluorouracil (5-FU, Adrucil), toxicity of, 525t–528t
Fluoxetine hydrochloride (Prozac, Sarafem)
  formulary entry for, 790
  for mental health disorders, 209t
Flurandrenolide (Cordran), for atopic dermatitis, 182t–183t
Flushing, poisoning diagnosis and, 20.e1t–20.e3t
Fluticasone propionate (Cutivate, Flonase HFA, Flovent Diskus, Veramyst)
  for allergic rhinitis, 335
  for asthma, 558.e1t–558.e2t
  for atopic dermatitis, 182t–183t
  dosage recommendations for, 558.e1t–558.e2t
  for EE, 275
  formulary entry for, 791–792
Fluticasone propionate and salmeterol (Advair)
  for asthma, 558.e1t–558.e2t
  dosage recommendations for, 558.e1t–558.e2t
  formulary entry for, 792–793
Fluvoxamine (Luvox), formulary entry for, 793–794
Focalin. See Dexmethylphenidate
Folex. See Methotrexate
Folic acid (Folvite)
  DRIs for, 502t–503t
  formulary entry for, 794
  reference values for, 621t–623t
  for sickle cell disease, 312t
Folinic acid, for congenital toxoplasmosis, 388t
Follicle-stimulating hormone (FSH)
  in delayed puberty, 236–237, 237t, 238f
  normal levels of, 237t
Follicular eczema, CP6
Folvite. See Folic acid
Fomepizole (Antizol)
  for ethylene glycol/methanol poisoning, 21t, 795
  formulary entry for, 795
Fontan procedure, 161
Food allergies
  diagnosis of, 337–339, 338f
  epidemiology of, 336
  formula for, 518t–519t

Food allergies (Continued)
  manifestations of, 336–337
  natural history of, 339
  treatment of, 339
Food intolerance, 339
Food-induced enterocolitis, 337
Foradil Aerolizer. See Formoterol
Forced expiratory flow between 25% and 75% of FVC (FEF_{25-75}), 553, 555f, 555t
Forced expiratory volume in 1 second (FEV_1), 553, 555f, 555t
Forced vital capacity (FVC), 553, 555f, 555t
Foreign countries
  immunoprophylaxis for travel to, 363
  infection in children adopted from, 413
Foreign-body aspiration
  emergency management of, 13, 14f
  imaging of, 576
Formoterol (Foradil Aerolizer, Perforomist)
  for asthma, 558.e1t–558.e2t
  formulary entry for, 795–796
Formulas
  mixing instructions for, 510t
  nutrition components of, 509
  for special clinical circumstances, 518t–519t
  websites for, 485
Fortamet. See Metformin
Fortaz. See Ceftazidime
Fortical Nasal Spray. See Calcitonin–salmon
Forward bending test, 95.e1, 95.e2f
Foscarnet (Foscavir)
  formulary entry for, 796–797
  renal failure dosage adjustments for, 995t–1007t
Fosinopril, for hypertension, 463t–464t
Fosphenytoin (Cerebyx)
  formulary entry for, 797
  for status epilepticus, 16t
FPG. See Fasting blood glucose
Fractional excretion of bicarbonate ($FeHCO_3$), 457
Fractional excretion of sodium (FENa), 447
Fractional excretion of urea (FEurea), 447
Fractures
  birth trauma causing, 419
  in child abuse patients, 84, 85t

Fractures *(Continued)*
  imaging of
    stress, 590
    traumatic, 589
  long bone, 66, 67f, 67t
  patterns in children, 67f
  skeletal survey for, 597, 599f–600f
Fragile X syndrome, 303
Francisella tularensis, antibiotic
  sensitivity of, 385t
Free T$_4$
  age-based normal values for, 221t
  in preterm and term infants, 221t
  thyroid function test interpretation
    and, 220t
Free testosterone, normal levels of,
  240t
Free water deficit (FWD), repletion of,
  252
Fresh frozen plasma (FFP), 330
Frostbite, 79t
Frovatriptan (Frova), for migraine
  headaches, 473t
FSH. *See* Follicle-stimulating hormone
FSS. *See* Familial short stature
5-FU. *See* Fluorouracil
Full thickness burns, 79t
Function studies, liver, 276, 277t
Functional constipation,
  272–273, 273t
Funduscopic exam, for ROP, 433
Fungal infections. *See also specific
  fungal infections*
  common community-acquired, 410,
    411t
  diagnosis of, 410
Fungizone. *See* Amphotericin B
Furadantin. *See* Nitrofurantoin
Furosemide (Lasix)
  formulary entry for, 798
  for hydrocephalus, 480
  for hypercalcemia, 261
  for hyperparathyroidism, 225
  for hypertension, 463t–464t
  neonate dosages of, 435
  renal failure dosage adjustments for,
    1008t–1016t
Fusobacterium spp., antibiotic sensitivity
  of, 386t
FVC. *See* Forced vital capacity
FWD. *See* Free water deficit

G
G6PD deficiency. *See* Glucose-6-
  phosphate dehydrogenase
  deficiency
Gabapentin (Neurontin, Gralise,
  Horizant)
  formulary entry for, 798–799
  renal failure dosage adjustments for,
    1008t–1016t
  for seizures, 479t
Gabitril. *See* Tiagabine
Gablofen. *See* Baclofen
Galactose, reference values for, 621t–623t
Galactosemia, 293–294
  formula for, 518t–519t
Galzin. *See* Zinc salts
GamaSTAN. *See* Intramuscular
  immunoglobulin
Gamma benzene hexachloride. *See*
  Lindane
Gammagard. *See* Intravenous
  immunoglobulin
Gamma-glutamyl transpeptidase (GGT)
  liver function testing with, 277t
  reference values for, 621t–623t
Gammaked. *See* Intravenous
  immunoglobulin
Gammaplex. *See* Intravenous
  immunoglobulin
Gamunex-C. *See* Intravenous
  immunoglobulin
Ganciclovir (Cytovene, Vitrasert, Zirgan)
  for CMV, 388t
  formulary entry for, 800
  renal failure dosage adjustments for,
    995t–1007t
Garamycin. *See* Gentamicin
Gardasil. *See* Human papilloma virus
  vaccine
Gardnerella vaginalis, antibiotic
  sensitivity of, 386t
Gas exchange, evaluation of
  acid-base disturbance analysis, 551,
    552f, 552t
  blood gases, 550–551, 552f
  capnography, 550
  pulse oximetry, 549–550, 551f
Gastrocrom. *See* Cromolyn
Gastroenteritis
  allergic eosinophilic, 337
  management of, 393t–399t

Gastroenterology. *See also*
Gastrointestinal tract
emergencies in
acute abdominal pain, 269–270,
270t
GI bleeding, 268–269, 268t, 675
liver conditions in
ALF, 276–278, 278t
function studies for, 276, 277t
hyperbilirubinemia, 278, 279t
miscellaneous tests in
occult blood, 281
quantitative fecal fat, 281
newborn disease in
abdominal wall defects, 431.e1t, 431
bilious emesis, 431.e1t, 431
necrotizing enterocolitis, 431.e1t,
431, 584
pancreatitis in
acute, 278–280, 280t
chronic, 280–281, 281.e1t
websites for, 268
Gastrointestinal reflux disease (GERD),
274
evaluation/diagnosis of, 274–275
management of, 275
Gastrointestinal (GI) tract
burns of, 82
conditions of
bleeding, 268–269, 268t, 675
celiac disease, 276
constipation and encopresis,
272–273, 273t
diarrhea, 270–272
EE, 275
GERD, 274–275
IBD, 274
vomiting, 270, 271t
food allergy syndromes involving, 337
obstruction of
formula for, 518t–519t
imaging of, 584–588, 586f
in newborns, 431.e1t
Gastroschisis, 431.e1t
Gas-X. *See* Simethicone
Gatifloxacin ophthalmic (Zymar),
991t–992t
GBS infection. *See* Group B
streptococcal infection
G-CSF. *See* Filgrastim
Gemcitabine, toxicity of, 525t–528t

Gender identity, 98
Gene sequencing, for dysmorphology,
299
Gene testing, for dysmorphology, 299
General anesthetics
ketamine as, 824
for status epilepticus, 16t
Generalized seizures, 478b
Generic names, trade names
corresponding to, 648–666
Genetic disorders
with dysmorphology
chromosome microarray for, 299
connective tissue diseases,
301–302
FISH for, 299
fragile X syndrome, 303
gene testing for, 299
history for, 295
imaging for, 295
karyotyping for, 299
NF1, 302
physical examination for, 295
trisomy 13, 300–301
trisomy 18, 300
trisomy 21, 299–300
Turner syndrome, 301
22q11 syndrome, 302–303
whole-exome sequencing for, 299
workup for, 295–299
with metabolism errors
clinical presentation of, 285, 285b
disorders of carbohydrate
metabolism, 293–294
evaluation of, 285–290, 286t,
286b, 287f–289f
FAO disorders, 290–291
GSD, 294–295
HT1, 292
hypotonia, 295, 296f–298f
lysosomal storage diseases, 293
mitochondrial diseases, 292–293
newborn screening for, 284–285
organic acidemias, 291
PKU, 292
treatment of metabolic crisis in, 290
urea cycle defects, 291–292
Genetic studies, for developmental
disorder evaluation, 205
Genetics, websites/databases for, 284
Gengraf. *See* Cyclosporine modified

Genital herpes, 106t–107t

Genital ulcers, 104, 106t–107t

Genital warts, 104, 106t–107t

Genitalia
adolescent
development of, 91, 93t
physical examination of, 95
ambiguous, 239–242

Genitourinary (GU) system
burns of, 82
imaging of
uterine and ovarian pathology, 589
UTIs, 589
trauma to, secondary survey of, 62t

Gentamicin (Garamycin)
formulary entry for, 801
for neonatal pneumonia, 392t
for neonatal septic arthritis, 392t
for pelvic inflammatory disease,
400t–401t
renal failure dosage adjustments for,
995t–1007t
sensitivity-based selection of, 385t
for spinal fusion infections, 393t–399t
for UTI, 393t–399t

GERD. See Gastrointestinal reflux
disease

Germinal matrix hemorrhage, 572

Gesell block skills, 202, 204f

Gesell figures, 202, 203f

Gestational age
expected birth weight by, 415.e2,
416t
fetal assessment for estimation of,
415.e1
New Ballard Score for estimation of,
416, 418f

GFR. See Glomerular filtration rate

GGT. See Gamma-glutamyl
transpeptidase

GI tract. See Gastrointestinal tract

Giant cell arteritis, 613t

Giardia lamblia, antibiotic sensitivity
of, 386t

Glargine insulin (Lantus), 218t

Glasgow Coma Scale, 15t

Glaucoma, 668–669

Gleevec. See Imatinib

Glenn shunt, 160f, 161

Glomerular filtration rate (GFR)
CCr measurement of, 445
normal values of, 445, 445t

Glomerular function tests, 445–446,
445t–446t

Glomerular hematuria, 451

Glomerulonephritis. See Nephritis

Glucagon HCl (GlucaGen, Glucagon
Emergency Kit)
for beta blocker poisoning, 21t
for calcium channel blocker
poisoning, 21t
formulary entry for, 802

Glucagon stimulation test, newborn
screening with, 242–243

Glucerna 1.0 Cal, 511t–517t

Glucocorticoids
for adrenal insufficiency, 229t, 230
for sarcoidosis, 616
for scleroderma, 616.e1
for Sjögren syndrome, 616.e3

Glucophage. See Metformin

Glucose
in CSF, 631t
for hypoglycemia, 242, 421t, 422f
monitoring of, 219
newborn requirements for, 420, 421t,
422f
reference values for, 621t–623t
testing of
FPG, 214, 219
OGTT, 214–215
for tet spells, 160t
in transudate vs. exudate, 630t

Glucose reabsorption, 447

Glucose-6-phosphate dehydrogenase
(G6PD) deficiency, 308, 993

Glucosuria, 439

Glulisine insulin (Apidra), 218t

Glycate. See Glycopyrrolate

Glycerin (Pedia-Lax, Sani-Supp, Fleet
Liquid Supp), formulary entry
for, 802

Glycerol phenylbutyrate, for urea cycle
defects, 292

Glycogen storage disease (GSD),
294–295

Glycolic acid, for acne vulgaris, 188t

Glycopyrrolate (Robinul, Cuvposa,
Glycate), formulary entry for,
802–803

Glycosade, for GSD, 294–295

GnRH stimulation test. See
Gonadotropin-releasing hormone
stimulation test

Goiter, 223
GoLYTELY. *See* Polyethylene glycol, electrolyte solution
Gonadal tumors, 523t–524t
Gonadotropin-releasing hormone (GnRH) stimulation test, delayed puberty evaluation with, 237, 238f
Gonorrhea
  adolescent screening for, 96
  management of, 400t–401t, 694–695
  perinatal, 392t
Good Start 2 Gentle PLUS, 511t–517t
Good Start 2 Protect PLUS, 511t–517t
Good Start 2 Soy PLUS, 511t–517t
Good Start Gentle PLUS, 511t–517t
Good Start Premature 24, 511t–517t
Good Start Protect PLUS, 511t–517t
Good Start Soy PLUS, 511t–517t
Goodenough-Harris Draw-a-Person Test, 202.e1b–202.e2b, 202
Graded challenge, for drug allergy management, 340f, 341
Graft-*versus*-host disease, after bone marrow transplantation
  acute, 534.e1t, 534
  chronic, 534–535
Gralise. *See* Gabapentin
Gram stain, urine, 440
Granisetron (Kytril, Granisol, Sancuso)
  formulary entry for, 803
  for nausea and vomiting, 537
Granulomatous disease
  differential diagnosis of, 615
  sarcoidosis, 615–616
Graves disease, 223–224
Gray patch tinea capitis, 185
Great arteries, transposition of, 158t–159t
Griseofulvin (Grifulvin V, Grisactin, Griseofulvin Microsize, Gris-PEG)
  formulary entry for, 804
  for tinea capitis, 185
  for tinea infections, 411t
Gross hematuria, 450
Gross motor skills, 196, 197t–198t
Group B streptococcal (GBS) infection
  ampicillin for, 686
  perinatal, 386, 391f, 392t
Growth. *See also* Nutrition
  energy needs for, 497, 498t
    catch-up growth, 499–500, 500b
    estimation of, 497–498, 499t
    in stressed conditions, 498–499

Growth *(Continued)*
  as indicator of nutritional status, 486
  of newborns, 423
  obesity and, 235–236
  PCOS and, 236
  short stature, 233–235, 234f, 235t
  tall stature, 235
  target height range in, 233
  websites for, 485
Growth charts
  BMI
    boys, 494f
    girls, 492f
  head circumference
    boys, 486.e3f, 490f
    girls, 486.e3f, 488f
    preterm infants, 495f–496f
  height velocity
    boys, 486.e2f
    girls, 486.e1f
  interpretation of, 486
  length
    boys, 489f
    boys with Down syndrome, 486.e5f
    girls, 487f
    girls with Down syndrome, 486.e4f
    preterm infants, 495f–496f
  length-to-weight ratio
    boys, 490f
    girls, 488f
  stature
    boys, 493f
    boys with Down syndrome, 486.e7f
    girls, 491f
    girls with Down syndrome, 486.e6f
  weight
    boys, 489f
    boys with Down syndrome, 486.e5f, 486.e7f
    girls, 487f, 491f
    girls with Down syndrome, 486.e4f, 486.e6f
    preterm infants, 495f–496f
Growth failure, 499–500
Growth-plate injuries, 66, 67t, 589
GSD. *See* Glycogen storage disease
GU system. *See* Genitourinary system
Guanfacine (Intuniv, Tenex), formulary entry for, 804–805
Gynecomastia, in males, 91
Gyne-Lotrimin. *See* Clotrimazole

H

Habit spasms, 474t
Haemophilus influenza type b,
    351f–358f, 360–361, 362.e1t,
    362t, 366–367
Haemophilus influenza type b (Hib)
    conjugate vaccine, 366–367
    for children at high risk for Hib
        disease, 360–361
    for oncology patients, 362.e1t, 362t
    recommended schedules for,
        351f–358f
Haemophilus influenzae, antibiotic
    sensitivity of, 383t–385t
Hair loss, diagnosis and treatment of
    alopecia areata, CP8, 185–186
    telogen effluvium, CP8, 186
    tinea capitis, CP8, 185
    traction alopecia, CP8, 186
    trichotillomania, 186
Halcinonide (Halog), for atopic
    dermatitis, 182t–183t
Haldol. *See* Haloperidol
Haldol Decanoate. *See* Haloperidol
Halobetasol propionate (Ultravate), for
    atopic dermatitis, 182t–183t
Halog. *See* Halcinonide
Haloperidol (Haldol, Haldol
    Decanoate)
    formulary entry for, 805–806
    for mental health disorders, 209t
    palliative care with, 546t
Hand, splinting of, 58–59
Haptoglobin, 307
    reference values for, 621t–623t
Hashimoto thyroiditis, 224
HAV. *See* Hepatitis A virus
Havrix, 367
Hb. *See* Hemoglobin
HbA$_{1c}$. *See* Hemoglobin A$_{1c}$
HBIG. *See* Hepatitis B Ig
HBV. *See* Hepatitis B virus
hCG stimulation test. *See* Human
    chorionic gonadotropin
    stimulation test
HCT. *See* Hematocrit
HCTZ. *See* Hydrochlorothiazide
HCV. *See* Hepatitis C virus
HDL cholesterol. *See* High-density
    lipoprotein cholesterol
Head, imaging of, 572–573

Head circumference, growth charts for,
    486.e3f
    boys, 490f
    girls, 488f
    preterm infants, 495f–496f
Head trauma
    abusive, 84
    imaging of, 573
    minor closed, 61–64, 62t, 63b
    secondary survey of, 62t
Headaches
    evaluation of
        classification, 470
        differential diagnosis, 470b
        history, 471b
        lumbar puncture, 471, 471b
        neuroimaging, 470
        physical and neurologic
            examination, 470.e1t
    migraines
        classification of, 472
        diagnosis of, 471–472, 472b
        precursors to, 472
        seizure with, 474t
        treatment of, 472–473, 473t,
            680–681
HEADSSS assessment, 93.e1b, 93,
    93b–94b
Heart and vessel imaging
    blood flow, 583
    cardiac catheterization, 155.e1f,
        155
    cardiology radiography, 154–155,
        154f, 157t–159t
    congenital heart disease, 583, 584f
    echocardiography, 155, 583
    vessel abnormalities, 584
Heart block, 149f, 149t
Heart disease. *See* Cardiology
Heart murmurs
    benign, 137
    examination of, 128–139, 139t,
        139b–140b
    grading of, 136
    likely pathologic, 139
    systolic and diastolic, 139,
        139b–140b
Heart rate (HR)
    assessment of, 8, 128, 142t
    on ECG, 140, 142t
    monitoring of fetal, 415.e2–415.e3

Heart rhythm
   assessment of, 8
   on ECG, 140–141
Heart sounds
   abnormal, 138b
   examination of, 128
Heat rash. See Miliaria
Hecoria. See Tacrolimus
Heelstick, 27–28
Height
   growth charts for
     boys, 493f
     boys with Down syndrome, 486.e7f
     girls, 491f
     girls with Down syndrome, 486.e6f
   short stature, 233–235, 234f, 235t
   tall stature, 235
   target range of, 233
Height velocity, growth charts for
   boys, 486.e2f
   girls, 486.e1f
Heinz body preparation, 309
Helicobacter pylori
   antibiotic sensitivity of, 385t–386t
   bismuth subsalicylate for, 702–703
Hemangiomas
   clinical presentation of, 172–175
   complications of, 175–176
   diagnosis of, 175
   incidence of, 175
   management of, 176–177
   natural history of, 175
   pathogenesis of, CP3, 172
Hematocrit (HCT), age-specific values
   for, 306t
Hematology
   anemia in
     cancer patients with, 536
     causes of, 305–309
     classification of, 308t
     darbepoetin alfa for, 748–750
     diagnosis of, 305, 308t
     epoetin alfa for, 772–773
     general evaluation of, 305, 306t,
       307f
     microangiopathic hemolytic, CP12,
       315
   blood component replacement in
     blood product components,
       325–331
     blood volume, 325, 329t

Hematology *(Continued)*
     for cancer patients, 536
     complications of, 331–332
     direct donors for, 332
     for hyperleukocytosis/leukostasis,
       529
     immunoprophylaxis for patients
       treated with, 363.e1t, 363
     PRBC exchange transfusion, 331
   blood smear interpretation in, CP11,
     CP12, 332–333
   cancer care and complications in, 536
     anemia, 536
     neutropenia, 537
     thrombocytopenia, 536–537
   coagulation in
     age-specific values for, 317t–318t
     bleeding disorders, 325, 326f,
       327t–328t, 327b
     cascade, 316f
     hypercoagulable states, 319–324,
       319b–320b, 321t–324t, 325b
     tests of, 316–319, 317t–318t,
       322–324
   hemoglobinopathies in
     Hb electrophoresis for screening of,
       309, 310t
     sickle cell anemia, 309–310,
       311t–312t, 361
     thalassemias, 310–313
   neutropenia in, 313, 314t, 314b
     cancer patients with, 531–532,
       533f, 537
   newborn hematologic diseases in
     conjugated hyperbilirubinemia,
       429–430
     polycythemia, 430–431
     unconjugated hyperbilirubinemia,
       428–429, 428t, 429f–430f
   thrombocytopenia in, 313–316, 327b,
     536–537
Hematopoietic stem cell transplantation
   (HSCT)
   complications of
     aGVHD, 534.e1t, 534
     cGVHD, 534–535
     hemorrhagic cystitis, 536
     mucositis, 536
     thrombotic microangiopathy, 535
     veno-occlusive disease, 535
   goal of, 532

Hematopoietic stem cell transplantation *(Continued)*
immunoprophylaxis after, 361–362, 362.e1t
types of, 532
vaccination after, 538.e2
Hematuria, 450–451
etiology of, 451, 451t
evaluation of, 451–453, 452f
management of, 453, 453f
Hemodialysis, 450
drug dosage adjustments for, 994
for metabolic crisis, 290
Hemoglobin (Hb)
age-specific values for, 306t, 307f
electrophoresis of, 309, 310t
in urine, 439
Hemoglobin A_{1c} (HbA_{1c})
diabetes diagnosis/screening with, 214, 219
monitoring of, 219
reference values for, 621t–623t
Hemoglobin Bart, 313
Hemoglobin F, reference values for, 621t–623t
Hemoglobin SC disease, CP11
Hemoglobin SS disease, CP11
Hemoglobinopathies
Hb electrophoresis for screening of, 309, 310t
sickle cell anemia, 309–310
complications of, 310, 311t–312t
health maintenance in, 310, 312t
immunoprophylaxis for children with, 361
thalassemias, 310–313
α, 310–313
β, 313
Hemolytic anemia, 307–309
microangiopathic, CP12, 315
Hemolytic uremic syndrome (HUS), 535
Hemolytic-uremic syndrome/thrombotic thrombocytopenic purpura (HUS/TTP), 315
Hemophilia A, 326f, 327t–328t
Hemorrhage
categorization of, 72t
in child abuse patients, 84
germinal matrix, imaging of, 572
intraventricular, 431–432
subgaleal, 419f, 419t

Hemorrhagic cystitis, after bone marrow transplantation, 536
Hemothorax, 66
Henoch-Schönlein purpura (HSP), 612–614, 613t
HepA vaccine. *See* Hepatitis A vaccine
Heparin sodium. *See also* Low molecular weight heparin; Unfractionated heparin
antidote for, 920–921
formulary entry for, 806–807
for Kawasaki disease, 167.e1t
for stroke, 482–483, 531
Hepatic toxicity, of acetaminophen, 23, 24f
Hepatitis A (HepA) vaccine, 367
for oncology patients, 362.e1t
recommended schedules for, 351f–358f
Hepatitis A virus (HAV)
immunoprophylaxis for, 344, 351f–358f, 362.e1t, 367
postexposure prophylaxis for, 344, 367
Hepatitis B Ig (HBIG), 367, 368t, 389t–390t
Hepatitis B (HepB) vaccine, 367–368
for oncology patients, 362.e1t, 362t
for perinatal infection, 389t–390t
for postexposure prophylaxis, 368t
for preterm and LBW infants, 363, 364f
recommended schedules for, 351f–358f
Hepatitis B virus (HBV)
immunoprophylaxis for, 362.e1t, 351f–358f, 362t, 363, 364f, 367–368, 368t, 389t–390t
perinatal, 389t–390t
postexposure prophylaxis for, 368t, 412–413
serologic markers of, 278t
Hepatitis C virus (HCV)
perinatal, 389t–390t
postexposure prophylaxis for, 413
Hepatoblastoma, 523t–524t
Hepatocytes, injury to, liver function studies demonstrating, 276, 277t
HepB vaccine. *See* Hepatitis B vaccine
Hereditary tyrosinemia (HT1), 292

Herpes simplex virus (HSV)
    acyclovir for, 670–671
    in adolescents, 106t–107t
    in atopic dermatitis, 183
    perinatal, 389t–390t
Herpes zoster
    acyclovir for, 670–671
    reactive erythema caused by, CP11
Herpetic gingivostomatitis, reactive
        erythema caused by, CP3
Hexadrol. See Dexamethasone
Hexaxial reference system, ECG, 141f
HFOV. See High-frequency oscillatory
        ventilation
Hib and Neisseria meningitidis
        serogroups C and Y
        (Hib MenCY) vaccine series,
        371–372
    for children at high risk for
        meningococcal disease, 360
Hib vaccine. See Haemophilus
        influenza type b conjugate
        vaccine
Hiberix, 366
HIE. See Hypoxic-ischemic
        encephalopathy
High-density lipoprotein (HDL)
        cholesterol
    management of, 170
    reference values for, 621t–623t
High-frequency jet ventilation,
        75.e1–75.e2
High-frequency oscillatory ventilation
        (HFOV), 71.e2, 75
High-frequency ventilation, 71,
        75.e1, 75
Hip disorders, imaging of, 590,
        591f–593f
Histamine-1 receptor antagonists
    for anaphylaxis, 10
    for nausea and vomiting, 537
Histamine-2 receptor antagonists
    for anaphylaxis, 10
    for burns, 82
    cimetidine as, 735
    famotidine as, 781–782
    for GERD, 275
    for GI bleeding, 269
    for prolonged NSAID use, 113
    ranitidine HCl as, 927–928
Histiocytic disease, 523t–524t

History
    family, of adolescents, 94
    medical
        for allergic rhinitis, 334
        AMPLE, 61
        for developmental disorder
            evaluation, 202
        for dysmorphology, 295
        for food allergies, 337
        for headaches, 471b
        for poisoning evaluation, 19
        for PPE, 97
        for procedural sedation, 120
        for UTIs, 440
    medicosocial, adolescent, 93.e1b,
        93, 93b–94b
    natural, of food allergies, 339
    psychosocial, adolescent, 93.e1b, 93,
        93b–94b
HIV/AIDS. See Human
        immunodeficiency virus/acquired
        immunodeficiency syndrome
Hizentra. See Subcutaneous
        immunoglobulin
HLA-B27, 608
HN₂. See Mechlorethamine
Holliday-Segar method, maintenance
        fluid volume calculation with,
        247, 248t, 248b
Home, palliative care in, 543
Homocystinemia, 319b
Homovanillic acid, normal values of,
        243.e1t
Horizant. See Gabapentin
Horizontal reference system, ECG,
        141f
Hormonal contraception. See Combined
        hormonal contraception
Hospice care, 540
Howell-Jolly body, CP12
HPV. See Human papillomavirus
HPV vaccine. See Human papilloma
        virus vaccine
HR. See Heart rate
HSCT. See Hematopoietic stem cell
        transplantation
HSP. See Henoch-Schönlein purpura
HSV. See Herpes simplex virus
HT1. See Hereditary tyrosinemia
Humalog. See Lispro insulin
Human albumin. See Albumin

Human bites, 77t
  in child abuse patients, 84
  HIV transmission through, 412
  management of, 393t–399t
Human chorionic gonadotropin (hCG)
      stimulation test, cryptorchidism
      evaluation with, 242
Human immunodeficiency virus/
      acquired immunodeficiency
      syndrome (HIV/AIDS), 401–406
  adolescent screening for, 96, 402
  counseling and testing for, 402
  diagnosis of, 403t–404t
  exposure to
    nonoccupational, 411–412
    occupational, 411
    PEP for, 412
  perinatal, 389t–390t, 402–405,
      403t–404t
  immunoprophylaxis for children with,
      351f, 361, 406
  IVIG for, 341
  management of, 403t–404t,
      405–406
  opportunistic infections in,
      405.e1t–405.e2t, 405, 694–695
  revised pediatric classification system
      for, 406
Human milk, 511t–517t
Human papilloma virus vaccine (HPV
      vaccine, Gardasil, Cervarix), 368
  recommended schedules for,
      351f–358f
Human papillomavirus (HPV)
  in adolescents, 97.e1t, 97, 106t–107t
  immunoprophylaxis for, 351f–358f,
      368
  skin warts caused by, 177
Humatin. *See* Paromomycin sulfate
Humulin N. *See* Isophane insulin
Hunter syndrome, 293
Hurler syndrome, 293
HUS. *See* Hemolytic uremic syndrome
HUS/TTP. *See* Hemolytic-uremic
      syndrome/thrombotic
      thrombocytopenic purpura
Hyaluronidase (Amphadase, Hylenex,
      Vitrase), formulary entry for, 807
Hycamtin. *See* Topotecan
Hydralazine hydrochloride (Apresoline)
  formulary entry for, 807–808
  for hypertension, 463t–464t

Hydralazine hydrochloride *(Continued)*
  for hypertensive emergency, 69t
  renal failure dosage adjustments for,
      1008t–1016t
Hydrea. *See* Hydroxyurea
Hydrocephalus
  diagnosis of, 480
  treatment of, 480, 668–669
Hydrochlorothiazide (HCTZ, Hydrodiuril,
      Microzide)
  formulary entry for, 808
  for hypertension, 463t–464t
Hydrocodone, analgesic properties of,
      113.e1t
Hydrocortisone (Cetacort, Colocort,
      Cortaid, Cortef, Cortenema,
      Cortifoam, Hytone, Locoid,
      Micort-HC, NuCort, Nutracort,
      Pandel, Solu-Cortef, Synacort)
  for adrenal crisis, 230–231
  for adrenal insufficiency, 229t, 230
  for atopic dermatitis, 182t–183t
  formulary entry for, 808–809
  for hyperparathyroidism, 225
  potency of, 229t
  for shock, 73f
Hydrocortisone valerate (Westcort), for
      atopic dermatitis, 182t–183t
Hydrodiuril. *See* Hydrochlorothiazide
Hydromorphone HCl (Dilaudid, Exalgo)
  analgesic properties of, 113.e1t, 114t,
      809–810
  formulary entry for, 809–810
  PCA with, 117t
  tapering of, 118t
Hydrops fetalis, 313
Hydroxychloroquine (Plaquenil)
  for arthritis, 608.e1t, 608
  formulary entry for, 810
  for SLE, 611
21-Hydroxylase deficiency, 228–229, 228t
17-Hydroxyprogesterone (17-OHP),
      228–229, 228t
Hydroxyurea (Hydrea)
  for sickle cell disease, 312t
  toxicity of, 525t–528t
25-Hydroxyvitamin D, suggested ranges
      of, 226t
Hydroxyzine (Vistaril)
  analgesic properties of, 113.e1t
  formulary entry for, 811
  procedural sedation with, 121b–122b

Hylenex. *See* Hyaluronidase
Hyoscyamine, palliative care with, 546t
Hyperammonemia, 285, 287f
Hyperbilirubinemia, 278
  differential diagnosis of, 279t
  in newborns
    conjugated, 429–430
    unconjugated, 428–429, 428t,
      429f–430f
Hypercalcemia, 261, 261b
  calcitonin–salmon for, 707
  ECG effects of, 151t–152t
  urine calcium for diagnosis of, 447,
    447t
Hypercoagulable states, 319b
  laboratory evaluation for, 319–320,
    320b
  treatment of, 320–324, 321t–324t,
    325b
Hypercyanotic spells, 160t
Hyperglycemia, in newborns, 420, 421t,
  422f
Hypergonadotropic hypogonadism, 236
Hyperimmune globulins, 345
Hyperkalemia, 259, 259t, 260f
  ECG effects of, 151t–152t, 153, 259,
    260f
Hyperleukocytosis, 529
Hyperlipidemia, 170
Hypermagnesemia, 262, 262b
  ECG effects of, 151t–152t
Hypernatremia, 257, 258t
Hypernatremic dehydration
  deficit repletion in, 250f, 252–253
  replacement strategy for, 253.e3t, 253
Hyperparathyroidism, 225.e1b, 225
Hyperphosphatemia, 263, 263b, 675
  calcium acetate for, 708
Hyperpigmentation, post inflammatory,
  CP6
Hyperpyrexia, poisoning diagnosis and,
  20.e1t–20.e3t
Hypersal. *See* Sodium chloride, inhaled
  preparations
Hypersensitivity, insect bite-induced,
  183–184
Hypertension
  acute, 68, 69t
  chronic, 460
    antihypertensive drugs for (*See*
      Antihypertensives)
    classification of, 461, 462t

Hypertension *(Continued)*
    etiologies of, 460, 461t
    evaluation of, 460–461
    treatment of, 461
  poisoning diagnosis and,
    20.e1t–20.e3t
Hypertensive emergency, 68, 69t
Hypertensive urgency, 68, 69t
Hyperthyroidism
  characteristics of, 223
  Graves disease, 223–224
  Hashimoto thyroiditis, 224
  neonatal thyrotoxicosis, 224
  thyroid function tests demonstrating,
    220t
  thyroid storm, 224
Hypertrophic cardiomyopathy, 163–164
Hyperviscosity, hypercoagulable state
  caused by, 319b
Hypnotics. *See* Sedative-hypnotics
Hypoalbuminemia, 672
Hypocalcemia, 259–261, 261b
  ECG effects of, 151t–152t
Hypochloremia, 688
Hypogammaglobulinemia, 341
Hypoglycemia
  evaluation of, 285, 288f
  newborn screening for, 242–243
  in newborns, 420, 421t, 422f
  poisoning diagnosis and, 20.e1t–20.e3t
Hypoglycemic agents, for type II
  diabetes, 220f
Hypogonadotropic hypogonadism, 236
Hypokalemia, 257, 258t
  ECG effects of, 151t–152t
Hypomagnesemia, 262, 262b
  ECG effects of, 151t–152t
Hyponatremia
  management of, 256–257, 257t
  SIADH causing, 231–232
Hyponatremic dehydration
  deficit repletion in, 250f, 252
  replacement strategy for, 253.e2t,
    253
Hypoparathyroidism, 224–225
Hypoperfusion, poisoning diagnosis
  and, 20.e1t–20.e3t
Hypophosphatemia, 263, 263b
Hypoplastic left heart syndrome, 161
Hypotension, 8
  asthma-associated, 11
  poisoning diagnosis and, 20.e1t–20.e3t

Hypothermia
  for HIE in newborn, 419–420
  poisoning diagnosis and, 20.e1t–20.e3t
Hypothyroidism
  characteristics and types of, 219, 222t
  newborn screening for, 223
  obesity and, 219–223, 235
  thyroid function tests demonstrating,
    220t
Hypotonia, 295, 296f–298f
Hypotonic fluids, 248–249
Hypovolemia, 672
Hypovolemic shock, 71.e1t, 71
Hypoxia, poisoning diagnosis and,
    20.e1t–20.e3t
Hypoxic-ischemic encephalopathy
    (HIE), in newborns, 419–420
Hytone. See Hydrocortisone

I

131I. See Radioactive iodine
IBD. See Inflammatory bowel disease
IBIH. See Insect bite-induced
    hypersensitivity
Ibuprofen (Advil, Caldolor, Children's
    Advil, Children's Motrin, Motrin,
    NeoProfen)
  analgesic properties of, 113
  for arthritis, 608
  formulary entry for, 811–812
  neonate dosages of, 435
  for PDA, 428
ICF deficit. See Intracellular fluid deficit
Ichthyosis, CP7, 184
ICP. See Intracranial pressure
ID. See Intellectual disability
Idarubicin (Idamycin), toxicity of,
    525t–528t
IDEA. See Individuals with Disabilities
    Education Act
Idiopathic thrombocytopenic purpura
    (ITP), 313–315
Ifosfamide (Isophosphamide, Ifex)
  late effects of, 538.e1t
  toxicity of, 525t–528t
Ig. See Immunoglobulin
IGF-1. See Insulin-like growth factor 1
IGF-BP3. See Insulin-like growth factor
    binding protein
IGRA. See Interferon gamma release
    assay
IIV. See Inactivated influenza vaccine

IL-1 receptor antagonists. See
    Interleukin-1 receptor
    antagonists
Ilotycin. See Erythromycin preparations
IM injection. See Intramuscular injection
Imaging. See Radiology
Imatinib (Gleevec), toxicity of, 525t–528t
Imidazole carboxamide. See
    Dacarbazine
IMIG. See Intramuscular
    immunoglobulin
Imipenem, sensitivity-based selection of,
    383t–384t
Imipenem and cilastin (Primaxin)
  formulary entry for, 812–813
  renal failure dosage adjustments for,
    995t–1007t
Imipramine (Tofranil), formulary entry
    for, 813–814
Imiquimod, for genital warts, 106t–107t
Imitrex. See Sumatriptan succinate
Immune thrombocytopenic purpura, 341
Immunization. See also specific
    vaccines
  administration of, 350–359
    by intramuscular injection, 54
    by subcutaneous injection, 53
  for animal bites, 78
  for burns, 82
  after cancer treatment, 538.e2
  in children with HIV disease, 406
  with combination vaccines, 378
  general indications and precautions
    for, 359–360
  informed consent for, 350
  misconceptions regarding, 359
  recommended schedules for, 350,
    351f–358f
  for sickle cell disease, 312t
  vaccine types used in, 359
Immunocompetent children, 360
Immunocompromised children, 360
Immunodeficiency
  congenital, immunoprophylaxis for
    children with, 361
  evaluation for, 341, 342t–343t
Immunoglobulin (Ig)
  IgA, 342t–343t, 345t–346t
  IgE, 345t–346t
    allergen-specific, 334, 338–339
  IgG, 345t–346t
  IgM, 345t–346t

Immunoglobulin therapy
  formulary entry for, 814–815
  for HBV, 367, 368t, 389t–390t
  hyperimmune globulins, 345
  IMIG (*See* Intramuscular
    immunoglobulin)
  immunoprophylaxis for patients
    treated with, 363.e1t, 363
  IVIG (*See* Intravenous
    immunoglobulin)
  for measles, 344, 370–371
  monoclonal antibody preparations,
    345
  for rabies, 344, 373–374, 374t
  $RH_O(D)$ immune globulin intravenous
    as, 929
  for RSV, 374–375
  for rubella, 344, 371
  subcutaneous (*See* Subcutaneous
    immunoglobulin)
  for tetanus, 365
  for varicella, 376–377, 389t–390t,
    405.e1t–405.e2t
Immunology. *See also* Immunoglobulin
    therapy
  allergic reactions
    dermatitis, CP10, 194
    drug, 339–341, 340f
    food, 336–339, 338f, 518t–519t
    rhinitis, 334–336, 336t, 693–694
  complement pathway, 348f
  evaluation of suspected
    immunodeficiency, 341,
    342t–343t
  reference values for
    lymphocyte enumeration, 347t
    serum complement levels, 347t
    serum IgG, IgM, IgA, and IgE
      levels, 345t
    serum IgG, IgM, IgA, and IgE levels
      for LBW preterm infants, 346t
    serum IgG subclass levels, 346t
Immunoprophylaxis. *See also*
    Immunization
  combination vaccines for, 378
  for special hosts
    children at high risk for Hib
      disease, 360–361
    children at high risk for
      meningococcal disease, 360
    children at high risk for
      pneumococcal disease, 360

Immunoprophylaxis *(Continued)*
    children with asplenia, 361
    children with congenital
      immunodeficiency disorders, 361
    children with HIV disease, 351f,
      361, 406
    oncology patients, 361–362,
      362.e1t, 362t
    patients on biological response
      modifier therapy, 363
    patients on corticosteroids, 362,
      362t
    patients treated with
      immunoglobulin or other blood
      products, 363.e1t, 363
    patients with solid organ
      transplants, 362
    pregnant patients, 363
    preterm and LBW infants, 363,
      364f
    travelers to foreign countries, 363
  for specific diseases
    diphtheria, 351f–358f, 362.e1t,
      362t, 363
    haemophilus influenza type b,
      351f–358f, 360–361, 362t,
      362.e1t, 366–367
    HAV, 344, 351f–358f, 362.e1t, 367
    HBV, 351f–358f, 362.e1t, 362t,
      363, 364f, 367–368, 368t,
      389t–390t
    HPV, 351f–358f, 368
    influenza, 312t, 351f–358f, 362t,
      362.e1t, 363, 366–370, 676
    measles, 344, 351f–358f, 361,
      362t, 362.e1t, 363, 363.e1t,
      370–371
    meningococcal infection, 312t,
      351f–358f, 360, 362t, 362.e1t,
      371–372
    mumps, 351f–358f, 361, 362t,
      362.e1t, 363.e1t, 363,
      370–371
    pertussis, 351f–358f, 362t,
      362.e1t, 363
    pneumococcal infection, 362.e1t,
      312t, 351f–358f, 360, 362t,
      372
    poliomyelitis, 351f–358f, 362t,
      362.e1t, 373
    rabies, 78, 344, 373–374, 374t
    rotavirus, 351f–358f, 375–376

Immunoprophylaxis *(Continued)*
  RSV, 374–375
  rubella, 344, 351f–358f, 361,
    362t, 362.e1t, 363, 363.e1t,
    370–371
  tetanus, 362.e1t, 78, 82,
    351f–358f, 362t, 363
  tuberculosis, 376
  typhoid fever, 376
  varicella, 362.e1t, 363.e1t,
    351f–358f, 361, 362t, 363,
    376–377
  yellow fever, 377–378
  websites for, 350
Immunosuppressants
  for arthritis, 608.e1t, 608
  azathioprine as, 693
  cyclosporine as, 745–746
  for GVHD prevention, 534
  for HSP, 614
  for IBD, 274
  mycophenolate as, 867–868
  for pemphigus vulgaris, 193
  pimecrolimus as, 907
  for scleroderma, 616.e2
  sirolimus as, 941–942
  for SLE, 611
  tacrolimus as, 954–955
Immunotherapy, for allergic rhinitis,
    336
Imodium. *See* Loperamide
Impaired glucose tolerance, 518t–519t
Impetigo, 192
Imuran. *See* Azathioprine
IMV. *See* Intermittent mandatory
    ventilation
Inactivated influenza vaccine (IIV),
    368–370
  during pregnancy, 363
  recommended schedules for,
    351f–358f
Inactivated poliovirus (IPV) vaccine, 373
  for oncology patients, 362.e1t, 362t
  recommended schedules for,
    351f–358f
Inapsine. *See* Droperidol
Inches, conversion formulas for, 633
Incidence, 639
Inderal. *See* Propranolol
Indirect Coombs test, 307
Individuals with Disabilities Education
    Act (IDEA), 212

Indomethacin (Indocin)
  formulary entry for, 815–816
  for IVH, 432
  for PDA, 427–428
Infant formulas
  mixing instructions for, 510t
  nutrition components of, 509
  for special clinical circumstances,
    518t–519t
  websites for, 485
Infantile eczema, CP6, 180
Infantile proctocolitis, 337
Infantile spasms, 476t–477t
Infants. *See also* Neonates/newborns.
  age-appropriate behavioral issues in,
    196, 199t–200t
  catch-up growth requirements for,
    499–500, 500b
  constipation in, 273
  DRIs for, 501t–503t, 507t–509t
  EER for, 498
  HIV exposure and diagnosis in,
    403t–404t, 405
  HIV management in, 403t–404t
  mean TSH and T$_4$ of, 221t
  multivitamins for, 504t
  pain assessment for, 111, 112t
  physiologic anemia of, 309
Infasurf. *See* Surfactant, pulmonary/
    calfactant
Infection. *See also specific infectious
    diseases*
  of animal bite wounds, 78
  in atopic dermatitis, 183
  blood transfusion transmission of, 332
  bloodborne pathogen exposure
    HBV prophylaxis after, 368t,
      412–413
    HCV prophylaxis after, 413
    HIV prophylaxis after, 411–412
  common pediatric, 393t–399t
  ear, 393t–399t, 682, 694–695
  fever without localizing source,
    380–382, 387f
  granulomatous disease with, 615
  immunodeficiency indicated by, 342t
  impetigo, 192
  in internationally adopted children,
    413
  intrauterine, 382, 388t, 572–573,
    386.e1t
  of lymph node, 524

Infection *(Continued)*
  microbiology studies for
    rapid identification of aerobic
      bacteria, 381f–382f
    sensitivity-based antibiotic
      selection, 380, 383t–386t
    specimen collection for blood
      culture, 380
    urine culture, 442
  as oncologic emergency, 531–532,
    533f
  opportunistic, 405.e1t–405.e2t, 405,
    694–695
  perinatal *(See* Perinatal infection)
  red cell aplasia caused by, 309
  STIs *(See* Sexually transmitted
    infection)
  tickborne *(See* Tickborne illnesses)
  UTIs *(See* Urinary tract infections)
Infectious rhinitis, 335
INFeD. *See* Iron, injectable preparations
Infertility, in CF patients, 568
Infiltrate, imaging of, 580
Inflammation
  acute phase reactant laboratory
    studies for, 602–603
  anemia caused by, 309
Inflammatory bowel disease (IBD)
  classification of, 274
  evaluation of, 274
  management of, 274
Infliximab, for arthritis, 608
Influenza
  chemoprophylaxis for, 369–370, 676
  immunization for, 366–370
    for oncology patients, 362.e1t, 362t
    during pregnancy, 363
    recommended schedules for,
      351f–358f
    for sickle cell disease, 312t
  management of, 393t–399t, 676
Informed consent. *See* Consent
INH. *See* Isoniazid
Inhalation injury, 79t, 80–82
Inhaled anesthetics, for asthma, 11
Inhaled corticosteroids, for asthma,
  558.e1t–558.e2t, 562f–564f
Injectable local anesthetics, analgesic
    properties of, 113–116, 115t
Injections
  intramuscular, 54
  subcutaneous, 53

Inotropes
  digoxin as, 758
  for hypertrophic cardiomyopathy, 164
  milrinone as, 861
  for PPHN, 425
  for shock, 71.e1t, 73f
INR. *See* International normalized ratio
Insect bite-induced hypersensitivity
    (IBIH), 183–184
Inspiratory time (Ti), 74
Inspired oxygen concentration (Fi_{O_2}), 74
Insulin
  currently available products of, 218t
  for diabetic ketoacidosis, 216, 217f,
    218t
  dosing of, 218t
  formulary entry for, 816
  for hyperkalemia, 260f
  neonate dosages of, 435
  renal failure dosage adjustments for,
    1008t–1016t
  in type I compared with type II
    diabetes, 215
  for type II diabetes, 220f
Insulin/dextrose
  for beta blocker poisoning, 21t
  for calcium channel blocker
    poisoning, 21t
Insulin-like growth factor 1 (IGF-1),
    normal levels of, 235t
Insulin-like growth factor binding protein
    (IGF-BP3), normal values of,
    243.e2t, 243
Intal. *See* Cromolyn
Intellectual disability (ID), 205
  severity levels for, 206t–207t
Interferon alfa-2a, for Behçet disease,
    616.e2
Interferon gamma release assay (IGRA),
    for TB testing, 406
Interleukin-1 (IL-1) receptor antagonists,
    for arthritis, 608
Intermittent mandatory ventilation
    (IMV), 74
Internal jugular vein, catheter placement
    in, 31, 33, 34f–35f
International normalized ratio (INR),
    age-specific values for,
    317t–318t
Internationally adopted children,
    infection in, 413
Intervals, on ECG, 141, 142t

Intestinal obstruction
 formula for, 518t–519t
 imaging of, 584–586, 586f
 in newborns, 431.e1t
Intraabdominal infections, 393t–399t
Intracellular fluid (ICF) deficit,
  electrolyte replacement based
  on, 249–252, 251t
Intracranial pressure (ICP)
 increased
  critical care of, 69–70
  minor CHT with, 63
  as oncologic emergency, 530
 lumbar puncture and, 42
Intramuscular immunoglobulin (IMIG,
  GamaSTAN)
 administration of, 344
 adverse reactions to, 344
 doses of, 344
 formulary entry for, 814–815
 indications for, 343–344
 precautions for, 344
Intramuscular (IM) injection, 54
Intraosseous (IO) infusion, 37–38, 37f
Intrapartum FHR monitoring,
  415.e2–415.e3
Intrapulmonary shunt fraction (Qs/Qt),
  76.e1
Intrauterine device (IUD), 103
Intrauterine infections, 382, 386.e1t,
  388t, 572–573
Intravaginal antifungals, for yeast
  infections, 105t
Intravenous fluids (IVFs), 246
Intravenous immunoglobulin (IVIG,
  Carimune NF, Flebogamma
  DIF, Gamunex-C, Gammagard,
  Gammaked, Gammaplex,
  Octagam, Privigen)
 adverse reactions to, 343
 for antibody-deficient disorders, 341
 for bone marrow transplantation,
  341
 for CMV, 405.e1t–405.e2t
 for enterovirus, 389t–390t
 formulary entry for, 814–815
 for immune thrombocytopenic
  purpura, 341
 immunoprophylaxis for patients
  treated with, 363.e1t, 363
 indications for, 341
 for Kawasaki disease, 167–168, 341

Intravenous immunoglobulin (Continued)
 for pediatric HIV infection with
  antibody deficiency, 341
 for pemphigus vulgaris, 193
 precautions for, 343
 for thrombocytopenia, 315
 for unconjugated hyperbilirubinemia
  in newborns, 428
 for varicella, 389t–390t,
  405.e1t–405.e2t
Intraventricular hemorrhage (IVH), in
  newborns, 431–432
Intropin. See Dopamine
Intubation, 4–7
 for asthma, 11
 drugs used for, 4, 5f, 6t–7t,
  691–692
 treatment algorithm for, 5f
Intuniv. See Guanfacine
Intussusception, 588, 588f
Invanz. See Ertapenem
Invasive bacterial infection,
  405.e1t–405.e2t
IO infusion. See Intraosseous infusion
Iodine, DRIs for, 507t–508t
Iohexol (Omnipaque), formulary entry
  for, 816–817
Iosat. See Potassium iodide
Ipratropium bromide (Atrovent)
 for allergic rhinitis, 336
 for asthma, 10
 formulary entry for, 817–818
IPV vaccine. See Inactivated poliovirus
  vaccine
Iquix. See Levofloxacin
Irbesartan, for hypertension, 463t–464t
Irinotecan (Camptosar, IRN), toxicity of,
  525t–528t
Iron
 deferoxamine mesylate for overload
  of, 750–751
 deficiency of, blood smear
  demonstrating, CP11
 DRIs for, 507t–508t
 newborn requirements for, 423
 poisoning with, 21t
 reference values for, 621t–623t
 supplementation of, 504, 820
Iron, injectable preparations
  (DexFerrum, Ferrlecit, INFeD,
  Venofer), formulary entry for,
  818–819

Iron, oral preparations (Feosol, Fergon, Fer-In-Sol, Niferex, Slow FE), 504t
  formulary entry for, 820
  neonate dosages of, 435
Iron dextran. *See* Iron, injectable preparations
Iron sucrose. *See* Iron, injectable preparations
Iron-deficiency anemia, 305
Irradiated blood products, 330
Irritant contact dermatitis, 193
Islet cell autoantibodies, 215
Isoflurane, for asthma, 11
Isomil Advance, 511t–517t
Isomil DF, 511t–517t
IsonaRif. *See* Isoniazid with rifampin
Isonatremic dehydration
  deficit repletion in, 249–252, 250f, 251t
  replacement strategy for, 253.e1t, 253
Isoniazid (INH, Laniazid, Nydrazid)
  formulary entry for, 820–821
  for tuberculosis, 405.e1t, 407. e1t–407.e2t, 407–408
Isoniazid with rifampin (Rifamate, IsonaRif), formulary entry for, 820–821
Isoniazid with rifampin and pyrazinamide (Rifater), formulary entry for, 820–821
Isophane insulin (NPH, Humulin N, Novolin N), 218t
Isophosphamide. *See* Ifosfamide
Isoproterenol (Isuprel), formulary entry for, 821
Isoptin. *See* Verapamil
Isopto Carpine. *See* Pilocarpine HCl
Isopto Hyoscine. *See* Scopolamine hydrobromide
Isosexual precocious puberty, 238
Isosource formulas, 511t–517t
Isotonic fluid, fluid replacement with, 253
Isotretinoin (Absorica, Accutane, Amnesteem, Claravis, Myorisan, Zenatane)
  for acne vulgaris, 188, 189t
  formulary entry for, 822
Isradipine, for hypertension, 463t–464t
Isuprel. *See* Isoproterenol
ITP. *See* Idiopathic thrombocytopenic purpura

Itraconazole (Onmel, Sporanox)
  formulary entry for, 822–823
  for tinea infections, 411t
IUD. *See* Intrauterine device
Ivermectin, for scabies, 178
IVFs. *See* Intravenous fluids
IVH. *See* Intraventricular hemorrhage
IVIG. *See* Intravenous immunoglobulin

J

Jantoven. *See* Warfarin
Jaundice
  poisoning diagnosis and, 20.e1t–20.e3t
  transient neonatal, 279t
JE. *See* Japanese encephalitis
Jevity formulas, 511t–517t
JIA. *See* Juvenile idiopathic arthritis
Joint Commission, do not use list of, 667, 667t–668t
Joint fluid analysis, 605, 605f, 632t
Joint pain, differential diagnosis of, 609t
Jones criteria, 169b
JRA. *See* Juvenile rheumatoid arthritis
Jugular vein
  external
    catheter placement in, 28f, 31, 33
    puncture of, 28–29, 28f
  internal, catheter placement in, 31, 33, 34f–35f
Junctional rhythm, 145t–146t
Junctional SVT, 145t–146t
Juvenile dermatomyositis, 614–615
Juvenile idiopathic arthritis (JIA), 606
  autoantibodies associated with, 603t
  classical divisions of, 607t
Juvenile myoclonic epilepsy, 476t–477t
Juvenile rheumatoid arthritis (JRA), 606
  autoantibodies associated with, 603t
  joint fluid analysis for, 605f

K

Kadian. *See* Morphine sulfate
Kanamycin (Kantrex)
  formulary entry for, 823
  renal failure dosage adjustments for, 995t–1007t
Kaopectate. *See* Bismuth subsalicylate
Kao-Tin. *See* Bismuth subsalicylate; Docusate
Kapvay. *See* Clonidine

Karyotyping
  for dysmorphology, 299
  fetal, 415.e1
Kasabach-Merritt phenomenon, 175
Kawasaki disease, 613t
  acquired heart disease with,
      166–168, 167.e1t, 167f
  IVIG for, 167–168, 341
Kayexalate. *See* Sodium polystyrene
      sulfonate
Keflex. *See* Cephalexin
Kemstro. *See* Baclofen
Kenalog. *See* Triamcinolone
Keppra. *See* Levetiracetam
Keratolytics, for warts, 177
Keratosis pilaris, CP5
Kerion, CP8, 185
Ketamine (Ketalar)
  analgesic properties of, 113.e1t, 125t
  formulary entry for, 824
  procedural sedation with, 119,
      121b–122b, 125t
  for RSI, 5f, 6t–7t
  for tet spells, 160t
Ketoacidosis. *See also* Diabetic
      ketoacidosis.
  in type I compared with type II
      diabetes, 215
KetoCal, nutrition components in,
      511t–517t
Ketoconazole (Nizoral, Extina, Xolegel),
      formulary entry for, 824–825
Ketogenic diet, for seizure, 476t–477t,
      480
Ketones, in urine, 439
Ketorolac (Toradol, Acular, Acuvail)
  analgesic properties of, 113.e1t, 113
  formulary entry for, 825
Ketotifen fumarate (Zaditor), for allergic
      conjunctivitis, 336t
Kidney failure. *See* Renal failure
Kidney function tests
  for distal tubular function, 447, 447t
  for glomerular function, 445–446,
      445t–446t
  for proximal tubular function,
      446–447
Kidney stones. *See* Nephrolithiasis
Kidneys. *See also* Nephrology.
  imaging of, 443–444, 443f
Kilograms, conversion formulas for, 633
Kindercal TF Vanilla, 511t–517t

Kinrix, 378
Kionex. *See* Sodium polystyrene
      sulfonate
Klebsiella spp., antibiotic sensitivity of,
      383t–385t
Klonopin. *See* Clonazepam
Klout. *See* Pyrethrins
Klumpke paralysis, 433t
Kondremul. *See* Mineral oil
Konsyl. *See* Psyllium
K-PHOS Neutral. *See* Phosphorus
      supplements
Kristalose. *See* Lactulose
Kytril. *See* Granisetron

L

LABAs. *See* Long-acting beta$_2$-agonists
Labetalol (Normodyne, Trandate)
  formulary entry for, 826
  for hypertension, 463t–464t
  for hypertensive emergency, 69t
Labor, preventing HIV transmission
      during, 405
Laboratory studies. *See also* Blood
      chemistries.
  for developmental disorder evaluation,
      203–205
  for diabetic ketoacidosis, 216, 217f
  for metabolic disorders
    initial tests, 285, 286b
    sample collection for, 286t
  for rheumatologic disease
    acute phase reactants, 602–603
    autoantibodies, 603–604, 603t
    complement, 604
    joint fluid analysis, 605, 605f
    serum muscle enzymes, 605
    UA, 604
Laceration repair
  skin staples, 56–57
  suturing, 54–56, 55f, 56t
  tissue adhesives, 57
Lacosamide (Vimpat)
  formulary entry for, 826–827
  renal failure dosage adjustments for,
      1008t–1016t
  for seizures, 479t
Lactate, reference values for, 621t–623t
Lactate dehydrogenase (LDH)
  in hemolytic anemia, 307
  reference values for, 621t–623t
  in transudate *vs.* exudate, 630t

Lactated Ringers (LR), fluid replacement
    with, 253
Lactation. *See* Breastfeeding
Lactose intolerance, formula for,
    518t–519t
Lactulose (Cephulac, Chronulac,
    Enulose, Kristalose)
    for constipation, 272–273
    formulary entry for, 827
LAIV. *See* Live, attenuated influenza
    vaccine
Lamictal. *See* Lamotrigine
Lamivudine (Epivir, 3TC)
    formulary entry for, 828
    for PEP, 412
    renal failure dosage adjustments for,
        995t–1007t
Lamotrigine (Lamictal)
    formulary entry for, 828–831
    for seizures, 479t
Language, 196
    developmental milestones in,
        197t–198t
    disorders of, 205
Laniazid. *See* Isoniazid
Lanoxin. *See* Digoxin
Lansoprazole (Prevacid, First-
    Lansoprazole), formulary entry
    for, 831
Lantus. *See* Glargine insulin
Lariam. *See* Mefloquine HCl
Laryngeal mask airway (LMA), 4
Laryngoscope blade, 4
Laryngotracheobronchitis. *See* Croup
Lasix. *See* Furosemide
L-Asp. *See* Asparaginase
L-asparaginase, in cancer-related
    stroke, 531
Last menstrual period (LMP), 415.e1
Lateral chest radiograph, normal
    anatomy on, 581f–582f
Laxatives
    bisacodyl as, 702
    for constipation, 272–273
    docusate as, 762–763
    glycerin as, 802
    lactulose as, 827
    magnesium citrate as, 843
    magnesium hydroxide as, 844
    mineral oil as, 862
    polyethylene glycol, electrolyte
        solution as, 908–909

Laxatives *(Continued)*
    psyllium as, 922
    senna/sennosides as, 938
    sodium phosphate as, 944
Lax-Pills. *See* Senna/sennosides
Lazanda. *See* Fentanyl
LBBB. *See* Left bundle-branch block
LBW infants. *See* Low-birth-weight
    infants
L-Carnitine. *See* Carnitine
LDH. *See* Lactate dehydrogenase
LDL cholesterol. *See* Low-density
    lipoprotein cholesterol
LDs. *See* Learning disabilities
Lead, reference values for, 621t–623t
Lead placement, for ECG, 140, 141f
Lead poisoning, 23, 25t
    EDTA calcium disodium for, 767
Learning disabilities (LDs), 205–207
Leflunomide, for arthritis, 608.e1t
Left bundle-branch block (LBBB), 150t
Left ventricular hypertrophy (LVH), 145b
Legacy, palliative care and, 543
Legg-Calvé-Perthes disease, 590, 592f
Legionella spp., antibiotic sensitivity
    of, 385t
Legs. *See* Extremities
Leishmaniasis, 685
Length
    conversion formulas for, 633
    growth charts for
        boys, 489f
        boys with Down syndrome, 486.e5f
        girls, 487f
        girls with Down syndrome, 486.e4f
        preterm infants, 495f–496f
Length-to-weight ratio, growth charts for
    boys, 490f
    girls, 488f
Lennox-Gastaut syndrome, 476t–477t
Leptospirosis, 383t–384t
Leucovorin
    toxicity of, 525t–528t
    for *Toxoplasma gondii* infection,
        405.e1t–405.e2t
Leukemia
    hyperleukocytosis/leukostasis in, 529
    signs and symptoms of, 523t–524t
Leukemic blasts, blood smear
    demonstrating, CP12
Leukocyte adhesion deficiency,
    342t–343t

Leukocyte esterase test, 439
  for UTIs, 441
Leukocyte-poor platelets, 330
Leukocyte-poor PRBCs, 329
Leukocytes, age-specific values of, 314t
Leukostasis, 529
Leukotriene receptor antagonists
    (LTRAs)
  for allergic rhinitis, 335
  for asthma, 563f–564f
  montelukast as, 865
  zafirlukast as, 982
Leuprolide, GnRH stimulation test with,
    237
Leustatin. *See* Cladribine
Levalbuterol (Xopenex), formulary entry
    for, 832
Levamisole, for nephrotic syndrome, 456
Levaquin. *See* Levofloxacin
Levemir. *See* Detemir insulin
Levetiracetam (Keppra)
  formulary entry for, 832–833
  renal failure dosage adjustments for,
    1008t–1016t
  for seizure, 476t–477t, 479t
  for status epilepticus, 16t
Levocarnitine. *See* Carnitine
Levocetirizine, for allergic rhinitis, 335
Levofloxacin (Iquix, Levaquin, Quixin)
  formulary entry for, 833–834
  for meningitis, 393t–399t
  renal failure dosage adjustments for,
    995t–1007t
  sensitivity-based selection of, 385t
  for sinusitis, 393t–399t
Levonorgestrel (Plan B One Step, Next
    Choice), for adolescents, 102–103
Levophed. *See* Norepinephrine
    bitartrate
Levothyroxine (T₄, Synthroid, Tirosint,
    Unithroid), formulary entry for,
    834–835
Lexapro. *See* Escitalopram
LH. *See* Luteinizing hormone
Lialda. *See* Mesalamine
Licide. *See* Pyrethrins
Lidex. *See* Fluocinonide
Lidocaine (Xylocaine, L-M-X, Lidoderm)
  analgesic properties of, 115t, 116,
    125t
  formulary entry for, 835–836
  for RSI, 5f, 6t–7t

Lidocaine and prilocaine (Oraqix)
  analgesic properties of, 115t, 125t
  formulary entry for, 836–837
Lidoderm. *See* Lidocaine
Likelihood ratio (LR), 641
Lindane (Gamma benzene hexachloride),
    formulary entry for, 837
Linear morphea, 616.e1
Linezolid (Zyvox)
  formulary entry for, 838
  sensitivity-based selection of, 386t
Lioresal. *See* Baclofen
Lipase
  reference values for, 621t–623t
  supplementation of, 989t
Lipids
  monitoring of
    goals for levels in childhood, 169
    hyperlipidemia management, 170
  screening of children and
    adolescents, 168–169
  reference values for, 621t–623t
Liquid diets, formula for, 518t–519t
Liquid Pred. *See* Prednisone
Lisdexamfetamine (Vyvanse), formulary
    entry for, 839
Lisinopril (Prinivil, Zestril)
  formulary entry for, 839–840
  for hypertension, 463t–464t
  renal failure dosage adjustments for,
    1008t–1016t
Listeria monocytogenes, perinatal
    infection with, 392t
Listeria spp., antibiotic sensitivity of,
    383t–384t, 386t
Literacy, Reach Out and Read
    milestones of, 196, 198t
Lithium (Lithobid, Eskalith)
  formulary entry for, 840
  renal failure dosage adjustments for,
    1008t–1016t
Live, attenuated influenza vaccine
    (LAIV), 368–370
  for children with HIV disease, 361
  recommended schedules for, 351f–358f
Liver
  acetaminophen toxicity and, 23
  acute failure of, 276
    etiologies of, 276–277
    evaluation of, 277–278, 278t
    presentation of, 277

Liver *(Continued)*
coagulopathy caused by, 327b
function studies of, 276, 277t
hyperbilirubinemia of, 278, 279t
LMA. *See* Laryngeal mask airway
LMP. *See* Last menstrual period
LMWH. *See* Low molecular weight heparin
L-M-X. *See* Lidocaine
Lobular capillary hemangioma. *See* Pyogenic granuloma
Local anesthetics
analgesic properties of, 113.e1t, 113–116, 115t, 125t
lidocaine and prilocaine as, 115t, 125t
lidocaine as, 835–836
Localized scleroderma, 616.e1
Locoid. *See* Hydrocortisone
Lodoxamide tromethamine ophthalmic (Alomide), 991t–992t
Lomustine (CCNU), toxicity of, 525t–528t
Long arm posterior splint, 58, 58f
Long bones, trauma to, 66, 67f, 67t
in child abuse patients, 85t
imaging of, 589
Long QT, 150–153
Long-acting beta$_2$-agonists (LABAs)
for asthma, 562f–564f
fluticasone propionate and salmeterol as, 792–793
formoterol as, 705, 795–796
salmeterol as, 936
Loniten. *See* Minoxidil
Loperamide (Imodium), formulary entry for, 841
Lopinavir, for PEP, 412
Lopressor. *See* Metoprolol
Loratadine
for allergic rhinitis, 335
renal failure dosage adjustments for, 1008t–1016t
Loratadine and pseudoephedrine (Alavert, Claritin), formulary entry for, 841–842
Lorazepam (Ativan)
analgesic properties of, 113.e1t
formulary entry for, 842
for nausea and vomiting, 537
neonate dosages of, 435
palliative care with, 546t
procedural sedation with, 123t
for status epilepticus, 16t

Losartan (Cozaar)
formulary entry for, 843
for hypertension, 463t–464t
for Marfan syndrome, 302
Lotrimin AF. *See* Clotrimazole; Miconazole
Lovenox. *See* Enoxaparin
Low molecular weight heparin (LMWH), 320–322
enoxaparin as, 769–770
for Kawasaki disease, 167.e1t
for stroke, 482–483
Low-birth-weight (LBW) infants, 415
immunoprophylaxis for, 363, 364f
serum IgG, IgM, IgA, and IgE reference values for, 346t
Low-density lipoprotein (LDL) cholesterol
goal levels of, 169
management of, 170
reference values for, 621t–623t
Lower airway, foreign bodies in, 576
Lower motor neuron examination, 469t
L-PAM. *See* Melphalan
LR. *See* Lactated Ringers; Likelihood ratio
L-thyroxine, for hypothyroidism, 220t
LTRAs. *See* Leukotriene receptor antagonists
Lubricants, mineral oil as, 862
Lucinactant. *See* Surfactant therapy
Lumbar puncture, 42–44, 43f
for headache evaluation, 471, 471b
for seizure, 475
Luminal. *See* Phenobarbital
Lung volumes, 553, 555f, 555t
Lungs. *See also* Pulmonology.
chest radiography of, 154–155, 157t–159t
Luride. *See* Fluoride
Luteinizing hormone (LH)
in delayed puberty, 236–237, 237t, 238f
normal levels of, 237t
in precocious puberty, 237t, 239
Luvox. *See* Fluvoxamine
Luxiq. *See* Betamethasone
LVH. *See* Left ventricular hypertrophy
Lyme disease, 408–409
acquired heart disease with, 168
antibiotic selection for, 383t–384t, 682
joint fluid analysis for, 605f

Lymph nodes
  infection of, 524
  palpation of, 525
  reactive, 524
  size of, 525
Lymphadenitis, 393t–399t
Lymphadenopathy
  etiologies of, 524–525
  initial workup for, 525
  physical findings of, 525
Lymphocytes
  age-specific values of, 314t
  reference count values for, 347t
Lymphoma, 523t–524t
Lyrica. *See* Pregabalin
Lysosomal storage diseases, 293

M

M mode echocardiography, 155.e1
Maalox. *See* Aluminum hydroxide with magnesium hydroxide
Macrobid. *See* Nitrofurantoin
Macrocytic anemia, 308t
Macrodantin. *See* Nitrofurantoin
Macrolides
  azithromycin as, 694–695
  clarithromycin as, 737–738
  erythromycin ethylsuccinate and acetylsulfisoxazole as, 776
  erythromycin preparations as, 776–777
  sensitivity-based selection of, 385t
Macule, 172, 173f–174f
MAG-3. *See* Mercaptoacetyl triglycine
Mag-200. *See* Magnesium oxide
Magnesium. *See also* Hypermagnesemia; Hypomagnesemia.
  DRIs for, 507t–508t
  for migraine headaches, 472
  reference values for, 621t–623t
  serum disturbances in, 262, 262b
Magnesium citrate
  for constipation, 272
  formulary entry for, 843
Magnesium hydroxide (Milk of Magnesia)
  for constipation, 272–273
  formulary entry for, 844
Magnesium oxide (Mag-200, Mag-Ox 400, Uro-Mag), formulary entry for, 844

Magnesium sulfate (Epsom salts)
  for asthma, 11
  formulary entry for, 845
  for TCA poisoning, 21t
Magnetic resonance imaging (MRI)
  head imaging with, 572–573
  for neck injury, 65
  in place of CT, 572
  for seizures, 475
Mag-Ox 400. *See* Magnesium oxide
Maintenance dose, adjustments for renal failure, 994
Maintenance fluids, 246
  requirements for, 246, 247f
    caloric calculations of maintenance volume, 247–248, 248b, 248t
Maintenance solute, requirements for, 248–249, 248t, 256t
Major depressive disorder
  assessment of, 210
  epidemiology of, 210
  treatment of, 209t, 210–211
Malabsorption
  formula for, 518t–519t
  syndromes of, 339
Malaria, blood smear demonstrating, CP12
Malignancy. *See* Cancer
Malnourished children, catch-up growth requirements for, 499–500, 500b
Manganese, DRIs for, 507t–508t
Mannitol (Aridol, Osmitrol, Resectisol)
  formulary entry for, 845–846
  for hyperphosphatemia, 263
  for increased ICP, 70, 530
MAP. *See* Mean arterial pressure
Marfan syndrome, 301–302
Marinol. *See* Dronabinol
Maroteaux-Lamy syndrome, 293
Mast cell stabilizers
  for allergic rhinitis, 335
  cromolyn as, 743–744
Mastoiditis, 393t–399t
Maternal AFP, assessment of, 415.e1, 415.e1b
Matulane. *See* Procarbazine
Maturity-onset diabetes of youth (MODY), 215
Matzim. *See* Diltiazem
Maxalt. *See* Rizatriptan
Maxidex. *See* Dexamethasone

Maximal inspiratory pressure (MIP), 553
Maximum expiratory pressure (MEP), 553
Maxipime. *See* Cefepime
Maxivate. *See* Betamethasone
Maxolon. *See* Metoclopramide
MCAD deficiency. *See* Medium-chain acyl-CoA dehydrogenase deficiency
M-CHAT. *See* Modified Checklist for Autism in Toddlers
MCHC. *See* Mean cell hemoglobin concentration
MCNS. *See* Minimal change nephrotic syndrome
MCT oil. *See* Medium chain triglyceride oil
MCV. *See* Mean corpuscular volume
MCV vaccine. *See* Meningococcal conjugate vaccine
MDRD equation. *See* Modification of Diet in Renal Disease equation
Mean airway pressure, 74
Mean arterial pressure (MAP), 128
  percentiles, for infants 26-44 weeks postconceptional age, 128.e1t
Mean cell hemoglobin concentration (MCHC), age-specific values for, 306t
Mean corpuscular volume (MCV), age-specific values for, 306t, 307f
Measles
  immunoprophylaxis for, 362.e1t, 344, 351f-358f, 361, 362t, 363, 363.e1t, 370-371
  reactive erythema caused by, CP6
Measles, mumps, and rubella (MMR) vaccine, 370-371
  for children with HIV disease, 361
  for oncology patients, 362.e1t, 362t
  for patients treated with immunoglobulin or other blood products, 363.e1t, 363
  recommended schedules for, 351f-358f
Measles Ig, 344, 370-371
Mebendazole (Vermox), formulary entry for, 846
Mechlorethamine (Nitrogen mustard, HN$_2$, Mustine, Mustargen), toxicity of, 525t-528t

Meckel diverticulum, 588
Mediastinal masses, 580
Medical history. *See* History
Medical Orders for Life-Sustaining Treatment (MOLST) forms, 544
Medicosocial history, of adolescents, 93.e1b, 93, 93b-94b
Medium chain triglyceride (MCT) oil, 510t
Medium-chain acyl-CoA dehydrogenase (MCAD) deficiency, 290
Medrol. *See* Methylprednisolone
Medroxyprogesterone (Depo-Provera, Depo-Sub Q Provera 104, DMPA, Provera)
  formulary entry for, 846-847
  instructions for, 101f, 102
Mefloquine HCl (Lariam), formulary entry for, 847-848
Mefoxin. *See* Cefoxitin
Mellaril. *See* Thioridazine
Melphalan (L-PAM, Alkeran), toxicity of, 525t-528t
Memory making, in palliative care, 543
MEN. *See* Multiple endocrine neoplasia
Menactra. *See* Meningococcal conjugate vaccine
Meningitis
  emergency management of, 15
  management of, 393t-399t
  neonatal, 392t
  tuberculous, 407.e1t
Meningococcal conjugate vaccine (MCV vaccine, Menactra, Menveo), 371-372
  for children at high risk for meningococcal disease, 360
  for oncology patients, 362.e1t, 362t
  recommended schedules for, 351f-358f
Meningococcal immunoprophylaxis, 371-372
  for children at high risk, 360
  for oncology patients, 362.e1t, 362t
  recommended schedules for, 351f-358f
  for sickle cell disease, 312t
Men's Rogaine Extra Strength. *See* Minoxidil
Mental changes, as death approaches, 545

Mental health
of adolescents
anxiety, depression, and bipolar
disorder, 104
school problems, 108
substance use, 93b–94b, 108
suicidality, 93b, 104–108
screening tools for, 201t
Mental health disorders
ADHD, 201t, 208–209, 209t, 690
anxiety disorders, 209–210, 209t
depressive disorders, 201t, 209t,
210–211
referral and intervention for, 212
screening for, 201t, 208
substance abuse disorder, 211–212,
211b
websites for, 195
Mental status examination, 467
Mentzer index, 305
Menveo. *See* Meningococcal conjugate
vaccine
MEP. *See* Maximum expiratory pressure
Meperidine
in opioid tapering, 118t
renal failure dosage adjustments for,
1008t–1016t
Mephyton. *See* Phytonadione
Mepron. *See* Atovaquone
Mercaptoacetyl triglycine (MAG-3), 444
Mercaptopurine (6-MP)
late effects of, 538.e1t
toxicity of, 525t–528t
Meropenem (Merrem)
formulary entry for, 848
renal failure dosage adjustments for,
995t–1007t
sensitivity-based selection of,
383t–384t
Mesalamine (5-Aminosalicylic acid,
5-ASA, Asacol, Canasa, Lialda,
Pentasa, Rowasa, sfRowasa),
formulary entry for, 849
Mesna, toxicity of, 525t–528t
Mestinon. *See* Pyridostigmine bromide
Meta-analysis, 638t–639t
Metabolic acidosis, 264
arterial blood gas interpretation and,
552f
compensatory responses to, 552t
determination of, 264
etiology of, 265f–266f

Metabolic acidosis *(Continued)*
evaluation of, 285, 289f
poisoning diagnosis and, 20.e1t–20.e3t
Metabolic alkalosis, 264
arginine chloride for, 688
arterial blood gas interpretation and,
552f
compensatory responses to, 552t
determination of, 264
etiology of, 265f–266f
in PPHN, 425
Metabolic crisis, 290
Metabolic studies, for developmental
disorder evaluation, 205
Metabolism, genetic disorders of
clinical presentation of, 285, 285b
disorders of carbohydrate
metabolism, 293–294
evaluation of, 285–290, 286b, 286t,
287f–289f
FAO disorders, 290–291
GSD, 294–295
HT1, 292
hypotonia, 295, 296f–298f
lysosomal storage diseases, 293
mitochondrial diseases, 292–293
newborn screening for, 284–285
organic acidemias, 291
PKU, 292
treatment of metabolic crisis in, 290
urea cycle defects, 291–292
Metadate. *See* Methylphenidate HCl
Metamucil. *See* Psyllium
Metanephrines
normal values of, 243.e1t
pheochromocytoma detection with,
231
Metformin (Glucophage, Fortamet,
Riomet)
formulary entry for, 850
for type II diabetes, 220f
Methadone HCl (Dolophine, Methadose)
analgesic properties of, 113.e1t, 114t
formulary entry for, 851
neonate dosages of, 435
renal failure dosage adjustments for,
1008t–1016t
tapering of, 117, 118t
Methadose. *See* Methadone HCl
Methanol poisoning, 21t, 795
Methemoglobin, reference values for,
621t–623t

Methemoglobinemia, 852
Methicillin-resistant *Staphylococcus aureus* (MRSA)
  antibiotic selection for, 383t–384t
  antibiotic sensitivity of, 385t–386t
Methicillin-sensitive *Staphylococcus aureus* (MSSA)
  antibiotic selection for, 383t–384t
  antibiotic sensitivity of, 385t–386t
Methimazole (Tapazole)
  formulary entry for, 851
  for Graves disease, 223–224
  for hyperthyroidism, 224
Methohexital, procedural sedation with, 119, 123t
Methotrexate (MTX, Amethopterin, Folex, Mexate)
  for arthritis, 608.e1t, 608
  for GVHD prevention, 534
  for IBD, 274
  late effects of, 538.e1t
  for SLE, 611
  toxicity of, 525t–528t
Methyldopa
  formulary entry for, 852
  renal failure dosage adjustments for, 1008t–1016t
Methylene blue, formulary entry for, 852
Methylphenidate HCl (Ritalin, Methylin, Metadate, Concerta, Daytrana), formulary entry for, 853–854
Methylprednisolone (Depo-Medrol, Medrol, Solu-Medrol)
  for anaphylaxis, 10
  for asthma, 10
  formulary entry for, 854–855
  potency of, 229t
Methylxanthines
  aminophylline as, 678–679
  for asthma, 11
  caffeine citrate as, 707
  theophylline as, 956–957
Metoclopramide (Reglan, Maxolon, Metozolv)
  formulary entry for, 855
  for GERD, 275
  for nausea and vomiting, 537
  neonate dosages of, 435t
  renal failure dosage adjustments for, 1008t–1016t
Metolazone (Zaroxolyn), formulary entry for, 856

Metoprolol (Lopressor, Toprol-XL)
  formulary entry for, 856–857
  for hypertension, 463t–464t
Metozolv. *See* Metoclopramide
Metronidazole (Flagyl, MetroCream, MetroGel, MetroLotion, Noritate, Protostat)
  for acne vulgaris, 188t
  for bacterial vaginosis, 105t, 393t–399t
  formulary entry for, 857–858
  for gastroenteritis, 393t–399t
  for intraabdominal infections, 393t–399t
  neonate dosages of, 435t
  for pelvic inflammatory disease, 400t–401t
  renal failure dosage adjustments for, 995t–1007t
  sensitivity-based selection of, 386t
  for trichomonas, 400t–401t
  for trichomoniasis, 105t
Mexate. *See* Methotrexate
MI. *See* Myocardial infarction
Miacalcin. *See* Calcitonin–salmon
MIC. *See* Minimum inhibitory concentration
Micafungin sodium (Mycamine), formulary entry, 859
Miconazole (Lotrimin AF, Micatin, Monistat, M-Zole, Vagistat-3)
  for candidiasis, 411t
  for diaper candidiasis, 192
  formulary entry for, 860
  for tinea infections, 411t
  for tinea versicolor, 184
Micort-HC. *See* Hydrocortisone
Microalbuminuria, 454
Microangiopathic hemolytic anemia, CP12, 315
Microbiology
  rapid identification of aerobic bacteria, 381f–382f
  sensitivity-based antibiotic selection, 380
    aminoglycosides, 385t
    beta-lactams, 383t–384t
    fluoroquinolones, 385t
    macrolides, 385t
    single drug class, 386t
    tetracyclines, 385t
  specimen collection for blood culture, 380
  urine culture, 442

Microcytic anemia, 308t
Microlipid, 510t
Microscopic hematuria, 450
Microscopic polyangiitis, 613t
Microzide. *See* Hydrochlorothiazide
Midazolam (Versed)
    analgesic properties of, 113.e1t, 125t
    formulary entry for, 860–861
    procedural sedation with, 123t, 125t
    renal failure dosage adjustments for,
        1008t–1016t
    for RSI, 5f, 6t–7t
    for status epilepticus, 16t
Midsystolic click, 138b
Migergot. *See* Ergotamine tartrate with
        caffeine
Migraine headache
    classification of, 472
    diagnosis of, 471–472, 472b
    precursors to, 472
    seizure with, 474t
    treatment of, 472–473, 473t,
        680–681
Mild sedation, 118
Milestones
    developmental, 196, 197t–198t
    of early literacy, 196, 198t
Milia, CP9, 190
Miliaria, CP9, 190
Milk
    cow's
        formulas based on, 511t–517t
        formulas for allergies to, 518t–519t
        nutrition components in, 511t–517t
    evaporated, 511t–517t
    human, 511t–517t
Milk of Magnesia. *See* Magnesium
        hydroxide
Millipred. *See* Prednisolone
Milrinone (Primacor)
    formulary entry for, 861
    renal failure dosage adjustments for,
        1008t–1016t
    for shock, 71.e1t
Mineral oil (Kondremul, Fleet Mineral
        Oil), formulary entry for, 862
Mineralocorticoids
    for adrenal insufficiency, 229t, 230
    deficiency of, 227
Minerals
    DRIs for, 504–509, 507t–508t
    newborn requirements for, 420–423

Minimal change nephrotic syndrome
        (MCNS), 455–456
Minimum inhibitory concentration
        (MIC), 380
Minocycline (Arestin, Dynacin, Minocin,
        Solodyn)
    for acne vulgaris, 187, 188t
    formulary entry for, 862–863
Minoxidil (Loniten, Men's Rogaine Extra
        Strength, Rogaine)
    for alopecia areata, 186
    formulary entry for, 863
    for hypertension, 463t–464t
    for hypertensive urgency, 69t
Minute ventilation (V_E), 75
Miosis, poisoning diagnosis and,
        20.e1t–20.e3t
MIP. *See* Maximal inspiratory pressure
MiraLax. *See* Polyethylene glycol,
        electrolyte solution
Mirtazapine (Remeron), for mental
        health disorders, 209t
Mites. *See* Scabies
Mitochondrial diseases, 292–293
Mitoxantrone (Dihydroxyanthracenedione
        dihydrochloride, Novantrone),
        toxicity of, 525t–528t
Mixed connective tissue disease, 603t
MMF. *See* Mycophenolate mofetil
MMR vaccine. *See* Measles, mumps,
        and rubella vaccine
Mobitz type I block, 149f, 149t
Mobitz type II block, 149f, 149t
Moderate sedation, 119
Modification of Diet in Renal Disease
        (MDRD) equation, 446
Modified Checklist for Autism in Toddlers
        (M-CHAT), 201t, 207–208
Modified Coma Scale for Infants, 15t
MODY. *See* Maturity-onset diabetes of
        youth
Molluscum contagiosum, CP3,
        177–178
MOLST forms. *See* Medical Orders
        for Life-Sustaining Treatment
        forms
Molybdenum, DRIs for, 507t–508t
Mometasone furoate (Asmanex
        Twisthaler, Elocon, Nasonex)
    for allergic rhinitis, 335
    for asthma, 558.e1t–558.e2t
    for atopic dermatitis, 182t–183t

Mometasone furoate *(Continued)*
  dosage recommendations for,
      558.e1t–558.e2t
  formulary entry for, 864–865
Mometasone furoate and formoterol
      fumarate (Dulera)
  for asthma, 558.e1t–558.e2t
  formulary entry for, 864–865
Mongolian spots, 190–192
Monistat. *See* Miconazole
Monobactams
  aztreonam as, 696
  sensitivity-based selection of,
      383t–384t
Monoclonal antibody preparations, 345
Monoclonal factor VIII, 331
Monocytes, age-specific values of,
      314t
Monogen, 511t–517t
Monogenic diabetes, 215–216
Montelukast (Singulair)
  for allergic rhinitis, 335
  for asthma, 562f
  formulary entry for, 865
Moraxella catarrhalis, antibiotic
      sensitivity of, 383t–384t
Morphea, 616.e1
Morphine sulfate (Avinza, Kadian, MS
      Contin, Oramorph SR, Roxanol)
  analgesic properties of, 113.e1t, 113,
      114t
  formulary entry for, 866–867
  neonate dosages of, 435
  palliative care with, 546t
  PCA with, 117t
  renal failure dosage adjustments for,
      1008t–1016t
  tapering of, 117–118, 118t, 119b
  for tet spells, 160t
Morquio syndrome, 293
Motor examination, 467, 468b
Motor neuron examination, 469t
Motor skills, 196
  developmental and mental health
      screening tools for, 201t
  developmental milestones in,
      197t–198t
  for early literacy, 198t
Motrin. *See* Ibuprofen
Mouth-to-mouth breathing, 8
Mouth-to-nose breathing, 8
Movement, examination of, 468

Moxatag. *See* Amoxicillin
Moxifloxacin, sensitivity-based selection
      of, 385t
Moxifloxacin hydrochloride ophthalmic
      (Vigamox), 991t–992t
6-MP. *See* Mercaptopurine
MRI. *See* Magnetic resonance imaging
MRSA. *See* Methicillin-resistant
      Staphylococcus aureus
MS Contin. *See* Morphine sulfate
MSSA. *See* Methicillin-sensitive
      Staphylococcus aureus
MTX. *See* Methotrexate
Mucolytics
  acetylcysteine as, 669
  dornase alfa as, 764
Mucomyst. *See* Acetylcysteine
Mucopolysaccharidoses, 293
Mucositis, after bone marrow
      transplantation, 536
Mucosol. *See* Acetylcysteine
Mucous membranes, HIV exposure
      of, 411
Multiple endocrine neoplasia (MEN)
  hyperparathyroidism in, 225.e1b, 225
  syndromes of, 225.e1b
Multiple regression, 637
Multivitamins, 504t–506t
Mumps. *See also* Measles, mumps, and
      rubella vaccine.
  immunoprophylaxis for, 351f–358f,
      361, 362.e1t, 362t, 363,
      363.e1t, 370–371
Mupirocin (Bactroban)
  for bacterial superinfection in atopic
      dermatitis, 183
  formulary entry for, 867
  for impetigo, 192
Murine Ear. *See* Carbamide peroxide
Muscle enzymes, laboratory studies
      of, 605
Muscle stretch reflexes, 468.e1t
Muscles, examination of, 467, 468b
Musculoskeletal procedures
  basic splinting, 57–58
  long arm posterior splint, 58, 58f
  posterior ankle splint, 59
  radial head subluxation reduction, 60
  sugar tong forearm splint, 58, 59f
  thumb spica splint, 58–59
  ulnar gutter splint, 58
  volar splint, 59

Mustargen. *See* Mechlorethamine
Mustine. *See* Mechlorethamine
Myambutol. *See* Ethambutol HCI
Mycamine. *See* Micafungin sodium
Mycobacterium avium complex, in HIV/
　　AIDS patients, 405.e1t–405.e2t,
　　694–695
Mycobacterium spp.
　　antibiotic sensitivity of, 385t–386t
　　in HIV/AIDS patients, 405.e1t–405.e2t
Mycobacterium tuberculosis. See
　　Tuberculosis
Mycobutin. *See* Rifabutin
Mycophenolate mofetil (CellCept, MMF)
　　for arthritis, 608
　　formulary entry for, 867–868
　　for GVHD prevention, 534
　　for nephrotic syndrome, 456
　　for SLE, 611
Mycophenolate sodium (Myfortic),
　　formulary entry for, 867–868
Mycoplasma spp., antibiotic sensitivity
　　of, 383t–386t
Mycostatin. *See* Nystatin
Mydriasis, poisoning diagnosis and,
　　20.e1t–20.e3t
Mydriatic agents
　　cyclopentolate as, 745
　　cyclopentolate with phenylephrine
　　　as, 745
Myelocele, 574
Myelomeningocele, 574
Myfortic. *See* Mycophenolate sodium
Mylanta. *See* Aluminum hydroxide with
　　magnesium hydroxide
Mylanta Gas. *See* Simethicone
Myleran. *See* Busulfan
Mylicon. *See* Simethicone
Myocardial disease
　　dilated cardiomyopathy, 162–163
　　hypertrophic cardiomyopathy,
　　　163–164
　　myocarditis, 164
　　restrictive cardiomyopathy, 164
Myocardial infarction (MI), 153–154, 153f
Myocarditis, 164
Myoclonic seizures, 478b
Myoclonus, 474t
Myoglobin, in urine, 439
Myorisan. *See* Isotretinoin
Mysoline. *See* Primidone
M-Zole. *See* Miconazole

N
Nafcillin (Nallpen)
　　formulary entry for, 869
　　for neonatal septic arthritis, 392t
　　for osteomyelitis, 393t–399t
　　for parotitis, 393t–399t
　　sensitivity-based selection of, 383t–384t
　　for septic arthritis, 393t–399t
Nägele rule, 415.e1
NAIT. *See* Neonatal alloimmune
　　thrombocytopenia
Nallpen. *See* Nafcillin
Naloxone (Narcan)
　　coma treatment with, 13
　　formulary entry for, 869–870
　　for opioid poisoning, 21t
　　PCA with, 117
　　for procedural sedation reversal, 120,
　　　121b–122b, 122, 124b
　　for status epilepticus, 16t
NALS. *See* Neonatal advanced life
　　support
Nano-VM, 505t–506t
Naprelan. *See* Naproxen
Naproxen (Aleve, Anaprox, EC-Naprosyn,
　　Naprelan, Naprosyn DR)
　　analgesic properties of, 113
　　for arthritis, 608
　　formulary entry for, 870–871
Naratriptan (Amerge), for migraine
　　headaches, 473t
Narcan. *See* Naloxone
Narcolepsy, 474t
Narcotics. *See* Opioids/opiates
Nasacort AQ. *See* Triamcinolone
Nasal rinsing, 336
NasalCrom. *See* Cromolyn
Nasarel. *See* Flunisolide
Nascobal. *See* Cyanocobalamin
Nasoduodenal (ND) tube, 589
Nasogastric tube (NGT), 4
Nasonex. *See* Mometasone
Nasopharyngeal airway, 3
National Early Childhood Technical
　　Assistance Center, 212
Natural history, of food allergies, 339
Nausea and vomiting
　　differential diagnosis of, 271t
　　as GI tract condition, 270, 271t
　　treatment of cancer patients with,
　　　537–538
Navelbine. *See* Vinorelbine

ND tube. *See* Nasoduodenal tube
NDI. *See* Nephrogenic diabetes insipidus
NDM. *See* Neonatal diabetes
Nebcin. *See* Tobramycin
NebuPent. *See* Pentamidine isethionate
NEC. *See* Necrotizing enterocolitis
Neck injury, 65
  secondary survey of, 62t
Necrotizing enterocolitis (NEC), in newborns, 431.e1t, 431, 584
Nedocromil, for asthma, 563f–564f
Nedocromil sodium 2%, benzalkonium chloride (Alocril), for allergic conjunctivitis, 336t
Needle cricothyrotomy. *See* Percutaneous cricothyrotomy
Needle decompression, 44
Needlesticks, HIV exposure with, 411
Negative predictive value (NPV), 641
Neisseria spp., antibiotic sensitivity of, 383t–385t
Nembutal. *See* Pentobarbital
Neo To Go. *See* Neomycin/polymyxin B and bacitracin
NeoBenz Micro. *See* Benzoyl peroxide
Neocate Infant, 511t–517t
Neocate Junior, 511t–517t
Neomycin sulfate (Neo-Fradin), formulary entry for, 871
Neomycin/polymyxin B (Neosporin GU Irrigant), formulary entry for, 871–872
Neomycin/polymyxin B and bacitracin (Neo-Polycin, Neosporin, Neo To Go), formulary entry for, 871–872
Neonatal acne, CP9, 190
Neonatal advanced life support (NALS), 415, 417f
Neonatal alloimmune thrombocytopenia (NAIT), 315
Neonatal diabetes (NDM), 216
Neonatal Infant Pain Scale (NIPS), 111
Neonatal thyrotoxicosis, 224
Neonates/newborns
  antibiotic dosing for, 435t
  apnea in, 426–427, 426f
  assessment of
    APGAR scores, 415, 417t
    for birth trauma, 416–419, 419f, 419t

Neonates/newborns *(Continued)*
  HIE management, 419–420
  New Ballard Score, 416, 418f
  for selected anomalies, syndromes, and malformations, 420
  vital signs and birth weight, 415
  bradycardia in, 427
  cardiac disease in, 427–428
  common dermatologic conditions in
    acne, CP9, 190
    diaper candidiasis, CP10, 192
    ETN, CP9, 190
    evaluation algorithm for, 191f
    milia, CP9, 190
    miliaria, CP9, 190
    Mongolian spots, 190–192
    seborrheic dermatitis, CP10, 190
    transient neonatal pustular melanosis, CP9, 190
  congenital heart disease in
    acyanotic, 156, 157t–158t
    cyanotic, 156.e1t, 156, 158t–160t
    exercise recommendations for, 168.e1t, 168
    pulse oximetry screening for, 155–156
    surgeries and interventions for, 160–161, 160f
    syndromes associated with, 156, 156t
  cyanosis in
    differential diagnosis of, 423
    evaluation of, 423
  electrolyte requirements of, 420, 422t
  fluid requirements of, 420, 421t
  GI disease in
    abdominal wall defects, 431.e1t, 431
    bilious emesis, 431.e1t, 431
    necrotizing enterocolitis, 431.e1t, 431, 584
  glucose requirements of, 420, 421t, 422f
  Hb electrophoresis patterns of, 309, 310t
  hematologic disease in
    conjugated hyperbilirubinemia, 429–430
    polycythemia, 430–431
    unconjugated hyperbilirubinemia, 428–429, 428t, 429f–430f

Neonates/newborns *(Continued)*
  infection of
    bacterial, 386, 391f, 392t
    congenital, 386.e1t, 382, 388t,
        572–573
    syphilis, 386.e1t
    viral, 386, 389t–390t
  intensive care medications commonly
      used for, 435, 435t
  mineral and vitamin requirements of,
      420–423
  neonatology websites for, 415
  neurologic disease in
    abstinence syndrome, 432, 433b
    IVH, 431–432
    peripheral nerve injuries, 432, 433t
    periventricular leukomalacia, 432
    seizure, 289, 432, 476t–477t
  nutrition for
    growth and caloric requirements, 423
    total parenteral nutrition, 423
  respiratory disease in
    exogenous surfactant therapy for,
        423–424
    PPHN, 424–426
    RDS, 424
    spontaneous pneumothorax, 426
  resuscitation of
    endotracheal tube size and
        insertion depth, 415, 416t
    NALS algorithm for, 415, 417f
  ROP in, 433–435, 434f, 435t
  screening of
    for CF, 567
    for congenital adrenal hyperplasia,
        228t, 229
    Hb electrophoresis, 309, 310t
    for HIV infection, 402
    hypoglycemia and glucagon
        stimulation test, 242–243
    hypothyroidism, 223
    for IVH, 432
    metabolic, 284–285
    for ROP, 433–434
  seizure in, 289, 432, 476t–477t
  SLE in, 611–612
  thrombocytopenia in, 315
  transient jaundice in, 279t
  water loss in, 420, 421t
Neo-Polycin. *See* Neomycin/polymyxin
    B and bacitracin

NeoProfen. *See* Ibuprofen
Neoral. *See* Cyclosporine microemulsion
Neosporin. *See* Neomycin/polymyxin
    B and bacitracin; Polymyxin B
    sulfate, bacitracin zinc, neomycin
    sulfate ophthalmic
Neosporin GU Irrigant. *See* Neomycin/
    polymyxin B
Neostigmine (Bloxiverz, Prostigmin)
    formulary entry for, 872–873
    renal failure dosage adjustments for,
        1008t–1016t
Neosure, 511t–517t
Neo-Synephrine. *See* Oxymetazoline;
    Phenylephrine HCl
Nephritis
  in HSP, 614
  in SLE, 611.e1t, 611
Nephrogenic diabetes insipidus (NDI),
    232–233, 458
Nephrolithiasis
  diagnosis of, 462–464
  epidemiology of, 462
  management of, 464
  presentation of, 462
  prevention of, 465
  risk factors for, 462
  workup for, 464–465
Nephrology. *See also* Urinalysis.
  AKI in, 448
    ATN, 448–449
    clinical presentation of, 449, 449t
    complications of, 449
    dialysis for, 450
    etiology of, 448, 448t
    treatment considerations for, 449
  chronic hypertension in, 460
    antihypertensive drugs for (*See*
        Antihypertensives)
    classification of, 461, 462t
    etiologies of, 460, 461t
    evaluation of, 460–461
    treatment of, 461
  CKD in, 458–460, 459t
  hematuria and associated disorders
      in, 450–451
    etiology of, 451, 451t
    evaluation of, 451–453, 452f
    management of, 453, 453f
  kidney function tests in
    for distal tubular function, 447, 447t

Nephrology *(Continued)*
for glomerular function, 445–446, 445t–446t
for proximal tubular function, 446–447
nephrolithiasis in
diagnosis of, 462–464
epidemiology of, 462
management of, 464
presentation of, 462
prevention of, 465
risk factors for, 462
workup for, 464–465
proteinuria and associated disorders in, 454
detection of, 439, 454
etiologies of, 454, 455b
evaluation of, 455, 455b
nephrotic syndrome, 454–456, 456b, 456t
renal failure in (*See* Renal failure)
tubular disorders in
Fanconi syndrome, 458
NDI, 458
RTA, 456–458, 457t
UTIs in
diagnosis of, 441–442
history for, 440
imaging of, 589
management of, 393t–399t, 442–444, 443f
physical examination for, 441
risk factors for, 441
urine sampling for, 441
websites for, 438
Nephrotic syndrome, 454–456, 456b, 456t
Nephrotic-range proteinuria, 454
Nepro, 511t–517t
Nervous system instability, poisoning diagnosis and, 20.e1t–20.e3t
Neupogen. *See* Filgrastim
Neuroblastoma, 523t–524t
Neurofibromatosis type I (NF1), 302
Neurogenic shock, 71.e1t, 71
Neuroimaging, for developmental disorder evaluation, 205
Neurokinin-1 receptor antagonists, for nausea and vomiting, 537
Neurologic deficit. *See* Stroke

Neurology
ataxia in, 480
differential diagnosis of, 481b
evaluation of, 481b
poisoning diagnosis and, 20.e1t–20.e3t
emergencies in
altered states of consciousness, 13–15, 14b, 15t
status epilepticus, 15–16, 16t
examination in
coordination and movement, 468
cranial nerves, 468t
for developmental disorders, 203.e1t–203.e2t, 203
for headaches, 470.e1t
mental status, 467
motor, 467, 468b
sensory, 467, 469f, 469t
tendon reflexes, 467–468, 468.e1t, 469b
headaches in
evaluation of, 470.e1t, 470–471, 470b–471b
migraines, 471–473, 472b, 473t–474t, 680–681
hydrocephalus in
diagnosis of, 480
treatment of, 480, 668–669
newborn conditions in
abstinence syndrome, 432, 433b
IVH, 431–432
peripheral nerve injuries, 432, 433t
periventricular leukomalacia, 432
seizure, 289, 432, 476t–477t
paroxysmal events in
differential diagnosis of, 474t
first and recurrent seizures, 474–480, 476t–477t, 478b, 479t, 668–669
special seizure syndromes, 476t–477t, 480
stroke in
differential diagnosis of, 482, 482b
etiology of, 481
initial workup of, 482, 482b
management of, 482–483
as oncologic emergency, 530–531
trauma in, secondary survey of, 62t
websites for, 467

Neuromuscular blockers
  antidote for, 768
  pancuronium bromide as, 892
  rocuronium as, 935–936
  for RSI, 6t–7t
  succinylcholine as, 947
  vecuronium bromide as, 975
Neuromuscular disturbances, poisoning
    diagnosis and, 20.e1t–20.e3t
Neuromuscular maturity, of newborn,
    416, 418f
Neurontin. *See* Gabapentin
Neut. *See* Sodium bicarbonate
Neutropenia, 313, 314b, 314t
  care for cancer patients with, 537
  febrile, 685
  as oncologic emergency, 531–532,
    533f
Neutropenic enterocolitis, 531
Neutrophils, age-specific values of,
    314t
Nevirapine (NVP, Viramune)
  formulary entry for, 873
  neonate dosages of, 435
  for perinatal HIV exposure, 403t–404t
New Ballard Score, 416, 418f
Newborns. *See* Neonates/newborns
Nexiclon. *See* Clonidine
Nexium. *See* Esomeprazole
Next Choice. *See* Levonorgestrel
Nexterone. *See* Amiodarone HCl
NF1. *See* Neurofibromatosis type I
NGT. *See* Nasogastric tube
NH₃. *See* Ammonia
Niacin (Niacor, Niaspan, Slo-Niacin,
    Vitamin B₃)
  DRIs for, 502t–503t
  formulary entry for, 874
Nicardipine (Cardene)
  formulary entry for, 874–875
  for hypertensive emergency, 69t
Nicotinic acid. *See* Niacin
Nifedipine (Adalat CC, Nifediac CC,
    Procardia)
  formulary entry for, 875–876
  for hypertension, 463t–464t
Niferex. *See* Iron, oral preparations
Night feeding, 199t–200t
Night terrors, 199t–200t, 474t
Night walking, 199t–200t
Nightmares, 199t–200t
Nilstat. *See* Nystatin

NIPPV. *See* Noninvasive positive-pressure
    ventilation
Nipride. *See* Nitroprusside
NIPS. *See* Neonatal Infant Pain Scale
Nitric oxide (NO), for PPHN, 425
Nitrite test, 439
  for UTIs, 441
Nitro-Bid. *See* Nitroglycerin
Nitro-Dur. *See* Nitroglycerin
Nitrofurantoin (Furadantin,
    Macrodantin, Macrobid)
  formulary entry for, 876
  for UTI, 393t–399t
Nitrogen mustard. *See* Mechlorethamine
Nitroglycerin (Nitro-Bid, Nitro-Dur,
    NitroMist, Nitro-Time, Nitrostat),
    formulary entry for, 876–877
Nitroprusside (Nitropress, Nipride)
  formulary entry for, 877
  for hypertensive emergency, 69t
Nitrostat. *See* Nitroglycerin
Nitro-Time. *See* Nitroglycerin
Nix. *See* Permethrin
Nizoral. *See* Ketoconazole
NNRTIs. *See* Non-nucleoside reverse
    transcriptase inhibitors
NNT. *See* Number needed to treat
NO. *See* Nitric oxide
Nocardia spp., antibiotic sensitivity of,
    386t
Nodal escape, 145t–146t
Nodule, skin, 172, 173f–174f
Nonaccidental trauma, CP1, CP2,
    83–86, 85t
Nonanion gap metabolic acidosis,
    265f–266f
Noninvasive positive-pressure ventilation
    (NIPPV), 74
Non-nucleoside reverse transcriptase
    inhibitors (NNRTIs)
  nevirapine as, 873
  for PEP, 412
Nonopioid analgesics, 111–113
  acetaminophen as, 112, 113.e1t
  aspirin as, 112
  choline magnesium trisalicylate as, 113
  NSAIDs as, 113.e1t, 113
  quick reference for as, 113.e1t
Nonparametric statistical tests, 636t,
    637
Non-pegylated interferon-alpha-2b, for
    HCV, 389t–390t

Nonsteroidal antiinflammatory drugs
(NSAIDs)
analgesic properties of, 113.e1t, 113
for arthritis, 608
aspirin as, 689
choline magnesium trisalicylate as,
733
ibuprofen as, 811–812
indomethacin as, 815–816
ketorolac as, 825
for migraine headaches, 472
naproxen as, 870–871
poisoning with, 21t
for Sjögren syndrome, 616.e3
for SLE, 611
Nonventricular arrhythmias, 144,
145t–146t, 147f
Nonventricular conduction
disturbances, 144, 149f, 149t
Norcuron. See Vecuronium bromide
Norepinephrine
normal values of, 243.e1t
for shock, 71.e1t, 73f
Norepinephrine bitartrate (Levophed),
formulary entry for, 878
Norepinephrine reuptake inhibitors,
atomoxetine as, 690
Norfloxacin (Noroxin)
formulary entry for, 878
renal failure dosage adjustments for,
995t–1007t
Noritate. See Metronidazole
Normal saline (NS)
fluid maintenance with, 246
fluid replacement with, 253
for metabolic crisis, 290
Normal serum albumin. See Albumin
Normetanephrines, normal values of,
243.e1t
Normocytic anemia, 308t
Normodyne. See Labetalol
Noroxin. See Norfloxacin
Nortriptyline hydrochloride (Pamelor)
formulary entry for, 879
for migraine headaches, 473t
Norvasc. See Amlodipine
Norwood procedure, 161
Nostrilla. See Oxymetazoline
Novantrone. See Mitoxantrone
NovaSource Renal, 511t–517t
Novo Log. See Aspart insulin
Novolin N. See Isophane insulin

NPH. See Isophane insulin
NPO recommendations, for procedural
sedation, 119.e1f, 119, 120t
NPV. See Negative predictive value
NRTIs. See Nucleoside reverse
transcriptase inhibitors
NS. See Normal saline
NSAIDs. See Nonsteroidal
antiinflammatory drugs
5'-NT. See 5'-Nucleotidase
Nucleoside reverse transcriptase
inhibitors (NRTIs)
lamivudine as, 828
for PEP, 412
zidovudine as, 982–983
5'-Nucleotidase (5'-NT), liver function
testing with, 277t
NuCort. See Hydrocortisone
NuLYTELY. See Polyethylene glycol,
electrolyte solution
Number needed to treat (NNT), 640
Nummular eczema, CP6
Nursemaid's elbow, 60
Nutracort. See Hydrocortisone
Nutramigen AA Lipil, 511t–517t
Nutramigen LIPIL, 511t–517t
Nutramigen with Enflora LGG,
511t–517t
Nutren formulas, 511t–517t
Nutren Junior, 511t–517t
Nutr-E-Sol. See Vitamin E
Nutrition. See also Enteral nutrition.
DRIs
fat, 501t
fiber, 509t
measurement of, 500–501
minerals, 504–509, 507t–508t
in multivitamin examples,
504t–506t
protein, 501t
vitamins, 501–504, 502t–503t
energy needs, 497, 498t
for catch-up growth, 499–500,
500b
estimation of, 497–498, 499t
in stressed conditions, 498–499
for newborns, 423
parenteral
formulations for, 520, 520t–521t
indications for, 520
monitoring of patients on, 520, 521t
websites for, 485

Nutritional status
elements in assessment of, 485
indicators of, 485
BMI, 486
BMI percentile, 486
growth, 486
growth charts, 486.e1f–486.e3f,
486–497, 487f–494f
growth charts for special populations,
486.e4f–486.e7f, 497
recommendations for overweight
and obese children, 486.e8f, 486
waist circumference and waist-
height ratio, 497
NVP. *See* Nevirapine
Nydrazid. *See* Isoniazid
Nystagmus, poisoning diagnosis and,
20.e1t–20.e3t
Nystatin (Bio-Statin, Mycostatin, Nilstat)
for candidiasis, 411t
for diaper candidiasis, 192
formulary entry for, 879–880

O
O_2 extraction ratio, 76.e1
Obesity, 486
Cushing syndrome and, 236
hypothyroidism and, 219–223, 235
management of, 486.e8f, 486
normal growth and, 235–236
Obstructive airway disease, spirometry
in characterization of, 553,
554f–555f, 555t
Obstructive hypoventilation. *See*
Obstructive sleep apnea
syndrome
Obstructive shock, 71.e1t, 71
Obstructive sleep apnea syndrome
(OSAS)
clinical manifestations of, 568
diagnosis of, 569, 569b
treatment of, 569–570
Occult blood test, 281
Occupational exposure, to HIV, 411
Ocean. *See* Sodium chloride, inhaled
preparations
OCPs. *See* Oral contraceptive pills
Octagam. *See* Intravenous
immunoglobulin
Octreotide acetate (Sandostatin)
formulary entry for, 880
for sulfonylurea poisoning, 21t

Ocuflox. *See* Ofloxacin
Odds ratio (OR), 640
Odors, poisoning diagnosis and,
20.e1t–20.e3t
Ofirmev. *See* Acetaminophen
Ofloxacin (Floxin, Ocuflox), 991t–992t
formulary entry for, 880–881
OGTT. *See* Oral glucose tolerance test
17-OHP. *See* 17-Hydroxyprogesterone
OI. *See* Oxygenation index
Oligohydramnios, 415.e2b
Oliguria, 449, 449t
Olopatadine (Pataday, Patanase,
Patanol)
for allergic conjunctivitis, 336t
for allergic rhinitis, 335
formulary entry for, 881
Olsalazine (Dipentum, Di-mesalazine,
Di-5-ASA), formulary entry for,
882
Olux. *See* Clobetasol propionate
Omalizumab, for asthma, 564f
Omeprazole (First-Omeprazole,
Omeprazole and Syrspend SF
Alka, Prilosec), formulary entry
for, 882–883
Omnaris. *See* Ciclesonide
Omnicef. *See* Cefdinir
Omnipaque. *See* Iohexol
Omnipen. *See* Ampicillin
Omnipred. *See* Prednisolone
Omphalocele, 431.e1t
Oncology. *See* Cancer
Oncovin. *See* Vincristine
Ondansetron (Zofran)
formulary entry for, 883–884
for nausea and vomiting, 537
palliative care with, 546t
One-tailed statistical tests, 637
Onfi. *See* Clobazam
Onmel. *See* Itraconazole
Open comedo, 187
Open pneumothorax, 66
Ophthalmic agents, 991t–992t
for allergic conjunctivitis, 336, 336t
atropine sulfate as, 691–692
azelastine as, 693–694
azithromycin as, 694–695
Opioids/opiates
analgesic properties of, 113.e1t, 113,
114t, 125t
for burns, 82

Opioids/opiates *(Continued)*
  butorphanol as, 706
  codeine as, 742
  fentanyl as, 783–784
  hydromorphone as, 809–810
  methadone HCl as, 851
  morphine sulfate as, 866–867
  naloxone reversal of, 120, 121b–122b, 122, 124b, 869–870
  oxycodone and acetaminophen as, 889
  oxycodone and aspirin as, 890
  oxycodone as, 889
  palliative care with, 546t
  PCA with, 116–117, 117t
  poisoning with, 19, 20t–21t
  procedural sedation with, 114t, 121b–122b
  quick reference for, 113.e1t
  tapering of, 117–118, 118t, 119b
  toxidrome of, 20t–22t
  withdrawal from, 117
    neonatal, 432, 433b
Opportunistic infections
  in HIV/AIDS patients, 405.e1t–405.e2t, 405, 694–695
  immunodeficiency indicated by, 342t
Opticrom. *See* Cromolyn
Optimental, 511t–517t
Optivar. *See* Azelastine
OPV vaccine. *See* Oral poliovirus vaccine
OR. *See* Odds ratio
Oral airway, 3
Oral allergy syndrome, 337
Oral candidiasis, 411t
Oral contraceptive pills (OCPs)
  for acne vulgaris, 187
  for EC, 102–103
  instructions for, 100–102
Oral food challenges, 339
Oral glucose tolerance test (OGTT), 214–215
Oral poliovirus (OPV) vaccine, 373
Oral rehydration salts, 519t
Oral rehydration therapy (ORT)
  common solutions for, 509, 519t
  composition of fluids for, 254t–255t, 256
  for diarrhea, 271
Oralone. *See* Triamcinolone
Oramorph SR. *See* Morphine sulfate

Orapred. *See* Prednisolone
Oraqix. *See* Lidocaine and prilocaine
Orasone. *See* Prednisone
OraVerse. *See* Phentolamine mesylate
Orazinc. *See* Zinc salts
Orbital cellulitis
  imaging of, 573, 574f
  management of, 393t–399t
Organ transplantation, immunoprophylaxis for patients with, 362
Organic acidemias, 291
Organic milk based infant formula, 511t–517t
Organophosphate poisoning, 20t–22t, 691–692, 912–913
Ornithine transcarbamylase deficiency (OTCD), 291–292
ORT. *See* Oral rehydration therapy
Orthopedic evaluation, for adolescent PPE, 98.e1f, 98
Orthopedic trauma, 66, 67f, 67t
  in child abuse patients, 84, 85t
  imaging of, 589
Orthostatic proteinuria, 454
OSAS. *See* Obstructive sleep apnea syndrome
Os-Cal. *See* Calcium carbonate
Oseltamivir phosphate (Tamiflu)
  formulary entry for, 885–886
  for influenza chemoprophylaxis, 369–370
  renal failure dosage adjustments for, 995t–1007t
Osmitrol. *See* Mannitol
Osmolality
  reference values for, 621t–623t
  serum, 264
Osmolar gap
  serum, 264
  stool, 271
Osmolar gap disturbances, 264
  etiology of, 264, 265f–266f
  primary acid-base disorder determination, 264
Osmolite formulas, 511t–517t
OsmoPrep. *See* Sodium phosphate
Osmotic diarrhea, 271
Osmotic fragility test, 308
Osteochondroma, 590, 594f
Osteoma, 590, 595f
Osteomalacia, 225t

Osteomyelitis
 imaging of, 590
 management of, 393t–399t
Osteoporosis, calcitonin–salmon for, 707
Osteosarcoma, 590, 596f–597f
OTCD. *See* Ornithine transcarbamylase
  deficiency
Otic analgesia, 687
Otitis externa, 393t–399t
Otitis media, 393t–399t, 682,
  694–695
Ovarian pathology, imaging of, 589
Overweight, 486
 management of, 486.e8f, 486
Oxacillin
 for cellulitis, 393t–399t
 for dacryocystitis, 393t–399t
 formulary entry for, 886
 for lymphadenitis, 393t–399t
 for neonatal septic arthritis, 392t
 neonate dosages of, 435t
 for osteomyelitis, 393t–399t
 for parotitis, 393t–399t
 renal failure dosage adjustments for,
  995t–1007t
 sensitivity-based selection of,
  383t–384t
 for septic arthritis, 393t–399t
Oxcarbazepine (Oxtellar, Trileptal)
 formulary entry for, 886–888
 renal failure dosage adjustments for,
  1008t–1016t
 for seizures, 479t
Oxiconazole, for tinea versicolor, 184
Oxidizing agents, 993
Oxtellar. *See* Oxcarbazepine
Oxy-5. *See* Benzoyl peroxide
Oxy-10. *See* Benzoyl peroxide
Oxybutynin chloride (Ditropan, Oxytrol),
  formulary entry for, 888
Oxycodone (OxyContin, Roxicodone)
 analgesic properties of, 113.e1t, 114t
 formulary entry for, 889
Oxycodone and acetaminophen
  (Endocet, Percocet, Roxicet,
  Roxilox), formulary entry for, 889
Oxycodone and aspirin (Endodan,
  Percodan), formulary entry for,
  890
OxyContin. *See* Oxycodone
Oxygen challenge test, 156.e1t, 156
Oxygen content (Ca$_{O_2}$), 76.e1

Oxygen therapy
 for bronchiolitis, 565
 for inhalation injury, 82
 in newborns, 424
 for PPHN, 425
 for shock, 71.e1t, 73f
Oxygenation index (OI), 76
Oxyhemoglobin dissociation curve, 550,
  551f
Oxymetazoline (Afrin, Duramist, Neo-
  Synephrine, Nostrilla, Visine),
  formulary entry for, 890
Oxytrol. *See* Oxybutynin chloride

P
ΔP. *See* Power
P value, 637
P waves, 127f, 140–141
PA. *See* Physical activity coefficient
PAC. *See* Premature atrial contraction
Pacerone. *See* Amiodarone HCl
Packed RBCs (PRBCs), 329
 exchange transfusion with, 331
 leukocyte-poor, 329
Paclitaxel (Taxol), toxicity of, 525t–528t
Pain assessment
 for infants, 111, 112t
 for preschoolers, 111, 112t, 113f
 for school-age children and
  adolescents, 111, 112t
Pain relief. *See also* Analgesia.
 nonpharmacologic measures of, 116
Paired statistical tests, 637
PAL. *See* Physical activity level
Palgic. *See* Carbinoxamine
Palivizumab (Synagis)
 formulary entry for, 890–891
 for RSV, 374–375
Palliative care, 540, 540f
 communication and decision
  making in
   advance directive, 542
   child participation, 542, 542t
   decision-making tools, 541
   family meetings, 541–542
 death in
   autopsy consent after, 547
   bereavement after, 547
   certificate for, 547
   changes accompanying approach
    of, 544–545
   children's conceptualization of, 542t

Palliative care *(Continued)*
  documentation of, 546
  medication and management
    during last hours, 546t
  pronouncement of, 545–547
legacy and memory making in, 543
team members involved in, 540–541
treatment limits set in
  discontinuing current interventions,
    544
  DNAR decision, 543–544, 543b
  forgoing treatment escalation, 544
  state forms used for, 544
websites for, 540
Palliative superior vena cava-to-
    pulmonary artery shunts, 160f,
    161
Palliative systemic-to-pulmonary artery
    shunts, 160f, 161
Palonosetron, for nausea and vomiting,
    537
2-PAM. *See* Pralidoxime chloride
Pamelor. *See* Nortriptyline hydrochloride
Pamix. *See* Pyrantel pamoate
Panadol. *See* Acetaminophen
Panayiotopoulos syndrome, 476t–477t
Pancreatic disease, in CF patients, 568
Pancreatic enzyme replacement therapy
    (PERT), 568
Pancreatic enzymes
  formulary entry for, 891
  supplementation with, 989t
Pancreatitis
  acute, 278–280, 280t
  chronic, 280–281, 281.e1t
Pancrelipase, supplementation with,
    989t
Pancuronium bromide
  formulary entry for, 892
  neonate dosages of, 435
  renal failure dosage adjustments for,
    1008t–1016t
Pandel. *See* Hydrocortisone
Pantoprazole (Protonix), formulary entry
    for, 892–893
Pantothenic acid, DRIs for, 502t–503t
Papanicolaou (Pap) smear, 97.e1t, 97
Papular urticaria
  clinical presentation of, CP7, 183
  management of, 184
  pathogenesis of, 183
Papule, 172, 173f–174f

Papulosquamous lesions, diagnosis and
    treatment of
  atopic dermatitis, CP6, CP7, 180–183,
    182t–183t, 337, 339
  diagnosis algorithm, 181f
  ichthyosis, CP7, 184
  keratosis pilaris, CP5
  papular urticaria, CP7, 183–184
  pityriasis alba, CP6
  pityriasis rosea, CP5
  post inflammatory hyperpigmentation,
    CP6
  psoriasis, CP5
  tinea corporis, CP5, 184
  tinea pedis, CP5
  tinea versicolor, CP7, 184
Paracentesis, 47–49
Paracetamol. *See* Acetaminophen
Paralysis, poisoning diagnosis and,
    20.e1t–20.e3t
Paralytics, for RSI, 6t–7t
Parametric statistical tests,
    636t, 637
Paraplatin. *See* Carboplatin
Parapneumonic effusions and
    empyema, 580
Parathyroid gland function
  hyperparathyroidism, 225.e1b, 225
  hypoparathyroidism, 224–225
Parathyroid hormone (PTH), 224
Parenchymal findings, on chest
    imaging, 580
Parenteral iron. *See* Iron, injectable
    preparations
Parenteral nutrition (PN)
  formulations for, 520, 520t–521t
  indications for, 520
  monitoring of patients on,
    520, 521t
Parenteral rehydration fluids,
    254t–255t, 256
Parent's Choice Store Brand,
    511t–517t
Parents' Evaluation of Developmental
    Status (PEDS), 201t, 202
Parkland formula, 78, 81f
Paromomycin sulfate (Humatin),
    formulary entry for, 893–894
Parotitis, 393t–399t
Paroxetine (Brisdelle, Paxil, Pexeva),
    formulary entry for, 894–895
Paroxysmal dyskinesias, 474t

Paroxysmal events
  differential diagnosis of, 474t
  first and recurrent seizures
    causes of, 474–475
    disorders causing, 475, 476t–477t,
      478b
    evaluation of, 475
    febrile illness–associated, 475
    status epilepticus, 15–16, 16t, 478
    treatment of, 478–480, 479t,
      668–669
  special seizure syndromes,
    476t–477t, 480
Paroxysmal vertigo, 474t
PARS. See Pediatric Anxiety Rating
    Scale
Partial seizures, 478b
Parvovirus B19, congenital, 388t
Pataday. See Olopatadine
Patanase. See Olopatadine
Patanol. See Olopatadine
Patch, on skin, 172, 173f–174f
Patch contraceptives, 102
Patent ductus arteriosus (PDA),
    157t–158t
  diagnosis of, 427
  incidence of, 427
  management of, 427–428
  risk factors for, 427
Pathocil. See Dicloxacillin sodium
Pathologic short stature, 233–235, 234f
Patient-controlled analgesia (PCA),
    116–117, 117t
  weaning from, 117–118, 119b
Paxil. See Paroxetine
PCA. See Patient-controlled analgesia
PCOS. See Polycystic ovarian syndrome
PCP. See Phencyclidine; Pneumocystis
    jiroveci pneumonia
PCV13. See Pneumococcal conjugate
    vaccine
PDA. See Patent ductus arteriosus
PDE5 inhibitors. See Phosphodiesterase
    type 5 inhibitors
Peak expiratory flow rate (PEFR), 551
  normal predicted values for, 553t
Pearson's correlation coefficient, 637
Pediaflor. See Fluoride
Pedia-Lax. See Glycerin
Pediamycin. See Erythromycin
    preparations

Pediapred. See Prednisolone
Pediarix, 378
Pediasure 1.5, 511t–517t
Pediasure Enteral, 511t–517t
Pediasure Vanilla, 511t–517t
Pediasure with Fiber, 511t–517t
Pediatric Anxiety Rating Scale (PARS),
    210
Pediatric formulas. See Formulas
Pediatric Symptom Checklist (PSC),
    201t, 208
Pediazole. See Erythromycin
    ethylsuccinate and
    acetylsulfisoxazole
Pediculicides
  lindane as, 837
  pyrethrins as, 923
Pediotic. See Polymyxin B sulfate,
    neomycin sulfate, hydrocortisone
PEDS. See Parents' Evaluation of
    Developmental Status
PedvaxHIB, 366
PEEP. See Positive end-expiratory
    pressure
PEFR. See Peak expiratory flow rate
PEG-Asp. See Asparaginase
Pelvic inflammatory disease, 392–401,
    400t–401t
Pelvic trauma, secondary survey of, 62t
Pemphigus foliaceus, 193
Pemphigus vulgaris, CP10, 193
Penetrating abdominal trauma, 66
Penicillin G preparations (Pfizerpen)
  benzathine
    formulary entry for, 896
    for pharyngitis, 393t–399t
    for syphilis, 388t, 400t–401t
  benzathine and penicillin G procaine,
    formulary entry for, 896–897
  formulary entry for, 895
  for pharyngitis, 393t–399t
  procaine
    formulary entry for, 897
    for syphilis, 400t–401t
  renal failure dosage adjustments for,
    995t–1007t
  sensitivity-based selection of,
    383t–384t
  for syphilis, 106t–107t, 400t–401t
Penicillin V potassium (Veetids)
  formulary entry for, 898
  for pharyngitis, 393t–399t

Penicillin V potassium *(Continued)*
  renal failure dosage adjustments for, 995t–1007t
  sensitivity-based selection of, 383t–384t
Penicillins
  allergy to, 340–341, 340f
  amoxicillin as, 682
  amoxicillin–clavulanic acid as, 683
  ampicillin as, 686
  ampicillin/sulbactam as, 687
  for cancer patients, 538t
  dicloxacillin sodium as, 757
  for Lyme disease, 409, 682
  for maternal GBS prophylaxis, 386
  nafcillin as, 869
  for osteomyelitis, 393t–399t
  oxacillin as, 886
  penicillin G preparations as *(See* Penicillin G preparations)
  penicillin V potassium as *(See* Penicillin V potassium)
  piperacillin with tazobactam as, 907–908
  sensitivity-based selection of, 383t–384t
  for sickle cell disease, 312t
  ticarcillin and clavulanate as, 960
Penis, mean stretched length of, 243.e3t, 243
Pentacel, 378
Pentamidine isethionate (Pentam 300, NebuPent)
  for cancer patients, 538t
  formulary entry for, 898–899
  for perinatal HIV exposure, 403t–404t
  for *Pneumocystis jiroveci* pneumonia, 405.e1t–405.e2t
  renal failure dosage adjustments for, 995t–1007t
Pentasa. *See* Mesalamine
Pentobarbital (Nembutal)
  formulary entry for, 899
  procedural sedation with, 123t
  for status epilepticus, 16t
Pentostatin, for GVHD prevention, 534
PEP. *See* Postexposure prophylaxis
Pepcid. *See* Famotidine
Pepdite Junior, 511t–517t
Peptamen formulas, 511t–517t
Peptamen Junior, unflavored, 511t–517t

Peptamen Junior 1.5, 511t–517t
Peptamen Junior Fiber, 511t–517t
Peptamen Junior with Prebio, 511t–517t
Pepto-Bismol. *See* Bismuth subsalicylate
Peptostreptococcus spp., antibiotic sensitivity of, 386t
Perative, 511t–517t
Percocet. *See* Oxycodone and acetaminophen
Percodan. *See* Oxycodone and aspirin
Percutaneous (needle) cricothyrotomy, 13, 14f
Perforomist. *See* Formoterol
Perfusion
  assessment of, 8
  in PPHN, 425
  resuscitation with poor, 9
Periactin. *See* Cyproheptadine
Pericardial disease
  cardiac tamponade, 47, 48f–50f, 165
  Kawasaki disease, 166–168, 167.e1t, 167f
  Lyme disease, 168
  pericardial effusion, 165
  pericarditis, 164–165
  rheumatic heart disease, 168, 169b
Pericardial fluid, evaluation of, 630t
Pericardiocentesis, 47, 48f–50f
Pericarditis, 164–165
Perinatal infection
  bacterial, 386, 391f, 392t
  HIV, 389t–390t
    management of, 402–405, 403t–404t
    testing for, 402
  syphilis, 386.e1t
  viral, 386, 389t–390t
Periorbital cellulitis, 393t–399t
Periostat. *See* Doxycycline
Peripheral alpha antagonists, for hypertension, 463t–464t
Peripheral hypotonia, 295, 296f–297f
Peripheral intravenous placement, 31
Peripheral nerve injuries, in newborns, 432, 433t
Peripheral precocious puberty, 239
Peritoneal dialysis, 450
  drug dosage adjustments for, 994
Peritoneal fluid, evaluation of, 630t
Periventricular leukomalacia, in newborns, 432

Permethrin (Acticin, Elimite, Nix)
  formulary entry for, 899–900
  for scabies, 178
Persistent hematuria, 450
Persistent pulmonary hypertension of
  newborn (PPHN)
  diagnostic features of, 425
  etiology of, 424–425
  mortality of, 426
  therapy for, 425–426
PERT. *See* Pancreatic enzyme
  replacement therapy
Pertussis
  immunoprophylaxis for, 351f–358f,
    362.e1t, 362t, 363
  management of, 393t–399t, 694–695
Pexeva. *See* Paroxetine
Pfizerpen. *See* Penicillin G preparations
PGE₁. *See* Alprostadil
pH
  determination of, 264
  of transudate *vs.* exudate, 630t
  of urine, 438
PHACES syndrome, 175
Phagocytosis deficiency, 342t–343t
Pharyngitis, 393t–399t, 682,
  694–695
Phazyme. *See* Simethicone
Phenazopyridine HCl (Azo-Standard,
  Pyridium)
  formulary entry for, 900
  renal failure dosage adjustments for,
    1008t–1016t
Phencyclidine (PCP), poisoning with,
  20t–22t
Phenergan. *See* Promethazine
Phenobarbital (Luminal)
  formulary entry for, 900–901
  renal failure dosage adjustments for,
    1008t–1016t
  for seizures, 476t–477t, 479t
  for status epilepticus, 16t
Phenothiazines
  ECG effects of, 151t–152t
  for nausea and vomiting, 537
  poisoning with, 20t–22t
  prochlorperazine as, 917
  promethazine as, 918
  thioridazine as, 959
Phentolamine mesylate (OraVerse,
  Regitine), formulary entry for,
  901–902

Phenylalanine, reference values for,
  621t–623t
Phenylephrine HCl (Neo-Synephrine)
  formulary entry for, 902–903
  for increased ICP, 70
  for shock, 71.e1t
  for tet spells, 160t
Phenylketonuria (PKU), 292
Phenytoin (Dilantin, Dilantin Infatab,
  Phenytek)
  ECG effects of, 151t–152t
  formulary entry for, 903–904
  for seizures, 479t
  for status epilepticus, 16t
Pheochromocytoma, 231
Phlexy-Vits, 505t–506t
PhosLo. *See* Calcium acetate
Phoslyra. *See* Calcium acetate
PHOS-NaK. *See* Phosphorus
  supplements
Phospha 250 Neutral. *See* Phosphorus
  supplements
Phosphate. *See also* Hyperphosphatemia;
  Hypophosphatemia.
  serum disturbances in,
    263, 263b
Phosphate binders, aluminum
  hydroxide as, 675
Phosphodiesterase type 5
  (PDE5) inhibitors, sildenafil as,
  939–940
Phosphorus
  DRIs for, 507t–508t
  formulas lower in, 518t–519t
  reference values for, 621t–623t
Phosphorus supplements (K-PHOS
  Neutral, Phospha 250 Neutral,
  PHOS-NaK, Potassium
  phosphate, Sodium phosphate),
  formulary entry for, 904–905
Phototherapy, for unconjugated
  hyperbilirubinemia, 428, 428t,
  429f
Physical activity coefficient (PA), 497,
  498t
Physical activity level (PAL), 497
Physical changes, as death approaches,
  544–545
Physical examination
  for acute hypertension, 68
  of adolescents, 94–95, 95.e2f
  for allergic rhinitis, 334

Physical examination *(Continued)*
  cardiac
    blood pressure, 128.e1t, 128,
      129t–135t, 136f–138f
    heart murmurs, 128–139,
      139b–140b, 139t
    heart rate, 128, 142t
    heart sounds, 128
  for CHT, 61–63, 62t
  for cyanosis in newborns, 423
  for developmental disorders,
    202–203, 203.e1t–203.e2t
  for dysmorphology, 295
  for food allergies, 337
  for headaches, 470.e1t
  for increased ICP, 69–70
  for PPE, 97–98, 98.e1f
  for procedural sedation, 120
  respiratory, 549, 549t–550t
  for UTIs, 441
Physical maturity, of newborn, 416, 418f
Physician Orders for Life-Sustaining
    Treatment (POLST) forms, 544
Physiologic anemia of infancy, 309
Physostigmine salicylate (Antilirium)
  for anticholinergic poisoning, 21t
  formulary entry for, 905
Phytonadione (Mephyton, Vitamin K)
  deficiency of, 326f, 327b
  DRIs for, 502t–503t
  formulary entry for, 905–906
  neonate dosages of, 435, 905–906
  warfarin interaction and management
    with, 322, 324t
  for warfarin poisoning, 21t, 905–906
Pilocarpine HCl (Isopto Carpine,
    Salagen, Pilopine HS)
  formulary entry for, 906
  for Sjögren syndrome, 616.e3
Pilocarpine iontophoresis test, 567
Pilopine HS. *See* Pilocarpine HCl
Pimecrolimus (Elidel)
  for atopic dermatitis, 180
  formulary entry for, 907
Pin-Rid. *See* Pyrantel pamoate
Pin-X. *See* Pyrantel pamoate
Piperacillin, renal failure dosage
    adjustments for, 995t–1007t
Piperacillin with tazobactam (Zosyn)
  for catheter-related bloodstream
    infections, 393t–399t
  formulary entry for, 907–908

Piperacillin with tazobactam *(Continued)*
  for intraabdominal infections,
    393t–399t
  renal failure dosage adjustments for,
    995t–1007t
  sensitivity-based selection of, 383t–384t
  for sinusitis, 393t–399t
  for spinal fusion infections, 393t–399t
  for tracheitis, 393t–399t
  for UTI, 393t–399t
PIs. *See* Protease inhibitors
Pitressin. *See* Vasopressin
Pituitary gland, posterior gland/
    vasopressin function of
  in DI, 232–233
  in SIADH, 231–232
Pityriasis alba, CP6
Pityriasis rosea, CP5
Pivot 1.5, 511t–517t
PKU. *See* Phenylketonuria
Plan B One Step. *See* Levonorgestrel
Plantar warts, 177
Plaque, on skin, 172, 173f–174f
Plaquenil. *See* Hydroxychloroquine
Plasbumin. *See* Albumin
Plasma AST, in hemolytic anemia, 307
Plasma catecholamines, normal values
    of, 243.e1t, 243
Plasma LDH, in hemolytic anemia,
    307
Plasma volume expanders, albumin
    as, 672
Platelet activation, hypercoagulable
    state caused by, 319b
Platelet function testing, 319
  age-specific values for, 317t–318t
Platelets. *See also* Thrombocytopenia.
  age-specific values for, 306t
  on blood smears, 333
  transfusion of, 330
Platinol. *See* Cisplatin
Pleural effusion, 580
Pleural fluid, evaluation of, 630t
Plexus injuries, 433t
PN. *See* Parenteral nutrition
Pneumococcal conjugate vaccine
    (PCV13), 372
  for children at high risk for
    pneumococcal disease, 360
  for oncology patients, 362.e1t, 362t
  recommended schedules for,
    351f–358f

Pneumococcal immunoprophylaxis, 351f–358f, 360, 362t, 362.e1t, 372
   for sickle cell disease, 312t
Pneumococcal polysaccharide vaccine (PPSV23), 372
   for children at high risk for pneumococcal disease, 360
   for oncology patients, 362.e1t, 362t
   recommended schedules for, 351f–358f
Pneumococci, antibiotic sensitivity of, 385t
Pneumocystis jiroveci, antibiotic sensitivity of, 386t
Pneumocystis jiroveci pneumonia (PCP)
   atovaquone for, 405.e1t–405.e2t, 691
   in HIV/AIDS patients, 405.e1t–405.e2t, 405
Pneumonia
   in HIV/AIDS patients, 405.e1t–405.e2t, 405
   imaging of, 577
   management of, 393t–399t, 686, 694–695
   neonatal, 392t
Pneumothorax
   blunt thoracic and abdominal trauma causing, 66
   chest tube placement for, 44–47, 45f–46f
   in newborns, 426
Podofilox, for genital warts, 106t–107t
Podophyllin, for genital warts, 106t–107t
Poison ivy, CP10, 194
Poisoning
   acetaminophen, 19, 24f, 669
   carbon monoxide, 80–82
   chemotherapeutic drug toxicities, 525t–528t
   clinical diagnostic aids for, 20.e1t–20.e3t, 20
   drug ingestion and antidotes, 20–23, 21t
   initial evaluation for
     history, 19
     laboratory findings, 19, 20t
   lead, 23, 25t, 767
   toxidromes, 20t–22t, 23
   websites for, 19

Poliomyelitis immunoprophylaxis, 373
   for oncology patients, 362.e1t, 362t
   recommended schedules for, 351f–358f
POLST forms. *See* Physician Orders for Life-Sustaining Treatment forms
Polyarteritis nodosa, 613t
Polychromatophilia, blood smear demonstrating, CP12
Polycitra. *See* Citrate mixtures
Polycose, 510t
Polycystic ovarian syndrome (PCOS), 236
Polycythemia, in newborns, 430–431
Polyethylene glycol, electrolyte solution (Colyte, Dulcolax Balance, GoLYTELY, MiraLax, NuLYTELY, TriLyte)
   for constipation, 272–273
   formulary entry for, 908–909
Polyhydramnios, 415.e2b
Polymox. *See* Amoxicillin
Polymyositis, 603t
Polymyxin B sulfate, bacitracin zinc, neomycin sulfate ophthalmic (Neosporin), 991t–992t
Polymyxin B sulfate, neomycin sulfate, hydrocortisone (Cortisporin Otic, AK-Spore H.C. Otic, Pediotic), formulary entry for, 910
Polymyxin B sulfate, neomycin sulfate, hydrocortisone ophthalmic (Cortisporin), 991t–992t
Polymyxin B sulfate and bacitracin. *See* Bacitracin and Polymyxin B
Polymyxin B sulfate and trimethoprim sulfate (Polytrim Ophthalmic Solution), 991t–992t
   for conjunctivitis, 393t–399t
   formulary entry for, 909
Poly-Pred. *See* Prednisolone acetate, neomycin sulfate, polymyxin B sulfate ophthalmic
Polysaccharide-iron complex. *See* Iron, oral preparations
Polysomnography, 569
Polysporin Ophthalmic. *See* Bacitracin and polymyxin B
Polysporin Topical. *See* Bacitracin and polymyxin B
Polytrim Ophthalmic Solution. *See* Polymyxin B sulfate and trimethoprim sulfate

Poly-Vi-Sol, 504t
Poractant Alfa. *See* Surfactant therapy
Porcelain, reference values for, 621t–623t
Portagen, 511t–517t
Positive end-expiratory pressure (PEEP), 71
Positive predictive value (PPV), 641
Post inflammatory hyperpigmentation, CP6
Posterior ankle splint, 59
Posterior pituitary gland function
  in DI, 232–233
  in SIADH, 231–232
Posterior tibial artery puncture, 31
Postexposure prophylaxis (PEP)
  for HBV, 368t, 412–413
  for HCV, 413
  for HIV, 411–412
Postmenstrual age, 415.e1
Postural reactions, 203.e2t
Posture-D. *See* Calcium phosphate, tribasic
Potassium. *See also* Hyperkalemia; Hypokalemia.
  deficit repletion of
    in hypernatremic dehydration, 252–253
    in hyponatremic dehydration, 252
    in isonatremic dehydration, 251–252, 251t
  for diabetic ketoacidosis, 217f
  newborn requirements for, 422t
  reference values for, 621t–623t
  serum disturbances in, 257–259, 258t–259t, 260f
Potassium iodide (Iosat, SSKI, ThyroShield, ThyroSafe)
  formulary entry for, 910–911
  for hyperthyroidism, 224
Potassium phosphate. *See* Phosphorus supplements
Potassium supplements, formulary entry for, 911–912
Potassium-removing resins, sodium polystyrene sulfonate as, 944–945
Pounds, conversion formulas for, 633
Power (ΔP), ventilator, 74
Power Doppler imaging, 583
Power of statistical tests, 637
PPE. *See* Preparticipation physical evaluation

PPHN. *See* Persistent pulmonary hypertension of newborn
PPIs. *See* Proton pump inhibitors
PPSV23. *See* Pneumococcal polysaccharide vaccine
PPV. *See* Positive predictive value
PR interval, 141, 142t
Pralidoxime chloride (2-PAM, Protopam)
  formulary entry for, 912–913
  for organophosphate poisoning, 21t, 912–913
Pralidoxime chloride with atropine (DuoDote), formulary entry for, 912–913
Prazosin, for hypertension, 463t–464t
PRBCs. *See* Packed RBCs
Prealbumin, reference values for, 621t–623t
Precedex. *See* Dexmedetomidine
Precocious puberty, 91, 237–239, 237t, 239t–241t
Pred Forte. *See* Prednisolone
Pred Mild. *See* Prednisolone
Prednicarbate (Derm Atop), for atopic dermatitis, 182t–183t
Prednisolone (Millipred, Omnipred, Orapred, Pediapred, Pred Forte, Pred Mild, Prelone, Veripred 20)
  for asthma, 10
  formulary entry for, 913
  ophthalmic, 991t–992t
  potency of, 229t
Prednisolone acetate, neomycin sulfate, polymyxin B sulfate ophthalmic (Poly-Pred), 991t–992t
Prednisone (Deltasone, Liquid Pred, Orasone, Rayos)
  for adrenal insufficiency, 229t, 230
  for anaphylaxis, 10
  for asthma, 10
  formulary entry for, 914
  for GVHD prevention, 534
  immunoprophylaxis for patients on, 362t
  for nephrotic syndrome, 455–456
  potency of, 229t
Pregabalin (Lyrica), for seizures, 479t
Pregestimil LIPIL, 511t–517t
Pregnancy
  adolescent, 93.e1b
  DRIs for, 501t–503t, 507t–509t
  drug categories for, 648

Pregnancy *(Continued)*
  EER for, 498
  immunoprophylaxis during, 363
  preventing HIV transmission during, 402–405
Prehypertension, 460
Prelone. *See* Prednisolone
Premature atrial contraction (PAC), 145t–146t, 147f
Premature ventricular contraction (PVC), 148f, 148t
Prenatal screening, for HIV infection, 402
Preparticipation physical evaluation (PPE), for adolescents, 97–98, 98.e1f
Preschoolers, pain assessment for, 111, 112t, 113f
Pressors, for shock, 71.e1t
Pressure limited ventilation, 71, 74
Pressure support ventilation (PSV), 74
Preterm infants
  formula for, 511t–519t
  glucose requirements of, 420
  growth charts for, 495f–496f
  immunoprophylaxis for, 363, 364f
  mean TSH and T₄ of, 221t
  metabolic screening in, 284
  mineral and vitamin requirements of, 420–423
  nutrition for, 423
  phototherapy in, 428, 428t
  ROP in, 433–435, 434f, 435t
  serum IgG, IgM, IgA, and IgE reference values for, 346t
  water loss in, 420, 421t
Prevacid. *See* Lansoprazole
Prevalence, 639
Prevalite. *See* Cholestyramine
Prevotella spp., antibiotic sensitivity of, 386t
Prickly heat. *See* Miliaria
Prilocaine, analgesic properties of, 115t
Prilosec. *See* Omeprazole
Primacor. *See* Milrinone
Primaquine phosphate, formulary entry for, 914–915
Primary acid-base disorders, 264
Primary adrenal insufficiency, 229
  evaluation of, 226–227, 227t
  management of, 229–230, 229t
Primary hypothyroidism, 220t

Primary skin lesions, 172, 173f–174f
Primary survey, 61
Primaxin. *See* Imipenem and cilastin
Primidone (Mysoline)
  formulary entry for, 915
  renal failure dosage adjustments for, 1008t–1016t
Primitive reflexes, 203.e1t
Principen. *See* Ampicillin
Prinivil. *See* Lisinopril
Privigen. *See* Intravenous immunoglobulin
ProAir HFA. *See* Albuterol
Probenecid
  formulary entry for, 916
  for syphilis, 400t–401t
Probiotics, for diarrhea, 272
Problem-solving skills, 196
  developmental milestones in, 197t–198t
Procainamide
  formulary entry for, 916–917
  renal failure dosage adjustments for, 1008t–1016t
Procaine penicillin G (Wycillin)
  formulary entry for, 897
  for syphilis, 400t–401t
Procarbazine (Matulane), toxicity of, 525t–528t
Procardia. *See* Nifedipine
Procedural sedation, 118–119
  discharge criteria for, 122–124
  example protocols for, 125t
  monitoring during, 120–121
  pharmacologic agents for, 114t, 121–122, 121b–122b, 123t
  preparation for, 119.e1f, 119–120, 120.e1t, 120t
  quick reference for, 113.e1t
  reversal of, 120, 121b–122b, 122, 124b
  websites for, 111
Procedures
  for basic laceration repair
    skin staples, 56–57
    suturing, 54–56, 55f, 56t
    tissue adhesives, 57
  for blood sampling
    dorsalis pedis artery puncture, 31
    external jugular puncture, 28–29, 28f
    femoral artery/vein puncture, 29–30, 29f

Procedures *(Continued)*
  heelstick and fingerstick, 27–28
  pericardiocentesis, 47, 48f–50f
  posterior tibial artery puncture, 31
  radial artery puncture and
    catheterization, 30–31
  for body fluid sampling
    chest tube placement and
      thoracentesis, 44–47, 45f–46f
    lumbar puncture, 42–44, 43f
    paracentesis, 47–49
    soft tissue aspiration, 51–53
    suprapubic bladder aspiration, 51,
      52f–53f
    urinary bladder catheterization,
      50–51
  consent for, 27
  for immunization and medication
    administration
    intramuscular injection, 54
    subcutaneous injection, 53
  musculoskeletal
    basic splinting, 57–58
    long arm posterior splint, 58, 58f
    posterior ankle splint, 59
    radial head subluxation reduction,
      60
    sugar tong forearm splint, 58, 59f
    thumb spica splint, 58–59
    ulnar gutter splint, 58
    volar splint, 59
  risks in, 27
  for vascular access
    central venous catheter placement,
      28f, 31–37, 32f, 34f–36f, 582,
      582f–583f
    IO infusion, 37–38, 37f
    peripheral intravenous placement,
      31
    UA and UV catheterization, 38–42,
      39f–41f
ProCentra. *See* Dextroamphetamine
Prochlorperazine (Compazine)
  formulary entry for, 917
  palliative care with, 546t
Procrit. *See* Epoetin alfa
Proctocolitis, 337
Progestin only EC
  for adolescents, 102–103
  medroxyprogesterone as,
    846–847
Proglycem. *See* Diazoxide

Prograf. *See* Tacrolimus
Prokinetic therapy
  for GERD, 275
  metoclopramide as, 855
Promethazine (Phenergan)
  formulary entry for, 918
  for nausea and vomiting, 537
Promote formula, 511t–517t
Pronto. *See* Pyrethrins
Prophylaxis. *See* Immunoprophylaxis
Propionibacterium acnes, antibiotic
    sensitivity of, 385t
Propofol
  procedural sedation with, 119,
    121b–122b
  for RSI, 6t–7t
Propranolol (Inderal)
  ECG effects of, 151t–152t
  formulary entry for, 918–919
  for hemangioma, 176–177
  for hypertension, 463t–464t
  for hyperthyroidism, 224
  for migraine headaches, 473t
  for tet spells, 160t
Propylthiouracil (PTU)
  formulary entry for, 920
  Graves disease and, 223–224
ProQuad, 378
Prosource protein powder, 510t
Prostaglandin E$_1$. *See* Alprostadil
Prostaglandin I$_2$, for PPHN, 425
Prostigmin. *See* Neostigmine
Prostin VR Pediatric. *See* Alprostadil
Protamine, 320
Protamine sulfate, formulary entry for,
    920–921
Protease, supplementation of, 989t
Protease inhibitors (PIs), for PEP, 412
Protein
  in CSF, 631t
  DRIs for, 501t
  in transudate *vs.* exudate, 630t
Protein allergy, 518t–519t
Protein C and S deficiency, 319b
Protein electrophoresis, reference values
    for, 621t–623t
Protein intolerance, 518t–519t
Proteinuria, 454
  detection of, 439, 454
  etiologies of, 454, 455b
  nephrotic syndrome with, 454–456,
    456b, 456t

Proteus spp., antibiotic sensitivity of, 383t–384t

Prothrombin time (PT), 316–319
  age-specific values for, 317t–318t

Proton pump inhibitors (PPIs)
  for burns, 82
  esomeprazole as, 778–779
  for GERD, 275
  for GI bleeding, 269
  lansoprazole as, 831
  omeprazole as, 882–883
  pantoprazole as, 892–893

Protonix. *See* Pantoprazole

Protopam. *See* Pralidoxime chloride

Protopic. *See* Tacrolimus

Protostat. *See* Metronidazole

Proventil. *See* Albuterol

Provera. *See* Medroxyprogesterone

Proximal tubule function tests, 446–447

Proximal tubule reabsorption, 446

Prozac. *See* Fluoxetine hydrochloride

PS. *See* Pulmonary stenosis

PsA. *See* Psoriatic arthritis

PSC. *See* Pediatric Symptom Checklist

Pseudoephedrine (Sudafed), formulary entry for, 921

Pseudomonas spp., antibiotic sensitivity of, 383t–385t

Pseudoprecocious puberty, 239

Pseudoseizure, 474t

Pseudotumor cerebri, 668–669

Psoralens, for GVHD prevention, 534

Psorcon. *See* Diflorasone diacetate

Psoriasis, CP5

Psoriatic arthritis (PsA), 606–607

PSV. *See* Pressure support ventilation

Psychogenic seizure, 474t

Psychosis, poisoning diagnosis and, 20.e1t–20.e3t

Psychosocial development, of adolescents, 91, 92.e1t

Psychosocial history, of adolescents, 93.e1b, 93, 93b–94b

Psyllium (Metamucil, Fiberall, Konsyl, Reguloid), formulary entry for, 922

PT. *See* Prothrombin time

PTH. *See* Parathyroid hormone

PTU. *See* Propylthiouracil

Puberty, 91, 92f, 92t–93t
  delayed, 236–237, 237t, 238f
  precocious, 91, 237–239, 237t, 239t–241t

Pubic hair, 91, 92t

Pulmicort. *See* Budesonide

Pulmicort DPI Flexhaler, dosage recommendations for, 558.e1t–558.e2t

Pulmicort Respules, dosage recommendations for, 558.e1t–558.e2t

Pulmocare, 511t–517t

Pulmonary blood flow, chest radiography of, 154–155, 157t–159t

Pulmonary ejection murmur, 139t

Pulmonary flow murmur of newborn, 139t

Pulmonary function tests
  MIP and MEP, 553
  PEFR, 551, 553t
  spirometry, 553, 554f–555f, 555t

Pulmonary stenosis (PS), 157t–158t

Pulmonary vasoconstriction, in PPHN, 425

Pulmonology
  ALTE in, 556
    differential diagnosis of, 556, 556b–557b
    workup for, 557
  asthma in
    clinical manifestations of, 558
    exacerbation prevention in, 558
    management of, 10–11, 558.e1t–558.e2t, 558, 559f–564f, 672–673, 678–679
    severity classification of, 559f–561f
  BPD in, 566
  bronchiolitis in, 565–566
  CF in
    clinical manifestations of, 567t
    diagnosis of, 566–567
    formula for, 518t–519t
    management of complications of, 568
    pulmonary therapies for, 567–568
  gas exchange evaluation in
    acid-base disturbance analysis, 551, 552f, 552t
    blood gases, 550–551, 552f
    capnography, 550
    pulse oximetry, 549–550, 551f
  newborns respiratory disease in
    exogenous surfactant therapy for, 423–424
    oxygen therapy for, 424

Pulmonology *(Continued)*
  PPHN, 424–426
  RDS, 424
  spontaneous pneumothorax, 426
  OSAS in
    clinical manifestations of, 568
    diagnosis of, 569, 569b
    treatment of, 569–570
  pulmonary function tests in
    MIP and MEP, 553
    PEFR, 551, 553t
    spirometry, 553, 554f–555f, 555t
  respiratory distress in, 531
  respiratory emergencies in
    asthma, 10–11
    upper airway obstruction,
      11–13, 14f
  respiratory failure in, 71–75, 75t
  respiratory physical examination in,
    549, 549t–550t
  SIDS in, 570, 570b
  websites for, 549
Pulmozyme. *See* Dornase alfa
Pulse oximetry, gas exchange evaluation
  with, 549–550, 551f
Pulse oximetry screening, for congenital
  heart disease, 155–156
Pulse pressure, 128
Pulsus paradoxus, 128
Puncture
  dorsalis pedis artery, 31
  external jugular, 28–29, 28f
  femoral artery/vein, 29–30, 29f
  lumbar, 42–44, 43f
  posterior tibial artery, 31
  radial artery, 30–31
Pustule, 172, 173f–174f
PVC. *See* Premature ventricular
  contraction
Pyelonephritis, 393t–399t, 442
Pyloric stenosis, 586, 587f
Pyogenic granuloma, CP3, 178
Pyrantel pamoate (Reese's Pinworm,
  Pamix, Pin-Rid, Pin-X), formulary
  entry for, 922
Pyrazinamide (Pyrazinoic acid amide)
  formulary entry for, 923
  for tuberculosis, 407.e1t
Pyrethrins (A-200, Klout, Licide, Pronto,
  Pyrinyl, RID, Tisit), formulary
  entry for, 923
Pyridium. *See* Phenazopyridine HCl

Pyridostigmine bromide (Mestinon,
    Regonol), formulary entry for, 924
Pyridoxine (Vitamin B$_6$)
  DRIs for, 502t–503t
  formulary entry for, 924–925
  for seizure, 476t–477t
Pyrimethamine (Daraprim)
  formulary entry for, 925
  for toxoplasmosis, 388t,
    405.e1t–405.e2t
Pyrinyl. *See* Pyrethrins
Pyruvate, reference values for,
  621t–623t
Pyuria, 441

Q

Q waves, 141
Qnasl. *See* Beclomethasone
    dipropionate
QRS axis, 141, 142t, 143f
QRS complex, 127f, 140, 142t
QRS interval, 141, 142t
Qs/Qt. *See* Intrapulmonary shunt
    fraction
QTc, 141, 142t
Quantitative fecal fat test, 281
Quelicin. *See* Succinylcholine
Questran. *See* Cholestyramine
Quetiapine (Seroquel), for mental health
    disorders, 209t
Quick-start contraception, 100, 101f
Quinapril, for hypertension, 463t–464t
Quinidine
  formulary entry for, 925–926
  renal failure dosage adjustments for,
    1008t–1016t
Quinolones
  ciprofloxacin as, 735–736
  levofloxacin as, 833–834
  norfloxacin as, 878
  ofloxacin as, 880–881
Quinupristin and dalfopristin (Synercid),
    formulary entry for, 927
Quixin. *See* Levofloxacin
QVAR. *See* Beclomethasone
    dipropionate

R

R waves, 141, 142t
Rabies Ig (RIG), 344, 373–374, 374t
Rabies immunoprophylaxis, 78, 344,
    373–374, 374t

Racemic epinephrine. *See* Epinephrine, racemic
Radial artery catheterization, 30–31
Radial artery puncture, 30–31
Radial head subluxation, 60
Radiation exposure, minimization of, 572
Radiation therapy, late effects of, 538.e1t, 538
Radioactive iodine (131I), for Graves disease, 223–224
Radiography. *See also* Chest radiography.
  of adolescent spine, 95.e1, 95.e2f
  of airway, 576, 576t, 577f–578f
  for blunt thoracic and abdominal trauma, 65
  of bone lesions
    Ewing sarcoma, 597, 598f
    fibroma, 590, 595f
    osteochondroma, 590, 594f
    osteoma, 590, 595f
    osteosarcoma, 590, 596f–597f
    unicameral bone cyst, 590, 594f
  C-spine films, 573–574, 575f
  hip disorders on, 590, 591f–593f
  for neck injury, 65
  SCIWORA on, 574
  of scoliosis, 576
  after UTI, 444
Radiology
  abdomen imaging
    biliary atresia, 589
    bowel obstruction, 586–588
    esophageal atresia and tracheoesophageal fistula, 584, 585f
    high intestinal obstruction, 584–586, 586f
    intussusception, 588, 588f
    Meckel diverticulum, 588
    ND tube placement, 589
    neonatal enterocolitis, 584
    pyloric stenosis, 586, 587f
    trauma, 589
    after UTI, 444
  adolescent spine imaging, 95.e1, 95.e2f
  airway imaging
    foreign bodies, 576
    lateral radiographs, 576, 576t, 577f–578f
    vascular rings, 576

Radiology *(Continued)*
  for blunt thoracic and abdominal trauma, 65–66
  chest imaging
    atelectasis, 579–580
    cardiology radiography, 154–155, 154f, 157t–159t
    central line placement, 582, 582f–583f
    ETT placement, 583
    infiltrate, 580
    mediastinal masses, 580
    parapneumonic effusions and empyema, 580
    parenchymal findings, 580
    for pneumonia, 577
    posteroanterior and lateral radiographs, 577, 579f–582f
  for child abuse patients, 85, 597, 599f–600f
  for developmental disorder evaluation, 203–205
  for dysmorphology, 295
  extremity imaging
    bone age, 597
    bone lesions, 590–597, 594f–598f
    hip disorders, 590, 591f–593f
    osteomyelitis, 590
    skeletal survey for suspected child abuse, 597, 599f–600f
    stress fractures, 590
    trauma, 589
  eye imaging, 573, 574f
  general principles of, 572
  genitourinary tract imaging
    uterine and ovarian pathology, 589
    UTIs, 589
  head imaging, 572–573
  for headaches, 470
  heart and vessel imaging
    blood flow, 583
    cardiac catheterization, 155.e1f, 155
    cardiology radiography, 154–155, 154f, 157t–159t
    congenital heart disease, 583, 584f
    echocardiography, 155, 583
    vessel abnormalities, 584
  for minor CHT, 63, 63b
  for neck injury, 65
  poisoning diagnosis and, 20.e1t–20.e3t

Radiology *(Continued)*
  for seizures, 475
  spine imaging
    in adolescent, 95.e1, 95.e2f
    cervical spine trauma, 573
    C-spine film reading, 573–574,
      575f
    SCIWORA, 574
    scoliosis, 576
    spinal dysraphism, 574
  for UTIs, 443–444, 443f
Radionuclide cystogram (RNC), after
    UTI, 444
Radiopaque agents, iohexol as,
    816–817
Rages, 474t
Rales, auscultation of, 550t
Raniclor. *See* Cefaclor
Ranitidine HCl (Zantac)
  formulary entry for, 927–928
  neonate dosages of, 435
  renal failure dosage adjustments for,
    1008t–1016t
Rapamune. *See* Sirolimus
Rapid sequence intubation (RSI), 4
  drugs used for, 4, 5f, 6t–7t, 691–692
  treatment algorithm for, 5f
Rasburicase (Elitek)
  formulary entry for, 928
  for tumor lysis syndrome, 529
Rash. *See* Dermatology
Rate. *See also* Heart rate.
  respiratory, 549t
  ventilator, 74
Rayos. *See* Prednisone
RBBB. *See* Right bundle-branch block
RBCs. *See* Red blood cells
RDA. *See* Recommended dietary
    allowance
RDS. *See* Respiratory distress syndrome
Reach Out and Read milestones of early
    literacy, 196, 198t
Reactions, postural, 203.e2t
Reactive arthritis, 607–608
  joint fluid analysis for, 605f
Reactive erythema, CP3, CP4, 178, 179f
Reactive lymph node, 524
Rebetol. *See* Ribavirin
Recombinant factor IX, 331
Recombinant factor VIII, 331
Recombinant human DNAase,
    for CF, 568

Recombinant human erythropoietin.
    See Epoetin alfa
Recombivax, 367
Recommended dietary allowance
    (RDA), 500
Recurrent headache, differential
    diagnosis for, 470b
Red blood cells (RBCs). *See also*
    Packed RBCs.
  age-specific values for, 306t
  on blood smears, 332
  transfusion of, 325–330
  in transudate *vs.* exudate, 630t
  in urine, 440
Red cell aplasias, 309
Reducing substances, urine, 289–290
Reduction, of radial head
    subluxation, 60
Reese's Pinworm. *See* Pyrantel pamoate
Refeeding syndrome, 500
Reflexes
  examination of, 467–468, 468.e1t,
    469b
  primitive, 203.e1t
Regitine. *See* Phentolamine mesylate
Reglan. *See* Metoclopramide
Regonol. *See* Pyridostigmine bromide
Regression, 637
Regular insulin, 218t
  for hyperkalemia, 260f
  renal failure dosage adjustments for,
    1008t–1016t
Reguloid. *See* Psyllium
Rehydration fluids. *See also* Oral
    rehydration therapy.
  common solutions of, 509, 519t
  composition of, 254t–255t, 256
Relative risk (RR), 639
Relative risk reduction (RRR), 640
Reliability, measurements of, 640–641,
    641t
Relpax. *See* Eletriptan
Remeron. *See* Mirtazapine
Renal failure
  dosage adjustments in
    antimicrobials requiring,
      995t–1007t
    darbepoetin alfa, 748–750
    methods of, 994
    nonantimicrobials requiring,
      1008t–1016t
  formula for, 518t–519t

Renal system. *See also* Nephrology.
  imaging of, 443–444, 443f
Renal tubular acidosis (RTA), 456–458,
    457t
Renal tubular disorders
  Fanconi syndrome, 458
  NDI, 458
  RTA, 456–458, 457t
Renalcal, 511t–517t
Renova. *See* Tretinoin
Replete formula, 511t–517t
Reporting, of child abuse, 85
Resectisol. *See* Mannitol
Resource Beneprotein, 510t
Resource formulas, 511t–517t
Respiratory acidosis, 264
  arterial blood gas interpretation and,
    552f
  compensatory responses to, 552t
  determination of, 264
  etiology of, 265f–266f
Respiratory alkalosis, 264
  arterial blood gas interpretation and,
    552f
  compensatory responses to, 552t
  determination of, 264
  etiology of, 265f–266f
  in PPHN, 425
Respiratory auscultation, 550t
Respiratory disease, in newborns
  exogenous surfactant therapy for,
    423–424
  oxygen therapy for, 424
  PPHN, 424–426
  RDS, 424
  spontaneous pneumothorax, 426
Respiratory distress, 531
Respiratory distress syndrome (RDS),
    424
Respiratory emergencies
  asthma, 10–11
  upper airway obstruction, 11–13, 14f
Respiratory failure, 71–75, 75t
Respiratory rates, normal values of, 549t
Respiratory stimulants, caffeine citrate
    as, 707
Respiratory syncytial virus (RSV)
  bronchiolitis caused by, 565
  immunoprophylaxis for, 374–375
Respiratory syndromes, food allergies
    causing, 337
Restasis. *See* Cyclosporine modified

Restrictive airway disease, spirometry
    in characterization of, 553,
    554f–555f, 555t
Restrictive cardiomyopathy, 164
Resuscitation. *See also* Emergency
    management.
  atropine sulfate for, 691–692
  newborn
    endotracheal tube size and
      insertion depth, 415, 416t
    NALS algorithm for, 415, 417f
Reticulocytes
  age-specific values for, 306t
  anemia classification and, 308t
  in hemolytic anemia, 307
Retin-A. *See* Tretinoin
Retinal hemorrhages, 84
Retinoblastoma, 523t–524t
Retinoic acid, isotretinoin as, 822
Retinoic acid derivatives, tretinoin as,
    965
Retinoids, for acne vulgaris, 187, 189t
Retinol. *See* Vitamin A
Retinopathy of prematurity (ROP)
  classification of, 434, 434f
  diagnosis of, 433
  etiology of, 433
  management of, 434–435, 435t
  timing of screening for, 433–434
Retrovir. *See* Zidovudine
Revatio. *See* Sildenafil
Reversal agents, for procedural
    sedation, 120
Reverse T$_3$, age-based normal values
    for, 221t
Revonto. *See* Dantrolene
RF. *See* Rheumatoid factor
R-Gene 10. *See* Arginine chloride
Rhabdomyosarcoma, 523t–524t
Rheumatic heart disease, 168, 169b
Rheumatoid arthritis. *See* Juvenile
    rheumatoid arthritis
Rheumatoid factor (RF), 603–604, 603t
  reference values for, 621t–623t
Rheumatology
  arthritis in
    JIA, 603t, 606, 607t
    JRA, 603t, 605f, 606
    management of, 608.e1t,
      608–609
    PsA, 606–607
    reactive, 605f, 607–608

Rheumatology *(Continued)*
  Behçet disease in, 616.e2
  granulomatous disease in
    differential diagnosis of, 615
    sarcoidosis, 615–616
  joint fluid analysis in, 605, 605f,
    632t
  laboratory studies for
    acute phase reactants, 602–603
    autoantibodies, 603–604, 603t
    complement, 604
    joint fluid analysis, 605, 605f
    serum muscle enzymes, 605
    UA, 604
  scleroderma in
    autoantibodies associated with,
      603t
    DCSS, 616.e1–616.e2
    localized, 616.e1
  Sjögren syndrome in, 616.e2–616.e3
    autoantibodies associated with,
      603t
  SLE in
    ACR classification criteria for, 609,
      610t
    autoantibodies associated with,
      603t, 611
    clinical features of, 611.e1t,
      610–611
    drug-induced, 603t, 611
    neonatal, 611–612
    treatment of, 611
  vasculitis in
    autoantibodies associated with,
      603t
    general characterization of, 612,
      613t
    HSP, 612–614, 613t
    juvenile dermatomyositis,
      614–615
  websites for, 602
Rhinaris. *See* Sodium chloride, inhaled
    preparations
Rhinitis. *See* Allergic rhinitis
Rhinitis medicamentosa, 335
Rhinocort. *See* Budesonide
$RH_O(D)$ immune globulin (WinRho)
  formulary entry for, 929
  for thrombocytopenia, 315
Rhonci, auscultation of, 550t
Rhythm. *See* Heart rhythm
Rib fracture, 85t

Ribavirin (Copegus, Rebetol,
    Ribasphere, Virazole)
  formulary entry for, 929–931
  for HCV, 389t–390t
Riboflavin (Vitamin B_2)
  DRIs for, 502t–503t
  formulary entry for, 931
  reference values for, 621t–623t
Rickets, 225t
Rickettsia spp., antibiotic sensitivity
    of, 385t
RID. *See* Pyrethrins
Rifabutin (Mycobutin)
  formulary entry for, 931–932
  renal failure dosage adjustments for,
    995t–1007t
Rifadin. *See* Rifampin
Rifamate. *See* Isoniazid with rifampin
Rifampin (Rimactane, Rifadin)
  formulary entry for, 932–933
  for haemophilus influenzae type b
    exposure, 367
  for meningococcal exposure, 372
  renal failure dosage adjustments for,
    995t–1007t
  for spinal fusion infections, 393t–399t
  for tuberculosis, 405.e1t,
    407.e1t–407.e2t, 408
Rifater. *See* Isoniazid with rifampin and
    pyrazinamide
RIG. *See* Rabies Ig
Right bundle-branch block (RBBB),
    150t
Right ventricular hypertrophy (RVH),
    145b
Rimactane. *See* Rifampin
Rimantadine (Flumadine)
  formulary entry for, 933
  for influenza chemoprophylaxis,
    369–370
Riomet. *See* Metformin
Risperidone (Risperdal)
  formulary entry for, 934–935
  for mental health disorders, 209t
Ritalin. *See* Methylphenidate HCl
Ritonavir, for PEP, 412
Rituals, in palliative care, 543
Rituximab
  for arthritis, 608
  for pemphigus vulgaris, 193
  for SLE, 611
  for thrombocytopenia, 315

Rizatriptan (Maxalt), for migraine
headaches, 473t
RNC. *See* Radionuclide cystogram
Robinul. *See* Glycopyrrolate
Rocaltrol. *See* Calcitriol
Rocephin. *See* Ceftriaxone
Rocky Mountain spotted fever, 409
Rocuronium (Zemuron)
formulary entry for, 935–936
for RSI, 6t–7t
Rodent bites, 77t
Rogaine. *See* Minoxidil
Romazicon. *See* Flumazenil
Romycin. *See* Erythromycin preparations
ROP. *See* Retinopathy of prematurity
Ropivacaine, analgesic properties of, 115t
Roseola, CP6
Ross procedure, 161
Rotarix (RV1), 375–376
RotaTeq (RV5), 375–376
Rotavirus (RV), immunoprophylaxis for,
375–376
recommended schedules for,
351f–358f
Rowasa. *See* Mesalamine
Roxanol. *See* Morphine sulfate
Roxicet. *See* Oxycodone and
acetaminophen
Roxicodone. *See* Oxycodone
Roxilox. *See* Oxycodone and
acetaminophen
RR. *See* Relative risk
R-R interval, 141, 142t
RRR. *See* Relative risk reduction
RSI. *See* Rapid sequence intubation
RSV. *See* Respiratory syncytial virus
RTA. *See* Renal tubular acidosis
Rubella
congenital, 388t
IMIG postexposure prophylaxis for,
344, 371
immunoprophylaxis for, 344,
351f–358f, 361, 362.e1t, 362t,
363, 363.e1t, 370–371
MMR vaccination for, 351f–358f,
362.e1t, 363.e1t, 361, 362t,
363, 370–371
Rufinamide (Banzel), for seizures, 479t
Rulox. *See* Aluminum hydroxide with
magnesium hydroxide
Rumack-Matthew nomogram, 23, 24f
RV. *See* Rotavirus

RV1. *See* Rotarix
RV5. *See* RotaTeq
RVH. *See* Right ventricular hypertrophy

S
S waves, 142t
S₁, 128, 138b
S₂, 128, 138b
S-2 Inhalant. *See* Epinephrine,
racemic
S₃, 128, 138b
S₄, 128, 138b
SABAs. *See* Short-acting
beta₂-agonists
Sabril. *See* Vigabatrin
Sacral syndrome, 176
Salagen. *See* Pilocarpine HCl
Salicylates
aspirin as, 689
mesalamine as, 849
olsalazine as, 882
oxycodone and aspirin as, 890
poisoning with, 21t
Salicylazosulfapyridine. *See*
Sulfasalazine
Salicylic acid, for warts, 177
Saline solution. *See also* Normal saline.
for allergic rhinitis, 336
Salmeterol (Serevent Diskus)
for asthma, 558.e1t–558.e2t
formulary entry for, 936
Salmonella infection, 393t–399t
Salter-Harris classification, 66, 67t, 589
Sal-Tropine. *See* Atropine sulfate
Sample collection, for metabolic
disorder evaluation, 286t
Sample size, 637
Sancuso. *See* Granisetron
Sandimmune. *See* Cyclosporine
Sandostatin. *See* Octreotide acetate
Sanfilippo syndrome, 293
Sani-Supp. *See* Glycerin
Sarafem. *See* Fluoxetine hydrochloride
Sarcoidosis, 615–616
SBP. *See* Systolic blood pressure
Scabicides
lindane as, 837
permethrin as, 899–900
Scabies, CP3, 178
SCAD deficiency. *See* Short-chain
acyl-CoA dehydrogenase
deficiency

Scald burns, 79t
Scale, on skin, 172, 173f–174f
Scar, 172, 173f–174f
SCARED tool, 210
Scarlet fever, CP4
SCFE. See Slipped capital femoral epiphysis
Schedules, immunization, 350, 351f–358f
School problems, adolescents with, 108
School-age children, pain assessment for, 111, 112t
Schwartz equation, 446, 446t
SCIWORA. See Spinal cord injury without radiographic abnormality
Scleroderma
  autoantibodies associated with, 603t
  DCSS, 616.e1–616.e2
  localized, 616.e1
Scoliometer, 95.e1
Scoliosis
  assessment and treatment of, 95.e2f, 95
  imaging of, 576
Scopolamine hydrobromide (Isopto Hyoscine, Transderm Scop), formulary entry for, 937
Scopolamine poisoning, 20t–22t
SCRATCH principles, 183
Screening
  adolescent, 95–97, 97.e1t, 402
  cardiovascular
    for ADHD patients, 170
    for sports, 170.e1b, 170
  for congenital heart disease, 155–156
  developmental
    guidelines for, 200
    tools used for, 200–202, 201t, 202.e1b–202.e2b, 203f–204f
  fetal anomaly, 415.e1
  of lipid levels, 168–169
  for mental health disorders, 201t, 208
  newborn
    for CF, 567
    for congenital adrenal hyperplasia, 228t, 229
    Hb electrophoresis, 309, 310t
    for HIV infection, 402

Screening (Continued)
    hypoglycemia and glucagon stimulation test, 242–243
    hypothyroidism, 223
    for IVH, 432
    metabolic, 284–285
    for ROP, 433–434
    prenatal, for HIV infection, 402
    toxicology, 19, 20t
    for type II diabetes, 219
Scurvy, 688
Seborrheic dermatitis. See also Gray patch tinea capitis.
    in neonates, CP10, 190
Secondary skin lesions, 172, 173f–174f
Secondary survey, 61, 62t
Second-degree heart block, 149f, 149t
Secretory diarrhea, 271
Sedation. See also Procedural sedation.
    risks of, 27
    for RSI, 4, 5f, 6t–7t
Sedative-hypnotics
    chloral hydrate as, 727
    procedural sedation with, 119, 121, 121b–122b
    quick reference for, 113.e1t
    for RSI, 6t–7t
    toxidrome of, 20t–22t
Sedatives
    dexmedetomidine as, 753–754
    droperidol as, 767
    fentanyl as, 783–784
Sediment, in urine, 440
Seizure
    differential diagnosis of, 474t
    after DTaP vaccination, 365
    emergency management of, 15–16, 16t
    first and recurrent
      causes of, 474–475
      disorders causing, 475, 476t–477t, 478b
      evaluation of, 475
      febrile illness–associated, 475
      status epilepticus, 15–16, 16t, 478
      treatment of, 478–480, 479t, 668–669
    neonatal, 289, 432, 476t–477t
    poisoning diagnosis and, 20.e1t–20.e3t
    special syndromes of, 476t–477t, 480
Seldinger technique, 32–33, 32f
Selective progesterone receptor modulator EC, 102–103

Selective serotonin reuptake inhibitors
(SSRIs)
  for depressive disorders, 210
  fluoxetine hydrochloride as, 790
  fluvoxamine as, 793–794
  paroxetine as, 894–895
  poisoning with, 20t–22t
  sertraline HCl as, 939
Selenium, DRIs for, 507t–508t
Selenium sulfide (Selsun)
  formulary entry for, 937–938
  for tinea capitis, 185
  for tinea infections, 411t
  for tinea versicolor, 184
Semi-elemental formulas, 511t–517t
Senna/sennosides (Senna-Gen,
    Lax-Pills, Senokot)
  for constipation, 272
  formulary entry for, 938
Sensitivity, 640
Sensory examination, 467, 469f, 469t
Separation anxiety, 199t–200t
Sepsis
  blood transfusion causing, 332
  neonatal, 392t
Septic arthritis
  joint fluid analysis for, 605f
  management of, 393t–399t
  neonatal, 392t
Septic shock, 71.e1t, 71
Septra. See
    Trimethoprim-sulfamethoxazole
Serevent Diskus. See Salmeterol
Seroquel. See Quetiapine
Serotonin agonists, sumatriptan
    succinate as, 951
Serotonin antagonists
  dolasetron as, 763
  granisetron as, 803
  for nausea and vomiting, 537
  ondansetron as, 883–884
  risperidone as, 934–935
Serotonin syndrome, 20t–22t
Serratia spp., antibiotic sensitivity of,
    383t–384t
Sertraline HCl (Zoloft)
  formulary entry for, 939
  for mental health disorders, 209t
Serum androstenedione, normal values
    of, 243.e3t, 243
Serum complement levels, reference
    values of, 347t

Serum electrolyte disturbances
  calcium, 259–261, 261b
  magnesium, 262, 262b
  phosphate, 263, 263b
  potassium, 257–259, 258t–259t, 260f
  sodium, 256–257, 257t–258t
Serum IgA levels, reference values for,
    345t–346t
Serum IgE levels, reference values for,
    345t–346t
Serum IgG levels, reference values for,
    345t–346t
Serum IgM levels, reference values for,
    345t–346t
Serum muscle enzymes, laboratory
    studies of, 605
Serum osmolality, 264
Serum osmolar gap, 264
  poisoning diagnosis and,
    20.e1t–20.e3t
Serum testosterone, normal levels of,
    240t
Severe combined immunodeficiency,
    342t–343t
Sexual abuse, 84–85
Sexual development
  ambiguous genitalia in, 239–242
  cryptorchidism in, 241–242
  delayed puberty in, 236–237, 237t,
    238f
  precocious puberty in, 237–239,
    237t, 239t–241t
Sexual health, of adolescents
  contraception use, 98–104,
    99f, 101f
  follow-up recommendations, 104
  gender identity, 98
  orientation, 98
  STIs, 93.e1b, 93b, 96, 104
  vaginal infections, genital ulcers, and
    warts, 104, 105t–107t
Sexuality, adolescent, 93.e1b, 93b
Sexually transmitted infection (STI).
    See also specific STIs
  adolescent, 93.e1b, 93b, 104
    screening for, 96
  common, 400t–401t
  pelvic inflammatory disease and,
    392–401, 400t–401t
SFD. *See* Solute fluid deficit
sfRowasa. *See* Mesalamine
Shigella infection, 393t–399t

Shock
  categorization of, 72t
  critical care for, 71.e1t, 71, 72t, 73f
  resuscitation with, 9
Short stature, 233–235, 234f, 235t
Short-acting beta$_2$-agonists (SABAs), for
    asthma, 562f–564f
Short-chain acyl-CoA dehydrogenase
    (SCAD) deficiency, 290
Shortening fraction echocardiography,
    155.e1, 155
Shuddering attacks, 474t
Shunts, cardiac, 160f, 161
SIADH. *See* Syndrome of inappropriate
    antidiuretic hormone secretion
Siblings, new, 199t–200t
Sickle cell anemia, 309–310
  complications of, 310, 311t–312t
  health maintenance in, 310, 312t
  immunoprophylaxis for children with,
    361
SIDS. *See* Sudden infant death
    syndrome
Significance level of statistical tests
    (α), 637
Sildenafil (Revatio, Viagra), formulary
    entry for, 939–940
Silver sulfadiazine (Silvadene,
    Thermazene, SSD Cream)
  for burns, 83.e1b
  formulary entry for, 940
Silver-impregnated products, for burns,
    83.e1b
Simethicone (Gas-X, Mylanta Gas,
    Mylicon, Phazyme), formulary
    entry for, 941
Similac Advance Early Shield, 511t–517t
Similac Go and Grow Milk-Based
    Formula, 511t–517t
Similac Go and Grow Soy-Based
    Formula, 511t–517t
Similac HMF with preterm human milk,
    511t–517t
Similac Organic, 511t–517t
Similac PM 60/40, 511t–517t
Similac Sensitive, 511t–517t
Similac Sensitive RS, 511t–517t
Similac Special Care 20, 511t–517t
Similac Special Care 24 High Protein,
    511t–517t
Similac Special Care 30, 511t–517t
Simple febrile seizure, 475

Simple partial seizures, 478b
Simply Saline. *See* Sodium chloride,
    inhaled preparations
SIMV. *See* Synchronized IMV
Singulair. *See* Montelukast
Sinus bradycardia, 145t–146t
Sinus rhythm, 140
Sinus tachycardia, 145t–146t
Sinusitis, 393t–399t, 694–695
Sinusoidal obstruction syndrome, after
    bone marrow transplantation,
    535
Sirolimus (Rapamune)
  formulary entry for, 941–942
  for GVHD prevention, 534
6 Ps, of compartment syndrome, 66
Sjögren syndrome, 616.e2–616.e3
  autoantibodies associated with,
    603t
Skeletal anomalies, cardiology imaging
    with, 155
Skeletal injury, in child abuse patients,
    84, 85t
Skeletal muscle relaxants
  baclofen as, 697–698
  dantrolene as, 747
Skeletal survey, in suspected child
    abuse, 597, 599f–600f
Skin lesions. *See also* Dermatology.
  primary, 172, 173f–174f
  secondary, 172, 173f–174f
Skin staples, 56–57
Skin syndromes, food allergies causing,
    336–337, 339
Skin testing
  for allergic rhinitis, 334
  for drug allergies, 340f, 341
  for food allergies, 337
Skin trauma, secondary survey of, 62t
Skull fracture, in child abuse
    patients, 85t
SLE. *See* Systemic lupus erythematosus
Sleep apnea. *See* Obstructive sleep
    apnea syndrome
Slipped capital femoral epiphysis
    (SCFE), 590, 593f
Slo-Niacin. *See* Niacin
Slow FE. *See* Iron, oral preparations
Sly syndrome, 293
Smears. *See* Blood smears
SOAP. *See* Suction, oxygen, airway
    supplies, pharmacology

Social skills, 196
    developmental milestones in,
        197t–198t
Sodium. *See also* Hypernatremia;
        Hyponatremia.
    deficit repletion of
        in hypernatremic dehydration,
            252–253
        in hyponatremic dehydration, 252
        in isonatremic dehydration,
            249–251, 251t
    for diabetic ketoacidosis, 217f
    newborn requirements for, 422t
    reference values for, 621t–623t
    serum disturbances in, 256–257,
        257t–258t
Sodium benzoate
    for metabolic crisis, 290
    for urea cycle defects, 292
Sodium bicarbonate (Neut)
    for diabetic ketoacidosis, 217f
    formulary entry for, 942–943
    for hyperkalemia, 260f
    for local anesthetic injection, 116
    for metabolic crisis, 290
    neonate dosages of, 435
    for TCA poisoning, 21t
Sodium chloride
    for increased ICP, 70
Sodium chloride, inhaled preparations
        (Ayr Saline, Hypersal, Ocean,
        Rhinaris, Simply Saline),
        formulary entry for, 943
Sodium phenylacetate
    for metabolic crisis, 290
    for urea cycle defects, 292
Sodium phenylbutyrate, for urea cycle
        defects, 292
Sodium phosphate (Fleet Enema, Fleet
        Pedia-Lax, Fleet Phospho-Soda,
        OsmoPrep). *See also* Phosphorus
        supplements.
    formulary entry for, 944
Sodium polystyrene sulfonate
        (Kayexalate, Kionex, SPS)
    formulary entry for, 944–945
    for hyperkalemia, 260f
Soft tissue aspiration, 51–53
Solodyn. *See* Minocycline
Solu-Cortef. *See* Hydrocortisone
Solu-Medrol. *See* Methylprednisolone
Solute fluid deficit (SFD), 252–253

Solute maintenance, requirements for,
        248–249, 248t, 256t
Solute repletion
    based on excess electrolyte deficits,
        252
    based on FWD, 252
    based on SFD, 252–253
    based on solute fluid deficit,
        249–252, 251t
    calculation of appropriate fluids for,
        253–256, 254t–255t
    replacement strategy for, 250f,
        253.e1t–253.e3t, 253
Somatostatin analogs, octreotide acetate
        as, 880
Sorbitol, for constipation, 272–273
Source CF, 505t–506t
Soy formulas
    mixing instructions for, 510t
    nutrition components in, 511t–517t
Spastic CP, 208t
Specific gravity, of urine, 438
Specificity, 640
Specimen collection
    for blood culture, 380
    for metabolic disorder evaluation, 286t
    urine, 441
Spence Children's Anxiety Scale, 210
Spherocytosis, blood smear
        demonstrating, CP11
Spinal cord compression, 530
Spinal cord injury without radiographic
        abnormality (SCIWORA), 574
Spinal fusion infections, 393t–399t
Spine
    adolescent, assessment and
        treatment of, 95.e2f, 95
    imaging of
        in adolescent, 95.e1, 95.e2f
        cervical spine trauma, 573
        C-spine film reading, 573–574, 575f
        SCIWORA, 574
        scoliosis, 576
        spinal dysraphism, 574
Spiritual changes, as death approaches,
        545
Spirometry, 553, 554f–555f, 555t
Spironolactone (Aldactone)
    formulary entry for, 945
    for hypertension, 463t–464t
    renal failure dosage adjustments for,
        1008t–1016t

Spleen, evaluation of, 342t–343t
Splenic sequestration, in sickle cell disease, 311t–312t
Splinting
    basic, 57–58
    long arm posterior, 58, 58f
    posterior ankle, 59
    sugar tong forearm, 58, 59f
    thumb spica, 58–59
    ulnar gutter, 58
    volar, 59
Spontaneous pneumothorax, in newborns, 426
Sporanox. *See* Itraconazole
Sports participation
    cardiovascular screening for, 170.e1b, 170
    congenital heart disease and, 168.e1t
    PPE for, 98.e1f, 97–98
Sports-related injuries, 64
SPS. *See* Sodium polystyrene sulfonate
SSD Cream. *See* Silver sulfadiazine
SSKI. *See* Potassium iodide
SSRIs. *See* Selective serotonin reuptake inhibitors
Stadol. *See* Butorphanol
Staphylococcus spp.
    antibiotic sensitivity of, 383t–386t
    perinatal infection with, 392t
Staples, skin, 56–57
State support, for children with developmental or mental disorders, 212
Statins, 170
Statistics. *See* Biostatistics
Stature, growth charts for
    boys, 493f
    boys with Down syndrome, 486.e7f
    girls, 491f
    girls with Down syndrome, 486.e6f
Status epilepticus, 478
    emergency management of, 15–16, 16t
Stavzor. *See* Valproic acid
Stem cell transplantation. *See* Hematopoietic stem cell transplantation
Stenotrophomonas spp., antibiotic sensitivity of, 386t
Steroid hormones, biosynthesis of, 227, 227f

Steroids. *See also* Corticosteroids.
    for alopecia areata, 186
    for asthma, 10, 559f–564f
        dosages for inhaled steroids, 558.e1t–558.e2t
    for atopic dermatitis, 180, 182t–183t
    body surface area nomogram for dosing of, 988f
    for contact dermatitis, 194
    for EE, 275
    for hypercalcemia, 261
    immunoprophylaxis for patients on, 362, 362t
    late effects of, 538.e1t
    for migraine headaches, 472
    potency of, 182t–183t, 229t
    for RDS, 424
    for seizure, 476t–477t
    topical, 182t–183t
STI. *See* Sexually transmitted infection
Still's murmur, 139t
Stimate. *See* Desmopressin acetate
Stimulants. *See also* Respiratory stimulants.
    bisacodyl as, 702
    dexmethylphenidate as, 754–755
    dextroamphetamine as, 755–756
    doxapram HCL as, 765
    lisdexamfetamine as, 839
    methylphenidate HCl as, 853–854
Stomach Relief. *See* Bismuth subsalicylate
Stool osmolar gap, 271
Stool softeners, docusate as, 762–763
Stranger anxiety, 199t–200t
Strattera. *See* Atomoxetine
Strength, examination of, 467, 468b
Streptococcus spp. *See also* Group B streptococcal infection.
    ampicillin for, 686
    antibiotic sensitivity of, 383t–386t
Streptogramins, quinupristin and dalfopristin as, 927
Streptomycin sulfate
    formulary entry for, 946
    renal failure dosage adjustments for, 995t–1007t
    sensitivity-based selection of, 385t
Stress fractures, 590
Stretch reflexes, 468.e1t
Stridor, auscultation of, 550t

Stroke
  differential diagnosis of, 482, 482b
  etiology of, 481
  initial workup of, 482, 482b
  management of, 482–483
  as oncologic emergency, 530–531
ST-segment, 143, 143t
Study designs, comparison of,
    638t–639t
Stunting, 486
Subclavian vein, catheter placement in,
    31, 33, 35f
Subcutaneous immunoglobulin
    (Hizentra)
  adverse reactions to, 344
  considerations for, 344
  doses of, 344
  formulary entry for, 814–815
  indication for, 344
  precautions for, 344
Subcutaneous injection, 53
Subcutaneous insulin, 218t
Subgaleal hemorrhage, 419f, 419t
Sublimate. See Fentanyl
Subluxation, radial head, 60
Substance abuse disorders
  assessment of, 211, 211b
  epidemiology of, 211
  treatment of, 211–212
Substance use, adolescent, 93b–94b,
    108
Succimer (Chemet, Dimercaptosuccinic
    acid, DMSA)
  formulary entry for, 946
  for lead poisoning, 23
Succinylcholine (Anectine, Quelicin)
  in burn patients, 80
  formulary entry for, 947
  for RSI, 6t–7t
Sucralfate (Carafate), formulary entry
    for, 948
Sucrose (Sweet Ease), for pain relief,
    116
Suction, oxygen, airway supplies,
    pharmacology (SOAP), 4
Sudafed. See Pseudoephedrine
Sudden cardiac arrest, 3
Sudden infant death syndrome (SIDS),
    570, 570b
Sugar tong forearm splint, 58, 59f
Sugars, in urine, 439
Suicide, adolescent, 93b, 104–108

Sulfacetamide sodium ophthalmic
    (Bleph 10), 991t–992t
  formulary entry for, 948
Sulfadiazine
  formulary entry for, 949
  for toxoplasmosis, 388t
Sulfamethoxazole and trimethoprim. See
    Trimethoprim-sulfamethoxazole
Sulfasalazine (Azulfidine,
    Salicylazosulfapyridine,
    Sulfazine)
  for arthritis, 608.e1t, 608
  formulary entry for, 950–951
Sulfatrim. See
    Trimethoprim-sulfamethoxazole
Sulfazine. See Sulfasalazine
Sulfisoxazole, renal failure dosage
    adjustments for, 995t–1007t
Sulfonamides
  erythromycin ethylsuccinate and
    acetylsulfisoxazole as, 776
  sulfacetamide sodium ophthalmic
    as, 948
  sulfadiazine as, 949
  TMP-SMX as, 949–950
Sulfonylurea poisoning, 21t
Sumatriptan succinate (Imitrex)
  formulary entry for, 951
  for migraine headaches, 472,
    473t
Sumycin. See Tetracycline HCl
Sunkist Vitamin C. See Ascorbic acid
Superficial burns, 79t
Superficial partial thickness burns, 79t
Superior vena cava syndrome, 531
Superior vena cava-to-pulmonary artery
    shunts, 160f, 161
Suplena, 511t–517t
Supplements
  fluoride, 504–509
  iron, 504
  pancreatic enzymes, 989t
  vitamin, 501–504, 504t–506t
Suprapubic bladder aspiration, 51,
    52f–53f
Supraventricular arrhythmias
  adenosine for, 671
  ECG of, 145t–146t, 147f
Supraventricular tachycardia (SVT)
  adenosine for, 671
  ECG of, 145t–146t, 147f
Suprax. See Cefixime

Surfactant, pulmonary/beractant (Survanta), formulary entry for, 952

Surfactant, pulmonary/calfactant (Infasurf), formulary entry for, 952–953

Surfactant, pulmonary/lucinactant (Surfaxin), formulary entry for, 953

Surfactant, pulmonary/poractant alfa (Curosurf), formulary entry for, 954

Surfactant therapy, 423–424
  for RDS, 424

Surfaxin. See Surfactant, pulmonary/ lucinactant

Surgery, endocarditis prophylaxis for, 162, 162t, 163b, 694–695

Sur-Q-Lax. See Docusate

Survanta. See Surfactant, pulmonary/ beractant

Suturing
  for animal bites, 77–78
  techniques and procedure for, 54–56, 55f, 56t
  vertical mattress, 54, 55f

SVT. See Supraventricular tachycardia

Sweat chloride test, 567

Sweet Ease. See Sucrose

Symbicort. See Budesonide and formoterol

Symbols, Joint Commission do not use list for, 667, 667t–668t

Symmetrel. See Amantadine hydrochloride

Sympathomimetics
  cyclopentolate with phenylephrine as, 745
  dobutamine as, 762
  dopamine as, 764
  epinephrine as, 771–772
  pseudoephedrine as, 921
  racemic epinephrine as, 772
  toxidrome of, 20t–22t

Synacort. See Hydrocortisone

Synagis. See Palivizumab

Synalar. See Fluocinolone acetonide

Synchronized IMV (SIMV), 74

Syncope, 474t

Syndrome of inappropriate antidiuretic hormone secretion (SIADH), 231–232

Synercid. See Quinupristin and dalfopristin

Synovial fluid, characteristics of, 605, 605f, 632t

Synthroid. See Levothyroxine

Syphilis
  in adolescents, 96, 106t–107t
  congenital, 386.e1t, 388t
  management of, 400t–401t
  serology of mothers and infants with, 386.e1t

Systemic illness, ECG effects of, 150, 151t–152t

Systemic lupus erythematosus (SLE)
  ACR classification criteria for, 609, 610t
  autoantibodies associated with, 603t, 611
  clinical features of, 611.e1t, 610–611
  drug-induced, 603t, 611
  neonatal, 611–612
  treatment of, 611

Systemic-to-pulmonary artery shunts, 160f, 161

Systems review
  for adolescents, 94
  for PPE, 97–98, 98.e1f

Systolic blood pressure (SBP)
  assessment of, 128.e1t, 128, 129t–135t, 136f–138f
  definition of normal, 460
  linear regression by postconceptional age, 138f
  percentiles
    for boys 1-17 years by height, 133t–135t
    for boys from birth to 12 months, 136f
    for girls 1-17 years by height, 129t–132t
    for girls from birth to 12 months, 137f
    for infants 26-44 weeks postconceptional age, 128.e1t

Systolic heart murmurs, 139, 139b–140b

Systolic heart sounds, 128

T

T cell count, reference values for, 347t

T waves, 127f, 140, 143, 143t, 144f

T_3. See Triiodothyronine

T₄. *See* Levothyroxine; Thyroxine

Tachyarrhythmia, 679–680

Tachycardia, poisoning diagnosis and, 20.e1t–20.e3t

Tachypnea, poisoning diagnosis and, 20.e1t–20.e3t

Tacrolimus (Astagraf XL, FK506, Hecoria, Prograf, Protopic)
   for atopic dermatitis, 180
   for Behçet disease, 616.e2
   formulary entry for, 954–955
   for GVHD prevention, 534
   for IBD, 274

Tagamet. *See* Cimetidine

Takayasu arteritis, 613t

Tall stature, 235

Tambocor. *See* Flecainide acetate

Tamiflu. *See* Oseltamivir phosphate

Tanner staging
   breast development, 92f
   pubic hair, 92t

Tapazole. *See* Methimazole

Tapering, opioid, 117–118, 118t, 119b

Taxol. *See* Paclitaxel

Tazicef. *See* Ceftazidime

Tazidime. *See* Ceftazidime

TB. *See* Tuberculosis

TBG. *See* Thyroxine-binding globulin

TBSA. *See* Total body surface area

3TC. *See* Lamivudine

TCAs. *See* Tricyclic antidepressants

Td vaccine. *See* Tetanus toxoid vaccine

Tdap vaccine. *See* Tetanus and diphtheria toxoids and acellular pertussis vaccine

TEC. *See* Transient erythroblastopenia of childhood

Technetium uptake
   thyroid function testing with, 219
   after UTI, 444

TEE. *See* Total energy expenditure; Transesophageal echocardiography

TEF. *See* Thermic effect of food

Tegretol. *See* Carbamazepine

Telogen effluvium, CP8, 186

Temodar. *See* Temozolomide

Temovate. *See* Clobetasol propionate

Temozolomide (Temodar), toxicity of, 525t–528t

Temper tantrums, 199t–200t

Temperature, conversion formulas for, 633

Temporal arteritis, 613t

Tempra. *See* Acetaminophen

Tendon reflexes, 468.e1t, 467–468, 469b

Tenex. *See* Guanfacine

Teniposide (VM-26), toxicity of, 525t–528t

Tenormin. *See* Atenolol

Tensilon. *See* Edrophonium chloride

Tension pneumothorax
   blunt thoracic and abdominal trauma causing, 66
   needle decompression for, 44

Teratogens, 648

Terazosin, for hypertension, 463t–464t

Terbinafine
   for tinea capitis, 185
   for tinea corporis, 184
   for tinea infections, 411t

Terbutaline (Brethine)
   for asthma, 11
   formulary entry for, 956
   renal failure dosage adjustments for, 1008t–1016t

Testicles
   normal size and volume of, 241t
   in precocious puberty, 239, 241t

Testosterone
   biosynthesis of, 227f
   cryptorchidism evaluation with, 242
   normal levels of, 240t
   in precocious puberty, 239, 240t

Tet spells, 160t

Tetanus, immunoprophylaxis for, 351f–358f, 362.e1t, 78, 82, 362t, 363
   for animal bites, 78
   for burns, 82

Tetanus and diphtheria toxoids and acellular pertussis (Tdap, Boostrix, Adacel) vaccine, 363–366, 366t
   for oncology patients, 362t
   during pregnancy, 363
   recommended schedules for, 351f–358f
   side effects of, 365

Tetanus Ig (TIG), 365

Tetanus toxoid (Td) vaccine, 363–366, 366t

Tetracaine, analgesic properties of, 115t
Tetracycline HCl (Sumycin)
  formulary entry for, 956–957
  renal failure dosage adjustments for, 995t–1007t
Tetracyclines
  for acne vulgaris, 188t
  doxycycline as, 765–766
  for gastroenteritis, 393t–399t
  minocycline as, 862–863
  sensitivity-based selection of, 385t
  for syphilis, 400t–401t
Tetrahydrocannabinol. See Dronabinol
Tetralogy of Fallot, 158t–160t
6-TG. See Thioguanine
Thalassemias, 310–313
  α, 310–313
  β, 313
THC. See Dronabinol
Theophylline (Elixophyllin, Theo-24, Theochron)
  for asthma, 563f–564f
  formulary entry for, 956–957
Thera-Ear Gly-Oxide. See Carbamide peroxide
Thermal injury. See Burns
Thermazene. See Silver sulfadiazine
Thermic effect of food (TEF), 497
Thiamine (Vitamin B_1)
  coma treatment with, 13
  DRIs for, 502t–503t
  formulary entry for, 958
  reference values for, 621t–623t
  for status epilepticus, 16t
Thioguanine (6-TG, 6-Thioguanine)
  late effects of, 538.e1t
  toxicity of, 525t–528t
Thiopental
  procedural sedation with, 119
  renal failure dosage adjustments for, 1008t–1016t
  for RSI, 5f, 6t–7t
Thiopurines, for IBD, 274
Thioridazine (Mellaril), formulary entry for, 959
Thiotepa, toxicity of, 525t–528t
Third-degree heart block, 149f, 149t
Thoracentesis, 44–47, 45f–46f
Thoracic trauma
  blunt, 65–66
  secondary survey of, 62t

Thorazine. See Chlorpromazine
3232A formula, 511t–517t
Thrombocytopenia, 313–316, 327b, 536–537
Thrombolytic therapy, 324
  alteplase as, 674–675
  for stroke, 483
Thromboses
  as oncologic emergency, 530–531
  treatment of
    coagulation tests and, 322–324
    LMWH, 320–322
    thrombolytic therapy, 324
    UFH, 320–322, 321t–322t
    warfarin, 322, 323t–324t, 325b
Thrombotic microangiopathy, after bone marrow transplantation, 535
Thrombotic thrombocytopenic purpura (TTP), after bone marrow transplantation, 535
Thrush, 411t
Thumb spica splint, 58–59
Thyroid function
  hyperthyroidism, 220t, 223–224
  hypothyroidism, 219–223, 220t, 222t, 235
  tests of, 219, 220t–221t
Thyroid scan, 219
Thyroid storm, 224
Thyroid-stimulating hormone (TSH)
  age-based normal values for, 221t
  management of, 222t
  in obesity, 219–223
  in preterm and term infants, 221t
  thyroid function test interpretation and, 220t
ThyroSafe. See Potassium iodide
ThyroShield. See Potassium iodide
Thyrotoxicosis, neonatal, 224
Thyroxine (T_4)
  age-based normal values for, 221t
  formulary entry for, 834–835
  for hypothyroidism, 220t
  management of, 222t
  in obesity, 219–223
  in preterm and term infants, 221t
  thyroid function test interpretation and, 220t

Thyroxine-binding globulin (TBG), age-based normal values for, 221t

Ti. *See* Inspiratory time

Tiagabine (Gabitril) formulary entry for, 959–960 for seizures, 479t

Tiazac. *See* Diltiazem

TIBC. *See* Total iron-building capacity

Ticarcillin, renal failure dosage adjustments for, 995t–1007t

Ticarcillin and clavulanate (Timentin) formulary entry for, 960 for intraabdominal infections, 393t–399t renal failure dosage adjustments for, 995t–1007t sensitivity-based selection of, 383t–384t

Tickborne illnesses anaplasmosis, 410 ehrlichiosis, 409–410 Lyme disease, 408–409 acquired heart disease with, 168 antibiotic selection for, 383t–384t, 682 joint fluid analysis for, 605f Rocky Mountain spotted fever, 409

Tics, 474t

Tidal volume (V$_T$), 74

TIG. *See* Tetanus Ig

Tigan. *See* Trimethobenzamide HCl

Timentin. *See* Ticarcillin and clavulanate

Timolol, for hemangioma, 177

Tinactin. *See* Tolnaftate

Tinea capitis etiology and treatment of, 411t skin lesions of, CP8, 185

Tinea corporis etiology and treatment of, 411t skin lesions of, CP5, 184

Tinea cruris, 411t

Tinea pedis etiology and treatment of, 411t skin lesions of, CP5

Tinea unguium, 411t

Tinea versicolor, CP7, 184

Tinidazole, for trichomoniasis, 105t

Tirosint. *See* Levothyroxine

Tisit. *See* Pyrethrins

Tissue adhesives, 57

Tissue plasminogen activator (tPA), formulary entry for, 674–675

TIV. *See* Trivalent inactivated influenza vaccine

TMP-SMX. *See* Trimethoprim-sulfamethoxazole

TNF inhibitors. *See* Tumor necrosis factor inhibitors

Tobramycin (Bethkis, Nebcin, Tobrex, AKTob, TOBI Podhaler) formulary entry for, 961–962 ophthalmic, 991t–992t renal failure dosage adjustments for, 995t–1007t sensitivity-based selection of, 385t

Tofranil. *See* Imipramine

Toilet training, 199t–200t

Tolerable upper intake level (UL), 501

Tolerex, 511t–517t

Tolnaftate (Tinactin), formulary entry for, 963

Tonic seizures, 478b

Tonic-clonic seizures, 478b

Topamax. *See* Topiramate

Topical local anesthetics analgesic properties of, 113–116, 115t lidocaine and prilocaine as, 115t, 125t

Topical steroids, 182t–183t

Topicort. *See* Desoximetasone

Topiramate (Topamax, Topiragen, Trokendi XR) formulary entry for, 963–964 for migraine headaches, 473t for seizures, 476t–477t, 479t

Topotecan (Hycamtin), toxicity of, 525t–528t

Toprol-XL. *See* Metoprolol

Toradol. *See* Ketorolac

TORCH infections, 382, 388t

Totacillin. *See* Ampicillin

Total anomalous pulmonary venous return, 158t–159t

Total body surface area (TBSA), 78, 80f

Total cholesterol, 169

Total energy expenditure (TEE), 497

Total hemolytic complement level (CH$_{50}$), 604

Total iron-building capacity (TIBC), reference values for, 621t–623t

Total palsy, 433t

Total parenteral nutrition, for newborns, 423

Total protein, reference values for, 621t–623t

Total triglyceride, reference values for, 621t–623t

Toxic granulations, blood smear demonstrating, CP12

Toxicology. See Poisoning

Toxicology screens, 19, 20t

Toxidromes, 20t–22t, 23

Toxoplasma gondii
    antibiotic sensitivity of, 386t
    atovaquone for, 405.e1t–405.e2t, 691
    congenital infection with, 388t
    in HIV/AIDS patients, 405.e1t–405.e2t

tPA. See Tissue plasminogen activator

Trachea, chest radiography of, 155

Tracheitis, 393t–399t

Tracheoesophageal fistula, 584, 585f

Traction alopecia, CP8, 186

Trade names, generic names corresponding to, 648–666

Trained night feeding, 199t–200t

Trandate. See Labetalol

Transaminase. See Alanine aminotransferase; Aspartate aminotransferase

Transderm Scop. See Scopolamine hydrobromide

Transdermal contraceptives, 102

Transesophageal echocardiography (TEE), 155

Transferrin, reference values for, 621t–623t

Transfusion. See Blood component replacement

Transfusion reactions
    acute, 331–332
    delayed, 332

Transient erythroblastopenia of childhood (TEC), 309

Transient neonatal jaundice, 279t

Transient neonatal pustular melanosis, CP9, 190

Transplantation. See also Hematopoietic stem cell transplantation.
    solid organ, 362

Transposition of great arteries, 158t–159t

Transthoracic echocardiography (TTE), 155

Transudate, 630t

Trauma
    abdominal, 62t, 65–66, 589
    AMPLE history of, 61
    cervical, 65
        imaging of, 573
        secondary survey of, 62t
    extremity, 66, 67f, 67t
        in child abuse patients, 84, 85t
        imaging of, 589
        secondary survey of, 62t
    head
        abusive, 84
        imaging of, 573
        minor closed, 61–64, 62t, 63b
        secondary survey of, 62t
    neck injury, 62t, 65
    nonaccidental, CP1, CP2, 83–86, 85t
    orthopedic/long bone, 66, 67f, 67t
        imaging of, 589
    primary survey of, 61
    secondary survey of, 61, 62t
    thoracic, 62t, 65–66

Traumatic head injury, acute assessment of, 13

Travelers, immunoprophylaxis for, 363

Trazodone (Desyrel), formulary entry for, 964–965

Treatment effect, measurements of, 638t–639t, 639–640

Treponema spp., antibiotic selection for, 383t–385t

Tretinoin (Avita, Renova, Retin-A), formulary entry for, 965

Trial elimination diet, food allergy evaluation with, 339

Triamcinolone (Aristospan, Kenalog, Nasacort AQ, Oralone, Trianex, Triderm)
    for allergic rhinitis, 335
    for atopic dermatitis, 182t–183t
    formulary entry for, 965–966
    potency of, 229t

Triamterene (Dyrenium)
    formulary entry for, 966–967
    for hypertension, 463t–464t
    renal failure dosage adjustments for, 1008t–1016t

Trianex. See Triamcinolone

Trichomonas vaginalis, antibiotic
  sensitivity of, 386t
Trichomoniasis, 105t, 400t–401t
Trichotillomania, 186
Tricuspid atresia, 158t–159t
Tricyclic antidepressants (TCAs)
  amitriptyline as, 680–681
  ECG effects of, 151t–152t
  imipramine as, 813–814
  nortriptyline hydrochloride as,
    879
  poisoning with, 20t–22t
Triderm. *See* Triamcinolone
Trifluridine ophthalmic (Viroptic),
    991t–992t
Triglycerides
  management of, 170
  reference values for, 621t–623t
TriHIBit, 378
Triiodothyronine (T₃)
  age-based normal values for, 221t
  in obesity, 219–223
Trileptal. *See* Oxcarbazepine
Trilisate. *See* Choline magnesium
    trisalicylate
TriLyte. *See* Polyethylene glycol,
    electrolyte solution
Trimethobenzamide HCl (Tigan),
    formulary entry for, 967
Trimethoprim-sulfamethoxazole (TMP-
    SMX, Bactrim, Co-trimoxazole,
    Septra, Sulfatrim)
  for acne vulgaris, 188t
  for bite infections, 393t–399t
  for cancer patients, 538t
  for cellulitis, 393t–399t
  formulary entry for, 949–950
  for gastroenteritis, 393t–399t
  for osteomyelitis, 393t–399t
  for perinatal HIV exposure, 403t–404t
  for pertussis exposure, 366
  for *Pneumocystis jiroveci* pneumonia,
    405.e1t–405.e2t, 405
  renal failure dosage adjustments for,
    995t–1007t
  sensitivity-based selection of, 386t
  for *Toxoplasma gondii* infection,
    405.e1t–405.e2t
  for UTI, 393t–399t
Trimox. *See* Amoxicillin
Trisomy 13, 300–301
Trisomy 18, 300

Trisomy 21
  dysmorphology in, 299–300
  growth charts for, 497
    length and weight for boys,
      486.e5f, 486.e7f
    length and weight for girls, 486.e4f,
      486.e6f
    stature for boys, 486.e7f
    stature for girls, 486.e6f
Trivalent inactivated influenza vaccine
    (TIV), 368–370
Tri-Vi-Sol, 504t
Trokendi XR. *See* Topiramate
Troponin-I, reference values for, 621t–623t
Trousseau sign, poisoning diagnosis
    and, 20.e1t–20.e3t
True precocious puberty, 238
TSH. *See* Thyroid-stimulating hormone
TST. *See* Tuberculin skin test
TTE. *See* Transthoracic
    echocardiography
TTP. *See* Thrombotic thrombocytopenic
    purpura
Tube feeding, formula for, 518t–519t
Tuberculin skin test (TST), 406, 407b
Tuberculosis (TB)
  drug therapy for, 407.e1t, 407–408
  in HIV/AIDS patients,
    405.e1t–405.e2t
  immunoprophylaxis for, 376
  testing for, 406–407, 407b
Tubular disorders
  Fanconi syndrome, 458
  NDI, 458
  RTA, 456–458, 457t
Tubular function tests
  distal tubule, 447, 447t
  proximal tubule, 446–447
Tumor lysis syndrome, 529–530, 673
Tumor necrosis factor (TNF) inhibitors
  for arthritis, 608.e1t, 608
  for Behçet disease, 616.e2
  for IBD, 274
Tumors
  bone
    imaging of, 590–597, 594f–598f
    sarcoma signs and symptoms,
      523t–524t
  mediastinal masses, 580
  signs and symptoms of, 523t–524t
  skin, 172, 173f–174f
Tums. *See* Calcium carbonate

Turbidity, of urine, 438
Turner syndrome (45,X), 301, 497
22q11 syndrome, 302–303
Twinrix, 378
TwoCal HN, 511t–517t
Two-dimensional echocardiography, 155.e1
Two-tailed statistical tests, 637
Tylenol. *See* Acetaminophen
Type I diabetes, 215, 215t
Type II diabetes
    characteristics of, 215, 215t
    etiology of, 216
    presentation of, 219
    prevalence of, 216
    screening for, 219
    treatment of, 219, 220f
Typhilitis, 531
Typhoid fever, 376
Tyrosinemia, hereditary, 292

U
U waves, 127f, 140
UA. *See* Urinalysis
UA catheterization. *See* Umbilical artery catheterization
UAG. *See* Urine anion gap
UC. *See* Ulcerative colitis
Uceris. *See* Budesonide
UFH. *See* Unfractionated heparin
UGI series. *See* Upper gastrointestinal series
UL. *See* Tolerable upper intake level
Ulcerative colitis (UC), 274
Ulcers
    gastrointestinal, 702–703
    genital, 104, 106t–107t
    on skin, 172, 173f–174f
Ulipristal, 102–103
Ulnar gutter splint, 58
Ultrasound. *See also* Echocardiography.
    blood flow imaging with, 583
    for blunt thoracic and abdominal trauma, 66
    gestational age estimation with, 415.e1
    intussusception on, 588, 588f
    in place of CT, 572
    pyloric stenosis on, 586, 587f
Ultravate. *See* Halobetasol propionate
Umbilical artery (UA) catheterization, 38–42, 39f, 41f

Umbilical vein (UV) catheterization, 38–42, 40f–41f
Unasyn. *See* Ampicillin/sulbactam
Unconjugated DHEA, normal levels of, 240t
Unconjugated hyperbilirubinemia, in newborns
    evaluation of, 428
    management of, 428–429, 428t, 429f–430f
Underweight, 486
Unfractionated heparin (UFH), 320–322
    dose adjustment algorithm for, 321t–322t
    dose initiation guidelines for, 321t
Unicameral bone cyst, 590, 594f
Unithroid. *See* Levothyroxine
Unpaired statistical tests, 637
Upper airway, emergency management of, 11–13
    croup, 12
    epiglottitis, 12
    foreign-body aspiration, 13, 14f
Upper airway resistance syndrome. *See* Obstructive sleep apnea syndrome
Upper gastrointestinal (UGI) series, 584–586, 586f
Upper motor neuron examination, 469t
Urea cycle disorders, 291–292, 688
Urea nitrogen, reference values for, 621t–623t
Urecholine. *See* Bethanechol chloride
Uric acid
    allopurinol for, 673
    probenecid for, 916
    reference values for, 621t–623t
Urinalysis (UA)
    bilirubin and urobilinogen, 439, 440t
    color, 438
    epithelial cells, 440
    Gram stain, 440
    hemoglobin and myoglobin, 439
    ketones, 439
    leukocyte esterase, 439, 441
    nitrite, 439, 441
    pH, 438
    protein, 439, 454
    RBCs, 440
    in rheumatology studies, 604
    sediment, 440
    specific gravity, 438

Urinalysis *(Continued)*
  sugars, 439
  turbidity, 438
  WBCs, 440
Urinary bladder
  catheterization of, 50–51
  suprapubic aspiration of, 51, 52f–53f
Urinary tract infections (UTIs)
  diagnosis of, 441–442
  history for, 440
  imaging of, 589
  management of, 393t–399t,
    442–444, 443f
  physical examination for, 441
  risk factors for, 441
  urine sampling for, 441
Urine
  acidification of, 447, 682
  alkalinization of, 668–669
  concentration of, 447
  obtaining samples of, 441
Urine anion gap (UAG), 457
Urine calcium, 447, 447t
Urine catecholamines, normal values of,
    243.e1t, 243
Urine cultures, for UTIs, 442
Urine protein/creatinine ratio, 454
Urine reducing substances, 289–290
Urine toxicology screen, 19, 20t
Urobilinogen, 439, 440t
Uro-Mag. *See* Magnesium oxide
Ursodiol (Actigall, Urso 250, Urso Forte)
  for conjugated hyperbilirubinemia in
    newborns, 430
  formulary entry for, 967–968
  neonate dosages of, 435
Urticaria
  blood transfusion causing, 331–332
  food allergies causing, 336, 339
Uterine pathology, imaging of, 589
UTIs. *See* Urinary tract infections
UV catheterization. *See* Umbilical vein
    catheterization
Uveitis
  atropine sulfate for, 691–692
  JIA with, 606, 607t

V
Vaccination. *See* Immunization
Vaccine information statement (VIS), 350
Vaginal infections, 104, 105t
Vaginal ring, 102

Vaginitis, 105t
Vaginosis, 105t, 393t–399t
Vagistat-3. *See* Miconazole
Valacyclovir (Valtrex)
  for eczema herpeticum
    superinfection, 183
  formulary entry for, 968–969
  for genital herpes, 106t–107t
  renal failure dosage adjustments for,
    995t–1007t
Valganciclovir (Valcyte)
  for CMV, 388t, 405.e1t–405.e2t
  formulary entry for, 969–970
  renal failure dosage adjustments for,
    995t–1007t
Validity, measurements of, 640–641,
    641t
Valium. *See* Diazepam
Valproate
  for migraine headaches, 472
  for status epilepticus, 16t
Valproic acid (Depakene, Depacon,
    Stavzor)
  formulary entry for, 970–971
  for seizures, 476t–477t, 479t
Valsartan (Diovan), formulary entry for,
    971
Valtrex. *See* Valacyclovir
Vancomycin (Vancocin)
  for catheter-related bloodstream
    infections, 393t–399t
  for cellulitis, 393t–399t
  formulary entry for, 972–973
  for gastroenteritis, 393t–399t
  for meningitis, 393t–399t
  for neonatal pneumonia, 392t
  neonate dosages of, 435t
  renal failure dosage adjustments for,
    995t–1007t
  sensitivity-based selection of, 386t
  for septic arthritis, 393t–399t
  for spinal fusion infections, 393t–399t
  for ventriculoperitoneal shunt
    infection, 393t–399t
Vanderbilt Assessment Scales, 201t,
    209
Vanillylmandelic acid, normal values of,
    243.e1t
Vanos. *See* Fluocinonide
Vantin. *See* Cefpodoxime
Vaqta, 367
VAR vaccine. *See* Varicella vaccine

Varicella
  immunoprophylaxis for, 351f–358f, 361, 362.e1t, 362t, 363.e1t, 363, 376–377
  perinatal, 389t–390t
  reactive erythema caused by, CP4
Varicella (VAR) vaccine, 376–377
  for children with HIV disease, 361
  for oncology patients, 362.e1t, 362t
  for patients treated with immunoglobulin or other blood products, 363.e1t, 363
  recommended schedules for, 351f–358f
Varicella zoster virus (VZV)
  acyclovir for, 670–671
  in HIV/AIDS patients, 405.e1t–405.e2t
Varicella-zoster Ig (VariZIG, VZIG), 405.e1t–405.e2t, 376–377, 389t–390t
  formulary entry for, 973–974
Vascular access
  central venous catheter placement, 28f, 31–37, 32f, 34f–36f, 582, 582f–583f
  IO infusion, 37–38, 37f
  peripheral intravenous placement, 31
  UA and UV catheterization, 38–42, 39f–41f
Vascular rings, 576
Vasculitis
  autoantibodies associated with, 603t
  general characterization of, 612, 613t
  HSP, 612–614, 613t
  juvenile dermatomyositis, 614–615
Vasoconstrictors, oxymetazoline as, 890
Vasodilators
  alprostadil as, 674
  hydralazine hydrochloride as, 807–808
  for hypertension, 463t–464t
  nitroglycerin as, 876–877
  nitroprusside as, 877
  for PPHN, 425
Vasomotor rhinitis, 335
Vaso-occlusive crisis, 311t–312t
Vasopressin (Pitressin, 8-Arginine Vasopressin). See also Desmopressin acetate.
  in DI, 232–233
  formulary entry for, 974
  in SIADH, 231–232
Vasopressin test, for DI, 232–233

Vasotec. See Enalapril maleate; Enalaprilat
VATER association, 420
VBG. See Venous blood gas
VCFS. See Velocardiofacial syndrome
VCR. See Vincristine
VCUG. See Voiding cystourethrogram
V_E. See Minute ventilation
Vecuronium bromide (Norcuron)
  formulary entry for, 975
  for RSI, 6t–7t
Veetids. See Penicillin V potassium
Vegetable oil, 510t
Vegetarian formulas, 518t–519t
Veins
  external jugular
    catheter placement in, 28f, 31, 33
    puncture of, 28–29, 28f
  femoral
    catheter placement in, 31, 33–37, 36f
    puncture of, 29–30, 29f
  internal jugular, catheter placement in, 31, 33, 34f–35f
  subclavian, catheter placement in, 31, 33, 35f
  umbilical, catheterization of, 38–42, 40f–41f
Velban. See Vinblastine
Velocardiofacial syndrome (VCFS), 302–303
Venofer. See Iron, injectable preparations
Veno-occlusive disease (VOD), after bone marrow transplantation, 535
Venous blood gas (VBG), gas exchange evaluation with, 551
Venous congestion, chest radiography of, 155, 157t–159t
Venous hum, 139t
Ventilation
  for asthma, 11
  bag-mask, 3, 8
  for respiratory failure
    initial settings for, 74–75
    modes of operation for, 74
    parameters for, 71–74
    setting changes in, 75t
    types of, 71
Ventolin HFA. See Albuterol
Ventricular arrhythmias
  amiodarone for, 679–680
  ECG of, 144, 148f, 148t

Ventricular conduction disturbances, 144, 150t
Ventricular fibrillation, 148f, 148t
Ventricular hypertrophy, 142t, 144, 145b
Ventricular septal defect (VSD), 157t–158t
Ventricular tachycardia, 148f, 148t
Ventriculoperitoneal (VP) shunt
  for hydrocephalus, 480
  imaging of, 573
  infection of, 393t–399t
VePesid. See Etoposide
Veramyst. See Fluticasone propionate
Verapamil (Calan, Isoptin, Verelan)
  ECG effects of, 151t–152t
  formulary entry for, 975–976
  renal failure dosage adjustments for, 1008t–1016t
Verdeso Foam. See Desonide
Verelan. See Verapamil
Veripred 20. See Prednisolone
Vermox. See Mebendazole
Versed. See Midazolam
Vertical mattress suturing, 54, 55f
Vesicle, on skin, 172, 173f–174f
Vesicoureteral reflux (VUR)
  imaging for, 443–444, 443f
  management of, 444
Vessel imaging. See Heart and vessel imaging
Vfend. See Voriconazole
Viagra. See Sildenafil
Vibramycin. See Doxycycline
Vibrio spp., antibiotic sensitivity of, 385t
Vigabatrin (Sabril)
  formulary entry for, 976–977
  renal failure dosage adjustments for, 1008t–1016t
  for seizures, 476t–477t, 479t
Vigamox. See Moxifloxacin hydrochloride ophthalmic
Vimpat. See Lacosamide
Vinblastine (Vincaleukoblastine, Velban), toxicity of, 525t–528t
Vincristine (VCR, Oncovin), toxicity of, 525t–528t
Vinorelbine (Navelbine), toxicity of, 525t–528t
Viramune. See Nevirapine
Virazole. See Ribavirin
Viroptic. See Trifluridine ophthalmic
VIS. See Vaccine information statement
Visceral hemangiomas, 175–176

Viscous lidocaine, analgesic properties of, 115t
Visine. See Oxymetazoline
Vistaril. See Hydroxyzine
Vistide. See Cidofovir
Visual-motor skills, 196
  developmental milestones in, 197t–198t
Vital formulas, 511t–517t
Vital jr, 511t–517t
Vital signs
  monitoring of, during procedural sedation, 120–121
  newborn, assessment of, 415
  poisoning diagnosis and, 20.e1t–20.e3t
Vitamax, 505t–506t
Vitamin A (Aquasol A)
  DRIs for, 502t–503t
  formulary entry for, 977
  neonate dosages of, 435
  reference values for, 621t–623t
Vitamin B₁. See Thiamine
Vitamin B₂. See Riboflavin
Vitamin B₃. See Niacin
Vitamin B₆. See Pyridoxine
Vitamin B₁₂. See Cobalamin
Vitamin C. See Ascorbic acid
Vitamin D
  deficiency of, 225–226, 225t–226t
  DRIs for, 502t–503t
  neonate dosages of, 435
  reference values for, 621t–623t
  suggested ranges of, 226t
  supplementation of, 501–504, 708, 731–732, 774
  for hypoparathyroidism, 225
Vitamin D₂. See Ergocalciferol
Vitamin D₃. See Cholecalciferol
Vitamin E (Alpha-tocopherol, Aquasol E, Aquavit-E, Nutr-E-Sol)
  DRIs for, 502t–503t
  formulary entry for, 978
  neonate dosages of, 435
  reference values for, 621t–623t
Vitamin K. See Phytonadione
Vitamins. See also specific vitamins
  DRIs for, 501–504, 502t–503t
  newborn requirements for, 420–423
  supplementation of, 501–504, 504t–506t
Vitrase. See Hyaluronidase
Vitrasert. See Ganciclovir
Vivonex formulas, 511t–517t

VM-26. *See* Teniposide
VOD. *See* Veno-occlusive disease
Voiding cystourethrogram (VCUG), after
    UTI, 443–444, 589
Volar splint, 59
Volume. *See* Water volume
Volume limited ventilation, 71, 74
Vomiting. *See* Nausea and vomiting
von Willebrand disease, 326f,
    327t–328t
Voriconazole (Vfend)
    for cancer patients, 538t
    formulary entry for, 979–980
VoSpire ER. *See* Albuterol
VP shunt. *See* Ventriculoperitoneal shunt
VP-16. *See* Etoposide
VSD. *See* Ventricular septal defect
V_T. *See* Tidal volume
VUR. *See* Vesicoureteral reflux
Vyvanse. *See* Lisdexamfetamine
VZIG. *See* Varicella-zoster Ig
VZV. *See* Varicella zoster virus

W

Waist circumference (WC), 497
Waist-height ratio, 497
Warfarin (Coumadin, Jantoven), 322
    dose adjustment and monitoring of,
        323t
    formulary entry for, 980–981
    heparin with, 320–322
    for Kawasaki disease, 167.e1t
    management of excessive, 324t
    medications influencing, 325b
    poisoning with, 21t
    for stroke, 482–483, 531
Warts
    genital, 104, 106t–107t
    skin
        clinical presentation of, 177
        management of, 177
        pathogenesis of, 177
Washed RBCs, 329
Water deprivation test, for DI, 232
Water loss. *See* Dehydration
Water management. *See* Fluid and
    electrolyte management
Water volume
    caloric calculations for maintenance
        of, 247–248, 248b, 248t
    deficit repletion for, 249, 251t
WBCs. *See* White blood cells

WC. *See* Waist circumference
Wegener granulomatosis, 613t
Weight
    classification of, 486
    conversion formulas for, 633
    growth charts for
        boys, 489f, 493f
        boys with Down syndrome,
            486.e5f, 486.e7f
        girls, 487f, 491f
        girls with Down syndrome, 486.e4f,
            486.e6f
        preterm infants, 495f–496f
    management of, 486.e8f, 486
Wenckebach block, 149f, 149t
Westcort. *See* Hydrocortisone valerate
Wheal, 172, 173f–174f
Wheezes, auscultation of, 550t
Whey formulas, 511t–517t
White blood cells (WBCs)
    age-specific values for, 306t
    on blood smears, 333
    in CSF, 631t
    in transudate *vs.* exudate, 630t
    in urine, 440
Whole-exome sequencing, for
    dysmorphology, 299
Wide QRS complex, poisoning diagnosis
    and, 20.e1t–20.e3t
Wilms tumor, 523t–524t
WinRho. *See* $RH_O(D)$ immune globulin
Withdrawal, opioid, 117
    neonatal, 432, 433b
Wolff-Parkinson-White syndrome
    (WPW), 147f, 150t
Wounds
    animal bite, 76–78, 77t
    tetanus prophylaxis considerations for,
        365–366, 366t
WPW. *See* Wolff-Parkinson-White
    syndrome
Wycillin. *See* Procaine penicillin G
Wymox. *See* Amoxicillin

X

Xanthine oxidase inhibitors, allopurinol
    as, 673
X-linked agammaglobulinemia, 342t–343t
Xolegel. *See* Ketoconazole
Xopenex. *See* Levalbuterol
Xylocaine. *See* Lidocaine

Y

Yeast infections. *See also specific yeast infections*
in adolescents, 105t
common community-acquired, 410, 411t
diagnosis of, 410
Yellow fever, 377–378
Yersinia infection, 393t–399t
Yuzpe method, for EC, 102–103

Z

Zaditor. *See* Ketotifen fumarate
Zafirlukast (Accolate), formulary entry for, 982
Zantac. *See* Ranitidine HCl
Zarontin. *See* Ethosuximide
Zaroxolyn. *See* Metolazone
Zemuron. *See* Rocuronium
Zenatane. *See* Isotretinoin
Zenzedi. *See* Dextroamphetamine
Zestril. *See* Lisinopril
Zetonna. *See* Ciclesonide
Zidovudine (AZT, Retrovir)
formulary entry for, 982–983
for PEP, 412
for perinatal HIV exposure, 402–405, 403t–404t

Zileuton, for asthma, 564f
Zinacef. *See* Cefuroxime
Zinc
DRIs for, 507t–508t
reference values for, 621t–623t
Zinc salts (Galzin, Orazinc), formulary entry for, 983–984
Zirgan. *See* Ganciclovir
Zithromax. *See* Azithromycin
Zmax. *See* Azithromycin
Zofran. *See* Ondansetron
Zolicef. *See* Cefazolin
Zolmitriptan (Zomig), for migraine headaches, 473t
Zoloft. *See* Sertraline HCl
Zomig. *See* Zolmitriptan
Zonisamide (Zonegran)
formulary entry for, 984–985
for seizures, 479t
Zosyn. *See* Piperacillin with tazobactam
Zovirax. *See* Acyclovir
Zyloprim. *See* Allopurinol
Zymar. *See* Gatifloxacin ophthalmic
Zyrtec. *See* Cetirizine
Zyrtec-D 12 Hour. *See* Cetirizine and pseudoephedrine
Zyvox. *See* Linezolid

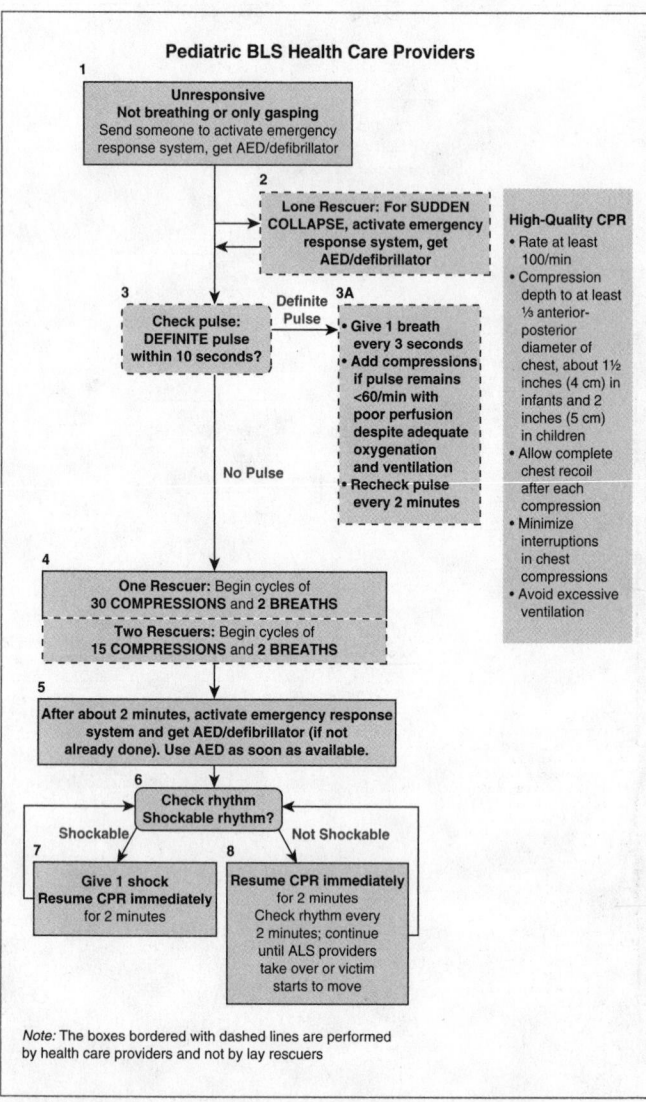

Pediatric BLS health care providers algorithm. *Reprinted with permission. 2010 American Heart Association Guidelines for Cardiopulmonary Resuscitation and Emergency Cardiovascular Care. Part 13.* Circulation. *2010;122:S862-S875.* © 2010 American Heart Association, Inc.

Pediatric Cardiac Arrest

Shout for Help/Activate Emergency Response

1
Start CPR
• Give oxygen
• Attach monitor/defibrillator

Rhythm shockable?

Yes → **2** VF/VT

3 Shock

4
CPR 2 min
• IO/IV access

Rhythm shockable?

No →

Yes → **5** Shock

6
CPR 2 min
• Epinephrine every 3–5 min
• Consider advanced airway

Rhythm shockable?

Yes → **7** Shock

No →

8
CPR 2 min
• Amiodarone
• Treat reversible causes

No →

9 Asystole/PEA

10
CPR 2 min
• IO/IV access
• Epinephrine every 3–5 min
• Consider advanced airway

Rhythm shockable?

Yes →

No →

11
CPR 2 min
• Treat reversible causes

Rhythm shockable?

No →

Yes → **Go to 5 or 7**

12
• Asystole/PEA →10 or 11
• Organized rhythm → check pulse
• Pulse present (ROSC) → postcardiac arrest care

Doses/Details

CPR Quality
• Push hard (≥⅓ of anterior-posterior diameter of chest) and fast (at least 100/min) and allow complete chest recoil
• Minimize interruptions in compressions
• Avoid excessive ventilation
• Rotate compressor every 2 minutes
• If no advanced airway, 15:2 compression-ventilation ratio. If advanced airway, 8–10 breaths per minute with continuous chest compressions

Shock Energy for Defibrillation
First shock 2 J/kg, second shock 4 J/kg, subsequent shocks ≥4 J/kg, maximum 10 J/kg or adult dose.

Drug Therapy
• **Epinephrine IO/IV Dose:** 0.01 mg/kg (0.1 mL/kg of 1:10 000 concentration). Repeat every 3–5 minutes. If no IO/IV access, may give endotracheal dose: 0.1 mg/kg (0.1mL/kg of 1:1000 concentration).
• **Amiodarone IO/IV Dose:** 5 mg/kg bolus during cardiac arrest. May repeat up to 2 times for refractory VF/pulseless VT.

Advanced Airway
• Endotracheal intubation or supraglottic advanced airway
• Waveform capnography or capnometry to confirm and monitor endotracheal tube placement
• Once advanced airway in place give 1 breath every 6–8 seconds (8–10 breaths per minute)

Return of Spontaneous Circulation (ROSC)
• Pulse and blood pressure
• Spontaneous arterial pressure waves with intra-arterial monitoring

Reversible Causes
– Hypovolemia
– Hypoxia
– Hydrogen ion (acidosis)
– Hypoglycemia
– Hypokalemia/hyperkalemia
– Hypothermia
– Tension pneumothorax
– Tamponade, cardiac
– Toxins
– Thrombosis, pulmonary
– Thrombosis, coronary

Pediatric cardiac arrest algorithm. *Reprinted with permission. 2010 American Heart Association Guidelines for Cardiopulmonary Resuscitation and Emergency Cardiovascular Care. Part 14: Pediatric advanced life support. Circulation. 2010;122:S885.* © 2010 American Heart Association, Inc.

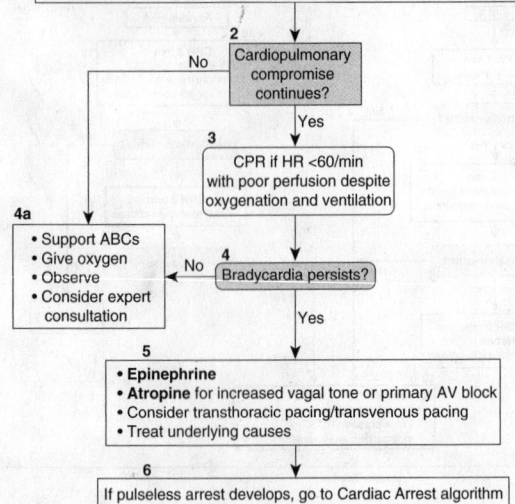

Pediatric Bradycardia
With a Pulse and Poor Perfusion

1

Identify and treat underlying cause
- Maintain patent airway; assist breathing as necessary
- Oxygen
- Cardiac monitor to identify rhythm; monitor blood pressure and oximetry
- IO/IV access
- 12-lead ECG if available; do not delay therapy

2
Cardiopulmonary compromise continues?

No

3
CPR if HR <60/min with poor perfusion despite oxygenation and ventilation

Yes

4a
- Support ABCs
- Give oxygen
- Observe
- Consider expert consultation

4
Bradycardia persists?

No

Yes

5
- **Epinephrine**
- **Atropine** for increased vagal tone or primary AV block
- Consider transthoracic pacing/transvenous pacing
- Treat underlying causes

6
If pulseless arrest develops, go to Cardiac Arrest algorithm

Cardiopulmonary Compromise
- Hypotension
- Acutely altered mental status
- Signs of shock

Doses/Details
Epinephrine IO/IV Dose: 0.01 mg/kg (0.1 mL/kg of 1:10,000 concentration). Repeat every 3–5 minutes. If IO/IV access not available but endotracheal (ET) tube in place, may give ET dose: 0.1 mg/kg (0.1 mLkg of 1:1000).
Atropine IO/IV Dose: 0.02 mg/kg. May repeat once. Minimum dose 0.1 mg and maximum single dose 0.5 mg.

Pediatric bradycardia algorithm. *Reprinted with permission. 2010 American Heart Association Guidelines for Cardiopulmonary Resuscitation and Emergency Cardiovascular Care. Part 14: Pediatric advanced life support. Circulation. 2010;122:S887.* © 2010 American Heart Association, Inc.